Jean W. Keeling (Ed.)

Fetal and Neonatal Pathology

Second Edition

With 662 Figures

Springer-Verlag
London Berlin Heidelberg New York
Paris Tokyo Hong Kong
Barcelona Budapest

Jean W. Keeling, MBBS, FRCPath, FRCP (Edin),
Consultant Paediatric Pathologist,
Department of Paediatric Pathology and Cytogenetics
Royal Hospital for Sick Children
Edinburgh EH9 1LF

Honorary Senior Lecturer in Pathology, University of Edinburgh

ISBN 3-540-19711-7 2nd edition Springer-Verlag Berlin Heidelberg New York
ISBN 0-387-19711-7 2nd edition Springer-Verlag New York Berlin Heidelberg

ISBN 3-540-16211-9 1st edition Springer-Verlag Berlin Heidelberg New York
ISBN 0-387-16211-9 1st edition Springer-Verlag New York Berlin Heidelberg

British Library Cataloguing in Publication Data
Fetal and Neonatal Pathology—2 Rev. ed
I. Keeling, Jean W.
618.32
ISBN 3-540-19711-7

Library of Congress Cataloging-in-Publication Data
Fetal and neonatal pathology/[edited by] Jean W. Keeling.—2nd ed.
p. cm.
Includes bibliographical references and index.
ISBN 0-387-19711-7.—ISBN 3-540-19711-7
1. Fetus—Diseases. 2. Infants (Newborn)—Diseases. 3. Fetus—Abnormalities.
4. Infants (Newborn)—Abnormalities. 5. Pediatric pathology. I. Keeling, Jean.
[DNLM: 1. Fetal Diseases—pathology. 2. Infant, Newborn, Diseases—pathology.
WQ 211 F4192]
RG626.F45 1993
618.3′2—dc20
DNLM/DLC 92-2323
for Library of Congress CIP

Printed in Great Britain

Typeset by Best-set Typesetter Ltd., Hong Kong
Printed by BAS Printers Limited, Over Wallop, Hampshire, UK
2128/3830-543210 Printed on acid-free paper

Preface to the First Edition

This book is primarily intended for the histopathologist who is called upon to provide a perinatal necropsy service. It will help the junior pathologist to achieve competence in the performance of perinatal necropsies and fetal examination. It does not attempt to provide an exhaustive review of every aspect of fetal pathology but concentrates on common problems, particularly where recognition of morbid anatomical abnormalities indicates the direction of subsequent investigations.

Some years ago, I was advised to consider a move away from paediatric pathology because both birth rate and perinatal mortality were falling and there would be a dramatic reduction in workload and interest. Nothing could have been further from the truth. The downward trend in birth rate has reversed, and, although in Europe, Australia and North America perinatal mortality has continued to fall, the effect has been to direct more attention to those deaths which still occur. Neonatal Paediatrics has emerged as a field for specialisation. The availability of non-invasive techniques for fetal assessment and the rapid expansion of prenatal diagnosis of malformations and inherited disorders have increased the demand for detailed pathological examination of the deceased fetus and infant. Obstetricians and neonatalogists have become increasingly aware that information obtained from post-mortem examination can make a useful contribution to clinical management. It has an important audit function and provides the most reliable basis for parental counselling about future pregnancies.

The histopathologist is almost the last generalist in hospital practice. The development of specialised areas of interest and expertise within the major medical specialties has made heavy demands on pathology departments. It is difficult to keep abreast of new methodology and changing views about the interpretation of pathological findings in every specialist field. As most births take place away from teaching centres, in hospitals where pathologists with particular interests in perinatal pathology are unlikely to be based, it is the general histopathologist, often with no specific training in this field, who is expected to investigate the majority of fetal and perinatal deaths.

Provision of satisfactory answers for clinicians depends as much on an understanding of their day-to-day problems, so that answers may be provided to fundamental questions which may have gone unasked, as it does on answering questions related to the specific case in hand. The first part of this book (Chapters 1–15) aims to provide essential clinical and physiological information related to currently important problems in fetal and neonatal pathology as well as a guide to their investigation. Chapter 1 discusses the relevance of post-mortem examination to obstetric and neonatal practice and the need to resist preoccupation with a cause of death as the only reason for necropsy. Details of necropsy technique appropriate to the fetal and neonatal periods are described and the necessity for modifications in technique discussed. Chapter 2 describes the normal progression of implantation of the ovum and placentation in the human, together with methods of placental examination and normal findings as well as its appearance in abnormal pregnancies and specific pathological states.

The following four chapters discuss particular aspects of fetal pathology in the first and second trimesters of pregnancy. Chapter 3 addresses the pathology and pathogenesis of spontaneous abortions. Chapter 4 examines some of the problems related to examination of the fetus from terminated pregnancies. This is a new and important area of morbid anatomy, and fetal examination is particularly valuable following ultrasound diagnosis of fetal anomaly. Chapters 5 and 6 examine the pathologist's contribution to the investigation of malformations and inherited metabolic disease.

The remainder of this problem-orientated section relates largely to the second half of pregnancy, beginning with epidemiological analyses and related problems. The topics covered in subsequent chapters are those where clinical information is particularly relevant to the appropriate direction of pathological investigations.

The second part of the book (Chapters 16–28) is system orientated and describes and illustrates those pathological abnormalities which are likely to be encountered in the fetus and neonate. Each chapter is prefaced by a concise account of the development of the particular system and, where relevant, a description of the changes which occur at birth or an account of normal function in the neonatal period. Cross-referencing between sections by chapter and page number provides ready access to relevant pathological detail or related conditions.

Acknowledgements to the First Edition

It is a pleasure to acknowledge the generosity of colleagues in Britain and Europe who have made available photographs and material for illustrations or have read chapters during their preparation. I am particularly grateful to Drs. Ashley King, Simon Knowles and Helen Porter who read my own contributions. Miss Sheila Moore patiently prepared sections for illustrations and Geoffrey Richardson and Julian Markham produced illustrations for several chapters.

Mr. Michael Jackson and Mrs. Judy Watt of Springer-Verlag have generously given help, advice and encouragement throughout the preparation of this book.

Particular thanks are owed to Miss Shirley Martin, who has cheerfully typed and kept track of the manuscripts throughout.

Oxford, 1987 Jean W. Keeling

Preface to the Second Edition

It is five years since the publication of the first edition. During this time clinical practices have been modified and changes in the content of the second edition reflect this. Some contributors to the first edition have moved to new positions, or have developed new interests. The effect of these changes is two new chapters, the loss of one, and an amalgamation of two others. The perinatal mortality amongst twins is five to six times that of singletons, many problems are specific to multiple pregnancy. A new chapter seemed appropriate. The development and pathology of the Reproductive System has been separated from that of the Urinary Tract. Immunological aspects of pregnancy are covered in the chapters on Placenta, Spontaneous abortion and Reticuloendothelial system. The previous chapters on Fetal Examination after Termination of Pregnancy and Congenital Malformations have been amalgamated, the sections on causes of malformations and diagnostic methods have been expanded. There is change of authorship of many chapters with nine new contributors. Some chapters have been updated but retain their original form. Many have been completely rewritten either because of change of authorship or because the extent of changes in a particular field necessitates changes in emphasis.

The book retains the overall format of the first edition, the first half presenting problems encountered in fetal/perinatal pathology with some essential clinical background, the second describing systemic pathology in a more detailed and orderly fashion. The aim remains the same, to provide an easy to read book to answer day to day problems encountered during examination of fetal and perinatal deaths within a single volume. It is not an exhaustive text but refers the reader to appropriate sources for more detailed information of the unusual.

Edinburgh, 1992 Jean W. Keeling

Acknowledgements to the Second Edition

Colleagues in Scotland have given their time, material and much encouragement during the preparation of this second edition. The staff of Springer-Verlag have responded promptly and effectively when problems arose, and Michael Jackson gave sound advice and encouragement throughout. My secretary, Miss Ann Burns has patiently and efficiently translated endless amendments into comprehsible copy, and introduced much-needed humour into trying situations.

Edinburgh, 1992 Jean W. Keeling

Contents

Chapter 7 Macerated Stillbirth
Isabella E. Moore

Chapter 8 Prematurity
Gillian Batcup

Chapter 9 Pathology of Twinning
Geoffrey A. Machin

Chapter 10 Intrapartum Asphyxia and Birth Trauma
Jean W. Keeling

Chapter 11 Fetal Hydrops
Jean W. Keeling

Chapter 15 The Gastrointestinal Tract and Exocrine Pancreas
Dick Variend

Chapter 16 Liver and Gall Badder
D. Ian Rushton

Chapter 17 The Respiratory System
Steve J. Gould

Chapter 18 The Cardiovascular System
Jerry N. Cox and Jakob Briner

Contributors

J. Patrick Barbet, MD, PhD,
Pathologist and Forensic Pathologist, Service d'Anatomie Pathologique, Hôpital Saint-Vincent-de-Paul, 74 Avenue Denfert-Rochereau, F-75014 Paris, France

Gillian Batcup, BSc, MB, MRCPath,
Senior Lecturer in Paediatric and Perinatal Pathology, Department of Pathology, Clarendon Wing, General Infirmary, Belmont Grove, Leeds LS2 9NS

Colin L. Berry, MD, PhD, FRCPath,
Professor of Morbid Anatomy, The London Hospital Medical College, Whitechapel, London E1 1BB

P. Jeremy Berry, BA, MBBChir, MRCP, MRCPath,
Professor of Paediatric Pathology, Bristol Royal Hospital for Sick Children, St Michael's Hill, Bristol BS2 8BJ and Bristol Maternity Hospital, Southwell Street, Bristol BS2 8EG

Patricia A. Boyd, MD,
Associate Specialist in Prenatal Diagnosis, Oxford Regional Prenatal Diagnosis Service, Maternity Department, John Radcliffe Hospital, Headington, Oxford OX3 9DU

Jakob Briner, MD,
Professor, Head of Paediatric Pathology Section, Institut für Pathologie der Universität Zürich, Schmelzbergstrasse 12, CH-8091 Zürich, Switzerland

Jerry N. Cox, BSc, MD, FRCPath,
Paediatric Pathologist, Institute of Pathology, CMU, 1 rue Michel-Servet, 1211 Geneva 4, Switzerland

Jean Golding, MA, PhD,
Professor of Paediatric and Perinatal Epidemiology, Institute of Child Health, Royal Hospital for Sick Children, St Michael's Hill, Bristol BS2 8BJ

Steve J. Gould, BSc, MBBS, MRCPath,
Consultant in Paediatric and Perinatal Histopathology, Paediatric Pathology, Maternity Department, John Radcliffe Hospital, Headington, Oxford OX3 9DU

Elizabeth S. Gray, MBChB, FRCPath,
Senior Lecturer in Pathology, Hon. Consultant Perinatal and Paediatric Pathologist, University Medical School, Forresterhill, Aberdeen AB9 2ZD

Niels Græm, MD,
Consultant Pathologist, Pathological-Anatomical Institute, Herlev Hospital, DK-2730 Herlev, Denmark

Helen S. Holzel, MSc, MBChB, FRCPath,
Consultant Medical Microbiologist, The Hospital for Sick Children, Great Ormond Street, London WC1N 3JH

Jean W. Keeling, MBBS, FRCPath, FRCP (Edin),
Consultant Paediatric Pathologist, Department of Paediatric Pathology, Royal Hospital for Sick Children, 2 Rillbank Crescent, Edinburgh EH9 1LF

T. Yee Khong, MD, MCRPath, MSc,
Consultant Pathologist, Adelaide Medical Centre for Women and Children, Queen Victoria Hospital, 160 Fullarton Road, Rose Park, South Australia 5067

Simon Knowles, BSc, MBBS, MRCPath,
Director of Laboratory Services, King Edward Memorial Hospital for Women, 374 Bagot Road, Subiaco, Western Australia 6008

K. Michael Laurence, MA, MBChB, DSc, FRCP, FRCPath,
Springside, Pen-y-Turnpike, Dinas Powys CF6 4HG, Wales

Brendan McDonald, BSc, MBChB,
Senior Registrar in Neuropathology, Department of Neuropathology, Radcliffe Infirmary, Oxford OX2 6HE

Geoffrey A. Machin, BA, PhD, BM, BCh, FRCPath, FRCP(C),
Professor of Paediatric Pathology, Department of Pathology, University of Alberta Hospital, 8440-112 Street, Edmonton, Alberta, Canada T6G 2B7

Peter R. Millard, MD, FRCPath,
NHS Consultant Histopathologist, Department of Histopathology, John Radcliffe Hospital, Headington, Oxford OX3 9DU

Isabella E. Moore, DM, MRCPath,
Consultant Paediatric Pathologist, Department of Histopathology, Southampton General Hospital, Southampton SO9 4XY

Jørn Müller,
Department of Growth and Reproduction, Rigshospitalet, 9 Blegdamsvej, DK-2100 Copenhagen Ø, Denmark

R. Anthony Risdon, MD, FRCPath,
Professor in Histopathology, The Hospital for Sick Children, Great Ormond Street, London WC1N 3JH

D. Ian Rushton, MBChB, FRCPath,
Senior Lecturer in Pathology, University of Birmingham, Hon. Consultant Pathologist, Birmingham Maternity Hospital, Queen Elizabeth Medical Centre, Edgbaston, Birmingham B15 2TG

Marian V. Squier, MRCP, MRCPath,
Consultant Neuropathologist, Department of Neuropathology, Radcliffe Infirmary, Oxford OX2 6HE

Hans J. van der Harten, MD,
Paediatric Pathologist, Pathology Department, Free University Hospital, De Boelelaan 1117, 1007 MB Amsterdam, The Netherlands

Dick Variend, MD, MRCP, FRCPath, DCH,
Consultant Paediatric Pathologist, Department of Pathology, Children's Hospital, Western Bank, Sheffield S10 2TH

Chapter 1

The Perinatal Necropsy

Jean W. Keeling

Introduction

The importance to clinical practice of information obtained by adequate necropsy examination of babies dying in the perinatal and neonatal periods (Alberman 1980) is often not fully appreciated by histopathologists providing a biopsy-orientated service for adult patients. Examination of stillborn infants has been particularly neglected. This is probably related both to the unattractive nature of the material and to negative expectations concerning the likelihood of being able to make specific diagnoses.

Necropsy information is of practical importance at three different levels of clinical practice. Firstly, it is important to the family of the dead baby and to the clinicians involved in their care. Secondly, necropsy findings are necessary for adequate audit of unit policies and practices. Lastly, data derived from post-mortem examination make an important contribution to regional or national statistics by complementing clinical data collection. Some necropsy data are appropriate to all three levels of enquiry, but each requires answers to more specific questions.

In developed countries, where perinatal mortality rates are low, the anticipated outcome of pregnancy is a normally formed healthy infant, and the possibility of perinatal death is not seriously entertained unless there has been such a death in the immediate family. The parents want to know what and how things went wrong, without necessarily wanting to attach blame to a particular individual or institution. Of even greater concern is the need to know the risks of repetition of perinatal death in subsequent pregnancies and, particularly when death occurs in a first pregnancy, their chances of achieving their desired family size.

From the point of view of providing optimal management in the next and subsequent pregnancies, the obstetrician needs to know whether clinical estimates of gestation and fetal growth were correct and if the results of prenatal investigations accurately predicted fetal growth and maturity and the presence or absence of malformations. He will also want to know whether uterine response to gestation was appropriate and whether there was evidence of infection in either fetus or gestation sac. In some circumstances he will be particularly concerned about the possibility of asphyxial or mechanical insult during labour. He will want to know about the presence of any clinically unsuspected malformation, as well as details of dysmorphic features and anomalies accompanying a malformation recognised before or at delivery, so that the correct risk of recurrence is calculated and so that he can institute an appropriate plan for surveillance of subsequent pregnancies. The neonatologist will want confirmation of diagnoses made during life and will want to know whether any treatable conditions went unrecognised. He will be concerned about complications of treatment and will welcome information about gestation-related characteristics to compare with clinical estimates of maturity.

National perinatal mortality data are an important index of the nation's health. Accurate collection of information, both in respect of completeness of ascertainment and causes of death, is a necessary part of this process. Accurate completion of death certificates and their subsequent registration are essential, and it is important that causes of death are verified by post-mortem examination. Remittance of information for analysis at national level often seems far removed from unit practice. We should remember that it is often on the basis of such data that decisions concerning staffing levels and funding of services are made. It is in the local interest to cooperate with national statistical agencies to improve the accuracy of perinatal mortality data.

In many countries perinatal mortality rates are currently below 15 per 1000 births. This means that the number of deaths in individual units and even regional totals are so low that detailed analyses are readily distorted by events which, in the long term, are of little relevance to practice. Because of these low levels of perinatal mortality, we are sometimes urged to measure morbidity rates instead (Chamberlain 1985). Whilst it is important to try to collect this sort of information, it should be an adjunct to the collection of mortality data and not an alternative method of measuring clinical practice. Some of the problems related to the accuracy of perinatal mortality data are discussed in Chapter 6 (see p. 165). They are small when set beside the difficulties in obtaining accurate information concerning morbidity. The worst of these are related to imprecision of definition and the need to follow children for several years in order to approach "complete" ascertainment. Death rates have enormous merit in that the end point is precise!

An aspect of necropsy examination which is often forgotten is its importance to the continuing education of doctors and other hospital staff, irrespective of seniority. Most benefit accrues to those in training, but even the most senior pathologist or clinician can learn something by being present during the performance of the most "routine" perinatal necropsy examination. To this end, it is important that perinatal necropsies are not just delegated to junior staff and then forgotten. Such necropsy experience should be part of the training of all junior histopathologists, but careful supervision and demonstration of appropriate techniques by a senior pathologist, preferably with experience in perinatal pathology, is essential.

When clinicians take time to attend post-mortem examinations on their patients, it does a great deal to encourage the pathologist concerned and to educate him about current clinical practice and the clinical relevance of information which he can readily obtain. In this way, both clinician and pathologist gain satisfaction and the value of necropsy examination is enhanced. Attendance of senior clinical staff in the mortuary demonstrates to junior doctors the importance of post-mortem examination in a way that no amount of exhortation from pathologists can ever do.

Importance of Negative Findings

For a pathologist accustomed to the plethora of manifestations of degenerative disease evident at adult necropsy, the lack of findings during perinatal post-mortem examination is often a disappointment. It is used as justification for a cavalier approach to perinatal work, which is then accorded low priority. This attitude is quite inappropriate. Often, the most useful contribution that the pathologist can make is to report negative findings after a carefully executed necropsy.

When a baby dies, the parents contemplate many theoretical abnormalities which, in their view, remove entirely the possibility of successful pregnancy. Clinicians may be worried about the possibility of birth injury or of missed, treatable abnormalities. Careful recording of negative necropsy findings does a great deal to reassure all those involved. To this end, negatives should be clearly and unambiguously stated in the necropsy report, a copy of which is usually filed in the mother's notes. In subsequent pregnancies it may be consulted by relatively junior members of both medical and nursing staff to answer specific parental queries or as a basis for management decisions. There must be no room for doubt about negative findings. For this reason too, the significance of the presence or absence of necropsy findings should be clearly stated, particularly those opinions formed after recourse to the literature or discussions with colleagues with particular experience in this field.

Adequate Clinical Information

The importance of the availability of clinical information before the start of any necropsy examination cannot be overstated. This is doubly important to necropsy examination of neonates, when information about the mother is always required and may in some circumstances be of equal or greater importance than that concerning the baby.

Maternal notes are frequently unavailable before a necropsy examination. This may be because the maternal condition necessitates constant recourse to her notes and their removal, even for a short time would be inappropriate. Sometimes necropsy examination is undertaken in a different building or in a hospital far removed from the place of delivery. In these circumstances, clinicians may be reluctant to allow removal of notes from the maternity unit because of the length of time of their absence and for fear of loss. In most cases, however, it is likely to be lack of awareness on the part of both clinician and pathologist concerning the relevance of information about the mother to satisfactory performance of necropsy examination. In this situation, no thought is given to the institution of an efficient routine to make notes available with minimal interference to clinical needs.

Ready availability of both infant and maternal notes does not negate the benefit to both sides of discussion between clinician and pathologist before necropsy commences. Direct communication between colleagues is without doubt the best way to ensure that important clinical questions are answered and unrealistic expectations modified before unproductive or even antagonistic attitudes are allowed to interfere. It is important to both clinical and pathological practice that questions are clearly formulated and that techniques are modified to realise the best chance of an unambiguous answer. Clinicians are often disappointed when they do not get answers to questions relevant to patient management following post-mortem examination. This disappointment pales into insignificance beside the irritation of the pathologist who is faced at the end of his examination with a question which he could have answered if it had been put to him at the appropriate time—before he started!

Essential information comprises date and outcome of previous pregnancies as well as details of the index pregnancy. The date of the mother's last menstrual period is the basis for assessment of length of gestation together with the method and reason for any revisions of the original assessment. A history of maternal problems during pregnancy should be sought, particularly hypertension, preeclamptic toxaemia, pyrexial illness, diabetes (mellitus or gestationis) and vaginal haemorrhage. A note of investigations undertaken during pregnancy and abnormal findings, particularly maternal serum alpha-fetoprotein levels and ultrasound examinations in the second trimester, are required.

Details of delivery should include date, time and mode of delivery, reasons for induction of labour or operative delivery and birthweight. These are all necessary to ensure that the appropriate investigations are undertaken. For livebirths, details should include condition at birth, appearance, clinical estimation of maturity, together with a brief postnatal history comprising problems, procedures undertaken and clinical opinions about causes of death. Because both positive and negative answers to these questions are important for the conduct of an appropriate necropsy examination, I find that a structured information sheet (Figs. 1.1; 1.2) is the best way of obtaining the information at the right time.

Place of Structured Request Forms in Perinatal Pathology

A carefully completed structured perinatal request form provides the pathologist with consistent, minimal clinical information which can always be available before necropsy examination begins. Such forms (Figs. 1.1; 1.2) are not a substitute for access to clinical notes and their use should not deter clinicians from submitting additional information which they consider relevant to a particular case.

Besides being a convenient means of transfer of essential information, structured request forms achieve other ends. The process of their completion affords an opportunity to junior staff in obstetric and neonatal units for critical review of individual patient management. It

DEPARTMENT OF PATHOLOGY, ROYAL HOSPITAL FOR SICK CHILDREN, EDINBURGH

REQUEST FOR EXAMINATION OF A FETUS OR PERINATAL NECROPSY

Unit No. DoB Baby's Name Sex Paediatrician

Name Hospital Ward

Address Obs GP

PREVIOUS PREGNANCIES

	Date	Gestation	Labour	Puerperium	Sex	Outcome
1						
2						
3						
4						

PRESENT PREGNANCY Booked/Unbooked, Contraception Yes/No Type

INFECTION RISK High/Low Reason ....

LMP / / EDD / / Gestation Clinical w. USS w.

Threatened Abortion : Yes/No When? w. Amniocentesis : Yes/No Why? ....

Hypertension : Yes/No US Scan : Yes/No Why? ....

Pre-Eclamptic Toxaemia : Yes/No AFP : Normal/High/Low/Not Done

I.U.G.R. : Yes/No Blood Group :

Polyhydramnios : Yes/No Maternal Pyrexia : Yes/No When? ....

Antepartum Haemorrhage : Yes/No Source .... When? w.

Other Problem ....

TYPE OF ABORTION : Spontaneous/Induced for IUD/Social Reasons/Fetal Anomaly Specify ....

....

ONSET OF LABOUR : Spontaneous/Induced/Why? ....

Last Evidence of Fetal Life : / / Time ....

Rupture of Membranes : Date : / / Time ....

Liquor: Amount : Normal/Little/Excess Colour ....

1st Stage : .... Hr .... Min 2nd : .... Hr .... Min

Fetal Distress : Yes/No Specify ....

Presentation : Vertex/Breech/Other .... Delivery ....

Delivery : Date : / / Time : .... Death : Date : / / Time : ....

Fig. 1.1. Structured information sheet provides minimal clinical data required by the pathologist before perinatal necropsy. Pregnancy and Labour.

NEONATE : Birth Weight g Gestation Wk APGAR Score .... at 1 min .... at 5 min

RESUSCITATION : Nil/Mucus Extraction/0_2 Mask/Intubation

NEONATAL PROBLEMS

1

2

3

4

PROCEDURES

1

2

3

4

SUSPECTED CAUSES OF DEATH

1

2

3

4

ANY OTHER RELEVANT INFORMATION

MEDICAL OFFICER TO BE CONTACTED FOR DISCUSSION OF CASE/VERBAL REPORT

....

Block Capitals

PLACE SPECIMEN WITH PLACENTA IN A SEALED CONTAINER OR POLYTHENE BAG IN FRIDGE
DO NOT ADD PRESERVATIVE
WHERE VAN SERVICE NOT AVAILABLE, TELEPHONE 031-667 1991 EXT 271 DAY OR NIGHT (ANSAFONE)
GIVING YOUR NAME, HOSPITAL AND UNIT, AND REQUEST THAT SPECIMEN BE COLLECTED

Fig. 1.2. Structured information sheet, neonatal details.

may be their first opportunity to look at the case as a whole and observe the way in which problems inter-relate at a time when they are no longer distracted by a stressful clinical situation. A structured request form also serves to guide the pathologist through the complexities of management of a baby who has received prolonged intensive care, when his notes are likely to be voluminous.

Growth and Development

The fetal and neonatal periods are ones of continuing development at both organ and tissue level, first by a process of cell division (hyperplasia) and then by growth of individual cells (hypertrophy). There is rapid somatic growth, which is roughly linear for most of the second and third trimesters, slowing down from about 38 weeks' gestation until delivery. Knowledge of the length of gestation is an important yardstick against which the appropriateness of developmental markers and somatic growth are measured. Assessment of normality and uniformity of organ development is also important for interpretation of findings at perinatal necropsy. Growth and development advance concurrently and, whilst they are inter-related, they may be affected together or independently by environmental factors. An awareness of developmental criteria and normal fetal growth is essential to the performance and interpretation of necropsy examination of fetus and neonate. Particular patterns of deviation from the normal might indicate the way in which investigations should proceed or alert the pathologist to commonly associated abnormalities.

In obstetric practice the duration of pregnancy is commonly measured from the start of the mother's last menstrual period. The relationship of this method of measurement to conceptional (gestational) age is dependent on the length of the individual's menstrual cycle and also on her memory. Despite these reservations, menstrual dating usually permits the best estimate of the length of gestation. Ultrasound measurement of fetal parts in early pregnancy is performed very frequently at the present time. It is particularly useful in women with irregular menstrual cycles or poor memory. Current standards for ultrasound dating of pregnancy are as good as menstrual dating (Campbell and Pearce 1985). However, these standards are derived from fetal measurements in a population of women of "certain" menstrual dates; a machine-generated number to several decimal places does not imply a dating accuracy down to fractions of a week!

Many of the babies who die in the fetal and neonatal period are of low birthweight. The term "premature" used to be applied indiscriminately to this group of babies and discrepant historical evidence about the length of gestation was ignored. Current practice (Working Party of Obstetricians and Paediatricians in Europe 1970) defines prematurity as duration of pregnancy of less than 37 weeks from last menstrual date. This group defines "term" as pregnancy duration of 37–41 weeks and designates those pregnancies of 42 weeks and longer as "post term". Babies who weigh less than or equal to 2500 g at birth are designated "low birthweight". Thus babies of low birthweight may be preterm and appropriately grown, preterm and growth retarded (small-for-dates) or mature and growth retarded.

Birthweight is affected by many different factors, both constitutional (e.g. genetic factors, chromosome abnormality) and environmental. The latter may act directly on the fetus (e.g. first trimester infection affects fetal cell mass), on the placenta (e.g. haematogenous infection compromises fetomaternal transfer of oxygen and nutrients) or via the mother (e.g. chronic undernutrition or poor uteroplacental perfusion from any cause). Small women tend to have small babies as do women with some inherited abnormalities such as phenylketonuria (PKU). Babies from multiple gestations are of lower birthweight than those from singleton pregnancies. Low birthweight is a feature of many malformation syndromes with major somatic defects such as dwarfism, anencephaly and Meckel–Gruber syndrome. Fetal growth and factors which adversely affect it are discussed by Kliegman and King (1983). Recently published birthweight data (Lucas et al. 1986; Yudkin et al. 1987) demonstrate the way in which our concept of the normal weight of preterm infants is altered if standards are based on the weights of all babies delivered. Both groups of workers have shown that babies delivered electively before 34 weeks' gestation are lighter than babies born spontaneously at the same gestation (see Fig. 1.7).

Fetal growth retardation may be of early onset, when it is characteristically "symmetrical", so that fetal organs are smaller but proportionally unchanged (Fig. 1.3). Serial measurements of

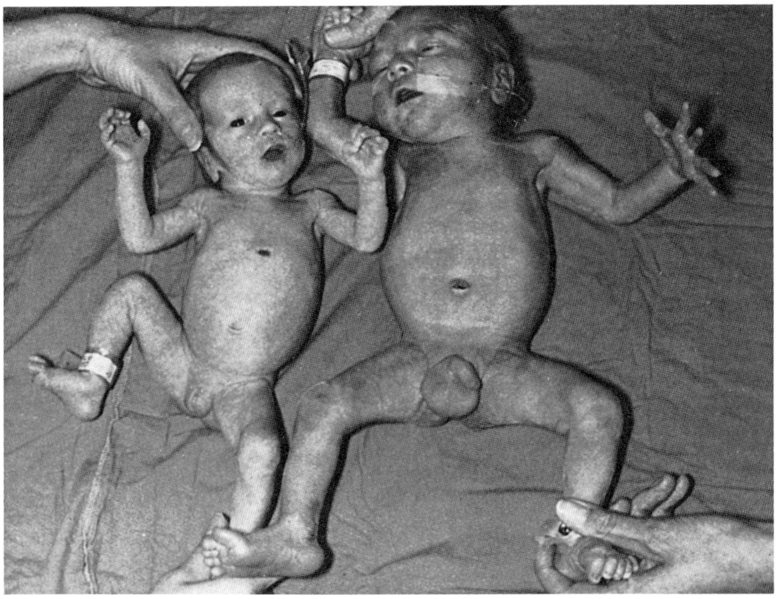

Fig. 1.3. Growth-retarded baby (*left*), birthweight 1180 g at 35 weeks' gestation compared with a normally grown baby (median birthweight 2630 g). Growth retardation is symmetrical (early onset).

biparietal diameter (BPD) show that it grows below, but parallel to, the centile lines. This type of growth retardation may be the result of intrauterine infection (TORCH organisms, see Chap. 13, p. 295), genetic constitution, chromosome abnormality (Fig. 1.4) or malformation syndromes such as renal agenesis (Table 1.1). Late-onset growth retardation results in "asymmetric" growth disturbance with relative sparing of brain growth and therefore of head circumference and BPD (Cooke et al. 1977; Fig. 1.5). Disturbance of organ weight ratios is observed, for example an increase in brain to liver weight ratio. Serial BPD measurements are initially within the normal range but progressively fall below normal values in late pregnancy. The causes of this type of growth retardation are usually environmental. It may be the result of reduced uteroplacental perfusion in conditions such as maternal hypertension or preeclampsia, maternal diabetes mellitus or non-availability of nutrients as seen in chronic maternal undernutrition. Prematurity and its related problems are discussed in Chapter 8, p. 199.

Some babies are inappropriately large for gestational age (heavy-for-dates). These babies tend to be born to taller, heavier mothers who are older and of higher parity. Excessive maternal weight gain may be observed during the pregnancy. Maternal diabetes mellitus (Fig.

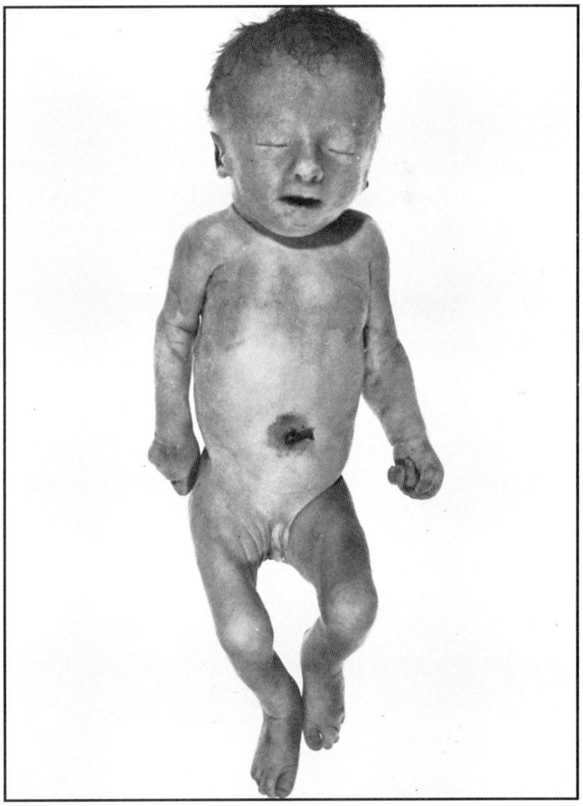

Fig. 1.4. Growth-retarded baby, trisomy 18, weighed 1790 g at 39 weeks' gestation (median birthweight 3220 g).

Table 1.1. Features of fetal growth retardation

Characteristics	
Symmetrical: early onset constitutional reduced growth potential organ weight ratios normal	*Asymmetric*: late onset environmental late growth arrest brain relatively large
Causes	
Early fetal infection: rubella CMV toxoplasmosis malaria syphilis	*Reduced uteroplacental perfusion*: pre-eclampsia maternal hypertension diabetes mellitus maternal smoking
Chromosome abnormalities: trisomy 13, 18, 21 triploidy sex chromosome abnormalities	*Undernutrition*: evidence of malnutrition adolescent mother chronic infection alcoholism; drug ingestion dietary faddism materal PKU
Metabolic abormalities: agenesis of pancreas/absent islets of Langerhans gangliosidosis I I cell disease hypophosphatasia Menkes' syndrome	

1.6) and gestational diabetes are associated with large babies. Macrosomia is a feature of Wiedemann–Beckwith syndrome and Soto's syndrome. Large babies are at risk of birth injury and intrapartum asphyxia (see Chap. 10, p. 244).

Equipment for Perinatal Necropsy

Necropsy examination of fetuses and neonates requires few facilities beyond those which one would expect to find in a well-equipped mortuary. Any pathology department which routinely undertakes examination of babies must have equipment which will allow easy recording of body measurements and structural abnormalities.

Measurement

Accurate weighing scales for measurement of both body and organ weights are essential. Mature babies can usually be weighed on scales suitable for adult organ weighing. For organ weights and the weighing of fetuses less than 20 weeks' gestation, scales accurate to 0.5 g are needed. An electronic balance with digital display is very convenient.

A metric ruler and calipers or measuring board with one fixed end (Langley 1971) are required for measurement of body and foot lengths and skull diameters. Circumferential measurements are best made with string and read off against a ruler; a tape measure is less accurate. Techniques of mensuration are illustrated by Valdes-Dapena and Huff (1983).

Dissection Instruments

Instruments of appropriately small size make fetal dissection much easier to carry out without damage to structures before examination is complete. Scissors with tapering blades and rounded ends (Mayo) reduce frequency of inadvertent perforation, which often occurs when pointed scissors are used. Iridectomy scissors are a useful size for dissection of second trimester abortuses. Non-toothed forceps are less damaging to fetal tissues than those with

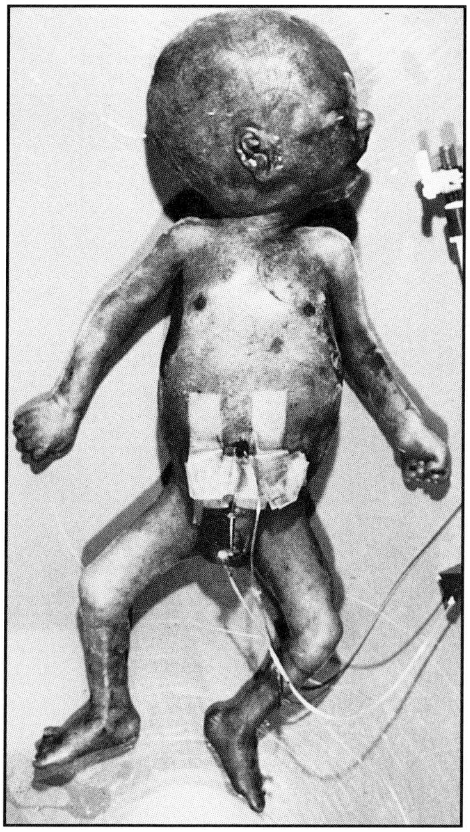

Fig. 1.5. Asymmetric growth retardation, birthweight 595 g at 27 weeks' gestation (median birthweight 930 g). Head size is relatively normal.

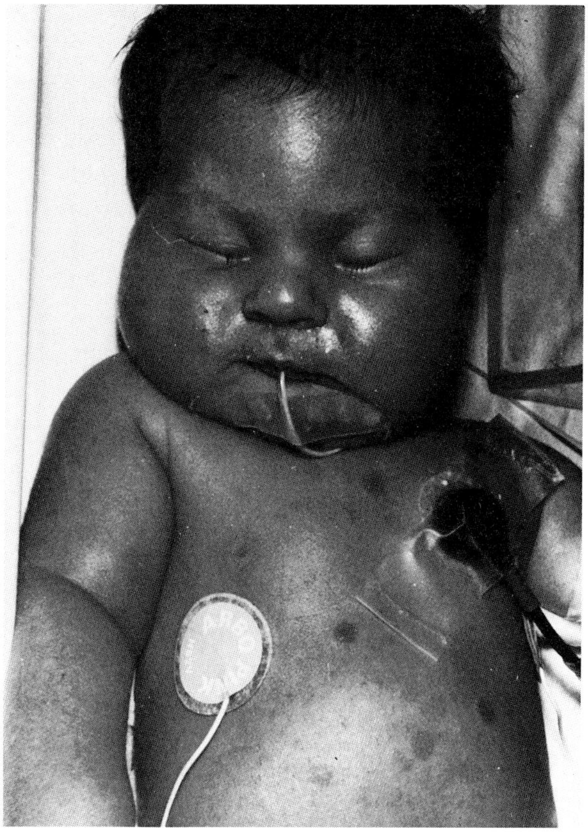

Fig. 1.6. Infant of diabetic mother is both large and obese, birthweight 3614 g at 36 weeks' gestation (median birthweight 2940 g). (Courtesy of Dr. A.R. Wilkinson, Oxford)

teeth. A range of models is available and a selection of round-ended, tapering-blade forceps of different lengths, such as 10 cm–17 cm (4 in–7 in), is useful.

A size 3 scalpel handle and a range of blades to fit will suit most purposes during fetal examination. Trainees will find neck dissection in the neonate a great deal easier with a narrow scalpel blade of small size.

A selection of probes, down to small lachrymal duct size, makes demonstration of abnormal anatomy easier, and a pair of 20 cm (8 in) straight, sprung bone forceps will cut ribs, vertebral bodies and femoral shafts, and open middle ears. A domestic fish slice is invaluable for handling brain slices.

A mounted magnifying lens, perhaps with an integral light source, is especially useful in departments where second trimester fetuses are examined regularly.

Post-mortem Examination

The post-mortem examination of fetuses and babies dying in the neonatal period follows a similar pattern to examination of adults but differs in certain important respects. Neglect of these modifications will result in failure to obtain important information or cause unnecessary difficulty in the performance of necropsy examination. It is better to adopt modifications of adult necropsy technique which are appropriate to the demonstration of the range of pathological and developmental abnormalities one is likely to encounter and to use them for all perinatal necropsies than to use a variety of minor modifications of technique when a particular abnormality is suspected. This will promote familiarity with the variations in technique and means that abnormalities which were

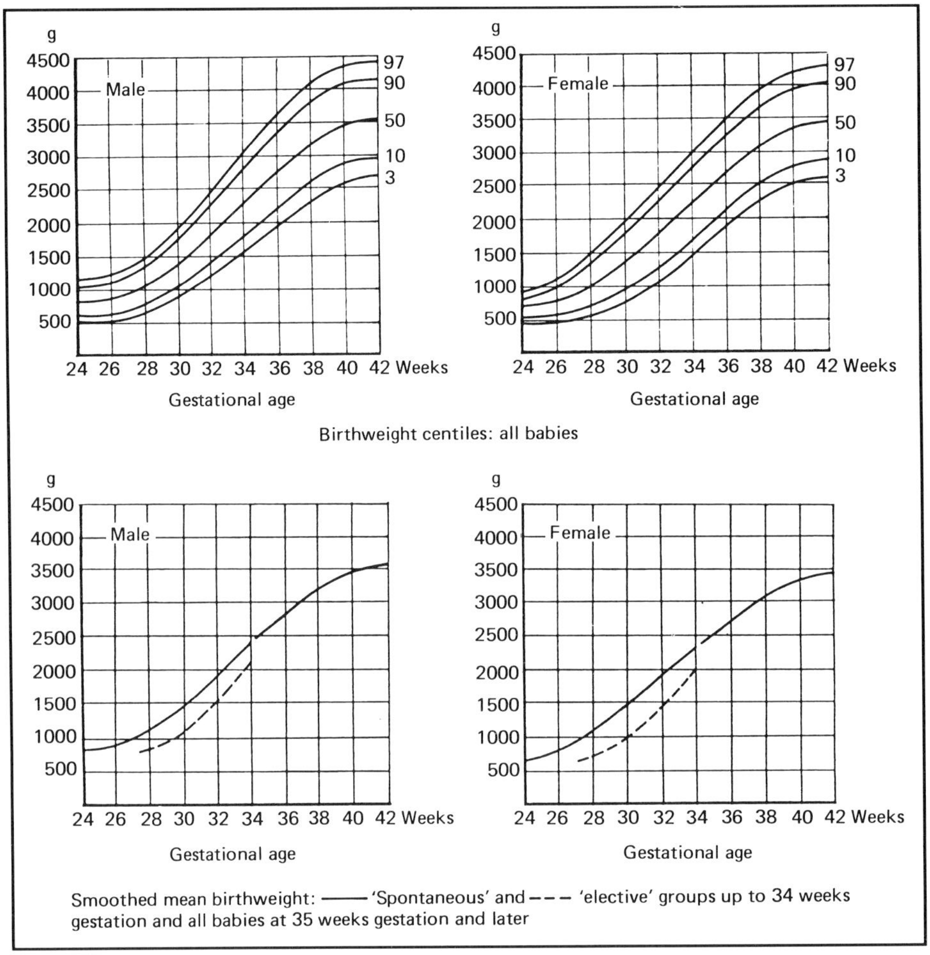

Fig. 1.7. Smoothed percentiles of birthweight by sex and gestation. (Yudkin et al. 1987)

not diagnosed during life are less likely to be missed.

Measurements

The body weight and external measurements should be recorded and compared with standard weight charts. The best comparisons are data sets compiled from the local population (Fig. 1.7), but such data are not often available. Standards used by local clinicians are the best compromise. Charts based on data of Gairdner and Pearson (1971) and Milner and Richards (1974) are available commercially. It is important that weights and measurements are assessed against appropriate gestation-related normal values. The frequency of growth retardation amongst babies who die in the perinatal period can influence the pathologist's concept of normality (Fig. 1.8) to the extent that significant growth retardation may be ignored. Crown–rump, crown–heel and foot lengths are useful for assessment of fetal growth. Foot length (Table 1.2) is a useful gestation-related measurement to supplement menstrual dating and for comparison with ultrasound measurements made during pregnancy or clinical assessment of maturity undertaken at birth. Both crown–rump and crown–heel lengths are prone to inaccuracy, particularly following intrauterine death, when joint ligaments are lax and permit excessive stretching. Foot length has the advantage that it is less open to manipulation of this type, but its range is small and this measurement should be carefully performed.

Information about other measurements at different gestations, such as head and abdominal circumference (Campbell and Pearce 1985) and BPD and femoral length (Yagel et al. 1986) have

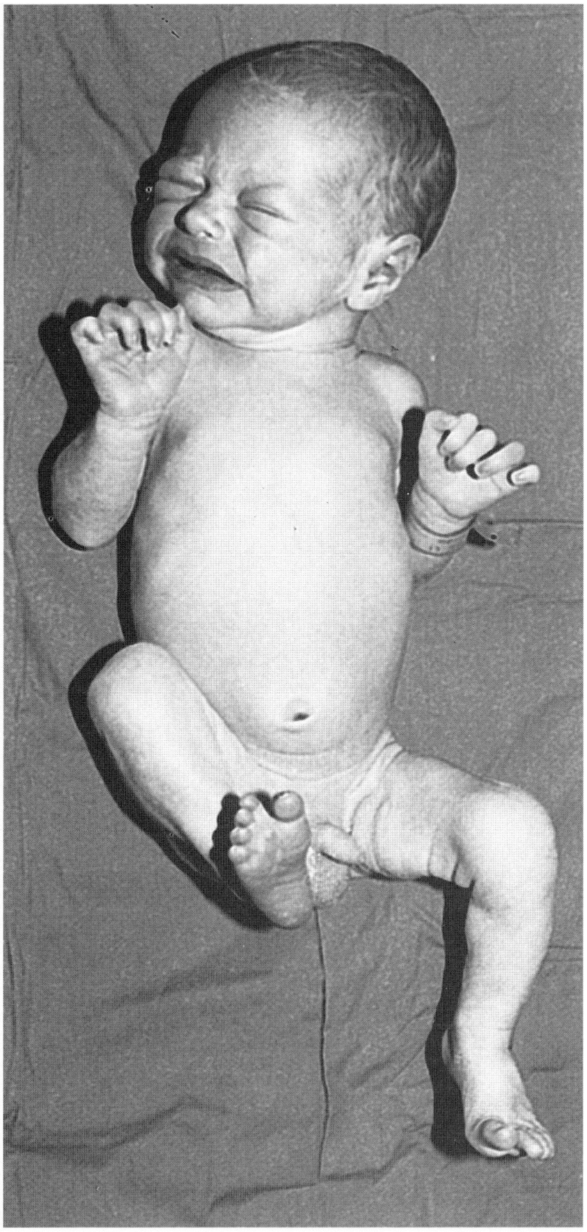

Fig. 1.8. A mature baby of normal birthweight, 3005 g at 38 weeks' gestation (median 3020 g). Compare this baby with Figs. 1.3–1.6.

become available as a result of prenatal ultrasound fetal measurement.

Head circumference should be recorded. It is approximately equal to crown–rump length during the second and third trimester of pregnancy (Fig. 1.9) and provides a useful indication of the appropriateness of head size and may also draw attention to growth retardation.

Radiographic Examination

A whole-body radiograph is a useful adjunct to perinatal necropsy (Russell 1981) and mandatory in the investigation of generalised skeletal disorders and skeletal deformity (Kalifa et al. 1989). An anteroposterior radiograph of the whole body will detect disproportion between trunk and limbs, and between the different components of limbs, more reliably than visual assessment. It can also provide information pertaining to maturity (Table 1.3; Russell 1981). The appearance of ossification centres is not sufficiently reliable to be used to assess gestational age but permits examination of the relationship between skeletal development and other parameters of gestation. Some of the factors which affect the appearance of ossification centres are discussed by Pryse-Davies et al. (1974). A radiograph will detect local skeletal abnormalities (Fig. 1.10), extraskeletal calcification (Fig. 1.11), air embolism and abnormal accumulations of gas such as pneumothorax (Fig. 1.12).

Contrast studies provide a useful record of some sorts of malformation (Fig. 1.13; Foote et al. 1978) and may be valuable for direction of subsequent dissection (Fig. 1.14).

Access to the radiography department for post-mortem radiographs is sometimes difficult, and appropriate apparatus sited within the pathology department usually means that radiographs are obtained regularly. A self-contained unit, such as the Faxitron (Hewlett-Packard) is ideal for pathologists' use, and gives the best results for fetal radiography and examination of individual bones (Kjær et al. 1991). An old portable X-ray machine, discarded by the radiography department because of the high dose of radiation per exposure compared with new machines, is quite suitable for pathology department use. Xeroradiography shows good fetal skeletal detail (Elejalde et al. 1985) but it is very expensive. Good results can be obtained with mammography or fine grain industrial film. Radiography of stillbirths or neonatal deaths in the labour ward or neonatal unit before transfer to the mortuary may be the easiest solution for some departments.

Photography

A photographic record of dysmorphic features and other external abnormalities provides both a quicker and a more accurate record than a

Table 1.2. Fetal crown-rump and foot lengths (Streeter 1921)

End of week	Mean sitting height (mm)	Mean foot length (mm)	Minimum foot length (mm)	Maximum foot length (mm)	Percentage mean foot length: sitting height
$8\frac{1}{2}$	27	4.2	3.8	4.6	15.6
9	31	4.6	4.2	5.0	15.0
10	40	5.5	5.0	6.0	13.8
11	50	6.9	6.0	7.8	13.8
12	61	9.1	7.5	10.8	15.0
13	74	11.4	9.8	13.0	15.4
14	87	14.0	12.5	15.5	16.0
15	101	16.8	15.2	18.5	16.6
16	116	19.9	18.2	21.6	17.0
17	130	23.0	21.0	25.0	17.7
18	142	26.8	24.8	28.8	18.9
19	153	30.7	28.5	33.0	20.0
20	164	33.3	31.0	35.7	20.0
21	175	35.2	32.5	38.0	20.0
22	186	39.5	36.0	43.0	21.0
23	197	42.2	39.0	45.5	21.4
24	208	45.2	42.0	48.5	21.8
25	218	47.7	44.5	51.0	22.0
26	228	50.2	47.0	53.5	22.0
27	238	52.7	49.0	56.5	22.0
28	247	55.2	51.5	59.0	22.3
29	256	57.0	53.0	61.0	22.3
30	265	59.2	55.5	63.0	22.3
31	274	61.2	57.5	65.0	22.3
32	283	63.0	59.0	67.0	22.3
33	293	65.0	61.0	69.0	22.2
34	302	68.2	64.0	72.5	22.6
35	311	70.5	66.0	75.0	22.6
36	321	73.5	69.0	78.0	23.0
37	331	76.5	72.0	81.0	23.0
38	341	78.5	74.0	83.0	23.0
39	352	81.0	76.0	86.0	23.0
40	362	82.5	77.5	87.5	23.0

Table 1.3. Times of appearance of bone centres on postnatal radiograph film (derived from Russell 1981)

Calcaneus	25 weeks
Talus	27 weeks
Lower femoral centre	36 weeks
Upper tibial centre	37 weeks

lengthy written description. Such photographs are particularly useful when further opinion is sought in difficult cases. It is particularly important to photograph the fetus from pregnancies terminated for malformation. Regular photographic recording of dysmorphic detail is a useful educational tool for the individual pathologist as well as being of enormous value for teaching trainees. Serial photographs during the course of organ dissection, often before the organs are removed from the body, are commonly required during examination of the fetus and neonate. This need is best met by a mounted camera with adjustable light source located within the mortuary. The equipment should be easy to use. Split screen focusing and automatic illumination monitoring ensures success for the photographically inept. Such equipment is a sound investment; good recording of dysmorphic features results in a high proportion of firm diagnoses and better parental counselling, as well as more interesting clinical meetings and lectures.

External Examination

Dysmorphic features should be sought in an orderly fashion prior to dissection during the examination of all fetal and neonatal deaths. These features, taken in combination with major malformations, permit accurate syndrome diagnosis which enables specific recurrence risks to be given to parents (see Chap. 4). Recognition of typical external abnormalities

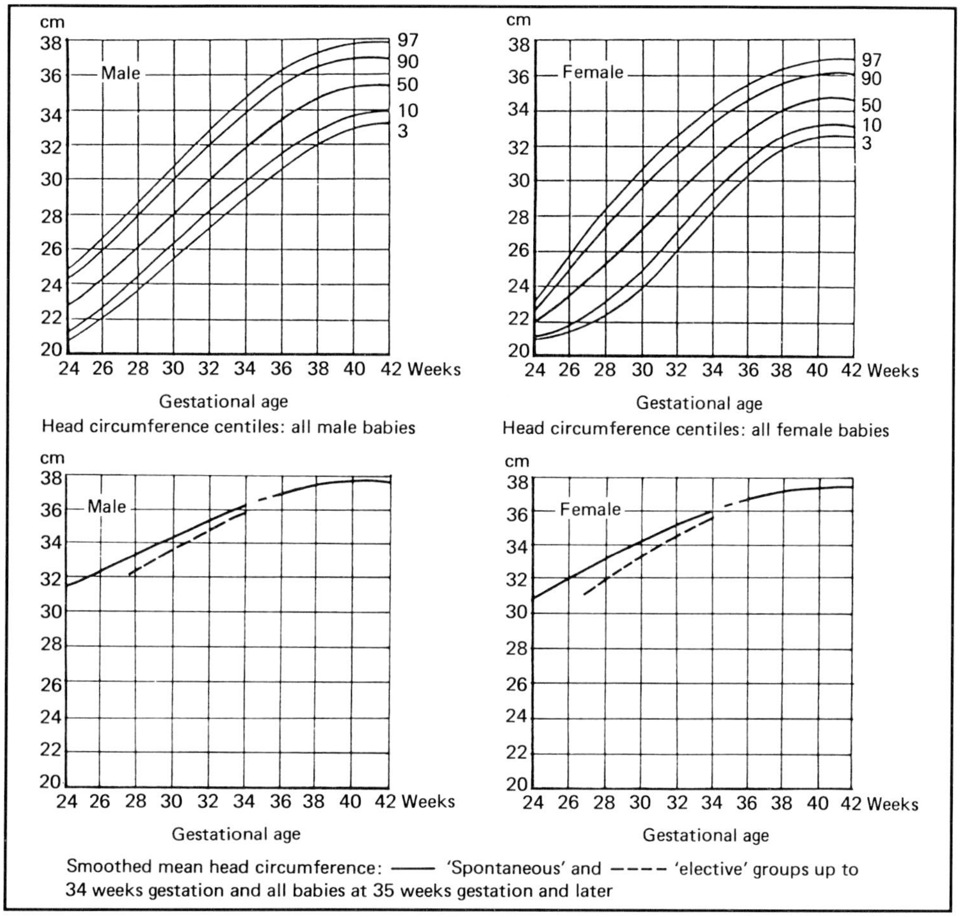

Fig. 1.9. Centiles of head circumference by sex and gestational age. (Yudkin et al. 1987)

(Figs. 1.15–1.19; see also Fig. 19.2) alerts the prosector to the likely type or range of internal malformations as well as giving an indication of the type of investigations such as chromosome culture or biochemical assay which might be necessary for a firm diagnosis to be reached.

The presence of other external abnormalities, including the site of drains or catheters or surgical incisions, should be noted. Evidence of injury related to birth or prenatal investigation or to intensive care in the neonatal period should be carefully sought.

The appearance and colour of the skin may give clues about time of death (maceration), maturity (bright pink in the very preterm baby, wrinkled and peeling in postmaturity). Extreme pallor might alert one to the possibility of haemorrhage, and the presence of jaundice, bruising or petechial haemorrhages which are not explained clinically require further investigation.

Examination of Body Cavities

Before the body cavities are opened, it is appropriate to look for pneumothorax, if a radiograph has not been done, in all livebirths who die in the neonatal period, even if survival has been very brief. This can be done by immersing the whole body in water and inserting a trocar and cannula into each hemithorax in turn. The sixth intercostal space in the midaxillary line is a convenient entry point. When a pneumothorax is present, a stream of gas bubbles will issue from the cannula when the trocar is removed.

The skin can be opened with a straight, midline incision skirting to the left of the umbilicus or with Y or inverted Y-shaped incisions. The first makes for easy dissection of neck structures; the second is useful when further viewing of the baby is likely after necropsy. An inverted Y allows forward reflection of the bladder and umbilical vessels, and

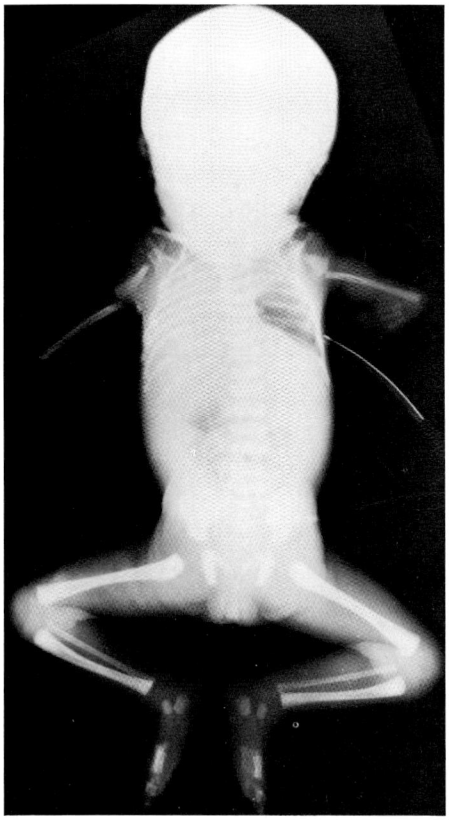

Fig. 1.10. Post-mortem radiograph. Bilateral radial aplasia.

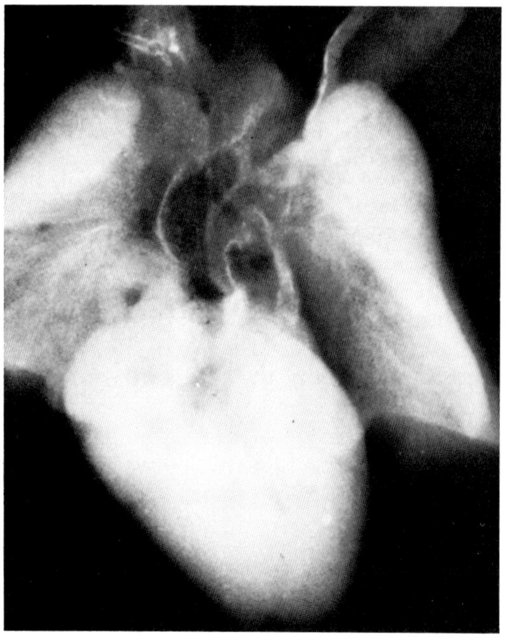

Fig. 1.11. Radiographic demonstration of calcification in the walls of aorta and large arteries.

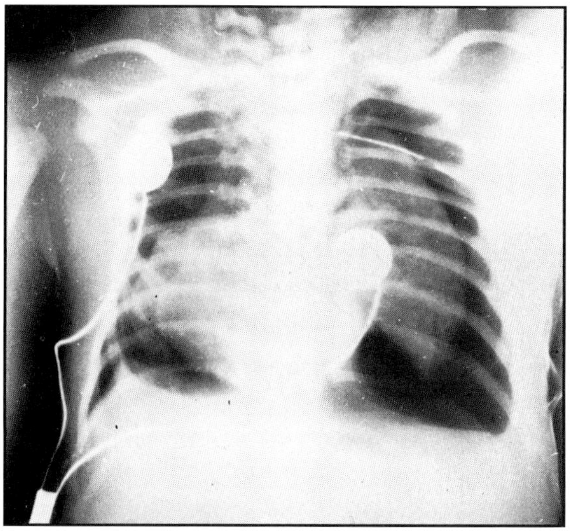

Fig. 1.12. Post-mortem radiograph; large pneumothorax.

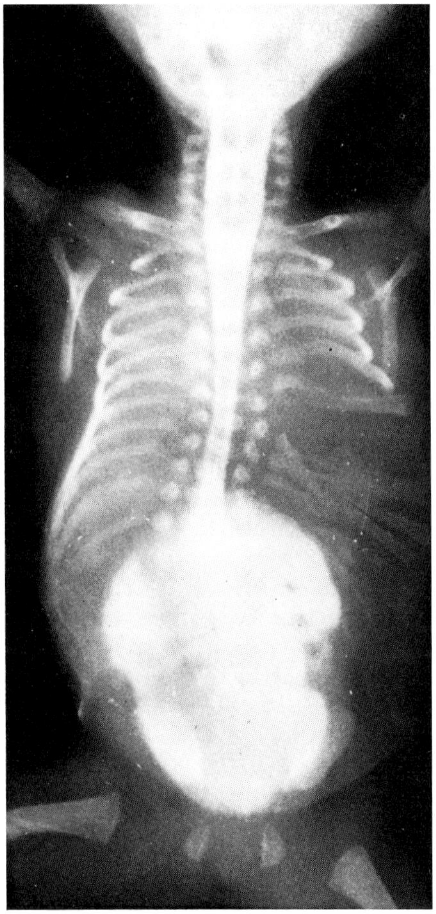

Fig. 1.13. Gastrografin injected into the lateral ventricles of a fetus with meningomyelocoele outlines the spinal cord and lumbar defect.

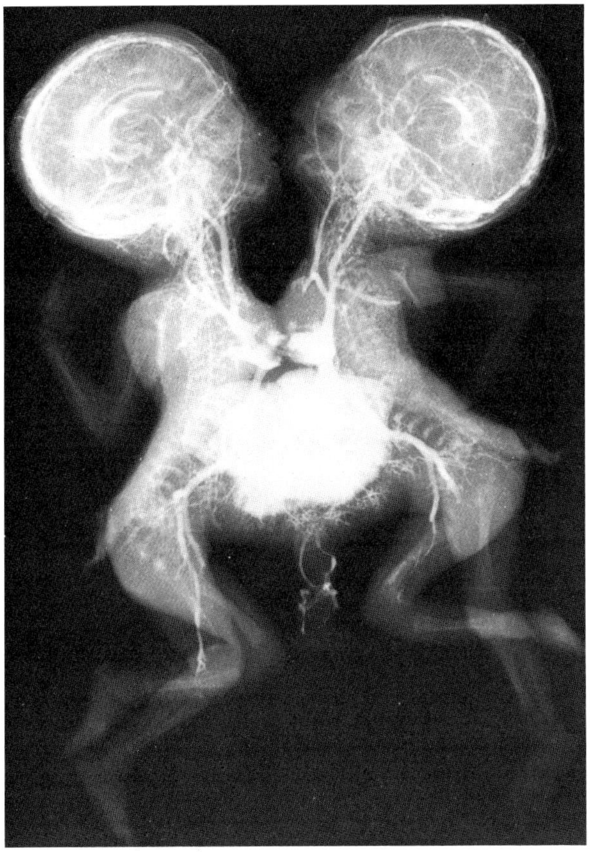

Fig. 1.14. Contrast radiograph of conjoined twins at 20 weeks' gestation indicates the site of vascular connection.

one limb of the Y can be continued down the thigh to the level of the knee medial to the patella to facilitate removal of the femur.

Skin and subcutaneous tissues are dissected off the rib cage, note being taken of the amount of subcutaneous fat and the colour and volume of muscle, which may be pale and reduced in amount in neuromuscular disorders. The abdominal viscera are examined in situ. The presence of ascites, blood, pus or fecal material in the cavity is sought and any adhesions between viscera are noted. Intestinal rotation and the presence of herniae, volvulus or intussusception is noted. The size, position and contour of the liver are inspected, and its colour, surface appearance and presence of haematomas are recorded.

The sternum is removed either by cutting through costal cartilages about 0.5 cm medial to the costochondral junction or cutting through the ribs in the anterior axillary line. Either method will ensure that costochondral junc-

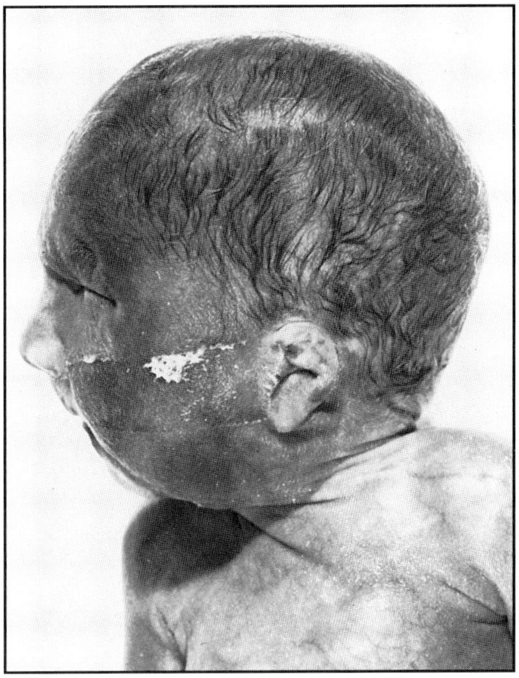

Fig. 1.15. Trisomy 13: there is microcephaly, sloping forehead, micrognathia and low-set ears with abnormal helix.

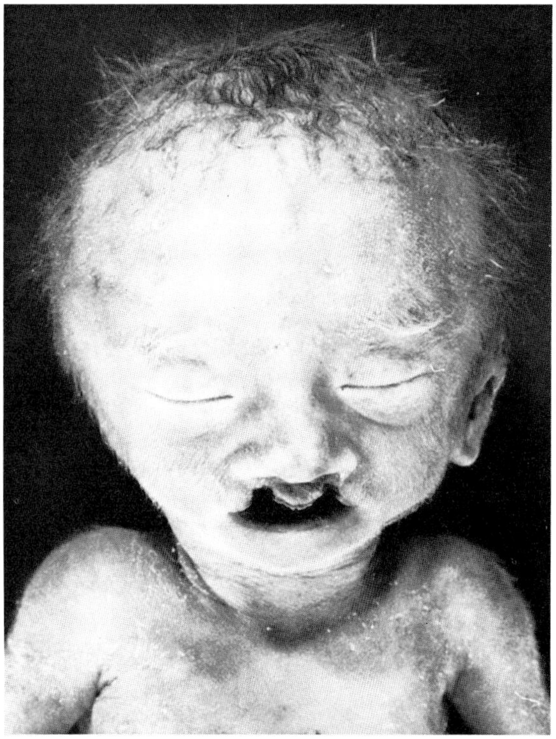

Fig. 1.16. Trisomy 18: the head is rather globular; there is hypertelorism, bilateral cleft lip and palate and micrognathia.

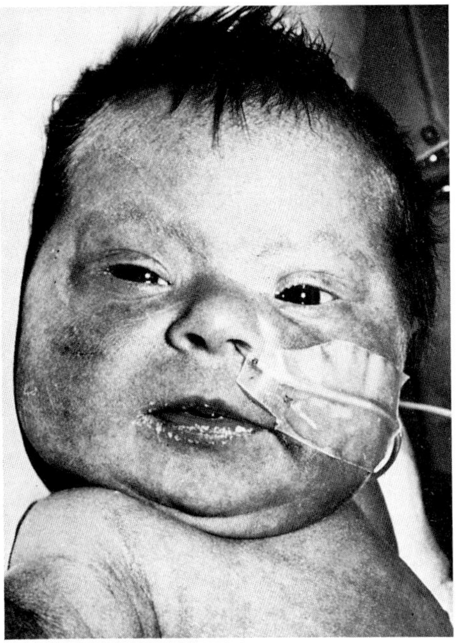

Fig. 1.17. Trisomy 21: upslanting palpebral fissures, inner epicanthal folds, small nose.

tions are intact for subsequent histological examination. Dividing the ribs gives wide access to the thoracic cavity, facilitating inspection and photography of thoracic viscera in situ.

The relative size of heart, lungs and thoracic diameter are observed, and the presence of pleural and pericardial effusions sought. The level and completeness of the diaphragm are noted. The route of chest drains is explored, looking particularly at the position of the drain tip and searching for visceral injury, particularly in the presence of haemothorax.

The thymus lies in the upper part of the anterior mediastinum. It is bilobed with narrow extensions up through the thoracic inlet into the neck. It is a large organ weighing 12–18 g at term but is relatively smaller in preterm infants. When of normal size, it overlies the aorta and pulmonary arteries. Petechial haemorrhages within it suggest an episode of hypoxia. Its size is much reduced following long-standing stress of any sort. It is convenient to dissect the thymus off the pericardium, taking care not to

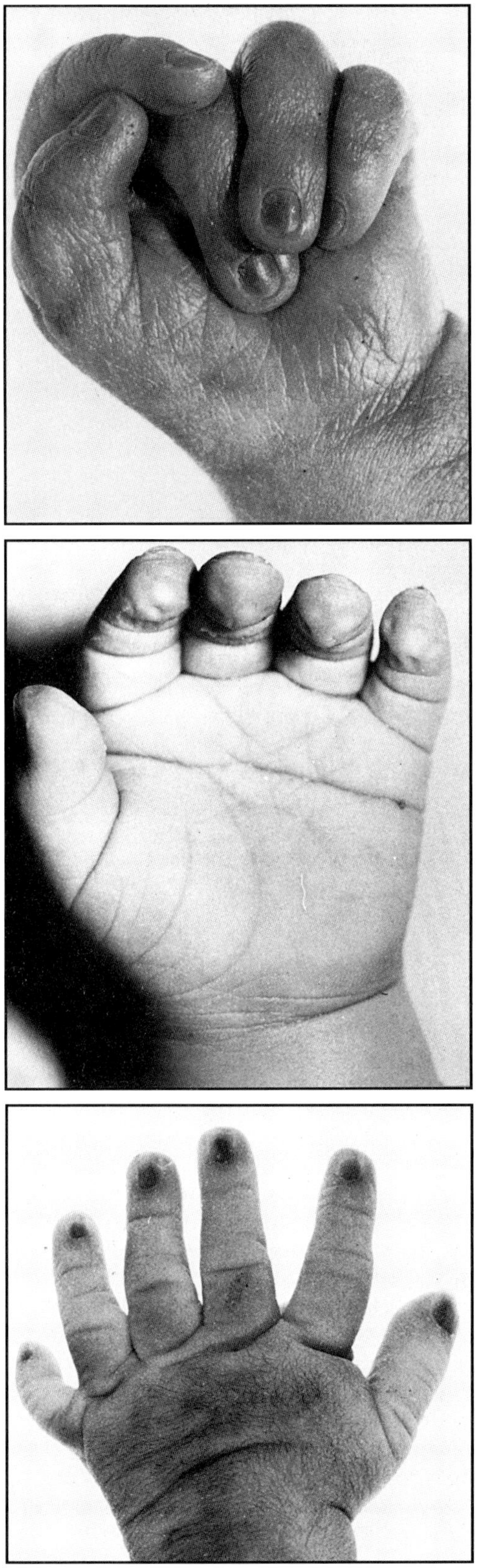

a

b

c

Fig. 1.18. **a** Trisomy 18; overfolding of fingers is usually present. **b** Trisomy 21; transverse palmar crease. **c** Meckel–Gruber syndrome; postaxial polydactyly.

a 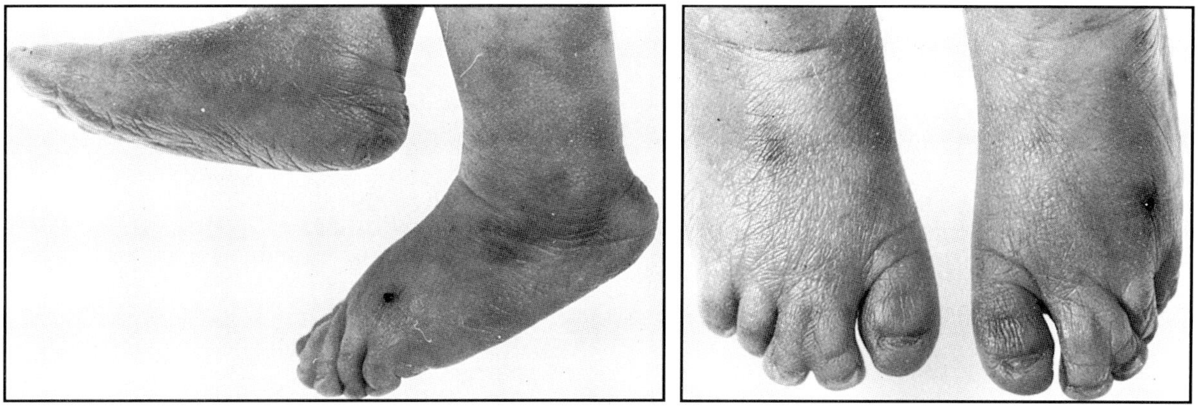 b

Fig. 1.19a,b. Trisomy 18. **a** Rocker bottom feet; **b** syndactyly of 2nd and 3rd toes.

damage the innominate vein which runs behind it at the thoracic inlet. The thymus is usually absent in Di George syndrome, although a nodule of thymic tissue may be found on the lateral border of the pericardial sac in that condition. The thymus of the sick preterm baby who dies in the late neonatal period is often very small and easily overlooked. This situation should not be confused with Di George syndrome. If in doubt, re-examine the face; a backwards sloping forehead and small nose are characteristic of Di George syndrome.

Incise the pericardium in the midline, noting the appearance and amount of any effusion or haemorrhage. The exterior of the heart and its vascular connections should be examined in situ. Note the shape and size of the atria and their appendages to determine atrial situs. The right atrium is dilated in heart failure and when there is anomalous pulmonary venous return; it may be small when the tricuspid valve is stenosed or atretic. The left atrium is small when there is mitral atresia or stenosis and in the presence of pulmonary hypoplasia or total anomalous pulmonary venous return.

Inspect the distribution of the coronary arteries. The anterior descending branch of the left coronary artery is the surface marking of the interventricular septum. Its position indicates the relative contribution of each ventricle to the ventricular mass. At term the right ventricle is relatively larger and its wall relatively thicker than in later life. Abnormal coronary artery distribution, particularly a leash of small vessels running obliquely across the anterior surface of the ventricles, should alert one to the possibility of a defective interventricular septum or abnormalities of the origin or relationships of great arteries. The relative size and position of the aorta and pulmonary artery are noted; they should be of approximately equal size, with the pulmonary artery crossing in front of the aorta. The distribution of the aortic arch branches and configuration of the superior vena cava and its tributaries are noted. The heart should be pulled to the right; observe the course of the left pulmonary veins, which can be observed running to the back of the heart. Where pulmonary venous drainage is abnormal, the pulmonary veins join to form a trunk which may run to join a superior vena cava or downwards through the diaphragm to join the portal venous system (Fig. 1.20) or, occasionally, the inferior vena cava.

Evisceration

At this point, the prosector has a number of options for evisceration of the body. One of the important differences between necropsy examination of babies and adults is that organs should not be removed individually but rather in continuity as one, two or three large blocks. Barson (1981) and Valdes-Dapena and Huff (1983) advocate the removal of the thoracic and abdominal organs together, beginning with separation of neck structures and after bringing down the tongue; midline thoracic structures are freed from prevertebral fascia; the diaphragm is cut through and all the abdominal viscera are removed in continuity with thoracic organs, cutting through the bladder neck and rectum. The viscera are then dissected from the back. I adopt this method in those cases where there are pathological abnormalities of the intestines,

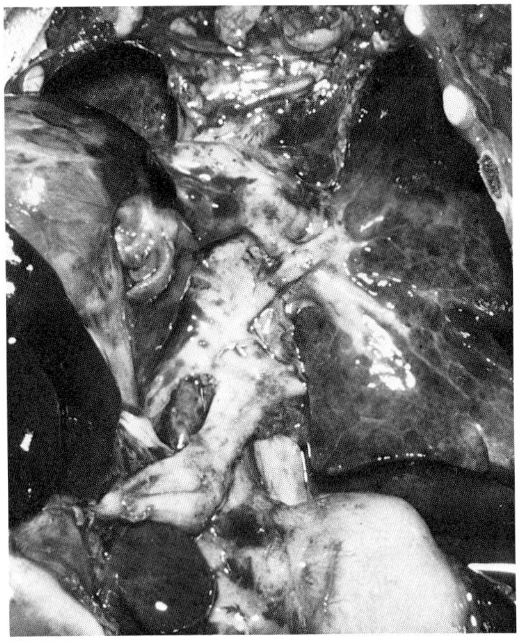

Fig. 1.20. Traction of the heart to the right shows confluence of pulmonary veins and an anomalous venous trunk descending through the diaphragm.

particularly if genitourinary abnormalities are also present; however, I do not like the scheme for cardiac dissection proposed by Barson, from the point of view of photography of abnormal hearts.

Pryse-Davies (1981) and Wigglesworth (1984) advocate routine removal of viscera in four blocks: neck structures and thoracic viscera, small and large intestines, upper abdominal viscera and urogenital tracts and related vessels. I favour the removal of thoracic and upper abdominal viscera in one block for all perinatal necropsies as advocated by Langley (1971) and Wigglesworth (1984) for cases where congenital heart disease is suspected. Adoption of this method as a routine reduces the number of decisions which need to be made during dissection and therefore reduces error; it also means that the prosector becomes familiar with the technique more quickly, and if he has failed to notice a hint in the clinical notes or forgotten to look at the pulmonary veins then all is not lost. It also enables one to open the oesophagus in continuity with the stomach, an opportunity which is lost with four-block evisceration. Individual organs are weighed after dissection. Weights of fetal organs grouped by body weight and gestation are detailed in Tables 1.4 and 1.5.

Abdominal Vessels and Genitourinary System

The abdominal parts of the inferior vena cava and ascending aorta are opened in situ. It is convenient to leave aortic catheters in position until that vessel has been opened. The position of the catheter tip and any thrombus or endothelial damage is noted; renal vessels are opened. When there is no evidence of urinary tract obstruction, the adrenals and kidneys are dissected individually and weighed. The internal genitalia are inspected. If the scrotum is empty, testes are sought in the abdomen or inguinal canal. Should lower urinary tract obstruction be evident, then the whole urinary tract should be removed in continuity (Fig. 1.21). Lower urinary tract obstruction usually occurs in males. The pubic symphysis is divided with strong scissors.

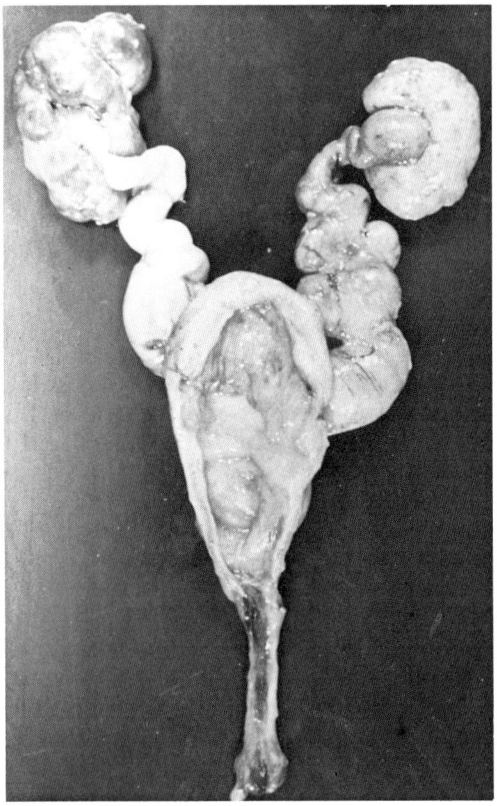

Fig. 1.21. Lower urinary tract obstruction (posterior urethral valves). The urinary tract has been removed in continuity and the urethra opened from below; part of the wall of the bladder and prostatic urethra has been removed.

Table 1.4. Lengths and organ weights of newborn infants grouped by body weight (Gruenwald and Minh 1960)

Body weight (g)	Number of cases	Body length (cm)	Heart (g)	Lungs combined (g)	Spleen (g)	Liver (g)	Adrenal glands, combined (g)	Kidneys combined (g)	Thymus (g)	Brain (g)	Gestational age	
											Weeks	Days
500	317	29.4	5.0	12	1.3	26	2.6	5.4	2.2	70	23,	5
		±2.5	±1.6	±5	±0.8	±10	±1.7	±2.1	±0.8	±18	±2,	3
750	311	32.9	6.3	19	2.0	39	3.2	7.8	2.8	107	26,	0
		±3.0	±1.8	±6	±1.2	±12	±1.5	±2.6	±1.3	±27	±2,	6
1000	295	35.6	7.7	24	2.6	47	3.5	10.4	3.7	143	27,	5
		±3.1	±2.0	±8	±1.5	±12	±1.6	±3.4	±2.0	±34	±3,	1
1250	217	38.4	9.6	30	3.4	56	4.0	12.9	4.9	174	29,	0
		±3.0	±3.3	±9	±1.8	±21	±1.7	±3.9	±2.1	±38	±3,	0
1500	167	41.0	11.5	34	4.3	65	4.5	14.9	6.1	219	31,	3
		±2.7	±3.3	±11	±2.0	±18	±1.8	±4.2	±2.7	±52	±2,	3
1750	148	42.6	12.8	40	5.0	74	5.3	17.4	6.8	247	32,	4
		±3.1	±3.2	±13	±2.5	±20	±2.0	±4.7	±3.0	±51	±2,	6
2000	140	44.9	14.9	44	6.0	82	5.3	18.8	7.9	281	34,	6
		±2.8	±4.2	±13	±2.7	±23	±2.0	±5.0	±3.4	±56	±3,	2
2250	124	46.3	16.0	48	7.0	88	6.0	20.2	8.2	308	36,	4
		±2.9	±4.3	±15	±3.3	±24	±2.3	±4.9	±3.4	±49	±3,	0
2500	120	47.3	17.7	48	8.5	105	7.1	22.6	8.3	339	38,	0
		±2.3	±4.2	±14	±3.5	±21	±2.8	±5.5	±4.4	±50	±3,	2
2750	138	48.7	19.1	51	9.1	117	7.5	24.0	9.6	362	39,	2
		±2.9	±3.8	±15	±3.6	±26	±2.7	±5.4	±3.8	±48	±2,	2
3000	144	50.0	20.7	53	10.1	127	8.3	24.7	10.2	380	40,	0
		±2.9	±5.3	±13	±3.3	±30	±2.9	±5.3	±4.3	±55	±2,	1
3250	133	50.7	21.5	59	11.0	145	9.2	27.3	11.6	395	40,	4
		±2.6	±4.3	±18	±4.0	±33	±3.4	±6.6	±4.4	±53	±1,	6
3500	106	51.8	22.8	63	11.3	153	9.8	28.0	12.8	411	40,	4
		±3.0	±5.9	±17	±3,6	±33	±3.5	±6.5	±5.1	±55	±1,	5
3750	57	52.1	23.8	65	12.5	159	10.2	29.5	13.0	413	40,	6
		±2.3	±5.1	±15	±4.1	±40	±3.3	±6.8	±4.8	±55	±2,	3
4000	31	52.4	25.8	67	14.1	180	10.8	30.2	11.4	420	41,	4
		±2.7	±5.3	±20	±4.0	±39	±3.4	±6.2	±3.2	±62	±1,	3
4250	15	53.2	26.5	68	13.0	197	12.0	30.7	11.7	415	41,	2
		±2.5	±5.3	±16	±2.5	±42	±3.7	±5.8	±3.7	±38	±2,	1

Kidneys, ureters and bladder, with aorta and iliac vessels, are freed from the top. The bladder neck is freed and the rectum divided just above the anus. The urethra is freed around its perimeter and pulled upwards so that the penis is progressively invaginated using blunt dissection in a subcutaneous plane. When invagination is complete, the urethra is divided immediately proximal to its external meatus.

Thoracic and Upper Abdominal Viscera

Dissection of the thoracoabdominal block is begun from the back with organs resting on a sponge to reduce their mobility. The spleen is dissected free and weighed and the pancreas identified. Gross evidence of pancreatic involvement in mucoviscidosis is unusual in the neonate, and part of the pancreas should always be removed for histological examination. The oesophagus is opened along its posterior wall and the stomach round the greater curvature, then through the pylorus and duodenum. Oesophageal atresia will be obvious in the early part of this manoeuvre (see Fig. 15.3, p. 349). The contents of viscera are noted. Meconium may be present in oesophagus and stomach following birth asphyxia, and gastric ulceration is sometimes seen following tolazoline medication (see Fig. 14.18, p. 338). In duodenal atresia the relationship of the head of the pancreas to the duodenum should be carefully observed. Continuity of the bile ducts and appearance of the gall bladder are noted and the oesophagus and stomach dissected off remaining viscera.

The larynx and trachea are opened down the posterior wall and their contents noted. The larynx should be carefully opened with forceps and the presence and site of ulceration or fibrous scarring noted. Laryngeal atresia is an occasional cause of respiratory distress at birth; the entrance to the larynx is surprisingly

Table 1.5. Weight and length of newborn infants and their organ weights at different gestational ages (Gruenwald and Minh 1960)

Gestational age[a]	Number of cases	Body length (cm)	Body weight (g)	Heart (g)	Lungs combined (g)	Spleen (g)	Liver (g)	Adrenal glands, combined (g)	Kidneys combined (g)	Thymus (g)	Brain (g)
24	108	31.3 ±3.7	638 ±240	4.9 ±1.6	17 ±6	1.7 ±1.1	32 ±15	2.9 ±1.4	6.4 ±2.6	2.7 ±1.4	92 ±31
26	143	33.3 ±3.6	845 ±246	6.4 ±2.0	18 ±6	2.2 ±1.5	39 ±15	3.4 ±1.5	7.9 ±2.9	3.0 ±2.3	111 ±39
28	139	36.0 ±4.2	1020 ±340	7.6 ±2.3	23 ±7	2.6 ±1.4	46 ±16	3.7 ±1.7	10.4 ±3.6	3.8 ±2.1	139 ±48
30	148	37.8 ±3.7	1230 ±340	9.3 ±3.3	28 ±11	3.4 ±2.0	53 ±19	4.2 ±2.2	12.3 ±3.9	4.6 ±2.3	166 ±55
32	150	40.5 ±4.5	1488 ±335	11.0 ±3.7	34 ±11	4.1 ±2.1	65 ±22	4.3 ±2.3	14.5 ±4.8	5.5 ±2.3	209 ±44
34	104	42.8 ±4.5	1838 ±530	13.4 ±3.9	40 ±13	5.2 ±2.1	74 ±27	5.5 ±2.3	17.7 ±5.3	7.5 ±3.8	246 ±58
36	87	45.0 ±4.6	2165 ±600	15.1 ±4.8	46 ±16	6.7 ±3.0	87 ±33	6.4 ±3.0	21.6 ±6.7	8.1 ±4.2	288 ±62
38	102	47.2 ±4.6	2678 ±758	18.5 ±5.5	53 ±15	8.8 ±4.2	111 ±40	8.4 ±3.5	23.8 ±7.0	9.7 ±4.8	349 ±56
40	220	49.8 ±3.9	3163 ±595	20.4 ±5.3	56 ±15	10.0 ±3.9	130 ±45	8.6 ±3.4	25.6 ±6.5	9.5 ±4.4	362 ±55
42	112	50.3 ±3.6	3263 ±573	21.9 ±6.2	56 ±18	10.2 ±4.3	139 ±45	9.1 ±4.0	25.8 ±7.5	10.4 ±4.4	405 ±54
44	42	52.8 ±2.8	3690 ±800	25.8 ±4.5	60 ±17	11.2 ±4.1	149 ±35	9.3 ±4.4	28.4 ±7.5	10.3 ±4.7	417 ±55

[a] Gestational age is expressed in weeks from the last menstrual period.

normal in these cases. The inferior vena cava can be incised just above the diaphragm, and the incision continued downwards to open the intrahepatic course of the inferior vena cana, the hepatic veins and ductus venosus. This should be done with care when an umbilical venous catheter has been passed (Fig. 1.22).

Examination of the Heart

It is now most convenient to turn over the remaining viscera and continue dissection in the front. The apex of the heart is lifted up and the entry of the inferior vena cava into the heart noted. If pulmonary venous return is to the heart, the inferior vena cava is divided, and the liver removed and weighed.

It is always easier to open the heart whilst it is attached to the lungs from the point of view of both stability and chamber identification, and this method is obligatory in those cases where congenital heart disease is suspected. Definitions of cardiac structures are detailed in Chapter 18. The general sequence of examination of the heart described by Langley (1971) is, with minor modifications, suitable for examination of all infant hearts. Direction and sequence of incisions are displayed in Fig. 1.23. I find that it is easier to examine the heart in the fresh state than after fixation; manipulation is easier and the anatomy can be demonstrated to attendant clinicians at the same time. The right atrium is opened by cutting from inferior vena cava to superior vena cava along the right border of the heart; closed scissors or a probe may be passed between the two veins to visualise the cutting line. Care should be taken to preserve the junction of the superior vena cava and atrial

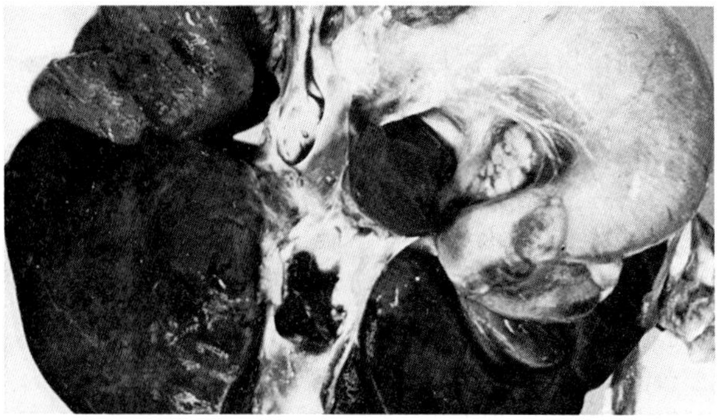

Fig. 1.22. Liver from behind. Opening the inferior vena cava reveals the presence of thrombus in the hepatic veins; umbilical venous catheterisation had been undertaken.

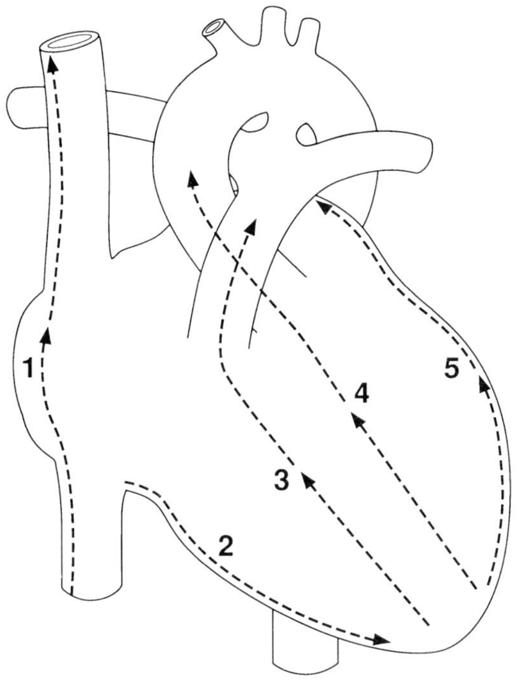

Fig. 1.23. Diagrammatic representation of incision lines to display the infant heart. The heart is opened whilst it is attached to the lungs.

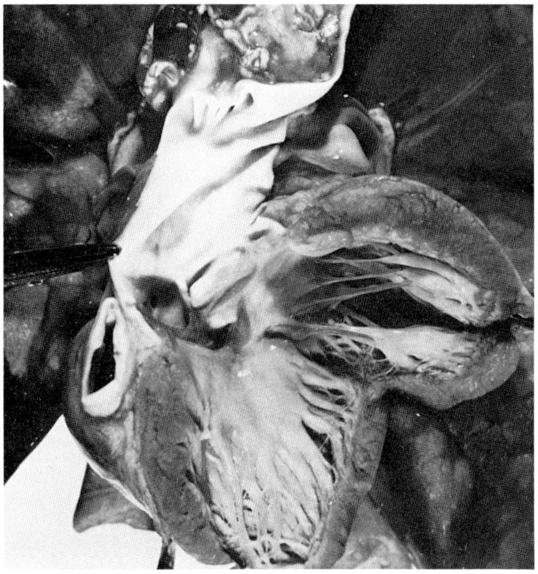

Fig. 1.24. Ventricular septal defect observed from the left ventricle. The view of septal defects from the left side is not obstructed by valve cusps or coarse trabecular pattern.

appendage when examination of the cardiac conduction system is proposed. Remove blood clot from the atrium and appendage and identify the fossa ovalis and coronary sinus. Note the presence and site of any septal defects and test the patency of the foramen ovale with a probe. Inspect the tricuspid valve from the atrial chamber for dilatation, atresia or stenosis. Open the right ventricle by cutting down the right lateral border of the heart to the apex and then upwards along the outflow tract through the pulmonary valve. Examine the configuration of the tricuspid valve and note any nodularity of the free border. Trabecular pattern should be noted. The pulmonary valve is then examined. The three cusps should be equal in size and pliable. Look for obstruction to pulmonary outflow at valvar level and both above and below it. Look for aberrant coronary artery origins. Note the size and origin of the right and left pulmonary arteries and examine the presence and patency of the ductus arteriosus. It will be widely patent in stillbirths and neonates dying within 6 h of birth. Thereafter, constriction of the vessel is observed, and anatomical closure is apparent by 10 days of age. The ductus arteriosus may remain open or re-open in very preterm babies (see Chap. 18, p. 455).

Turn the heart to the right, identify the left superior pulmonary vein, incise it and extend the incision into the left atrial appendage. Open the left border of the heart down through the mitral valve and down the lateral border of the left ventricle to the apex and then cut upwards towards the base of the heart to the left of the interventricular septum. Put the scissors through the aortic valve into the aorta to visualise the cutting line and then open the aorta by cutting through the pulmonary trunk and aortic valve. Extend the incision round the arch of the aorta to the descending thoracic aorta. Examine the mitral valve and configuration of the left ventricle. Inspect the interventricular septum for defects from the left side (Fig. 1.24). It is easier to see small muscular ventricular septal defects from the left side; they may be obscured by the coarse trabeculation of the right ventricle. Inspect the aortic valve. The three cusps should be equal in size, pliable and translucent. The coronary artery origins should be identified; they are usually at the level of the superior limit of the aortic valve commissures at the midpoint of the anterior and left posterior

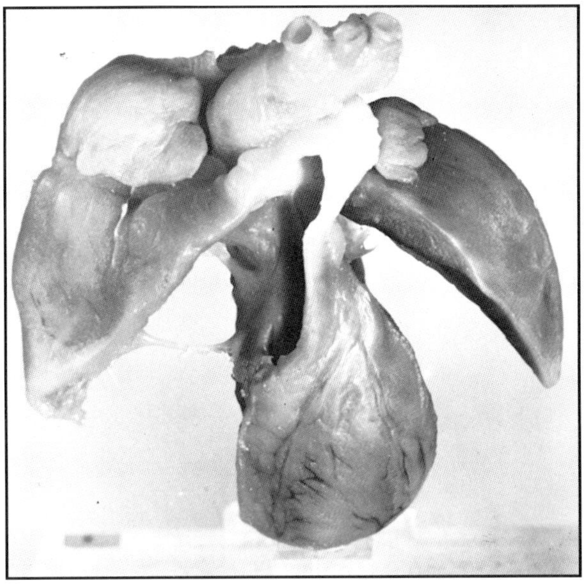

Fig. 1.25. Wax-impregnated heart. Position of ventricular flaps is achieved by the use of orange sticks during processing.

valve cusps. The aorta narrows between the aortic valve and the ductus arteriosus, and the distal part of the arch is approximately two-thirds of the diameter of the ascending aorta. A localised coarctation is usually sited proximal to the ductus arteriosus.

Wax impregnation of hearts after fixation provides useful teaching models (Fig. 1.25). When this is contemplated, the heart should not be fully dissected in the fresh state. I incise both atria and wash out blood clot from all chambers and great vessels and stuff them with wet cotton wool to ensure satisfactory post-fixation contour. After fixation for 3–4 weeks, dissection is completed; care should be taken to remove all traces of pericardium and connective tissue from the surface of vascular trunks. Muscle flaps can be kept in position during processing by use of orange sticks, which are then easily removed. A programme for dehydration and clearing is detailed by Russell and Berry (1986), but large specimens may require a longer time in each solution.

Head and Cranial Contents

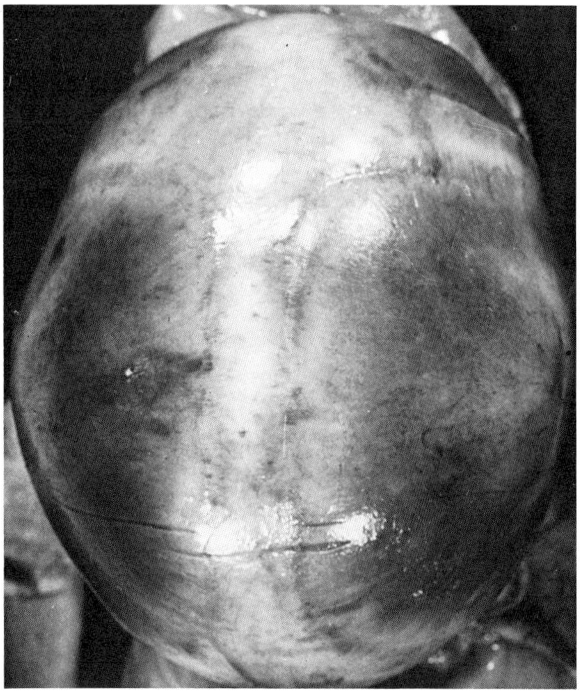

Fig. 1.26. Bulging anterior fontanelle and tense, wide suture lines; post-haemorrhagic hydrocephalus.

Examination of the brain and its coverings in the newborn requires a different approach to that used when examining older children and adults. The scalp is incised coronally starting behind one ear, cutting posterior to the vertex towards the other ear. This incision permits satisfactory reconstruction of the head should further viewing of the body be required; it also imparts a degree of stability should skull bones be retained for examination. The scalp flaps are reflected forwards and backwards and examined for the presence of oedema or haemorrhage (see Chap. 10, p. 245). The size of the anterior fontanelle and width of suture lines are noted. Where there is increased intracranial pressure, particularly of recent origin, the fontanelle is tense and bulging (Fig. 1.26) and the suture lines may be wider than normal. When there is long-standing increased intracranial pressure then the anterior fontanelle often extends forwards so that the frontal bones are widely separated along their whole length. This appearance is seen in some dysmorphic syndromes such as trisomy 18 as well as hydrocephalus of long standing. The appearance of skull bones and the position of any fractures or skull deformity are noted. Central or oval areas of thinning in the bone, sometimes with a central defect (craniolacunae), may accompany long-standing hydrocephalus.

The posterior scalp flap should be reflected to the level of the cervical spine so that the whole of the occipital bone is exposed (Wigglesworth and Husemeyer 1977); any dislocation of its component parts will be apparent because of interruption of the normal contour of the bone and undue mobility between the squamous and lateral parts. The posterior margin of the foramen magnum is identified and the atlanto-occipital membrane incised. A sample of cerebrospinal fluid (CSF) for bacteriological culture is conveniently taken at this point with sterile pipette or needle and syringe; the CSF sample should be examined for blood staining or opacity. Herniation of the cerebellar tonsils is sometimes seen when the brain is swollen. If there is hydrocephalus, the upper cervical vertebral arches may be removed to look for malformation and downward displacement of the cerebellum and medulla oblongata, which usually accompany meningomyelocoele.

The upper cervical cord may be divided horizontally from the back. The cranial cavity is now opened. It is here that necropsy technique differs most from that appropriate to the examination of adults because of the need to examine the supporting dural membrane, which may be damaged during delivery. The anterior fontanelles are incised parasagittally with a scalpel, taking care that the sagittal sinus is not damaged. Incisions are extended forwards and backwards on each side in turn (Fig. 1.27). Right-handed prosectors will find this part of the examination easier if they start with the left side, as they will be able to support the opened side of the head more efficiently when examining the second side. The scissor point should be kept up against the bone to avoid injury to the brain. This is often difficult when brain swelling reduces the subdural space. The frontoparietal and parieto-occipital suture lines are incised on each side.

The frontal and parietal bone flaps can be deflected laterally and the surface of the brain inspected on each side in turn. The presence, site and size of any haemorrhages are noted, together with the appearance of the surface of the dura and arachnoid membranes. The size of the subdural space is noted; this is relatively large in the preterm baby and will be obliterated by cerebral oedema or hydrocephalus. When the dura and leptomeninges have been in contact for a few days, the shiny surface is lost and instead appears roughened.

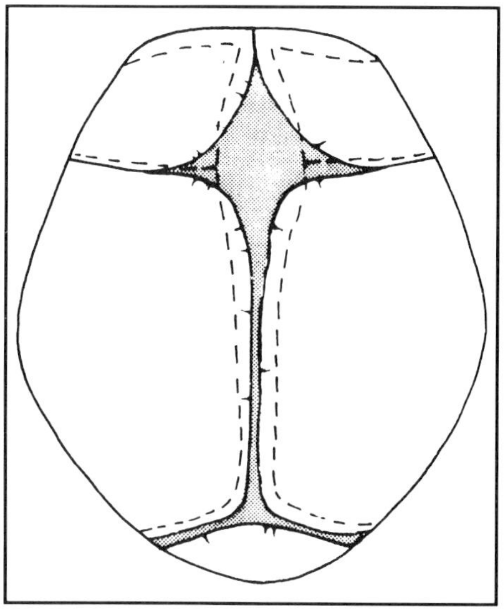

Fig. 1.27. Cutting lines used to expose the brain without injury to dural folds or venous sinuses. (Courtesy of Dr. S.A.S. Knowles, Adelaide)

The cerebral gyral pattern is observed. It is a useful marker of maturity as cerebral development is usually maintained despite the presence of growth retardation of sufficient severity to affect body measurements and even head circumference. The appearance of the normal gyral pattern is surprisingly uniform and its increasing complexity with fetal maturity is well documented by Dorovini-Zis and Dolman (1977; Fig. 1.28). Observation of cerebral gyral pattern in macerated stillbirths (see Chap. 7, p. 186) may assist the dating of fetal death when it has occurred some weeks before delivery. The cerebral gyral pattern may be abnormal when there is major cerebral malformation and obliterated by severe hydrocephalus; such abnormal appearances will alert the prosector to these possibilities.

The head is then tipped forwards and laterally and the occipital pole gently lifted with a finger or scalpel handle so that the falx and tentorium can be inspected for haemorrhage and tears. Congestion and focal haemorrhage within the dural folds are often seen and are usually insignificant. Tearing of the supporting membranes of the brain may occur when excessive deformity of the head has occurred during rapid spontaneous or instrumental delivery. It is possible to examine the whole of the falx and tentorium in this way. The usual site of traumatic injury is the junction of the two folds

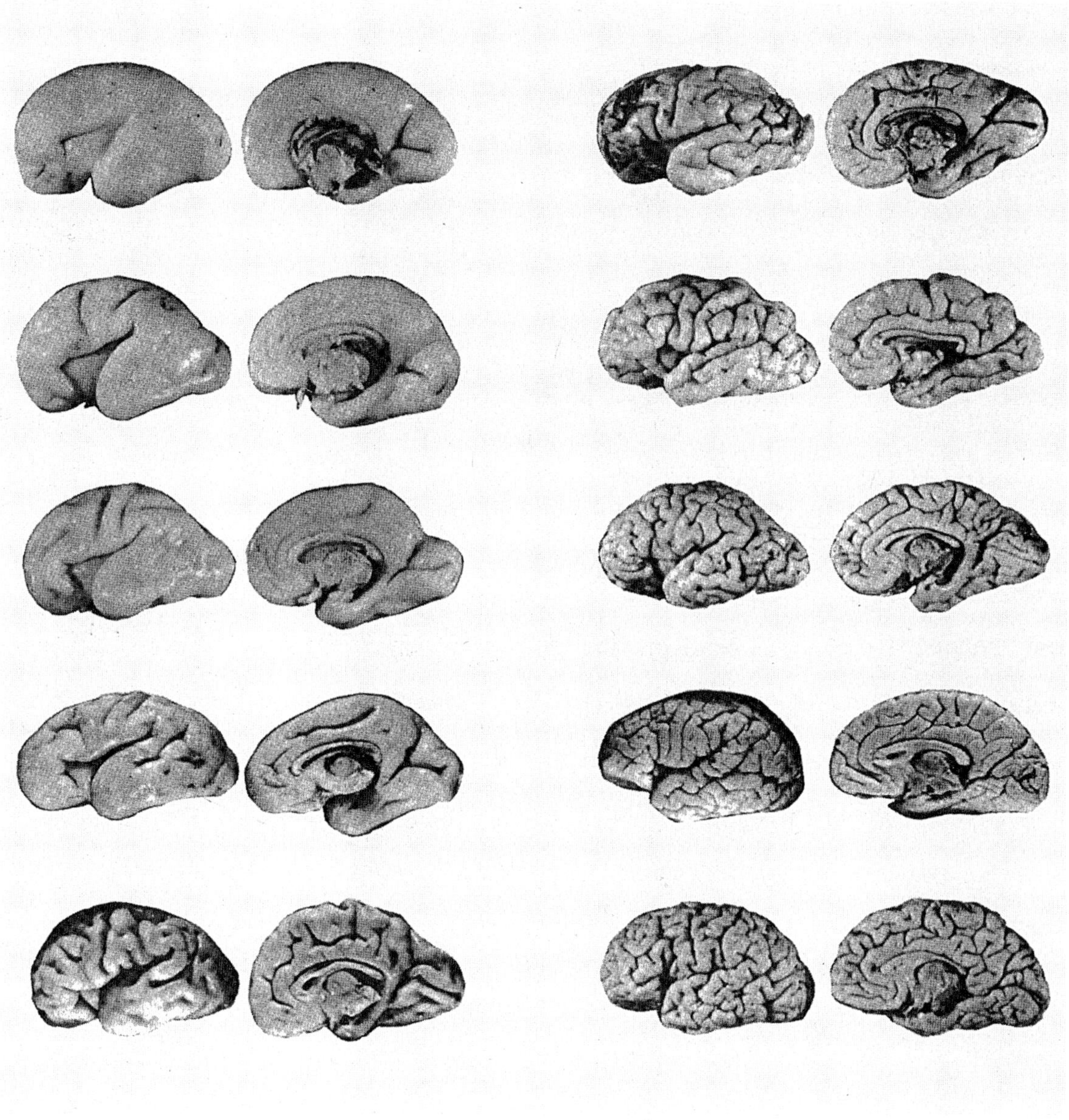

Fig. 1.28. Characteristic gyral pattern of the fetal brain from 22 to 40 weeks' gestation (brains brought to same size). (Dorovini-Zis and Dolman 1977)

(see Fig. 10.11, p. 249); it may be partial, when tearing of the surface fibres is seen, or complete, with disruption of the concave margin of the tentorium. The vein of Galen and its tributaries are seen at the confluence, when they are intact. It is not necessary to remove the cerebral hemispheres to make this examination unless photography is contemplated. Following this manoeuvre, the skull flaps are returned to their original position and kept in place with the hand whilst the procedure is repeated on the other side.

The brain may now be removed. The sagittal sinus is divided anteriorly and lifted up and backwards. It should be inspected for the presence of antemortem thrombus, which may be secondary to severe brain swelling. The head is tipped backwards so that the frontal poles can be lifted out of the anterior cranial fossa. The nerves and vessels are divided in turn and the tentorium is incised in the same manner as that adopted for removal of the adult brain. Because of the soft consistency of the infant brain as the result of incomplete myelination, especially marked in preterm babies, removal of the brain may be facilitated if the body is supported by an assistant and the brain removed on to a board (Langley 1971) or if the head is immersed in a wide bucket or bowl of hypertonic saline so that the brain is supported on all sides as removal proceeds. I have found the latter method satisfactory for the removal of brains of prematures, where post-haemorrhagic hydrocephalus and cystic change following ischaemia make the brain softer than normal. If a wide bucket is used, some of the saline can be removed with a ladle and replaced by formalin to permit fixation without the need for transfer to another container, thus minimising the risk of damage. The base of the brain can be inspected through this supporting fluid and the need for suspension of the brain to maintain its normal contour during fixation is removed by maintaining the hypertonicity of the solution.

Isaacson (1984) describes a similar method for removal of infant brains under water. He also suggests injecting gelatin mixture into the ventricles after fixation and immersing the whole brain in gelatin solution. This is allowed to set in refrigeration overnight and then sliced with a hot knife. This method would certainly support the brain well, although ventricular injection should be undertaken with care so that pathological abnormalities are not disturbed. Wigglesworth (1984) describes removal of the brain of macerated stillbirths within the protection of the dural membrane, which is removed only after fixation.

The base of the skull is inspected following removal of the brain. Dural sinuses are incised and the pituitary inspected and removed by incising the posterior clinoid processes and dissecting free the gland anteriorly, while grasping a posterior clinoid process to prevent crushing of the gland.

The middle ears may be opened with bone forceps to permit bacteriological samples to be taken or the squamous bone removed intact (Kelehan 1984). The middle and inner ears are examined after fixation.

Much useful information is lost if the infant brain is cut in the fresh state, although much of the yellow staining of kernicterus will be eluted by formalin fixation, particularly if this is prolonged. Incomplete myelination allows slices to collapse and the extent of ischaemic injury is difficult to evaluate. Any blood in the ventricles spills out and its amount may go unnoticed when the prosector is distracted by collapse of the brain. It is not possible to slice the fresh brain thinly and focal pathological abnormalities may go unobserved. After fixation, a second inspection of the brain surface is made, and the cerebellum and brain stem are detached by dividing the cerebral peduncles. The cerebrum may be sliced coronally in the traditional manner, the first slice being made from the basal aspect at the level of the mamillary bodies. A method of blocking the neonatal brain for histological examination is described by Gruenwald and Laurence (1968). A device to facilitate brain cutting to produce slices in the planes of any premortem computerised tomographic (CT) scan is described by Muller and McCombs (1984). This could also be used to produce slices which correspond with the progressive obliquity of plane of ultrasound scans performed through the anterior fontanelle.

A technique for the removal of the brain and cord in continuity, protected by skull bones and spinal column, is described by Laurence and Martin (1959). This method is particularly useful for removal of the brain when there is marked hydrocephalus from any cause (Fig. 1.29), particularly when myelination is incomplete. The authors suggest that the best results are achieved when prior fixation of the brain by perfusion of the carotid arteries with 10% formol saline is undertaken. This is generally unacceptable because of its effect on the face. I have found that replacement of some of the CSF with formalin by needling the anterior fontanelle several hours before necropsy is a satisfactory alternative. Although the procedure sounds like a formidable undertaking, it is not difficult and the dissection is very clearly described. A modification I use is to leave the superior orbital margin intact by sawing through the frontal bones and the orbital roof. The brain does not prolapse through this small space, and the technique facilitates circulation of fixative in the subdural space (Fig. 1.30). Dissection is continued after fixation (see Chap. 23, p. 545). In the absence of appropriately skilled assistance to ensure the accuracy of a parasagittal saw cut to expose brain and cord, I find that nibbling bone away with bone forceps and cutting with heavy scissors is satisfactory. Particular attention should be paid to the CSF pathway from the

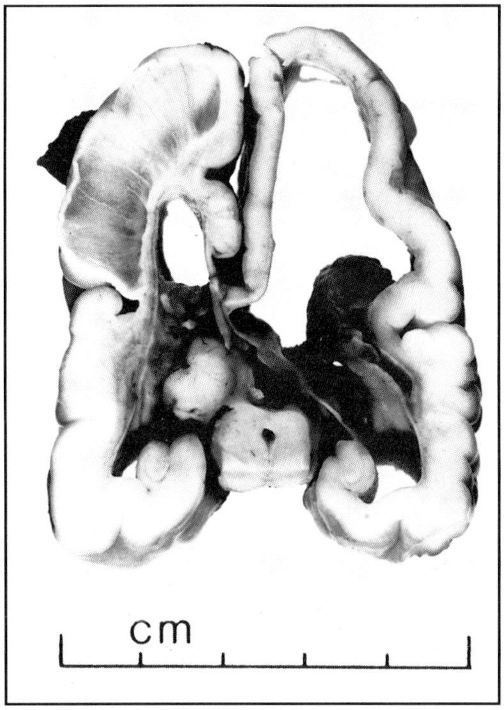

Fig. 1.29. Brain slice from an infant born at 28 weeks' gestation, died at 58 days. Removal within the skull ensured good fixation and minimal distortion despite hydrocephalus and cystic leukomalacia.

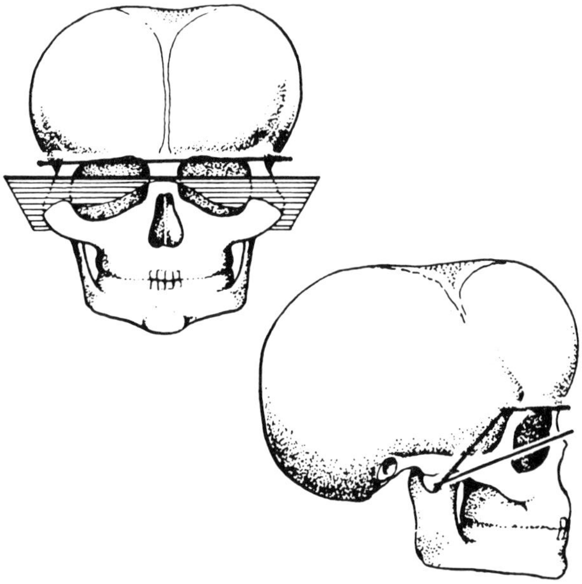

Fig. 1.30. Plane of saw cut to divide the calvarium from the facial skeleton. The upper plane is the one I use, the lower is that described by Laurence and Martin (1959).

third ventricle to the upper cervical region of the spinal cord. It may be appropriate to block all slices of tissue through the aqueduct region if it cannot be followed easily.

Should one be presented with a stillbirth where hydrocephalus was recognised prenatally and decompression of the head undertaken to facilitate vaginal delivery, the above technique is inappropriate. The cranium can be opened in the usual way. The hemispheres will be collapsed but not extensively disrupted and there is usually much haemorrhage. The inferior parts of the cerebral cortex, midbrain, cerebellum and brain stem are usually undamaged. They can be removed in continuity and fixed in formalin, together with part of the cortical mantle. After fixation the appearance of the cortex is noted, looking for ependymal granularity and cortical necrosis as evidence of infection and for brown staining or organising thrombus as evidence of past haemorrhage. The rest of the brain is sliced vertically in 2–3 mm slices, the CSF pathway is traced and samples taken for histological examination.

Spinal Cord

The neonatal spinal cord is most easily approached from the front. An intervertebral disc is incised in the lower lumbar region and the pedicles are divided on each side with heavy scissors. When two or three pedicles have been divided, the vertebral bodies may be elevated to facilitate further dissection. The pedicles are divided on each side in turn up to the high cervical region and the freed vertebral bodies held by an assistant. The filum terminale is divided and elevated with forceps and the spinal nerve roots divided in turn upwards on either side with a sharp scalpel. As the brain has been removed there is no tethering at the level of the atlas.

When traumatic injury to the cervical cord is suspected, it is better to remove the cervical part of the cord within its bony coverings as described by Yates (1959). The intervertebral disc at C–8/T–1 is divided, and the muscle attachments on both sides of the spinal column are divided with scissors and dissection continued round to the back, keeping close to the vertebral arches. The atlas is separated from the skull from the posterior aspect. After fixation and brief decalcification, the whole specimen can be sliced at 2–3 mm intervals using a sharp knife (Fig. 1.31). The surface of

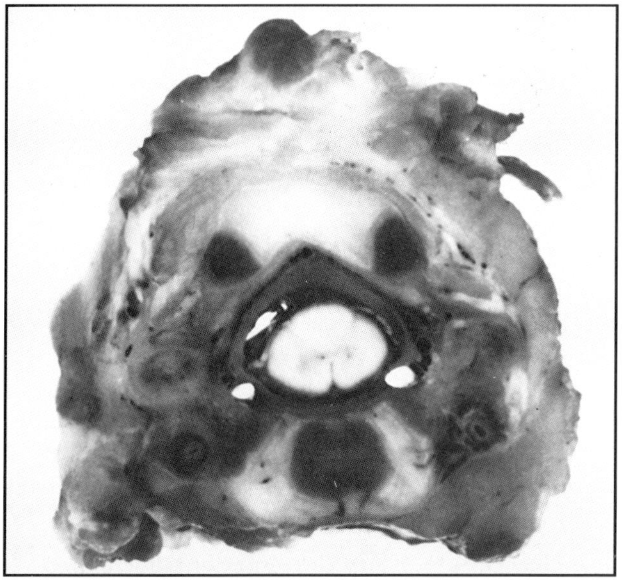

Fig. 1.31. Slice through the cervical vertebral block after fixation and decalcification. Appropriate slices for histological examination can be selected with a hand lens.

each block is examined with a magnifying lens. This permits evaluation not only of cord injury but also of the site of any haemorrhage and injury to joints or vertebral arteries. Yates (1959) described arterial dissection and thrombosis as a result of birth injury.

Skeleton

Radiography is a more efficient technique than dissection for the recognition and documentation of skeletal malformation or injury. However, dissection of parts of the skeleton may be required in order to examine a particular joint, e.g. following recognition of congenital dislocation of the hip, or, more usually, to obtain samples of long bones for histological or biochemical examination.

The femur may be removed in a similar manner to that used in adults. The ventral abdominal incision is extended through one groin, down the anteromedial border of the thigh to the medial aspect of the knee. The anterior thigh muscles are divided vertically down to the bone, and the knee ligaments divided. The lower end of the femur is elevated and posterior muscle attachments divided progressively in a cephalad direction. Muscles around the hip joint are divided. The joint capsule is incised. When the hip has dislocated, division of the ligament of the head of the femur and posterior part of the capsule can be done easily by displacing the femoral head downwards and laterally. When the joint is normal, the ligament of the femoral head is exposed by elevation and lateral rotation of the femur and incision of the joint capsule inferiorly; the remaining ligaments are then divided.

In babies with osteochondrodystrophies or osteogenesis imperfecta (see Chap. 26, p. 621) it may be desirable to remove several long bones. In the interests of reconstruction and aesthetics, the following method for removal of bones is preferred. The proximal limb joint (hip or shoulder) is approached by lateral reflection of the skin from the ventral incision and division of muscles vertically downwards onto the joint, which is then disarticulated. The proximal end of the bone is grasped and muscle attachments divided progressively in a peripheral direction, invaginating the "sleeve" of muscle, subcutaneous fat and skin. The next joint may be left intact and dissection continued to ankle or wrist, which is then disarticulated. The bones are then fixed in formalin and the limb reconstructed by filling the bone space with wadding. Radiographic examination of individual bones is desirable (Fig. 1.32) before histological examination is undertaken. The bones may be usefully divided longitudinally so that undecalcified and conventional sections of the same bone can be compared.

Histological Examination

I have found that routine sampling of fetal organs for histological examination has been a useful part of the investigation of perinatal death, producing essential information about the likely cause or mode of death in 20% of both stillbirths and neonatal deaths (Porter and Keeling 1987). Naeye (1983) analysed his department's experience of the value of routine histology in normally formed perinatal deaths and found a high return for such examination amongst their cases. He also stressed the need to look beyond the cause of death when undertaking post-mortem examination of babies; many positive findings in his analysis had clear indications for unit audit and patient management. Pryse-Davies (1981) found routine histological examination to be useful for confirmation of necropsy diagnoses in 80% of his cases, where a diagnosis was reached after

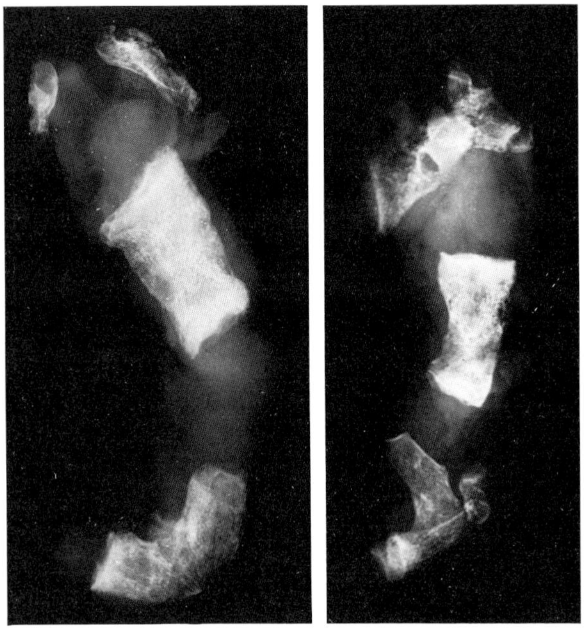

Fig. 1.32. Radiograph following fixation of arm and leg bones from a neonate with osteogenesis imperfecta shows fine detail of bone pathology.

Table 1.6. Samples for routine histological examination at perinatal necropsy

All perinatal deaths	Additional blocks in neonatal deaths
Both lungs	Larynx (vertical through vocal cords)
Thymus	Trachea
Ventricular myocardium	Pituitary
Both lobes of liver	Thyroid
Kidney	Intestine
Pancreas	Gonads
Adrenals	Brain (after Gruenwald and Laurence 1968)
Diaphragm	
Costochondral junction	
Cerebral cortex	
Placenta × 2	
Extraplacental membranes	
Umbilical cord	

gross examination of fetus and placenta, and essential in the remaining 20%, where no conclusion was reached after gross examination.

Usefulness of histological examination in macerated stillbirths is often questioned, even by those who recognise routine histology as an essential part of perinatal necropsy (Langley 1971; Pryse-Davies 1981). I find that routine blocking of major organs and the use of trichrome stains often yields useful information in such cases.

Routine samples for histological examination at perinatal necropsy are listed in Table 1.6. Examination of the costochondral junction provides evidence of regularity of pre- or postnatal growth (Emery and Kalpaktsoglou 1967) and diagnostic information in osteochondrodysplasias (see Chap. 26, p. 621). Blocking of the brain, as described by Gruenwald and Laurence (1968), may be accomplished in fewer blocks in the very small preterm baby. These blocks are additional to those taken from any abnormality which is recognised during dissection.

Interpretation of histological appearances in the fetus and neonate requires an understanding of the normal appearance at that particular stage of development. Changes in appearance which are developmentally related occur to a different degree and at different gestational ages in individual organs. Some are sufficiently specific, e.g. kidney, to provide further evidence of gestational age. In other organs, e.g. lung, the stage of development to some extent determines the likely type of pathological abnormality. The histological appearances of fetal organs at different gestational ages are illustrated in the appendix to this chapter. The histological appearance of the placenta at different gestations is illustrated in Chapter 2. A reference collection of histological sections of normal organs from babies of known gestational ages is very useful for purposes of comparison.

Microbiological Examination

Pryse-Davies and Hurley (1979) examined the usefulness of cysternal CSF, heart swab and bronchial swab as microbiological screening procedures as part of routine examination in 835 perinatal necropsies. Positive cultures were obtained from 12.1%, 12.1% and 41.3% of samples, respectively. They did not find that post-mortem delay increased the proportion of positive cultures and found a significant correlation between positive bronchial cultures and histological evidence of pneumonia.

The role of routine microbiological sampling during perinatal necropsy was questioned by Mueller et al. (1983) and found by them to be a cost-effective investigation. They obtained positive cultures in 4% of stillbirths and 15% of neonatal deaths. Barson (1990) found microbiological evidence of infection in only 1.8% of stillbirths but 28% of neonates had pneumonia and 13% were septicaemic.

Naeye (1983) cited recovery of organisms from 72% of placentae with histological evidence of chorioamnionitis amongst preterm deliveries. Amongst our cases (Zaaijman et al. 1982), positive culture was obtained less frequently from placentae from both term and preterm deliveries, and correlation between histological evidence of inflammation and bacteriological isolation was poor. Langley (1971) advocates samples of lung and blood from a large subchorial placental vessel for routine microbiological examination.

Many units are selective in their requests for virological investigations post-mortem. This policy should extend to bacteriological examination as well (Billson et al. 1993).

Chromosome Examination

A counsel of perfection is that samples should be taken from all fetal and neonatal deaths for chromosome examination. There are few departments which are prepared to undertake this amount of routine work and some selection of cases has to be undertaken. The best return from chromosome examination is amongst malformed fetuses and perinatal deaths. Normally formed macerated stillbirths provide the next highest rate of abnormalities, followed by samples from normally formed fresh stillbirths and neonatal deaths (Alberman and Creasy 1977). Sutherland and Carter (1983) report a very low rate of chromosome abnormality when the only fetal malformation is anencephaly or spina bifida.

I take heart blood and tissue from lung or gonad from fresh fetuses. Lymphocyte transformation in blood samples gives a rapid answer. In the macerated fetus, placental amnion may be more rewarding than fetal tissue and less prone to contamination by maternal cells than placental parenchyma.

Sampling for Biochemical Investigations

When samples of body fluids or organs are needed for the investigation of possible inborn errors of metabolism, they should be obtained as soon as possible after death. When there is clinical suspicion of such abnormality, which has not been confirmed or excluded during life, then colleagues should be advised to seek consent for necropsy, or, failing that, for removal of specific tissue samples, before the baby dies so that delay in obtaining important diagnostic material is minimised. Delay reduces the reliability of investigations. Samples required will depend on the type of disorder suspected, but plasma, serum and urine together with skin for fibroblast culture are useful minima. Appropriate samples in particular circumstances are detailed by Benson and Fensom (1985), but prior discussion with chemical pathologist colleagues may avert disappointment and unnecessary effort.

It is advisable to obtain these samples together with liver, heart, brain and kidney in mature babies with symptoms of hypoglycaemia and acidosis, respiratory failure, central nervous system signs, vomiting, hepatomegaly or jaundice in whom no diagnosis was reached during life. The samples are then snap frozen and can always be discarded should symptomatology be explained during the course of necropsy or histological examination.

Examination of the Placenta

It is important that the placentae of fetuses, stillbirths and neonatal deaths be examined as part of necropsy examination. Additionally, placentae from some complicated pregnancies are worthy of examination, whatever the outcome of pregnancy in terms of fetal viability and wellbeing. It is not difficult to ensure that the placentae of fetuses and stillbirths are available for examination as they usually accompany the baby to the pathology department. Difficulties often arise in ensuring the availability of a placenta in the event of neonatal death. Few pathology departments are willing, or even able, to undertake the examination of all placentae delivered in their obstetric unit, even though this is the only way to ensure that useful information is not lost (Rushton 1982). Most of us find it necessary to invoke some degree of selection. One method is to hold all placentae from livebirths in refrigeration in individually labelled bags for 1 week. This method may have been useful when virtually all neonatal deaths occurred during the first 7 days; however, the proportion of late neonatal deaths has increased as a result of neonatal intensive care, so this method is no longer appropriate.

All placentae from babies who go to the intensive care nursery are sent to our pathology department, and the majority, particularly when the baby is preterm or growth retarded, are examined, irrespective of outcome. We also examine all placentae from multiple pregnancies and pregnancies complicated by maternal hypertension or pre-eclamptic toxaemia, when alpha-fetoprotein level was elevated in the second trimester in the absence of fetal malformation, in rhesus incompatability and maternal immunological disorders. Additionally, any placentae thought unusual by obstetric staff are sent for pathological evaluation. In this way those placentae which are likely to have pathological abnormality are selected for examination and it is probable that most neonatal deaths will have had one of these adverse factors during pregnancy. Only placentae from a few externally normal, mature babies, who are well at birth, are likely to evade examination when this selection procedure is used. In practice, 15% of delivered placentae are examined in the pathology department.

Macroscopic Examination

Placentae of infants at high risk of infection (i.e. cases of prematurity, maternal pyrexia or prolonged rupture of membranes) may have amniotic and chorionic smears and swabs taken, as described by Blanc (1980), as soon as possible after delivery. This procedure avoids problems of contamination, and examination of Gram-stained smears provides a quick diagnosis of bacterial infection. Should there be a history of maternal viral infection or if the baby is unexpectedly growth retarded, or the placenta is small and pale, a block of placental parenchyma is obtained for viral studies (see Chap. 2, p. 75).

Once samples have been taken, the placenta may be examined in a fresh state or fixed flat in formalin for a few days. Some lesions are easier to see in the fixed organ, whilst a recent infarct may be easier to detect in the fresh state.

Weight and Measurement

The gross weight of the placenta is not a good indication of its functional mass. Trimmed weight (membranes trimmed to the disc margin and cord cut within 2 cm of its insertion) is a better guide. Whilst accepting the limitations of placental weight in respect of placental function, comparison with the weight of the baby does serve to draw attention to excessively heavy or light placentae which are worthy of further examination (Table 1.7). Two placental diameters are measured at right angles and maximum thickness recorded.

Table 1.7. Placental weight and placental/fetal weight ratio at different gestations (Gruenwald and Minh 1961)

Weeks from LMP	Weight of placenta (g) mean	1 SD	Ratio of placenta to fetal weight
24	225	70	1:2.9
25	235	70	1:3.1
26	245	70	1:3.3
27	260	65	1:3.5
28	270	70	1:4.9
29	290	70	1:5.1
30	310	70	1:5.3
31	335	70	1:5.4
32	360	70	1:5.6
33	380	75	1:5.8
34	400	75	1:6.0
35	420	75	1:6.2
36	435	80	1:6.4
37	450	85	1:6.5
38	465	85	1:6.6
39	480	85	1:6.7
40	490	90	1:6.8
41	500	90	1:7.0
42	505	95	1:7.1
43	505	95	1:7.1
44	505	95	1:7.1

Abbreviation: LMP, last menstrual period

Membranes

The completeness of the membranes and point of rupture are noted. Membranes are often incomplete and ragged in cases of prolonged rupture. The distance from point of rupture to the disc margin may indicate placenta praevia.

The colour and fetal surface of the membranes are examined. Membranes are cloudy or opaque and greenish when there is bacterial infection, greenish following the passage of meconium and brownish in cases of old retroplacental haemorrhage. Surface irregularity may be observed when there is amnion nodosum, squamous metaplasia or certain infections such as *Candida albicans* or *Listeria monocytogenes*.

Umbilical Cord

Naeye (1985) provides gestation-related normal values of cord length (Table 1.8). Excessively long (greater than 90 cm) or short (less than 40 cm) cords are significant findings. The former predispose to entanglement, the latter may interfere with fetal descent through the birth canal.

Table 1.8. Umbilical cord length at various gestational ages from 35 779 neonates (Naeye 1985)

Gestational age (weeks)	*n*	Umbilical cord length (cm)
20–21	16	32.4 ± 8.6
22–23	27	36.4 ± 9.0
24–25	38	40.1 ± 10.1
26–27	59	42.5 ± 11.3
28–29	80	45.0 ± 9.7
30–31	113	47.6 ± 11.3
32–33	337	50.2 ± 12.1
34–35	857	52.5 ± 11.2
36–37	3 153	55.6 ± 12.6
38–39	10 083	57.4 ± 12.6
40–41	13 841	59.6 ± 12.6
42–43	4 797	60.3 ± 12.7
44–45	1 450	60.4 ± 12.7
46–47	492	60.5 ± 13.0

Data represent mean ± 1 SD.
n = number of cases.

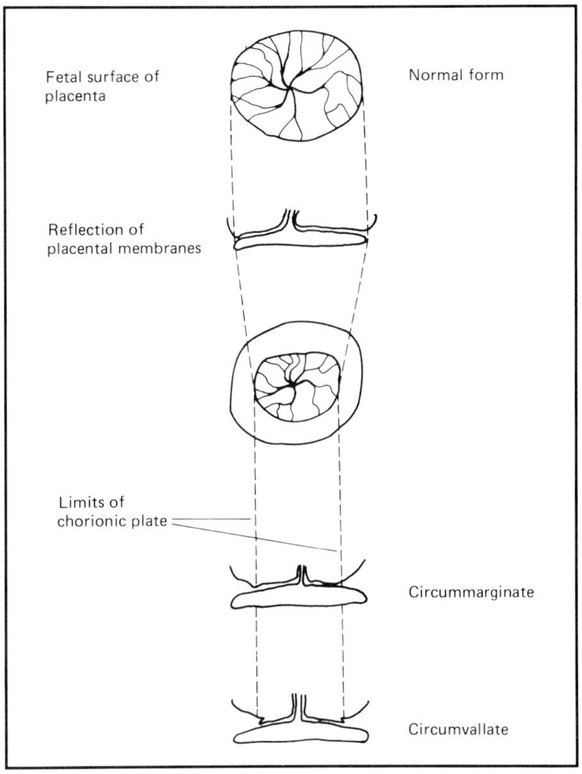

Fig. 1.33. Different types of placentation.

Oedema of the cord and focal abnormalities such as bruises or strictures, haematomas, haemorrhage as well as knots and varicosity, the number of cord vessels and the site of insertion are recorded. Where there is velamentous insertion, the distance from insertion to the disc margin and the length of the membranous course of the vessels is measured. Disruption of these vessels should be carefully sought.

Placental Surface

The fetal surface of the placenta is inspected. The course of large vessels is observed (arteries can be identified as they cross superficially to veins). Large vessels should extend to the disc margin (normal form) but stop short of it when the placenta is circummarginate or circumvallate in form (Fig. 1.33). Subchorial haemorrhage or fibrin deposition may be apparent but are of little significance. Occasional vascular thrombi or aneurysms are apparent.

The maternal surface is examined for completeness, adherent clot and surface depression which might have been caused by retroplacental haemorrhage. Focal calcification is often apparent in the maternal surface. It is of no significance in respect of placental function.

Slicing the Placenta

The placenta is sliced (easiest with maternal surface upwards) at approximately 1 cm intervals and the slices laid out in order for close inspection. Any lesions such as subchorionic fibrin, perivillous fibrin, infarcts or cysts should be noted. Many macroscopic abnormalities can be identified during this examination, but where there is any doubt blocks should be taken for histological confirmation. Blocks should be taken from apparently normal areas of the placenta (Fig. 1.34). Obtaining representative samples from placentae is a problem for there are quantitative structural differences between the edge and the centre of the placenta and between basal and sub-

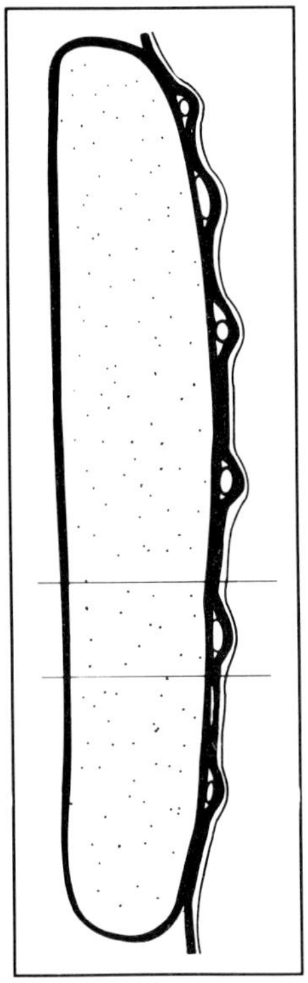

Fig. 1.34. Blocks of placenta for histological examination should include both the fetal and maternal surfaces.

chorionic areas (Boyd et al. 1980). For routine histological analysis, it is appropriate to take one or two full-thickness blocks from the placenta, avoiding the margins. If villitis is suspected then four blocks should be taken from different regions. A roll of membranes from the site of rupture and a block of umbilical cord complete placental sampling for histological examination.

The Post-mortem Report

All of the activity discussed in this chapter is of limited usefulness if it is not communicated to clinicians in a clear and timely fashion. It may be difficult to complete all necessary investigations and issue a report within one or two weeks. A useful compromise is to send a brief note to the clinician summarising gross necropsy findings on the day of examination and to ensure that a more detailed description with histological findings, radiology and bacteriology, preferably with gross inspection of the fixed brain is available for the maternal postnatal out-patient appointment and perinatal mortality meeting. Further details can be sent out later.

Is there a place for structured report forms in perinatal pathology? I don't think so. The amount of description in any particular system varies enormously from case to case, so structured forms are inappropriately constricting. It is helpful to set out one's reports in the same way so that clinicians find their way around easily. The report should include all weights and measurements with normal values or a comment about normality. An opinion about fetal maturity and appropriateness of size is important. Specific questions should be answered and the clinician's attention drawn to any lesion thought to result from treatment. All pathological diagnoses should be set out at the end of the report.

Appendix

Normal Histology at Different Stages of Development

An awareness of the normal histological appearance of organs as gestation progresses is essential for the correct interpretation of tissue samples obtained during fetal or neonatal necropsy. Pulmonary immaturity or hypoplasia are frequently encountered during perinatal necropsy. Often it is the extent of pulmonary maturation which determines viability. For this reason, normal pulmonary histology is illustrated at 5-week intervals from 10 weeks of gestation to term. The same intervals are used for the kidney. Renal maturation is distinctive, and the histological appearance of the kidneys is a useful marker of fetal maturity. Other organs are illustrated at three gestational ages, chosen to demonstrate changes which take place during the maturation of that particular organ.

Photographs of individual organs at different gestations have been taken at the same magnification to facilitate comparison and, with the exception of the gonad, illustrations at two different magnifications are presented for each gestation.

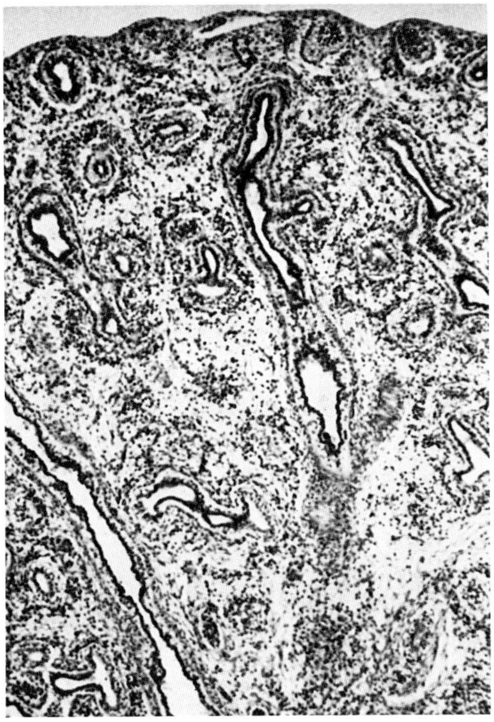

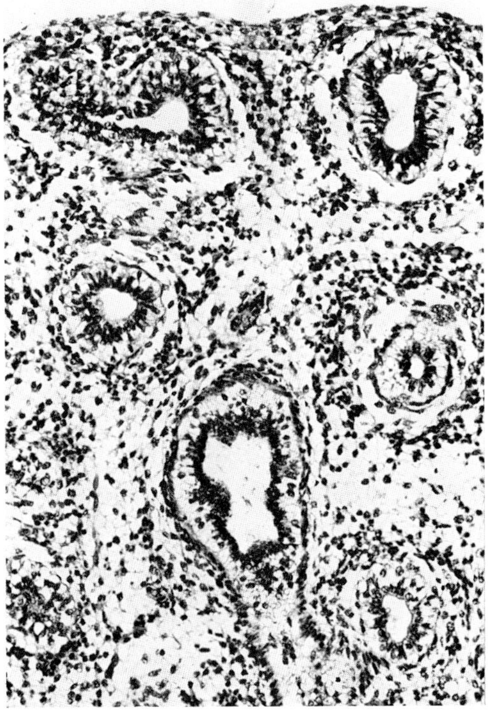

LUNG 10 weeks: Bronchi, lined by simple columnar epithelium, extend to the pleural surface. Airways are separated by large amounts of cellular mesenchyme. Poorly defined bars of cartilage are present adjacent to bronchi towards the hilus.

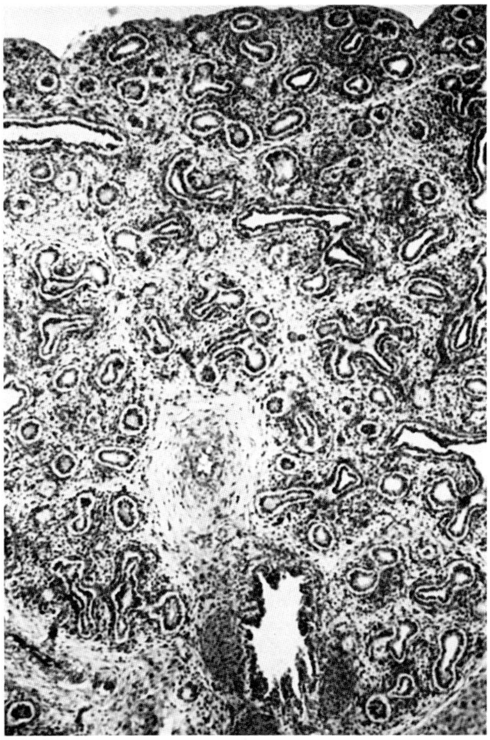

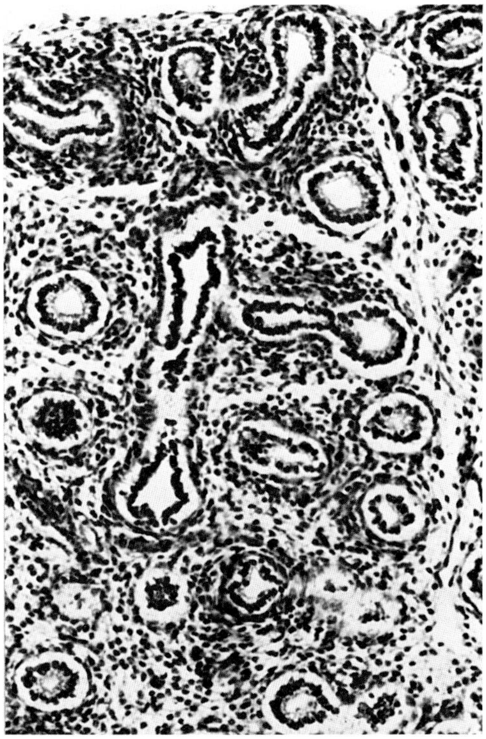

LUNG 15 weeks: Further bronchial branching has replaced some mesenchyme. Bronchial cartilages are more circumscribed. At this stage bronchial epithelium is ciliated.

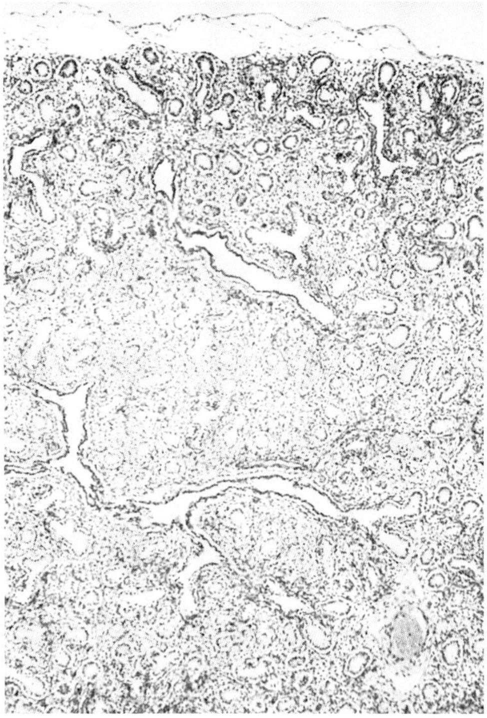 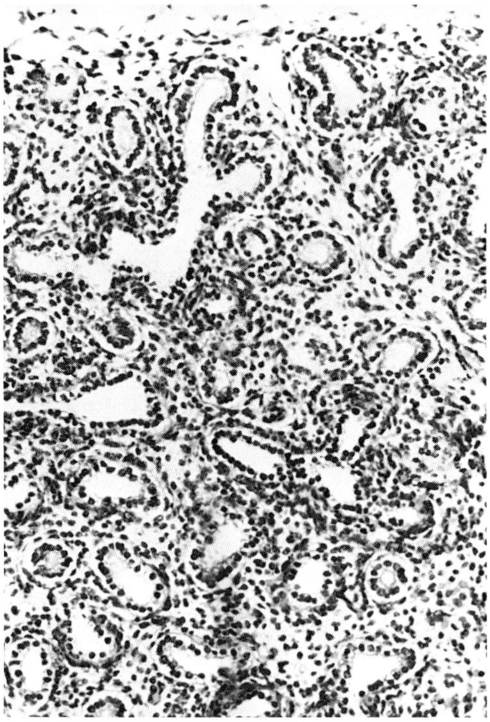

LUNG 20 weeks: Bronchi can be distinguished from bronchioles, which are proliferating rapidly at this stage.

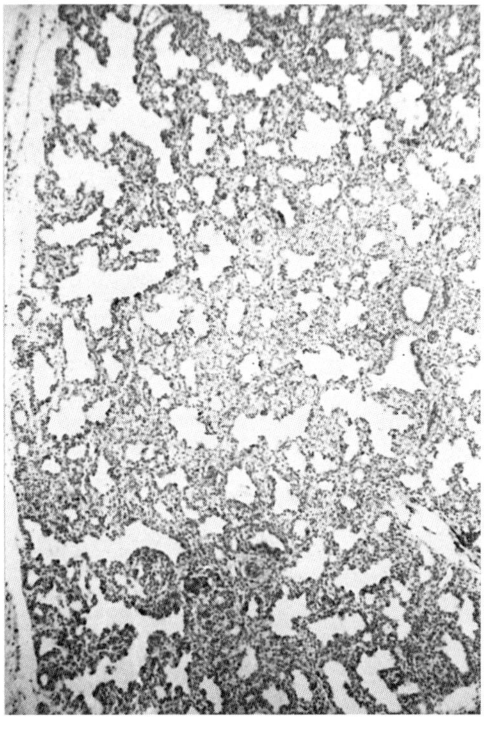 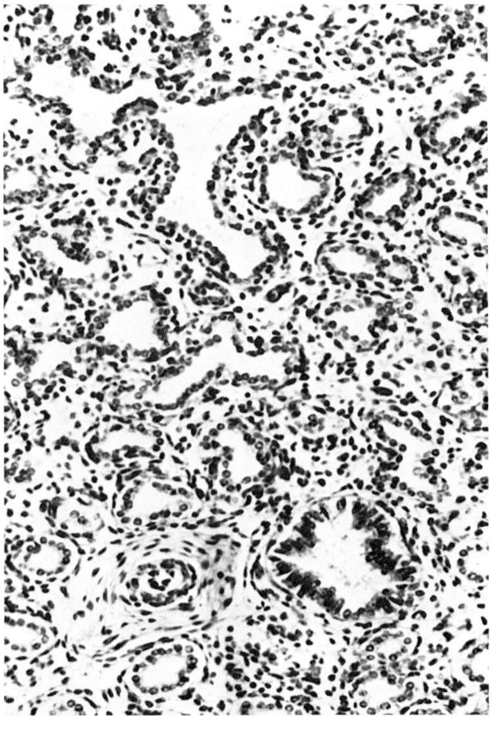

LUNG 25 weeks: Alveolar saccules are apparent. They are lined by cuboidal epithelium.

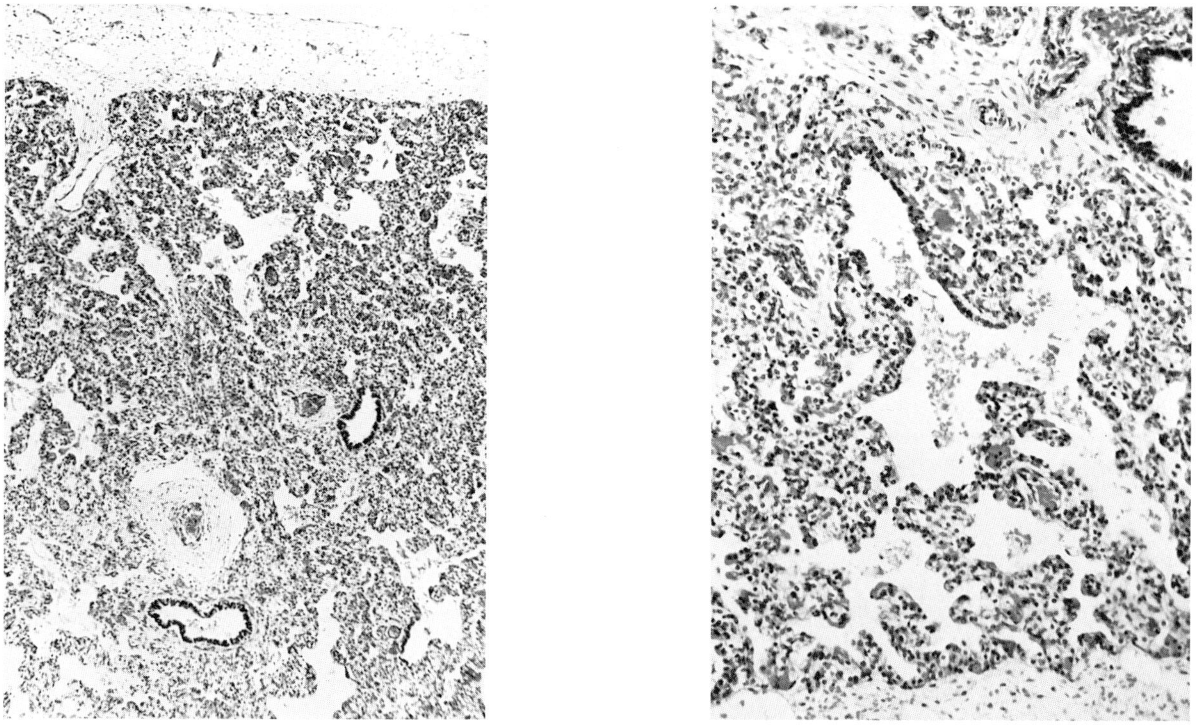

LUNG 30 weeks: Further generations of alveolar saccules have developed. Their lining epithelium is low cuboidal.

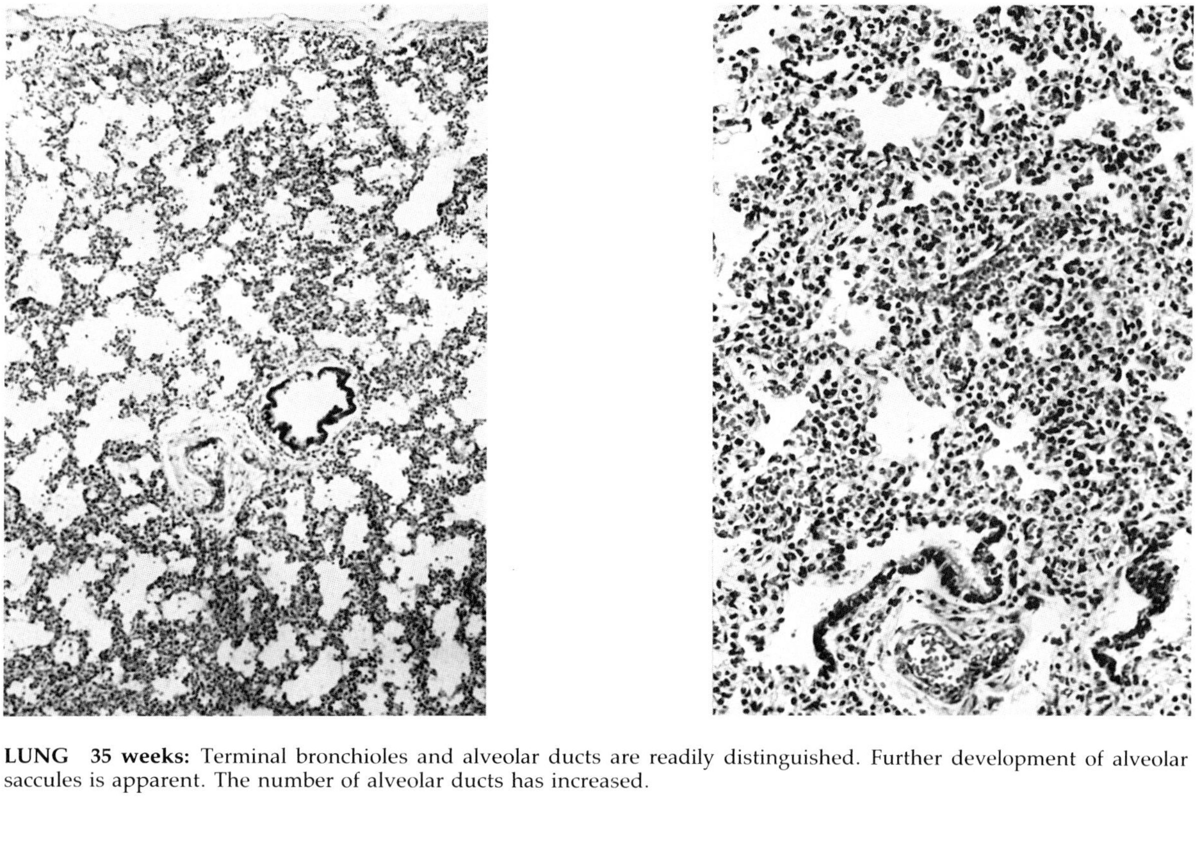

LUNG 35 weeks: Terminal bronchioles and alveolar ducts are readily distinguished. Further development of alveolar saccules is apparent. The number of alveolar ducts has increased.

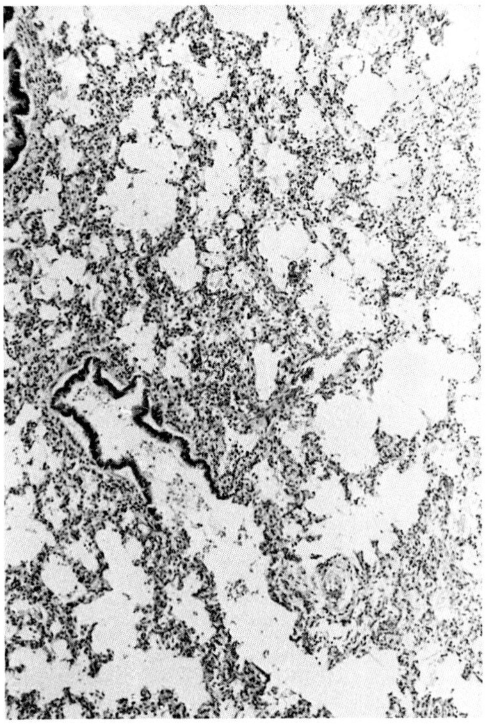
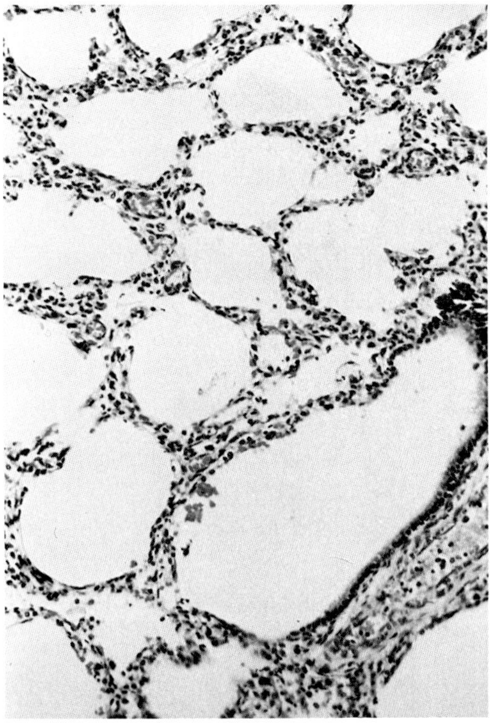

LUNG 40 weeks: There has been further growth of alveoli and marked thinning of alveolar walls. Alveoli are lined by flat, barely distinguishable epithelium.

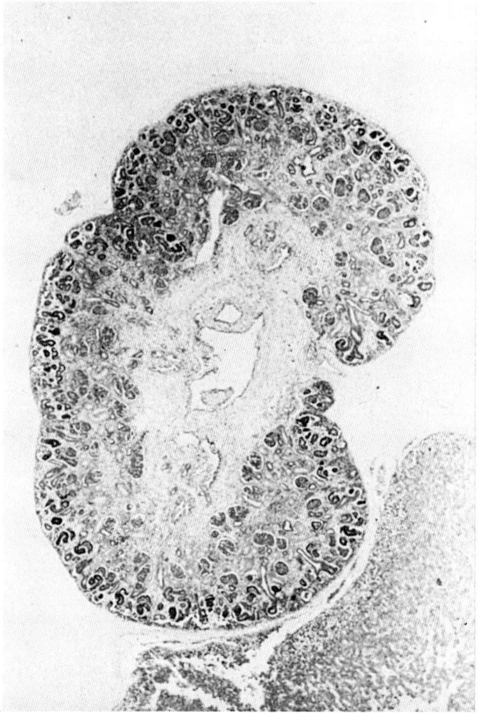
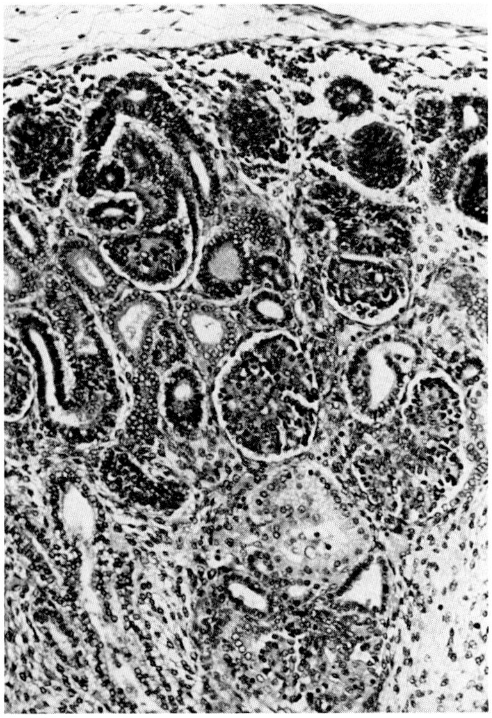

KIDNEY 10 weeks: Immature glomeruli and tubules are present in the deeper cortex and are easily distinguished from the subcapsular nephrogenic zone. The pelvis is surrounded by abundant loose mesenchyme.

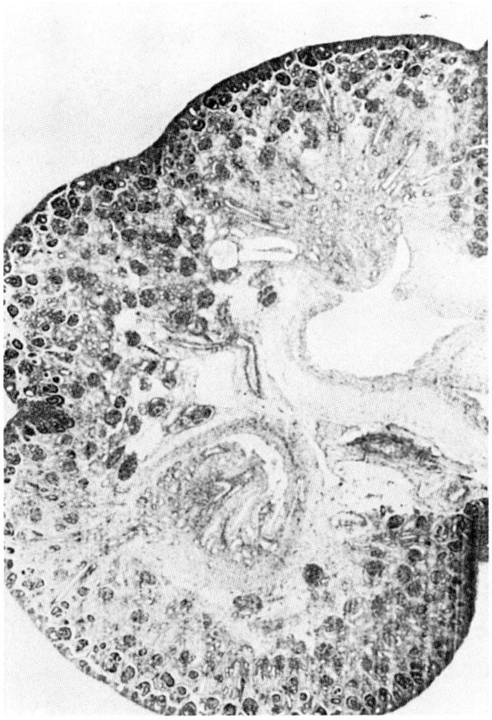

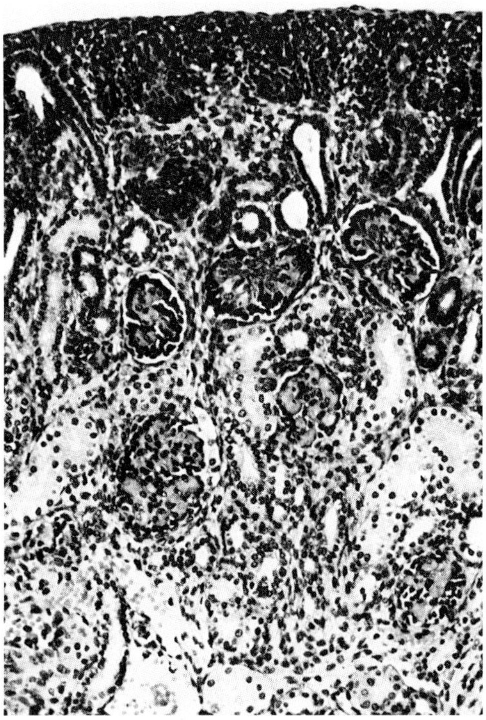

KIDNEY 15 weeks: Maturation of the deepest generations of glomeruli is apparent. Papillary development is well advanced.

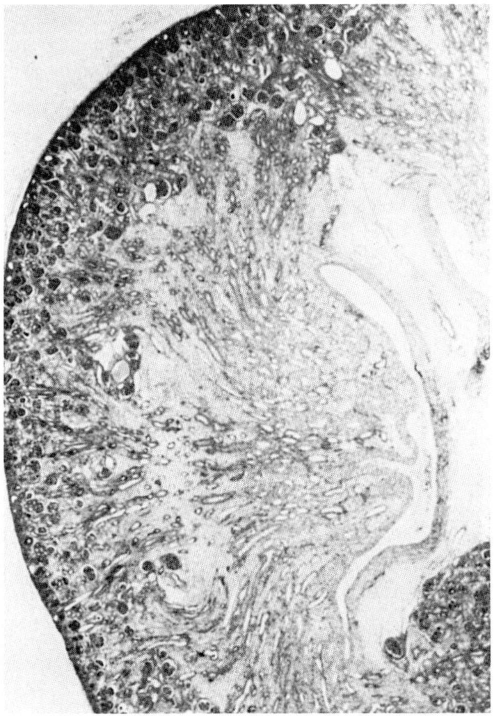

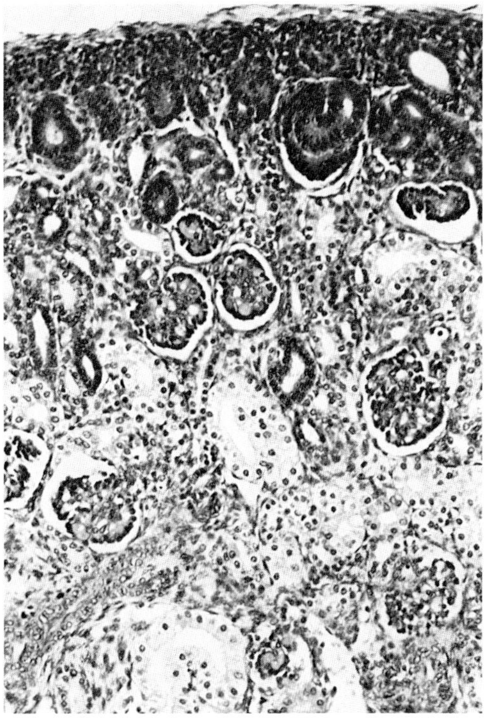

KIDNEY 20 weeks: Further elaboration of the collecting ducts and papillae has taken place. The plane of the arcuate arteries is clearly defined.

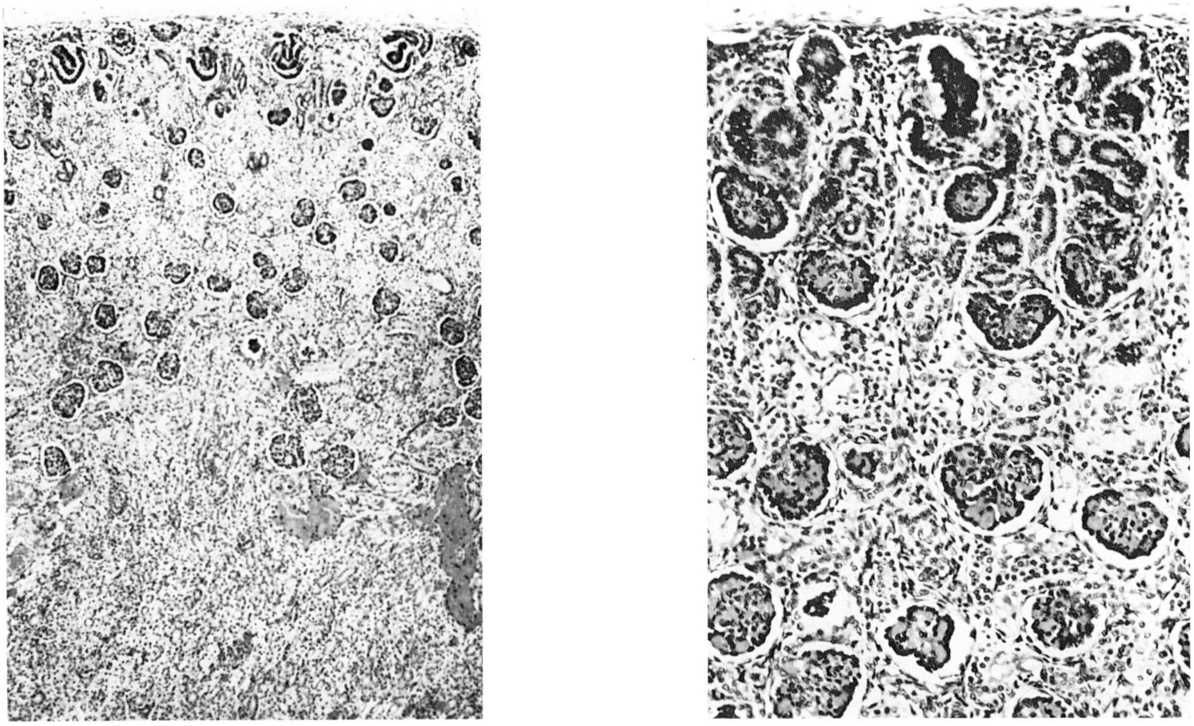

KIDNEY 25 weeks: The nephrogenic zone has narrowed but is still continuous. Maturation of juxtacortical glomeruli is readily apparent.

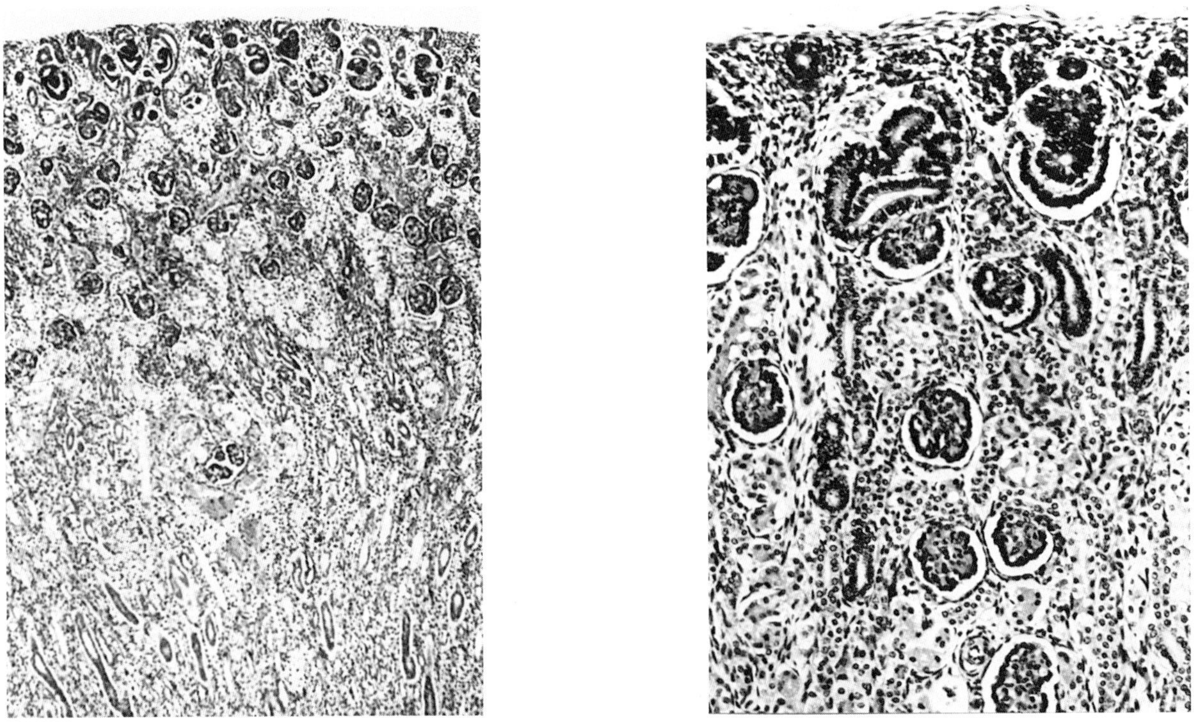

KIDNEY 30 weeks: The nephrogenic zone is prominent, but breaks are present where differentiated tubules abut on the capsular surface.

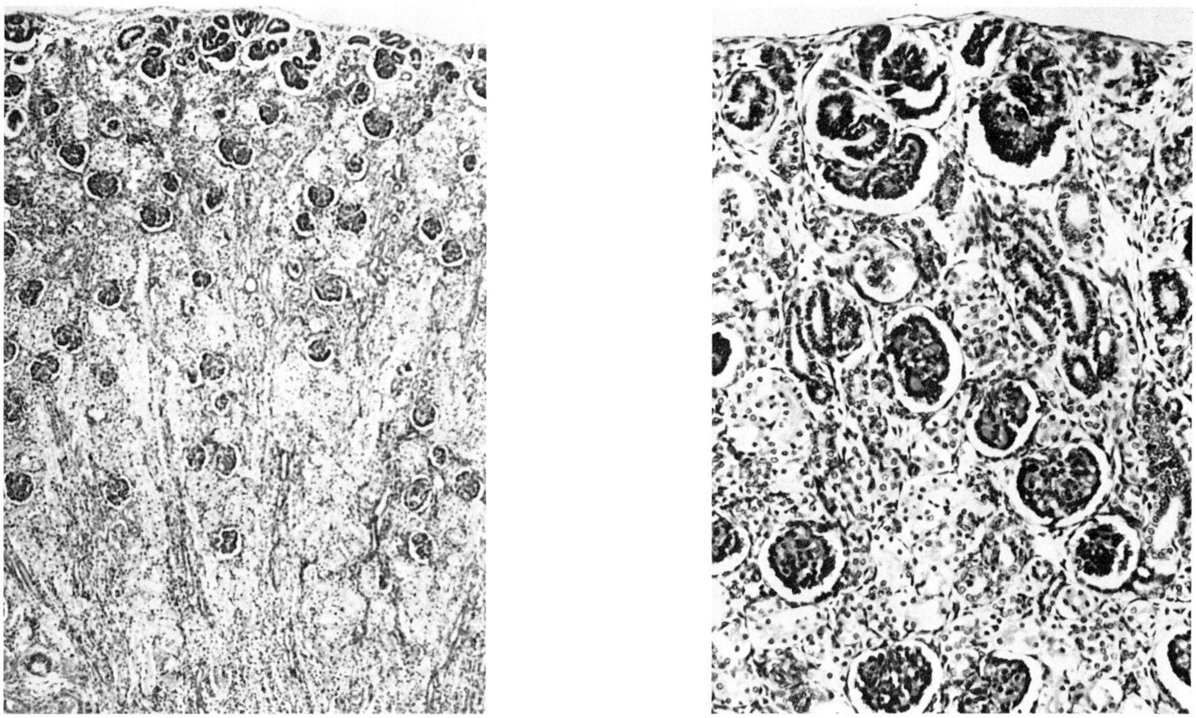

KIDNEY 35 weeks: Islands of nephrogenic structures normally persist. Rapid tubular growth has increased cortical depth and separated glomeruli.

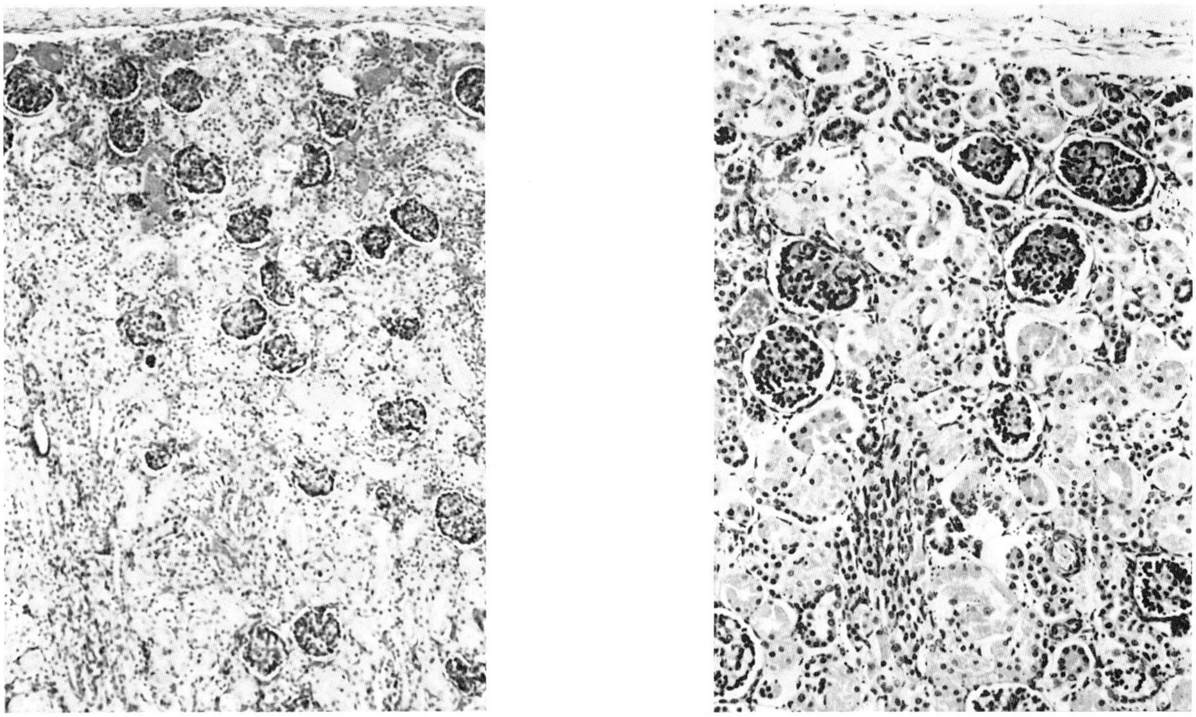

KIDNEY 40 weeks: Nephrogenic tissue has disappeared. Subcapsular glomeruli still have a halo of darkly staining epithelium.

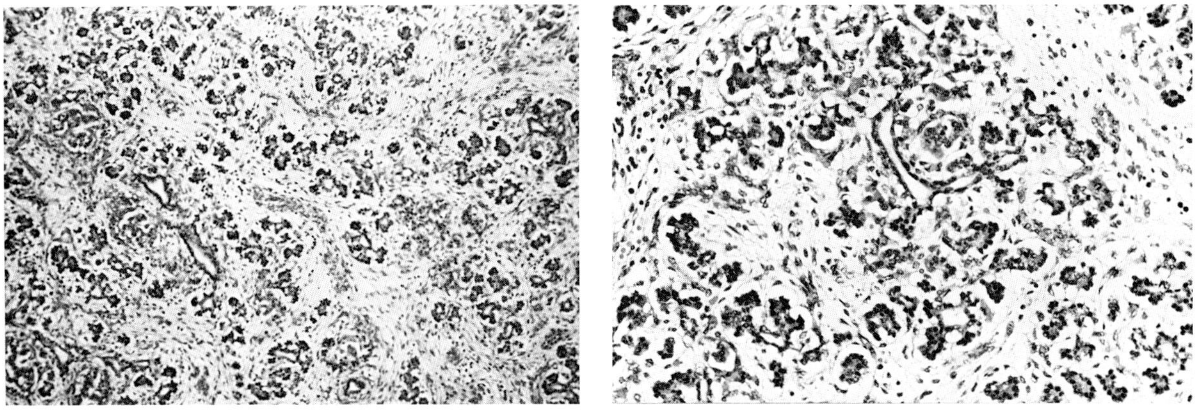

PANCREAS 15 weeks: Large ducts are easily distinguished. Clusters of branching ductules are widely spaced and separated from each other by mesenchyme.

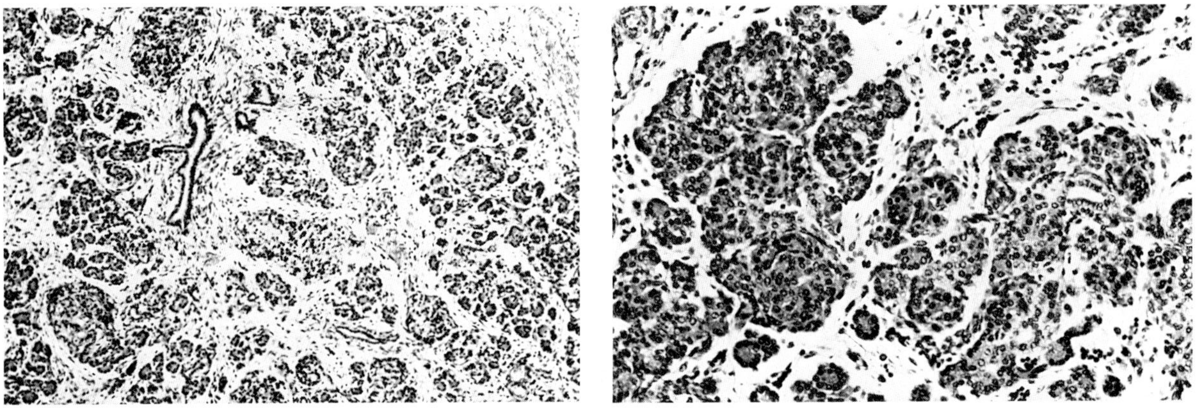

PANCREAS 25 weeks: Proliferation of ductules and growth in differentiation of acini results in a lobular structure. Lobules are still separated by cellular mesenchyme. Islets of Langerhans are centrilobular and poorly circumscribed.

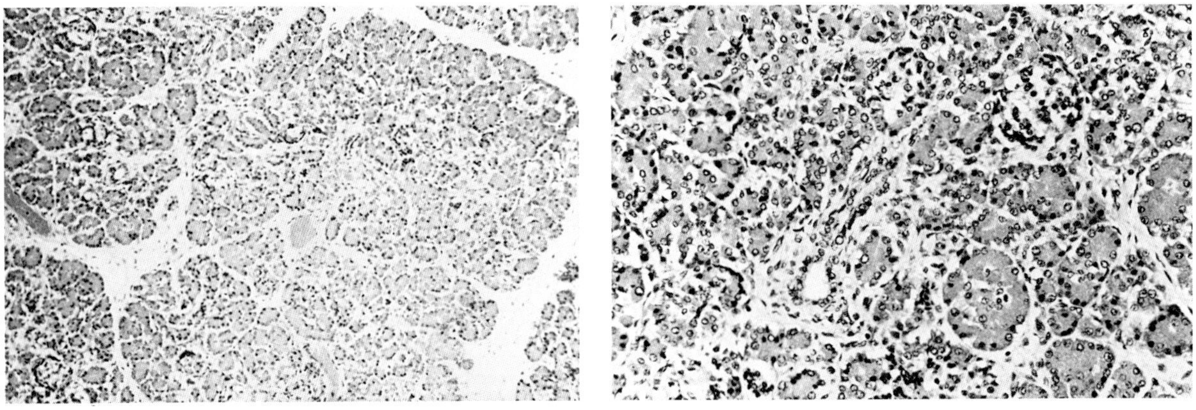

PANCREAS 40 weeks: Lobules comprise closely packed acini; fibrous septa are narrow. Islets are now compact structures in the body and tail of the pancreas and widely distributed within the lobule.

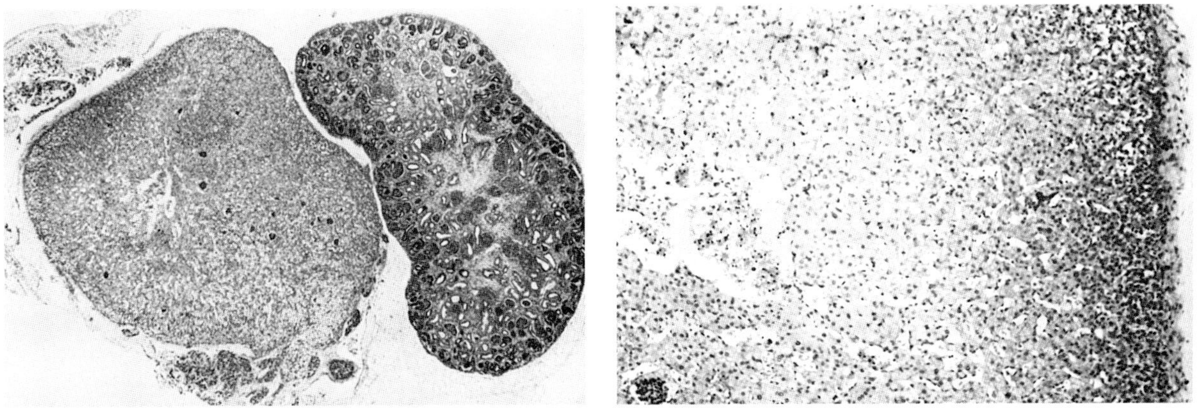

ADRENAL 10 weeks: The adrenal is larger than the adjacent kidney. Subcapsular cortical cells are smaller than those more centrally situated. Islands of darkly staining cells in the centre of the gland represent adrenal medulla.

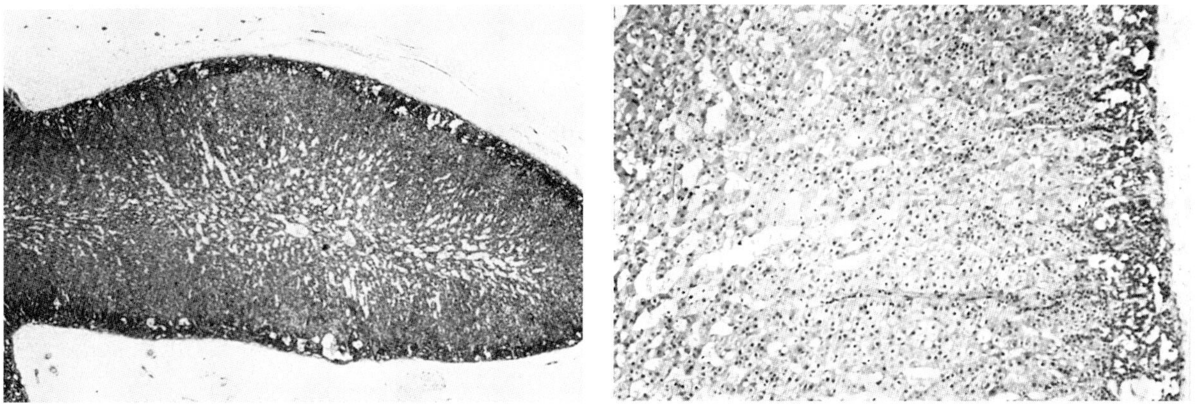

ADRENAL 25 weeks: The adrenal is invaginated by the adjacent kidney and large vessels present in the centre of the gland. The definitive cortex has a glandular structure; the larger cells of the fetal cortex are disposed in cords.

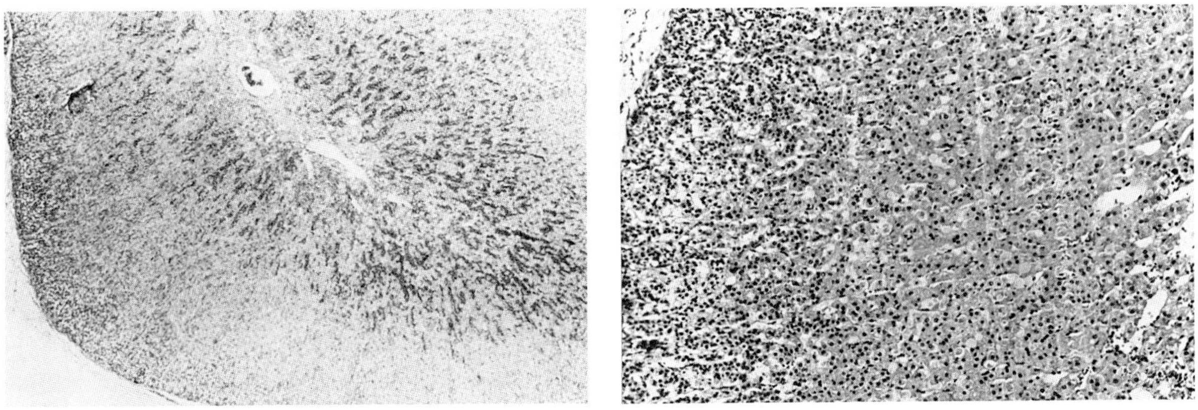

ADRENAL 35 weeks: Cortical width is increased and the definitive cortex is deeper. Islands of immature neural crest cells persist in the centre of the gland within the inner part of the fetal cortex; mature medullary cells are relatively sparse.

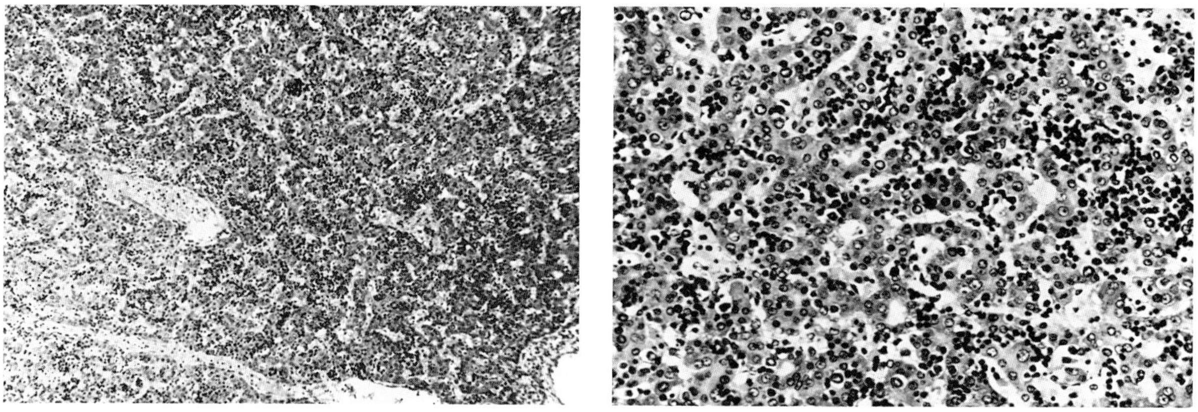

LIVER 10 weeks: Lobular structure is already present but small portal tracts are not easily distinguished. Hepatocytes have a high nuclear:cytoplasmic ratio; haemopoiesis is extensive.

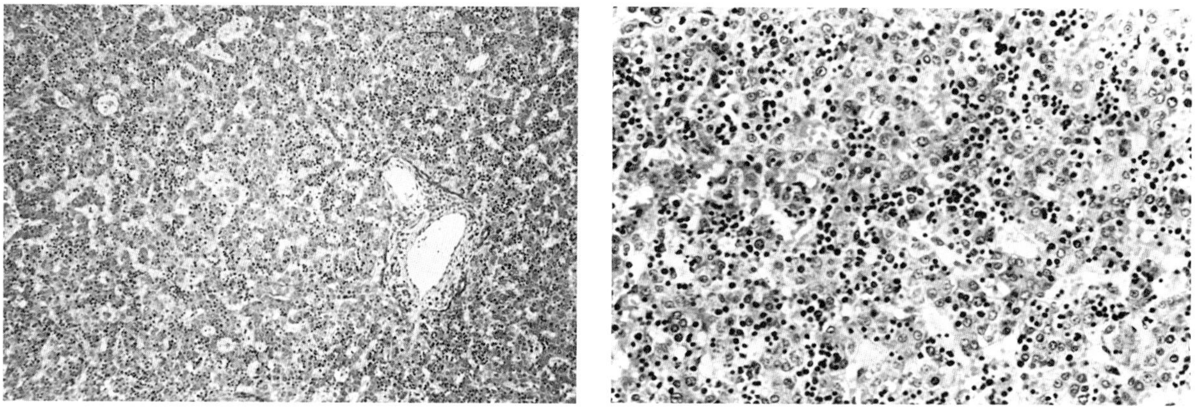

LIVER 20 weeks: Connective tissue in portal tracts is more mature, less cellular, and tracts are more easily distinguished. Haemopoiesis is still abundant but liver cell plates are apparent.

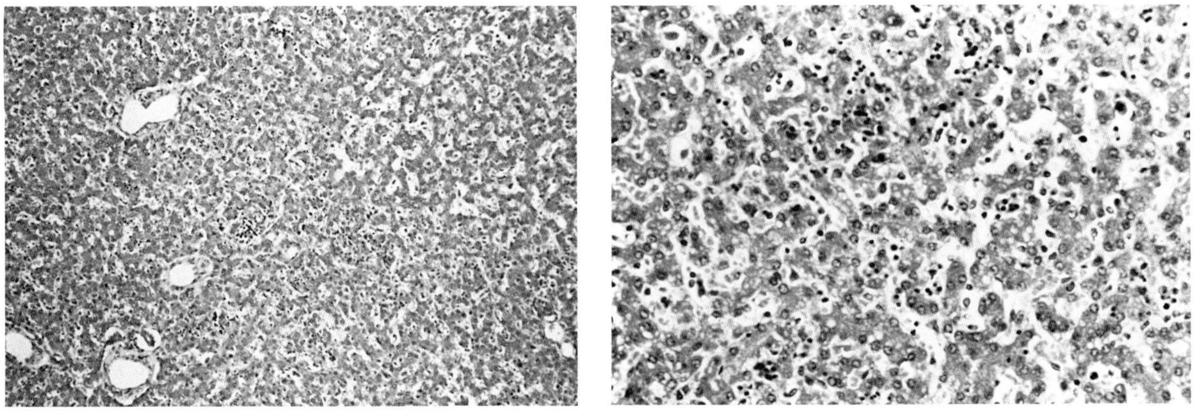

LIVER 30 weeks: Portal tracts and liver cell plates are easily distinguished; hepatocytes appear mature with high nuclear: cytoplasmic ratio.

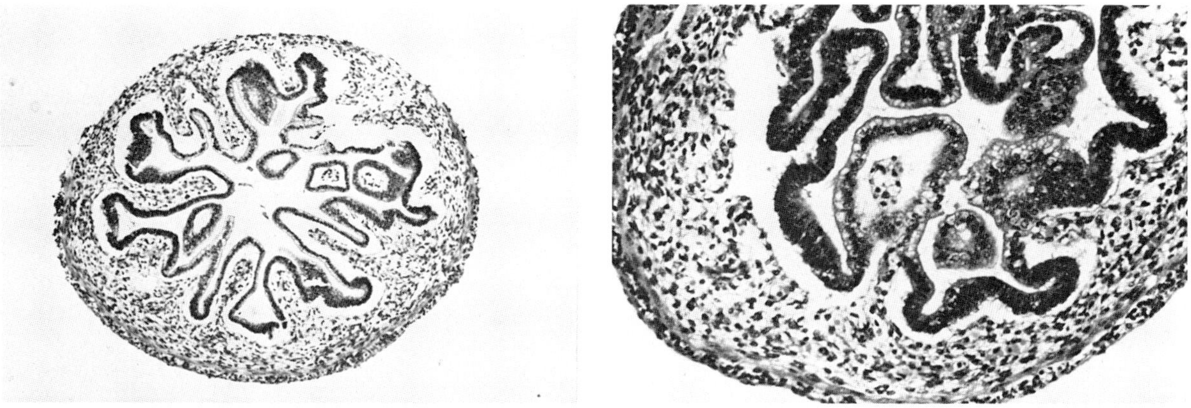

ILEUM 10 weeks: Intestinal villi are few in number and covered by a single layer of columnar cells. The muscularis externa is just distinguishable.

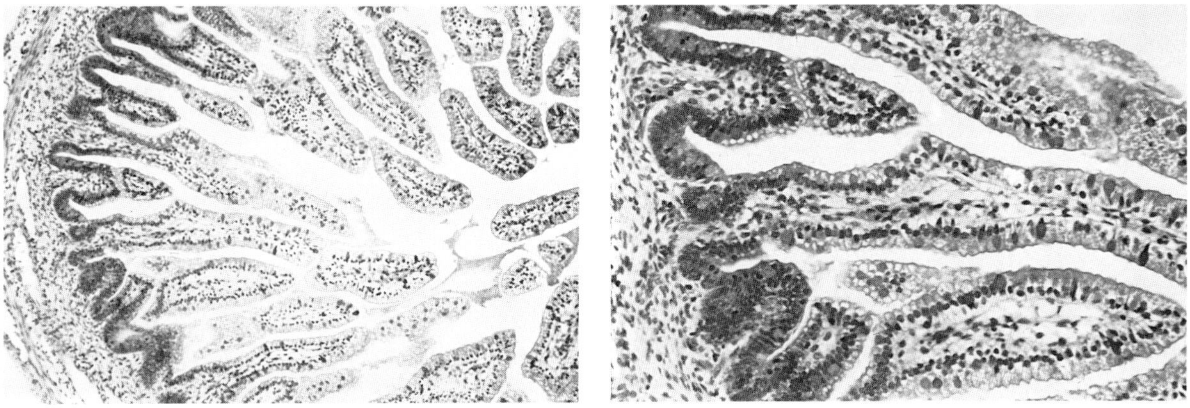

ILEUM 20 weeks: Villi are longer and more numerous. Crypts are shallow. Columnar, mucus-producing epithelial cells covering villi are readily distinguished from crypt-lining cells.

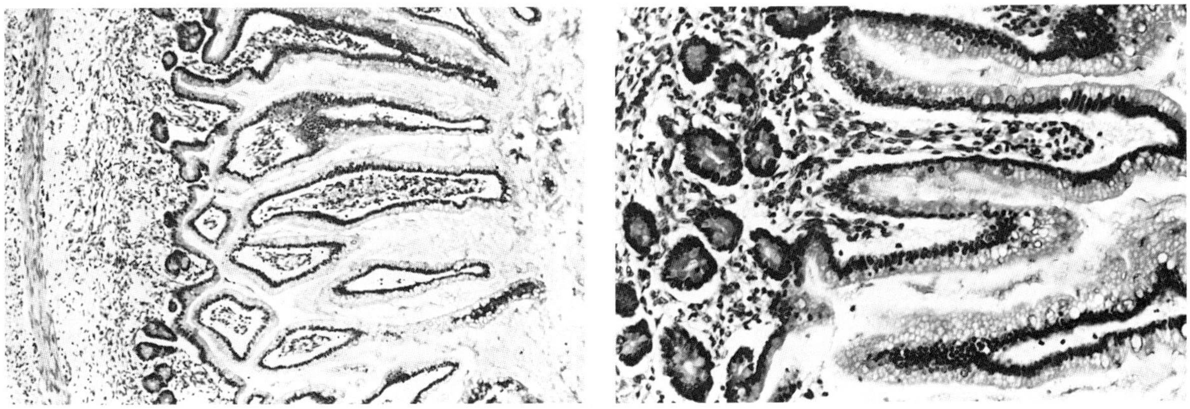

ILEUM 30 weeks: Villi are long and tapering. Glands are deeper and narrower. Lamina propria, muscularis mucosae and submucosa are easily distinguished. Lymphoid tissue is not prominent.

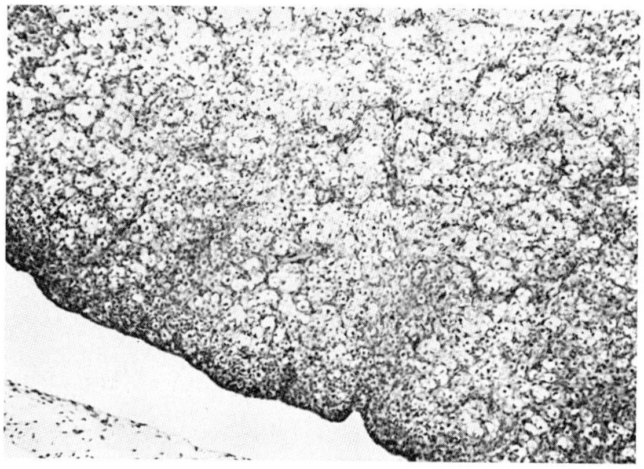

OVARY 15 weeks: Surface germinal epithelium and underlying stroma stain darkly. Abundant oocytes are separated by blood vessels which occupy the centre of the gonad.

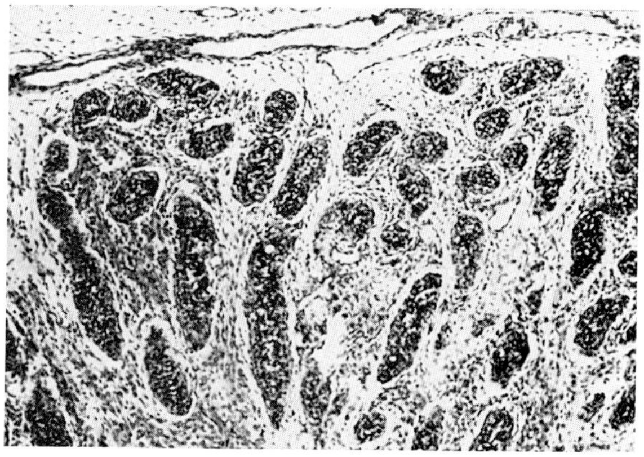

TESTIS 15 weeks: Darkly staining sex cord cell columns are separated by paler interstitial cells. The tunica albuginea is quite distinct.

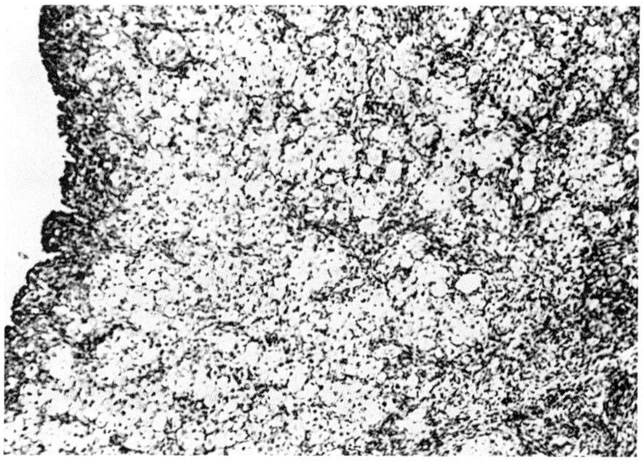

OVARY 25 weeks: Oocytes in the centre of the gonad are larger, surrounded by primordial follicular cells and separated by stroma.

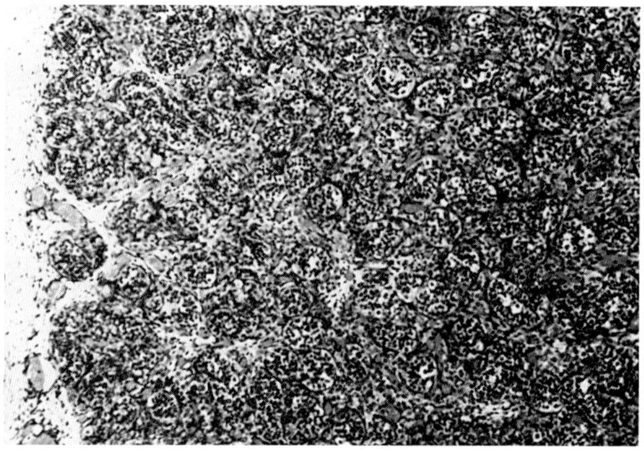

TESTIS 25 weeks: Tubules are numerous and have a flattened peripheral layer and are filled with spermatogonia. Clusters of interstitial cells are prominent.

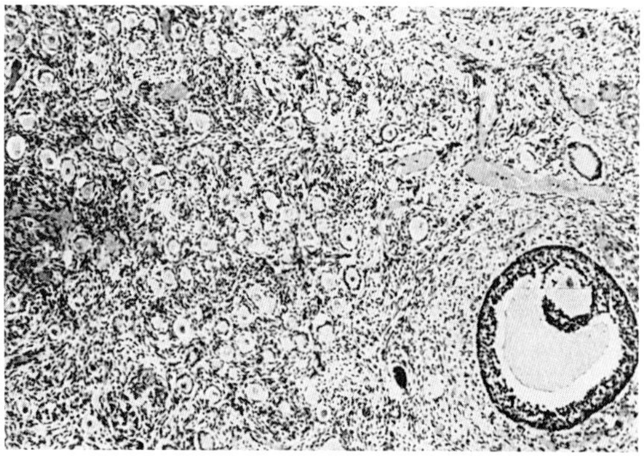

OVARY 40 weeks: A secondary follicle with fluid-filled follicular space and a cumulus containing an enlarged oocyte has matured under the influence of maternal hormones.

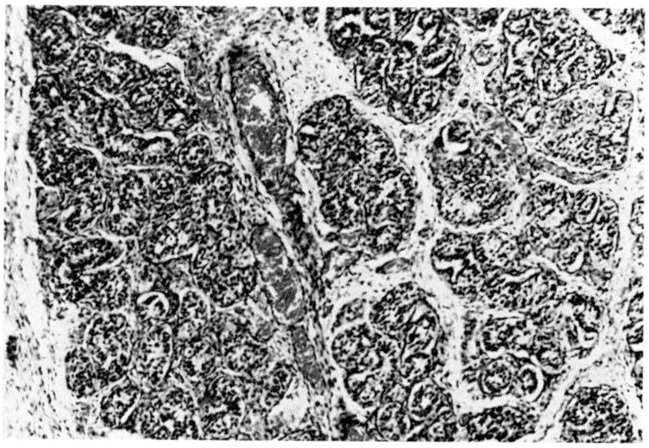

TESTIS 40 weeks: Groups of tubules are closely packed and separate a vascular fibrous stroma. Interstitial cells are infrequent.

References

Alberman E (1980) Prospects for better perinatal health. Lancet I: 189–192

Alberman ED, Creasy MR (1977) Frequency of chromosomal abnormalities in miscarriages and perinatal deaths. J Med Genet 14: 313–315

Barson AJ (1981) The perinatal postmortem. In: Barson AJ (ed) Laboratory investigation of fetal disease. Wright, Bristol, pp 476–497

Barson AJ (1990) A postmortem study of infection in the newborn from 1976 to 1988. In: de Louvois J, Harvey D (eds) Infection in the newborn. Wiley, Chichester, pp 13–34

Benson PF, Fensom AH (1985) Genetic biochemical disorders. Oxford monographs on medical genetics No 12. Oxford University Press, Oxford

Berry CL (1980) The examination of embryonic and fetal material in diagnostic histopathology laboratories. J Clin Pathol 33: 317–326

Billson V, Masterton RG, Keeling JW (1993) How useful is postmortem bacteriological investigation? J Pathol 169 suppl 120A

Blanc WA (1981) Pathology of the placenta, membranes and umbilical cord in bacterial, fungal and viral infections in man. In: Naeye RL, Kissane JM, Kaufman, N (eds) Perinatal disease. Williams and Wilkins, Baltimore, pp 67–132

Boyd PA, Brown RA, Stewart WJ (1980) Quantitative structural differences within the normal term human placenta: a pilot study. Placenta 1: 337–344

Campbell S, Pearce JMF (1985) Ultrasound in obstetrics and gynaecology. In: McDonald RR (ed) Scientific basis of obstetrics and gynaecology. Churchill Livingstone, Edinburgh, pp 304–349

Chamberlain GVP (1985) The length of labour. In: Crawford JW (ed) Risks of labour. Wiley, Chichester, pp 1–10

Cooke RWI, Lucas A, Yudkin PLN, Pryse-Davies J (1977) Head circumference as an index of brain weight in the foetus and newborn. Early Hum Dev 1: 145–149

Dorovini-Zis K, Dolman CL (1977) Gestational development of brain. Arch Pathol Lab Med 101: 192–195

Elejalde BR, Mercedes de Elejalde M, Gilman M (1985) Analysis of the human fetal skeleton and organs with xeroradiography. Am J Obstet Gynecol 151: 666–670

Emery JL, Kalpaktsoglou PK (1967) The costochondral junction during later stages of intrauterine life, and abnormal growth patterns found in association with perinatal death. Arch Dis Child 42: 1–13

Foote GA, Wilson AJ, Stewart JH (1978) Perinatal postmortem radiography—experience with 2500 cases. Br J Radiol 51: 351–356

Gairdner D, Pearson J (1971) A growth chart for premature and other infants. Arch Dis Child 46: 783–794

Gruenwald P, Laurence KM (1968) A method of examining the brain of the newborn. Dev Med Child Neurol 10: 64–68

Gruenwald P, Minh HN (1960) Evaluation of body and organ weights in perinatal pathology. Am J Clin Pathol 34: 247–253

Gruenwald P, Minh HN (1961) Evaluation of body and organ weights in perinatal pathology. Am J Obstet Gynecol 82: 312–319

Isaacson G (1984) Postmortem examination of infant brains. Arch Pathol Lab Med 108: 80–81

Kalifa G, Barbet JP, Labbe F, Houette A, Sellier N (1989) Value of systematic post mortem radiographic examinations of fetuses—400 cases. Pediatr Radiol 19: 111–113

Kelehan P (1984) Technique for removal of the newborn middle and inner ear. In: Wigglesworth JS (ed) Perinatal pathology. Saunders, Philadelphia, pp 431–433

Kjær I, Keeling JW, Græm N (1991) The midline craniofacial skeleton in holoprosencephalic fetuses. J Med Genet 28: 846–855

Kliegman RM, King KC (1983) Intrauterine growth retardation: determinants of aberrant fetal growth. In: Fanaroff AA, Martin RJ (eds) Behrman's neonatal–perinatal medicine: diseases of the fetus and infant, 3rd edn. Mosby, St Louis, pp 49–80

Langley FA (1971) The perinatal postmortem examination. J Clin Pathol 24: 159–169

Laurence KM, Martin D (1959) A technique for obtaining undistorted specimens of the central nervous system. J Clin Pathol 12: 188–190

Lucas A, Cole TJ, Gandy GM (1986) Birthweight centiles in preterm infants reappraised. Early Hum Dev 13: 313–322

Milner RDG, Richards B (1974) An analysis of birth weight by gestational age of infants born in England and Wales, 1967 to 1971. J Obstet Gynaecol Br Common 81: 956–967

Mueller RF, Sybert VP, Johnson J, Brown ZA, Chen WJ (1983) Evaluation of a protocol for post-mortem examination of stillbirths. N Engl J Med 309: 586–590

Muller J, McCombs RV (1984) Brain-cutting device for correlation with CT-scan planes of section. Acta Neuropathol (Berl) 62: 257–258

Naeye RL (1983) The investigation of perinatal deaths. N Engl J Med 309: 611–612

Naeye RL (1985) Umbilical cord length: clinical significance. J Pediatr 107: 278–281

Porter HJ, Keeling JW (1987) The value of the perinatal post-mortem examination. J. Clin Pathol 40: 180–184

Pryse-Davies J (1981) The perinatal autopsy. In: Anthony PP, MacSween RNM (eds) Recent advances in histopathology. Churchill Livingstone, Edinburgh, pp 65–82

Pryse-Davies J, Hurley R (1979) Infections and perinatal mortality. J Antimicrob Chemother 5 (Suppl A): 59–70

Pryse-Davies J, Smitham JH, Napier KA (1974) Factors influencing development of secondary ossification centres in the fetus and newborn. Arch Dis Child 49: 425–431

Rushton DI (1981) Examination of products of conception from previable human pregnancies. J Clin Pathol 34: 819–835

Rushton DI (1982) Resource implications of examination of the placenta. In: Organisation of perinatal pathology services. Harrogate seminar reports 6. Crown Copyright 1981.

Russell GA, Berry PJ (1986) Approaches to the demonstration of congenital heart disease. J Clin Pathol 39: 503–507

Russell JGB (1981) Radiological assessment of age, retardation and death. In: Barson AJ (ed) Laboratory investigation of fetal disease. Wright, Bristol, pp 3–16

Streeter GL (1921) Weight, sitting height, head size, foot length, and menstrual age of the human embryo. Contrib Embryol Carnegie Inst 55: 143–170

Sutherland GR, Carter RF (1983) Cytogenetic studies: an essential part of the paediatric necropsy. J Clin Pathol 36: 140–142

Valdes-Dapena M, Huff DS (1983) Perinatal autopsy manual. Armed Forces Institute of Pathology, Washington DC

Wigglesworth JS (ed) (1984) Performance of the perinatal autopsy. In: Perinatal pathology. Saunders, Philadelphia, pp 48–83

Wigglesworth JS, Husemeyer RP (1977) Intracranial birth trauma in vaginal breech delivery: the continued importance of injury to the occipital bone. Br J Obstet Gynaecol 84: 684–691

Working Party of Obstetricians and Paediatricians in Europe (1970) Report of working party to discuss nomenclature based on gestational age and birth weight. Arch Dis Child 45: 730

Yagel S, Adoni A, Oman S, Wax Y, Hochner-Celnikier D (1986) A statistical examination of the accuracy of combining femoral length and biparietal diameter as an index of fetal gestational age. Br J Obstet Gynaecol 93: 109–115

Yates PO (1959) Birth trauma to the vertebral arteries. Arch Dis Child 34: 436–441

Yudkin PL, Aboualfa M, Eyre JA, Redman CWG, Wilkinson AR (1987) The influence of elective preterm delivery on birthweight and head circumference standards. Arch Dis Child 62: 24–29

Zaaijman J du T, Wilkinson AR, Keeling JW, Mitchell RG, Turnbull AC (1982) Spontaneous premature rupture of the membranes: bacteriology, histology and neonatal outcome. J Obstet Gynaecol 2: 155–160

Chapter 2

Placenta and Umbilical Cord and the Immunology of Pregnancy

T. Yee Khong

Introduction

The placenta and extraplacental membranes are an apposition of fetal and maternal tissues for the purposes of physiological exchange. The gestation sac has a finite lifespan and is the body's largest biopsy, yet its examination is often neglected, even from fetal and neonatal deaths, sick and premature neonates and maternal complications of pregnancy. This is perplexing because its function is embodied in its definition. It may be that placental pathology is considered complex since the organ is evolving rapidly over a short period of time, or that lesions found may be quantitative rather than qualitative. The response of the placenta to injury is limited and there is a need to correlate the macroscopic and microscopic findings with clinical and laboratory investigations.

The introduction of non-invasive techniques to investigate fetal wellbeing early in pregnancy, including prenatal diagnosis, has made it important for the pathologist to be familiar with the development and structure of the placenta through all stages of pregnancy. This is necessary also to validate newer techniques such as Doppler ultrasound assessment of fetal, umbilical and maternal vessels.

Development of the Placenta

Embryology of Early Development

Fertilisation of the ovum usually occurs in the ampullary region of the fallopian tube and results in the restoration of the diploid number of chromosomes. Cleavage begins at once and by three days after fertilisation a cluster of 12 cells, called a morula, is formed. This is the state in which the fertilised ovum enters the uterine cavity, the endometrium being in a luteal phase. Fluid then accumulates within the morula and trophoblast differentiation results in the formation of the blastocyst which begins to attach to the uterine mucosa about 6 days following fertilisation.

During the second week the outer layer of the blastocyst proliferates to form the trophoblastic or chorionic shell while the inner layer differentiates into a bilaminar embryonic disc, which then separates from the trophoblastic layer by the formation of a cavity that ultimately becomes the amniotic space. The primitive trophoblast differentiates into an inner layer composed of mononuclear cells known as the cytotrophoblast and an outer layer consisting of multinucleated cells known as the syncytio-

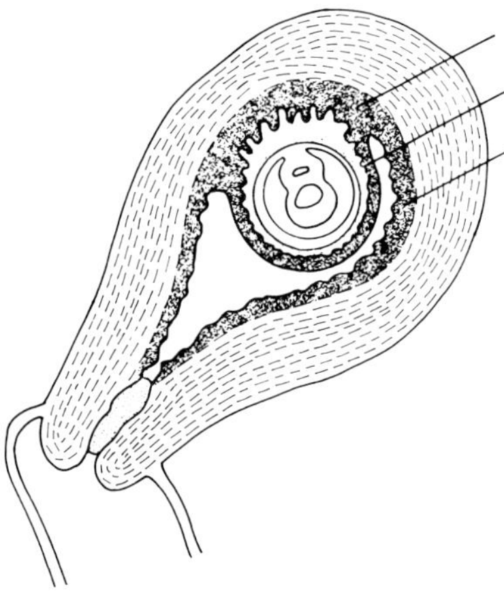

Fig. 2.1. Development of the decidua in early pregnancy.

trophoblast. Intercommunicating fluid-filled spaces appear in the rapidly enlarging trophoblastic mass from the 8th day. These coalesce to form a lacunar system which opens into maternal sinusoids, presumably derived from endometrial capillaries. With the involvement of more capillaries and, later, venous sinusoids the lacunae fill with maternal blood and endometrial glandular secretions to form a primitive intervillous space.

Invasion of the endometrium which began on the 7th day after fertilisation is completed by the 12th day. The initial site of implantation is covered by a plug of blood clot and cellular debris but by the 12th day the endometrial epithelium is reconstituted resulting in an interstitial implantation. The endometrial stromal cells around the conceptus enlarge and accumulate glycogen and lipid. The vascular and glandular changes in the endometrium together with the stromal cellular changes are known as the decidual reaction and soon spread to involve the entire endometrium. Until the 4th month of gestation three regions of the decidua are identified according to their relation to the implantation site. The decidua basalis is the part underlying the conceptus while the decidua capsularis is the superficial portion of the decidua overlying the conceptus. The remainder of the uterine cavity is lined by the decidua parietalis or decidua vera which ultimately fuses with the decidua capsularis at about the 4th month of gestation, thus obliterating the uterine cavity (Fig. 2.1).

The last two days of the second week are characterised by the appearance of chorionic villi. The lacunae are incompletely separated from each other by columns of syncytiotrophoblast. Although the system is labyrinthine rather than villous and none of the trabeculae have free ends, nevertheless they are called primary villous stems. They possess a central core of cells derived from proliferation of cytotrophoblast at the chorionic base. With continuing development and expansion of the implantation site the primary villous stems increase in length and their cytotrophoblastic cells extend distally toward the attachment of the syncytium to the endometrium (Fig. 2.2).

During the third week after fertilisation the bilaminar disc is converted into a trilaminar embryo composed of three definitive germ cell layers. It also includes the development of the primitive streak, notochord and somites. The primary villi develop mesenchymal cores, converting them into secondary villi. These branch and cover the entire surface of the chorionic shell. Differentiation of the mesenchymal cells into vascular capillaries converts the villi into tertiary villi. These villous vessels soon become connected with the embryonic heart via vessels that differentiate in the mesenchyme of the chorion and connecting stalk. By the end of the 3rd week, completion of the development of arteriocapillary–venous network within the villi and contraction of the embryonic heart result in a true embryonic and villous circulation. Nutrients are absorbed from maternal blood in the intervillous space and products from the fetus are excreted back across the villi into the intervillous space (Fig. 2.2).

Concurrent with the development of the secondary and tertiary villi, cytotrophoblastic cells derived from the tips of the villi break through the syncytiotrophoblastic layer and expand laterally to meet and fuse with adjacent columns to form a cytotrophoblastic shell that completely surrounds the conceptus. Thus, the primitive syncytium is split into an inner layer, the definitive syncytium, and an outer layer separating the cytotrophoblastic shell from the decidua. The outer layer eventually degenerates, being replaced by fibrinoid material known as Nitabuch's layer.

Development of the Definitive Form

During the 4th to 8th weeks the embryo develops limbs and all internal organs are formed. By the end of the 16th week the external genitalia are well defined and ossification has commenced. During this period the placenta attains its definitive form and thereafter undergoes no

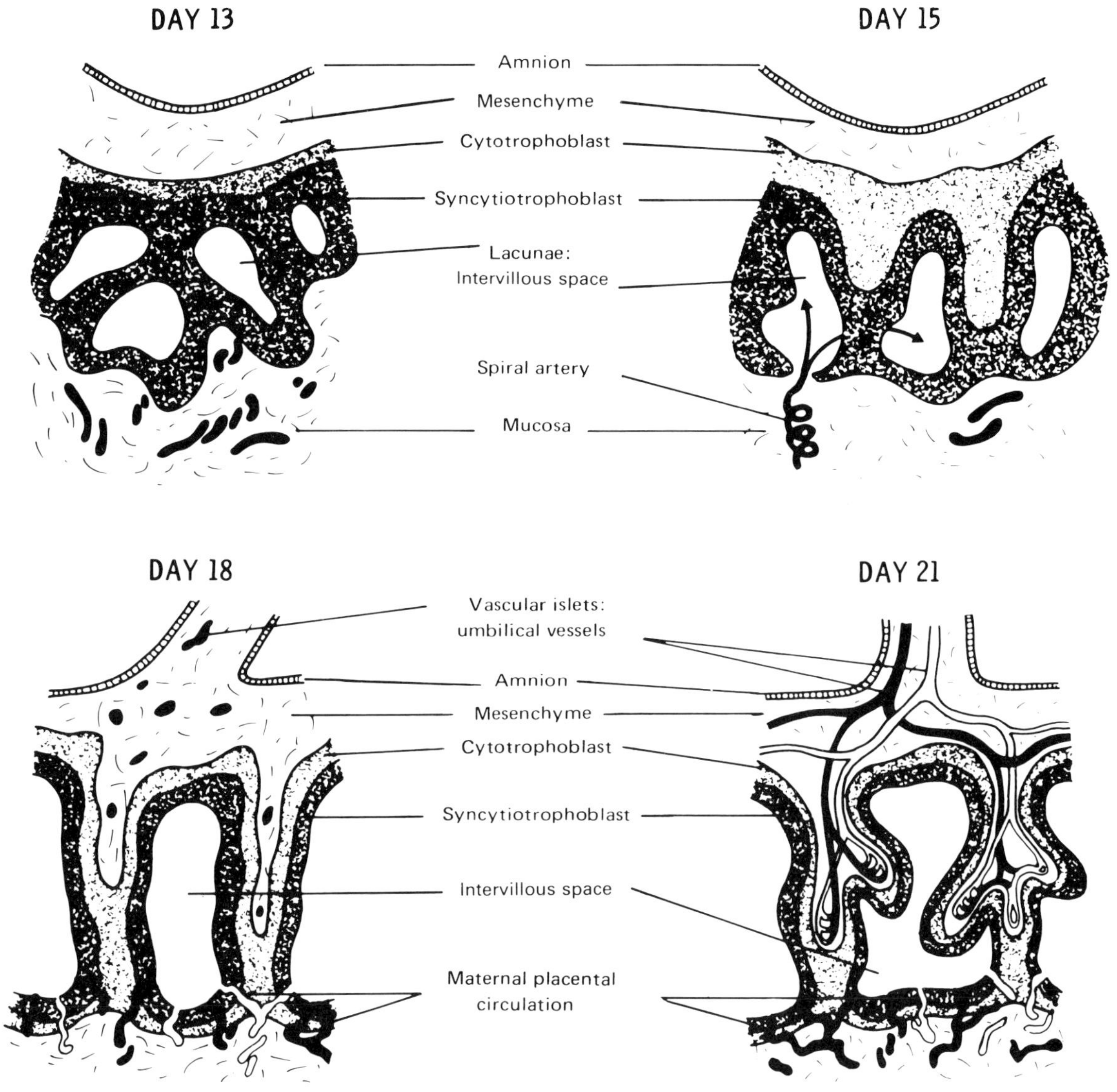

Fig. 2.2. Development of the chorionic villous tree from day 13 to day 21 (after Tuchmann-Duplessis et al. 1971).

further major modifications. Establishment of the cytotrophoblastic shell results in a rapid circumferential extension of the implantation site. The intervillous space expands and the primary stem villi now branch. Like their predecessors, these branches initially consist of syncytiotrophoblast but are rapidly invaded by cytotrophoblast, mesenchymal core and fetal vessels.

Initially the entire chorion is villous but differential growth results in the formation of the definitive placenta. The villi on the side of the chorion toward the decidua basalis continue to proliferate to form the chorion frondosum, which becomes the definitive placental parenchyma. The villi of the decidua capsularis regress leaving a smooth relatively avascular area known as the chorion laeve. The regression of these villi is accompanied by the loss of associated intervillous space in this area. As the conceptus enlarges, the chorion laeve bulges into the uterine cavity to fuse with the decidua parietalis thus obliterating the uterine cavity.

During this period there is some regression of the cytotrophoblastic elements in the cytotrophoblastic shell and chorionic plate but remnants of cells are found in the former location to form the cytotrophoblastic cell islands in the layer of Nitabuch. Cytotrophoblast derived from these remnants in the cytotrophoblastic shell and from tips of anchoring villi continue to migrate into the decidua basalis and myometrium to play a key role in the development of the uteroplacental circulation (see below).

The chorion frondosum continues to grow rapidly. Placental septa first appear in the 3rd month of gestation. It is now generally accepted that the septa are formed partly as a result of differential growth of villi relating to a given stem villus with compression of decidua in the regions where villous growth is more vigorous, and partly by the pulling up of the basal plate into the intervillous space by relative diminished growth of some anchoring villi. The septa are formed of variable amounts of maternal and fetal tissue making up the basal plate and have no functional significance. These septa partially divide the placenta into 15 to 20 lobes.

By the end of the 4th month of pregnancy the placenta has attained its definitive form. Growth continues by further arborisation of the stem villi and production of new villi. The proportion and size of the fetal components of the placenta increase as gestation proceeds. There is continuous growth until term although the rate of increase gradually decreases from approximately 34 to 36 weeks' gestation; this has been confirmed by ultrasound determination of placental volume (Bleker et al. 1977; Geirsson et al. 1985). Morphometric studies indicate that the villous surface area continues to increase till term (Teasdale 1980; Boyd 1984) while the quantity of DNA as an indicator of nuclear (not cell) number in the placenta continues to rise linearly until term (Sands and Dobbing 1985) thus dispelling the concept of placental senescence.

Mature Placenta

Macroscopically the placenta shows wide variation in shape, size and weight. The fetal surface is normally shiny and bluish. The most superficial layer is the amnion through which large vessels running to the umbilical cord insertion are seen. Arteries and veins may be distinguished as arteries lie superficial to the veins. A small white plaque is commonly seen beneath the amnion surface; this is the yolk sac remnant and is of no clinical significance although the presence of two in a singleton placenta may alert one to the possibility of a vanishing twin syndrome. Insertion of the umbilical cord is variable. The chorionic plate lies beneath the amnion. Subchorionic fibrin deposition is variable and may obscure the subchorial lake. Blood vessels course perpendicularly through the chorionic plate towards the decidua. Beneath the chorionic plate lie chorionic villi and the intervillous space.

Calcium deposition is commonly seen near term and is usually at or near the maternal surface, within old infarcts, septa and subchorionic fibrin plaques. Remnants of the maternal decidua may be adherent to the basal plate. The basal plate forms the floor of the placenta. Extraplacental membranes extend from the lateral margin of the placenta and form, in utero, a closed cavity containing the fetus and approximately 500 ml of amniotic fluid.

Villous Structure: Vasculature and Histology

Wilkin (1965) believes that each primary stem villus gives off several secondary stem villi, each of which forms a lobule by division into tertiary stem villi which are arranged in a circular manner running towards the basal plate and leaving a central, relatively villus-free area in the centre of the lobule. The tertiary stem villi turn back from the basal plate and break up into terminal villi (Fig. 2.3).

Kaufmann (1982) proposed the intermediate villus as an additional type to the stem and terminal villi. The stem villi, responsible for the mechanical stability of the villous tree, are defined on the basis of containing blood vessels with media and detailed studies have shown that these ramify further peripherally than originally thought. Branches arising from these stem villi are either smaller stem villi or intermediate villi. Intermediate villi are defined on the basis of a reticular stroma with vessels lacking media and are located between the stem and terminal villi. Two types of intermediate villi are distinguished: the mature intermediate villus, seen in the mature placenta, which is slender and bears a large number of terminal villi, and the immature intermediate villus, which is thicker and with fewer terminal villi arising from its surface. The immature intermediate villus corresponds to the immature villus that was thought to be a not yet fully developed terminal villus. In the schema of

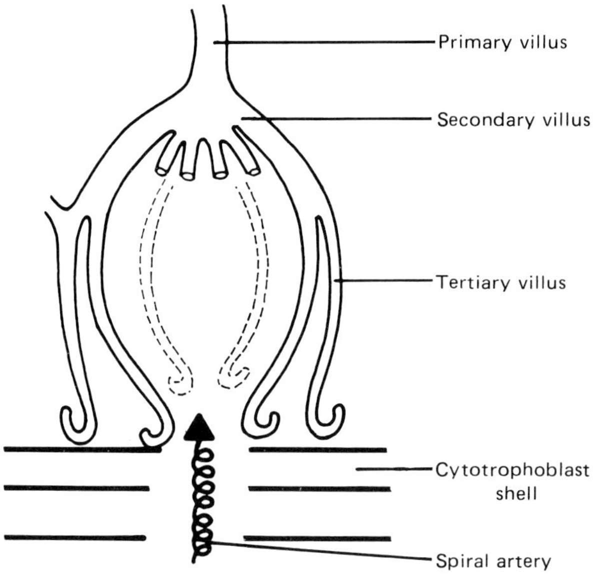

Fig. 2.3. Structure of a placental lobule.

this classification, as pregnancy progresses, the number of immature intermediate villi is reduced with only a few persisting to term, tending to be in the centres of functional placental circulatory units (Schuhmann and Wynn 1980), to act as growth centres and the growth of the placenta slows down accordingly.

The terminal villi are the sites for maternofetal and fetomaternal exchanges and are the final branchings of the villous tree. In early pregnancy the villi are relatively few and large (approximately 170 μm in diameter). There is a regular double layer of trophoblast, the outer syncytiotrophoblast and inner cytotrophoblast (Langhans' layer) enclosing a loose stroma. At this stage fetal capillaries are small and centrally placed. The villous core also contains stellate mesenchymal and Hofbauer cells, the latter acting as fetal macrophages. As pregnancy and placental growth proceed new terminal villi form by the development of trophoblastic sprouts which are then invaded by stroma and fetal capillaries. Those sprouts that do not form villi tend to become pedunculated and break off to be deported and lodge in the maternal pulmonary vasculature.

As pregnancy proceeds, terminal villi become more numerous and smaller (average diameter of 70 μm and 40 μm in second and third trimesters respectively). The cytotrophoblast becomes less numerous and has largely disappeared by term although its regenerative potential remains. The syncytiotrophoblastic layer becomes gradually thinner and fetal capillaries occupy an increasing proportion of the cross-sectional area of the villus and move more peripherally to eccentric positions beneath the syncytiotrophoblast (Fig. 2.4). In some areas the fetal capillaries appear to fuse with the overlying attenuated syncytiotrophoblast to form vasculosyncytial membranes that are believed to be the optimal area for gaseous exchange (Fig. 2.5). While the vascularity of the villus increases the villous stroma becomes increasingly condensed and Hofbauer cells, though present at term, may be difficult to visualise because of compression by vessels and stromal tissue.

Syncytial knots formed by the sequestration of nuclei of the syncytiotrophoblast increase in number in the last two months of gestation. They may bulge into the intervillous space where they meet similar knots from adjacent villi to form an intervillous bridge. Towards the end of pregnancy fibrinoid is deposited increasingly on the surface of the villi.

Electron Microscopy

The villous cytotrophoblast is relatively simple at the ultrastructural level, with few cytoplasmic organelles. It has a large nucleus with prominent nucleolus, and the cytoplasm contains large mitochondria, a few well-developed Golgi bodies and abundant free ribosomes. This ultrastructure is appropriate for its role in growth and differentiation. Syncytiotrophoblast is electron-dense with many organelles related to its role in steroid and protein synthesis and transport. It contains abundant dilated rough endoplasmic reticulum, pinocytotic vacuoles, free ribosomes and numerous glycogen granules. Well-developed Golgi apparatus and mitochondria are present. The surface has a microvillus border associated with pinocytotic vesicles and vacuoles. Scanning electron microscopy has revealed large numbers of densely packed microvilli in the first trimester. As pregnancy proceeds they become less dense, blunter and variable in size and focally absent. They are reduced in number over vasculosyncytial membranes.

Morphometry

Morphometry allows macroscopic and microscopic appearances to be quantified (Aherne and

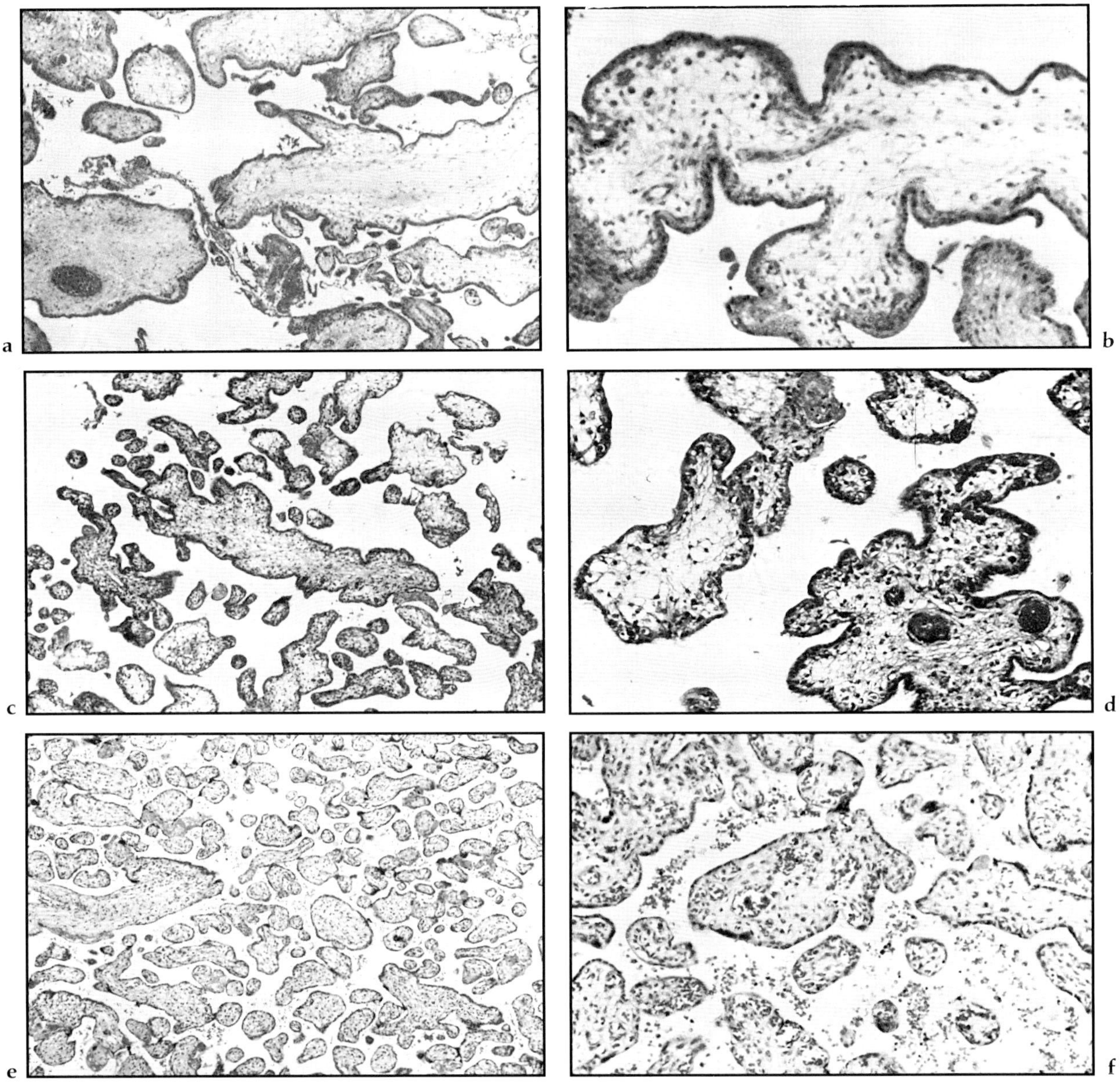

Fig. 2.4a–f. Placental villi at different stages of gestation from uncomplicated pregnancies. **a,b** 10 weeks: inner layer of cytotrophoblast and syncytiotrophoblast are apparent; blood vessels are inconspicuous and Hofbauer cells are present in the loose mesenchymal core. **c,d** 24 weeks: villi are more numerous and the vessels more centrally situated. **e,f** 32 weeks: numerous villi which are well vascularised with thinning of syncytiotrophoblast and inconspicuous cytotrophoblast.

Dunnill 1982). Whilst measurements on the fixed delivered placenta may not relate directly to the organ in vivo, they provide useful information for comparative analysis during ontogeny and in normal and abnormal pregnancies (Boyd 1984; Boyd and Scott 1985; Boyd et al. 1980, 1986). The latter is of particular utility as the pathological abnormality may be quantitative rather than qualitative. Mayhew and Burton (1988) have laid out requirements for meaningful morphometric studies in placentas based on standardised sampling and preparative steps. They stressed that the extant data on abnormal pregnancies are not comparable from centre to centre because of different sampling and preparative methods. The main criticism is that many investigators have relied on immersion fixation of the placenta

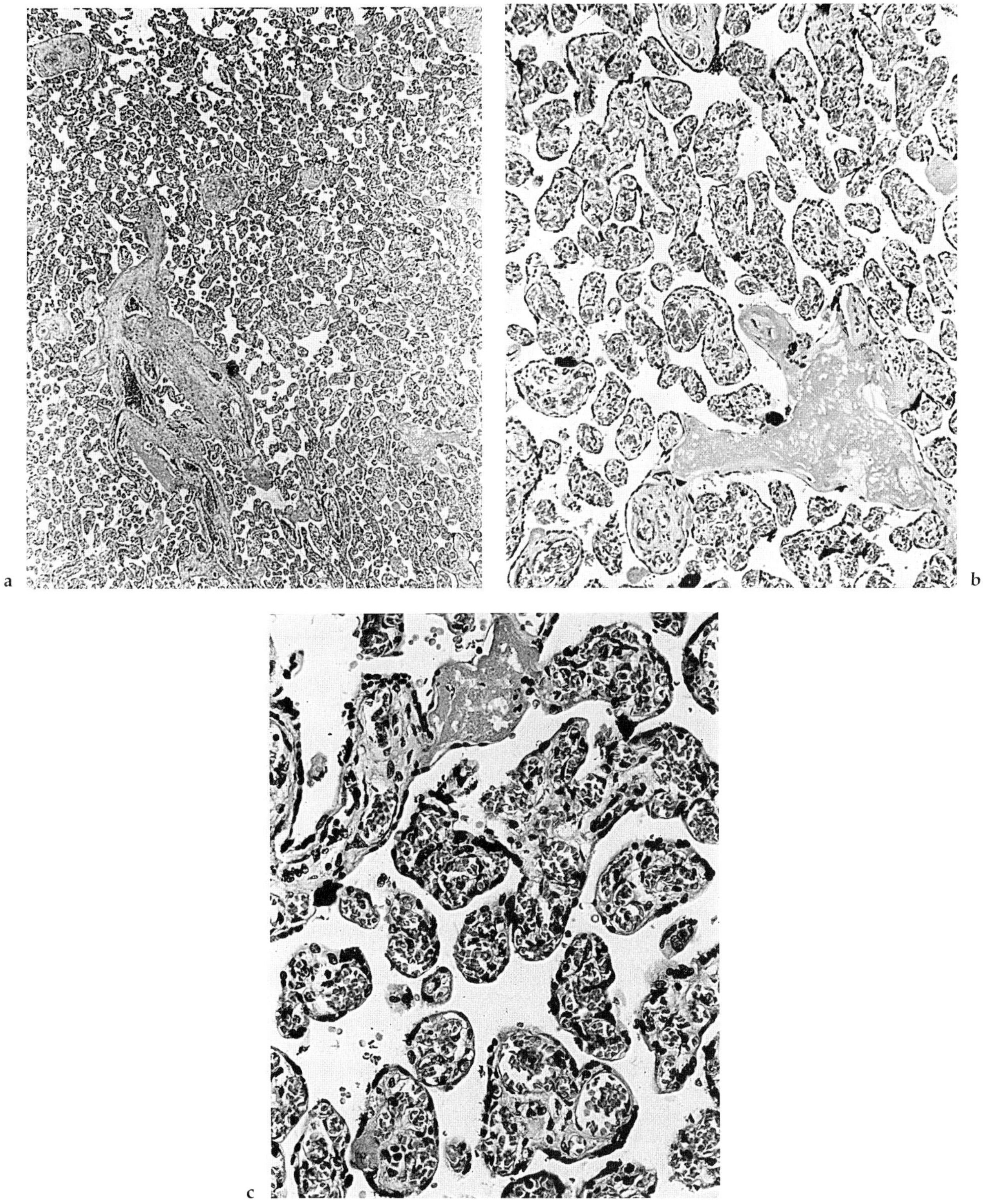

Fig. 2.5. Mature placenta. **a** At low power, well-vascularised small villi crowd round a stem villus. **b** At higher magnification, villous vessels are prominent. Syncytial knots are present in the trophoblast and fibrin is present in the intervillous space. **c** Many vasculosyncytial membranes are present.

while they advocate perfusion fixation, ideally dual-perfusion fixation, of the placenta for any morphometric study.

In general, however, the villous surface area seems to be significantly lower in placentas from women with severe pre-eclampsia or with small-for-gestational age infants uncomplicated by hypertensive diseases. A larger surface area was found in those with diabetes mellitus.

Development of the Membranes

By the 8th day following fertilisation a slit-like cavity destined to be the amniotic cavity, is formed superior to the bilaminar embryonic disc while inferior, a cavity that initially is the blastocyst cavity and later the primitive yolk sac cavity is formed. With formation of the extraembryonic coelom, the primitive yolk sac decreases in size and a secondary yolk sac develops. These sacs are surrounded by the developing extraembryonic coelom, extraembryonic mesoderm and trophoblast. The embryo, amnion and yolk sac suspended by the connecting stalk are thus contained within the chorionic sac. As the amniotic sac enlarges it obliterates the chorionic cavity and adheres to the chorion, covers the umbilical cord and displaces the receding yolk sac to the base of the umbilical cord, this process being completed by 12 weeks' gestation.

The amnion is multilayered with a cuboidal epithelium lying on a well-defined basement membrane, deep to which are the compact, fibroblast and spongy layers. The compact layer is relatively resistant to leucocyte infiltration and confers the strength of the amnion while the fibroblast layer permits distensibility. The spongy layer consists of collagen fibres, mucus, fibroblasts and macrophages. The chorion is also multilayered comprising cellular and reticular layers, pseudomembrane and trophoblast. Although the cytotrophoblastic cells in the chorion laeve do not appear to have marked secretory activity, there is increased rough endoplasmic reticulum suggesting continued functional capacity (Ho et al. 1982) The amnion and chorion grow till approximately 28 weeks' gestation after when mitotic activity is rare. Subsequent enlargement of the chorioamniotic sac takes place by stretching.

Development of the Umbilical Cord

At the beginning of fetal development there are two stalks: the yolk sac stalk containing the vitelline duct and vitelline vessels and the connecting stalk containing the allantois and umbilical vessels. These two stalks fuse to form the umbilical cord. The umbilical cord is covered by amnion that is continuous with the outer layer of the embryo. The blood vessels in the allantois become the umbilical vein and arteries and are supported by Wharton's jelly. Anastomoses between the arteries often occur close to the placenta and occasionally the arteries fuse.

Development of the Uteroplacental Circulation

The early involvement of the subepithelial capillaries and, later, the arterioles and veins in the lacunar and early intervillous stages of development of the placenta has been described. Concurrent with the formation and development of the placenta, there is an invasion of maternal decidua basalis and subjacent myometrium by trophoblast proliferating from the cytotrophoblastic shell and, later, from the tips of anchoring villi. There are two types of placental bed extravillous cytotrophoblast: interstitial and endovascular trophoblast.

Interstitial trophoblast tends to be concentrated around spiral arteries at both the decidual and myometrial levels and its migration continues for the first 6 months of pregnancy although invasion of the myometrium is probably most prolific during the first 18 weeks of gestation (Pijnenborg et al. 1981). There is a relative absence of mononuclear cytotrophoblast in the myometrium at term, suggesting that many such cells have either disappeared or the majority have been transformed into characteristic syncytial placental bed giant cells by symplasmic fusion, leading the unwary to the erroneous diagnosis of "syncytial endometritis".

Cytotrophoblastic migration into the spiral arteries appears to occur in two waves, the first wave from about 6 weeks to about 12 weeks' gestation and the second wave from about 16 to 22–24 weeks' gestation. Spatially the first wave affects predominantly decidual segments while the second wave of trophoblastic migration colonises the myometrial segments of the spiral arteries. The endovascular trophoblast penetrates the vessel wall through the endothelial lining, disrupting the intima, internal elastic lamina and much of the muscular media, the process being accompanied by the deposition of fibrinoid material. These extensive structural alterations in the walls of invaded arteries result in their conversion to uteroplacental arteries and as these changes are obviously adaptations to pregnancy, the term physiological changes was used to describe them. While the veins draining the intervillous space must be opened up, presumably by trophoblast, intravascular trophoblast migration has not been seen in decidual veins.

In the final stages of transformation of the spiral arteries into fully developed uteroplacental arteries the trophoblastic cells become entirely incorporated into the wall of the vessel and there is no longer direct contact with intraluminal trophoblast, the endothelial lining being reconstituted. During the third trimester the affected vessels undergo progressive distension resulting in a series of dilated, funnel-shaped, tortuous vessels opening into the intervillous space (Fig. 2.6). It is assumed that the fully developed uteroplacental arteries lose their ability to respond to vasomotor influences because of the loss of their musculoelastic tissue and probably their autonomic nerve supply. There is certainly a significant drop in peripheral resistance at the opening of the uteroplacental arteries into the intervillous space allowing greater conductance and, hence, an increased blood flow at a low pulse pressure into and through the intervillous space. In this way the tenfold increase in blood supply required by the fetoplacental unit in the third trimester can be accommodated.

Multiple Pregnancy

Placentation in multiple pregnancy is reviewed at length by Benirschke and Driscoll (1967), Strong and Corney (1967), Boyd and Hamilton (1970) and MacGillivray et al. (1975). Geographical differences in the incidence of twinning are noted (Strong and Corney 1967). The incidence of multiple pregnancy is increased by the use of fertility drugs and by in vitro fertilisation involving multiple embryo transfer.

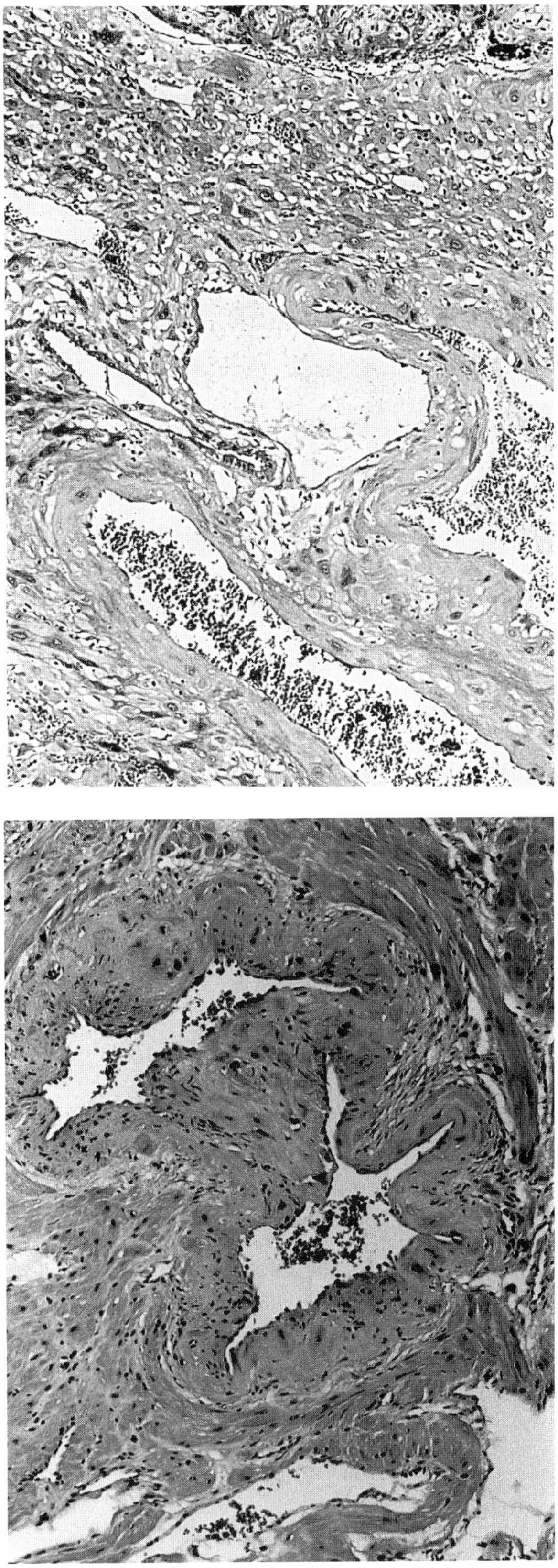
a

b

Fig. 2.6a,b. Uteroplacental artery in **a** the basal plate and **b** in the decidua–myometrial junction at term. **b** reproduced from Khong et al. 1986.

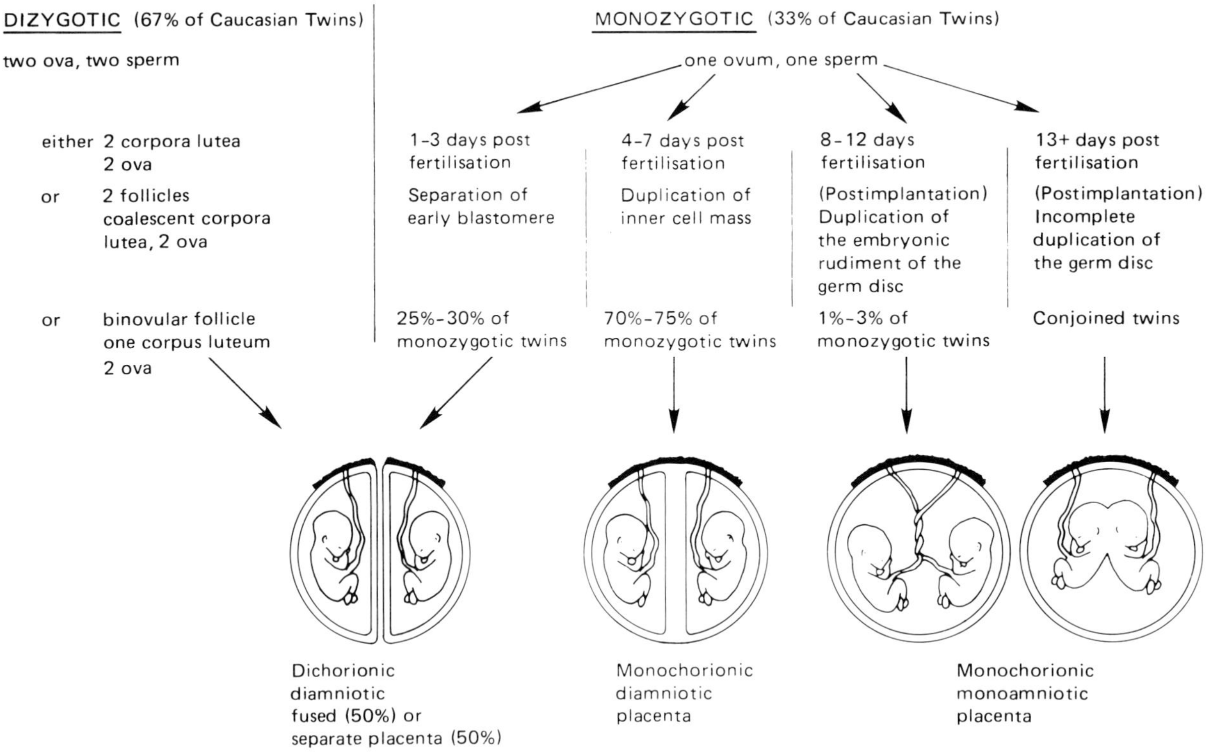

Fig. 2.7. Twinning mechanisms and placentation.

The incidence of twin conceptions is higher than that of twin births (Bryan 1986). Ultrasound examination early in pregnancy not uncommonly identifies two fetuses; however, death of one twin may ensue, with complete or partial resolution (fetus papyraceous).

Monozygotic Twins

Monozygotic twins arise when one fertilised ovum subsequently divides, the type of placentation produced being related to the timing of the division of the embryo in relation to development of the amniotic cavity (Fig. 2.7).

Monozygotic diamniotic twins have a much higher perinatal mortality than dichorionic twins. This is in part related to the twin transfusion syndrome. Vascular anastomoses between the circulations of both fetuses are present in monochorionic diamniotic placentas but are less common in monochorionic monoamniotic placentas (Wharton et al. 1968). Anastomoses may be superficial, occurring in the large vessels between the placental membranes, or deep, occurring within the placental parenchyma. The methods that may be employed to demonstrate vascular anastomoses are discussed by Strong and Corney (1967). Injection of milk or coloured saline can be used for the routine demonstration of anastomoses.

Although anastomoses between the two circulations are very common, uncompensated transfusion between the circulations is a much less frequent occurrence. A difference in cord haemoglobin of greater than 5 g% or a birthweight difference greater than 20% is required for diagnosis. In evaluating these criteria, Danskin and Neilson (1989) emphasised the need to interpret them in the light of knowledge of placental morphology and whether the heavier or lighter twin had the higher haemoglobin as it was possible that some cases could represent growth retardation in association with polycythaemia. Uncompensated twin–twin transfusions may be acute or chronic. One twin is usually pale while the other is plethoric and polycythaemic. If transfusion is chronic then there may be large differences between the size and weight of the infants. Changes in the placenta are observed; the part supplying the anaemic donor twin will be pale and that associated with the recipient will be very congested. The relative size of the two parts is related to the chronicity of transfusion. When the donor twin is hydropic, that part of the placenta is likely to be unduly large (Fig. 2.8).

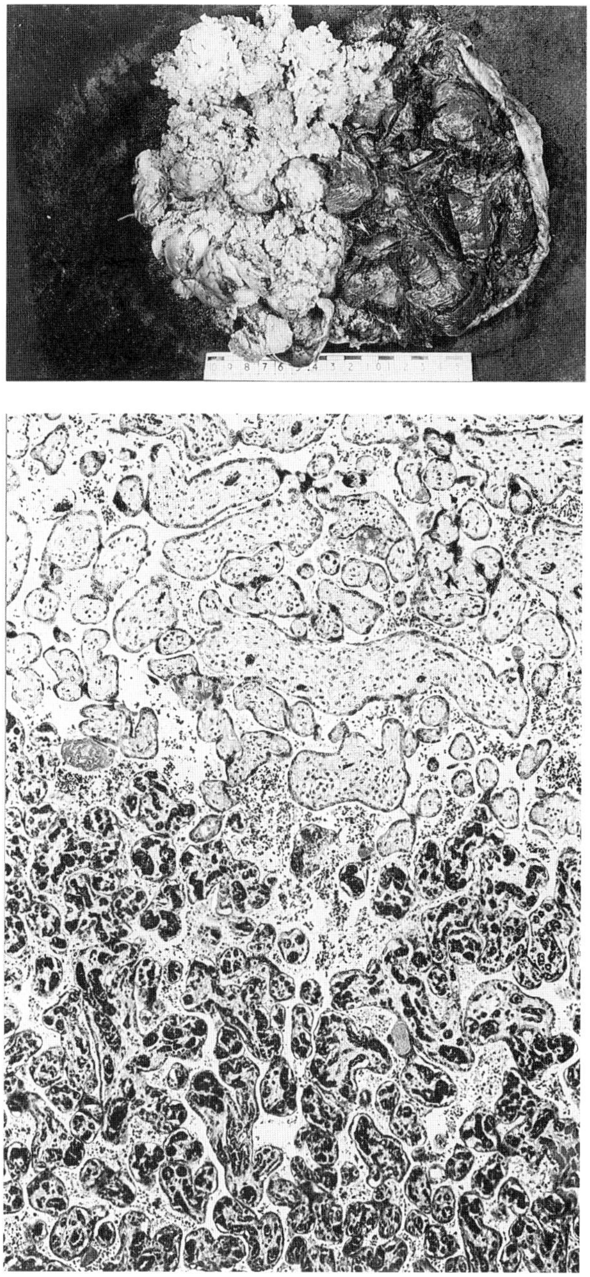

a b

Fig. 2.8a,b. Twin–twin transfusion syndrome: plethoric donor half (right) and pale recipient hydropic half (left).

Monoamniotic twins have an even higher fetal and neonatal mortality than monochorionic diamniotic twins. Mortalities of between 30% and 50% have been described (Benirschke and Driscoll 1967; Wharton et al. 1968). These are due to a combination of cord entanglement, inequality of functional division of the placenta, mechanical difficulties during delivery and a high incidence of malformation, particularly anencephaly, holoprosencephaly sequence and sirenomelia (Jones 1988).

Triplets and Higher Multiple Births

Detailed discussion of triplets and higher multiple births is given by Boyd and Hamilton (1970) and MacGillivray et al. (1975). Triplet pregnancies may be trizygotic, resulting from fertilisation of three ova, or dizygotic, resulting from fertilisation of two ova, followed by replication of one, or monozygotic, resulting from fertilisation of a single ovum, which undergoes replication, followed by a further division of one of the zygotes. It follows that in higher multiple births, zygosity may necessarily be more complex.

Examination of the Placenta in Multiple Pregnancy

The zygosity of twins may not necessarily be determined from examination of the placenta. If twins are of different sex then they are dizygotic. Twins with monochorionic placentation are monozygotic. Monochorionic diamniotic and dichorionic diamniotic placentas may be distinguished from each other by examination of the membranes. The septum between the two amniotic cavities is usually transparent in the former and relatively more opaque and thicker in the latter. Histologically, chorionic tissue is absent from monochorionic placentas whereas it is present in dichorionic placentas. Unless the twins are differently sexed when dizygosity is assured, the dichorionic diamniotic placenta may derive from monozygous or dizygous fertilisation.

When twins are same-sexed and information about placentation is either lacking or confirms dichorionicity, then examination of red cell antigens, enzymes and genetic markers will be required to establish zygosity if this is deemed essential, for example if an inherited disorder is observed in one of the infants. Unequivocal determination of zygosity is now possible using highly polymorphic minisatellite DNA.

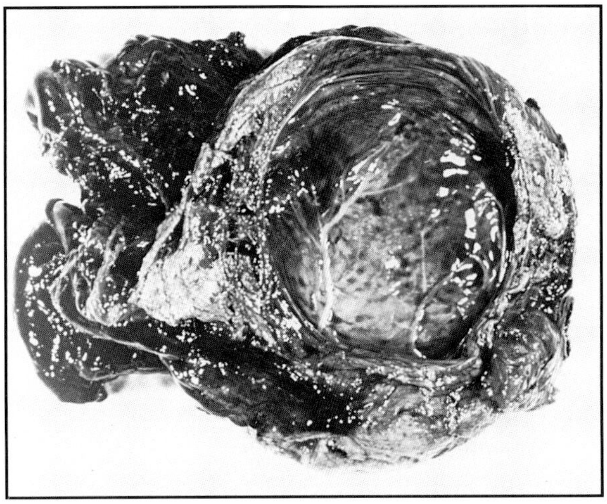

Fig. 2.9. Fetal aspect of complete circumvallate placenta. Thrombus is adherent to the margin of the placental disc.

Abnormalities in Development and Placentation

There is wide variation in placental shape with no effect on the outcome of pregnancy. Accessory lobes occur in 3%–8% of pregnancies and are the result of non-involution of chorion laeve in the membranes. They are usually of no clinical significance except when retained in utero after delivery or associated with vessels running a velamentous course and situated near the cervical os when there is danger of vessel rupture during labour and fetal exsanguination. Bilobate placentas are uncommon and are not associated with any effect on perinatal morbidity. Fenestrate placenta with central absence of villous growth is very rare.

Extrachorial placentation is present in 24% of pregnancies (Fox and Sen 1972). In this situation, the chorionic plate from which the villi arise is smaller than the basal plate, i.e. where the transition from villous to non-villous chorion takes place within the circumference of the fetal surface of the placenta (see Fig. 1.33). Where the membranes form a flat ring comprising only amnion and chorion with fibrin, the placenta is classified as circummarginate and this is without clinical significance. Where the transition is raised and contains decidual tissue, ghost villi, functioning villi and blood clot, the placenta is classified as circumvallate (Fig. 2.9). This is associated with low birthweight and a high rate of threatened abortion and premature onset of labour (Fox and Sen 1972). It is not uncommon to find partially circumvallate or circummarginate placentas or a mixture of both. Circumvallate placentas are found more commonly in multigravida.

Placenta praevia occurs when implantation is in the lower uterine segment, lying in advance of the presenting fetal part. This may be total, where the placenta covers the internal os completely; partial, where part of the internal os is covered; or marginal, where the placental edge just reaches the internal os. The incidence of this disorder is approximately 1 in 250 births, the majority occurring in parous women. It is associated with severe antepartum haemorrhage and delivery by caesarean section is required. Placenta praevia is a clinical diagnosis and cannot usually be diagnosed by examination of the placenta although the finding of the site of rupture of the membranes at the placental edge is supportive evidence.

Placenta accreta is rare and occurs when there is direct apposition of placental villi to myometrium which may be complete or partial. It has been argued that many pregnancies necessitating manual removal of placenta represent minor degrees of this condition. Predisposing factors are placenta praevia, previous uterine surgery including curettage and caesarean section and previous manual removal of placenta. It is associated with antepartum haemorrhage, uterine inversion and rupture and post-partum haemorrhage. A missing piece of tissue from the maternal surface may indicate a degree of accreta and, even in fragmented tissues following manual removal of the placenta, the diagnosis may be confirmed histologically by the finding of myometrial fibres pulled up into placental septa (Fig. 2.10) or immediately subjacent to Nitabuch's fibrinoid layer without an intervening layer of decidua basalis (Khong and Robertson 1987).

In placenta membranacea there is persistence of villous growth over the whole surface of the placental membranes. It is very rare (1 in 3300 to 1 in 21 500 deliveries) and said to be associated with low birthweight, recurrent bleeding in the first and second trimesters, often leading to spontaneous abortion or premature labour, retained placenta and post-partum haemorrhage. Good outcome has also been described (Hurley and Beischer 1987).

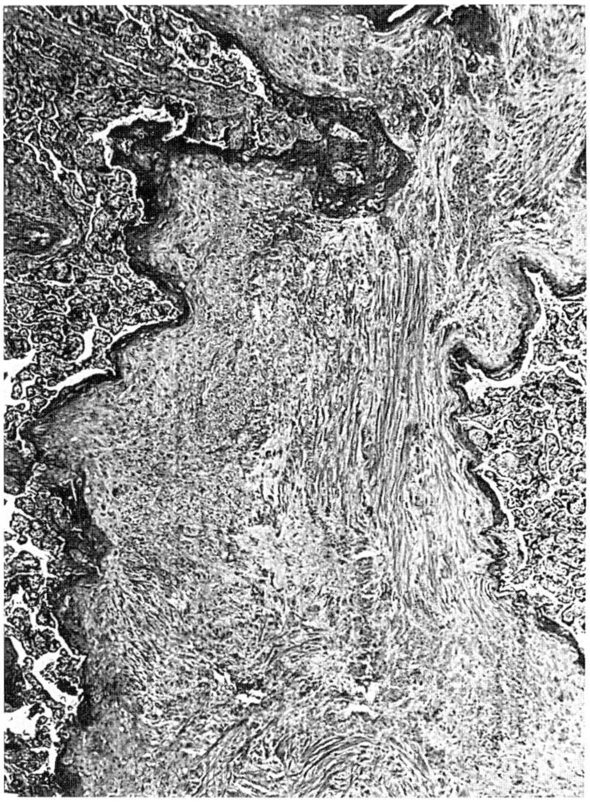

Fig. 2.10. Placenta accreta showing myometrial fibres in placental septum (reproduced from Khong and Robertson 1987).

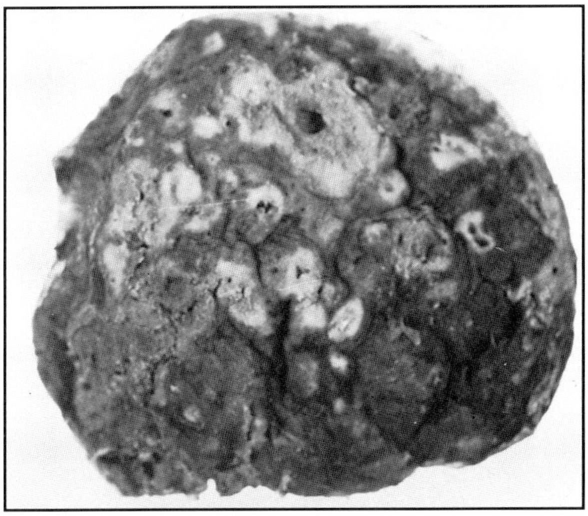

Fig. 2.11. Maternal surface of placenta: many areas of infarction are seen. Aneurysmal dilatation of the maternal arteries entering the centre of the placental lobules is clearly seen in the infarcted areas.

Placental Macroscopic Abnormalities

Many of the pathological abnormalities apparent on naked eye examination of the placenta are related to disturbances in either maternal or fetal circulations. These abnormalities may be difficult to distinguish from each other and may require histological examination for identification.

Infarction

Single small infarcts are common while numerous multiple infarcts occur most commonly in placentas from pre-eclamptic women. Cessation of the fetal circulation following fetal demise is not accompanied by discrete areas of infarction within the placenta. A fresh infarct seen in the cut surface of the placenta is dark red and moderately soft. As the infarct ages it appears brownish then yellow and finally white and firm (Figs. 2.11 and 2.12). The histological appearance of an infarct is characterised by villous crowding, narrowing of the intervillous space, congestion of the fetal vessels and pyknosis of the syncytiotrophoblast nuclei. As the infarct ages, villi undergo necrosis and an old infarct consists of "ghost" villi (Fig. 2.13).

It is generally accepted that infarcts occupying less than 10% of the parenchyma are insignificant. Infarction of a larger proportion of the placenta is associated with a high incidence of intrauterine growth retardation and intrauterine death. Infarction is not the primary cause of fetal problems but an indication of reduced maternal blood supply to the placenta (see below) (Fig. 2.14) and the use of the term "uteroplacental insufficiency" has been advocated (Wigglesworth 1964).

Haematoma – Retroplacental and Marginal

Retroplacental haematomas were described in 4.5% of placentas (Wilkin 1965) and were three times more common in placentas from pre-eclamptic women. The cause of the haemorrhage may be arterial, venous or both. Retroplacental haematomas are often accompanied by adjacent placental infarction and decidual necrosis.

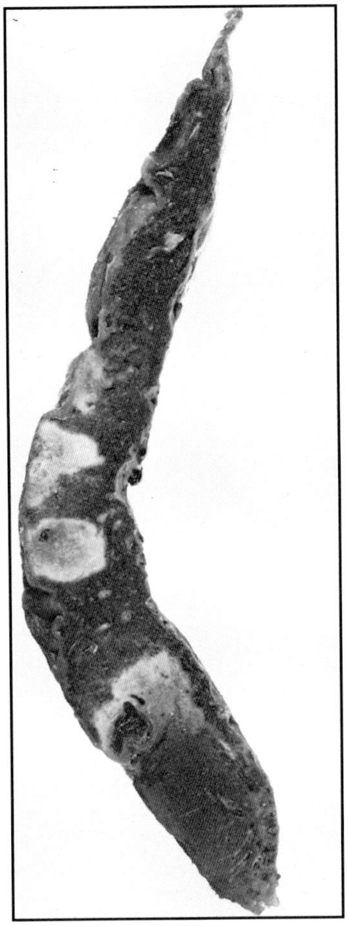

Fig. 2.12. Slice from Fig. 2.11. There is an area of fresh infarction (*bottom*) with older infarcts *centrally*.

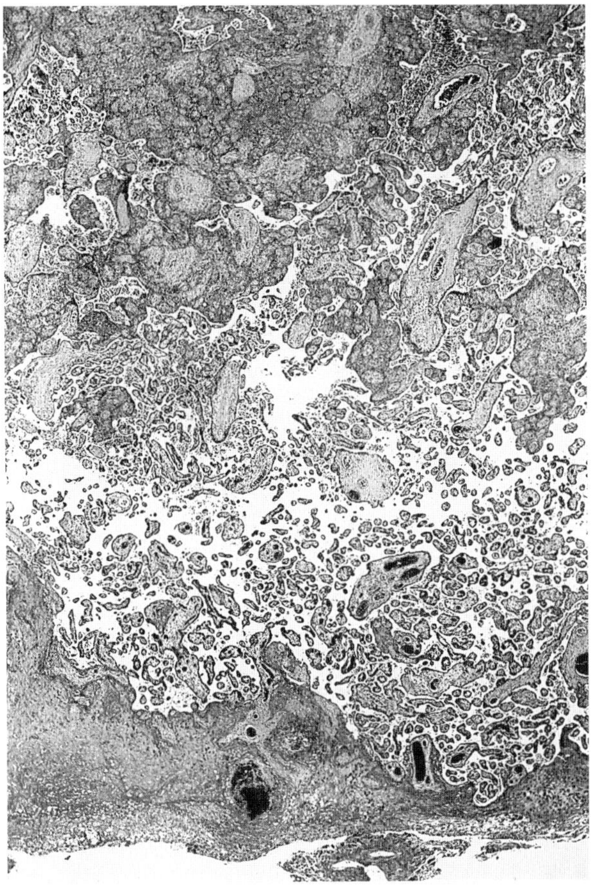

Fig. 2.14. Thrombosis in a maternal vessel in the basal plate with overlying placental infarction.

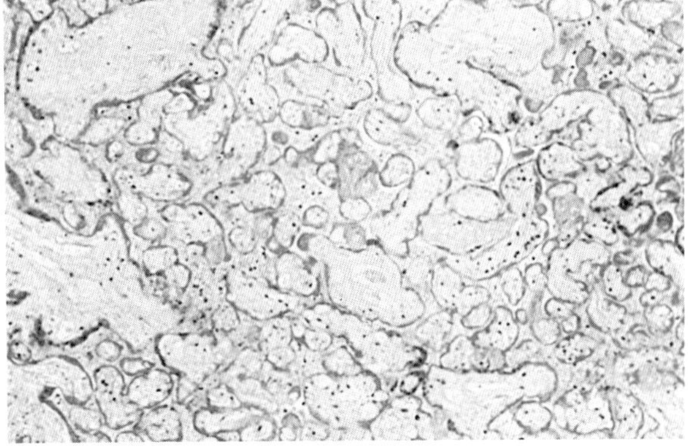

Fig. 2.13. Old placental infarct. The villi are crowded and ghost-like: the trophoblast has undergone necrosis.

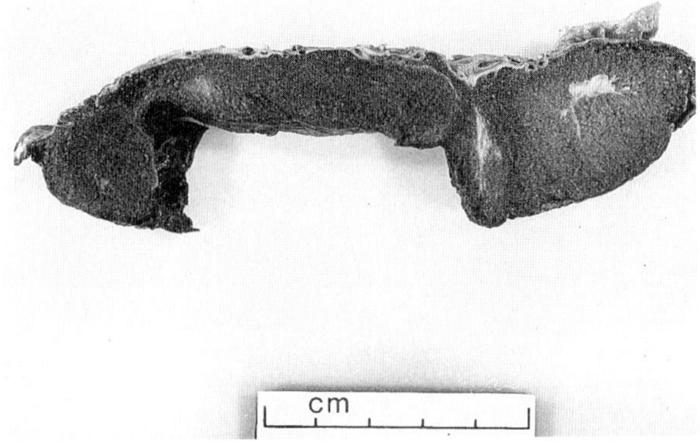

Fig. 2.15. Retroplacental haematoma with excavation of the clot to leave an indented placental parenchyma.

Haematomas vary in size from less than 10 mm, only apparent when the placenta is sliced, to large lesions which may involve much of the maternal surface. On the cut surface of the placenta the haematoma may be seen bulging into placental tissue, compressing it and causing infarction (Fig. 2.15). The clot when newly formed is soft and red in colour and may become separated from the placenta during delivery. Careful inspection of the maternal surface will reveal a depression at the site of haematoma formation, and adherent strands of fibrin give the surface a dull rough appearance. This enables distinction from insignificant blood clot which may be delivered with the placenta but which does not indent the maternal surface. The histological appearance of haematomas is age related. Fresh clots consist entirely of red blood cells. With age, there is increasing fibrin deposition, degeneration of red blood cells and infiltration by polymorphonuclear leucocytes and macrophages.

Peripheral or marginal haematomas form at the lateral margin of the placenta and may spread onto the maternal surface but do not compress it. An association has been noted between premature delivery, premature rupture of the membranes and peripheral placental haemorrhage (Harris et al. 1985).

Intervillous Thrombosis

Thrombi in the intervillous space are more frequent as pregnancy progresses and are seen in 36% of placentas from uncomplicated term pregnancies (Fox 1978). Grossly, they are roughly spherical. As a thrombus ages it changes from soft to firm and from dark-red to brown in colour and eventually becomes a laminated white lesion. Their aetiology is not clear but fetal and maternal cells are seen in thrombi. Their increased frequency near term when fetomaternal haemorrhage is most frequent, suggests that thrombosis may occur at the site of fetomaternal haemorrhage.

Subchorial Thrombosis

Accumulation of blood between the chorionic plate and underlying villous parenchyma protruding into the amniotic cavity may be identified in mid-trimester missed abortions. Slicing shows a mass of red thrombus dissecting the chorionic plate from the underlying villi (Fig. 2.16). The thrombus is maternal in origin and histologically consists of villous-free laminated thrombus. The belief that they occur only after fetal death has been discounted by the finding of similar lesions in liveborn infants (Shanklin and Scott 1975).

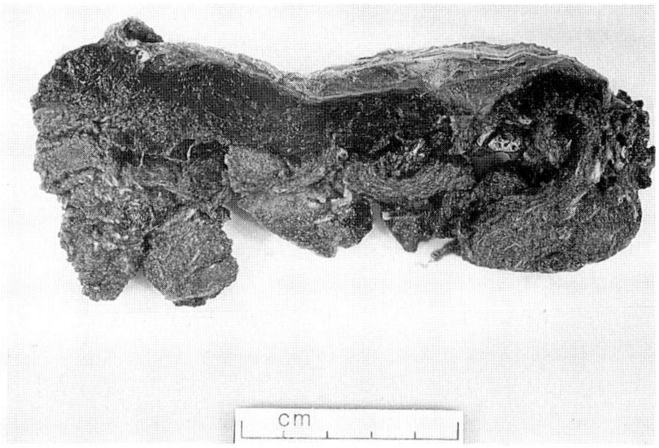

Fig. 2.16. Subchorial thrombosis. Early lamination is evident.

Perivillous Fibrin Deposition

Some deposition of fibrin can be seen around villi on histological examination of all placentas at term and may be associated with some villous atrophy. It is of no clinical significance. Massive perivillous fibrin deposition, sometimes affecting up to 30% of placental parenchyma, can be detected macroscopically as irregular white areas and may be indistinguishable from infarcts. It is thought that turbulence of blood in the intervillous space leads to fibrin deposition. When villi are entrapped they become secondarily infarcted.

Maternal floor infarction is characterised by a thickened layer of perivillous fibrin deposition involving villi at the maternal surface and grossly the furrows of the lobes are lost as the maternal surface becomes encased within fibrin. Thought by some to be a post-mortem artefact because of the strong association with fetal loss (Fox 1978), liveborn outcomes have been described (Clewell and Manchester 1983) suggesting either the lesion occurs late in the disease process or else develops rapidly. The lesion may recur in subsequent pregnancies; this is associated with abortion and stillbirth (Naeye 1985a; Andres et al. 1990).

Abruptio Placentae

Abruptio placentae implies a premature separation of the placenta from the maternal surface with decidual haemorrhage. Most studies report a perinatal death rate following abruption of approximately 50% while infants born after abruption were significantly smaller-for-gestation than controls (Krohn et al. 1987). Cigarette smoking has been associated with abruptio placentae , presumably as a result of decidual necrosis (Naeye 1980). The incidence of abruptio placentae is increased in pre-eclampsia and diabetes mellitus. However, in many cases no cause of placental abruption can be identified. It is suggested that aneurysmal dilatation of the spiral artery leads to rupture and bleeding. In cases of abruption the placenta may show no abnormality or a mass of retro-placental haematoma with depression of the maternal surface. Obliteration of the intervillous space and infarction may be seen.

Chorangioma

Chorangiomas are haemangiomas occurring within villi and they occur in 1% of all placentas (Fox 1978). Most are small, single, discrete and intraplacental; because of their characteristic red colour they may be indistinguishable from fresh infarcts on gross examination. Small chorangiomas are clinically insignificant. Larger chorangiomas (larger than 50 mm in diameter) may be intraplacental and elevate the fetal surface. They may lie on the maternal surface or within membranes, or may be attached to the placental disc by a vascular pedicle. They may be visualised antenatally by ultrasound examination. Large or numerous chorangiomas may affect the fetus by inducing high-output cardiac failure due to arterio-venous anastomoses. Polyhydramnios, fetal hydrops, anaemia, thrombocytopaenia and cardiomegaly, premature labour and ante-partum haemorrhage are described. Haemangiomas of the fetus are occasionally found in association with large placental haemangiomas.

Large haemangiomas are usually purplish-red, encapsulated, of variable shape and frequently divided by fibrous septa. Histologically they resemble a capillary haemangioma or with a predominant spindle-cell pattern or both. Degenerative changes such as necrosis, calcification, hyalinisation or myxoid change are frequently present.

Fetal Stem Artery Thrombosis

Fetal stem artery thrombosis is usually a single lesion and produces a sharply defined zone of avascular villi and is found in 4.5% of placentas from full term uncomplicated pregnancies, but in 10% of placentas from diabetic women. The lesion is easy to distinguish as a pale triangular area with its base in the basal plate. Histological examination shows a sharp division between avascular and uninvolved villi and no villous crowding is observed. Villous vessels are constricted and sclerosed and connective tissue is fibrous with a hyalinised appearance. There is an excess of syncytial knots but no cytotrophoblast proliferation. A large thrombosed stem artery can be identified at the apex of the lesion. Organisation and recanalisation of the thrombus may be seen. Vessels distal to the occlusion show progressive fibromuscular sclerosis.

Other Macroscopic Abnormalities

An intraplacental multilobulated tumour, termed chorangiocarcinoma, showing vascular proliferation similar to that of a chorangioma but surrounded by a neoplastic trophoblastic proliferation, was recently reported (Jauniaux et al. 1988b). Maternal and fetal outcome were normal. Intraplacental choriocarcinoma presenting as red friable masses, either recognised immediately or retrospectively, have been reported also (Fox and Laurini 1988; Hallam et al. 1990) and can be associated with markedly elevated maternal serum alpha-fetoprotein levels (Ollendorf et al. 1990).

Placental Microscopic Abnormalities

Teratoma

Placental teratomas are rare tumours of disputed histogenesis. Some believe them to be a separate entity while others believe that they are extreme examples of fetus amorphus. They are histologically benign with no organisation of tissue components and no umbilical cord. They are clinically insignificant.

Placental Lesions of Uncertain Significance

Chorangiosis. Altshuler (1984) has attempted to define quantitatively the lesion called chorangiosis as present when, with a ×10 objective, there are 10 villi each with 10 vascular channels in 10 or more non-infarcted and non-ischaemic zones in at least three different placental areas. The incidence in normal uncomplicated pregnancy was not evaluated. Of 1350 placentas examined for a limited defined range of maternal and fetal disorders, he found 5.5% had evidence of chorangiosis. Since these placentas had been examined because of maternal reproductive failure, intrauterine infection, dysmaturity, congenital abnormalities, diabetes or erythroblastosis, it is not surprising that his conclusion was that chorangiosis is associated with incidences of neonatal death and major congenital malformations as high as 39% and 42% respectively.

Haemorrhagic endovasculitis. Collapse of fetal vessels after fetal death is followed by progressive obliterative fibromuscular sclerosis. There may be recanalisation and reorganisation of thrombi with neutrophils or nuclear debris in the vessel walls. These features have been termed haemorrhagic endovasculitis and thought to be a unique lesion strongly associated with stillbirth and intrauterine growth retardation (Sander et al. 1986). However, they are seen following fetal death and the morphological features may be the result of endothelial disintegration and degeneration of blood constituents.

Umbilical Cord and Membranes

Cord Length

The length of the umbilical cord varies widely (Mills et al. 1983; Naeye 1985b). Cord length is dependent on the stretch provided by fetal intrauterine motor activity. Accordingly, short cords may be a marker of abnormal fetal brain development (Moessinger et al. 1982), secondary to maternal ingestion of β-blockers (Katz et al. 1987) or intrauterine constraint, such as twin pregnancy (Soernes and Bakke 1987), uterine abnormalities or reduced amniotic fluid volume (Ogita et al. 1989). A length of less than 30 cm is insufficient to permit unrestricted fetal descent during labour, and fetal hypoxia may result from stretching with obstruction of vessels (Bain and Elliot 1976), placental separation or cord rupture. Long cords (greater than 100 cm) predispose to prolapse, knots and fetal entanglement and thus to fetal morbidity and mortality. The umbilical cord is often oedematous when there is fetal or placental hydrops, in maternal diabetes and Wiedemann–Beckwith syndrome.

Single Umbilical Artery

Single umbilical artery may result from primary aplasia of one vessel or secondary atrophy. The incidence varies from 0.2% to 1.1% of births with a higher incidence among white compared to black women in the USA (Peckham and Yerushalmy 1965) and higher in girls than in boys (Lilja 1991a). Single umbilical artery is associated with maternal diabetes (Haust 1981) and maternal smoking (Lilja 1991b) and with low birthweight and preterm births (Lilja 1991a). An increase in fetal malformation is reported in association with single umbilical artery in between 20% and 50% of cases. Frequently associated malformations are sirenomelia sequence, VACTERL complex and anorectal atresia and oesophageal atresia (Lilja 1991c). Single umbilical artery is seen more frequently in trisomy 13, trisomy 18 and Zellweger syndromes and is said not to occur with trisomy 21 and sex chromosome abnormalities (Saller et al. 1990) but a recent study has shown associations also with trisomy 21 and gonosomal abnormalities (Khong and George 1992).

Umbilical Cord Insertion

The umbilical cord may be inserted into the placental disc centrally, eccentrically, marginally (battledore) or velamentously (via the membranes). There is no association between the first three types of insertion and premature delivery or other abnormality of fetus or pregnancy (Uyanwah-Akpom and Fox 1977; Bruyniks et al. 1988). Velamentous insertion carries the danger of vessel rupture during labour, especially if vessels run across the internal os (vasa praevia), or of compression during delivery (Fig. 2.17). Both these complications are associated with a high perinatal mortality rate quoted as 75%–100% and 50%–

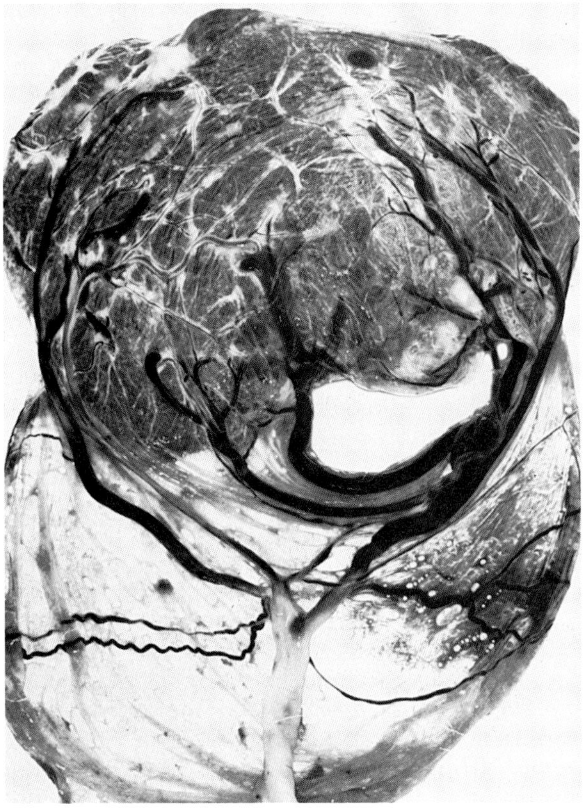

Fig. 2.17. Velamentous insertion of the umbilical cord. Large vessels run around the hole through which delivery took place.

60% respectively (Dougall and Baird 1987). An excess of fetal deformity, but not malformation or disruption, is described in association with velamentous insertion of the cord (Robinson et al. 1983).

Cord Knots and Entanglements

"False knots" of the cord are localised accumulations of Wharton's jelly or vascular dilatation producing asymmetrical cord expansion. They are insignificant.

True knots are present in between 0.1% and 2.1% of cords at delivery and are more frequent in long umbilical cords, in male fetuses and in multiparous women (Blickstein et al. 1987). No significant association with fetal distress, Apgar scores or cord blood analysis, cardiotocographic abnormalities or perinatal mortality and neonatal morbidity was found (Matorras et al. 1990). They are significant only if tight enough to obstruct fetal circulation. The structure of the cord in respect of both spiralling of vessels and the physical characteristics of Wharton's jelly diminishes the likelihood of obstruction of cord vessels by torsion and entanglement. Knots that have been present for some time produce grooving and kinking of the cord, with localised loss of Wharton's jelly, constriction and sometimes thrombosis of the vessels. Knots which tighten just before or during labour may also cause asphyxia. Oedema and congestion or thrombosis of vessels should be sought in the vicinity of a knot.

A long cord predisposes to fetal entanglement. It is commonplace to find the cord around the fetal neck, and sometimes division is required to complete delivery. Entanglement around a limb or the neck with looping of the cord around itself is more likely to produce sufficient kinking to affect the fetal circulation. Oedema and congestion on one side of the alleged obstruction should be sought. Haemorrhage into Wharton's jelly and thrombosis of vessels and grooving of fetal parts increase the significance of cord entanglement.

Cord Torsion and Constriction

Torsion of the cord is the result of active or passive rotation of the fetus and is normally present throughout pregnancy. Marked cord torsion may be observed at delivery of an uncompromised infant or following termination of pregnancy for fetal anomaly. It is when excessive cord torsion is observed following intrauterine fetal death that its significance is overemphasised. Following fetal death, fluid is lost from Wharton's jelly leading to loss of turgor. Autolytic change in the cord may be accelerated in the 30–40 mm close to the umbilical cord insertion to the fetus. The generalised loss of turgor will serve to make any torsion more apparent and unopposed asymmetrical uterine action may produce further fetal torsion. Twists in the cord are often most apparent in the narrow segment of cord at the umbilical insertion to the fetus when torsion leading to cord constriction may be blamed for fetal demise. It is more likely that the twists collect in the constricted part of the cord as a purely mechanical phenomenon. Cord torsion per se is rarely the cause of fetal demise.

Constriction of the umbilical cord usually occurs close to the fetal insertion and is much less commonly recorded elsewhere. In the constricted segment vessels are collapsed or contracted and the stroma appears dense. It has been suggested that such constrictions are the result of congenital absence of Wharton's jelly. Such a view is erroneous. Cord constriction at the fetal end is exceptionally described with livebirth when the constricted segment is very short. It is more likely that it is the result of more rapid autolysis occurring close to the fetus. Labarrere et al. (1985b) described three rare cases where there was complete absence of Wharton's jelly around the umbilical cord arteries but present around the umbilical vein; these three cases were associated with perinatal death.

Localised constrictions elsewhere in the cord are the result of localised pressure. They are seen much more frequently in the presence of localised physical constriction such as amniotic bands (Heifetz 1984) or significant cord knot than as isolated lesions.

Localised Cord Swelling

Haematomas in the cord arise from focal haemorrhage from an umbilical vessel, usually a vein. A minority are associated with delivery trauma, vascular thrombosis or iatrogenic injury. The majority appear to accumulate before the onset of labour. Their significance is unclear.

Remnants of the allantois and omphalomesenteric duct may be found, the former situated between the two umbilical arteries and generally lined by transitional epithelium while the latter is located more peripherally in the cord and shows an intestinal, often mucinous, lining. Abscess of an allantoic duct remnant has been described (Baill et al. 1989). Cysts of the umbilical cord may arise from these remnants, usually situated at the fetal end of the cord and found by chance. An occasional cyst reaches 40–50 mm in diameter when there is a risk of vascular tamponade.

Tumours of the cord are exceedingly rare (Clausen 1989). Angiomas may give rise to cord haemorrhage and are a known cause of elevated maternal alpha-fetoprotein levels. Teratomas of the cord are extremely rare.

Abnormalities of Umbilical Cord Vessels

The prevalence of thrombosis of umbilical cord vessels is 1 in 1290 among prospectively

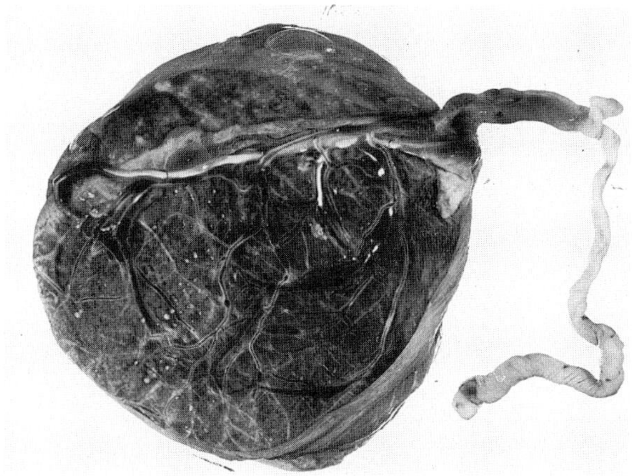

Fig. 2.18. Amnion nodosum. The placental also illustrates thrombosis of a major branch of an umbilical artery and marginal umbilical cord insertion.

examined placentas. There is a slight male predominance and venous thrombosis occurs more frequently than thrombosis of one or both umbilical arteries. In a review, Heifetz (1988) did not find an association between cord thrombosis and perinatal mortality and morbidity and thought that, when present, it was related to additional umbilical cord abnormalities, obstetrical complications or systemic fetal conditions that were likely cause of both the thrombosis and poor fetal outcome.

Calcification of umbilical cord vessels is thought to be rare and two different lesions have been described (Khong and Dilly 1989). In one there is complete calcification of arterial lumen resulting in total obliteration while in another, so-called sclerosing funisitis, there is sclerosis of the wall associated often with inflammation in the umbilical cord and its vessels, membranes and decidua suggesting intrauterine infection. Knowles and Frost (1989) described two cases of the latter variant in pregnancies complicated by maternal syphilis.

Amnion Nodosum

Amnion nodosum accompanies chronic oligohydramnios from any cause. It is evident as numerous raised, shiny, greyish nodules measuring up to 5 mm lying on the amniotic surface of the placenta (Fig. 2.18). The nodules are easily dislodged leaving a depression. This helps to distinguish amnion nodosum from

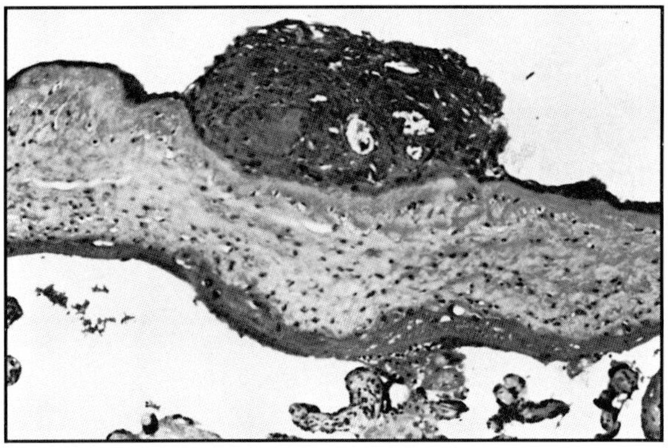

Fig. 2.19. Amnion nodosum. Granular material containing squamae becoming incorporated into amnion.

squamous metaplasia of the amnion which is not easily displaced and which has no clinical significance.

Amnion nodosum consists of granular material containing fetal cells and debris with occasional hair fragments and may be covered by amniotic epithelium (Fig. 2.19). The nodules derive from close contact between fetus and amnion and consist of vernix caseosa. The presence of amnion nodosum is evidence of oligohydramnios so that associated abnormality such as urinary tract obstruction, renal agenesis or a history of prolonged rupture of membranes should be sought. Bendon and Ray (1986) described subchorionic accumulation of squames, presumably from cells shed into amniotic fluid, in prolonged amniotic fluid leakage not occurring over the cervical os.

Placenta Following Intrauterine Fetal Death

Following the death of the fetus in utero, the fetal circulation ceases. However, the placenta survives as maternal circulation within the intervillous space continues. Characteristic changes take place in the placenta post mortem and it is important to recognise them so as not to implicate them in fetal demise.

Macroscopically the placenta appears pale and feels firm. A striking histological feature is progressive fibromuscular sclerosis of fetal stem arteries. The villi appear avascular because of capillary collapse and become increasingly fibrotic. There is an increase in villous syncytial knots, thickening of the trophoblast basement membrane and cytotrophoblast hyperplasia. Patchy villous oedema is common with an apparent increase in Hofbauer cells.

Placental Oedema

Shen-Schwarz et al. (1989) found villous oedema in 11% of unselected term placentas, with significant associations with fetal and neonatal death. The placenta is often oedematous in those conditions which give rise to fetal hydrops, particularly when hydrops is the result of chronic fetal anaemia. In these conditions severe fetal oedema is usually accompanied by a similar degree of placental oedema, but this is not always the case and placental oedema may be the more striking change, particularly in rhesus incompatibility. Some abnormalities which produce fetal hydrops are rarely accompanied by placental oedema. Conversely, the placenta may be hydropic while the fetus is normal, as in congenital nephrotic syndrome.

The hydropic placenta is pale, friable and bulky, often weighing more than 1 kg. Fluid exudes from the cut or damaged surface, and intervillous thrombi or septal cysts are frequently seen. Because of its friability, manual removal of the placenta is often necessary and post-partum haemorrhage may occur (Gough et al. 1986). Histological examination reveals oedema affecting immature intermediate villi (Shen-Schwarz et al. 1989); the change may be focal or uniform. Hofbauer cells and cytotrophoblast appear prominent. Villous syncytiotrophoblast is usually normal and thickening of the basement membrane may be seen. Fibrinoid necrosis of the villi is frequently seen. When there is severe fetal oedema, focal erythropoiesis is present within fetal capillaries (Fig. 2.20). The overall impression in this condition is one of crowding of immature and oedematous villi. Striking differences in villous appearance are seen in different areas of the same placenta, and focal villous hypercellularity is often present.

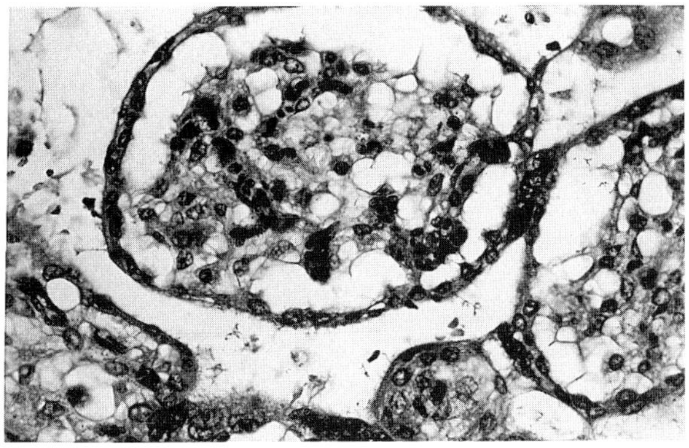

Fig. 2.20. Extramedullary haemapoiesis in fetal vessel and stroma in villus from rhesus incompatibility.

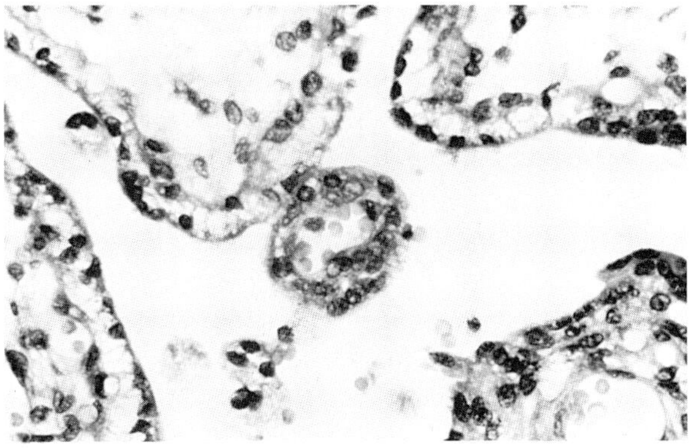

Fig. 2.21. Placental villi at 20 weeks gestation in G_{M1} gangliosidosis; large vacuoles distend the syncytiotrophoblast.

Placenta in Genetic and Congenital Abnormalities of the Fetus

Some chromosome abnormalities are commonly seen in spontaneous abortion but are rarely seen amongst pregnancies which continue to term. Placentas from mature trisomic pregnancies are often small, as is the fetus, but appear grossly normal. Villi may be normal or immature for gestation with patchy hydropic change. Philippe and Boué (1969) regard intravillous trophoblast as diagnostic for placental trisomy but this is not universally present and may be seen in normal pregnancies.

Turner's syndrome (monosomy X0). Massive subchorial thrombosis is frequently present in the placenta in Turner's syndrome. This is particularly common when mid-trimester intrauterine death occurs.

Triploidy. Triploidy of the fetus and placenta usually leads to abortion in the first half of pregnancy although a few continue to term. Partial molar change with villous hydrops and scattered vesicles may be seen when the additional haploid complement is paternally derived.

Inborn errors of metabolism. Lysosomal storage disorders are all very rare. Vacuolation of the syncytiotrophoblast was reported in the placenta of a fetus with G_{M1} gangliosidosis (Lowden et al. 1973) (Fig. 2.21). Powell et al. (1976) described a foamy appearance of the cytoplasm of syncytiotrophoblast, extravillous trophoblast and Hofbauer cells in the placenta in mucolipidosis type II. Histochemically confirmed sphingomyelin was demonstrated and described in the placentas from fetuses with Niemann–Pick disease type A (Schoenfeld et al. 1985). Ultrastructural evidence of accumulation of metabolites was found in specimens from pregnancies complicated by Niemann–Pick, Hurler's, Pompe's and sialic acid storage diseases as early as 10 weeks' gestation. The use of electron microscopy on one or two villi from chorionic villus sampling to provide expedient prenatal diagnosis has been proposed (Jones et al. 1990). Demonstration by electron microscopy of characteristic densely packed cytoplasmic filaments and lamellar inclusions has also allowed diagnosis of heretofore unsuspected maternal carrier status of Fabry's disease (Popli et al. 1990).

Anencephaly. The placenta is usually normal in anencephaly but there may be delay in villous maturation.

Fetal tumours. Metastases from fetal tumours, especially neuroblastoma and leukaemia, are well documented. The placenta appears large, pale and oedematous. Histological examination reveals tumour cells plugging villous capillaries.

Placenta in Sudden Infant Death Syndrome

A careful case-controlled study has not found any predictive pathology in placental examin-

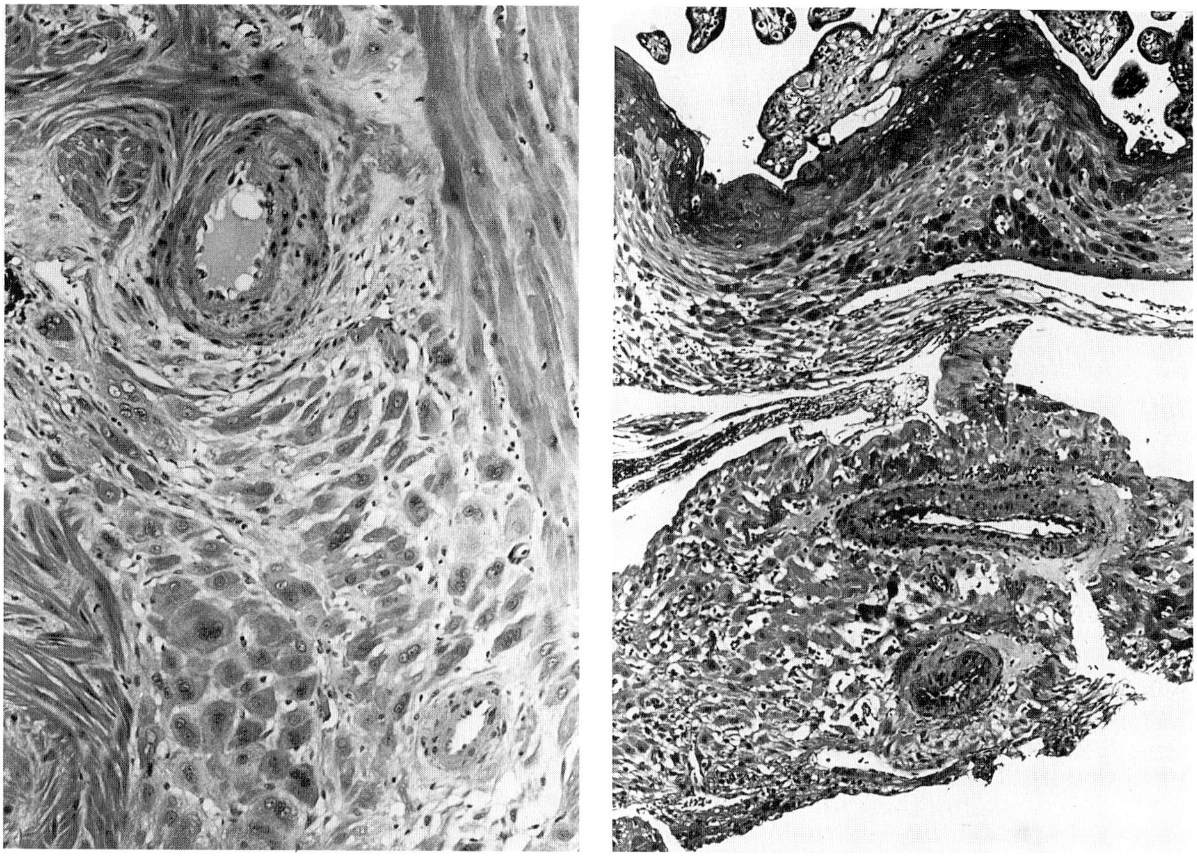

a b

Fig. 2.22a,b. Maternal spiral arteries showing absence of physiological changes. **a** Decidual segments underlying the basal plate. **b** Myometrial segments in placental bed (reproduced from Khong et al. 1986).

ation for sudden infant death syndrome (SIDS) when birthweight and gestational age were controlled (Denmead et al. 1987). The higher incidence of both chorioamnionitis and SIDS among preterm infants may account for Naeye's finding (1977) of a higher incidence of chorioamnionitis in SIDS cases. Prematurity as a confounding risk factor was not analysed in his study.

Placenta in Maternal Disorders

Pre-eclampsia and Eclampsia

Pre-eclampsia is a disorder characterised by maternal hypertension, proteinuria and oedema. In eclampsia fitting occurs although women do not necessarily go through a prodromic pre-eclamptic phase. Both syndromes are important clinically because of their association with high perinatal mortality and intrauterine fetal growth retardation and maternal morbidity and mortality. There is a general lack of uniformity of definition of these conditions. Recently formulated definitions from an international study group have done much to rectify this problem (Davey and MacGillivray 1988).

There is a defect in the normal invasion of the spiral arteries by the two waves of endovascular cytotrophoblast leading to absence of physiological vascular changes in the myometrial segments of all spiral (uteroplacental) arteries and in the decidual segments of many of these arteries (Fig. 2.22). This defect is not specific to pre-eclampsia and eclampsia and has been described in a number of cases of growth-retarded or small-for-dates infants from normotensive pregnancies (Khong et al. 1986). Where the spiral arteries have not undergone physiological changes the undisturbed vascular anatomy would render them responsive to vasomotor influences. A further vascular abnormality in pre-eclampsia and eclampsia is acute atherosis which is defined as fibrinoid necrosis of the smooth muscle arterial wall accompanied by lipid-laden macrophages and a perivascular round cell infiltrate (Labarrere 1988; Khong 1991) (Fig. 2.23).

These vascular abnormalities explain the reduction in uteroplacental blood flow, placental infarction and low birthweight. Because the number of physiologically converted decidual segments of spiral arteries varies from case to case the degree of non-conversion may be a factor in determining the volume of blood flow into the intervillous space and, together with the maternal blood pressure driving the blood flow, may explain why some babies in pre-eclamptic pregnancies are of normal birth weight.

Placentas from women with pre-eclampsia are usually smaller than those from uncomplicated pregnancies and contain numerous infarcts; retroplacental haematomas are common. Cytotrophoblast proliferation, thickening of the basement membrane and an excess of syncytial knots are characteristic of placentas associated with pre-eclampsia. These findings are not specific and are all associated with poor uteroplacental blood flow. The villous pattern may appear inappropriately mature for gestation. Villi may be hypovascular because of obliterative endarteritis of fetal stem arteries. Fibrinoid necrosis of villi is often seen.

Essential Hypertension

In pregnancies in which there is antecedent hypertension, the spiral arteries in the placental bed show hyperplastic arteriosclerosis but uteroplacental arteries are developed in the normal way. In the absence of other complications essential hypertension does not seem to have an adverse effect on placental and fetal growth, and, because of the increased driving blood pressure, may actually result in a baby with a birthweight higher than from a normotensive pregnancy. However, in women with established hypertension who develop superimposed pre-eclampsia, a defective maternal vascular response to placentation also exists and this is complicated by arteriosclerosis, the consequence of the pre-existing hypertension, to which acute atherosis may be superimposed.

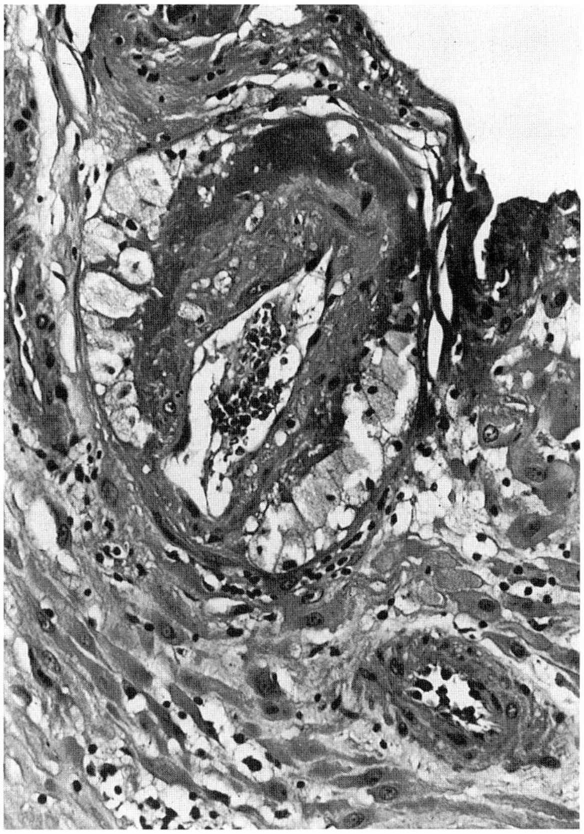

Fig. 2.23. Acute atherosis in pre-eclampsia showing lipid-laden macrophages, fibrinoid necrosis and a perivascular lymphocytic infiltrate (reproduced from Khong et al. 1987b).

Diabetes Mellitus

The many studies of placentas in diabetes mellitus have produced contradictory and confusing results owing to failure to take account of confounding variables such as severity of disease, degree of control of hyperglycaemia, premature delivery and related abnormalities such as pre-eclampsia.

Reassessment of the claim that placentas from diabetics are, on average, heavier than those from non-diabetic mothers has not been confirmed on a recent series of well-controlled diabetics but an association of larger placentas with maternal glycosylated haemoglobin levels is noted (Clarson et al. 1989). The placenta may be oedematous. Umbilical cord oedema is frequent and the incidence of single umbilical artery is increased. Although fetal artery thrombosis is common there is no increase in infarction.

The range of histological abnormality in placentas from diabetic women may be related to inadequate sampling. Fox (1969) found groups of immature villi interspersed with areas of accelerated maturity although 40% of placental villi were of appropriate maturity. Villous oedema with prominent stromal Hofbauer cells, fibrosis of the villous stroma, villous fibrinoid necrosis and increase in cytotrophoblast and syncytial knots, thickening of the trophoblast basement membrane, proliferative and tortuous fetal capillaries and proliferative endarteritis of fetal stem arteries have been described in placentas from diabetic pregnancies. None of these findings is specific and many placentas are histologically normal. Björk and Persson (1982) found increased numbers of vasculosyncytial membranes and syncytial knots in the placentas of diabetics with imperfect metabolic control between the 12th and 32nd weeks of pregnancy.

Morphometric study of the placentas of diabetics (Boyd et al. 1986) showed a significant increase in the volume of parenchyma and a decrease in non-parenchyma. The villous surface area was significantly increased even after correction for fetal weight. Björk and Persson (1984) found increased branching of peripheral villi in the placentas of diabetic mothers. Electron microscopy has confirmed the light microscopic findings of increased cytotrophoblast, focal syncytial necrosis and thickening of the trophoblast basement membrane and has shown increased surface density of microvilli.

Intrahepatic Cholestasis of Pregnancy

Intrahepatic cholestasis of pregnancy is rare but perinatal mortality, probably due to increased preterm delivery, is increased. No specific placental abnormality was noted but there was villous oedema, cytotrophoblastic proliferation, increased syncytial sprout formation but no histochemical staining for bilirubin (Costoya et al. 1980).

Collagen Vascular Disease

Much of the literature pertaining to collagen vascular diseases, such as scleroderma and systemic lupus erythematosus, is confused by inclusion of confounding complications such as hypertension and growth retardation. There is an increased incidence of placental infarction in pregnancies where there is maternal lupus anticoagulant or anticardiolipin antibody but the degree of placental infarction is often insufficient to account for fetal death. Abramowsky et al. (1980) claimed that there is a vasculopathy similar to acute atherosis in placentas from women with lupus erythematosus but confounding complications of pregnancies that may give a similar morphological feature were not allowed for.

Sickle Cell Disease and Other Haematological Disorders

Sickle crises are more common during pregnancy and spontaneous abortion and perinatal loss may exceed 50%. It was said that if the fetus survives it is usually growth-retarded but this is now disputed (Baill and Witter 1990). The reduced oxygen tension in the intervillous space predisposes to infarction, and placental weight may be increased as a nonspecific adaptation to severe maternal anaemia (O'Herlihy and O'Driscoll 1987). Microscopically, sludging and characteristic sickling of cells in the intervillous space may be seen, even in sickle cell trait (Fig. 2.24).

Routine histochemical staining revealed iron deposits at the trophoblastic basement membrane in a term placenta from a woman with homozygous β thalassaemia although successful pregnancy in this condition is rare (Birkenfeld et al. 1989).

Maternal Malignant Disease

Placental metastases from maternal neoplasms have been reviewed (Fox 1978; Dildy et al. 1989). The commonest tumour to metastasise to the placenta is malignant melanoma. Carcinoma of the breast, bronchus, gastrointestinal tract, cervix and ovary, Ewing's sarcoma and leukaemias occasionally metastasise to the placenta. Tumour deposits may be visible macroscopically and histological examination reveals clumps or sheets of tumour cells in the intervillous space. Villous involvement is uncommon but cases of fetal involvement have been reported, including one with survival at 6 months' follow-up (Moller et al. 1986).

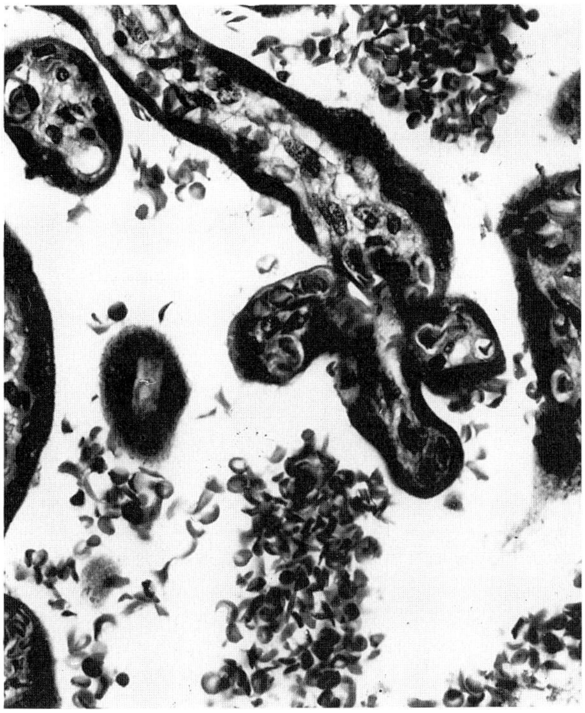

Fig. 2.24. Sickle cell trait. Sickling of cells in intervillous space.

Cigarette Smoking

The association between maternal cigarette smoking and low birthweight is well established. Placental weights from smokers have been found to be increased (Naeye 1978), smaller (Kullander and Kallen 1971) or not different (Van der Velde et al. 1983) when compared with those from non-smoking mothers. An increase in placenta praevia and abruption amongst smoking mothers, the latter condition being ascribed to decidual ischaemia and necrosis, have also been reported (Naeye 1978). Histological evidence of hypoxia in the form of atrophic and hypovascular changes in placental villi in heavy but not in moderate smokers is presented by Mochizuki et al. (1984). Using perfusion-fixed placentas Burton et al. (1989) showed that there was an increased thickness of the vasculosyncytial membrane separating maternal and fetal circulations and a reduction in capillary volume but these changes were less severe than those found in studies using immersion-fixed placentas.

Van der Veen and Fox (1982) suggest that placental ischaemia may be the result of nicotine-induced constriction of uterine vessels. Alternatively, cadmium toxicity or accumulation of polycyclic aromatic hydrocarbons may inhibit placental oxidative enzyme systems.

Intrauterine Growth Retardation

Many factors are related to poor fetal growth but when no cause is found it is tempting to attribute the cause of intrauterine growth retardation to "placental insufficiency", a term that has been deprecated. Gruenwald (1975) argues that as the placenta is a fetal organ it cannot be responsible for poor fetal growth but its growth and development will be affected by factors suppressing or promoting fetal growth. Should the placenta fail in its nutritive function, it is rarely a primary placental problem.

Van der Veen and Fox (1983) examined placentas from "idiopathic" intrauterine growth retardation and found an excess of villous cytotrophoblast. Electron microscopy revealed cytotrophoblast hyperplasia, focal syncytial necrosis, microvillous abnormalities, reduced syncytial secretory activity, irregular thickening of trophoblastic basement membrane and the presence of small fetal villous vessels with multilayered basement membranes. These changes are consistent with uteroplacental ischaemia. This is in accordance with recent studies demonstrating inadequate physiological changes in the maternal spiral arteries, implicating a failure of extravillous trophoblast migration during placentation, and the finding of acute atherosis (Althabe et al. 1985; Khong et al. 1986). There is an increased incidence of villitis in placentas complicated by small-for-dates infants (Russell 1980; Althabe and Labarrere 1985) and the birthweight appears to correlate with the degree of severity of villitis (Altshuler and Russell 1975; Russell 1980; Garcia 1982).

Infection

Infection of the placenta or membranes may adversely affect the fetus in several ways. It may be associated with mid-trimester abortion, premature onset of labour or intrauterine fetal

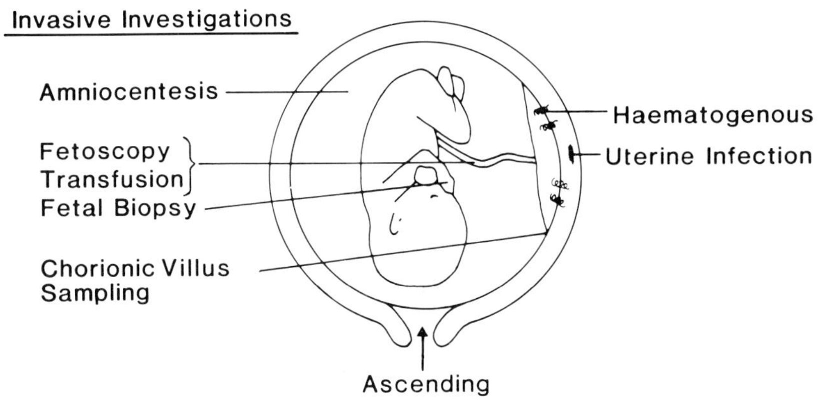

Fig. 2.25. Sources of placental infection.

infection. Ascending infection may complicate prolonged rupture of membranes at any time of pregnancy and so may contribute to intrapartum and neonatal morbidity and mortality. Whilst most infection is the result of vaginal contamination by intestinal organisms or an extension of maternal systemic infection, it can be introduced by a medical attendant during the course of invasive investigations or vaginal examination before or during labour.

The possible routes of infection are illustrated (Fig. 2.25). The ascending route is common, giving rise to chorioamnionitis which, when severe, is accompanied by contamination of the liquor amnii and inflammation of the cord (funisitis) but does not usually involve the villi. Chorioamnionitis is the result of infection by organisms which are frequently present in the vagina, usually bacteria but sometimes fungi, mycoplasma or viruses and are not the result of pH change or meconium in the amniotic fluids or response to hypoxia. The transplacental route involves haematogenous spread from an overt or subclinical infection and leads to villitis with little or no inflammation of the membranes. Organisms spread by this route are usually viruses, occasionally certain bacteria, protozoa and parasites (Table 2.1). In the majority of cases, villitis is a histological diagnosis and no pathogen is isolated. This group has been designated "villitis of unknown aetiology" (VUE) (Russell 1980).

Infections affecting the placenta can now be confirmed using established pathological techniques such as immunofluorescence, immunocytochemistry, in-situ hybridisation and DNA analysis using restriction endonucleases (Herring et al. 1987).

Table 2.1. Organisms affecting the placenta

Ascending infection	Haematogenous infection
Group B streptococcus	Rubella virus
Escherichia coli	Poliomyelitis virus
Other enteric organisims	Enterovirus
Listeria monocytogenes	*Listeria monocytogenes*
Chlamydia	Chlamydia
Herpes simplex virus	Herpes simplex virus
Cytomegalovirus	Cytomegalovirus
	Hepatitis virus
	Varicella zoster virus
	Treponema pallidum
	Toxoplasma gondii

Chorioamnionitis

The reported incidence of chorioamnionitis varies widely and is related to selection of cases, criteria for positive diagnosis and the population studied. Fox and Langley (1971) found evidence of chorioamnionitis in 24.4% of 1000 consecutively delivered placentas. The incidence is increased among women of low socioeconomic status and in blacks (Naeye and Blanc 1970). Coitus, an incompetent cervix and maternal malnutrition are thought to increase the frequency and severity of amniotic infections. It has been suggested that reduction of the normal antibacterial activity of the amniotic fluid may predispose to ascending infection. A low level of a polypeptide linked to zinc may be important in malnourished women, as well as inadequate protein, vitamin and caloric intake.

Ascending infection frequently complicates premature rupture of the membranes, although chorioamnionitis can occur when membranes

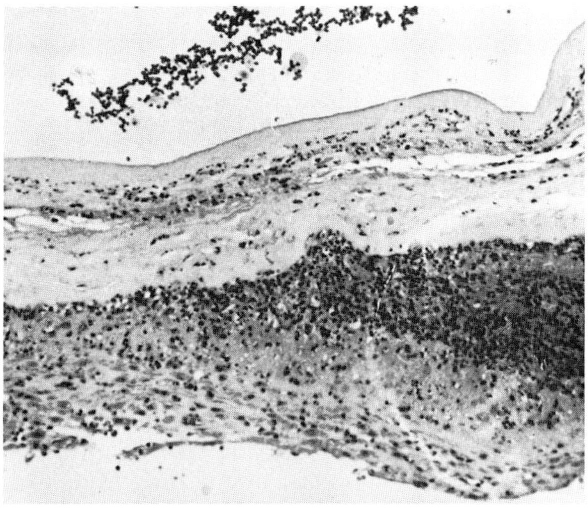

Fig. 2.26. Chorioamnionitis. There is loss of a amniotic epithelium. Maternal leucocytes are seen in the membrane and adhere to the chorionic plate.

are intact. Before term infection precedes rupture of the membranes and can initiate labour while near to term. Chorioamnionitis often is a consequence of spontaneous rupture of the membranes. Prematurity and not infection is responsible for adverse neonatal outcome (Garite et al. 1982; Zaaijmann et al. 1982; Zhang et al. 1985).

Microbiological investigation of chorioamnionitis is difficult. After vaginal delivery the significance of positive cultures from placental smears is difficult to evaluate and mixed isolates are common. A rapid method for diagnosis involves Gram stain examination of cells scraped from the amnion and examination for polymorphonuclear leucocytes in a smear of the chorionic plate (Blanc 1981). Numerous bacteria and leucocytes in the smear would indicate infection and the Gram stain permits appropriate antibiotic therapy to be given after early fetal samples have been taken.

There may be no macroscopic abnormality of the placental membranes in ascending infection. When infection is long standing there is loss of membrane translucency and the placenta may be foul-smelling. Meconium staining may obscure the appearance of chorioamnionitis. In some infections—listeriosis, candidiasis and herpes simplex—small white or yellowish spots may be seen on the amnion surface. The histological appearance is related to the duration and severity of the infection. In early infection polymorphonuclear leucocyte infiltration of maternal origin is present in the membranes nearest to the internal os (Fig. 2.26). This change becomes more widespread as infection spreads. Maternal leucocytes accumulate beneath the chorionic plate and become embedded in fibrin and infection may extend into the adjacent intervillous space. At first, polymorphs are maternal in origin but a fetal response develops which is first evident as a vasculitis in the chorionic plate. Similar changes may be seen in the umbilical cord: polymorphonuclear leucocytes are first seen in the arterial walls, then in the vein and finally spread into Wharton's jelly, the migration being preferentially towards the amniotic cavity (Fig. 2.27). A severe ascending infection will involve extraplacental membranes, amniotic fluid, chorionic plate and adjacent intervillous space and the umbilical cord. The amniotic infection sequence comprises

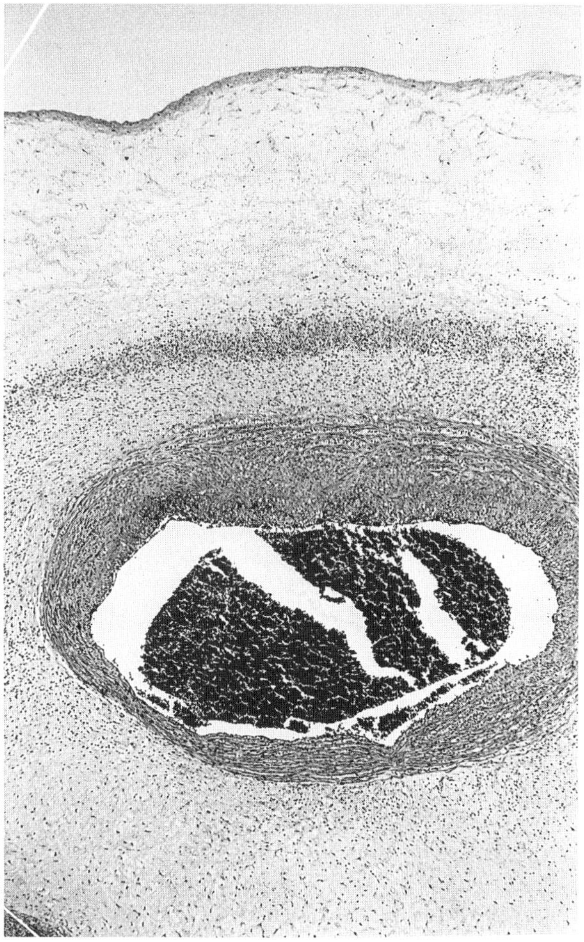

Fig. 2.27. Funisitis. Leucocyte migration is more apparent towards the amniotic cavity.

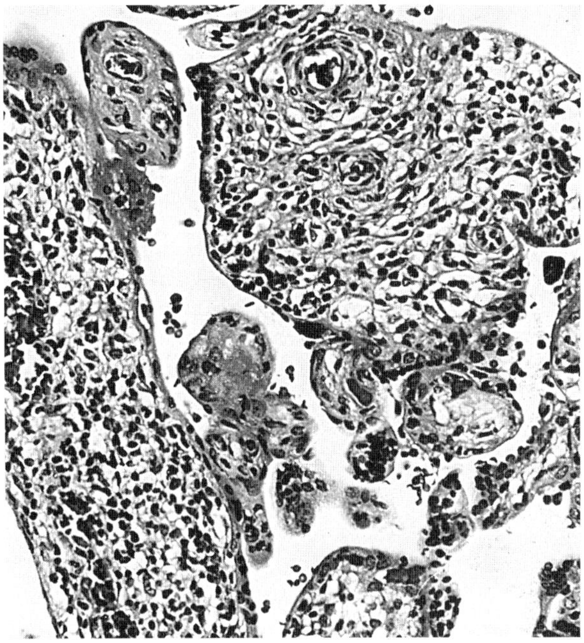

Fig. 2.28. Villitis of unknown aetiology. The villi are distended by fetal lymphocytes.

membranitis, chorionitis, funisitis and deglutition and inhalation of infected liquor; this gives rise to fetal infection, particularly pneumonia and otitis media.

Experimental evidence suggests that inflammation of the umbilical cord vessels may cause vasoconstriction and thus affect fetal perfusion (Hyde et al. 1989). Abnormal fetal heart rate patterns were associated with acute inflammation in the placental membranes, amniotic fluid or both (Salafia et al. 1989), lending support to the hypothesis that chorioamnionitis may have an effect on fetal cardiovascular haemodynamics.

Villitis

Inflammation of the villi is the result of haematogenous spread of infection from the mother or local extension of focal endometrial inflammation. Although many specific maternal infections can give rise to villitis, in 98% of cases no organism is isolated and serological investigation results are negative. In most instances, villitis is found during histological examination of the placenta by which time it is too late to instigate microbiological studies.

The reported incidence of villitis varies from 6% to 26% (Altshuler and Russell 1975; Labarerre et al. 1982). Although these studies differed in size and techniques, it seems likely that there are real geographical differences in the incidence of villitis.

Villitis seems to be associated with a history of reproductive failure (Russell et al. 1980; Knox and Fox 1984). Several groups have found a high incidence of fetal growth retardation. The degree of growth retardation appears to be related to the severity of the villitis. Villitis is known to occur in a variety of infections, particularly viral, and a questionable argument suggests that growth retardation is related to subclinical fetal infection rather than to villous injury, as in the majority of cases villitis is focal. Mortimer et al. (1985) found that villitis of unknown aetiology is truly idiopathic and is infective in only about 1%, as based on detection of IgM levels in the umbilical cord sera. Findings such as this have raised the idea that villitis of unknown aetiology may be a marker of defective maternofetal interaction (see below).

Villitis may be diffuse in distribution or largely parabasal, i.e. close to the decidual surface. Labarerre et al. (1982) have suggested this might be evidence of maternal immune-mediated response against placental tissue, but these workers have not demonstrated a maternal origin for the infiltrating cells. Blanc (1981) draws attention to the presence of villitis in the vicinity of haemorrhagic and ischaemic lesions within the placenta, although he regards most cases of villitis as being the result of undiagnosed infection.

Macroscopic abnormality may be present in the placenta in a few specific infections such as those due to *Mycobacterium tuberculosis* and *Listeria monocytogenes*. No specific features are reported for villitis of unknown aetiology although Russell (1980) noted pallor of the placental parenchyma in some cases of very severe villitis examined by him. Histologically, the inflammatory infiltrate of the placental villi may be lymphocytic or lymphocytic and histiocytic (Fig. 2.28). A spectrum of parenchymal involvement is observed from less than one focus of inflammation in two sections to an extensive lesion with large areas of every section examined being affected by villitis. The foci of inflammation may be randomly distributed throughout the parenchyma or be confined to the basal region. Collections of inflammatory cells within the villous stroma may elevate the trophoblast and necrosis is common. Villi are often adherent and surrounded by a mesh of fibrin. In some cases a concomitant vasculitis of stem arteries is present.

Findings in Some Specific Infections

Bacterial Infections

Group B streptococcus. The ascending infection caused by group B streptococcus can be diagnosed by the finding of clumps of bacteria on the surface of the amniotic epithelium and by gastric lavage in the neonate. Infection with this organism may progress so rapidly that fetal death ensues before an inflammatory response can be mounted.

Listeria monocytogenes. Listerial infection can reach the placenta by ascending or haematogenous routes, the latter probably being more common. Meconium-stained liquor appears to be a consistent finding when intrauterine listeriosis is present (Larsson et al. 1979). In haematogenous infection there may be soft grey or white necrotic foci in the maternal surface of the placenta and these may be apparent in the parenchyma when the placenta is sliced. Ascending infection can produce tiny foci of necrosis on the surface of the amnion, umbilical cord and fetal skin. The abnormalities recognised with the naked eye are seen histologically to be macro- and microabscesses (Fig. 2.29). In fatal cases similar lesions may be found in fetal organs. Older lesions are granulomatous with peripheral palisading of histiocytes and central necrosis. Focal villous abnormality comprises vasculitis and necrosis.

Treponema pallidum. The placenta in congenital syphilis is large and pale, and cord oedema is usual. The villi are oedematous with generalised increase in Hofbauer cells and proliferative endovasculitis and perivasculitis. Focal lymphocytic or plasmacytic infiltration is usually apparent.

Mycobacterium tuberculosis. The placenta may become infected when the mother has active tuberculosis, but such spread seems to be infrequent. Tiny white soft nodules may be seen within the parenchyma. Histological examination shows typical caseous granulomata and a non-specific mixed villitis.

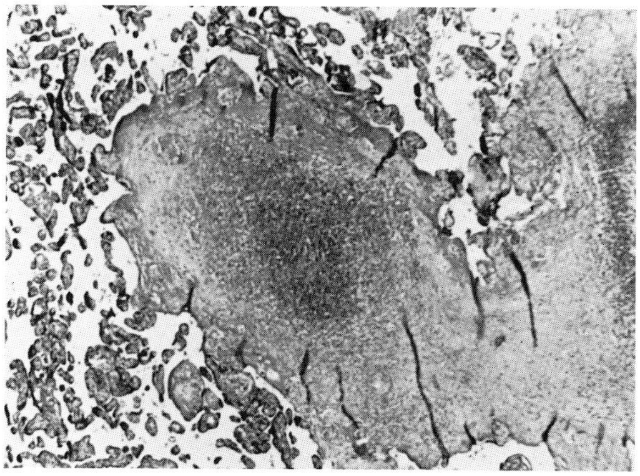

Fig. 2.29. Listeriosis. A microabscess with inflammation and necrosis close to the maternal surface is seen.

Campylobacter jejuni. Infection due to *Campylobacter jejuni* leads to mild maternal diarrhoea, with or without fever but can lead to abortion, predominantly in the second trimester (Simor et al. 1986). A severe villitis with prominent necrosis and massive perivillous fibrin deposition is seen (Coid and Fox 1983; Moscuna et al. 1989).

Viral Infections

Cytomegalovirus. The most frequently identified placental viral pathogen is cytomegalovirus (CMV). The gross appearance of the placenta varies widely. It may be normal, but is frequently small if there is concomitant fetal infection and intrauterine growth retardation, or may be large, pale and oedematous when there is fetal anaemia and hydrops. Samples of amnion and parenchyma will often yield positive viral cultures. Histological changes are a marked villitis, villous necrosis, intervillositis and patchy oedema (Fig. 2.30). Haemosiderin pigment may be apparent within the villi. Occasionally typical intranuclear inclusions may be seen in endothelial cells but more frequently these are encrusted with calcium and iron. In the normal placenta vascular and intravascular calcification is uncommon and this rare finding should raise the possibility of CMV infection. Chronic vasculitis may be apparent in umbilical vessels (Mostoufi-Zadeh et al. 1984).

Rubella virus. The placentitis which accompanies gestational rubella is well documented

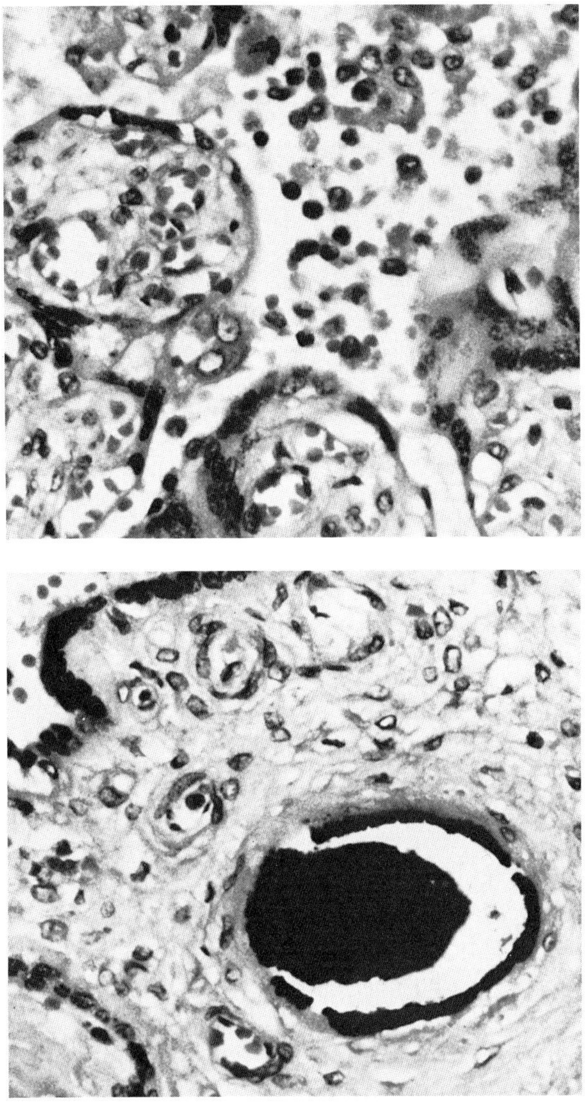
a

b

Fig. 2.30a,b. Cytomegalovirus infection. **a** Histiocytes are present in the intervillous space. **b** Calcification of vascular endothelium is seen.

and placental abnormalities are related to the time interval between infection and delivery. When infection is recent there is necrotising endarteritis in villous vessels and focal villitis. Viral inclusion may be present in endothelial cells or in trophoblast. Later, vasculitis leads to avascular atrophic villi. Vessels have prominent endothelial cushions and may contain calcified thrombus. Rubella infection interferes with villous development; there is hypoplasia with few terminal villi and an immature villous pattern.

Herpes simplex virus. This virus can cause ascending infection leading to chorioamnionitis or haematogenous spread producing villitis, or there may be a combination of both types of infection. Both may result in fatal fetal infection. Acute and chronic chorioamnionitis may be present within the placenta. Small abscesses with lymphocytic infiltration are seen. Sometimes viral inclusions may be demonstrated in the vicinity of microabscesses.

Varicella virus. When the mother contracts varicella during pregnancy there may be a lymphocytic villitis and diffuse epithelioid and multinucleate giant cell granulomata are seen within the parenchyma.

Coxsackie virus. The route of Coxsackie virus infection is haematogenous, occasionally as a complication of maternal illness (Batcup et al. 1985) but the mother is usually asymptomatic. Diffuse villitis with villous necrosis and intervillositis are apparent within the placenta.

Human immunodeficiency virus (HIV). The fate of infants born to HIV-seropositive mothers is unclear, but there is an increased incidence of intrauterine growth retardation (Minkoff et al. 1987). There is clinical, immunological and serological evidence for the vertical transplacental transmission of HIV (Sprecher et al. 1986), from as early as eight weeks' gestation (Lewis et al. 1990). There are no lesions specific for HIV infections but morphological studies suggest a high rate of chorioamnionitis contrasted with an absence of villitis and relative villous hypocellularity (Jauniaux et al. 1988). Retrovirus-like particles have been found at various sites, such as syncytiotrophoblast, fibroblast and endothelial cells, but their relation to the HIV is unclear.

Hepatitis virus. Extensive bilirubin deposition throughout membranes and villous tissue but no inflammation was seen in two placentas from mothers with HBsAg negative hepatitis delivered of normal infants (Khudr and Benirschke 1972).

Other Infections

Candida albicans. A common vaginal commensal, *C. albicans* may produce ascending infection. In some cases white spots may be identified on the surface of the amnion, cord or fetal skin; however, in many instances there is merely a membrane opacity and a purulent exudate in longstanding infection. Infection usually occurs in the presence of intact membranes. There is usually heavy mixed inflammatory cell infiltration within the amnion, often with loss of the epithelial layer. Focal or linear necrosis is frequently seen. Fungal hyphae may be missed unless special stains are used; this contributes in part to the alleged rarity of candidal infections. Sometimes necrosis within the membranes is very marked with microabscesses present. A funisitis may be present.

Toxoplasma gondii. The placenta is infected by *T. gondii* via the haematogenous route. It is frequently normal on macroscopic examination but there may be placental oedema if there is long-standing fetal infection. Focal mixed villitis may be apparent. Encysted parasites may be present within the membranes and chorionic plate with little surrounding inflammatory response.

Chlamydia psittaci. Infection by *Chlam. psittaci* is an occupational hazard of sheep farmers and infection in a pregnant woman may result in placental infection and fetal death. The placenta shows no macroscopic abnormality. There is a spectacular intervillositis and chlamydial inclusions can be demonstrated in trophoblast cells. Infection appears to be confined to the placenta and does not pass on to the fetus.

Mycoplasma and ureaplasma. An association of low birthweight with the isolation of ureaplasma and mycoplasma has been found. Isolation rates for *Ureaplasma urealyticum* in stillbirths and neonatal deaths were higher than in controls. However, *M. hominis* and *U. urealyticum* frequently colonise the placenta and vagina so that their isolation should be viewed with caution. It has been suggested that mycoplasma chorioamnionitis may result in premature onset of labour. Histologically chorioamnionitis but not villitis was seen in 60% of the placentas from which ureaplasma was isolated (Kundsin et al. 1984).

Plasmodium malariae. Malarial placentitis is very common in endemic areas, affecting up to one third of unselected placentas in one report. Histological features are those of a chronic intervillositis with macrophages, much perivillous fibrin deposition, brown pigment and parasites in the intervillous space. Trophoblast necrosis and basement thickening are universally present.

Immunological Aspects of Placentation

Pregnancy Immunology

It is quite impossible to cover every aspect of the maternofetal relationship, so the information presented has been selected to give an overview, inasmuch as that is possible. There is a bias towards the relationship between trophoblast and mother. The placental bed where maternal and fetal tissues are in contact and actually intermingle is thought to be the site of optimal fetomaternal communication (Mossman 1974). It may be that success or failure of normal development of the uteroplacental circulation is dependent on specific fetomaternal interactions in the placental bed.

Implicit in the assumption that immunological mechanisms are operating to allow the intrauterine survival of the allograft is that the fetoplacental unit bears fetal and paternal antigens capable of acting as transplantation antigens in the first instance. These mechanisms involve the afferent and efferent pathways of the maternal immune system and could be classified as (i) the recognition or otherwise of transplantation antigens on the fetoplacental unit, and (ii) the mounting or otherwise of an immune response by the mother.

Alloantigenicity of Trophoblast

Since trophoblast is the only component of the fetoplacental unit that is encountered by maternal cells, attention has focused on the alloantigenicity of trophoblast. The trophoblast population is heterogeneous topographically: there are different subsets, namely villous syncytiotrophoblast and cytotrophoblast, extravillous endovascular and interstitial trophoblast in the placental bed, and extravillous cytotrophoblast in the chorion laeve.

Major Histocompatibility Complex (MHC)

MHC antigens constitute the most potent transplantation antigens. They are encoded on chromosome 6 in the human and are divided into Class I (HLA-A, B and C), Class II (HLA-DR, DP, DQ, DX and DZ) and Class III (some complement factors). Several other loci and their products have been described, among which are molecules designated as HLA-E, F and G (Koller et al. 1989). Allograft recognition is dependent on Class II MHC antigens while cytotoxicity is directed towards Class I MHC antigens.

Class I MHC antigens are not found on syncytiotrophoblast or villous cytotrophoblast but are expressed on many but not all extravillous trophoblast at other sites. However, only monomorphic but not polymorphic determinants were detected (Redman et al. 1984) leading to the discovery and sequencing of non-classical or novel Class I MHC antigens (Ellis et al. 1986; 1990). It has been suggested that the role of Class I-like molecules on trophoblast may be to induce specific suppression of the maternal immune response (Bulmer and Johnson 1983), although the mechanism by which this could occur has not been satisfactorily explained. It may be that this novel antigen has taken on the immune system function of the classical Class I MHC antigens, and acts as "neutral" Class I MHC molecule to resist attack by natural killer cells or that it may be involved in the regulation of peptide hormones (Head et al. 1987).

Class II MHC antigens have not been found on syncytiotrophoblast, trophoblast cell columns or cytotrophoblast of the chorion laeve.

Other Antigen Systems

The TLX (trophoblast–lymphocyte cross-reactive) antigen system (Faulk et al. 1978) has yet to be characterised biochemically and has no defined function. It was defined serologically and is thought to be linked to the MHC antigens and encoded also on chromosome 6 (McIntyre and Faulk 1983). Their hypothesis is that maternal recognition of allotypic TLX antigens leads to production of blocking antibodies which block the trophoblast from immune attack against closely related antigens. Others have found blocking antibodies in maternal circulation with supposedly similar functions but their relation to each other is unclear (Rocklin et al. 1976; Fizet and Bousquet 1983).

The importance of other blood group antigens such as the P blood group system is highlighted by a recent publication of successful treatment of recurrent abortion by plasmapheresis to remove maternal anti-P antibodies (Rock et al. 1985).

Maternal Immune Response

The hypothesis that a decreased maternal immune response during pregnancy is the mechanism by which the fetal allograft survives has been proposed but the many studies on the level of immunocompetence in the pregnant female do not provide evidence for a consistent effect of pregnancy on immune responsiveness.

Measurements of peripheral blood lymphocytes are difficult to interpret because there are wide fluctuations in T and B lymphocytes with time even in the same individual. Studies have shown conflicting results with raised, normal or reduced levels in B or T lymphocytes, with or without variations through the gestation (see review by Carter 1984). There is appreciable natural killer (NK) cell activity during early pregnancy in the primigravid but not in the multigravid and activity declines during the later stages of pregnancy (Gregory et al. 1985). No clear role has been assigned to the peripheral leucocyte population and it is thought that they may be unrelated to the immunological interactions that are actually occurring in the placenta bed where maternal and fetal tissues are most intimately apposed.

Decidual Lymphocytes

First trimester decidua contains numerous bone marrow derived cells, including T cells, macrophages and granulated lymphocytes. These granulated lymphocytes (Kornchenzellen or "K" cells) are recognised immunologically by their reactivity to antibodies to various cluster differentiation (CD) antigens and are $CD2^+$ $CD7^+$ $CD38^+$ $CD56^+$ $CD3^-$ $CD5^-$ $CD8^-$ $CD25^-$ immunophenotypically (Ritson and Bulmer 1989). Most are also $CD16^-$ but some are $CD16^+$. Morphologically $CD16^-$ lymphocytes possess granules of more variable size and exhibit negligible cytotoxic activity against natural killer cell targets; $CD16^+$ lymphocytes express strong activity and it is suggested that natural cell activity of decidual leucocyte populations is mediated largely by the small numbers of $CD16^+$ cells (Christmas et al. 1990; Ferry et al. 1990). However, their role in vivo is unclear as cultured human trophoblast cells are resistant to the cytotoxic activity of decidual leucocytes or peripheral blood natural cells (King et al. 1989) and they respond poorly to mitogens or lymphokines (Ritson and Bulmer 1989). Furthermore, intradecidual lymphocytes lack T-cell antigen receptors (TCR) rendering them functionally anergic towards paternally derived antigens although mitogens and lymphokines could induce TCR expression in cultured lymphocytes (Marzusch et al. 1991).

Other workers have classified decidual lymphocytes morphologically into cells with large granules and large cells with small granules and found that normal pregnancies were associated with the former subtype while abortions were associated with the latter (Clark et al. 1987; Michel et al. 1990). No difference in numbers or immunophenotype of leucocytes has been detected in term human uterine tissue between normal and pre-eclamptic pregnancies (Khong 1987).

Decidual Macrophages

The putative role of macrophages in the uterine response to pregnancy has been reviewed recently (Hunt 1990). Macrophages are abundant throughout the entire uterus and express MHC Class II antigens—HLA-DR early in pregnancy with, additionally, DQ later (Lessin et al. 1988). Macrophage functions are numerous and include the synthesis of prostaglandin E2 which decreases lymphocyte proliferation and generation of cytotoxic T lymphocytes (Lala et al. 1988). This may in turn regulate synthesis of other substances and cytokines that may result in an immunosuppressive environment. The synthesis of cytokines by activated decidual macrophages has not been evaluated fully and their effect on human pregnancy in vivo remains to be elucidated. Interspecies differences make extrapolation difficult but animal experiments show production of interleukin-1 (IL-1) which can enhance, and TNF-α (tumour necrosis factor) and TGF-β1 (transforming growth factor) which can inhibit trophoblast cell DNA synthesis respectively (Hunt 1990). TNF-α and TGF-β originating from uterine macrophages may prevent exessive trophoblast invasion of the uterus (Hunt 1989).

Hormones

Immunomodulatory or immunosuppressive properties have been claimed for numerous proteins and hormones, such as hCG, progesterone and pregnancy-associated plasma protein A (PAPP-A) but while they are immunosuppressive in high concentrations in vitro, their role in vivo is unclear (Table 2.2).

Table 2.2. Substances with putative immunoregulative function during pregnancy

Hormones
progesterone
oestrogens
corticosteroids
prostaglandins
Placental proteins
human chorionic gonadotrophin (hCG)
human placental lactogen (hPL)
pregnancy-associated pregnancy protein A (PAPP-A)
Schwangerschaftsprotein 1 (SP1)
placental protein 14 (PP14)
Pregnancy-associated proteins
pregnancy zone protein (PZP, α-2-PAG)
pregnancy-associated α-2 macroglobulin
beta-1-macroglobulin (β-1-PAM)
early pregnancy protein (EPF)
Fetal proteins
carcinoembryonic antigen (CEA)
alpha-fetoprotein (AFP)
Other substances
transferrin
lactoferrin
isoferritin
interferons
interleukins
seromucoid

Evidence for Immunological Mechanisms in Abortion and Pre-eclampsia

Spontaneous Abortion

Successful pregnancy occurs in only 18%–28% of menstrual cycles in women having intercourse frequently without contraception (Roberts and Lowe 1975) while 62% of pregnancies recognised by hCG changes did not come to term (Edmonds et al. 1982). Whilst there are many causes of spontaneous abortion, much evidence has accumulated recently supporting the idea that many abortions, particularly recurrent spontaneous abortions, may be due to immunological processes (Mowbray and Underwood 1985). Women with three or more spontaneous abortions are deemed to be suffering from recurrent spontaneous abortions and this is defined on obstetrical history as being primary or secondary. Primary recurrent spontaneous aborters have never had a viable pregnancy with the mate who shares her spontaneous abortion history, whereas a secondary recurrent abortion follows a history of a livebirth or a stillbirth of more than 20 weeks' gestation. Occasionally, patients exhibit a mixture of viable births interspersed with two or more recurrent abortions.

There is no single increase in MHC antigen frequency between partners suffering recurrent abortions but an increased sharing of MHC antigens has been noted by some workers. It is thought that homozygosity at these loci themselves is not necessarily important but more probably that histocompatibility genes or analogues of developmental genes found in rodents, such as the T/t or the grc complex, close to or in genetic disequilibrium with these loci are responsible. These hypotheses are controversial and unproven. The histoincompatibility theory for fetal allograft survival and the importance of production of blocking antibodies has led to the introduction of immunotherapy, such as transfusion of partner's leucocytes, pooled third party leucocytes, seminal plasma and trophoblast microvillous preparations, to stimulate HLA antibodies as a treatment for recurrent abortions (Hill 1990). This is analogous to the use of pretransplantation transfusions to improve allograft survival in renal transplantation. Carefully controlled clinical trials are needed to evaluate their efficacy.

Pre-eclampsia

Pre-eclampsia is predominantly a disorder of first pregnancies and a change in partner increases the risk in the parous woman. The incidence is diminished by previous abortions and blood transfusions but these observations are being questioned. Nevertheless, the resulting suggestion is that prior exposure to histocompatibility antigens either on the major histocompatibility complex or linked to it leads to a protective immunological mechanism. The risk of developing pre-eclampsia is not associated with any specific major histocompatibility complex antigen and the finding of sharing of MHC antigens between mother and father is disputed.

The theory, therefore, is similar to that of recurrent abortions and while the speculation for an immunological basis for these disorders is strong, supportive evidence is either completely lacking or contradictory.

Morphological Correlates of Pregnancy Immunology

The development of trophoblast-induced morphological changes in the spiral arteries in the placental bed in normal pregnancy has been contrasted with their absence in pre-eclampsia (see above). These pregnancy-induced vascular changes and trophoblast migration are also deficient in spontaneous abortion (Khong et al. 1987a; Michel et al. 1990; Hustin et al. 1990). One argument proposes that maternofetal interaction, putatively immunologically mediated, operates either physiologically to allow trophoblast migration and interaction with the arteries or pathologically to impede it. Proof of this is lacking, however.

Complement activation and deposition on trophoblastic basement membrane has been reported in normal pregnancy and appears to be amplified in pre-eclampsia (Faulk 1988). Deposition of complement components has been described in the uteroplacental arteries as well as in the spiral arteries in pre-eclamptic or diabetic women (Wells et al. 1987). These findings suggest that immunological phenomena are part of the normal processes of pregnancy.

Two lesions thought to be histological hallmarks of "fetal immune aggression" are acute atherosis and villitis of unknown aetiology (Labarrere 1989). Acute atherosis has been reported in pre-eclampsia and has been claimed to be seen in normal pregnancies terminated in the first trimester but this has been disputed by others. The possibility of an immunological pathogenesis of the lesion is suggested by the morphological similarity of this lesion to that seen in allograft rejection (Khong 1991) and by clinical parameters (Khong et al. 1987b). Labarrere and his colleagues (1985a) have found immunoglobulin (IgM) and complement (C3) in acute atherotic lesions similar to the findings in atherosis-like lesions from rejected renal and cardiac transplants, leading them to speculate that acute atherosis is primarily an immunologically determined vasculopathy. They have suggested that development of acute atherosis is due to complement-fixing immune complexes along with a T-cell or natural killer maternal aggression on fetal tissues. However, the perivascular cell infiltrate is similar to that seen around vessels with physiological changes and those without physiological changes but also without acute atherosis (Khong 1987).

Villitis of unknown aetiology is seen frequently in placentas from pregnancies complicated by pre-eclampsia, intrauterine growth retardation and maternal autoimmune disease but have also been described in normal term placentas, again suggesting that immunopathology is part of the normal phenomenon in pregnancy (Labarrere et al. 1990). Villitis areas were found to be filled by activated macrophages and helper-T lymphocytes, the reasons for which could be infection, allogeneic recognition reactions or scavenger functions in putative areas of avascular necrosis.

Overall, therefore, while the theoretical basis for a role for immunology in pregnancy is attractive, the evidence is far from conclusive.

References

Abramowsky CR, Vegas ME, Swinehart G, Gyves MT (1980) Decidual vasculopathy of the placenta in lupus erythematosus. N Engl J Med 303: 668–672

Aherne W, Dunnill MS (1982) Morphometry. Arnold, London

Althabe O, Labarrere C (1985) Chronic villitis of unknown aetiology and intrauterine growth-retarded infants of normal and low ponderal index. Placenta 6: 369–373

Althabe O, Labarrere C, Telenta M (1985) Maternal vascular lesions in placentae of small-for-gestational-age infants. Placenta 6: 265–276

Altshuler G (1984) Chorangiosis. An important sign of neonatal morbidity and mortality. Arch Pathol Lab Med 108: 71–74

Altshuler G, Russell P (1975) The human villitides; a review of chronic intrauterine infection. Springer, Berlin, pp 63–112

Andres RL, Kuyper W, Resnik R, Piacquadio KM, Benirschke K (1990) The association of maternal floor infarction of the placenta with adverse perinatal outcome. Am J Obstet Gynecol 163: 935–938

Baill IC, Moore GW, Hendrick LA (1989) Abscess of allantoic duct remnant. Am J Obstet Gynecol 161: 334–336

Baill IC, Witter FR (1990) Sickle trait and its association with birthweight and urinary tract infections in pregnancy. Int J Gynaecol Obstet 33: 19–21

Bain C, Elliot BW (1976) Fetal distress in the first stage of labour associated with early fetal heart decelerations and a short umbilical cord. Aust NZ J Obstet Gynaecol 16: 51–56

Batcup G, Holt P, Hambling MH, Gerlis LM, Glass MR (1985) Placental and fetal pathology in Coxsackie virus A9 infection: a case report. Histopathology 9: 1227–1235

Bendon RW, Ray MB (1986) The pathologic findings of the fetal membranes in very prolonged amniotic fluid leakage. Arch Pathol Lab Med 110: 47–50

Benirschke K, Driscoll S (1976) The pathology of the human placenta. Springer, Berlin

Birkenfeld A, Mordel N, Okon E (1989) Direct demonstration of iron in a placenta in a case of β-thalassemia major. Am J Obstet Gynecol 160: 562–563

Björk O, Persson B (1982) Placental changes in relation to the degree of metabolic control in diabetes mellitus. Placenta 3: 367–378

Björk O, Persson B (1984) Villous structure in different parts of the cotyledon in placentas of insulin-dependent diabetic women. Acta Obstet Gynecol Scand 63: 37–43

Blanc WA (1981) Pathology of the placenta, membranes and umbilical cord in bacterial, fungal and viral infections in man. In: Naeye RL, Kissane JM, Kaufman N (eds) Perinatal disease. Williams and Wilkins, Baltimore, pp 67–132

Bleker OP, Kloosterman GJ, Breur W, Mieras DJ (1977) The volumetric growth of the human placenta: a longitudinal ultrasonic study. Am J Obstet Gynecol 127: 657–661

Blickstein I, Shoham-Schwartz Z, Lancet M (1987) Predisposing factors in the formation of true knots of the umbilical cord—analysis of morphometric and perinatal data. Int J Gynaecol Obstet 25: 395–398

Boyd JD, Hamilton WJ (1970) The human placenta. Heffer, Cambridge

Boyd PA (1984) Quantitative structure of the normal human placenta from ten weeks of gestation to term. Early Hum Dev 9: 297–307

Boyd PA, Scott A (1985) Quantitative structural studies in human placentas associated with pre-eclampsia, essential hypertension and intrauterine growth retardation. Br J Obstet Gynaecol 92: 714–721

Boyd PA, Brown R, Stewart W (1980) Quantitative structural differences within the normal term human placenta: a pilot study. Placenta 1: 337–344

Boyd PA, Scott A, Keeling JW (1986) Quantitative structural studies on placentas from pregnancies complicated by diabetes mellitus. Br J Obstet Gynaecol 93: 31–35

Bryan EM (1986) The intrauterine hazards of twins. Arch Dis Child 61: 1044–1045

Bruyniks N, Khong TY, Leong R (1988) Relation of site of umbilical cord insertion and birth weight. J Obstet Gynaecol 9: 34–35

Bulmer JN, Johnson PM (1983) Antigen expression by trophoblast populations in the human placenta and their possible immunobiological relevance. Placenta 6: 127–140

Burton GJ, Palmer ME, Dalton KJ (1989) Morphometric differences between the placental vasculature of nonsmokers, smokers and ex-smokers. Br J Obstet Gynaecol 96: 907–915

Carter J (1984) The maternal immunological response during pregnancy. In: Clarke JR (ed) Oxford reviews of reproductive biology, vol 6. Clarendon Press, Oxford, 47–128

Christmas SE, Bulmer JN, Meager A, Johnson PM (1990) Phenotypic and functional analysis of human CD3- decidual leucocyte clones. Immunology 71: 182–189

Clark DA, Mowbray J, Underwood J, Liddell H (1987) Histopathologic alteration in the decidua in human spontaneous abortion: loss of cells with large cytoplasmic

granules. Am J Reprod Immunol 13: 19–22
Clarson C, Tevaarwerk GJM, Harding PGR, Chance GW, Haust MD (1989) Placental weight in diabetic pregnancies. Placenta 10: 275–281
Clausen I (1989) Umbilical cord anomalies and antenatal fetal deaths. Obstet Gynecol Surv 44: 841–845
Clewell WH, Manchester DK (1983) Recurrent maternal floor infarction: a preventable cause of fetal death. Am J Obstet Gynecol 147: 346–347
Coid CR, Fox H (1983) Short review: campylobacters as placental pathogens. Placenta 4: 295–306
Costoya AL, Leontic EA, Rosenberg HG, Delgado MA (1980) Morphological study of placental terminal villi in intrahepatic cholestasis of pregnancy: histochemistry, light and electron microscopy. Placenta 1: 361–368
Danskin FH, Neilson JP (1989) Twin-to-twin transfusion syndrome: what are appropriate criteria? Am J Obstet Gynecol 161: 365–369
Davey DA, MacGillivray I (1988) The classification and definition of the hypertensive disorders of pregnancy. Am J Obstet Gynecol 158: 892–898
Denmead DT, Ariagno RL, Carson SH, Benirschke KB (1987) Placental pathology is not predictive for sudden infant death syndrome (SIDS). Am J Perinatol 4: 308–312
Dildy GA III, Moise KJ Jr, Carpenter RJ Jr, Klima T (1989) Maternal malignancy metastatic to the products of conception. Obstet Gynecol Surv 44: 535–540
Dougall A, Baird CH (1987) Vasa praevia—report of three cases and review of literature. Br J Obstet Gynaecol 94: 712–715
Edmonds DK, Lindsay KS, Miller JF, Williamson E, Wood PJ (1982) Early embryonic mortality in women. Fertil Steril 38: 447–453
Ellis SA, Sargent IL, Redman CWG, McMichael AJ (1986) Evidence for a novel HLA antigen found on human extravillous trophoblast and a choriocarcinoma cell line. Immunology 59: 595–601
Ellis SA, Palmer MS, McMichael AJ (1990) Human trophoblast and the choriocarcinoma cell line BeWo express a truncated HLA class I molecule. J Immunol 144: 731–735
Faulk WP (1988) Haemostasis and fibrinolysis in human normal placentae: possible role in early pregnancy failure. In: Beard RW, Sharp F (eds) Early pregnancy loss. Mechanisms and treatment. Peacock Press, Ashton-under-Lyne, pp 193–198
Faulk WP, Temple A, Lovins R, Smith NC (1978) Antigens of human trophoblast: a working hypothesis for their role in normal and abnormal pregnancies. Proc Natl Acad Sci USA 75: 1947–1951
Ferry BL, Starkey PM, Sargent IL, Watt GMO, Jackson M, Redman CWG (1990) Cell populations in the human early pregnancy decidua: natural killer activity and response to interleukin-2 of CD56-positive large granular lymphocytes. Immunology 70: 446–452
Fizet D, Bousquet J (1983) Absence of a factor blocking a cellular cytotoxicity reaction in the serum of women with recurrent abortions. Br J Obstet Gynaecol 90: 453–456
Fox H (1969) Pathology of the placenta in maternal diabetes mellitus. Obstet Gynecol 34: 792–798
Fox H (1978) Pathology of the placenta. Saunders, London
Fox H, Langley FA (1971) Leucocytic infiltration of the placenta and umbilical cord: a clinico-pathologic study. Obstet Gynecol 37: 451–458
Fox H, Laurini RN (1988) Intraplacental choriocarcinoma: a report of 2 cases. J Clin Pathol 41: 1085–1088
Fox H, Sen DK (1972) Placenta extrachorialis: a clinicopathological study. J Obstet Gynaecol Br Cmwlth 79: 32–35
Garcia AGP (1982) Placental morphology of low birth weight infants at term: gross and microscopic study of 50 cases. Contrib Gynecol Obstet 9: 100–112
Garite TJ, Freeman RK (1982) Chorioamnionitis in the preterm gestation. Obstet Gynecol 59: 538–545
Geirsson RT, Ogston SA, Patel NB, Christie AD (1985) Growth of total intrauterine, intra-amniotic and placental volume in normal singleton pregnancy measured by ultrasound. Br J Obstet Gynaecol 92: 46–53
Gough JD, Keeling JW, Castle B, Iliff PJ (1986) The obstetric management of non-immunological hydrops. Br J Obstet Gynaecol 93: 226–234
Gregory CD, Lee H, Rees GB, Scott IV, Shah LP, Golding PR (1985) Natural killer cells in normal pregnancy: analysis using monoclonal antibodies and single-cell cytotoxicity assays. Clin Exp Immunol 62: 121–127
Gruenwald P (1975) The supply line of the fetus: definitions relating to fetal growth. In: Gruenwald P (ed) The placenta and its maternal supply line. MTP, Lancaster, pp 1–7
Hallam LA, McLaren KM, El-Jabbour JN, Helm CW, Smart GE (1990) Intraplacental choriocarcinoma: a case report. Placenta 11: 247–251
Harris BA Jr, Gore H, Flowers CE (1985) Peripheral placental separation: a possible relationship to premature labour. Obstet Gynecol 66: 774–778
Haust MD (1981) Maternal diabetes mellitus—effects of the fetus and placenta. Monogr Pathol 22: 201–285
Head JR, Drake BL, Zuckermann FA (1987) Major histocompatibility antigens on trophoblast and their regulation: implications in the maternal-fetal relationship. Am J Reprod Immunol Microbiol 15: 12–18
Heifetz SA (1984) Strangulation of the umbilical cord by amniotic bands: report of 6 cases and literature review. Pediatr Pathol 2: 285–304
Heifetz SA (1988) Thrombosis of the umbilical cord: analysis of 52 cases and literature review. Pediatr Pathol 8: 37–54
Herring AJ, Anderson IE, McClenaghan M et al. (1987) Restriction endonuclease analysis of DNA from two isolates of *Chlamydia psittaci* obtained from human abortion. Br Med J 295: 1239
Hill JA (1990) Immunological mechanisms of pregnancy maintenance and failure: a critique of theories and therapy. Am J Reprod Immunol 22: 33–41
Ho PC, Haynes WDG, Ing RMY, Jones WR (1982) Histological, ultrastructural and immunofluorescence studies on the amniochorionic membrane. Placenta 3: 109–126
Hunt JS (1989) Macrophages in human uteroplacental tissues. A review. Am J Reprod Immunol 21: 119–122
Hunt JS (1990) Current topic: the role of macrophages in the uterine response to pregnancy. Placenta 11: 467–475
Hurley VA, Beischer NA (1987) Placenta membranacea. Case reports. Br J Obstet Gynaecol 94: 798–802
Hustin J, Jauniaux E, Schaaps JP (1990) Histological study of the materno-embryonic interface in spontaneous abortion. Placenta 11: 477–486
Hyde S, Smotherman J, Moore JI, Altshuler G (1989) A model of bacterially induced umbilical vein spasm, relevant to fetal hypoperfusion. Obstet Gynecol 73: 966–970
Jauniaux E, Nessmann C, Imbert MC, Meuris S, Puissant F, Hustin J (1988) Morphological aspects of the placenta in HIV pregnancies. Placenta 9: 633–642
Jauniaux E, Zucker M, Meuris S, Verhest A, Wilkin P, Hustin J (1988) Chorangiocarcinoma: an unusual tumour

of the placenta. The missing link? Placenta 9: 607–613
Jones CJP, Lendon M, Chawner LE, Jauniaux E (1990) Ultrastructure of the human placenta in metabolic storage disease. Placenta 11: 395–411
Jones KL (1988) Smith's recognizable patterns of human malformation. Saunders, London
Katz V, Blanchard G, Dingman C, Bowes WA, Cefalo RC (1987) Atenolol and short umbilical cords. Am J Obstet Gynecol 156: 1271–1272
Kaufmann P (1982) Development and differentiation of the human placental villous tree. Bibl Anat 22: 29–39
Khong TY (1987) Immunohistologic study of the leukocytic infiltrate in maternal uterine tissues in normal and pre-eclamptic pregnancies at term. Am J Reprod Immunol 15: 1–8
Khong TY (1991) Acute atherosis in pregnancies complicated by hypertension, small-for-gestational-age infants, and diabetes mellitus. Arch Pathol Lab Med 115: 722–725
Khong TY, Dilly SA (1989) Calcification of umbilical artery: two distinct lesions. J Clin Pathol 42: 931–934
Khong TY, George K (1992) Chromosomal abnormalities associated with single umbilical artery. Prenat Diagn, (in press)
Khong TY, Robertson WB (1987) Placenta creta and placenta praevia creta. Placenta 8: 399–409
Khong TY, De Wolf F, Robertson WB, Brosens I (1986) Inadequate maternal vascular response to placentation in pregnancies complicated by pre-eclampsia and by small-for-gestational-age infants. Br J Obstet Gynaecol 93: 1049–1059
Khong TY, Liddell HS, Robertson WB (1987a) Defective haemochorial placentation as a cause of spontaneous miscarriage: a preliminary study. Br J Obstet Gynaecol 94: 649–655
Khong TY, Pearce JM, Robertson WB (1987b) Acute atherosis in pre-eclampsia: maternal determinants and fetal outcomes in the presence of the lesion. Am J Obstet Gynecol 157: 360–363
Khudr G, Benirschke K (1972) Placental lesions in viral hepatitis. Obstet Gynecol 40: 381–384
King A, Birkby C, Loke YW (1989) Early human decidual cells exhibit NK activity against the K562 cell line but not against first trimester trophoblast. Cell Immunol 118: 337–344
Knowles S, Frost T (1989) Umbilical cord sclerosis as an indicator of congenital syphilis. J Clin Pathol 42: 1157–1159
Knox WF, Fox H (1984) Villitis of unknown aetiology: its incidence and significance in placentae from a British population. Placenta 5: 395–402
Koller BH, Geraghty DE, DeMars R, Duvick L, Rich SS, Orr HT (1989) Chromosomal organisation of the MHC class I gene family. J Exp Med 169: 469–480
Krohn M, Voigt L, McKnight B, Daling JR, Starzyk P, Benedetti TJ (1987) Correlates of placental abruption. Br J Obstet Gynaecol 94: 333–340
Kullander S, Kallen (1971) A prospective study of smoking and pregnancy. Acta Obstet Gynecol Scand 50: 83–94
Kundsin RB, Driscoll SG, Monson RR, Yeh C, Biano SA, Cochran WD (1984) Association of *Ureaplasma urealyticum* in the placenta with perinatal morbidity and mortality. N Engl J Med 310: 941–945
Labarrere CA (1988) Review article. Acute atherosis: a histopathological hallmark of immune aggression? Placenta 9: 95–108
Labarrere CA (1989) Allogeneic recognition and rejection reactions in the placenta. Am J Reprod Immunol 21: 94–99
Labarrere C, Althabe O, Telenta M (1982) Chronic villitis of unknown aetiology in placentae of idiopathic small for gestational age infants. Placenta 3: 309–318
Labarrere C, Alonso J, Manni J, Domenichini E, Althabe O (1985a) Immunohistochemical findings in acute atherosis associated to intrauterine growth retardation. Am J Reprod Immunol Microbiol 7: 149–155
Labarrere C, Sebastiani M, Siminovich M, Torassa E, Althabe O (1985b) Absence of Wharton's jelly around the umbilical arteries: an unusual cause of perinatal mortality. Placenta 6: 555–559
Labarrere CA, McIntyre JA, Faulk WP (1990) Immunohistologic evidence that villitis in human normal term placentas is an immunologic lesion. Am J Obstet Gynecol 162: 515–522
Lala PK, Kennedy TG, Parhar RS (1988) Suppression of lymphocyte alloreactivity by early gestational human decidua. II Characterization of the suppressor mechanisms. Cell Immunol 116: 411–422
Larsson S, Cronberg S, Winblad S (1979) Listeriosis during pregnancy and neonatal period in Sweden 1958–1984. Acta Paediatr Scand 68: 485–493
Lessin DL, Hunt JS, King CR, Wood GW (1988) Antigen expression by cells near the maternal-fetal interface. Am J Reprod Immunol Microbiol 16: 1–7
Lewis SH, Reynolds-Kohler C, Fox HE, Nelson JA (1990) HIV-1 in trophoblastic and villous Hofbauer cells, and haematological precursors in eight-week fetuses. Lancet 335: 565–568
Lilja M (1991a) Infants with single umbilical artery studied in a national registry. General epidemiological characteristics. Paediatr Perinat Epidemiol 5: 27–36
Lilja M (1991b) Single umbilical artery and maternal smoking. Br Med J 302: 569–570
Lilja M (1991c) Infants with single umbilical artery studied in a national registry 2. Survival and malformations in infants with single umbilical artery. Paediatr Perinat Epidemiol
Lowden JA, Cutz E, Conen PE, Rudd N, Doran TA (1973) Prenatal diagnosis of G_{M1} gangliosidosis. N Engl J Med 288: 225–228
MacGillivray I, Nylander PPS, Corney G (1975) Human multiple reproduction. Saunders, London
Marzusch K, Dietl J, Horny H-P et al. (1991) Tolerance and the fetal graft. Lancet 337: 52
Matorras R, Diez J, Pereira JG (1990) True knots in the umbilical cord: clinical findings and fetal consequences. J Obstet Gynaecol 10: 383–386
Mayhew TM, Burton GJ (1988) Methodological problems in placental morphometry: apologia for the use of stereology based on sound sampling practice. Placenta 9: 565–581
McIntyre JA, Faulk WP (1983) Recurrent spontaneous abortion in human pregnancy: results of immunogenetical, cellular and humoral studies. Am J Reprod Immunol 4: 165–170
Michel MZ, Khong TY, Clark DA, Beard RW (1990) A morphological and immunological study of human placental bed biopsies in miscarriage. Br J Obstet Gynaecol 97: 984–988
Mills JL, Harley EE, Moessinger AC (1983) Standards for measuring umbilical cord length. Placenta 4: 423–426
Minkoff H, Nanda D, Menez R, Fikrig S (1987) Pregnancies resulting in infants with acquired immunodeficiency syndrome or AIDS-related complex. Obstet Gynecol 69: 285–287
Mochizuki M, Maruo T, Masuko K, Ohtsu T (1984) Effects

of smoking on fetoplacental-maternal system during pregnancy. Am J Obstet Gynecol 149: 413–420

Moessinger AC, Blanc WA, Marone PA, Polsen DC (1982) Umbilical cord length as an indicator of fetal activity: experimental study and clinical implications. Pediatr Res 16: 109–112

Moller D, Ipsen L, Asschenfeldt P (1986) Fatal course of malignant melanoma during pregnancy with dissemination to the products of conception. Acta Obstet Gynecol Scand 65: 501–502

Mortimer G, MacDonald DJ, Smeeth A (1985) A pilot study of the frequency and significance of placental villitis. Br J Obstet Gynaecol 92: 629–633

Moscuna M, Gross Z, Korenblum R, Volfson M, Oetinger M (1989) Septic abortion due to *Campylobacter jejuni*. Eur J Clin Microbiol Infect Dis 8: 800–801

Mossman HW (1974) Structural changes in vertebrate fetal membranes associated with the adoption of viviparity. Obstet Gynecol Annu 3: 7–32

Mostofi-Zadeh M, Driscoll SG, Biano SA, Kundsin RB (1984) Placental evidence of cytomegalovirus infection of the fetus and neonate. Arch Pathol Lab Med 108: 403–406

Mowbray JF, Underwood JL (1985) Immunology of abortion. Clin Exp Immunol 60: 1–7

Naeye RL (1977) Placental abnormalities in victims of sudden infant death syndrome. Biol Neonate 32: 189–192

Naeye RL (1978) Effects of maternal cigarette smoking on the fetus and placenta. Br J Obstet Gynecol 85: 732–737

Naeye RL (1980) Placental disorders and smoking. Obstet Gynecol 55: 701–704

Naeye RL (1985a) Maternal floor infarction. Hum Pathol 16: 823–828

Naeye RL (1985b) Umbilical cord length: clinical significance. J Pediatr 107: 278–281

Naeye RL, Blanc W (1970) Relation of poverty and race to antenatal infection. N Engl J Med 283: 558–560

Ogita S, Oka T, Imanaka M et al. (1989) Effect of amniotic fluid volume on umbilical cord length. Asia Oceania J Obstet Gynaecol 15: 203–208

O'Herlihy C, O'Driscoll K (1987) Disease associated with abnormal placenta. In: The human placenta. Lavery JP (ed) Aspen Publishers, Rockville, pp 237–256

Ollendorff DA, Goldberg JM, Abu-Jawdeh GM, Lurain JR (1990) Markedly elevated maternal serum alphafetoprotein associated with a normal fetus and choriocarcinoma of the placenta. Obstet Gynecol 76: 494–497

Peckham CH, Yerulshamy J (1965) Aplasia of one umbilical artery: incidence by race and certain obstetric factors. Obstet Gynecol 26: 359–366

Philippe E, Boué JG (1969) Le placenta dans les abérrations chromosomiques léthales. Ann Anat Pathol 14: 249–266

Pijnenborg R, Bland JM, Robertson WB, Dixon G, Brosens I (1981) The pattern of interstitial trophoblast invasion of the myometrium in early human pregnancy. Placenta 2: 303–316

Popli S, Leehey DJ, Molnar ZV, Nawab ZM, Ing TS (1990) Demonstration of Fabry's disease deposits in placenta. Am J Obstet Gynecol 162: 464–465

Powell HC, Benirschke K, Favara BE, Pfluoger OH Jr (1976) Foamy changes of placental cells in fetal storage disorders. Virchows Arch [A] 369: 191–196

Redman CWG, McMichael AJ, Stirrat GM, Sunderland CA, Ting A (1984) Class I MHC complex antigens on human extravillous trophoblast. Immunology 52: 457–468

Ritson A, Bulmer JN (1989) Isolation and functional studies of granulated lymphocytes in first trimester human decidua. Clin Exp Immunol 77: 263–268

Roberts CJ, Lowe CR (1975) Where have all the conceptions gone? Lancet i: 498–499

Robinson LK, Jones KL, Benirschke K (1983) The nature of structural defects associated with velamentous and marginal insertion of the umbilical. Am J Obstet Gynecol 146: 191–193

Rock JA, Shirey RS, Braine HG, Ness PM, Kickler TS, Niebyl JR (1985) Plasmapheresis for the treatment of repeated early pregnancy wastage associated with anti-P. Obstet Gynecol 66 suppl 3: 57S–60S

Rocklin RE, Kitzmiller J, Carpenter B, Garovoy M, David JR (1976) Maternal-fetal reactions: absence of an immunologic blocking factor from the serum of women with chronic abortions. N Engl J Med 295: 1209–1213

Russell P (1980) Inflammatory lesions of the human placenta. III The histopathology of villitis of unknown aetiology. Placenta 1: 227–244

Russell P, Atkinson K, Krishnan L (1980) Recurrent reproductive failure due to severe placental villitis of unknown etiology. J Reprod Med 24: 93–98

Salafia CM, Mangam HE, Weigl CA, Foye GJ, Silberman L (1989) Abnormal fetal heart rate patterns and placental inflammation. Am J Obstet Gynecol 160: 140–147

Saller DN, Keene CL, Sun C-CJ, Schwartz S (1990) The association of single umbilical artery with cytogenetically abnormal pregnancies. Am J Obstet Gynecol 163:922–925

Sander CH, Kinnane L, Stevens NG, Echt R (1986) Haemorrhagic endovasculitis of the placenta: a review with clinical correlation. Placenta 7: 551–574

Sands J, Dobbing J (1985) Continuing growth and development of the third trimester human placenta. Placenta 6: 13–22

Schoenfeld A, Abramovici A, Klibanski C, Ovadia J (1985) Placental, ultrasonographic, biochemical and histochemical studies in fetuses affected with Niemann–Pick disease type A. Placenta 6: 33–44

Schuhmann RA, Wynn RM (1980) Regional ultrastructural differences in placental villi in cotyledons of a mature human placenta. Placenta 1: 345–353

Shanklin DR, Scott JS (1975) Massive subchorial thrombohaematoma (Breus' mole). Br J Obstet Gynaecol 82: 476–487

Shen-Schwarz S, Ruchelli E, Brown D (1989) Villous oedema of the placenta: a clinicopathological study. Placenta 10: 297–307

Simor AE, Karmali MA, Jadaviji T, Roscoe M (1986) Abortion and perinatal sepsis associated with campylobacter infection. Rev Infect Dis 8: 397–402

Soernes T, Bakke T (1987) The length of the human umbilical cord in twin pregnancies. Am J Obstet Gynecol 157: 1229–1230

Sprecher S, Soumenkoff S, Puissant F, Degueldre M (1986) Vertical transmission of HIV in 15-week fetus. Lancet ii: 288–289

Strong SJ, Corney G (1967) The placenta in twin pregnancy. Pergamon, Oxford

Teasdale F (1980) Gestational changes in the functional structural of the human placenta in relation to fetal growth. Am J Obstet Gynecol 137: 560–568

Tuchmann-Duplessis H, David G, Haezel P (1971) Illustrated human embryology, vol 1. Springer, New York; Chapman and Hall, London; Masson et Cie, Paris

Uyanwah-Akpom P, Fox H (1977) The clinical significance of marginal and velamentous insertion of the cord. Br J Obstet Gynaecol 84: 941–943

Van der Veen F, Fox H (1982) The effects of cigarette smoking on the human placenta: a light and electron microscopic study. Placenta 3: 243–256

Van der Veen F, Fox H (1983) The human placenta in idiopathic intrauterine growth retardation: a light and electron microscopic study. Placenta 4: 65–78

Van der Velde WJ, Peereboom-Stegeman JHJC, Treffers PE, James J (1983) Structural changes in the placenta of smoking mothers: a quantitative study. Placenta 4: 231–240

Wells M, Bennett J, Bulmer JN, Jackson P, Holgate CS (1987) Complement component deposition in uteroplacental (spiral) arteries in normal human pregnancy. J Reprod Immunol 12: 125–135

Wharton B, Edwards JH, Cameron AH (1968) Monoamniotic twins. J Obstet Gynaecol Br Cmwlth 75: 158–163

Wigglesworth J (1964) Morphological variations in the insufficient placenta. J Obstet Gynaecol Br Cmwlth 71: 871–884

Wilkin P (1965) Pathologie du placenta. Masson et Cie, Paris

Zaaijman J duT, Wilkinson AR, Keeling JW, Mitchell RG, Turnbull AC (1982) Spontaneous premature rupture of the membranes: bacteriology, histology and neonatal outcome. J Obstet Gynecol 2: 155–160

Zhang J, Kraus FT, Aquino TI (1985) Chorioamnionitis: a comparative histologic, bacteriologic, and clinical study. Int J Gynecol Pathol 4: 1–10

Chapter 3

Spontaneous Abortion and the Pathology of Early Pregnancy

Simon Knowles

Spontaneous Abortion

Careful pathological studies of spontaneous abortion material are few and our understanding of the pathogenesis of abortion is correspondingly poor. The examination of abortuses is often delegated to the most junior pathologist, hence the widespread belief that there is little to gain from such studies. However, pathology departments do have a useful role to play in the management of abortion. In cases of repeated abortion, pathological abnormalities in mother or fetus may point to a treatable cause. Some abortion specimens may yield information which will modify maternal management, in cases of infection or trophoblast neoplasia for example. Accurate description of aborted material may help to elucidate obscure mechanisms involved in this most common of pregnancy complications. With a trend towards smaller families, later in life and with earlier bonding to a fetus often visualised by ultrasound in the first trimester, the emotional impact of spontaneous abortion is greater than ever. For all these reasons, simple products of conception should perhaps be treated more seriously in the diagnostic pathology laboratory.

Frequency of Spontaneous Abortion

Spontaneous abortion is the commonest complication of pregnancy. Assessment of its incidence varies according to the method of ascertainment used in a given study. The peak gestational age for spontaneous abortion which is recognised by parents is between 8 and 12 weeks. Some 50% of abortions occur at this time, representing 10% of recognised pregnancies (Roman and Stevenson 1983). The reason for stressing recognition of pregnancy here is that there is evidence that many gestations abort before the pregnancy is clinically apparent. Careful examination of hysterectomy specimens (Hertig et al. 1936, Hertig et al. 1959, James 1970) or the estimation of chorionic gonadotrophic levels in women trying to become pregnant (Miller et al. 1980) suggest that approximately 50% of zygotes perish after conception (Opitz 1987). Since 20% of recognised pregnancies abort spontaneously, it is reasonable to assume that 30% of conceptuses have already been lost during the first 2 months after fertilisation. The accuracy of such figures is pivotal to the assessment of the safety of prenatal diagnostic techniques (Simpson 1990) but from a practical point of view, only products of recognised gestations are likely to come to the attention of the pathologist. The remainder of this section will therefore be largely limited to a discussion of studies on this population, although it should be understood that such cases represent less than half of early pregnancy wastage.

Recurrent Abortion

The term habitual or recurrent abortion is generally defined as where a couple has had three or more consecutive abortions. The risk of subsequent abortion in this population has been quoted as 80%–90% (Malpas 1938). This risk and the concept of the habitual aborter have been accepted as the basis for many trials of the management of recurrent abortion. However, there are cogent arguments for believing that this view is erroneous, and that the risk of abortion in a pregnancy following spontaneous abortion is independent of the number of preceding abortions (Warburton and Fraser 1964). This risk is about 25%–30% in women with one liveborn infant (Warburton and Fraser 1964) and over 40% where there is no living child (Poland et al. 1977). Nevertheless, the clinical problem of the couple who have suffered multiple miscarriage is a genuine and tragic one which demands special care and scrupulous investigation.

Recurrent abortion may occur before clinically apparent pregnancy and the condition blends imperceptibly with that of clinical infertility. Some of the causes of suboptimal pregnancy are also relevant to 'the study of infertility. Many factors have been implicated in the genesis of recurrent abortion; some of these are listed in Table 3.1.

The investigation of a women with recurrent abortion will depend on a variety of factors including the gestational age at the time of the abortions, maternal age, the presence of chromosome abnormalities in the abortuses and general maternal health (Elias and Simpson 1980). An important factor, emphasised by Simpson (1981), is that there is little point in invasive investigation of the maternal genital tract unless anatomical and genetic abnormalities of the conceptuses have been excluded. This highlights the need for careful examination of the products of conception from such women. Only after such an examination should endometrial biopsy and hysteroscopy or hysterosalpingography be contemplated. A scheme for the investigation of recurrent abortion is shown in Table 3.2. Although habitual abortion tends to be treated as a special problem, much of its pathobiology resembles that of miscarriage in general "only more so" and the issue of recurrent miscarriage is raised wherever indicated under the general discussion of the problem of spontaneous abortion below.

Table 3.1. Causes of repeated spontaneous abortion (after Simpson 1981)

Before pregnancy is apparent
Fetal anomaly (Hertig et al. 1936)
Luteal phase insufficiency (Cline 1979)
Ectopic pregnancy (Schenker et al. 1972; DeCherney et al. 1985)
Predominantly first trimester
Chromosome anomalies (Mennuti et al. 1978)
Luteal phase insufficiency (Tho et al. 1979)
Immunological factors (Mowbray et al. 1985)
Predominantly second trimester
Anatomical defects of uterus (Jones and Wheeless 1969)
Uterine leiomyomas (Malone and Ingersoll 1975)
Cervical incompetence (Hughey and McElin 1979)
First and second trimester
Mycoplasma and other infections (Stevenson 1977; Stray-Pedersen et al. 1977, 1978)

Table 3.2. Investigation of parents in recurrent abortion (modified from Mowbray et al. 1985)

Causes	Studies
Infective	Serology for Brucella and Toxoplasma
	Culture of cervical swab for cytomegalovirus, herpes simplex, Chlamydia and Mycoplasma
Metabolic/endocrine	Serum thyroxine
	Random blood glucose
	Endometrial biopsy for luteal phase insufficiency
Anatomical	Assessment of cervical incompetence, leiomyomas and anomalies of corpus uteri
Genetic	Parental chromosome examination with banding studies
Immunological	Maternal antibodies against paternal lymphocytes

N.B. These studies should only be initiated after detailed anatomical, chromosomal and microbiological examination of aborted material.

Criminal Abortion

With the present liberal attitude to legal termination of unwanted pregnancy, criminally procured abortion is uncommon in the UK and many other First World countries. However, this is not the case in many Third World countries and there is a sinister increase in illegal abortion even in more liberal countries due to an increasing demand for "feminist" abortion services that are seen to be more sympathetic to the mother than those provided by conventional public or private utilities.

Where there is any clinical suspicion of unauthorised interference, it is mandatory that the specimens, whether delivered "spontaneously" or by subsequent curettage, be sent to the pathology department unfixed. There is major risk of sepsis following criminal abortion, and the examination must include microbiological studies. A plan of investigations is outlined in Table 3.3.

Table 3.3. Examination in suspected criminal abortion (after Rushton 1981)

Exclude injection of foreign material into amniotic fluid
- Sample amniotic fluid
- Examine surface of fetus and placenta
- Take placenta and fetal lung for histological assessment

Exclude injury caused by introduction of instruments
- Examine placenta, membranes and fetus

Exclude infection with risk to mother
- Take bacteria samples of membranes, placental and fetal lungs

Assess gestational age
- Weigh and measure wherever possible
- Take fetal organs for histological assessment

Documentation
- Carefully describe and photograph specimens, including evidence of trauma etc.

Causes of Spontaneous Abortion

Chromosome Abnormality

Chromosome anomalies are a frequent finding in spontaneous abortions with or without demonstrable fetal abnormality. Although the mechanism of expulsion is far from clear, the vast majority of chromosome abnormalities result in abortion rather than progression to term. Those aneuploidies that are liveborn constitute a small and unrepresentative proportion of all chromosomally abnormal pregnancies. The literature of cytogenetics of pregnancy wastage has been reviewed elsewhere (Boué et al. 1985; Creasy 1988).

Aborted fetuses with chromosome abnormalities differ in two respects from the liveborn aneuploidies familiar to paediatricians. Firstly, phenotypic anomalies may be different in aborted specimens; for example, the phenotype of Turner syndrome survivors is characterised by features which are far removed from those of the grossly hydropic mid-trimester abortus (see Fig. 4.17). More importantly, the types of chromosome abnormality which dominate early fetal wastage are rarely seen at term. For example, trisomy 16 represents 15% of all chromosome defects in abortuses and 30% of all trisomic conceptuses but is not seen at term (Warburton et al. 1980).

Chromosome abnormality tends to cause abortion early in pregnancy. Over 50% of successfully karyotyped abortions in the first trimester are aneuploid, whereas after 20 weeks only about 10% of spontaneously aborted fetuses have chromosome anomalies (Creasy et al. 1976; Warburton et al. 1980). Survival beyond the first trimester depends upon the nature of the abnormality. One-third of trisomies persist beyond the 15th week, whereas only 10% of triploid pregnancies continue beyond this point (Creasy et al. 1976). There is evidence to suggest that chromosome anomalies do not commonly lead to expulsion until the 8th week of gestation or later. Analysis of very early abortuses from gestations of 7 weeks or less reveals few aneuploid karyotypes (Warburton et al. 1980).

Trisomy is generally due to an error in maternal gametogenesis. Such errors occur more frequently with advancing maternal age. Autosomal trisomies represent one-quarter of the abnormalities seen in younger women but three-quarters of those in the older mother. Interestingly, trisomy 16 does not show this age-related effect and the factors causing this condition are not clear. Cytogenetic analysis of consecutive miscarriages suggests that some couples have a higher tendency than expected for trisomic conception, though the trisomies may be of different chromosomes (Hassold 1980). If maternal age is taken into account, these effects are less definite (Warburton et al. 1987). Triploidy can result from dispermic fertilisation of a normal oocyte, fertilisation by a diploid spermatocyte or fertilisation of a diploid oocyte by a normal spermatozoon. The phenotype appears to depend on whether the fetus receives its double dose of chromosomes from the maternal or paternal side (Kalousek et al. 1990). The rarer structural abnormalities such as deletions and inversions generally seem to arise spontaneously or from balanced anomalies in either of the parents (Jacobs and Hassold 1980). In general, karyotyping of both parents is worthwhile in these cases. The origin of monosomy X is less clear.

Infection

Theoretically, infection could be introduced into the gestation by carriage in the spermatozoon or by direct spread from the endometrium or fallopian tubes. However, the common routes are haematogenous, causing villitis and fetal infection, or ascending infection of the maternal genital tract causing chorionamnionitis (Blanc 1981). An important and preventable cause of chorioamnionitis is the direct introduction of pathogens during chorionic villus sampling, amniocentesis or fetoscopy (Blanc 1981). It is difficult, particularly in early abortion, to separate the direct effects of pathogens on the gestation from the effects of pyrexial illness in the mother. It is also difficult to assess the quantitative impact of infection upon pregnancy wastage; however, in *Homo sapiens* it seems to be slight. Information on most infections is incomplete, and many of the studies have been based on clinical evidence of infection in either mother or fetus. Organisms which have been repeatedly isolated in cases of spontaneous abortion are listed in Table 3.4. This list is far from complete, and many other agents, particularly influenza and Coxsackie viruses and more recently Herpes simplex type 2 (Bujko 1988), have been implicated in spontaneous abortion. Based on a prospective study of intravenous drug users, there currently seems to be little reason to suppose that Human Immunodefficiency Virus causes miscarriage or other complications of pregnancy (Selwyn et al. 1989).

Parvovirus infection is becoming increasingly well recognised as a cause of non-rhesus hydrops fetalis and fetal death (Anand et al. 1987; Kinney et al. 1988) and transplacental infection by parvovirus B19 has been documented by electron microscopy (Caul et al. 1988) and in situ hybridization (Porter et al. 1988). From a numerical point of view, the most important virus to cause fetal wastage is rubella, not as a cause of spontaneous abortion but because of the number of pregnancies that continue to be terminated to prevent congenital anomaly. Infection in pregnancy, with examination of the roles of the more important agents, is well reviewed by Peckham and Marshall (1983).

Table 3.4. Placental infection

Chorionamnionitis—ascending infection	
Bacteria	*Escherichia coli*
	Staphylococcus aureus
	Haemophilus vaginalis
	Streptococcus sp
	Klebsiella
	Pseudomonas sp
	Listeria monocytogenes
Viruses	Herpes simplex
Other	Mycoplasma
	Ureoplasma
	Candida albicans
Villitis—haematogenous infection	
Bacteria	*Listeria monocytogenes*
	Mycobacterium tuberculosis
	Treponema pallidum
	(pyogenic cocci and Gram-negative organisms rarely)
Viruses	Rubella
	Cytomegalovirus
	Parvovirus
	Herpes simplex
	Hepatitis B
	Human immunodeficiency virus
	Epstein–Barr virus
Other	Toxoplasma
	Malaria
	Trypanosomes
	Filaria

The use of live vaccines during early pregnancy carries a theoretical risk of fetal infection and death. Transplacental passage has been shown for rubella vaccine (Banatvala et al. 1981). However, a series of 112 seronegative woman were vaccinated against rubella between 8 and 16 weeks of pregnancy and none of the gestations suffered ill effect (Preblud et al. 1981). With regard to other live vaccines, there are insufficient data on yellow fever; vaccinia is not in current use; rabies vaccine is mandatory in all cases of exposure irrespective of gravidity; and in polio a killed vaccine is available.

Listeria monocytogenes has been identified in the public eye with stillbirth and neonatal death but is less often recognised as a cause of midtrimester fetal loss although this is the period during which it has its major impact: the majority of cases occur between 14 and 30

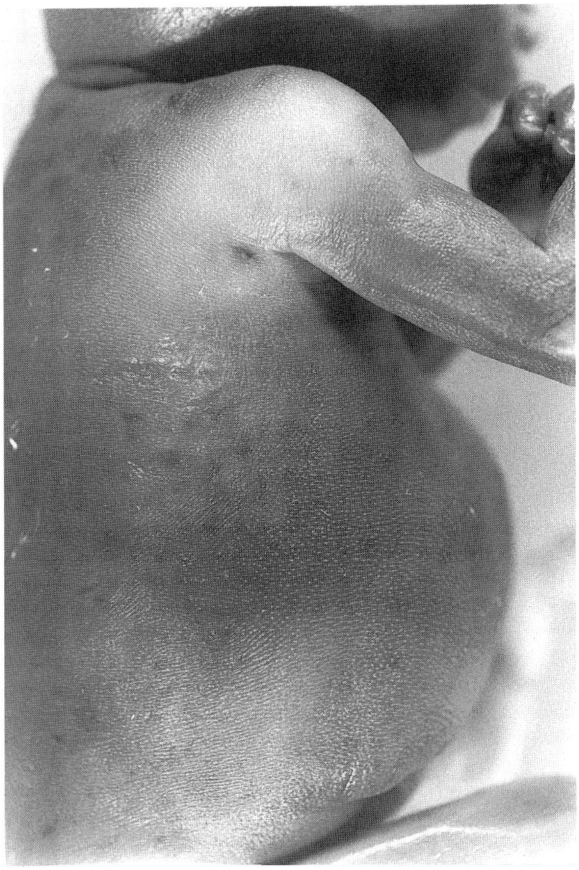

Fig. 3.1. An 18 week fetus with proven listeriosis showing only petechial skin haemorrhages with none of the more typical pustules asocaited with the disease.

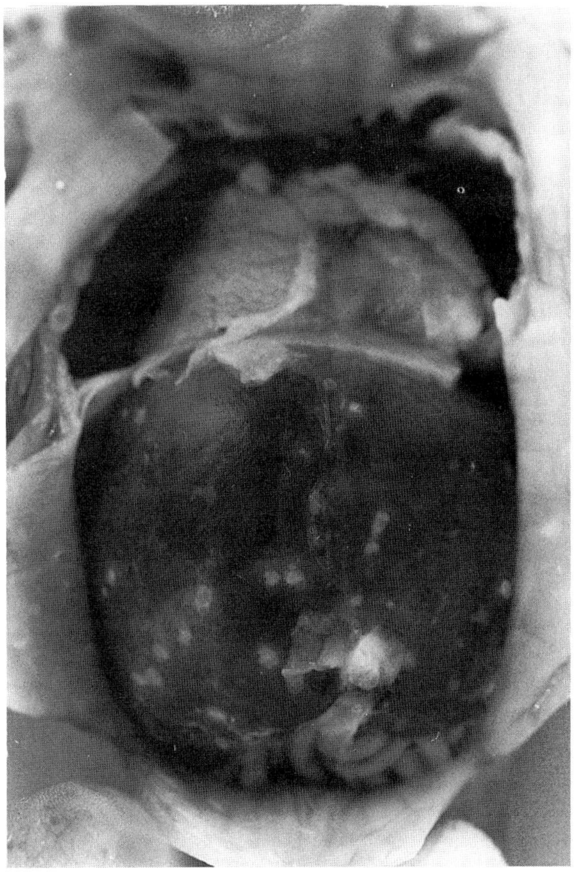

Fig. 3.2. Internal examination of the fetus from Fig. 3.1 shows hepatomagaly and well-defined foci of suppuration.

weeks' gestation (Bortolussi et al. 1990). Unless the possibility of listeria is considered in all midtrimester losses, some cases will escape detection. The fetuses may well be severely macerated and do not always show the characteristic skin lesions or lesions of the liver and lung that usually raise the pathologist's suspicion (Figs. 3.1 and 3.2). In order to avoid missing cases of listeria, it is good practice to swab placentas routinely and to set up cultures of swab and placental tissue for cold enrichment. Although the organism is not fastidious, it occasionally takes several weeks for a positive culture to reveal itself. Benirschke reports seeing a case of congenital listeriosis in the child of a microbiology technologist and makes a legitimate plea for special vigilance when laboratory staff are pregnant (Benirschke and Kaufman 1990). Anti-listeriolysin O titres are said to be of value in establishing the serodiagnosis (Berche et al. 1990).

Although it has been suggested that listeria is a blood-borne infection, because of the marked villositis that is generally present (Steele and Jacobs 1979), the precise route of infection has not been determined. It has been suggested that the initial route may be as an ascending infection with subsequent maternal haematogenous spread after a period of replication in the fetus (Spencer 1987; Bortolussi and Seeliger 1990). The disproportionately advanced autolysis seen in some fetuses and the presence of a heavy chorionamnionitis are both factors which lend weight to this argument. The particular susceptibility to listeria shown by the fetus may be related to low levels of fetal interferons (Bortolussi et al. 1989).

Helicobacter, previously named *Campylobacter jejuni*, has been associated with spontaneous abortion and stillbirth in case reports; its true role is not yet understood. In a series from North America, only 10 cases of clinical infection were seen in 24 000 pregnancies and only two of these led to premature labour or neonatal infection (Simor and Ferro 1990). This contrasts with the high carriage rate seen in the upper gastrointestinal tract of asymptomatic adults.

From the pathologist's point of view, few organisms cause specific or characteristic pathological changes in fetus or placenta, and unequivocal identification of an infective agent requires microbiological studies. The histological changes in the placenta in infection are discussed in Chapter 2.

Contraception

In a large prospective study (Harlap et al. 1980) of women on different contraceptives, a twofold increase in risk of first and second trimester abortion was seen where pregnancy had occurred in the presence of an intrauterine contraceptive device (IUCD). There was no demonstrable difference between different brands of IUCDs in this series. In this study there was also an increased risk associated with pregnancy resulting from oral contraceptive failure. In these cases the risk was to first trimester pregnancies only. Oral contraception, when discontinued at least 1 month prior to the last menstrual period was not associated with a statistically increased abortion risk and there is no increased risk of other pregnancy complications (Speroff 1989).

There is evidence that if an IUCD is removed shortly after pregnancy has been recognised, the rate of abortion falls (Tatum et al. 1976) but remains approximately twice that of non-users (Skjeldestad et al. 1988). The use of the sheath or rhythm methods has no impact on abortion, and the use of the diaphragm appears to reduce the incidence of second trimester pregnancy loss (Harlap et al. 1980).

Maternal Disease—General

Both essential hypertension and pre-eclampsia predispose to late abortion. Congenital heart disease in the mother, especially when she is cyanosed, is also associated with high fetal loss (Szekely and Snaith 1977). Untreated maternal tetrad of Fallot carries 30% fetal wastage (Batson 1974).

Most maternal endocrinological deficiencies interfere with normal ovulation and thus rarely complicate pregnancy. Where maternal hypothyroidism has been sufficiently well treated to permit pregnancy, medication need not be changed during pregnancy or after delivery. Interestingly, spontaneous abortion appears to be associated with the subsequent development of hypothyroidism (Othman et al. 1990). Thyrotoxicosis may be treated successfully in pregnancy (Montgomery and Harley 1977). Maternal diabetes may be complicated by intrauterine death, pre-eclampsia, polyhydramnios and infection. Such problems are more likely in the third trimester than early in pregnancy (see Chap. 21, p. 518). Where periconceptional metabolic control has been poor, as assessed by maternal glycosylated haemoglobin levels, the risk of spontaneous abortion is significantly increased compared with insulin-dependent diabetics under good control (Disker et al. 1988).

The Obstetric Lupus Syndrome

There is a well-established association between a circulating anticoagulant in maternal lupus erythematosus and poor pregnancy outcome (Nilsson et al. 1975) which may result in spontaneous abortion, often recurrent, or stillbirth (Branch et al. 1985; Cowchock et al. 1986). Pregnancy loss associated with the lupus anticoagulant is not restricted to women with active clinical autoimmune disease and indeed is more common in apparently asymptomatic women. Such patients are said to be suffering "obstetric lupus" (Prentice et al. 1984). The "lupus anticoagulant" in fact comprises a rather heterogeneous group of poorly defined antibodies (Triplett 1989). Although the activated partial thromboplastin time is generally used to screen for lupus anticoagulant, simple coagulation studies may be less satisfactory than measuring levels of anticardiolipin antibodies by ELISA or radioimmunoassay (Cowchock et al. 1986; Lazarchick and Kizer 1989).

Microscopic examination of the placenta in the presence of the lupus anticoagulant shows a somewhat variable picture although there is often a necrotising vasculopathy in the decidual vessels (Abramowski et al. 1980). Atherosis and other features more classically attributed to pre-eclampsia may also be seen (Gleicher and Friberg 1985), often at an earlier gestational age than is traditionally associated with hypertensive disease. These lesions and the variable immunological findings at a tissue level are somewhat non-specific and are not seen in all cases of fetal death associated with lupus, lupus anticoagulant or anticardiolipin antibody.

The severity of the effects of maternal lupus syndrome on the fetus seems to be related to the degree of decidual vasculopathy present. Although Trudinger et al. (1988) have demonstrated an apparent loss of fetal vessels in the tertiary villi in cases of maternal lupus, the existence of this lesion and the causal relationship between it and the presence of impaired umbilical artery velocity waveform has been disputed (Benirschke and Kaufman 1990b).

Abnormalities of the Maternal Genital Tract

Gynaecological disorders resulting in fetal loss include developmental and pathological abnormalities of uterine anatomy, cervical incompetence and disorders predisposing to ectopic pregnancy. Anatomical abnormalities of uterine development may cause repeated spontaneous abortion. Hydatidiform mole does not seem to predispose to subsequent abortion (Goldstein et al. 1984). However, spontaneous abortion, and particularly recurrent abortion, may be associated with the development of trophoblast neoplasia (Acaia et al. 1988).

Cervical incompetence is a significant factor in mid-trimester spontaneous abortion. The incidence of cervical incompetence has increased over the period that social termination of pregnancy by instrumentation in the first trimester has become widely practised but the relationship is not necessarily causal. In a prospective study of pregnancies in 520 women who had experienced vaginal termination, 8.1% suffered a spontaneous first or second trimester abortion. This compared with 2.4% in a control population of women who had previously had a spontaneous first trimester abortion (Ratten and Beischer 1979). A term pregnancy preceding the termination did not afford protection from the risk of post-termination abortion. However, conisation does not appear to predispose to miscarriage (Greene 1966). Histological studies of the cervix in cases of incompetence have provided little insight into the condition. Diethylstilboestrol (DES) exposure in utero has been implicated in the aetiology of some cases of cervical incompetence (Goldstein 1978).

Congenital uterine anatomical defects may lead to reproductive failure but quite major anomalies, including septate or double uteri may be associated with successful pregnancy although 20% of such patients will experience reproductive difficulties (Jones and Wheeless 1969; Rock and Jones 1977). Implantation of the placenta onto the septum of a bicornuate or septate uterus may lead to miscarriage and frequently such cases show evidence of placental hypoxia or infarction. Although anatomical defects of the uterus have been frequently reported in women exposed to DES (Kaufman et al. 1984), there is little evidence that such defects are associated with recurrent miscarriage (Barnes et al. 1980). Although the presence of leiomyomata is invoked as an explanation for miscarriage, there is considerable uncertainty as to the significance of fibroids since many pregnancies proceed unembarassed by the presence of often quite large tumours. Surgery may be indicated however (Malone and Ingersoll 1975).

Drugs—Social

Despite initial controversy, it is now generally accepted that heavy drinking during pregnancy is associated with growth and motor retardation and anatomical anomalies in the infant—fetal alcohol syndrome. It has been subsequently demonstrated that continued use of alcohol in pregnancy may also predispose to spontaneous abortion (Harlap and Shiono 1980; Kline et al. 1980a). Although both of these studies have been criticised, the study of Harlap and Shiono is both large and prospective. They demonstrated a threefold increase in the rate of second trimester abortions in women who admitted to having more than three drinks daily. A lower level of alcohol consumption carries a smaller risk. It is hypothesised that alcohol acts as a fetotoxin (Kline et al. 1980b), but to date there has been no description of morphological abnormalities in the products of these abortions and one study has shown no difference between rates of fetal anomaly in heavy drinkers and non-drinkers (Poland et al. 1981).

Although smoking during pregnancy is reported to increase the risk of abortion, growth retardation and stillbirth, many studies fail to separate the effects of alcohol from tobacco in women who use both. Once an attempt to isolate the effect of tobacco is made, its impact is diminished and risks appear less dose-dependent than those of alcohol (Harlap and Shiono 1980). A similar problem is seen in attempts to separate the effect of cannabis and LSD from other problems associated with their use. Neither has been shown unequivocally to increase the risk of spontaneous abortion, although LSD has been implicated in amniotic band syndrome (Blanc et al. 1971).

With rapidly increasing use of cocaine in the United States, there have now been reports associating the drug with spontaneous abortion, placental abruption and intrauterine growth retardation (Cregler and Mark 1986, Mercado et al. 1989). Of teratogenic interest is the apparent relationship between cocaine use and congenital anomalies that might legitimately be attributed to fetal vascular disruptions (Hoyme et al. 1990).

Drugs—Therapeutic

Reports from the 1970s that women working with anaesthetic gases suffered a high risk of spontaneous abortion (Spence and Knill-Jones 1978) underline a continuing theme in the investigation of the aetiology of spontaneous abortion, that of the need for great care in study design. Review of the original studies, which depended upon questionnaires, demonstrated that the incidence of spontaneous abortion in non-responders in the control group largely negated the relatively high incidence found in anaesthetists (Axelsson and Rylander 1982, 1984). However, some therapeutic agents have been unquestionably demonstrated to have clinically significant embryotoxicity.

The dose-dependent relationship between cytotoxic drugs and spontaneous abortion is well known and well proven. The risk ought to be sufficiently well recognised to present little problem in pratice but there is current evidence that woman regularly involved in the making up of cytotoxic perfusions experienced double the risk of miscarriage compared with a control population (Stucker et al. 1990).

Chloroquine is undoubtedly fetotoxic. Gentamicin, metronidazole, griseofulvin, beta-blockers and tricyclic antidepressants have all been cited in case reports as causes of fatal embryopathy. None of these are certain fetotoxins, although caution in their use during pregnancy seems prudent (Dukes 1980). For the majority of other therapeutic agents, there is little convincing evidence. For any student of developmental pathology, access to a well-informed drug advisory service or, at least, a compendium of teratogenics such as Shepard (1986), is indispensable.

Immunological Rejection

A striking feature of normal pregnancy is the retention within the mother, for 40 weeks, of tissue containing alien (paternal) antigens. Contradictory evidence has been collected concerning the importance of immunological mechanisms in the genesis of spontaneous abortion (Lauritsen et al. 1976; Purpura et al. 1980) but evidence suggests that an active maternal immune response to paternally derived antigens may facilitate the maintenance of pregnancy rather than militating against it. A popular current theory involves maternal "blocking antibodies". Possible actions might include IgG blocking antibodies to trophoblast/lymphocyte crossreactive antigens, antibodies to paternal HLA antigens, antibodies which block HLA receptors on maternal lymphocytes, T helper cell inhibitors or non-specific inhibitors of maternal lymphocyte proliferation. Allograft rejection is diminished following immunisation by blood transfusion. It has also been shown that women who have aborted spontaneously are less likely to have blocking antibodies than normal multiparous women (Tongio et al. 1972). An immunological basis for some cases of spontaneous abortion therefore seems plausible.

In a controlled trial (Mowbray et al. 1985), women who had experienced three or more abortions were given their own or paternal lymphocytes. The subsequent pregnancy rates in both groups were similar, but 78% of the women given paternal cells went to 28 weeks' gestation or beyond, compared with 37% of the women given their own cells. The couples selected for this trial were carefully screened for other causes of repeated abortion. The placebo effect in many series is well over 50%, suggesting that it is the control figure rather than the treatment figure that may be notable in this series. Other preparations used to stimulate a maternal response have included pooled donor lymphocytes (Taylor and Page-Faulk 1981) and syncytiotrophoblast membrane preparation (Johnson and Kirkpatrick 1984). A more recent study yielded an 83% livebirth incidence after paternal leucocyte immunisation (Beer 1988) but "tender loving care" may result in similar success rates (Stray-Pederson and Stray-Pederson 1984) and the situation remains far from clear at present. Furthermore, studies of HLA sharing have tended to concentrate on couples selected because of a history of repeated pregnancy loss. In a study of 111 couples in a Hutterite population, a community which is isolated and which proscribes contraception, recognised fetal loss rates did not differ between couples sharing or not sharing HLA antigens, although there was a significant association between HLA-DR sharing and increased pregnancy interval from the second pregnancy through to the sixth (Ober et al. 1988). The immunobiology of pregnancy is discussed more fully in Chapter 2.

Environmental Hazards to Early Pregnancy

The developing human fetus is vulnerable to external agents. Adverse effects will be manifested in abortion, growth retardation or anomaly shortly after exposure to a hazard. For this reason, the use of pregnancy surveillance as a means of monitoring the environment is very attractive. However, since the greatest number of fetuses is lost within the initial 12 weeks, the majority of abortions will be unperceived by the parents. Direct surveillance of unrecognised fetal loss is clearly costly, and the value of less stringent systems dependent upon parental reporting remains unproven (Wilcox 1983).

Despite the specific problems associated with reproductive epidemiology, several environmental hazards have been implicated in the genesis of abortion. Industrial exposure to organic solvents, copper smelting, soldering and sterilisation work using glutaraldehyde or ethylene oxide may all increase reproductive losses (Hemminki et al. 1983). Reports of clustering of spontaneous abortion in women exposed to prolonged use of word processors or other visual display units (VDUs) have led to several recommendations that pregnant women should be allowed to discontinue work on VDUs (Lee 1985). Allegations of reproductive hazards have provoked anxiety amongst VDU workers and it is this anxiety which justifies such recommendations, rather than the danger of the VDUs themselves. Preliminary work suggests that the quality of community drinking water may influence miscarriage rates (Aschengrau et al. 1989).

More contentious public issues such as the contamination caused by dumping chemical waste at the "Love Canal" site in New York county and the radioactive contamination after the Three Mile Island accident have been made even more difficult to study because of the sensationalism and litigation that have followed. The furore aroused by the Love Canal story has probably prejudiced any meaningful study (Editorial 1980), although tentative results suggest that there has been no significant impact on spontaneous abortion rates (Vianna 1980). A careful study of the population around Three Mile Island has failed to demonstrate an increased abortion rate (Goldhaber et al. 1983). Analysis of the aftermath of the Chernobyl accident of 1986 is still under way. There is a suggestion of increased rates of neural tube defect (Mocan et al. 1990), infant mortality (Luning et al. 1989) and induced abortion in Western Europe (Hubert 1990) following the disaster but the situation with regard to spontaneous miscarriage is less clear at present.

Other Factors

There is a statistically higher number of unsuccessful pregnancies amongst women with a history of early (under 12 years) and late (14 years or older) onset of menarche (Wyshak 1983). There is some dispute as to the importance of maternal age and birth order as separate factors in the genesis of spontaneous abortion. However, there seems little doubt that there are risks associated with both extremes of age. Very young women with a history of prior pregnancy appear to be at risk. Older women are, on the other hand, at greater risk if there has been no previous pregnancy (Roman and Stevenson 1983). There may be a relationship between suboptimal pregnancy outcome and luteal phase insufficiency (Cline 1979). Despite earlier reports, there appears to be no seasonal variation in the incidence of spontaneous abortion (Warren et al. 1980).

Pathological Classification of Spontaneous Abortion

It is axiomatic that a working classification of disease facilitates useful discussion of aetiology and pathogenesis. Because most busy pathology departments have little time or appetite for detailed embryological study, Rushton has

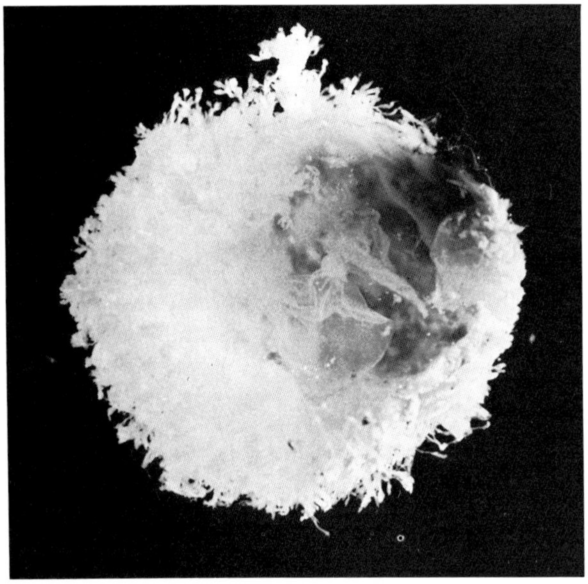

Fig. 3.3. A Group 1 blighted ovum. The sac has been opened to show strands of oedematous membrane but no recognisable fetal parts.

devised a classification which is not only simple in design but also easy to use (Rushton 1978, 1982, 1984). Table 3.5 shows the principal features of the system. The classification is based on simple macroscopic and microscopic findings only. It should therefore be within the ambit of even the most hard-pressed pathologist.

Table 3.5. Classification of spontaneous abortion

Group 1	*Blighted ova* (9.4 weeks)
	a) Most villi show microscopic oedema
	b) Intermediate between (a) and (c)
	c) Most villi show stromal fibrosis and vascular obliteration
Group 2	*Fetal death with maceration* (14.1 weeks)
	a) Embryo present
	b) Embryo absent
Group 3	*Non-macerated fetuses* (18.6 weeks)
	a) Fetus present
	b) Fetus absent

Numbers in parentheses indicate mean age after last ovulation (Rushton 1978).

Group 1: Blighted Ova

When delivered whole, the amniotic cavity in these gestations contains either no fetus or a small nodule of tissue on the end of a poorly formed umbilical cord (Fig. 3.3). When the specimen is fragmented or opened, the nubbin of fetal tissue may still be present or may have been lost. If a well-formed umbilical cord is present then the fetus was either lost during delivery or expelled earlier. These cases should be placed into Group 2 or 3. Where there is no convincing cord remnant, the specimen should be placed in Group 1. Group 1 contains the highest number of chromosomally abnormal conceptuses. The relative amount of villous oedema or stromal fibrosis on histological examination depends on the extent to which the fetal circulation had become established prior to fetal death and thus on gestational age.

Group 2: Macerated Fetuses

There is some overlap with Group 1. In many early cases the fetus or embryo appears well formed but shows marked autolysis on closer examination (Fig. 3.4). Gradual sludging of the maternal circulation through the placenta leads to the macroscopic appearance of "maternal floor infarction".

Aneuploidy is less common in this group but maternal factors seem not to play an important role either. Thus the majority of abortions in this category remain unexplained. Histological examination of the placenta shows vascular sclerosis and dystrophic calcification, and "ghost" fetal red cells are prominent. Syncytial knots may be striking and related to the length of time the fetus is retained after intrauterine death.

Group 3: Non-macerated Fetuses

Expulsion of a conceptus before maceration supervenes often implicates a maternal cause for abortion. This is the group in which chorionamnionitis and retroplacental haemorrhage are most likely to be found. The placenta should be examined carefully for evidence of these conditions and infarction should also be sought. Where the membranes are clouded or discoloured, microbiological examination should be undertaken.

Non-macerated fetuses are generally second trimester and may be large enough for a "mini-autopsy". Such examination is unlikely to reveal any anatomical anomaly but there may be evidence of aspiration of amniotic fluid containing maternal polymorphs and fetal squames

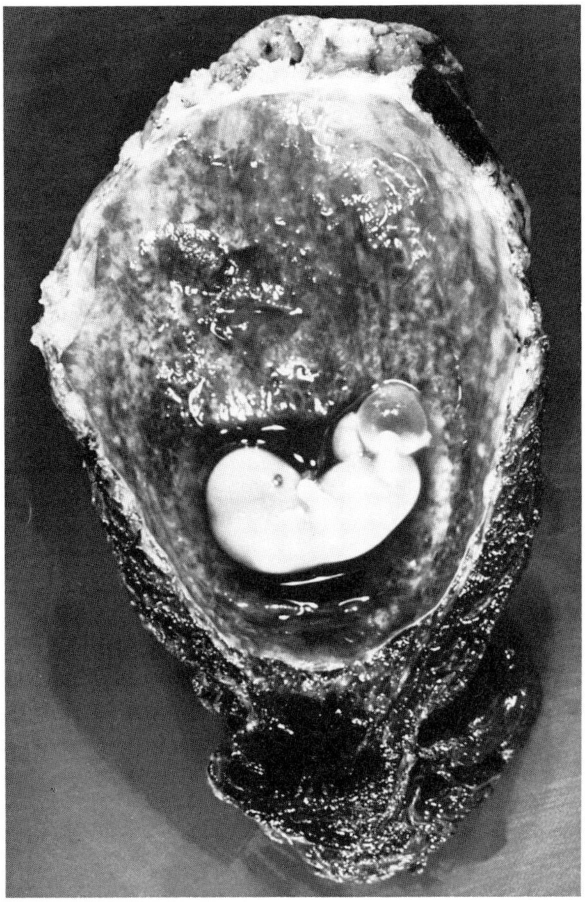

Fig. 3.4. A Group 2 abortus of about 12 weeks' gestation. The tear-shaped gestation sac has been opened. The fetus shows early maceration and there is a cyst of the cord.

on histological examination of the lungs. Polymorphs within airways do not indicate fetal infection. The histological diagnosis of fetal infection rests on the presence of interstitial inflammation in the lung parenchyma adjacent to airways.

Further classification of abnormally developed embryos is proposed by Poland et al. (1981) (Table 3.6).

Mechanisms of Spontaneous Abortion

Without medical intervention, fetuses with gross defects such as anencephaly may well proceed to term. This contrasts strongly with the high rate of spontaneous abortion seen in some "minor" anomalies such as cleft palate (Mikamo 1970). The conventional explanation for spontaneous abortion is abnormality of the

Table 3.6. Classification of abnormal embryonic development (after Poland et al. 1981)

Empty intact sac (GD1)—the equivalent to Rushton's group 1. The amnion is generally fused to the chorion, a situation abnormal before 8–10 weeks.

Nodular embryo (GD2)—a solid mass of embryonic tissue with no retinal pigment and feature to allow differentiation between cephalic and caudal poles.

Cylindrical embryo (GD3)—embryonic tissue up to 10 mm in length which includes retinal pigment but no limb buds.

Stunted embryo (GD4)—embryos in this category are longer than 10 mm but are small for gestational age and have disproportionately small heads which often show abnormal facial features.

conceptus, but this fails to explain a mechanism for expulsion of the gestation. Furthermore, pregnancies may continue in the presence of a dead fetus for weeks or months, thus it would appear unlikely that it is the fetus per se which initiates miscarriage. The establishment and maintenance of pregnancy demand a complex set of hormonal and anatomical interrelations between fetal and maternal tissues. Expulsion of a conceptus represents a "final common pathway" which may have been initiated by a failure of any of these factors or by a positive attempt by the maternal organism to expel an abnormal fetus with minimal risk to herself.

Although our understanding of the pathophysiology of abortion is poor, some clues as to its nature may be gleaned from clinical and pathological studies. Making some sense out of the pathological findings in abortion requires a basic understanding of the details of normal placentation (see Chap. 2, p. 47). It is sufficient to point out here that the three most important components in the development and maintenance of the gestation are first, trophoblast function, second, fetal circulation, and third, maternal circulation.

The evidence to date suggests that the single most important factor is the integrity of the trophoblast. Trophoblast function dictates implantation, fetal angiogenesis, maternal endocrine milieu and physiological adaptation of the uterine vasculature. The relative importance of each of these to abortion varies with gestational age. This is reflected in the gross and histological changes seen in abortions at different stages of pregnancy (Rushton 1988). The earliest, unperceived abortions occur as a consequence of implantation failure. In blighted ova (Group 1 above) histological evidence suggests incomplete or abnormal fetal angiogenesis within chorionic villi, especially in aneuploid embryos. Of particular interest are the findings of Kalousek et al. (1989) that the trophoblast of trisomy 13 and 18 infants that survive to term are mosaic for diploid and trisomic cells, suggesting that this has conferred an advantage on these fetuses over those with purely aneuploid placentas. In later abortion with retention of at least part of the conceptus after intrauterine death (macerated specimens, Group 2), the placental vasculature appears well established and the familiar changes of villous stromal fibrosis, sclerosis of villous vessels and maternal fibrin deposition are due to secondary change after fetal death and circulatory arrest. The expulsion may be related to a gradual onset of involutionary change in the uterus and enhanced uterine irritability.

In Group 3, where the product is fresh, following rapid expulsion, extrinsic influences such as cervical incompetence, uterine fibroids, retroplacental haemorrhage and placental infarction appear to play a primary role in abortion. However evidence of retroplacental haemorrhage, intrauterine growth retardation, placental infarction and spiral artery disease in the placental bed may all be seen in macerated and fresh midtrimester miscarriages. Acute atherosis in the uterine vessels has been considered to be pathognomonic of pre-eclampsia (Robertson et al. 1975) but can clearly arise in the placental bed before the onset of maternal symptoms (Khong et al. 1987). Thus miscarriage may represent one end-point in the spectrum of hypertensive disorders of pregnancy.

It seems reasonable to conclude that fetal inflammation, seen as interstitial pneumonitis in the presence of chorioamnionitis or villitis in the absence of membranous inflammation, is a genuine cause of fetal wastage. However, the association between chorionamnionitis and fetal death is not inevitably causal. Chorioamnionitis supervenes rapidly after rupture of the membranes and it may be that event, rather than the inflammation per se, which may lead to abortion (see Chap. 8, p. 202). However, there is good theoretical reason to suppose that infection may play a pivotal role in the pathogenesis of some cases of spontaneous abortion and indeed infection may be the cause of membrane rupture rather than the consequence. Bacterial organisms that commonly cause chorionamnionitis show high phospholipase A2 activity (Bejar et al. 1981). This may impact upon the pregnancy in two ways, by increasing the local production of prostaglandins and by converting amniotic fluid lecithin to lysolecithin which reduces membrane bursting pressure (Sbarra et al. 1985). Membrane weakness may be further exacerbated by the release of bacterial hydrogen peroxide. Interest in such mechanisms has been largely generated by the clinical problem of preterm rupture of the membranes rather than by miscarriage and no such studies are available for the previable pregnancy, but Rushton found evidence of chorionamnionitis in 29% of his group 3 cases, with one third of those cases showing evidence of an interstitial pneumonitis (Rushton 1988).

Pathological Examination of Abortion Material

A first trimester specimen received by the pathologist may vary from a gestation sac with attached decidua through to rather scrappy curettage material. It is possible to get useful information from most material, but the fullest information comes from the most complete specimens. A full history should accompany the specimen, including details of the present and previous pregnancies and relevant maternal gynaecological and medical history (Berry 1980). The principles of early abortion specimen handling and examination are comprehensively described and illustrated by Kalousek and co-authors (1990).

The specimen should be classified according to the Rushton system, based on macroscopic appearance (Table 3.5). The fetus, if present, and placental tissue can then be examined for clues to aetiological factors. At this time a decision should be made about sampling for microbiological or cytogenetic investigation or other laboratory studies. Failure to take specimens early in the examination may prejudice success. The examination of fetuses is discussed in Chapter 1.

Examination of Placental Tissue

On naked-eye and microscopic examination, it may be possible to detect evidence of chromosome abnormality, infection, hydatidiform change, retroplacental haemorrhage, infarction or infection. In addition, there may be evidence of iatrogenic intervention, and the placenta and membranes should be routinely searched for puncture marks, since the request form

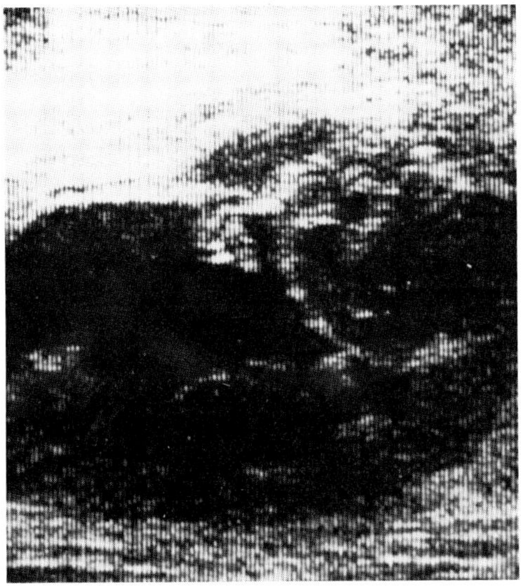

a

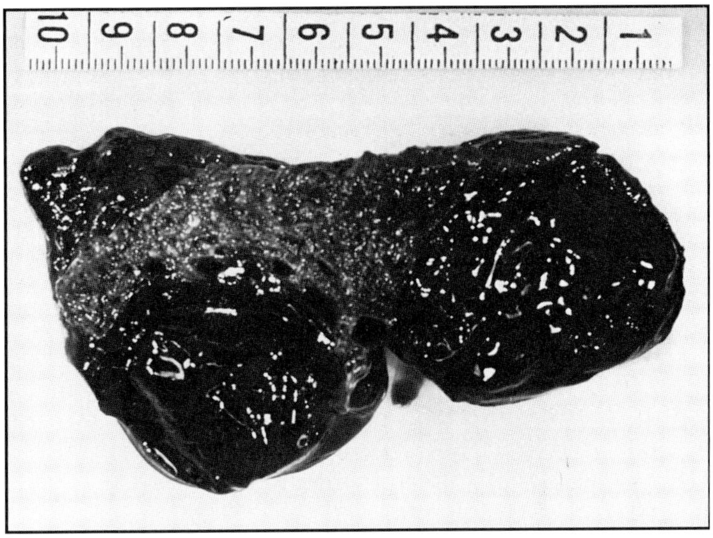

b

Fig. 3.5. Subchorionic haemorrhage may be detectable on ultrasound as large cystic spaces (**a**). This is characteristic of Breus' mole (**b**).

may omit details of previous amniocentesis or fetoscopy. There may be changes associated with retention of the conceptus after intrauterine death (Rushton 1981). In all spontaneous abortions, the pathologist should attempt to differentiate between placental pathology causing immediate abortion (e.g. retroplacental haemorrhage) or fetal death, and the placental changes which occur secondary to death of the fetus and cessation of the fetal circulation.

Placental Changes Following Fetal Death

Since the placenta received its oxygen and nutrients from the maternal circulation, cessation of the fetal circulation after intrauterine death does not cause placental infarction. The principal changes are sclerosis of the villous vessels and an increase in the quantity of villous stromal connective tissue.

A further change is an increase in villous fluid content—oedema or "hydropic degeneration" (see Fig. 3.9b). Although the latter term is an acceptable expression for this banal feature, the term "molar" is to be deprecated as it may lead to clinical confusion with true hydatidiform mole. Hydropic change is most commonly seen in early abortion, prior to establishment of the fetal circulation, often in the absence of fetal parts (Abaci and Aterman 1968). The oedema tends to be patchy, unlike that seen in hydatidiform mole. Although the swollen villi may be visible on careful macroscopic examination, the appearance is not so uniform nor so striking as that seen in hydatidiform mole. Microscopic hydropic degeneration without trophoblast excess may be apparent even when the fetus is absent. It is associated with chromosomal anomalies including trisomy and triploidy (see Chap. 2). Marked changes of this type (partial mole) may raise the possibility of trophoblast neoplasia (see p. 102).

In second trimester abortions, cessation of the fetal circulation leads to changes in the maternal compartment of the placenta. Gradual slowing of the maternal blood leads to deposition of fibrin in the maternal compartment. Perivillous fibrin deposition is most marked close to the placental floor. This change may be noted on naked-eye examination and has, erroneously, been referred to as "maternal floor infarction". The change is not infarction, neither is it implicated in the genesis of abortion, although the encroachment of intervillous fibrin on normal placental exchange may occur prior to fetal death. Another feature associated with, but not causally related to, fetal death is the striking condition of subchorial haemorrhage. The collections of blood may be sufficiently extensive to dominate the appearance of the placenta both on ultrasound and pathological examination (Fig. 3.5a,b). This appearance is known to gynaecologists as Breus' mole. It is not related in any way to hydatidiform mole.

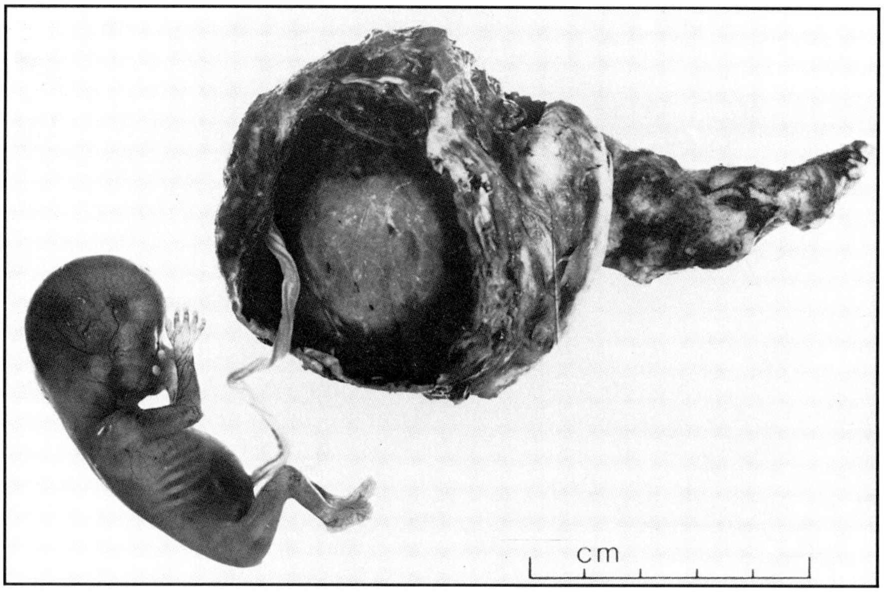

Fig. 3.6. A well-developed tubal gestation was detected after curettage demonstrated Arias-Stella reaction.

Retroplacental haemorrhage may occur as early as the second trimester. It usually results in precipitate expulsion of the conceptus. Pathological findings may be limited to the presence of clot on the maternal surface. For a full account of abruption see Chapter 2 (p. 59). If there is retention of the gestation, the placenta overlying the clot may be thin and show evidence of infarction. This is not a common feature in mid-trimester abortion. Placental infarction is not limited to the third trimester and may be seen in Group 3 second trimester abortion. As a significant indicator of uterine vascular insufficiency, 5%–10% of the placenta should be infarcted. Placental infarction is discussed in Chapter 2 (see p. 59).

Ectopic Gestation

The ovum, which is fertilised within the fallopian tube, generally implants in the upper portion of the corpus uteri. Implantation elsewhere is referred to as ectopic. The vast majority of ectopic pregnancies are found within the fallopian tubes (Fig. 3.6), but implantation may occur ectopically within the uterus in, for example, a poorly developed cornu of a bicornuate uterus. Primary implantation may be seen on the surface of the ovary or within the peritoneal cavity. However, most specimens located in these two sites have reimplanted after expulsion through the wall or fimbrial end of the fallopian tube (Budowick et al. 1980).

The precise incidence of ectopic pregnancy varies, depending on the rigour of the study. The incidence appears to be higher in the west and seems to be increasing (Rubin et al. 1983). An American study (DeCherney and Jones 1985) suggests a recent twofold increase from 1:67 live births to 1:21 livebirths. This may well represent an over-estimate, as the figures do not take into account changes in the incidence of pregnancy wastage through spontaneous or social termination; however, there seems little doubt that there is a recent and significant increase and ectopic pregnancy remains one of the leading causes of maternal death (Lawson et al. 1989). Legal abortion does not seem to have had an impact on the incidence of ectopic implantation (Holt et al. 1989).

The causative factors implicated in the genesis of ectopic pregnancy can be broken down into two main groups. Endosalpingeal damage, caused by pelvic inflammatory disease, abdominal surgery or previous ectopic pregnancy, appears to be the most important risk factor. Tubal pregnancy may also be seen in cases of endometriosis or the tubal equivalent, salpingitis isthmica nodosa (Fig. 3.7; Honore 1979; Green and Kott 1989). The

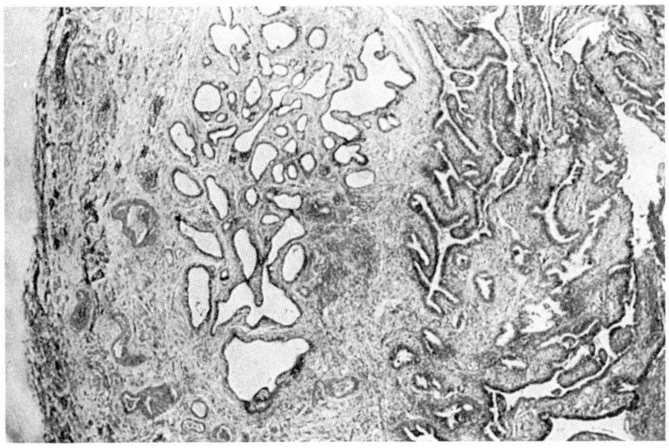

Fig. 3.7. Salpingitis isthmica nodosa: a focal collection of glands is situated underneath the tubal epithelium. The fallopian villi show much fusion and thickening, reflecting past inflammation.

current epidemic of venereally transmitted diseases might well explain the increase in incidence of ectopic pregnancy. Chlamydial infection in particular has been implicated. There is some evidence that the immune response of a particular woman with pelvic inflammatory disease may determine whether she develops chronic sequelae such as tubal pregnancy or infertility (Wagar et al. 1990).

The strongest associations with the increase in incidence of ectopic gestations in a recent Finnish study were previous pelvic surgery (including previous ectopic pregnancy), pelvic inflammatory disease and current use of an IUCD (Makinen et al. 1989). There is a higher incidence of ectopic pregnancy in patients with a history of miscarriage and particularly repeated spontaneous abortion (Fedele et al. 1989). Human immunodeficiency virus does not seem to have an independent impact on the disease (Selwyn et al. 1989).

The clinical features of ectopic pregnancy are well known. Amenorrhoea is followed by pain and bleeding in over 80% of cases. The diagnosis may be very obvious in cases admitted after severe intraperitoneal bleeding, but, not infrequently, the patient requires formal investigation in order to distinguish between ectopic pregnancy and inevitable or threatened abortion. Ultrasound is an increasingly important modality but there is also evidence that estimation of Ca-125 and oestradiol levels may be of value (Witt et al. 1990).

It must be stressed that Aria-Stella change may also be seen in curettings from women who are not pregnant. Uterine curettings in cases of proven tubal pregnancy may show changes ranging from extensive decidualisation through to normal proliferative endometrium. Thus, although suspicion of ectopic pregnancy may be raised by the pathologist who sees either Aria-Stella change or uninflamed decidual change, the absence of such features should not be used to reassure the physician in the presence of clinical features suggestive of ectopic gestation.

Combined tubal and fundal pregnancy is not uncommon. There are more than 600 reported cases (Bello et al. 1986). The uterine pregnancy may be salvageable in these cases, and subfertile women should probably not be routinely curetted at laparoscopy for ectopic pregnancy until ultrasonography has excluded a fundal gestation sac.

The sequelae of tubal implantation are as follows:

Absorption of the conceptus within the tube

Expulsion into the peritoneal cavity and absorption or mummification (fetus papyraceous), or reimplantation

Intraluminal or intramural haemorrhage and rupture

The chance finding of small nodules containing ghost villi within or outside the fallopian tubes in hysterectomy specimens suggests that clinically unapparent ectopic gestation is common.

Management of the tubal ectopic has become increasingly conservative recently with manipulations such as salpingotomy and simple massaging of the tube to expel the conceptus being used as alternatives to salpingectomy. Infusion of methotrexate is also being used with success as is infusion with prostaglandins. However, at least one study of multiple ectopic pregnancy suggests that fertility does not differ between conservatively treated patients and those who have had salpingectomy (Uotila et al. 1989).

Ovarian pregnancy is extremely rare (Hallatt 1982). For a diagnosis of ovarian ectopic gestation, the following criteria must be met:

1. Both fallopian tubes must be normal at laparotomy (i.e. there should be no possibility that the initial implantation was tubal)

2. There should be histological evidence of trophoblast (to exclude haemorrhagic corpus luteum)

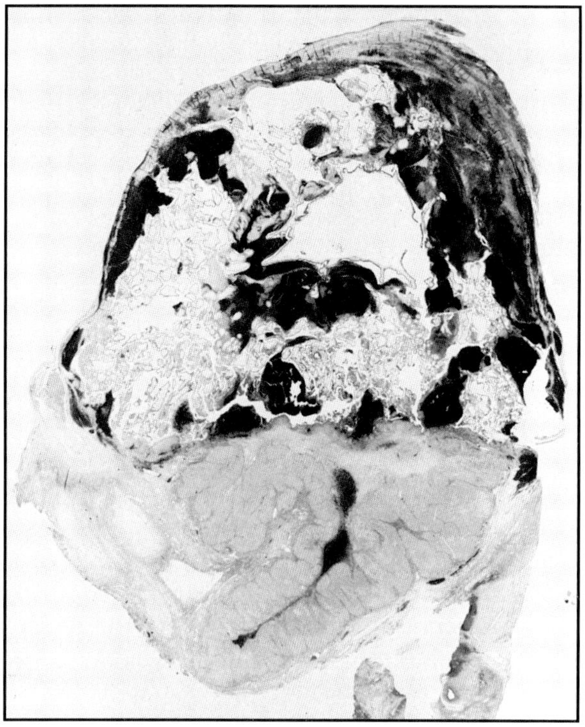

Fig. 3.8. A whole-mount preparation of an ovarian ectopic gestation. The gestation sac lies within the substance of the ovary, adjacent to the corpus luteum.

3. The gestation sac should be entirely surrounded by ovary, rather than simply adherent to it (Spiegelberg 1878).

Once these criteria have been satisfied, most specimens originally diagnosed as ovarian pregnancies may be discounted. However, the condition does occur (Fig. 3.8).

Genuine primary peritoneal pregnancy is sufficiently rare to warrant some doubt as to its existence. Ectopic intrauterine pregnancy is limited to women with developmental defects of their genital tract. From a practical point of view, ectopic pregnancy equates with tubal gestation.

Ectopic pregnancy remains an important cause of maternal mortality, although the death rate for ectopic pregnancy has fallen from 35.5 deaths per 10 000 ectopics in 1970 to 4.9 deaths per 10 000 ectopics in 1986, it still accounts for over 13% of maternal deaths overall (Lawson et al. 1989). In England and Wales, nearly half of the deaths from ectopic gestation occurred to women born in the New Commonwealth, although they only represented 6.3% of all maternities during the period under study (DHSS 1979). There is a similar bias towards minority races in the United States (Lawson et al. 1989).

Molar Placental Disease

Neoplasia of trophoblast traditionally includes three conditions—hydatidiform mole, invasive mole and chorioncarcinoma. To this list may be added the more recently described and uncommon placental site trophoblast tumour. Other conditions referred to loosely as "moles" do not carry unequivocal malignant connotations. In particular, "partial mole" is cytogenetically and behaviourally different from "complete mole" (Driscoll 1984) but, because it represents an important part of the differential diagnosis of trophoblast neoplasia, both ultrasonologically and pathologically, and because of some equivocal evidence that it may progress to overt neoplasia in a small number of cases, it is considered here.

Partial and Complete Hydatidiform Mole

Aetiology and Biology

Despite some questionable epidemiological studies, it is clear that the incidence of complete hydatidiform mole varies from country to country. The rate in Indonesia is quoted as 1 per 85 pregnancies, whereas in New York it is closer to 1 in 1700 (Buckley 1984). Although the variation has been attributed to racial differences, in Honolulu the local Asians have a low incidence. Similarly, in Singapore, there is no difference in rate between Indian, Chinese and Malays; the risk to all, using data from the 1960s, is 1:823.

No convincing environmental factor has been implicated in the genesis of complete mole. Epidemiological studies suggest a biphasic distribution with peaks under the age of 20 and over 40. The later peak is more dramatic, with an 80-fold increase in risk over the age of 50 when compared with 25- to 29-year-olds (Buckley 1984). These factors apply to Asian as well as European pregnancies. Indeed, with a marked decrease in teenage and elderly pregnancies in Singapore over the last 20 years, the local registry had difficulties finding any cases in 1987 (Teoh 1988). Although paternal age does not seem directly to affect the incidence of mole, the paternal genetic contribution to true mole is interesting and unique.

Using Q-banding for chromosomal polymorphism, Kajii and Ohama (1977) have demonstrated that hydatidiform mole is usually diploid (46XX) but that all the genetic material is paternal is origin. The hypothesis that mole results from dispermy (fertilisation by two sperm), or duplication of a haploid sperm after fertilisation of an "empty ovum", is supported by other banding studies and by the use of HLA antigen or enzyme marker studies (Jacobs et al. 1980). Thus hydatidiform mole and subsequent chorioncarcinoma are complete allografts, carrying no maternal genetic information, at least at a chromosomal level. Although most moles are 46XX, occasionally they may carry, through dispermy, a paternal 46XY genotype (Surti et al. 1982). The X chromosome appears to be essential to cellular survival; 46YY tumours are not seen. Suggestions that heterozygous complete moles may have a greater malignant potential (Wake et al. 1981) have not yet been validated Lawler and Fisher 1987) and it remains impossible to determine prognosis in hydatidiform mole on the basis of cytogenetic studies. Hyperdiploid cell lines demonstrated by flow cytometry may prove informative (Hemming et al. 1987). Flow cytometric demonstration of aneuploidy is associated with a higher risk of neoplastic sequelae than where a complete mole is uniformly diploid (Martin et al. 1989).

The absence of maternal genes in complete mole contrasts interestingly with the situation in "partial" mole, where the genotype is often triploid (one maternal and two paternal haplotypes), or occasionally tetraploid. Triploidy occurs in cases of fertilisation of a haploid ovum by two haploid spermatozoa or by a diploid sperm after paternal meiosis-1 error (Szulman and Surti 1984). The precise percentage of partial moles that are triploid or trisomic is not certain. A flow cytometric analysis of 35 partial moles showed 6 (17%) to be triploid and the remainder to be diploid. Only in the latter group were there any clinical sequelae (Davis et al. 1987). The bias of studies based on referral centre material downgrades the incidence of partial mole both in terms of its overall incidence and its impact upon overt trophoblast neoplasia (Bagshawe et al. 1990). Although histological differentiation from complete mole may prove problematical (see below), flow cytometry makes the distinction easier, even on paraffin-embedded material (Fisher et al. 1987, Lage et al. 1988).

Clinical Presentation

The paradigm clinical presentation of the partial mole is that of spontaneous or inevitable miscarriage early in the second trimester. Ultrasound may reveal a rather bulky placenta with a pattern of echogenicity suggestive of hydatidiform mole but a fetus, often dead or dying, is generally demonstrable. Where the conceptus is trisomic for chromosome 13, there may be severe pregnancy-induced hypertensive disease (Boyd et al. 1987, Bower et al. 1987).

Complete mole presents around the 16th week of pregnancy with vaginal bleeding, a bulky uterus and, in 10%–20% of cases, pre-eclampsia. Hyperemesis gravidarum occurs in approximately one quarter of all cases. Maternal serum human chorionic gonadotrophin (hCG) levels are usually grossly elevated. Approximately half of women with complete hydatidiform moles will show large (greater than 6 cm) theca lutein ovarian cysts. Rarely, maternal tachycardia may be the result of overproduction of chorionic thyrotrophin (Hertz 1978) and a few patients present with dyspnoea due to embolisation of trophoblast to the pulmonary vascular bed. Ultrasound examination is often specific, with a "snowstorm" appearance and amniography, although rarely used in the UK, may be diagnostic (Kohorn 1984).

Histopathology

Partial hydatidiform mole. Macroscopic examination of the products of conception is often unremarkable although occasional cystically dilated villi may be seen if the placental tissue is teased out under water (Fig. 3.9b). The villi are of variable size with a considerable number being of normal calibre. In triploid conceptuses where the extra haploid set is paternal, the placenta tends to be large for dates and is more frequently hydropic (Jacobs et al. 1982, Shepard et al. 1989).

Microscopic examination of the placental tissue in partial mole show focal villous oedema. The villi are frequently scalloped and contain trophoblast "inclusions" (Szulman

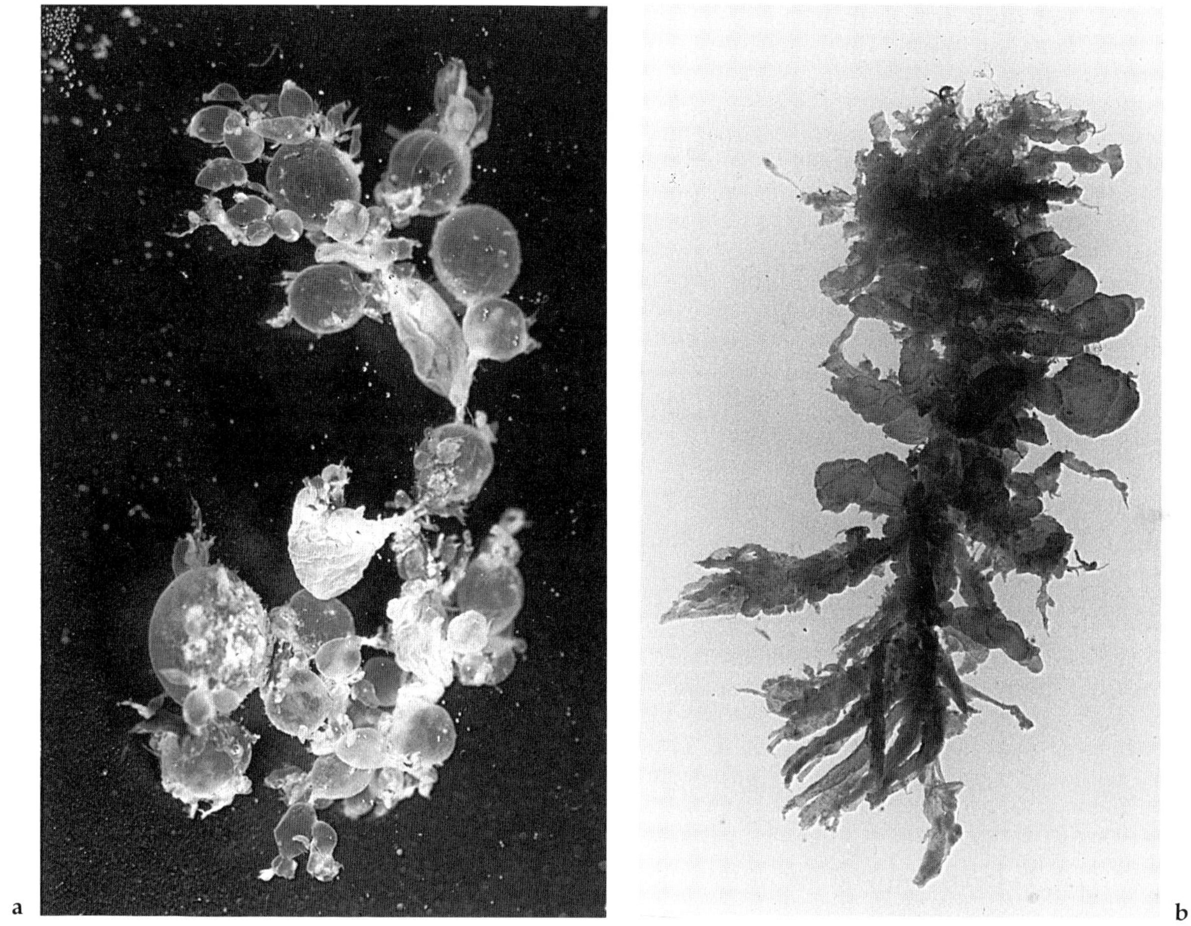

Fig. 3.9a,b. Villi from a hydatidiform mole photographed in saline, compared with those from a triploid abortus. In true hydatidiform mole (**a**), the grossly oedematous vesicles are connected by a very scanty stalk and all the villi show hydropic change. In the triploid placenta (**b**), only occasional villi are oedematous.

1988). Trophoblast inclusions appear as small, rather compact islands of trophoblast cells lying within the villous stroma and occasionally resembling involuting villous vessels. These inclusions in fact are cross-cut downgrowths of the surface trophoblast and continuity with the surface can often be demonstrated in other sections (Fig. 3.10). They are a particularly good pointer towards trisomic and triploid abortuses. Unlike complete hydatidiform mole, partial moles frequently show evidence of villous vascular development, although retention in utero following fetal death may lead to extensive involution.

Complete hydatidiform mole. Complete mole consists of masses of oedematous, grape-like vesicles strung together by scanty connective tissue (Fig. 3.9a). In most cases, neither fetus nor recognisable membrane is present. Only in multiple pregnancy may a well-formed fetus be found. In singleton pregnancies, when a fetus is present, hydropic change in the placental tissue is more likely to be the result of aneuploidy. Under these circumstances there is not the degree of proliferation seen in true mole and the uterus is unlikely to have been large for dates.

The histological picture of hydatidiform mole is characterised by distended, fluid-filled villi which have no recognisable vessels within them. The overlying trophoblast may be attenuated in some areas as a result of stromal oedema. Careful examination will almost always reveal areas of trophoblast excess (Elston and Bagshawe 1972). This change may be overdiagnosed by less experienced pathologists when examining the cross-cut ends of

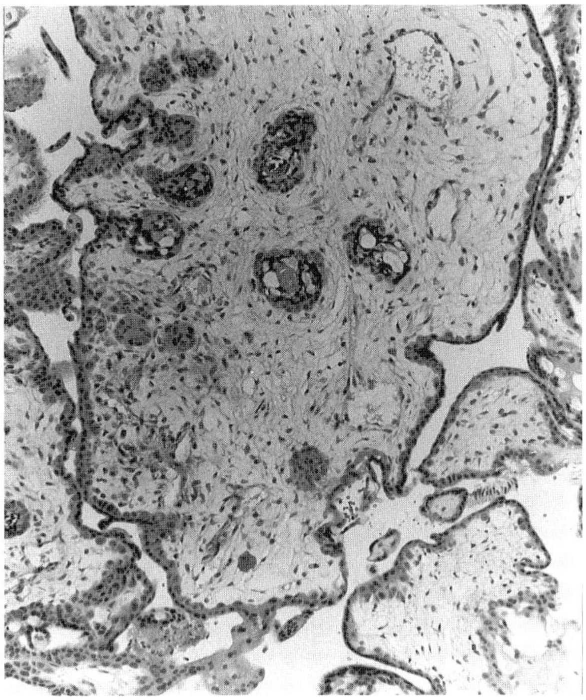

Fig. 3.10. Chorionic villi from a triploid conceptus. Note the scalloped outline to the villi, the minimal trophoblast proliferation and the trophoblast inclusions within the villous stroma. The largest of the villi is vascularised and a fetus was present in this case.

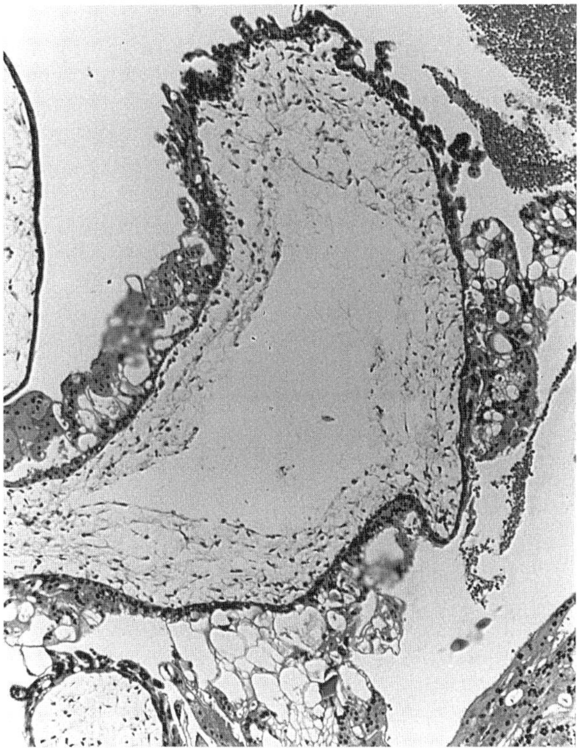

Fig. 3.11. Tissue from a complete hydatidiform mole showing cysterna formation in an avascular villus and circumferential trophoblast excess.

proliferating villi in cases of simple hydropic degeneration. Where there is trophoblast excess around the full circumference of the villus, it cannot be due to oblique sectioning and is diagnostic of hydatidiform mole (Fig. 3.11). The trophoblast seen here is composed of an admixture of cytotrophoblast and syncytiotrophoblast which often shows considerable nuclear pleomorphism (Fig. 3.12). Unlike partial mole, the hydropic change affects all villi, although variably. Most hydatidiform moles are suspected on naked eye examination. If the pathologist is agonising over dubious trophoblast proliferation in occasional villi from unremarkable uterine curettage, the lesion is probably not sinister.

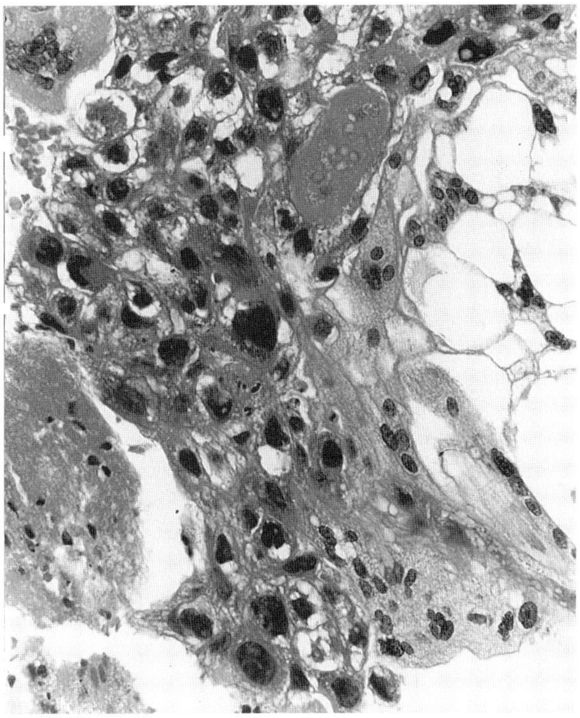

Fig. 3.12. High-power of trophoblast from the case shown in Fig. 3.11 with considerable nuclear pleomorphism.

Prognosis and Follow-up

Following a pregnancy complicated by complete hydatidiform mole, the majority of women suffer no sequelae. This reinforces the undesirability of overdiagnosis. However, 15% of moles develop evidence of local invasion ("invasive mole") and 5% of hydatidiform moles are followed by choriocarcinoma, whereas 50% of choriocarcinomata are preceded by hydatidiform mole (Elston 1981). Neoplastic sequelae are particularly common in older patients and this may be related to the higher incidence of aneuploidy in these cases. Current management involves careful follow-up to detect persistently raised hCG or persistent bleeding. Suction evacuation with or without chemotherapy is the treatment of choice. There is a 10-fold increase of further molar pregnancy after a hydatidiform mole (Yen and MacMahon 1968) with a risk between 1:150 and 1:50. Despite earlier reports, there is little increased risk of abortion, premature labour or congenital abnormality in subsequent pregnancies (Goldstein et al. 1984) although abortion seems to predispose to hydatidiform mole (Acaia et al. 1988). Careful hCG monitoring in patients with a history of known molar disease should permit optimistic counselling.

The prognostic significance of partial hydatidiform mole is moot. There are reports of persistent gestational trophoblastic tumour arising after the diagnosis of partial mole with suggestions that these cases are indistinguishable clinically and histologically from cases that do not progress (Rice et al. 1990). Bagshawe et al. (1990) quote a risk of neoplastic transformation in the order of 1:12 for complete mole and 1:200 for partial mole based on the data available to the United Kingdom hydatidiform mole registry. However, on this basis, the frequency of triploidy in spontaneous abortion suggests that all pregnancies would carry an overall risk of 1:58 of developing persistent molar disease not just partial mole alone. This is clearly an overestimate and may result from incomplete registration of partial moles to the UK registry.

There are potent arguments for dropping the term "partial mole" altogether in favour of identification of such abortuses by karyotype. The anxiety generated by a misapplied label of uncertain malignant connotation, in addition to the reproductive inconvenience of delaying subsequent pregnancies, lends power to the argument that all molar products of conception should be submitted to ploidy estimation (Benirschke 1989).

Invasive Mole, Placental Site Trophoblastic Tumour and Chorioncarcinoma

Invasive mole, placental site lesions and overt chorioncarcinoma present as gynaecological rather than reproductive problems and will only be covered briefly here. Excellent reviews are to be found in Benirschke and Kaufmann (1990c).

Invasive mole, sometimes still referred to as chorionadenoma destruens, can be differentiated histologically from chorioncarcinoma by the presence of recognisable villi amongst the proliferating trophoblast. A reasonable analogy is that it represents the molar equivalent of the morbidly adherent placenta. Presentation is generally as a persistently raised hCG level.

It has been recognised for some time that the condition referred to originally as "syncytial endometritis" is a normal infiltration of the decidua at the implantation site by intermediate trophoblast, occasionally referred to as X-cells (Boe 1967). The preferred term for this process is therefore "placental site reaction". However, a similar change may persist after pregnancy and indeed may metastasise with fatal results. Originally called "syncytioma" by Ewing and "atypical chorioncarcinoma" by Marchand, a more acceptable term for this condition is placental site trophoblast tumour (PSTT) (Elston 1984). Unlike chorioncarcinoma, few cases are preceded by hydatidiform mole; more commonly they follow abortion or preterm labour (Finkler et al. 1988). The uterus is generally bulky but gross pathological features vary from a discrete nodule to a polypoid mass filling the uterine cavity. Histological examination shows a largely mononuclear infiltrate of extravillous cytotrophoblast cells forming sheets between myometrial fibres. The biphasic appearance of chorioncarcinoma is not seen, the process closely resembling that of placental site reaction (Young and Scully 1984). Treatment and follow-up of PSTT may well depend upon an estimate of the mitotic index, fatal cases showing more than seven mitotic figures per high-power field. The histological finding of mitotic activity is interesting and may prove helpful in establishing the diagnosis as mitotic figures are rarely seen in normal extravillous trophoblast.

References

Abaci F, Aterman K (1968) Changes of the placenta and embryo in early spontaneous abortion. Am J Obstet Gynecol 102: 252–263

Abramowski CR, Vegas ME, Swineheart G, Gyves MT (1980) Decidual vasculopathy of the placenta in lupus erythematosus. N Engl J Med 303: 668–672

Acaia B, Parazzini F, La Vecchia C, Ricciardiello O, Fedele L, Battista Candidiani G (1988) Increased frequency of complete hydatidiform mole in women with repeated spontaneous abortion. Gynecol Oncol 31: 310–314

Anand A, Gray ES, Brown T, Clewley JP, Cohen BJ (1987) Human parvovirus infection in pregnancy and hydrops fetalis. N Engl J Med 316: 183–186

Aschengrau A, Zierler S, Cohen A (1989) Quality of community drinking water and the occurrence of spontaneous abortion. Arch Environ Health 44: 283–290

Axelsson G, Rylander R (1982) Exposure to anaesthetic gases and spontaneous abortion: response bias in a postal questionnaire study. Int J Epidemiol 11: 250–256

Axelsson G, Rylander R (1984) Validation of questionnaire reported miscarriage, malformation and birth weight. Int J Epidemiol 13: 94–98

Bagshawe KD, Lawler SD, Paradinas FG, Dent S, Brown P, Boxer GM (1990) Gestational trophoblast tumour following initial diagnosis of partial hydatidiform mole. Lancet 335: 1074–1076

Banatvala JE, O'Shea S, Best JM et al. (1981) Transmission of RA 27/3 rubella vaccine strain to products of conception. Lancet i: 392

Batson GA (1974) Cyanotic congenital heart disease and pregnancy. J Obstet Gynaecol Br Cwlth 81: 549–553

Barnes AB, Colton T, Gundersen J et al. (1980) Fertility and outcome of pregnancy in women exposed in utero to diethylstilbestrol. N Engl J Med 302: 609–613

Beer AE (1988) Pregnancy outcome in couples with recurrent abortions following immunological evaluation and therapy. In: Beard RW, Sharp F (eds) Early pregnancy loss—mechanisms and treatment. Springer Verlag, London, pp 337–349

Bejar R, Curbelo V, Davis C, Gluck L (1981) Premature labor. II. Bacterial sources of phospholipase. Obstet Gynecol 57: 479–482

Bello BV, Schonholz D, Moshirpur J, Jeng D-Y, Berkowitz RL (1986) Combined pregnancy: the Mount Sinai experience. Obstet Gynecol Surv 41: 603–613

Benirschke K (1989) Editorial: flow cytometry for ALL mole-like abortion specimens. Hum Pathol 20: 403–404

Benirschke K, Kaufmann P (1990a) Pathology of the human placenta, 2nd edn. Springer Verlag, New York, pp 568–572

Benirschke K, Kaufmann P (1990b) Pathology of the human placenta, 2nd edn. Springer Verlag, New York, pp 530–541

Benirschke K, Kaufmann P (1990c) Pathology of the human placenta, 2nd edn. Springer Verlag, New York, pp 782–840

Berche P, Reich KA, Bonnichon M et al. (1990) Detection of anti-listeriolysin O for serodiagnosis of human listeriosis. Lancet 335: 624–627

Berry CL (1980) The examination of embryonic and fetal material in diagnostic histopathology laboratories. J Clin Pathol 33: 317–326

Blanc WA (1981) Pathology of the placenta, membranes and umbilical cord in bacterial, fungal and viral infections in man. In: Naeye RL, Kissane JM, Kaufman N (eds) Perinatal diseases. Williams and Wilkins, Baltimore, pp 67–132

Blanc WA, Mattison DR, Kane R, Chauhan P (1971) LSD, intrauterine amputations and amniotic band syndrome. Lancet ii: 158–159

Boe F (1967) Studies on the human placenta I: The cell islands in the young placenta. Acta Obstet Gynecol Scand 46: 591–603

Bortolussi R, Seeliger HPR (1990) Listeriosis. In: Remington JS, Klein JO (eds) Infectious diseases of the fetus and newborn infant. Saunders, Philadelphia, pp 812–833

Bortolussi R, Issekutz T, Burbridge S, Schellekens H (1989) Neonatal host defence mechanisms against *Listeria monocytogenes* infection: the role played by lipopolysaccharidases and interferons. Pediatr Res 25: 311–315

Boué A, Boué J, Gropp A (1985) Cytogenetics of pregnancy wastage. Adv Hum Genet 14: 1–57

Boyd PA, Lindenbaum RH, Redman C (1987) Pre-eclampsia and trisomy 13: a possible association. Lancet ii: 425–427

Bower C, Stanley FJ, Walters BNJ (1987) Pre-eclampsia and trisomy 13. Lancet ii: 1032

Branch D, Scott J, Kochenour N, Hershgold E (1985) Obstetric complications associated with the Lupus Anticoagulant. New Engl J Med 313: 1322–1326

Buckley JD (1984) The epidemiology of molar pregnancy and chorioncarcinoma. Clin Obstet Gynecol 27(1): 153–159

Budowick M, Johnson TR, Genadry R, Parmley TH, Woodruff JD (1980) The histopathology of the developing tubal ectopic pregnancy. Fertil Steril 34: 169–171

Bujko M, Sulovik V, Zivanovic V, Dotlic R, Bardic I (1988) Herpes simplex virus infection in women with previous spontaneous abortion. J Perinat Med 16: 193–196

Caul EO, Usher MJ, Burton PA (1988) Intrauterine infection with human parvovirus B19: a light and electron microscopy study. J Med Virol 24: 55–66

Cline DW (1979) Unsuspected suboptimal pregnancies in patients with luteal phase defects. Am J Obstet Gynecol 134: 438–444

Cowchock S, Smith JB, Gocial B (1986) Antibodies to phospholipids and nuclear antigens in patients with repeated abortions. Am J Obstet Gynecol 155: 1002–1010

Creasy R (1988) The cytogenetics of spontaneous abortion in humans. In: Beard RW, Sharp F (eds) Early pregnancy loss—mechanisms and treatment. Springer Verlag, London, pp 293–308

Creasy MR, Crolla JA, Alberman ED (1976) A cytogenetic study of human spontaneous abortions using banding techniques. Hum Genet 31: 177–196

Cregler LL, Mark H (1986) Medical compications of cocaine abuse. New Engl J Med 315: 1495–1500

Davis JR, Kerrigan DP, Way DL, Weiner SA (1987) Partial hydatidiform moles: deoxyribonucleic acid content and course. Am J Obstet Gynecol 157: 969–73

DeCherney AH, Jones EE (1985) Ectopic pregnancy. Clin Obstet Gynecol 28: 365–374

DeCherney AH, Silidker JS, Hazer HC, Tariatzis BC (1985) Reproductive outcome following two ectopic gestations. Fertil Steril 28: 365–374

Disker D, Feldberg D, Samuel N, Yeshaya A, Karp M, Goldman JA (1988) Spontaneous abortion in patients with insulin dependent diabetes mellitus: the effect of preconceptional diabetic control. Am J Obstet Gynecol 158: 1161–1164

DHSS (1979) Confidential enquiry into maternal deaths in England and Wales 1973–1975. HMSO, London

Driscoll S (1984) Gestational trophoblastic neoplasia: surgical pathologic considerations with clinical emphasis. Clin Obstet Gynecol 27: 160–171

Dukes MNG (ed) (1980) Meyer's side effects of drugs. Excerpta Medica, Amsterdam

Editorial (1980) How not to cope with a pollution crisis. Lancet ii: 131–132

Elias S, Simpson JL (1980) Evaluation and clinical management of patients at apparent increased risk for spontaneous abortion. In: Porter IH, Hook EB (eds) Human embryonic and fetal death. Academic, New York, pp 331–354

Elston CW (1981) Gestational tumours of trophoblast. In: Anthony PP, MacSween RNM (eds) Recent advances in histopathology 11. Churchill Livingstone, Edinburgh, pp 149–161

Elston CW (1984) The pathology of trophoblastic disease: current status. Clin Obstet Gynaecol 11: 135–154

Elston CW, Bagshawe KD (1972) The diagnosis of trophoblastic tumours from uterine curettings. J Clin Pathol 25: 111–118

Fedele L, Acaia B, Parazzini F, Ricciardiello O, Candiani GB (1989) Ectopic pregnancy and recurrent spontaneous abortion: two associated reproductive failures. Obstet Gynecol 73: 206–208

Finkler NJ, Berkowitz RS, Driscoll SG, Goldstein DP, Bernstein MR (1988) Clinical experience with placental site trophoblastic tumours at the New England Trophoblastic Disease Center. Obstet Gynecol 71: 854–857

Fisher RA, Lawler SD, Ormerod MG, Imrie PR, Povey S (1987) Flow cytometry used to distinguish between complete and partial hydatidiform moles. Placenta 8: 249–256

Gleicher N, Friberg J (1985) IgM gammopathy and the lupus anticoagulant syndrome in habitual aborters. JAMA 253: 3278–3281

Goldhaber MK, Staub SL, Tokuhata GK (1983) Spontaneous abortion after the Three Mile Island nuclear accident: a life table analysis. Am J Public Health 73: 752–759

Goldstein DP (1978) Incompetent cervix in offspring exposed to diethylstilbestrol in utero. Obstet Gynecol 52 (suppl): 73S–75S

Goldstein DP, Berkowitz RS, Bernstein MR (1984) Reproductive performance after molar pregnancy and gestational trophoblast tumours. Clin Obstet Gynecol 27: 221–227

Green GH (1966) Pregnancy following cervical cancer in situ: a review of 60 cases. J Obstet Gynaecol Br Cwlth 73: 897–902

Green JK, Kott ML (1989) Histopathologic findings in ectopic tubal pregnancy. Int J Gynecol Pathol 8: 255–262

Hallatt JG (1982) Primary ovarian pregnancy: a report of 25 cases. Am J Obstet Gynecol 143: 55–60

Harlap S, Shiono PH (1980) Alcohol, smoking and incidence of spontaneous abortions in the first and second trimesters. Lancet ii: 173–176

Harlap S, Shiono PH, Ramcharan S (1980) Spontaneous fetal loss in women using different contraceptives around the time of conception. Int J Epidemiol 9: 49–56

Hassold TJ (1980) A cytogenetic study of repeated spontaneous abortion. Am J Human Genet 32: 723–730

Hemming JD, Quirke P, Womack C, Wells M, Elston CW, Bird CC (1987) Diagnosis of molar pregnancy and persistent trophoblastic disease by flow cytometry. J Clin Pathol 40: 615–620

Hemminki K, Axelson O, Niemi ML, Ahlborg G (1983) Assessment of methods and results of reproductive occupational epidemiology: spontaneous abortions and malformations in the offspring of working women. Am J Ind Med 4: 293–307

Hertig AT, Rock J, Adams EC (1936) A description of 34 human ova within 17 days of development. Am J Anat 98: 435–493

Hertig AT, Rock J, Adams EC, Menkin MC (1959) Thirty four human fertilised ova, good, bad and indifferent, recovered from 210 women of known fertility; a study of biological wastage in early human pregnancy. Pediatrics 23: 202–211

Hertz R (1978) Chorioncarcinoma and related gestational trophoblastic tumors in women. Raven, New York

Hotz VL, Daling JR, Voigt LF et al. (1989) Induced abortion and the risk of subsequent ectopic pregnancy. Am J Public Health 79: 1234–1238

Honore LH (1979) Salpingitis isthmica nodosa in female infertility and ectopic pregnancy. Fertil Steril 29: 164–168

Hoyme HE, Jones KL, Dixon SD et al. (1990) Prenatal cocaine exposure and fetal vascular disruption. Pediatrics 85: 743–747

Hubert D (1990) 4 years after Chernobyl: medical repercussions. Bull Cancer (Paris) 77: 419–428

Hughey MJ, McElin TW (1979) The incompetent cervix. In: Sciarra JJ (ed) Gynecology and obstetrics, vol 3. Harper and Row, Hagerstown, Chap 53

Jacobs PA, Hassold TJ (1980) The origin of chromosome abnormalities in spontaneous abortion. In: Porter IH, Hook EB (eds) Human embryonic and fetal death. Academic, New York, pp 289–298

Jacobs PA, Wilson CM, Sprenkle JA, Rosenshein NB, Migeon BR (1980) Mechanism of origin of complete hydatidiform mole. Nature 286: 714–716

Jacobs PA, Szulman AE, Funkhauser J, Matsuura JS, Wilson CC (1982) Human triploidy: relationship between parental origin of the additional haploid complement and development of partial hydatidiform mole. Ann Hum Genet 46: 223–231

James WH (1970) The incidence of spontaneous abortion. Pop Studies 24: 241–245

Johnson PM, Kirkpatrick DC (1984) HLA sharing in pregnancy. Lancet ii: 1122–1123

Jones HW Jr, Wheeless CR (1969) Salvage of the reproduction potential of women with anomalous development of the mullerian ducts: 1868–1968–2068. Am J Obstet Gynecol 104: 348–364

Kajii T, Ohama K (1977) Androgenic origin of hydatidiform mole. Nature 268: 633–634

Kalousek DK, Barret I, McGillivray B (1989) Confined chromosomal mosaicism in trophoblast and intrauterine survival of trisomies 13 and 18. Am J Hum Genet 44: 338–343

Kalousek DK, Fitch N, Paradice BA (1990a) Pathology of the human embryo and previable fetus. Springer Verlag, New York, pp 196–199

Kalousek DK, Fitch N, Paradice BA (1990b) Pathology of the human embryo and previable fetus. Springer Verlag, New York, pp 37–48, 226–236

Kaufman RH, Noller K, Adam E et al. (1984) Upper genital tract abnormalities and pregnancy outcome in diethylstilbestrol-exposed progeny. Am J Obstet Gynecol 148: 973–984

Khong TY, Liddell HS, Robertson WB (1987) Defective haemochorial placentation as a cause of miscarriage. A preliminary study. Br J Obstet Gynaecol 94: 649–655

Kinney JS, Anderson LJ, Farrar J et al. (1988) Risk of adverse outcomes of pregnancy after human parvovirus

B19 infection. J Infect Dis 157: 663–667
Kline J, Shrout P, Stein Z, Susser M, Warburton D (1980a) Drinking during pregnancy and spontaneous abortion. Lancet ii: 176–180
Kline J, Stein Z, Susser M, Warburton D (1980b) Environmental influence on early reproductive loss in a current New York City study. In: Porter IH, Hook EB (eds) Human embryonic and fetal death. Academic, New York, pp 225–240
Kohorn EI (1984) Molar pregnancy: presentation and diagnosis. Clin Obstet Gynecol 27: 181–191
Lage JM, Driscoll SG, Yavner DL, Olivier AP, Mark SD, Weinberg DS (1988) Hydatidiform moles: application of flow cytometry in diagnosis. Am J Clin Pathol 89: 596–600
Lauritsen JL, Grunnet N, Jensen OM (1976) Significance of HLA and blood group incompatibility in spontaneous abortion. Clin Genet 9: 575–582
Lawler SD, Fisher RA (1987) Genetic studies in hydatidiform mole with clinical correlations. Placenta 8: 77–88
Lawson HW, Atrash HK, Saftlas AF, Finch EL (1989) Ectopic pregnancy in the United States 1970–1986. MMWR CDC Surveillance Summ 38: 1–10
Lazarchick J, Kizer J (1989) The laboratory diagnosis of lupus anticoagulants. Arch Pathol Lab Med 113: 177–180
Lee WR (1985) Working with visual display units. Br Med J 291: 989–991
Luning G, Scheer J, Schmidt M, Ziggel H (1989) Early infant mortality in West Germany before and after Chernobyl. Lancet ii: 1081–1083
Makinen JI, Erkkola RU, Laippala PJ (1989) Causes of the increase in incidence of ectopic pregnancy. A study on 1017 patients from 1966 to 1985 in Turku, Finland. Am J Obstet Gynecol 160: 642–646
Malone LJ, Ingersoll FM (1975) Myomectomy in infertility. In: Behrman SJ, Kistner RW (eds) Progress in infertility, 2nd edn. Little Brown, Boston, pp 85–90
Malpas P (1938) A study of abortion sequences. J Obstet Gynaecol Br Cwlth 45: 932–949
Martin DA, Sutton GP, Ulbright TM, Sledge GW, Stehman FB, Ehrlich CE (1989) DNA content as a prognostic index in gestational trophoblast neoplasia. Gynecol Oncol 34: 383–388
May JW, Miller JB, Griers FC (1978) Maternal deaths from ectopic pregnancy in the South Atlantic region, 1960 through 1976. Am J Obstet Gynecol 132: 140–145
Mennuti MT, Jingeleski S, Schwarz RH, Mellman WJ (1978) An evaluation of cytogenetic analysis as a primary tool in the assessment of recurrent pregnancy wastage. Obstet Gynecol 52: 308–313
Mercado A, Johnson G, Calver D, Sokol RJ (1989) Cocaine, pregnancy and postpartum intracerebral haemorrhage. Obstet Gynecol 73: 467–468
Mikamo K (1970) Anatomic and chromosomal anomalies in spontaneous abortion. Possible correlation with overripeness of oocytes. Am J Obstet Gynecol 106: 243–254
Miller JF, Williamson E, Glue J, Gordon YB, Grudzinskas JG, Sykes A (1980) Fetal loss after implantation. A prospective study. Lancet ii: 554–556
Mocan H, Bozkaya H, Mocan MZ, Furtun EM (1990) Changing incidence of anencephaly in the Eastern Black Sea region of Turkey and Chernobyl. Paediatr Perinat Epidemiol 4: 264–268
Montgomery DAD, Harley JMG (1977) Endocrine disorders. Clin Obstet Gynaecol 4: 339–370
Mowbray JF, Gibbings C, Liddell H, Reginald PW, Underwood JL, Beard RW (1985) Controlled trial of treatment of recurrent spontaneous abortion by immunisation with paternal cells. Lancet i: 941–943
Nilsson IM, Astedt B, Hedner U, Berezin D (1975) Intrauterine death and circulating anticoagulant ("antithrombo-plastin"). Acta Med Scand 197: 153–159
Ober C, Elias S, O'Brien E, Kostyu DD, Hauck WW, Bombard A (1988) HLA sharing and fertility in Hutterite couples: evidence for prenatal selection against compatible getuses. Am J Reprod Immunol Microbiol 18: 111–115
Opitz JM (1987) Prenatal and perinatal death: the future of developmental pathology. Pediatr Pathol 7: 363–394
Othman S, Phillips DI, Parkes AB et al. (1990) A long term follow up of postpartum thyroiditis. Clin Endocrinol 32: 559–564
Peckham CS, Marshall WC (1983) Infections in pregnancy In: Barron SL, Thomson AM (eds) Obstetrical epidemiology. Academic, London, pp 209–262
Poland BJ, Miller JR, Jones DC, Trimble BK (1977) Reproductive counselling in patients who have had a spontaneous abortion. Am J Obstet Gynecol 127: 685–691
Poland BJ, Miller JR, Harris M, Livingston J (1981) Spontaneous abortion. A study of 1961 women and their conceptuses. Acta Obstet Gynecol Scand (Suppl) 102: 1–32
Porter HJ, Quantrill AM, Fleming KA (1988) B19 parvovirus infection of myocardial cells. Lancet i: 535–536
Potter EL, Craig JM (1976) Pathology of the fetus and the infant. Lloyd-Luke, London
Preblud SR, Stetler HC, Frank JA et al. (1981) Fetal risk associated with rubella vaccine. JAMA 246: 1413–1417
Prentice RL, Gatenby PA, Loblay RH, Shearman RP, Kronenberg H, Basten A (1984) Lupus anticoagulant and pregnancy. Lancet ii: 464
Purpura M, Coghi I, Nicotra M, Carapella E, Bottini E (1980) HLA Bw 35 antigen and human reproduction. J Med Genet 17: 157–158
Ratten GJ, Beischer NA (1979) The effect of termination of pregnancy on maturity of subsequent pregnancy. Med J Aust 1: 479–480
Rice LW, Berkowitz RS, Lage JM, Goldstein DP, Bernstein MR (1990) Persistent gestational trophoblast tumour after partial hydatidiform mole. Gynecol Oncol 36: 358–362
Robertson WB, Brosens I, Dixon G (1975) Uteroplacental vascular pathology. Europ J Obstet Gynecol Reprod Biol 5: 47–65
Rock JA, Jones HW (1977) The clinical management of the double uterus. Fertil Steril 28: 798–806
Roman E, Stevenson AC (1983) Spontaneous abortion. In: Barron SL, Thomson AM (eds) Obstetrical epidemiology. Academic Press London, pp 61–87
Rubin GL, Peterson HB, Dorfman SF et al. (1983) Ectopic pregnancy in the United States 1970 through 1978. JAMA 249: 1725–1729
Rushton DI (1978) Simplified classification of spontaneous abortion. J Med Genet 15: 1–9
Rushton DI (1981) Examination of products of conception from previable human pregnancies. J Clin Pathol 32: 819–835
Rushton DI (1982) Examination of abortions. In: Barson AJ (ed) Fetal and neonatal pathology. Praeger, New York, pp 27–64
Rushton DI (1984) The classification and mechanisms of spontaneous abortion. Perspect Pediatr Pathol 8: 269–287
Rushton DI (1988) Placental pathology in spontaneous miscarriage. In: Beard RW, Sharp F (eds) Early pregnancy loss—mechanisms and treatment. Springer Verlag, London, pp 149–158

Sbarra AJ, Selvaraj RJ, Cetrulo CL, Feingold M, Newton E, Thomas GB (1985) Infection and phagocytosis as possible mechanisms of rupture of the membranes. Am J Obstet Gynecol 153: 38–43

Schenker JG, Eyal F, Polishuk WZ (1972) Fertility after tubal pregnancy. Surg Gynecol Obstet 135: 74–76

Selwyn PA, Schoenbaum EE, Davenny K et al. (1989) Prospective study of human immunodeficiency virus infection and pregnancy outcomes in intravenous drug users. JAMA 291: 1289–1294

Shepard TH (1986) Catalog of teratogenic agents, 5th edn. John Hopkins University Press, Baltimore

Shepard TH, Fitzsimmons JM, Fantel AG, Pascoe-Mason J (1989) Placental weights of normal and aneuploid early human fetuses. Pediatr Pathol 9: 425–431

Simor AE, Ferro S (1990) *Campylobacter jejuni* infection occurring during pregnancy. Euro J Microbiol Inf Dis 9: 142–144

Simpson JL (1981) Repeated suboptimal pregnancy outcome. Birth defects XVII: 113–142

Simpson JL (1990) Incidence and timing of pregnancy losses: relevance to evaluating safety of early prenatal diagnosis. Am J Med Genet 35: 165–173

Skjeldstad FE, Hammervild R, Peterson DR (1988) Outcomes of pregnancy with an IUD in situ—a population based case-control study. Adv Contracept 4: 265–270

Slone D, Siskind V, Heinonen OP, Monson RR, Kaufman DW, Shapiro S (1976) Aspirin and congenital malformations. Lancet i: 1373–1375

Spence AA, Knill-Jones RP (1978) Is there a health hazard in anaesthetic practice? Br J Anaesth 50: 713–719

Spencer JAD (1987) Perinatal listeriosis. Br Med J 295: 349

Speroff L (1989) The effects of oral contraception on reproduction. Int J Fertil 34 (Suppl): 34–39

Spiegelberg O (1878) Zur Causistic der ovarial Schwangerschaft. Arch Gynecol 13: 73–79

Steele PE, Jacobs DS (1979) *Listeria monocytogenes*. Microabscesses of placenta. Obstet Gynecol 53: 124–127

Stevenson RE (1977) The fetus and newly born infant: influences of the prenatal environment. Mosby, St Louis

Stray-Pederson B, Stray-Pederson S (1984) Etiologic factors and subsequent reproductive performance in 195 couples with a prior history of habitual abortion. Am J Obstet Gynecol 148: 140–146

Stray-Pedersen B, Lorentzen-Styr A (1977) Uterine toxoplasma infections and repeated abortions. Am J Obstet Gynecol 128: 716–721

Stray-Pedersen B, Eng J, Reikvam TM (1978) Uterine T-mycoplasma colonisation in reproductive failure. Am J Obstet Gynecol 130: 307–311

Stucker I, Caillard JF, Collin R, Gout M, Poyen D, Hemon D (1990) Risk of spontaneous abortion amongst nurses handling antineoplastic drugs. Scand J Work Environ Health 16: 102–107

Surti U, Szulman AE, O'Brien S (1982) Dispermic origin and clinical outcome of three complete hydatidiform moles with 46XY karyotype. Am J Obstet Gynecol 144: 84–87

Szekely P, Snaith L (1977) Cardiac disorders. Clin Obstet Gynaecol 4: 265–286

Szulman AE (1988) Trophoblast disease: clinical pathology of hydatidiform moles. Obstet Gynecol Clin N Amer 15: 443–456

Szulman AE, Surti U (1984) The syndromes of partial and complete molar gestation. Clin Obstet Gynecol 27: 172–180

Tatum HJ, Schmidt FH, Jain AK (1976) Management and outcome of pregnancies associated with the Copper-7 intrauterine contraceptive device. Am J Obstet Gynecol 126: 869–879

Taylor C, Page Faulk W (1981) Prevention of recurrent abortion with leukocyte transfusions. Lancet ii: 68–69

Teoh E-S (1988) Asian approaches in the treatment of trophoblastic disease. Obstet Gynecol Clin N Amer 15: 545–564

Tho PT, Byrd JR, McDonough PG (1979) Etiologies and subsequent reproductive performance of 100 couples with recurrent abortion. Fertil Steril 32: 389–395

Tongio MM, Berrebi A, Mayer S (1972) A study of lymphocytotoxic antibodies in multiparous women having had at least four pregnancies. Tissue Antigens 2: 378–388

Triplett DA (1989) Antiphospholipid antibodies and recurrent pregnancy loss. Am J Reprod Immunol 20: 52–67

Trudinger BJ, Stewart GJ, Cook CM, Connelly A, Exner T (1988) Monitoring lupus anticoagulant pregnancies with umbilical artery flow velocity waveforms. Obstet Gynecol 72: 215–218

Uotila J, Heinonen PK, Punnonen R (1989) Reproductive outcome after multiple ectopic pregnances. Int J Fertil 34: 102–105

Vianna NJ (1980) Adverse pregnancy outcomes—potential endpoints of human toxicity in the Love Canal. Preliminary results. In: Porter IH, Hook EB (eds) Human embryonic and fetal death. Academic, New York, pp 165–168

Wagar EA, Schachter J, Bavoil P, Stephens RS (1990) Differential human serologic response to two 60 000 molecular weight *Chlamydia trachomatis* antigens. J Infect Dis 162: 922–927

Wake N, Tanaka K, Chapman V, Matsui S, Sandberg AA (1981) Chromosomes and cellular origin of chorioncarcinoma. Cancer Res 41: 3137–3143

Warburton D, Fraser FC (1964) Spontaneous abortion risks in man: data from reproductive histories collected in a medical genetics unit. Am J Hum Genet 16: 1–25

Warburton D, Stein Z, Kline J, Susser M (1980) Chromosome abnormalities in spontaneous abortion: data from the New York City Study. In: Porter IH, Hook EB (eds) Human embryonic and fetal death. Academic, New York, pp 261–287

Warburton D, Kline J, Stein Z, Hutzler M, Chin A, Hassold T (1987) Does the karyotype of a spontaneous abortion predict the karyotype of a subsequent abortion? Evidence from 273 women with two karyotyped spontaneous abortus? Am J Hum Genet 41: 465–483

Warren CW, Gold J, Tyler CW, Smith JC, Paris AL (1980) Seasonal variation in spontaneous abortions. Am J Public Health 70: 1297–1299

Wigglesworth JS (1984) Perinatal pathology. Major problems in pathology, vol 15. Saunders, Philadelphia, pp 130–167

Wilcox AJ (1983) Surveillance of pregnancy loss in human populations. Am J Ind Med 4: 285–291

Witt BR, Wolf GC, Wainwright CJ, Johnston PD, Thorneycroft IH (1990) Relaxin, Ca-125, progesterone, estradiol, Schwangerschaft protein, and human chorionic gonadotrophin as predictors of outcome of threatened and non-threatened pregnancies. Fertil Steril 53: 1029–1036

Wyshak G (1983) Age at menarche and unsuccessful pregnancy outcome. Ann Hum Biol 10: 69–73

Yen S, MacMahon B (1968) Epidemiological features of trophoblastic disease. Am J Obstet Gynecol 135: 597–600

Young RH, Scully RE (1984) Placental site trophoblastic tumor: current status. Clin Obstet Gynecol 27: 248–258

Chapter 4

Congenital Malformations, Prenatal Diagnosis and Fetal Examination

Jean W. Keeling and Patricia A. Boyd

Introduction

Congenital malformations are an important cause of perinatal and infant mortality and morbidity. Three per cent of newborns have a single major malformation and 0.7% have multiple major defects. They have fascinated curious individuals for centuries but during the past 50 years infants with major anomalies have become the focus of increasing and diverse professional expertise and consume a large slice of health budgets in developed countries. Their importance as a cause of perinatal mortality has grown as deaths from intrapartum problems have declined and better neonatal care has improved the survival of normally formed low birthweight babies (see Chapter 8). Clinical interest in malformations has been enhanced because sophisticated surgical and anaesthetic management makes correction of some major defects possible. This and the recognition of syndromes, their mode of inheritance and sometimes their aetiology requires detailed information from the pathologist in respect of those babies who die.

There has been rapid expansion of methods of prenatal diagnosis and of the many different types of disorder that can be detected prenatally. This, and increasing obstetric interest in the pathology of the spontaneously aborted fetus means that the pathologist needs to be acquainted with malformations in the fetus which will be at an earlier stage of development than previously encountered. He must also recognise that some disorders may have distinct, gestation-related manifestations, that a major malformation may have different aetiologies and thus, different recurrence risks and that coexisting minor dysmorphisms may indicate a syndrome diagnosis or a specific aetiology. Recognition of the difference between a collection of associated defects which may constitute a *syndrome* and a chain of events consequent on a single malformation which can produce a *sequence* of malformations or progressive deformity is important. Detailed observation of normal embryonic and fetal development and of structural abnormalities in the fetus has increased our awareness of the pathogenesis of many malformations. Our understanding of their aetiology has progressed at a much slower rate.

Definitions

An International Working Group (Benirschke et al. 1979; Spranger et al. 1982) addressed the problem of confusion of nomenclature. They defined some essential and widely used terms and concepts relating to malformations. The following definitions are those of Spranger et al. (1982):

Developmental field—a region or part of an embryo which responds as a coordinated unit to embryonic interaction and results in complex or multiple anatomic structures.

Malformation—a morphologic defect of an organ, part of an organ, or larger region of the body resulting from an intrinsically abnormal developmental process.

Disruption—a morphologic defect of an organ, part of an organ, or a larger region of the body resulting from the extrinsic breakdown of, or an interference with, an originally normal developmental process.

Deformation—an abnormal form, shape, or position of a part of the body caused by mechanical forces.

Dysplasia—an abnormal organisation of cells into tissue(s) and its morphologic result(s). In other words: a dysplasia is the process (and the consequence) of dyshistogenesis.

Polytopic field defect—a pattern of (widely separated) anomalies derived from the disturbance of a single developmental field.

Sequence—a pattern of multiple anomalies derived from a single known or presumed prior anomaly or mechanical factor.

Syndrome—a pattern of multiple anomalies thought to be pathogenetically related and not known to represent a single sequence or a polytopic field defect.

Association—a non-random occurrence in two or more individuals of multiple anomalies not known to be a polytopic field defect, sequence or syndrome.

In practice, it may be difficult to distinguish between malformations and disruptions, particularly when exposure to a teratogen occurred early in embryogenesis.

Causes of Congenital Malformations

The causes of malformations can be considered in five broad groups, mutant genes, chromosome anomalies, multifactorial disorders which are considered the result of interaction between genetic predisposition and presumed environmental factors, teratogenic agents and those of unknown cause. We know that in addition to their adverse effects on embryogenesis both chromosome anomalies and environmental teratogens have a range of effects on the developing human organism. These include loss of zygotes resulting in infertility, early abortion, fetal growth retardation, alterations of system function and predisposition to malignant neoplasms. Some of these other effects may also be present in the individual with a structural malformation. Exciting new developments in genetics such as evidence for genes involved in the regulation of development, awareness of microdeletion syndromes, imprinting mechanisms and uniparental isodisomy (the presence of two identical copies of the same chromosome from one parent) have given new insight into the aetiology of some of these conditions (Lancet 1991). For a fuller discussion of single gene defects, chromosome anomalies and genetic counselling see Gardner and Sutherland (1989), Emery and Rimoin (1990), Weatherall (1991).

Despite enormous advances in genetics over the last decade, particularly in gene mapping and the elucidation of specific structural changes within mutant genes, the aetiology of more than 60% of malformations is unknown. Mutant genes, chromosome anomalies or known teratogens can each be identified in about 6% of cases with a further 20% of malformations falling into the group of multifactorial disorders. Even when an aetiological agent is identified, their actual mode of action is usually not understood.

Single Gene Defects

These disorders are the result of a single mutant gene and are inherited in Mendelian fashion. Many individual disorders are rare and others do not result in anatomical defects. However a very large number of disorders have been identified: McKusick (1990) lists more than 4000. Together they account for 6%–8% of congenital malformations at term, roughly the same proportion as are caused by chromosome abnormalities.

Autosomal dominant genes give rise to recognisable effects in heterozygous individuals with an equal sex distribution. Some do not usually produce recognisable disease until adult life, e.g. Huntington's chorea and adult renal polycystic disease. Others such as achondroplasia are recognisable at birth and may be recognised prenatally by ultrasound examination. Although this disorder is not fatal, some parents opt to terminate the pregnancy. It is clearly important to distinguish this from other types of skeletal dysplasia (see Chap. 26). When an isolated autosomal dominant disorder occurs and the parents are unaffected it is likely to be a new mutation and not recur in siblings. However, the possibility of gonadal mosaicism, reduced penetrance and variable expression means that there may be a real but small recurrence risk.

Some dominant genes can be identified directly and others indirectly using molecular biological techniques, e.g. adult polycystic kidney and myotonic dystrophy genes (Reeders et al. 1985; Weatherall 1991).

Autosomal recessive genes occur in males and females equally and are only clinically manifest in the homozygous state. Thus affected individuals have healthy heterozygous parents. Unless an autosomal recessive gene is common in the population, (e.g. cystic fibrosis in western European Caucasians or Tay–Sachs disease in Ashkenazi Jews) there is often a history of consanguinous marriage. Because the recurrence risk for affected siblings is 1 in 4 it is important that these conditions be recognised rapidly so that families can be appropriately counselled.

Recessively inherited disorders likely to be encountered by pathologists amongst perinatal deaths are Meckel's syndrome, infantile polycystic renal disease (Chapter 19), short-ribbed dwarfing syndromes (Chapter 26), cystic fibrosis with meconium ileus (Chapter 15) and Werdnig–Hoffman syndrome (neurogenic muscular atrophy) (Chapter 25).

Some genetic metabolic disorders such as glutaric acidaemia type II and Zellweger's syndrome exhibit a range of malformations. These are thought to result from an autoteratogenic effect of the abnormal fetal biochemical milieu due to accumulation of metabolites because of enzyme deficiency.

X-linked recessive genes, carried on the X chromosome are expressed in the hemizygous state. Thus only males are affected and the disorder is transmitted from healthy female carriers. Examples are Duchenne muscular dystrophy and haemophilia. All daughters of affected males are obligate carriers and all sons unaffected. The sons of carrier females have a 1 in 2 chance of being affected and the daughters a similar chance of carrying the gene. In some of these conditions gene carriers can be identified biochemically or by using DNA techniques.

Chromosome Abnormalities

Normal human development is dependent on the correct chromosome complement, normally 22 homologous pairs of autosomes and a pair of sex chromosomes. Too much or too little chromosome material usually results from a fault occurring during meiosis. Sixty per cent of first trimester abortuses and 5% of stillbirths are chromosomally unbalanced. Karyotyping these groups and any dysmorphic fetus or baby is particularly important.

There is a huge range of chromosome disorders, many are outwith the remit of this Chapter but Schinzel (1984) provides a useful catalogue. Those involving whole extra haploid sets of chromosomes are *polyploidy* (e.g. triploidy, 69 chromosomes) and *aneuploidy*—the loss or gain of a whole chromosome (monosomy and trisomy respectively). Both polyploidy and monosomy are virtually lethal in humans. *Structural chromosome abnormalities* may involve translocations (exchange of material between chromosomes), deletions or duplications (loss or addition of chromosome material). Gardner and Sutherland (1989) describe aetiology and mechanisms of chromosome disorders.

Triploidy

Triploidy occurs in approximately 2% of recognised pregnancies. It usually results from an error at fertilisation, an ovum being fertilised by two spermatozoa, occasionally by a diploid sperm and less usually from fertilisation of a diploid egg. The karyotype is most commonly 69XXY. In those triploids resulting from a double paternal contribution (diandry) the placenta is abnormal and shows partial molar change; pregnancy rarely proceeds beyond the first trimester. Half of these pregnancies abort spontaneously, and most of the rest persist as missed abortions. Invasive mole is an infrequent sequel, choriocarcinoma is not described as a complication (Szulman and Surti 1982).

Triploids resulting from fertilisation of a diploid egg (digyny) do not have molar change in their placentas and pregnancy may continue beyond the first trimester. The difference in development of the embryo and of trophoblast growth and function is related to the parental origin of the extra set of chromosomes (Jacobs et al. 1982). This is the first recognised manifestation of genomic imprinting in the human. Ploidy and sex chromosome composition can be assessed on tissue sections using probes to specific regions on chromosomes and in situ hybridisation techniques (van de Kaa et al. 1991). This should prove useful when culture fails or when examining archival material.

Tetraploidy (92 chromosomes) is most uncommon. Warburton et al. (1991) found it in 2% of abortuses in their study.

Autosomal Trisomy

An additional chromosome is much more common than is its loss. Trisomy of most autosomes has been recorded but the incidence varies enormously. Overall, trisomy of chromosome 16 is the most common (Warburton et al. 1991), but the usual result of this anomaly is spontaneous or missed abortion towards the end of the first trimester. About 15% of cases have a disorganised embryo, more advanced embryonic development is present in less than 10% of cases. When liveborn trisomic infants are examined, trisomy 21 (Down's syndrome) is the most common followed by trisomy 18 (Edward's syndrome) and trisomy 13 (Patau's syndrome). It is important to remember that even amongst these karyotypes, miscarriage is the most common outcome. The majority of trisomic pregnancies perish between 10 and 15 weeks of gestation. Survival to term in trisomies 18 and 13 may only occur when there is placental mosaicism with some placental cells having a normal karyotype (Kalousek et al. 1989) (see p. 119). Ninety-five per cent of Down's syndrome, nearly all Edward's syndrome and 80% of Patau's syndrome are regular trisomies arising by non-disjunction at the first or second meiotic division. A small proportion of cases has a translocation either arising de novo or inherited from a parent who carries a balanced translocation. Mosaicism involving a normal and a trisomic cell line arises either by loss of an abnormal cell line in an abnormal conception by anaphase lag or from post-zygotic mitotic non-disjunction in a previously normal conceptus. Such individuals exhibit abnormalities which may be less severe than pure trisomic individuals (see Jones 1988 for details of phenotypes).

Structural Chromosome Abnormality

Structural chromosome rearrangements such as translocations, inversions, deletions may arise de novo or as a result of a parental chromosome rearrangement. Fusion at or near the centromere of the five acrocentric chromosomes (Robertsonian translocation) is one of the most common balanced structural rearrangements. Simple reciprocal translocations involve exchange of material between two chromosomes. A break occurs in one arm of each and chromosome material distal to the break swaps positions. Balanced carriers are entirely normal, having no gain or loss of chromosome material but they are at considerable risk of having chromosomally unbalanced offspring or miscarriages due to malsegregation at meiosis. The extent of the chromosome imbalance depends on the particular translocation.

Unbalanced structural chromosome rearrangements (arising de novo or resulting from an inherited rearrangement) often produce structural anatomical abnormalities which in a few cases (e.g. 4p−, Wolf Hirschorn syndrome) are sufficiently characteristic to suggest the nature of the chromosome defect.

Microdeletion syndromes such as Prader–Willi, Angelman, Di George, Wilms' tumour–aniridia syndrome, Miller–Dieker lissencephaly syndromes, are being recognised with increasing frequency as techniques for chromosome examination are improved. If one of these conditions is suspected and no visible deletion found on microscopic examination of a karyotype, DNA probes may identify one.

Genomic imprinting is the difference in phenotypic expression of a genetic disorder depending on the maternal or paternal origin of the mutation. It may go some way towards explaining observations which appear to contradict simple Mendelian inheritance (Hall 1990; Lancet 1991).

Examples of imprinting in humans include the different phenotype in triploids which depends on the parent contributing the extra haploid set, and Prader–Willi and Angelman syndromes which both have a microdeletion at 15q11-13. Phenotype here reflects the parental source of the missing genetic material. Other expressions of genetic imprinting are the clinical observations of difference in severity of inherited disorders such as Wiedemann–Beckwith syndrome, neurofibromatosis and Huntington's chorea when inherited through the father or mother (Hall 1990).

Sex Chromosome Abnormality

The common sex chromosome abnormalities are 47XXY (Klinefelter's syndrome), 47XXX (Triple X), 45XO (Turner's syndrome or monosomy X) and 47XYY. Turner's syndrome, although by far least common in liveborns, is the one most likely to be encountered by the pathologist because over 99% abort spontaneously. It is the commonest chromosome abnormality amongst spontaneously aborted second trimester fetuses (Kalousek et al. 1990; Warburton et al. 1991). The typical phenotype is described on page 133.

The other abnormalities listed above are phenotypically normal at birth and only likely to be encountered by pathologists if a termination of pregnancy is requested after an incidental finding of one of these abnormalities at amniocentesis. Most liveborn XXY males present in adult life for investigation of infertility. Girls with Turner's syndrome may be recognised at birth because of typical phenotype, during investigation of short stature or heart murmur in childhood, or at puberty with primary amenorrhoea. Most XYY males remain undiagnosed.

The fragile X mental retardation syndrome deserves special mention because a recent breakthrough in molecular biology has provided insight into the curious inheritance pattern of this condition (Fu et al. 1991; Oberlé et al. 1991; Yu et al. 1991). It is the most common form of inherited mental retardation and the second most common cause of mental retardation after Down's syndrome. The typical phenotype does not fully develop until adulthood. Although affected males are more severely retarded, 30% of female heterozygotes are retarded although usually mildly.

Multifactorial Disorders

Multifactorial inheritance suggests that a disease is caused by the interaction of several adverse genes and environmental factors. Under this heading fall those disorders which occur with increased frequency among family members of an affected individual in an inverse frequency to their relationship. Families share environments as well as genes and a thesis of environmental agents acting on a susceptible population was proposed (Carter 1963, 1969). A mathematical model invoking a threshold effect can be constructed and recurrence risks in the offspring of family members calculated. Malformations where this model of inheritance has been invoked include cleft lip and palate and neural tube defects. The protective effect of folic acid administration to women who have borne a fetus with neural tube defect (Medical Research Council 1991b) lends support ot this model.

Environmental Teratogens

From recognised environmental teratogens such as rubella infection or particular drugs, we can extrapolate to a much larger number of agents with the potential to adversely affect the human embryo or fetus. Demonstration of a causal relationship in respect of a putative agent is very difficult because of the multiplicity of compounding variables. These include the timing of the insult, the dose, interaction with other potential teratogens and individual susceptibility. Initial recognition of a teratogen is only likely to occur when the effect is strong, or when it produces an unusual defect in sufficient cases. Recognition is most likely when there is a particular geographical or temporal restriction which serves to highlight the problem.

Maternal Disorders

A variety of maternal diseases, either genetic or acquired, and deficiency states may directly affect the developing embryo. In other disorders, such as epilepsy, it is most likely that it is the therapy which is damaging. Maternal phenylketonuria is the best documented example of genetic disease in the mother affecting her offspring when her serum phenylalanine level is elevated during pregnancy. It is likely that the elevated phenylalanine level acts during both the embryonic and fetal periods. The effect is mental deficiency which is unrelated to the genetic makeup of the child.

Maternal connective tissue disorders, such as osteogenesis imperfecta and Ehlers–Danlos syndrome are risk factors for early amnion disruption syndrome leading to a variety of disruptions and deformity in the fetus (Young et al. 1985).

Poorly controlled maternal diabetes increases the risk of malformation, particularly congenital heart disease and caudal regression syndrome. It is clear that improved control of the diabetic state using glycosylated haemoglobin levels as well as blood sugar monitoring has reduced the incidence of malformation in the offspring of these women (see Chap. 21).

Drugs

Reliable prediction of drug teratogenicity in man is not possible. Clinical testing to the point of certainty is a time-consuming and costly activity and is rarely undertaken (Ornoy 1991). It is most important to remember that the effect of a drug (or lack of it) in animals is not direct evidence of its likely effect in humans.

The action of some drugs such as antimetabolites and alkylating agents used as chemotherapeutic agents in the management of malignant disease make a teratogenic effect likely. This has been observed with a variety of antineoplastic drugs; folic acid antagonists such as aminopterin have the highest risk. Central nervous system defects, renal and limb abnormalities are well recognised and there is an increased risk of early abortion with these drugs. Most reported defects follow maternal treatment but malformations have been reported in babies conceived some months after paternal chemotherapy.

Anticonvulsant drugs such as phenytoin and carbamazepine produce a recognised syndrome of craniofacial defects with or without microcephaly, mental retardation and hypoplastic nails. Sodium valproate can cause meningomyelocoele (Martinez-Frias 1991) and other defects have been recorded. The teratogenic effect of phenobarbitone is not so clear but it does seem to potentiate the teratogenic effects of other anticonvulsants. The management of epilepsy in pregnancy is complex as convulsions following withdrawal or reduction of therapy may cause fetal death from hypoxia.

Coumarin anticoagulants, e.g. warfarin, can affect both embryo and fetus. Embryopathic effects are chondrodysplasia punctata and nasal hypoplasia whilst their effect on the fetus can result in microcephaly, mental retardation and optic atrophy (Hall et al. 1980).

Vitamin A (retinol) affects neural tube development and closure in animals and a concern has been expressed about its inclusion in vitamin supplements aimed at reduction of neural tube defect in susceptible populations. There is increasing evidence that vitamin A and related compounds can produce malformations in humans. Craniofacial anomalies, hydrocephaly, posterior fossa cyst, cardiac and renal defects, and thymic hypoplasia are described. The facial appearance and related defects are similar to those described in Di George syndrome. Retinoids are available without prescription and currently advertised for treatment of common skin disorders such as acne. Some compounds have a half-life measured in weeks or months so that there is a risk to pregnancies conceived after cessation of treatment (Lammer et al. 1985).

Diethylstilboestrol is both a prenatal carcinogen and teratogen but there is little evidence to implicate other female sex hormone-like substances. Concern about the potential teratogenic effect of combined oral contraceptive pills in early pregnancy has abated. It was suggested that clomiphene and related ovulation inducers might predispose to some malformations, particularly Down's syndrome and neural tube defects. Careful scrutiny of data allowing for maternal age and pre-existing maternal disorders does not support this.

Social Drugs

Adverse effects on the offspring of women who abuse ethyl alcohol have been recognised for very many years. A variety of effects were described last century (Ballantyne 1902) but only during the last two decades has the pattern of dysmorphic features and major malformations which constitute the fetal alcohol syndrome been recognised (Jones et al. 1973). These comprise hypoplasia of the midfacial skeleton with narrow palpebral fissures, hypertelorism, broad upturned nose, long philtrum and smooth upper lip border. Microcephaly, cleft palate and atrial or ventricular septal defects are common. Growth retardation, neonatal jitteriness and failure to thrive are frequent problems. It seems likely that either periodic binge drinking or regular alcohol consumption at a level of about two units per day in early pregnancy can induce recognisable but mild abnormalities.

Despite extensive study of the effects of smoking in pregnancy, there is no clear evidence to support a teratogenic role for tobacco when alcohol ingestion and other factors are allowed for. The adverse effects of smoking on fetal growth is quite clear as is its relationship to spontaneous abortion, premature onset of labour and stillbirth.

There is no evidence of teratogenetic effect of opiates or marihuana but cocaine affects fetal vasculature which can result in disruptions.

Infection

A number of infectious agents affect the fetus producing a range of effects from structural anomalies to immunological disorders and mental retardation. Rubella virus is embryopathic as well as having a recognisable fetopathic effect. Evidence for embryopathic effects of other infectious agents is not so clear-cut and it is likely that some are lethal to the embryo and have a reducing effect compatible with continued survival as pregnancy progresses. The effects of intrauterine infection are discussed in detail in Chapter 13.

Physical Agents

Heat. Sources of elevated environmental temperature are maternal pyrexia for any reason and external sources such as thermal baths or saunas. It is difficult to dissociate the effects of fever during maternal illness from direct effect of the infectious agent on embryo or fetus. In some laboratory animals, hyperthermia may interfere with cranial neural tube closure. There is little evidence for this in humans but it has been suggested that hyperthermia may cause Moebius' syndrome (Graham et al. 1988).

Ionising radiation. Radiation at levels used for diagnostic purposes is unlikely to be of sufficient intensity to produce direct injury. However, it is clear that energy is liberated in all tissues exposed and that the chance of an ionising event at some critical place is proportional to the intensity, and is never zero.

The results of studies at Nagasaki and Hiroshima showed an increased incidence of childhood cancers and leukaemia among those exposed, as well as of microcephaly. In microcephaly the data are inadequate to exclude effects at the low levels used diagnostically and completely consistent with this being due to direct damage in those exposed to high levels.

Exposure before conception is likely to increase the risk of both numerical and structural chromosomal abnormalities, as has been established in mice. The premeiotic divisions in the male are particularly sensitive. The evidence relating paternal exposure to childhood leukaemia is weak and not readily explained by any well-established mechanism.

Ultrasound. When ultrasonographic examination was first introduced into obstetric practice much concern was expressed about possible disruptive effects on the embryo or fetus. Widespread and repeated use at all stages of gestation suggests that these early fears are unfounded.

Pregnancy reduction. Because of the high incidence of preterm labour with consequential perinatal mortality and morbidity, pregnancy reduction may be offered when in vitro fertilisation has resulted in successful implantation of three or more zygotes. An anencephaly-like syndrome in surviving fetuses following embryo reduction is described (Boulot et al. 1990). The authors suggest a direct effect of the hypertonic saline used for reduction.

Amniotic bands. Fetal disruption may result from direct pressure, entanglement or ischaemia because of the presence of amniotic bands (see p. 141).

Prenatal Diagnosis

Suspicion of congenital abnormality may arise on clinical grounds or because of an abnormal result from a routine prenatal investigation. A pregnancy may be known to be at high risk of abnormality because of a particular family history leading to appropriate search for a specific condition. High-risk groups for chromosome anomaly include women of high maternal age, those with a chromosomally

Table 4.1. Situations associated with raised levels of alpha-fetoprotein in maternal serum or amniotic fluid in the second trimester of pregnancy

Elevated alpha-fetoprotein	Pathogenesis	Association	Reference
Maternal serum	Physiological:		
	Increased production	Multiple pregnancy	Wald et al. (1978)
	Pathological:		
	Loss of placental surface integrity	Abdominal pregnancy	Stirrat et al. (1981)
		Fetomaternal haemorrhage	
		Placental angioma	Mann et al. (1983)
Maternal serum, amniotic fluid	Interruption of cutaneous integrity	Neural tube defects	Brock and Sutcliffe (1972)
		Omphalocoele	Laurence (1982)
		Gastroschisis	Laurence (1982)
		Amnion rupture sequence	Aitken et al. (1984)
		Meckel syndrome	Chemke et al. (1977)
		Scalp defect (trisomy 13)	Fitzsimons et al. (1976)
	Altered skin permeability	Missed abortion	Wisniewski et al. (1974)
	Altered skin permeability + ? local pressure effect	Teratoma	
		Cystic hygroma (45XO)	Seller et al. (1974)
		Fetal hydrops	
		Urethral (valvular) obstruction	Vinson et al. (1977)
		Urethral atresia	Nevin et al. (1978)
		Haemangioma of umbilical cord	Barson et al. (1980)
	Increased urine production	Monoamniotic (conjoined) twins	Seller et al. (1977)
	Defective renal function	Congenital nephrotic syndrome	Kjessler et al. (1975)
		Polycystic kidney	Koontz et al. (1983)
	Defective fetal swallowing and alpha-fetoprotein breakdown	Oesophageal atresia	Seppala (1973)
		Duodenal atresia	Weinberg et al. (1975)
		Hydrocephalus	
		Anencephaly	
	Concentration because of oligohydramnios	Renal agenesis	Balfour and Laurence (1980)
	Large/abnormal placental surface	Triploidy	

abnormal child or where one parent is a translocation carrier. These women are offered chorionic villus sampling (CVS) or amniocentesis routinely. An increasing number of single gene disorders are now identified at the molecular level, e.g. Duchenne muscular dystrophy, cystic fibrosis. For some families at risk for these disorders DNA diagnosis is feasible.

Population screening programmes may identify women at increased risk of fetal abnormality. Women with low serum alpha-fetoprotein (AFP), unconjugated oestriol and high human chorionic gonadotrophin levels have an increased risk of trisomy 21 and may be offered amniocentesis, fetal blood sampling or placental biopsy. Those with elevated AFP levels need detailed ultrasound examination to search for neural tube defects or other structural anomaly (see Table 4.1). The increasing use of routine ultrasound scanning at 18–20 weeks' gestation identifies many structural abnormalities in women previously thought of as "low risk".

Over the last 25 years different methods of assessing fetal wellbeing have come into use. Some, such as ultrasound scanning, are non-invasive and are offered to most pregnant women in the UK. Others, e.g. fetal blood sampling, are invasive, carry a risk to the fetus and are only offered if there is sufficient suspicion of abnormality to warrant the test. Maternal serum screening for neural tube defect (NTD) and Down's syndrome have become increasingly important in the last few years. The different tests and screening procedures commonly in use are outlined below. For a more complete review of invasive procedures see Arulkumaran and Rodeck (1990) and American Journal of Medical Genetics (1990) for a review of prenatal diagnosis.

Ultrasound Examination

Abdominal Ultrasound

This technique is commonly used for dating (best before 12 weeks), checking viability, monitoring fetal growth and wellbeing (biophysical profile), fetal sexing and diagnosis of multiple pregnancy. Anomaly scans are routinely offered in many hospitals at between 18 and 20 weeks' gestation. This gestation is preferred because the fetus is of a size when detailed examination becomes possible and termination of pregnancy is still feasible. Some abnormalities are not usually detectable until later in gestation (e.g. hydrocephaly, microcephaly). Ultrasound surveillance is essential during the performance of invasive techniques, e.g. chorion villus sampling, and for checking fetal viability before and after such procedures.

Vaginal Ultrasound

This is increasingly used in specialist departments for first trimester diagnosis of anomaly and checking viability.

Invasive Tests

Chorion Villus Sampling (CVS)

Although first performed in the late 1960s CVS only became widely available in the last decade when better ultrasound equipment and improved monitoring of the procedure have allowed development of techniques with a lower risk of complication.

The overwhelming advantage of CVS over amniocentesis is that it can be carried out during the first trimester with, in the event of a positive diagnosis, earlier termination of pregnancy. For many women this has made the decision to attempt another pregnancy possible.

Both the transcervical (usually performed between 8 and 12 weeks) and transabdominal (8 weeks onwards) routes are used. The route chosen usually reflects the experience of the operator. By aspiration or biopsy under ultrasound guidance, 5–25 mg of chorionic villi are obtained. Karyotyping can be performed both from direct examination or short-term culture of the cytotrophoblast and/or long-term culture of fibroblasts from the villus core.

Indications for CVS

1. Diagnosis using DNA techniques, e.g. cystic fibrosis, Duchenne muscular dystrophy. Chorionic villi are a good source of fetal DNA and are generally preferred to amniocytes because of the greater volume of tissue which can be obtained.
2. Inborn errors of metabolism, when the enzyme in question is known to be expressed in chorionic villi (see Chap. 5).
3. Karyotyping e.g. advanced maternal age for trisomies, fragile X, familial translocations, following abnormal scan.
4. Diagnosis of rubella infection (Terry et al. 1986). CVS is the method of choice for DNA diagnoses.

Complications of CVS

Reliability (see Gardner and Sutherland 1989).

Maternal cell contamination is a problem when only long-term culture is undertaken.

Confined placental mosaicism, where the chorionic villi have a different karyotype from the fetus, is more common in direct preparations. It can lead to false positive diagnoses (CVS abnormal, fetus normal) and false negative diagnoses (CVS normal, fetus abnormal). The risk of wrong diagnosis is reduced considerably if both direct and long-term cultures are karyotyped. The finding of a usually nonviable karyotype at CVS is an indication for amniocentesis. In most cases this will reveal a normal karyotype. Placental mosaicism is particularly associated with trisomies 13 and 18 liveborns. Kalousek et al. (1989) karyotyped 14 placentas from liveborns with trisomies 13 and 18 and found that all were mosaic. The mosaicism was confined to the cytotrophoblast. They suggested that livebirth of these trisomies was only possible in these circumstances. Caution is therefore essential in interpretation of karyotypes from CVS in the second trimester following an abnormal scan in order to obtain a rapid karyotype. Long-term villous culture should always be carried out.

From the point of view of the accuracy of chromosome analysis, CVS is inferior to amniocentesis.

Miscarriage risk—two randomised clinical trials, the Canadian multicentre trial and the MRC European trial compared the fetal loss of CVS to amniocentesis (Canadian Collaborative Group 1989; Medical Research Council 1991a). Both reported increased fetal loss in the CVS group with the MRC European trial reporting the higher loss rate. The European results show that a woman allocated CVS had a 4.6% (confidence limits 1.4% to 7.8%) less chance of a successful pregnancy outcome than a woman allocated to second trimester amniocentesis.

Fetal injury—Studies to date have concentrated on miscarriage risk rather than abnormalities of babies born following CVS and there are no long-term follow-up studies. There are isolated reports of abnormalities associated with CVS (Boyd et al. 1990), and more recently four babies were born with oromandibular/limb hypogenesis syndromes following CVS performed at less than 10 weeks' gestation (Firth et al. 1991). This report provoked reviews of the experience in other centres, several of which seem to confirm an increase in the number of cases of oromandibular/limb hypogenesis syndromes. Quintero et al. (1992) visualised haemorrhagic lesions which appeared on the calvarium, thorax, face and limbs by embryoscopy during CVS after 9 weeks of gestation. The need for follow-up after prenatal procedures and for careful documentation is emphasised by these reports.

Because of concern about safety and accuracy at CVS, this test may be used less often in future for pregnancies not considered at high risk of abnormality (Lilford 1991).

Amniocentesis

Amniocentesis has been performed for much longer than CVS and is a more routine procedure. Ten to 20 ml of amniotic fluid are taken under ultrasound guidance transabdominally usually between 15 and 18 weeks' gestation. Late second and third trimester amniocentesis is performed to assist management of pregnancy complicated by rhesus and other blood group incompatibilities. Currently, the safety and adequacy of earlier amniocentesis, from about 10 weeks' gestation, are being assessed (Elejalde et al. 1990) but there is at present no long-term follow-up of these pregnancies.

Indications for Amniocentesis

These are similar to those for CVS (apart from rubella diagnosis). In addition, sampling may be performed for AFP and acetylcholinesterase isoenzymes for diagnosis of NTD in cases with positive family history or raised serum AFP, although many centres now rely on ultrasound scanning to diagnose NTDs. Amniocentesis may also be performed following diagnosis of abnormality by ultrasound scan to enable karyotyping to be undertaken. The vast majority of amniocenteses are performed because of increased risk of Down's syndrome in women aged over 35 years or in younger women with a positive result from biochemical (AFP) screening.

Complications of Amniocentesis

Reliability—amniotic fluid cell culture is a very accurate means of providing a fetal karyotype (Gardner and Sutherland 1989). Maternal cell contamination occurs in 0.5%–1% of cultures, and in vitro chromosome changes giving rise to pseudomosaicism do occur.

Miscarriage risk after amniocentesis has been well studied (Canadian MRC 1977; NICHD 1976; MRC 1978; Tabor et al. 1987). A miscarriage rate of 0.5%–1.4% was found in these large studies.

Fetal damage during amniocentesis is rare, particularly in experienced hands under ultrasound control, but has been documented. In the UK study more skin marks and dimples were found in the control neonates. Limb abnormalities may be the result of direct fetal damage (Lamb 1975) or secondary to membrane damage (Rehder 1978) and amniotic bands in the case of distal constrictions and amputations.

Injury to thoracic organs (Rushton 1981), abdominal viscera (Swift et al. 1979; Therkensen

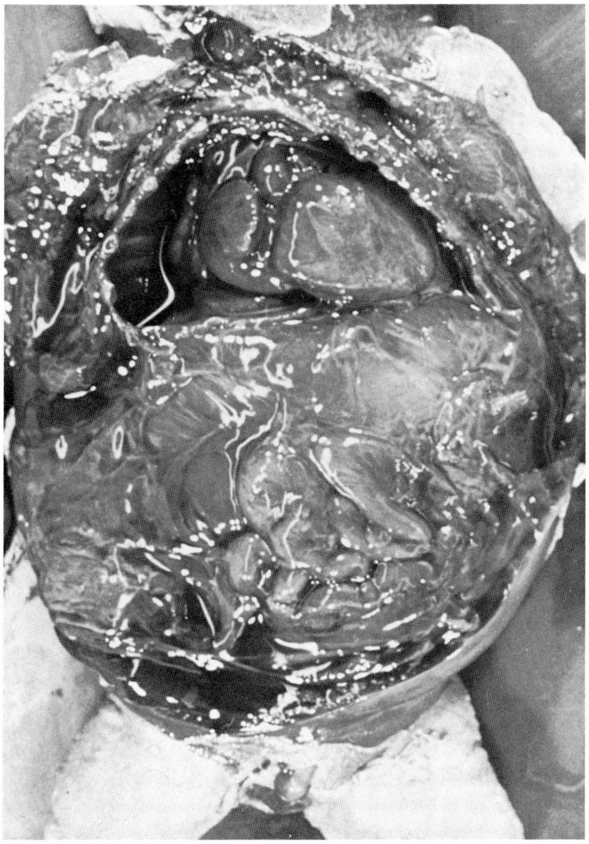

Fig. 4.1. Abdominal distension and peritonitis with adhesions; intrauterine death of fetus after amniocentesis.

and Rehder 1981) and brain (Youroukos et al. 1980) have been described. When intrauterine fetal death follows such injury, the puncture site may be difficult to identify because of supervening maceration (Fig. 4.1), and the possibility of injury is only raised by the nature of the internal abnormality.

Fetal Blood Sampling (FBS)

The use of the fetoscope to obtain fetal blood samples from the umbilical cord under direct vision has been superseded by ultrasound-guided transabdominal FBS, after 18 weeks' gestation. A transplacental route into an umbilical cord vessel at the placental insertion is used if the placenta is anterior. The transamniotic route if the placenta is posterior is technically more difficult. An alternative is puncture of the intrahepatic portion of the umbilical vein.

Indications for FBS

1. For the diagnosis of some haemoglobinopathies and clotting disorders, although most can now be diagnosed using DNA techniques on chorionic villi
2. Rapid karyotyping (three days)
   a. After a structural abnormality has been diagnosed on scan that has a high risk of chromosome abnormality (e.g. omphalocoele, hydrops fetalis, cystic hygroma)
   b. For women presenting too late for amniocentesis (e.g. after 19 weeks' gestation)
   c. Amniotic fluid culture failure or mosaicism
   d. Fragile X studies—these can now also be done on chorionic villi
3. Blood group incompatibility for grouping and haemoglobin level prior to intrauterine transfusion
4. A family history of severe combined immunodeficiency
5. The possibility of fetal rubella, CMV, parvovirus and toxoplasmosis infections.

Complications/Problems with FBS

FBS is not a routine test and is performed in relatively few specialist centres. As with all invasive procedures its safety is related to the experience of the operator. It is often carried out on fetuses with serious progressive disease, so that it is difficult to give accurate figures about the safety of the procedure.

Miscarriage risk—in experienced hands a procedure-related loss of 1.5% has been reported (Daffos et al. 1983).

Other Invasive Tests/Fetal Surgery

Aspiration and analysis of urine in male fetuses in some cases of urethral obstruction, usually due to urethal valves, together with careful renal ultrasound can provide useful information regarding long-term prognosis and possible shunting procedures. The outlook is usually poor and the benefit of shunting questionable. See Arulkmaran and Rodeck (1990) for discussion of this and other rarely performed invasive diagnostic tests such as liver and skin biopsy.

DNA Analysis and Prenatal Diagnosis

Prenatal diagnosis of many rare single gene disorders have been revolutionised by the fact that DNA analysis is now possible. The gene in question may have been cloned and sequenced and some mutations causing the disorder identified. The haemoglobinopathies, cystic fibrosis and Duchenne muscular dystrophy are amongst the more common disorders in which this has been achieved (Weatherall 1991). Many other disorders for which the gene has not yet been isolated have been mapped to a particular region of a chromosome. Prenatal diagnosis using linked DNA markers is possible for many families at risk of these disorders when DNA is available from appropriate family members. This includes fetuses from previously terminated pregnancies and the importance of storing tissue from any fetus at risk of single gene disorders *cannot be overemphasised*. Huntington's chorea and myotonic dystrophy are examples of disorders in this group. Following characterisation of the Fragile X mutation (Yu et al. 1991; Oberlé et al. 1991) the method of diagnosis is likely to move from cytogenetics to molecular genetics.

Prenatal Diagnosis and Cystic Fibrosis

Since identification of the cystic fibrosis (CF) gene in 1989 (Kerem et al. 1989; Rommens et al. 1989; Riordan et al. 1989) cystic fibrosis is known to be due to mutations in the CF transmembrane conductance regulator located on chromosome 7q31. The most frequent mutation, a three-base pair deletion, leads to the absence of a phenylalanine residue at position 508 (ΔF 508). This mutation occurs in approximately 75% of north European carriers. The remaining 25% of carriers have a variety of mutations. Approximately 5% of carriers have mutations still to be characterised at the molecular level so that population screening for carriers is not straightforward (Colten 1990).

Accurate prenatal diagnosis is now possible for many families at high risk by direct mutation detection in DNA from CVS samples. If parents are known to be carriers but have a mutation not yet identified, prenatal diagnosis is usually possible, if DNA from the affected child is available, by gene tracking with intragenic and extragenic RFLPs. If there is no DNA from the affected individual and one or both parents carry an uncharacterised mutation prenatal diagnosis can be offered by analysis of intestinal isoenzymes of alkaline phosphatase in the amniotic fluid (Brock et al. 1985).

Prenatal Maternal Serum Screening

Serum Screening for Neural Tube Defects

The observation by Brock and Sutcliffe (1972) of high levels of AFP in amniotic fluid of pregnancies complicated by open NTDs, followed by the finding that in most of these cases the maternal serum AFP (MSAFP) was also elevated has become the basis for an effective screening test for NTDs in high incidence areas (Ferguson-Smith 1983).

AFP is the major fetal plasma protein, initially manufactured by the yolk sac and later by the liver with maximum concentrations at 12 to 14 weeks' gestation (Gitlin 1975). AFP enters amniotic fluid initially by diffusion across poorly keratinised fetal skin, and after the development of glomerular filtration, comes mostly from fetal urine, with maximum levels at 14–15 weeks. AFP reaches the maternal circulation in normal pregnancies by diffusion across the placenta with a minor contribution from transmembrane transport. MSAFP rises from 13 weeks with a peak at approximately 32 weeks.

In pregnancies associated with an open NTD or certain other conditions (see Table 4.1) MSAFP and amniotic fluid AFP (AFAFP) are raised by leakage of fetal AFP from exposed fetal capillaries. For screening purposes MSAFP is measured at approximately 16 weeks' gestation. If the level is above a chosen cut-off level for that gestation (e.g. +2 MOMs) a detailed scan is performed to check for gestation, multiple pregnancy, fetal viability, and for NTDs and other anomalies associated with raised MSAFP. Sometimes amniocentesis is performed, in which case the pattern of cholinesterases in amniotic fluid by polyacrylamide gel electrophoresis is helpful in distinguishing causes of high MSAFP and AFAFP. Open NTDs always have a second faster band of acetylcholinesterases as do about 50% of anterior wall defects. Using MSAFP, ultrasound and sometimes amniocentesis approximately 100% of anencephalic fetuses and 88% of open NTDs are detected. In a high incidence area a reduction in NTD births of over 70% has been achieved (Ferguson-Smith 1983).

Fetal Abnormalities and Elevated AFP Levels in Amniotic Fluid or Maternal Serum

Conditions which interrupt the integrity of the fetal surface (meningomyelocoele or omphalocoele), increase skin permeability (fetal death, cystic hygroma), affect renal function (congenital nephrotic syndrome), or interfere with fetal swallowing (intestinal atresia, cerebral abnormality) are likely to increase the level of AFP in the amniotic fluid. AFAFP in normal pregnancies makes an insignificant contribution to MSAFP but when it is raised, transport across the placental membranes causes elevated levels in maternal serum. The amount of alphafetoprotein in maternal serum will also be increased when there is increased AFP production, as seen in multiple pregnancy and following damage to the placental surface which might result in fetomaternal haemorrhage.

When pregnancy is terminated because of raised MSAFP levels, the pathologist may expect to find a great variety of fetal anomalies (Table 4.1; Figs. 4.2, 4.14, 4.17, 4.19, 4.20). In the UK, and even in countries where the incidence of neural tube defect is low, anencephaly and meningomyelocoele are the commonest anomalies detected (Norgaard-Pedersen et al. 1985). When both ultrasound and amniocentesis are employed in the investigation of fetal abnormality in women identified by MSAFP screening programmes, inappropriate termination of a normal fetus is infrequent. However, when faced with an anatomically normal fetus it is important to exclude the possibility of congenital nephrotic syndrome by measurement of protein levels in fetal urine (Thom et al. 1977) and examination of the kidneys using PAS and lipid stains on frozen sections and electron microscopic examination of glomeruli from the corticomedullary junction.

Some urinary tract anomalies, renal agenesis (Balfour and Laurence 1980) and urethral obstruction (Vinson et al. 1977), which might be expected to result in a low AFAFP level, have also been detected because the AFP was elevated. Normally formed fetuses with raised MSAFP are at increased risk from a variety of antenatal complications, low birthweight, stillbirth and neonatal death (Boyd 1992). MSAFP is a useful placental function test and its value should be known to the pathologist performing autopsies on fetuses, stillbirths and neonates.

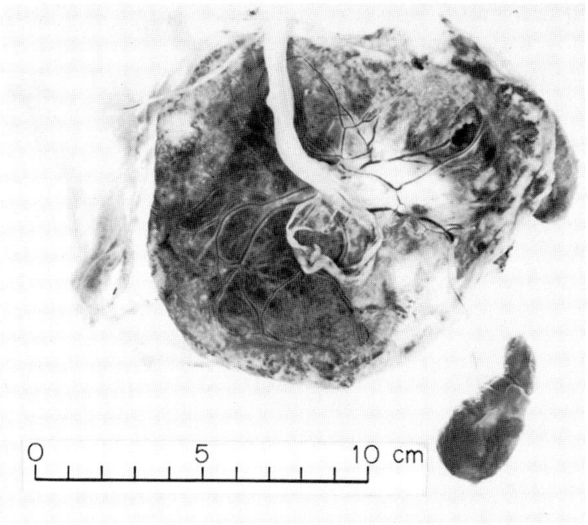

Fig. 4.2. Termination of pregnancy at 19 weeks' gestation because of raised maternal serum alpha-fetoprotein level. This twin was acardiac with a skin defect at one pole overlying a neural nodule; the other had unilateral cystic renal dysplasia.

Biochemical Screening for Down's Syndrome

Originally, screening for Down's syndrome (DS) was based on the knowledge that the incidence of DS increases with maternal age (Hook 1990). Theoretically, if all women aged over 36 years had amniocentesis performed for karyotyping, aproximately 30% of DS pregnancies would be detected. In practice, fewer are detected because of a low amniocentesis rate in older women for a variety of reasons.

In 1984, Merkatz et al. and Cuckle et al. reported an association between low MSAFP and fetal autosomal trisomy. Bogart et al. (1987) observed that human chorionic gonadotrophin (hCG) concentration in maternal serum was increased in trisomy 21 pregnancy and Canick et al. (1988) reported low maternal serum unconjugated oestriol in Down's syndrome pregnancies. Antenatal screening programmes have been set up using these observations. If all pregnant women were screened for AFP, hCG and unconjugated oestriol at 16 weeks' gestation and those with a risk calculated to be greater than 1 in 250 of giving birth to Down's syndrome baby had amniocentesis performed for karyotyping, 5% of all pregnant women would have amniocentesis and over 60% of Down's syndrome pregnancies would be identified (Wald et al. 1988).

Urea-resistant neutrophil alkaline phosphatase activity has been shown to be a very effective blood marker for Down's syndrome (Cuckle et al. 1990) and when a suitable method for measuring it in populations becomes available, serum screening will become even more effective.

Examination of Fetus and Placenta

When pregnancy terminates prematurely, either electively or spontaneously, following investigations for or diagnosis of fetal malformation, pathological examination of the fetus is essential. There are three important reasons for undertaking fetal examination. The first is confirmation of the nature of the abnormality for which termination of pregnancy was undertaken. The second is careful scrutiny of the fetus, placenta and membranes for any abnormality which might be related to the preceding investigations. Both of these points merit attention: together they comprise the quality control of antenatal diagnosis of malformation and are an essential, but often neglected, part of the antenatal diagnostic facility. The third, and perhaps the most important reason for fetal examination, is the careful documentation of all abnormalities which are present. It is the combination of external dysmorphic features and internal abnormalities which may accompany the major system anomaly identified prenatally that allows precise recurrence rates to be calculated. With some antenatally detectable anomalies, the contribution made by careful documentation of other abnormalities present may be the difference between no increase in risk of recurrence and a recurrence risk of one in four in every subsequent pregnancy.

Value of Fetal Examination

There is great variation in the accuracy of methods of prenatal diagnosis. Molecular, cytogenetic and biochemical techniques often allow very precise diagnosis, although the method of obtaining samples may introduce errors. Some methods of diagnosis are less specific. Ultrasound examination will demonstrate a major defect but may not identify it precisely (Fig. 4.3) nor will it identify many of the minor dysmorphisms which are necessary for syndrome diagnosis. Rutledge et al. (1986) compared ultrasound diagnosis with pathological findings and found an average of two additional malformations per case. They were unable to confirm some prenatal diagnoses. It is clearly most important to examine the fetus when conditions for ultrasound examination are suboptimal, for example when there is oligohydramnios or in the third trimester when fetal position is relatively fixed. Manchester et al. (1988) followed up 257 pregnancies referred for detailed ultrasound following prenatal suspicion of anomaly. Forty-six pregnancies were electively terminated and postnatal evaluation, clinical or postmortem or both, was undertaken in all cases. False positive diagnoses were made in 1.5% and false negatives in 2% of cases. Additional anomalies were present in 37% of malformed infants. Shen-Schwartz et al. (1989) found that postmortem examination of the fetus yielded clinically useful information in 46% of their cases. The pathologist's contribution was more likely where multiple malformations were present.

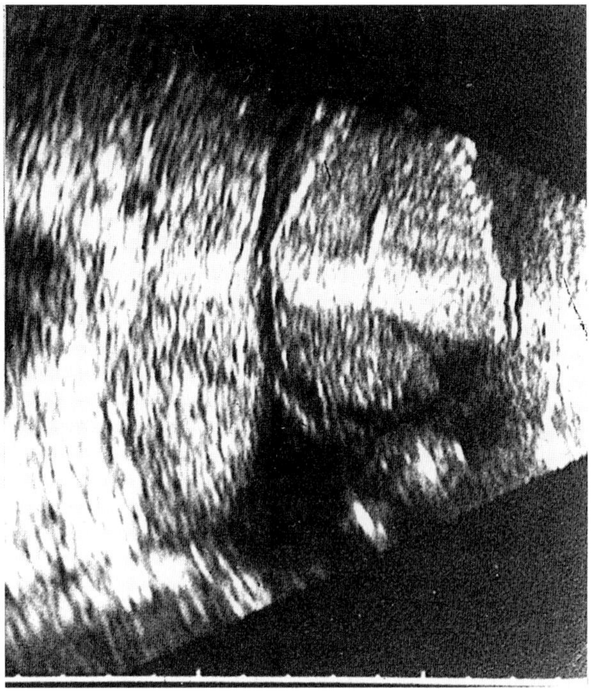

Fig. 4.3. Ultrasound scan of fetal trunk; there is oedema and ascites, diaphragms depressed; bright lungs. (Courtesy of Dr. B. Muir, Edinburgh)

UK studies are similar. Clayton-Smith et al. (1990) found that fetal examination changed or refined ultrasound diagnoses in 40% of cases and Keeling et al. (1990) found that 42% of prenatal diagnoses were modified or changed (Fig. 4.4) including 2% false negative diagnoses. Even following diagnosis based on amniotic fluid sampling clinically useful information may be derived from fetal examination. Clayton-Smith et al. (1990) found that it changed parental counselling in 3% of cases.

Information for the Pathologist

In order that the aims of examination of the fetus from the pregnancy terminated following the diagnosis of congenital abnormality or inherited disease may be accomplished, it is most important that the pathologist has sufficient clinical information before fetal examination is begun to ensure that the right investigations are undertaken. The minimum information required is identification, maternal age and past obstetric history, together with details of the terminated pregnancy including estimates of gestation, reasons for investigations, the nature, dates and results of scan reports, investigations undertaken with their results, and the clinical diagnosis, and method of termination. This information should accompany the unfixed fetus and placenta, which should be transferred to the laboratory as quickly as possible after delivery. A counsel of perfection is that the pathologist should be forewarned of all terminations of pregnancy undertaken for fetal anomaly, but this may be difficult in practice. However, this information is essential when confirmation of diagnosis demands recourse to techniques which require fresh tissue such as tissue culture, biochemical or DNA analysis, particularly if liaison with other laboratories is necessary.

Fetal Examination

At present, the majority of terminations of pregnancy following the prenatal diagnosis of fetal anomaly take place between 17 and 20 weeks' gestation, and most of this section will describe examination methods appropriate for the fetus at that stage of development. First trimester CVS is now the method of choice for the detecting of many inherited disorders, with suction evacuation used to terminate the affected pregnancy. Examination of such specimens with a hand lens or dissecting microscope permits the identification of tissues, limbs and sometimes whole organs in this sort of material (Markowski and Lawler 1977; Kalousek et al. 1990). It should be possible in most cases to retrieve material to enable confirmation of the antenatal diagnosis to be undertaken, and in some cases histological and electron microscopic examination may be possible.

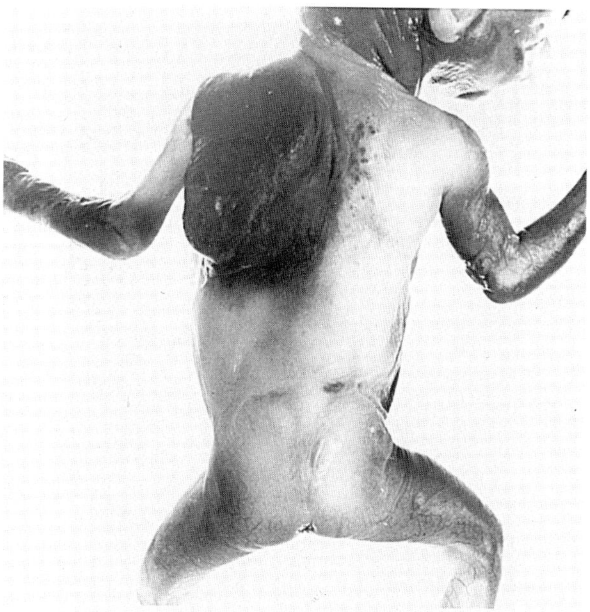

Fig. 4.4. 18-week gestation fetus with a large dorsal angioma, thought to be a meningocoele on ultrasound examination.

The fetus should be transported to the pathology department in a fresh state in a clean, dry container as quickly as possible following delivery. Immersion of the fetus in fixative rules out the possibility of tissue culture and biochemical studies, thereby preventing confirmation of the diagnosis in some cases.

Before dissection of the fetus is begun, weight and measurements should be recorded, and an anteroposterior radiograph (Fig. 4.5) and photographic record of all external abnormalities should be obtained (Fig. 4.6). When termination has been undertaken for skeletal dysplasia, radiographs or xerographs of individual bones may assist diagnosis. Should no dysmorphic features be apparent, then anterior and lateral views of the whole fetus are a useful minimum record.

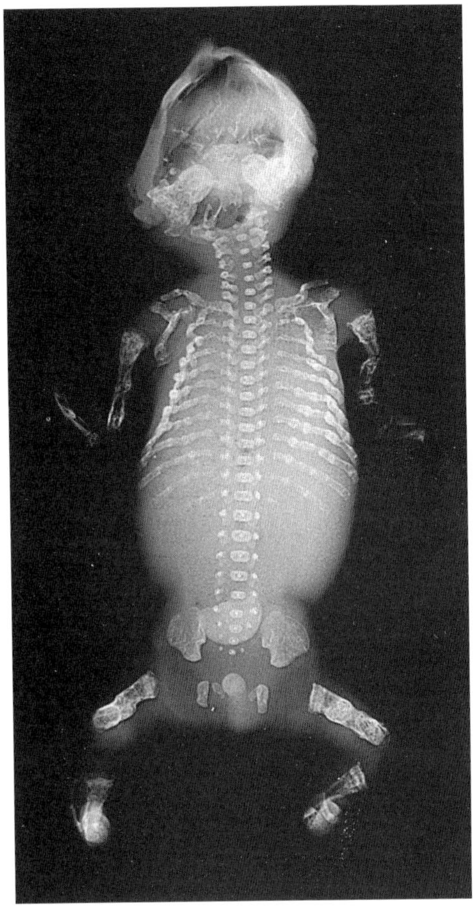

Fig. 4.5. Radiograph of a 20-week gestation fetus with osteogenesis imperfecta type II. There are multiple healing rib fractures and fractures, deformity and shortening of limb bones.

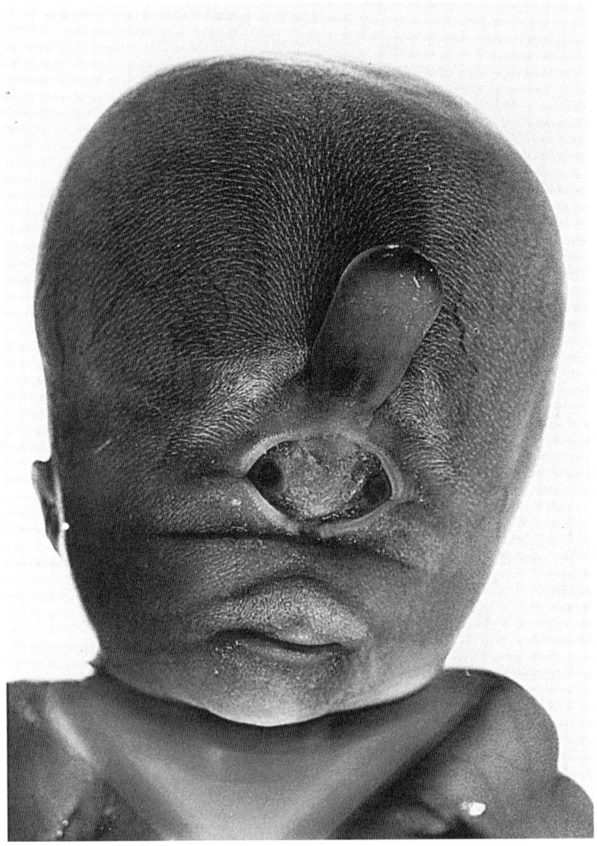

Fig. 4.6. Multiple external abnormalities: supraorbital proboscis, fused palpebral fissures, microphthalmia, long philtrum, smooth upper lip, large cranial vault. There was holoprosencephaly.

For geographical reasons, it is sometimes necessary to sample tissue for culture before pathological examination and photography of the fetus are undertaken. This should be done as inconspicuously as possible; the axilla and inner thigh are the least intrusive sites.

A detailed external examination is important with deliberate scrutiny and recording of each part of the body in an orderly fashion. A careful examination should be made of the head and the cervical region to record the shape of the head, the size and shape of the fontanelle, eyes, nose, mouth, palate and ears, with note being taken of proportions and whether there is any webbing of the neck. The length and proportions of limbs, the form of hands and feet, together with number, length and curvature of digits, are recorded. The trunk should be examined and particular attention given to the presence of abdominal wall defects. The back must be deliberately examined, recording the extent of rachischisis, size and site of any abnormality such as meningomyelocoele or skin pitting. Careful observation of external abnormalities may suggest the possibility of a particular syndrome and change the significance of major malformations in respect of subsequent genetic counselling.

Artefactual fetal distortion or injury may result from vaginal delivery or subsequent handling. Membranous sacs such as meningomyelocoele or omphalocoele are particularly vulnerable to delivery trauma. Care should be taken to distinguish spurious "abnormalities" from developmental defects and deformations which have occurred in utero (see p. 128).

Internal examination of the mid-trimester abortus requires examination of all organs in situ in a similar fashion to a perinatal necropsy (see Chap. 1, p. 9), and a positive search for those abnormalities which might be expected from the stated prenatal diagnosis. A detailed record should be made of all abnormalities found. Histological examination of organs which appear to be developmentally abnormal should be undertaken.

Fetal blood obtained by cardiac puncture and tissue samples such as skin, lung and gonad should be transported in tissue culture medium for chromosome studies. Samples for confirmation of genetic metabolic disease (see Chap. 5, p. 160) need to be tailored to specific diagnoses, but skin and lung for fibroblast cultures are usually required, and organ samples for biochemical analysis should be snap frozen. When termination of pregnancy has been undertaken for maternal illness such as rubella or varicella, then fetal blood for viral antibody levels and organ samples for virus culture should be attempted. Results of the latter are frequently negative.

When invasive investigations have been undertaken, injury to the fetus, cord and placenta should be carefully sought. The placenta, cord and membranes should be examined. The appearance and amount of membrane recorded, discoloration from haemorrhage or infection, perhaps related to amniocentesis, and nodularity of the amnion as an indication of long-standing oligohydramnios should be sought. Haematomas attached to the chorion or placenta or lying within placental tissue might be related to sampling procedures. Their appearance should be recorded and samples taken for histological examination to determine the age of the lesion.

Reconstruction and Disposal of the Fetus

Attitudes about the needs of the parents for support and an opportunity to mourn their aborted fetus have changed very much (Elder and Laurence 1991). It is important to be aware of parental wishes concerning fetal disposal before fetal examination begins. The need to reconstruct the body in a sensitive fashion for return to the parents for burial or cremation may conflict with dissection methods used to facilitate demonstration of anomalies. It is also sensible to check that photographs of the fetus have been taken for the parents (Batcup et al. 1989). Some parents may take several weeks to decide whether or not they wish to arrange a funeral ceremony. It is important that medical or nursing staff keep the pathology department fully informed about any indecision of this nature.

Problems with the need for extended fetal examination and subsequent reconstruction arise in two situations. First, the fetus with osteochondrodysplasia or other major skeletal abnormality when histological samples from long bones, often whole long bones, is essential. The second problem area is detailed examination of the central nervous system, particularly when there is hydrocephaly. The method of Laurence and Martin (1959) is inappropriate because of the difficulties encountered in reconstruction of the head, although one of the authors has successfully used this technique at 22 to 24 weeks' gestation when the skin is more robust. Parents may consent to fixation of the whole fetus for about one week so that the brain may be removed more easily. If this is not possible, then removal of the brain can be achieved (with difficulty) with the fetus immersed in a bowl of saline.

Difficulties in reconstruction are encountered even when examination is restricted to the thorax and abdomen. The skin of the second trimester abortus is poorly keratinised and collagen is immature so that sutures tend to cut out. Fine linen thread or silk with a fine needle may be adequate. Some report better cosmetic results using epoxy resin (Gau et al. 1991). Resin must be used with care, the hardening reaction is exothermic and over-generous application can result in burns to skin edges.

Artefactual Abnormalities

Artefactual abnormalities are present quite frequently in fetuses terminated in the second trimester of pregnancy. Such abnormalities may be the result of trauma during delivery or the effect of subsequent handling of the fetus (Knowles 1986).

The second trimester abortus has fragile skin and connective tissue so that delivery trauma is easily inflicted. Tearing of skin may occur, and in most sites, particularly limbs, groins and neck, its traumatic nature will be obvious; however, if it occurs over the trunk, particularly anteriorly or anterolaterally, then confusion with developmental defects of the abdominal

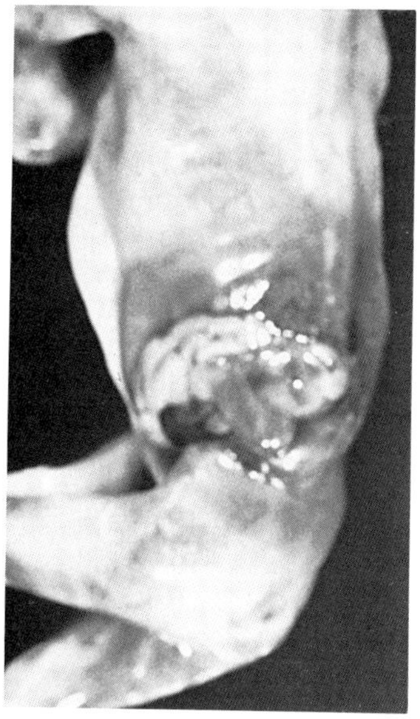

Fig. 4.7. Traumatic defect of the abdominal wall in the left flank. The margins of such defects are usually irregular.

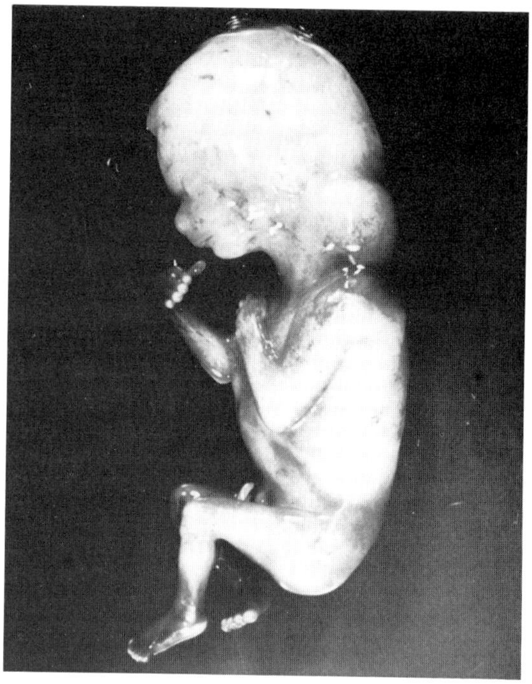

Fig. 4.9. Soft tissue swelling at the back of the neck is the result of brain being squeezed through vertebral foramina.

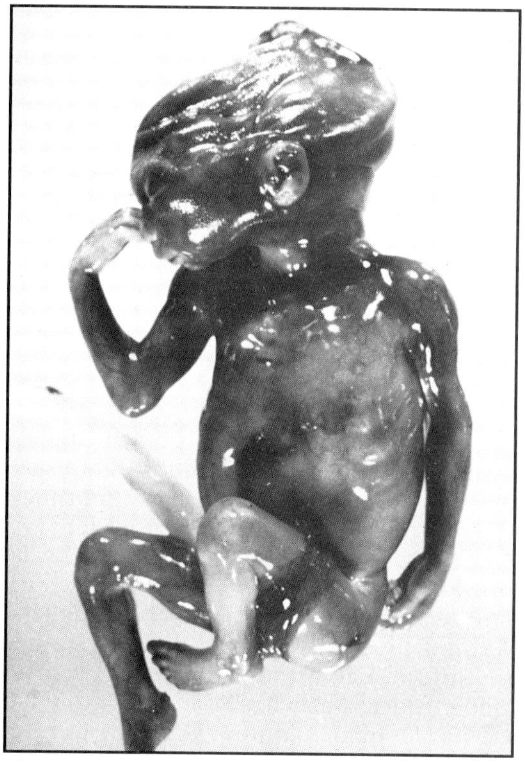

Fig. 4.8. Traumatic compression of the fetal head producing an illusion of microcephaly.

wall may arise. Traumatic defects are often in the lower quadrant or flank (Fig. 4.7) and have irregular margins within which different layers of the abdominal wall may be identified. There may be haemorrhage or necrosis of tissue in the margin of the defect. Intestines and occasionally other organs prolapse through the defect. Traumatic defects are also seen in spontaneous abortion and when termination of pregnancy has been undertaken for reasons other than recognised fetal anomaly.

Disruption of developmental anomalies may also occur during delivery. The flimsy sacs of meningomyelocoele or exomphalos are particularly vulnerable, and vestiges of the sac may be found only after careful scrutiny of the perimeter of the defect.

Compression of the head may result in cerebral tissue being forced backwards into a "sac" over the occiput (Fig. 4.8) or out through spinal foramina producing symmetrical thickening of the neck, resembling cystic hygroma (Fig. 4.9). Incision of the mass reveals semifluid, structureless white-grey brain tissue. Occasionally, cerebral tissue may be forced down the spinal canal and emerge retroperitoneally, when it may bear more than a passing resemblance to tumour.

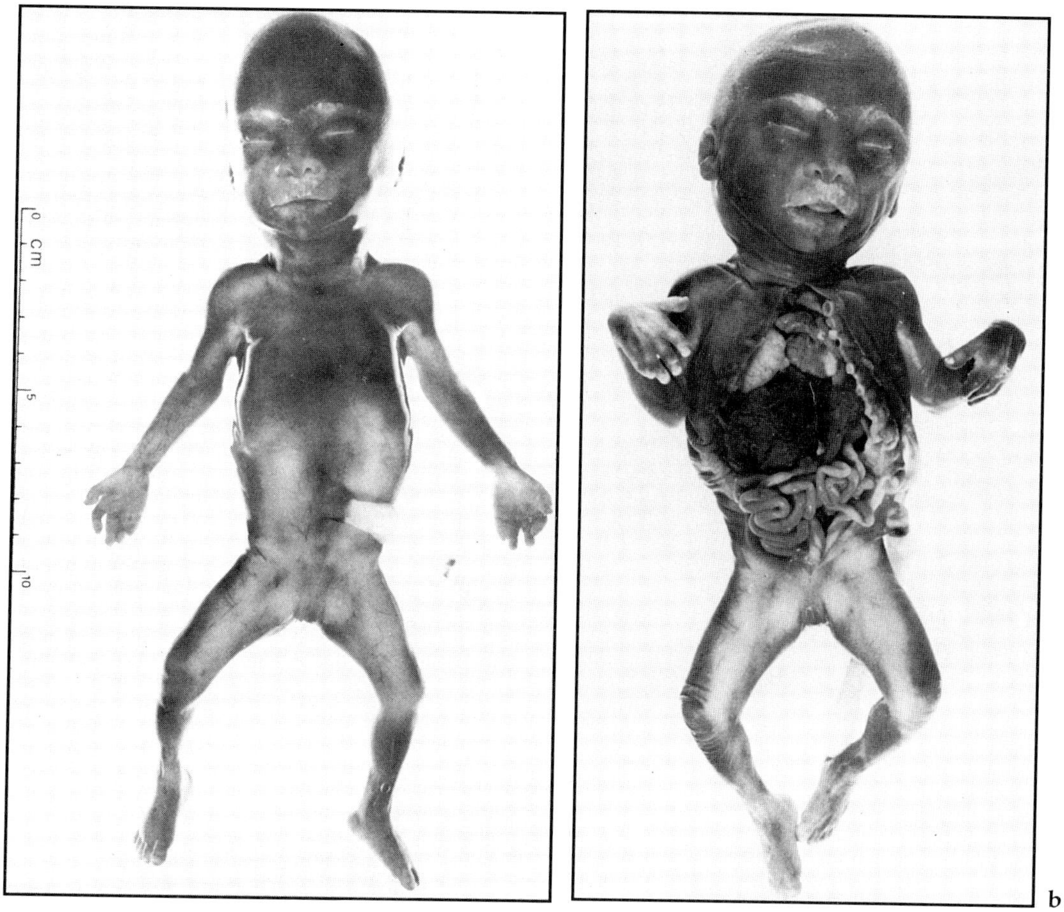

a b

Fig. 4.10a,b. Termination of pregnancy because of trisomy 21. **a** Fetus before fixation, prominent brow and broad nose. **b** Same fetus after fixation. Shrinkage of soft tissue results in spurious joint contractures and altered facies.

Dislocation of joints may occur during delivery. Whilst dislocations of large joints are easily recognisable, those affecting phalanges may evoke specific dysmorphic features, e.g. the hand deformities of trisomy 18 or triploidy.

A long interval between delivery and examination permits the combined effect of gravity and specimen container to affect fetal contour. Considerable facial asymmetry and distortion may result if the fetus remains in a lateral position for many hours. Such distortion may induce overdiagnosis or dysmorphism or make recognition of dysmorphic features rather difficult.

Immersion of the fetus in fixative may affect both facies and limbs. Soft tissue contraction induces facial deformity which was not previously present (Fig. 4.10) and produces contractures of limbs. This is particularly serious as it negates assessment of all but the most serious proximal limb contracture, where webbing may still be recognised (see Fig. 10.1, p. 243), and severe long-standing talipes, where the shape of the foot is quite abnormal (Fig. 4.11).

Specific Fetal Anomalies

Hydrocephalus

When hydrocephalus is detected antenatally, it may be an isolated finding or accompanied by other major defects, in particular by meningomyelocoele. The fetus terminated because of alleged hydrocephalus must be examined with care for two reasons: first, because there are particular pitfalls associated with the ultrasound diagnosis of the condition. A pregnancy may need to be monitored with scans for several weeks before a definite diagnosis can be made

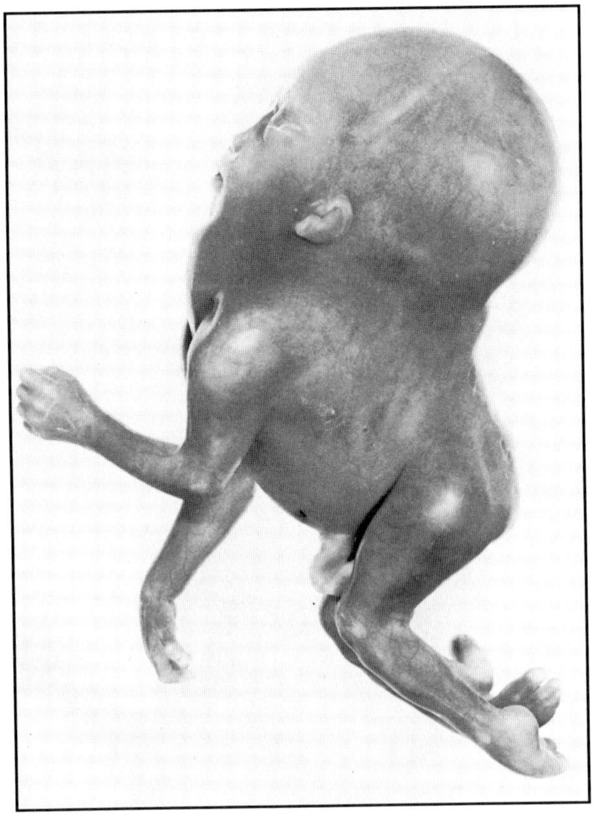

Fig. 4.11. Iniencephaly. There is gross spinal deformity and limitation of joint movements with marked talipes. Only gross deformity is unaffected by tissue fixation.

with confidence. Second, because a precise diagnosis of the cause of the hydrocephalus is required so that a reliable recurrence risk may be derived.

In order to achieve these aims, it is essential to fix the brain before examination. This may be done most conveniently by leaving the brain within the cranial cavity. Myelination is so poorly advanced at this stage that attempted removal may defeat all subsequent efforts to elucidate the cause for hydrocephalus. Fetal weight and measurements should first be recorded and any dysmorphic features and external malformations noted. The thoracic and abdominal viscera may be conveniently examined next, looking for structural anomalies and evidence of chronic inflammation. The scalp should be incised and reflected and the anterior fontanelles incised carefully. These incisions may be extended along the sagittal suture line anteriorly or down the frontoparietal suture to permit unobstructed access to fixative. The whole fetus is then immersed in a generous quantity of buffered formalin. Prior to immersion, ventricular puncture may be undertaken and some cerebrospinal fluid (CSF) carefully removed and replaced with fixative in order to enhance preservation of the ependyma and adjacent tissue.

After 1–2 weeks' fixation, the brain will be sufficiently hardened to permit careful handling. It may be removed in the conventional manner (see Chap. 1, p. 22). Alternatively, individual skull bones may be removed with scissors along a line from the supraorbital ridge to the occiput and a horizontal cut made through both hemispheres with a thin, broad-bladed sharp knife to remove the rostral portions of the cerebrum (Fig. 4.12) and permit direct comparison of the ventricular contour and ultrasound record.

The cortical mantle and the ependyma should be examined and blocks taken for histological examination. The critical region, from a diagnostic standpoint, is the pons, midbrain and medulla. It is safest to divide the whole of this region into 2 mm slices and submit the whole for histological examination. In this way, perhaps involving examination of several levels within a block, a firm diagnosis is likely to be achieved.

In the second trimester of pregnancy, the cerebral ventricles are much wider compared with overall cerebral and cortical width than they are at term, so that an impression of hydrocephalus may be obtained on initial examination of the fetal head. This is when observation of ventricular contour (Fig. 4.12) may be useful; this contour is lost early in the development of hydrocephalus. Ultrasound studies (Hobbins et al. 1979) have shown that before 24 weeks of gestation hydrocephalus may be marked, whilst biparietal diameter is within the normal range. This reflects the normally large subdural space at this stage of development which permits considerable increase in cerebral size before the cerebrum impinges on the inner table of the skull bones.

In the UK, the commonest cause for mid-trimester hydrocephalus is coexistent meningomyelocoele or myelocoele and Chiari type II malformation, where the medulla oblongata is displaced caudally into the spinal canal (see Chap. 23, p. 548).

Deformity of the aqueduct, which may be X-linked in some families, has been identified as a cause for hydrocephalus in the second trimester of pregnancy (Harrod et al. 1984). Other causes found by these authors were intra-

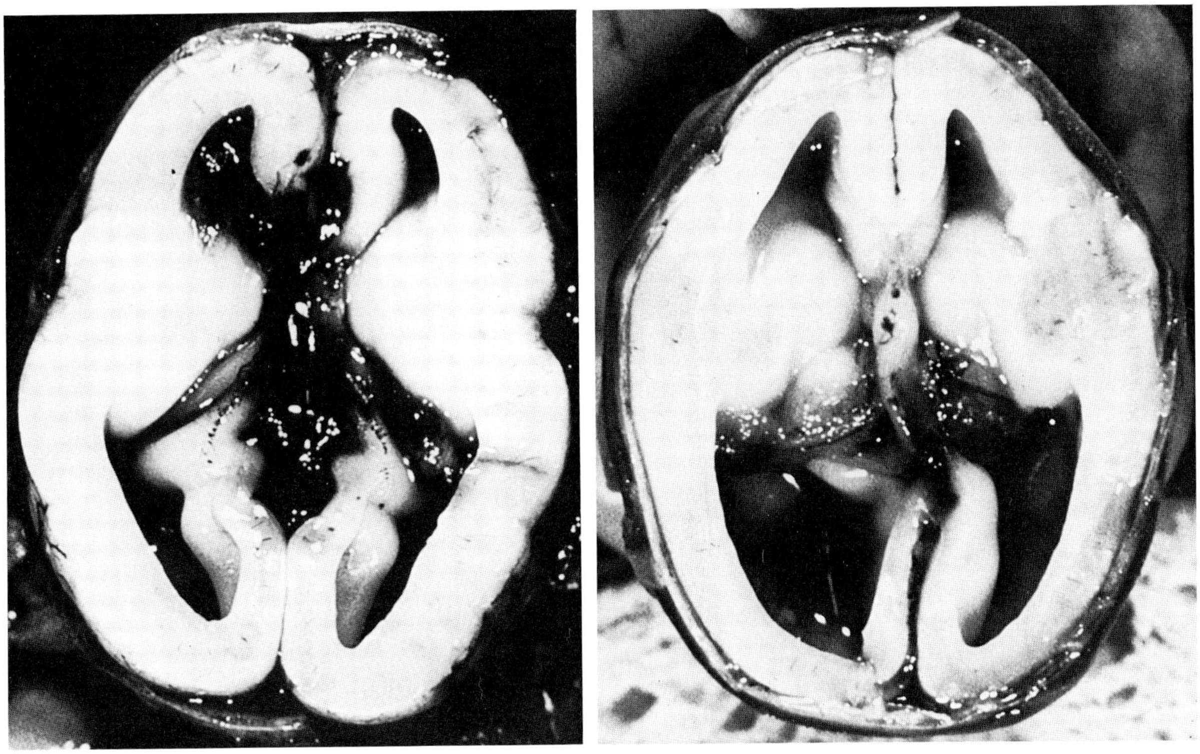

a b

Fig. 4.12a,b. Horizontal slice through fetal brain at 19–20 weeks' gestation. **a** Normal. Note relatively large size of lateral ventricles at this stage. **b** Hydrocephalus with meningomyelocoele. Ventricular dilatation is asymmetric and more marked posteriorly.

uterine infection and isolated hydrocephalus with no aqueduct deformity. Forking of the aqueduct is sometimes seen (Fig. 4.13).

A search for malformation in other systems is important; hydrocephalus with camptomelic dwarfism or renal anomaly may be inherited as an autosomal-recessive condition.

Encephalocoele

Encephalocoele may be covered by normal hair-bearing skin or by membranes (Fig. 4.14). The former type are accompanied by normal maternal serum alpha-fetoprotein levels and often diagnosed later in pregnancy. Although usually occipital in position, encephalocoele may be frontal or nasal. The anomaly may comprise a CSF-filled sac or may contain brain tissue (see Chap. 23, p. 555). There may be an accompanying hydrocephalus, or microcephaly may be present (Fig. 4.15), Encephalocoele, one variant of neural tube defect, may be a manifestation of the amnion rupture sequence, when strings of membranes may be adherent to the membranous sac; it may also be part of the manifestation of Meckel's syndrome, and kidneys and liver should be examined carefully in all fetuses with encephalocoele.

Occasionally, delivery trauma may produce a spurious appearance of encephalocoele when brain is squeezed out of the cranial cavity into the soft tissues of the scalp. No sac lining can be identified and the cerebral material is without structure. More importantly there is no defect in the occipital bone (Fig. 4.16).

Anencephaly

Anencephaly is discussed fully in Chapter 23 (see p. 553). It is frequently diagnosed in the second trimester of pregnancy either because of raised maternal alpha-fetoprotein levels or on ultrasound examination. When there is a family history of anencephaly, first trimester diagnosis may be possible using vaginal ultrasound. Whilst the majority are defects of neural tube closure, and are single defects, a full examina-

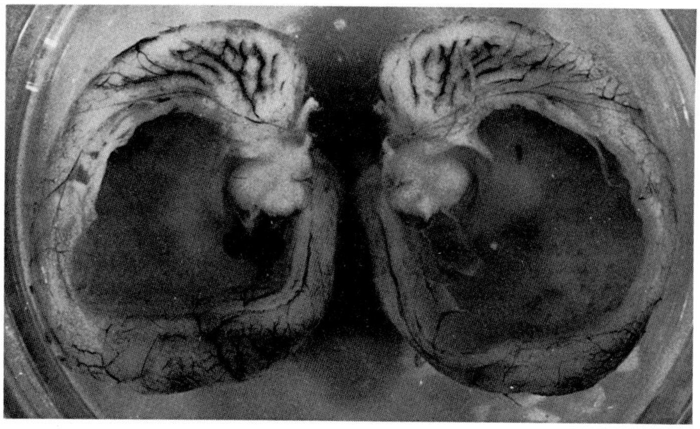

a

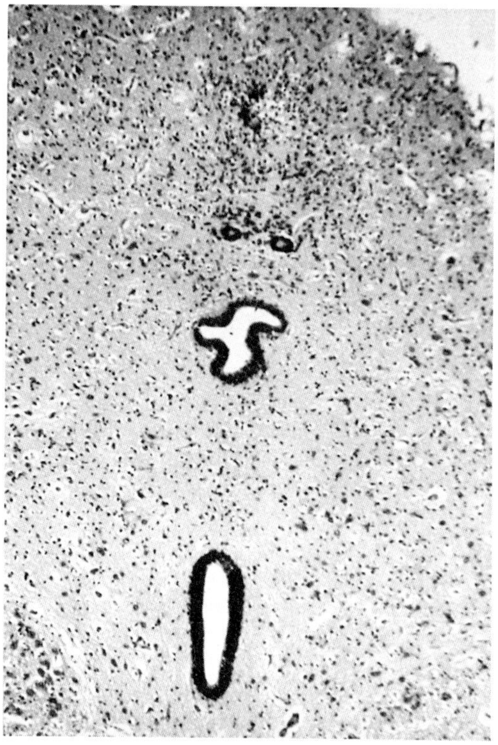

b

Fig. 4.13a,b. a Gross hydrocephalus diagnosed on ultrasound examination at 18 weeks' gestation; brain fixed in situ and supported in fluid for photography. **b** Histology of aqueduct which is divided into several ependymal lined channels.

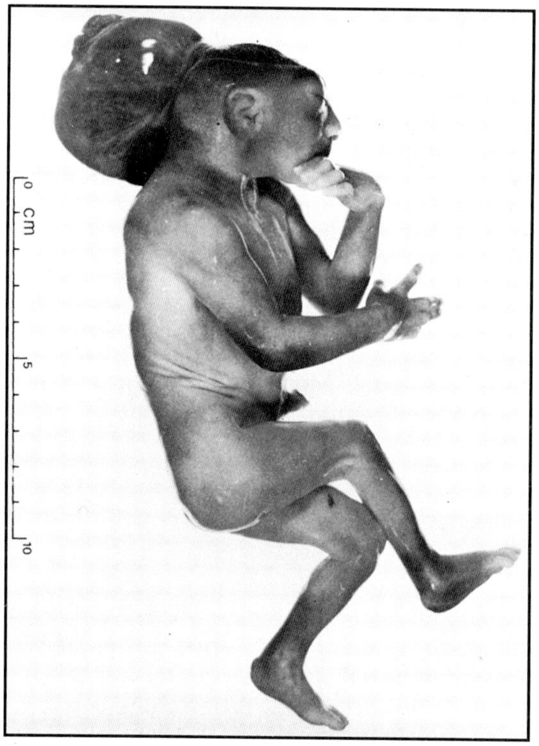

Fig. 4.14. Encephalocoele found on ultrasound examination in second trimester. The calvaria is very small, and most of the brain lies within the membranous encephalocoele sac.

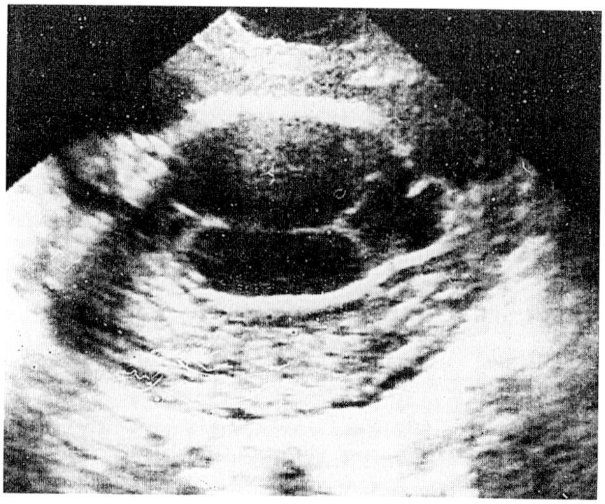

Fig. 4.15. Ultrasound scan, horizontal cut through fetal head. Head is small and narrow. There is an occipital bone defect and an encephalocoele. (Courtesy of Dr. A.J. Thompson, Kettering)

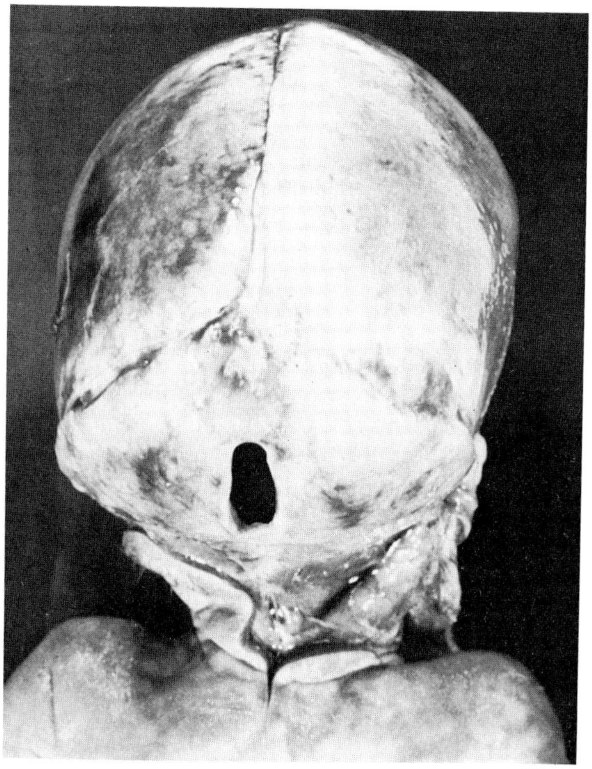

Fig. 4.16. Fetus with encephalocoele; a defect is present in the underlying bone.

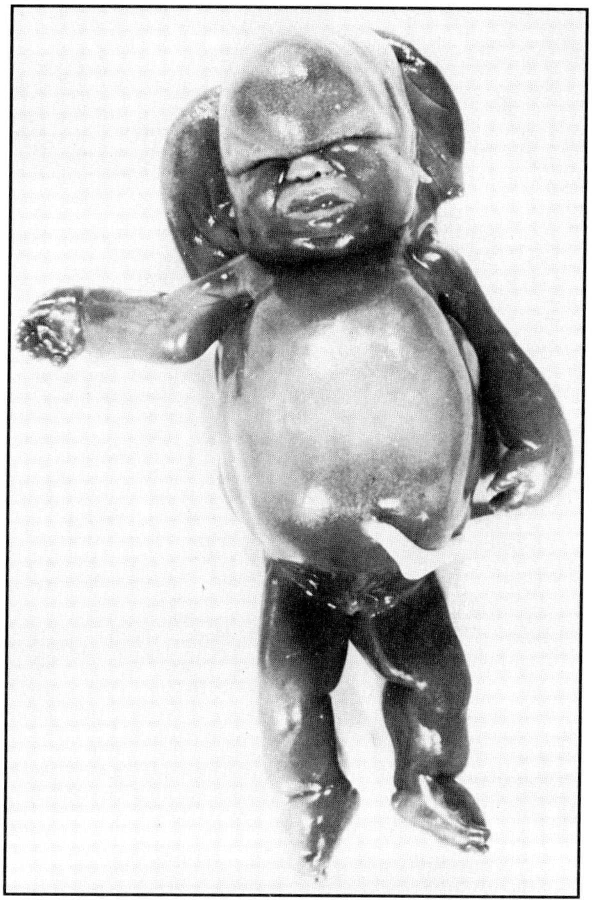

Fig. 4.17. 45 XO fetus at 19 weeks' gestation. A large fluid-filled sac is present over the occipital region, and there is generalised oedema and abdominal distension.

tion of the fetus is warranted. Trisomy 10q has been demonstrated in recurrent anencephaly with renal abnormalities (Singer et al. 1987). A few are the result of amnion rupture sequence. This possibility should be borne in mind when there are other abnormalities of the head, in particular facial clefts which are not explicable on developmental grounds, or gross facial asymmetry.

Cystic Hygroma

"Cystic hygroma" is quite commonly described on ultrasound examination from 10 weeks' gestation onwards. This is not the same lesion as the circumscribed, anterolateral hamartomatous malformation described by paediatric and plastic surgeons which is rarely diagnosed in the second trimester. The term cystic hygroma or nuchal swelling or thickening described by ultrasonographers is an echodense abnormality in the posterior or posterior-lateral nuchal and occipital area (Fig. 4.17). It is frequently accompanied by generalised fetal hydrops. The swelling is probably due to failure to establish communication between lymphatic channels of the head and neck and jugular vein (van der Putte 1977). Spontaneous resolution of the swelling has been reported with redundant skin webbing persisting in some survivors.

Kalousek et al. (1990) found that 85% of fetuses with cystic hygroma have a chromosome abnormality and Eydoux et al. (1989) found chromosome anomaly in 70% when cystic hygroma was the only malformation diagnosed on scan and in 22% when there were associated malformations. Monosomy X (Turner's syndrome) is the commonest chromosome abnormality and these fetuses also have general-

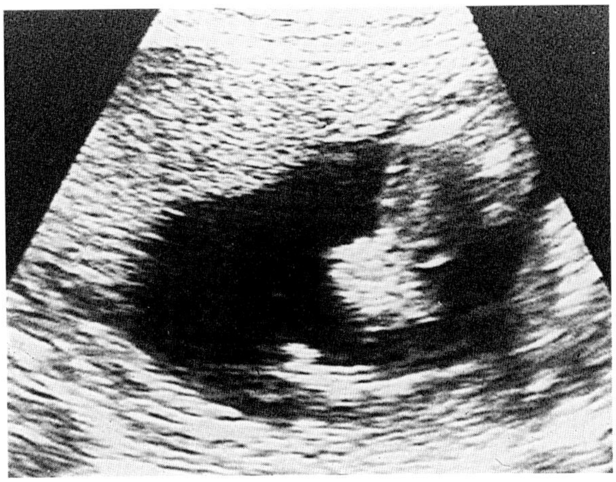

Fig. 4.18. Ultrasound scan, horizontal cut through fetal trunk. Gastroschisis, loops of bowel float freely in the amniotic cavity. (Courtesy of Dr. B. Muir, Edinburgh)

ised oedema and hypoplasia of the distal aortic arch. Trisomies 13, 18 and 21 and some structural chromosome abnormalities may also present with cystic hygroma. Rare single gene defects such as the lethal multiple pterygium syndrome, Noonan, Robert's and Cumming's syndromes also occur with cystic hygroma (Marchese et al. 1985). Cowchock et al. (1982) describe postnuchal fluid accumulation accompanied by cleft palate in second trimester sibling fetuses with normal chromosomes and Bieber et al. (1979) reported cystic hygroma in siblings with ascites and oedema. A dominant form has been reported (Graham and Smith 1981) and an entirely normal liveborn after diagnosis of cystic hygroma in the second trimester (Macken et al. 1989).

Chitayat et al. (1989) studied the structure and number of lymph vessels in 12 spontaneous abortions of fetuses with posterior cystic hygroma and generalised oedema of variable aetiology and compared them to five therapeutically aborted apparently normal fetuses. They found that in the non-Turner's fetus there was an increase in number and dilatation of lymphatic vessels whereas the Turner's fetus had no recognisable lymph vessels in the oedematous cutaneous tissues of the limbs, and sparse dilated vessels in the wall of the cystic hygroma and lungs. In the event of failure of cytogenetic analysis these histological findings may enable a diagnosis to be made.

Cervical teratoma may be mistakenly diagnosed on ultrasound as cystic hygroma but causes little diagnostic problem for the pathologist. Postnuchal fluid accumulation has been inadvertently diagnosed as occipital encephalocoele (Nevin et al. 1983) and must also be distinguished from cervical meningocoele. Minor degrees of postnuchal fluid accumulation are seen in spontaneous abortion, both fresh and macerated, and in the presence of a variety of apparently unrelated abnormalities.

Abdominal Wall Defects

There are three types of anterior abdominal wall defect: gastroschisis, omphalocoele (exomphalos) and body stalk defect (Mann et al. 1984). Attention may be drawn to their presence during the second trimester because of raised maternal serum alpha-fetoprotein level, or they may be visualised by ultrasound examination.

It is usually possible to distinguish between the three types of defects in utero (Fig. 4.18) and the distinction should most certainly be made postnatally.

The defect in gastroschisis lies above and to the right of the umbilicus, separated from it by a strip of abdominal wall. It does not have a membranous covering (Fig. 4.19). It is thought to be the result of secondary rupture of the abdominal wall with subsequent prolapse of viscera. The incidence of associated defects is lower in gastroschisis (5%–24%) than with omphalocoele (30%–75%) (Torffs et al. 1990). Many of the defects are local, intestinal atresia, presumably the result of volvulus of abnormally mobile bowel loops which are able to float about in the amniotic cavity. Mann et al. (1984) observed neural tube defect in two of their 16 cases.

Omphalocoele is the result of failure of reduction of the physiological extraembryonic mid-gut herniation. Abdominal contents remain in a membranous sac composed of amnion and peritoneum, the umbilical cord arises from the apex of the sac (Fig. 4.20). The sac may rupture in utero and undergo degeneration, although careful examination of the margin of the defect usually reveals some sac remnant. It may rupture during vaginal delivery of the fetus. Associated major defects are frequent. Hauge et al. (1983) estimated that chromosome abnormalities are likely in about 13% of cases. Trisomy 18 was most frequent in their cases, a further 6% had neural tube defects. Mann et al. (1984) found that 53% of their cases had other major defects and one-third of those karyotyped had autosomal trisomy, six of the

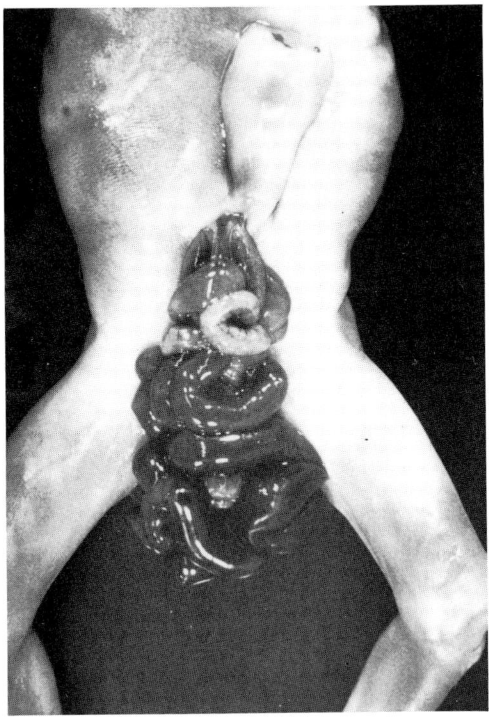

Fig. 4.19. Gastroschisis identified because of raised maternal serum alpha-fetoprotein level. An abdominal wall defect with well-defined, rounded margins lies to the right of the umbilicus. No sac remnants are present.

seven so diagnosed being born to young women. Nicolaides et al. (1986) found chromosome abnormalities in two-thirds of fetuses karyotyped because of prenatal diagnosis of exomphalos but referral patterns may have introduced bias towards cases with multiple anomalies. Torfs et al. (1990) reported that one-third of 81 cases of omphalocoele had recognisable syndromes, particularly trisomies 13 and 18 and Wiedemann–Beckwith syndromes.

Body stalk defect is a manifestation of the amnion rupture sequence with adhesions between the fetal abdomen and placenta and amnion (Fig. 4.21). Most examples of this defect are accompanied by major skeletal anomalies, often hypoplasia of lower limbs, pelvic deformity and major spinal distortion; neural tube defect is a common association.

When an anterior abdominal wall defect is detected prenatally, every effort to distinguish the type of defect should be made. A careful ultrasound search for associated anomalies should be undertaken and chromosome culture performed in all those cases thought to be exomphalos and perhaps in those where the type of defect cannot be specified, before parental counselling can be undertaken.

When pathological examination is performed, a search for minor dysmorphic features as well

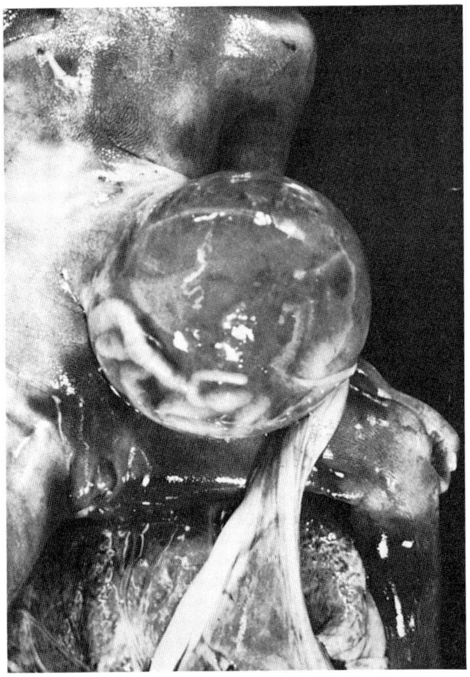

Fig. 4.20. Exomphalos in the second trimester. Protruding viscera lie within a sac of amnion and peritoneum.

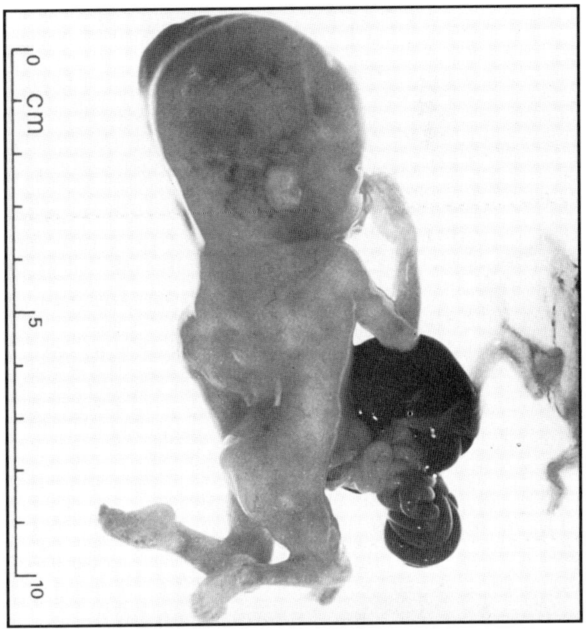

Fig. 4.21. Body stalk defect. Most of the viscera lie outside the abdomen. The covering sac has torn away from placental membranes. The umbilical cord is very short, and spinal deformity is apparent.

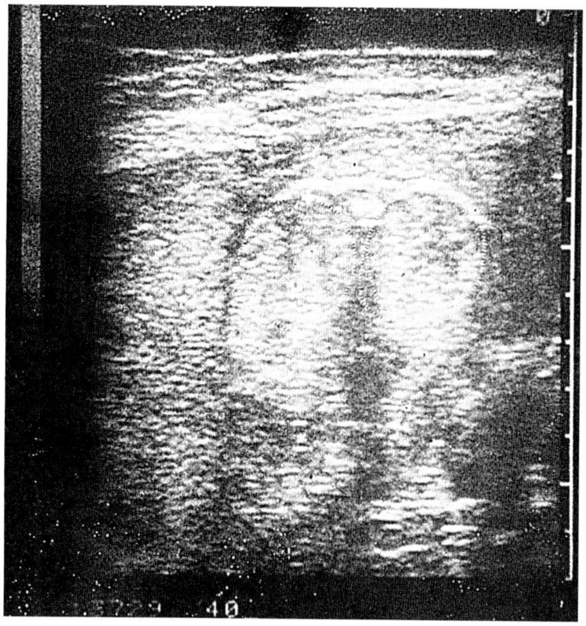

Fig. 4.22. Ultrasound scan, horizontal cut through fetal trunk. Large, paired oval bright objects are cystic kidneys.

as major defects should be undertaken and blood and tissue sent for chromosome analysis on the slightest suspicion of dysmorphism.

Intrapartum traumatic rupture of the abdominal wall may occur. This type of defect rarely occurs in the midline and is often in the flank (see p. 128).

Cystic Kidneys

Cystic enlargement of the fetal kidney may be discovered during routine ultrasound examination, when attention may be drawn to the possibility of renal malformation by oligohydramnios; during a deliberate search for cystic renal disease; or during the investigation of certain metabolic abnormalities in women at risk. Cystic kidneys may be identified because of raised maternal serum alpha-fetoprotein level caused either by impaired renal function or the presence of an associated anomaly.

It is important to distinguish between the different types of renal cystic disease so that accurate risks of recurrence are given to parents and appropriate investigations undertaken in subsequent pregnancies. Renal cystic disease is discussed in Chapter 20, p. 473. Different types of cystic dysplasia may be distinguished in the second trimester. Both the fetus with infantile polycystic disease (Figs. 4.22, 4.23) and the one with Meckel's syndrome (Fig. 4.24) have symmetrical reniform enlargement by 18 weeks of gestation. In both cases, small cysts can be seen through the renal capsule. The bladder is usually rudimentary as the volume of urine secreted by the kidneys is very small. It is unusual to detect liver cysts during dissection in the 18–20-week fetus, although the liver may be enlarged, but liver involvement may be apparent on histological examination. By the second trimester, cystic enlargement of the kidney may be apparent in some metabolic disorders such as cerebrohepatorenal syndrome (Powers et al. 1985) and glutaric aciduria (Boué et al. 1984) (Fig. 4.25).

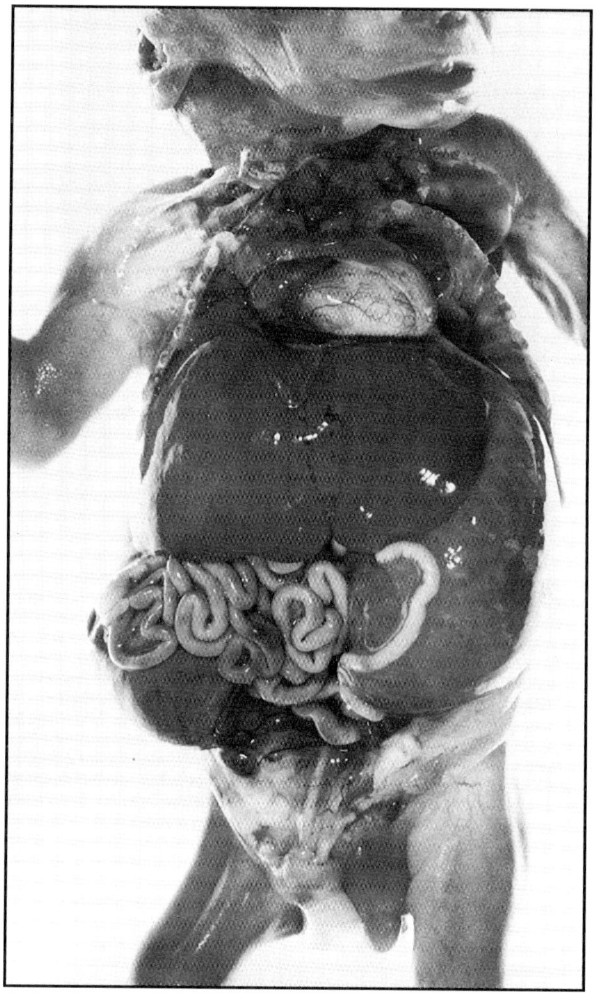

Fig. 4.23. Infantile polycystic disease of kidneys. There is enormous renal enlargement by 19 weeks' gestation.

Cystic renal dysplasia presents with oligohydramnios when it is bilateral or accompanied

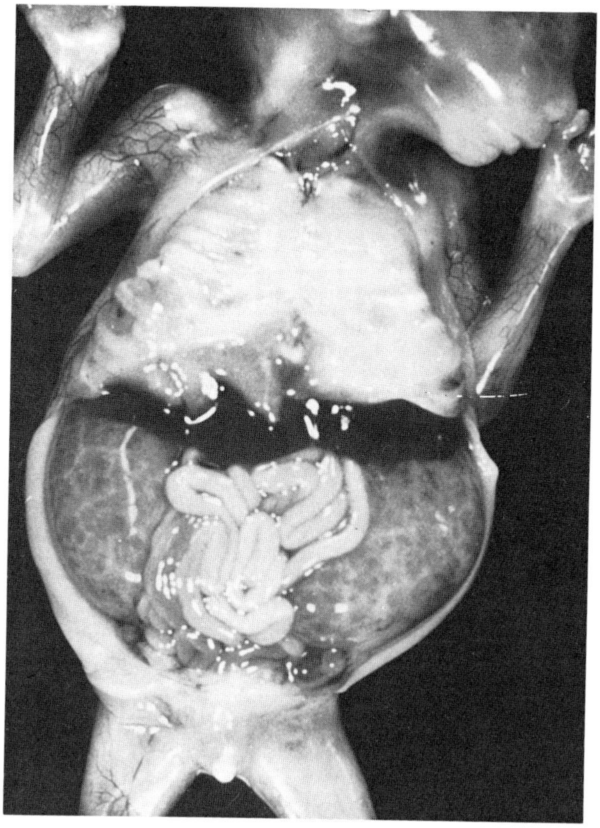

Fig. 4.24. Meckel's syndrome; symmetrical enlargement of kidneys at 18 weeks' gestation.

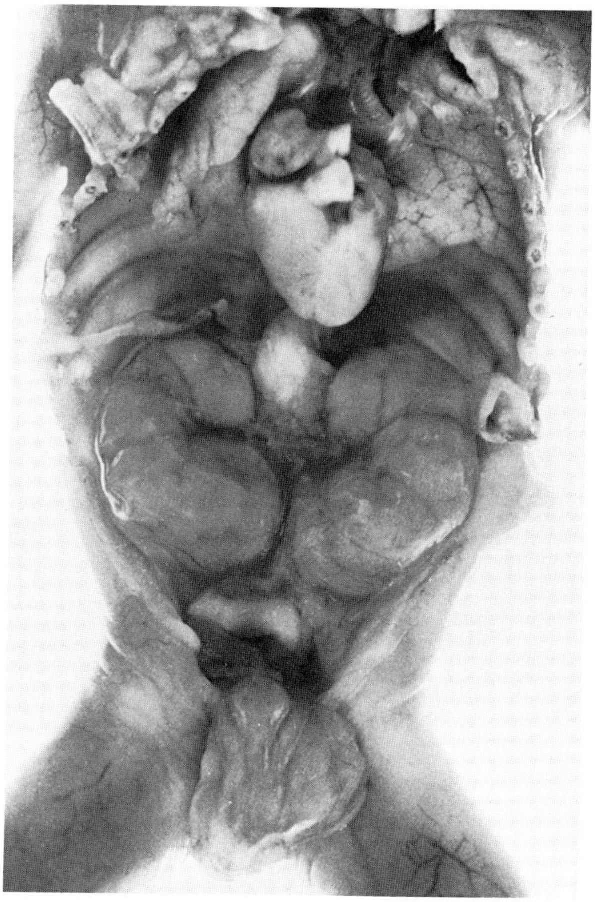

Fig. 4.25. Glutaric aciduria type II. Renal enlargement was apparent on pre-amniocentesis ultrasound examination in at-risk pregnancy. It is not as gross as in the two previous cases.

by agenesis of the contralateral kidney, which often makes detailed ultrasound examination difficult. This type of renal abnormality may be seen both with and without lower urinary tract obstruction (Fig. 4.26). It may be the first intimation of a recognised syndrome, e.g. Frazer syndrome (Boyd et al. 1988) or autosomal trisomy. Detailed examination of the fetus may elicit a pattern of dysmorphic features to back up this suspicion.

Renal Abnormalities Accompanying Urethral Obstruction

Urethral obstruction (Fig. 4.27) is usually detected in the second trimester of pregnancy during ultrasound examination undertaken for dating purposes or during the investigation of raised maternal serum alpha-fetoprotein levels. Reduced amniotic fluid volume leads to concentration of AFP.

Bladder drainage has been effected in utero and vesicoamniotic cavity communication established (Manning et al. 1983), but, nevertheless, some babies have died in infancy because of renal malfunction. It is important to realise that a range of urological abnormalities may already be present at 18–20 weeks' gestation. These range from cystic dysplasia (Fig. 4.28a), through hypoplasia, medullary hypoplasia, hydronephrosis (Fig. 4.28b) and hydroureter to relative normality of the urinary tract, when vesicoureteric insertions are able to withstand the considerable increase in intravesical pressure. It is necessary to examine both kidneys from these fetuses in order to

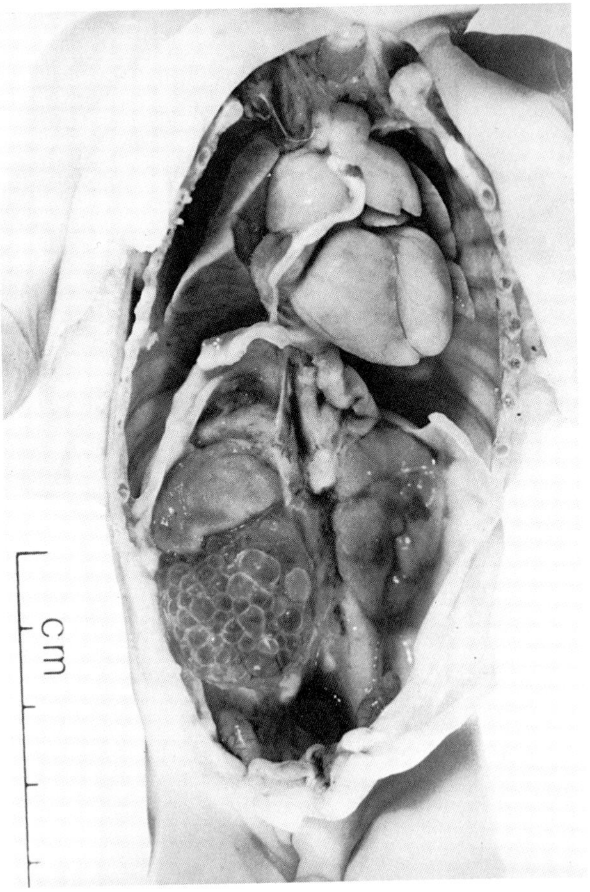

Fig. 4.26. Right cystic renal dysplasia and left renal agenesis. The left adrenal is discoid and the urinary bladder very small.

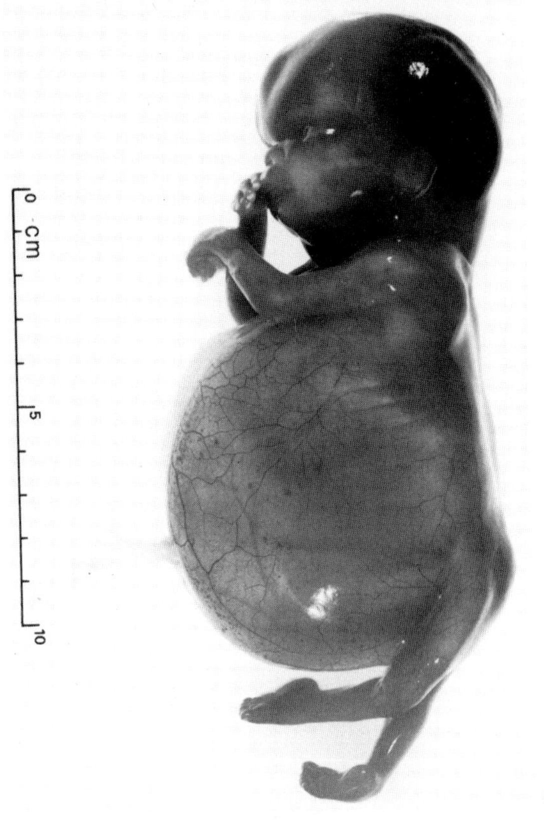

a

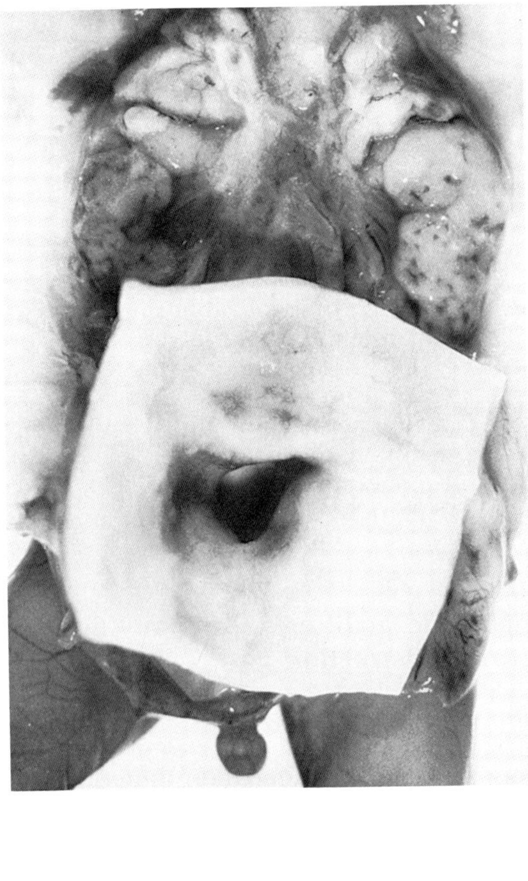

b

Fig. 4.27. Urethral obstruction. **a** The abdomen is distended because of cystomegaly, and there is oedema of the upper abdominal wall. **b** The front wall of the urinary bladder has been removed to display dilatation of the internal urethral orifice and prostatic urethra.

a
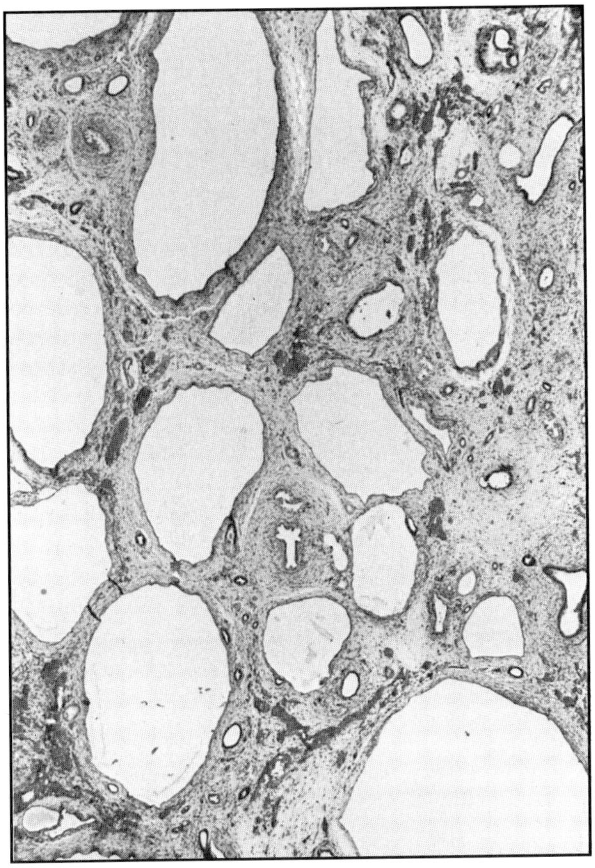

b
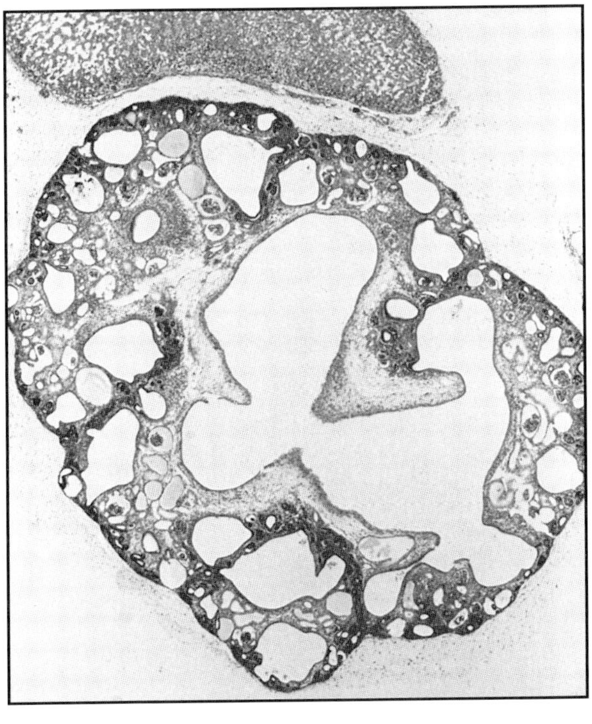

establish the frequency with which renal normality is likely to be found and to correlate any abnormality discovered with ultrasound appearances so that the appropriate surgical intervention can be undertaken in other pregnancies. It should not be forgotten that urethral obstruction may be the earliest manifestation of a chromosome abnormality (Hoagland et al. 1988). Examination for characteristic dysmorphic features and karyotyping should be performed on the smallest suspicion of a syndrome diagnosis.

Table 4.2 indicates the types of renal anomaly seen in fetuses from pregnancies terminated following the diagnosis of urethral obstruction.

Table 4.2. Renal anomalies in 14 fetuses terminated for urethral obstruction

Bilateral renal dysplasia	2
Bilateral renal dysplasia and hydronephrosis	1
Unilateral renal dysplasia + renal agenesis	2
Bilateral renal hypoplasia	2
Bilateral renal hypoplasia + hydronephrosis	2
Bilateral medullary hypoplasia	2
Bilateral medullary hypoplasia + hydronephrosis	3
Bilateral tubular and Bowman's capsular dilatation	1
Normal	—

Chromosome Anomalies

The most commonly encountered chromosome anomalies amongst fetuses from deliberately terminated pregnancies are trisomies 21 and 18 and monosomy X. When pregnancy is being terminated for chromosome anomaly, confirmation of fetal karyotype is an important part of fetal assessment and samples of blood and tissue should be taken as soon as possible after termination.

When trisomy 18 is present, characteristic dysmorphic features are always identifiable. A globular head with hypertelorism, broad nose and micrognathia is usual. Overlapping of

Fig. 4.28a,b. Kidneys from 18-week gestation fetuses with urethral obstruction. **a** Cystic dysplasia. **b** Hypoplasia and hydronephrosis.

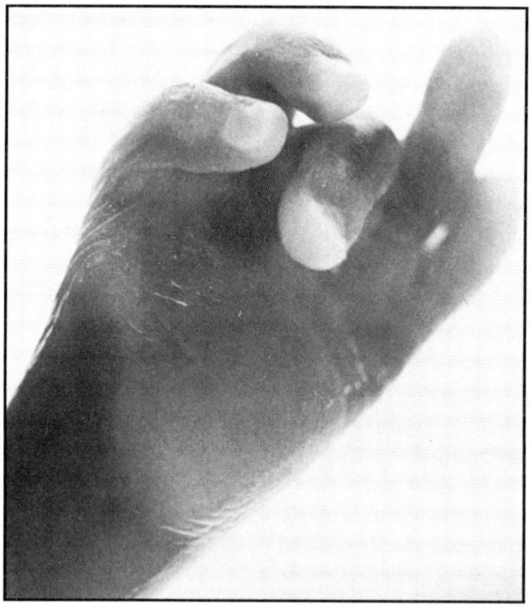

Fig. 4.29. Trisomy 18. Overlapping fingers apparent at 19 weeks' gestation.

fingers (Fig. 4.29) is easily distinguished and almost always present. Flexion deformities of lower limbs with abnormalities of the feet are usual. Major anomalies of viscera are frequently found. Table 4.3 shows the dysmorphic features and visceral anomalies found in locally

Table 4.3. Dysmorphic features and visceral malformations in 17 fetuses with trisomy 18 karyotype

Globular head	11
Hypertelorism/broad nose	8
Micrognathia	14
Low set/simple ears	15
Overlapping fingers	15
Transverse palmar crease	3
Short fingers	1
Rocker bottom feet	7
Talipes	4
Scoliosis	1
Limb flexion deformities	1
Hypospadias	1
Cleft lip and palate	5
Exomphalos	5
Incomplete intestinal rotation	6
Diaphragmatic eventration	2
Tracheo-oesophageal fistula	2
Cerebral anomaly	5
Meningomyelocoele	3
Renal tract anomaly	5
Ventricular septal defect	5
Double-outlet right ventricle	3
Bicuspid pulmonary valve	2
Anomalous aortic arch branching	1

examined material. It is possible, in the case of trisomy 18 to confirm prenatal diagnosis by naked-eye inspection of the fetus; nevertheless, karyotyping should be undertaken.

The fetus with trisomy 21 does not have such easily recognisable abnormalities in the second trimester. The typical facies associated with the infant with Down's syndrome has not developed (see Fig. 4.10), and whilst some fetuses with trisomy 21 have abnormalities of the face and head, they are neither so marked nor so consistent as those seen in trisomy 18; indeed, some fetuses appear normal even to the experienced observer. Bilateral transverse palmar creases are present in one-half to two-thirds of cases and a single palmar crease in a few of the remainder. A vertical plantar cleft between first and second toes is frequently present. In some fetuses, short digits and broad hands may be apparent. Visceral anomalies (Table 4.4) are not seen as frequently as in trisomy 18 and are usually single (Fig. 4.30).

Table 4.4. Dysmorphic features and visceral malformations in 26 fetuses with trisomy 21 karyotype

Coarse features	16
Low set/simple ears	14
Short neck	2
Transverse palmar crease:	
bilateral	12
unilateral	5
Abnormal palmar crease	3
Short fingers	2
Vertical plantar crease	11
Prominent heels	3
Talipes	1
Ventricular septal defect	3
Atrioventricular canal defect	2
Atrial septal defect	1
Fetal hydrops	2
Duodenal atresia	2
Duodenal duplication and ectopic pancreas	1
Hydrocephalus	1
Abnormal lung lobation	1

Monosomy X is sometimes picked up because of prenatal chromosome examination but is more usually identified during ultrasound examination in the second trimester or because of raised maternal serum alpha-fetoprotein levels. Disproportionate postnuchal fluid accumulation and fetal hydrops are apparent on examination of the fetus (see Fig. 4.17), and anomalies of great vessels, particularly hypoplasia of the third part of the aortic arch and aberrant origin of the large artery, are the most frequently identified abnormalities. A mem-

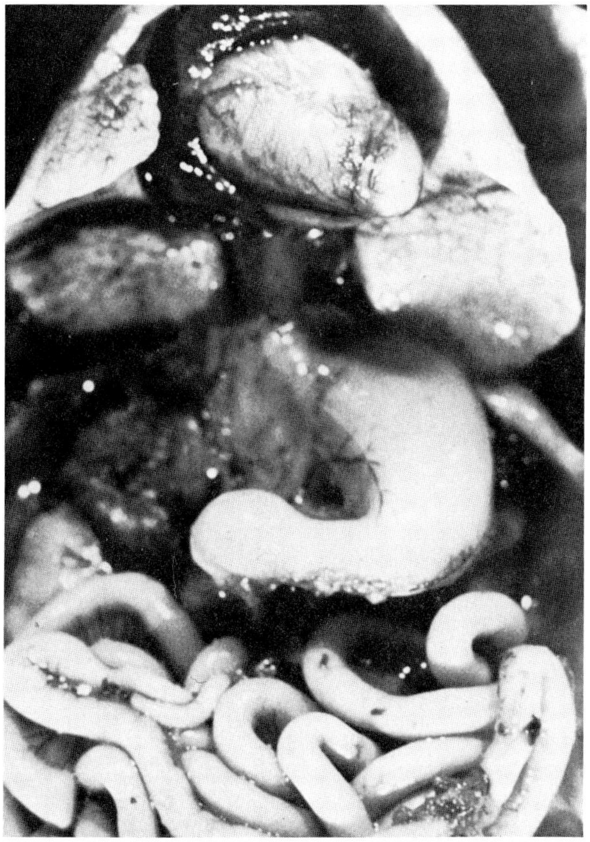

Fig. 4.30. Trisomy 21. Duodenal atresia; dilatation of the duodenum is apparent beyond the pylorus.

branomuscular ventricular septal defect may be present. The ovaries are normal at this stage of development.

Dysmorphic features found in other chromosome anomalies (Fig. 4.31) are detailed by Smith (1982) and Wiedemann et al. (1985). The fetus is often severely growth retarded (see Fig. 7.12) and intrauterine death in the second or third trimester is common. Some triploid babies are liveborn. Common malformations include meningomyelocoele, hydrocephaly, cardiac defects, cleft lip and palate and a variety of dysmorphic features (Jones 1988) (Fig. 4.31a).

Amnion Rupture Sequence

Rupture of the amnion in the first half of pregnancy gives rise to a range of anomalies which seem to be related to the time of amnion rupture, which in some cases may be deduced from the anomalies perceived (Higginbottom et al. 1979). It is important to recognise the results of amnion rupture, which may include disruption and deformity of major proportions (Fig. 4.32), because the recurrence risk is negligible. Amnion rupture sequence is frequently misdiagnosed when attention is paid only to the most striking anomaly, which sometimes resembles a defect with accurately assessed recurrence risk. Associated anomalies and atypical features of the major abnormality, which could indicate the correct diagnosis are often ignored (Seeds et al. 1982). Some of the names given to this sequence (Table 4.5) reflect ideas about the pathogenesis, whilst others concentrate on observed anomalies.

Table 4.5. Synonyms for amnion rupture sequence (after Seed et al. 1982)

Amniotic band syndrome
Aberrant tissue bands
"Adam complex" (amniotic deformity, adhesion, mutilations)
Amniochorionic mesoblastic fibrous strings
Amniogenic bands
Amniotic band disruption complex
Congenital annular bands
Congenital annular constrictions
Congenital constriction band syndrome
Congenital ring constrictions
Congenital transverse defects
Body wall defects with reduction limb deformities (Pagon et al. 1979)
Early amnion rupture spectrum (Smith 1982)

A spectrum of defects is described. The important observations which emerge are:

1. Striking asymmetry of defects
2. A combination of defects which both can and cannot be explained by our knowledge of normal development
3. No two individuals have the same combination of anomalies

Whilst it is generally accepted that amnion rupture is the common factor in the development of this group of defects, the cause for such rupture is not clear. Physical trauma in early pregnancy has been recognised in a very few cases (Smith 1982). Sequelae of amnion rupture are described in infants with connective tissue disorders such as Ehlers–Danlos syndrome and severe osteogenesis imperfecta (Young et al. 1985). In these disorders, de-

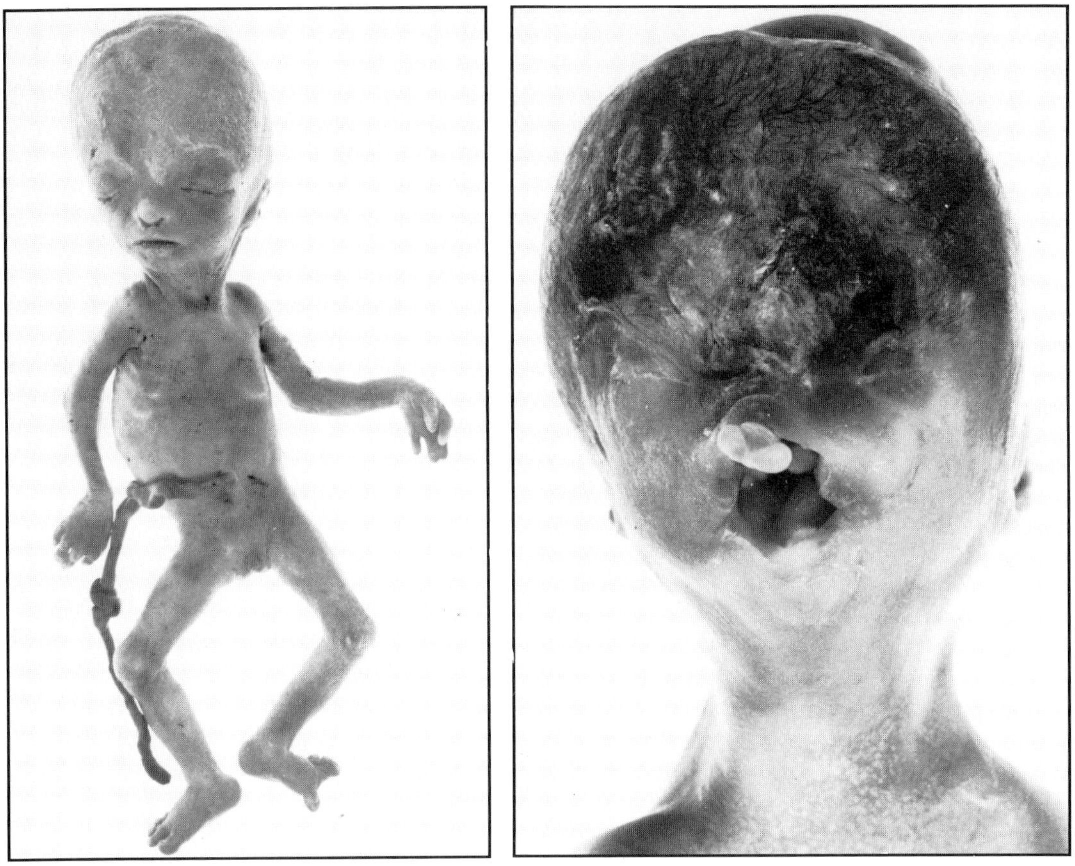

Fig. 4.31. **a** Triploidy. Growth-retarded fetus with globular head and abnormalities of hands and feet; "hitch-hiker" toe is striking. **b** 13 deletion. Dysmorphic features include microphthalmia, bilateral cleft lip and palate and micrognathia.

fective collagen probably reduces the load-bearing capacity of the placental membranes. A small excess of summer conceptions and continued ingestion of oral contraceptives in early pregnancy are also described (Ossipoff and Hall 1977). Amniotic bands are described following amniocentesis (Rehder and Weitzel 1978). Pregnancy complications among locally examined cases include maternal drug abuse, anorexia nervosa and in vitro fertilisation of the ovum. Infection does not seem to be a factor in the aetiology of amnion rupture.

The major defects associated with amnion rupture are frequently diagnosed because of raised maternal serum alpha-fetoprotein levels (see Fig. 4.21), and some are identified by ultrasound examination. The range of anomalies resulting from amnion rupture is shown in Table 4.6. Observed anomalies arise as a result of a combination of mechanisms which cause physical interruption of normal development, tethering, compression and injury to previously formed structures. Major defects arise early in gestation and are often accompanied by reduction of fetal movements because of firm attachment of fetal parts to the chorion which results in a very short umbilical cord. Visceral defects are only found in relation to disruption of the fetal surface and are not seen in those regions of the body where skin continuity is not breached.

Damage to the amnion is followed by loss of amniotic fluid. Torpin (1965) ascribes this to absorption by the chorion. This results in fetal deformity affecting the limbs in a fairly symmetrical fashion, as is seen in oligohydramnios from any cause and may exacerbate the effect of fetal tethering and produce gross spinal deformity.

When pregnancy terminates in the second trimester, intact bands of amnion may be identified running between the defect and the chorionic sac. In the more mature fetus, con-

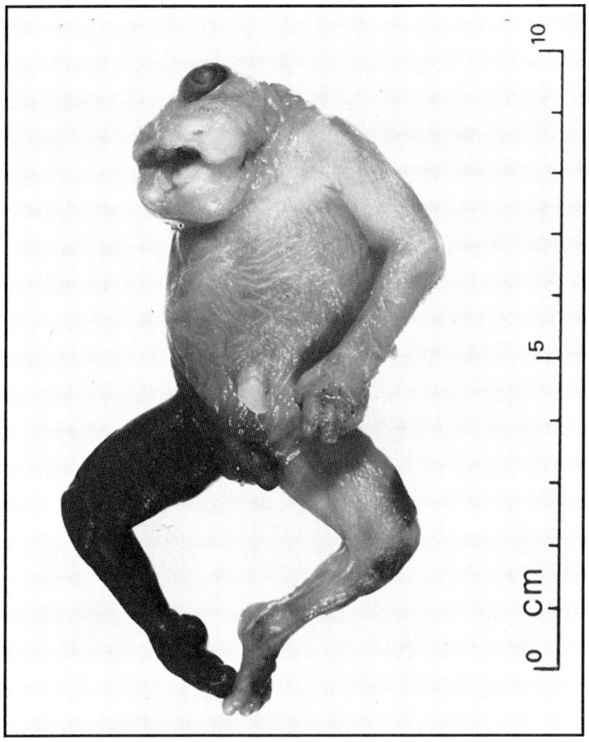

Fig. 4.32. Amnion rupture sequence; there is anencephaly, facial clefting and absence of right arm.

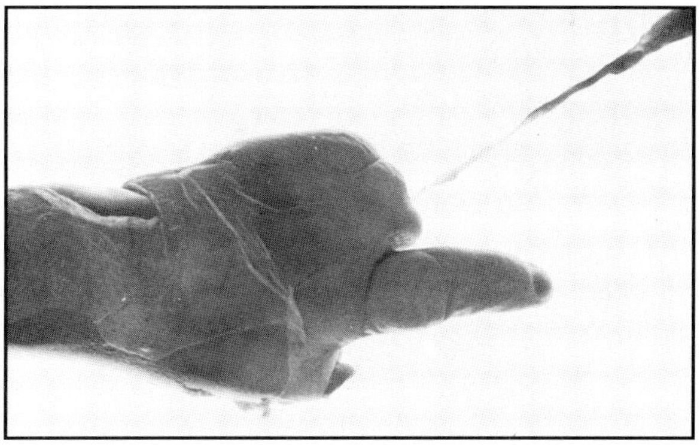

Fig. 4.33. Amputation of fingers; amnion string is still adherent. Stillbirth at 30 weeks' gestation.

tinuity is usually lost, particularly if the fetus is stillborn (Fig. 4.33), and a few degenerate threads remain, although a complete encircling band may be seen applied to a limb constriction defect (Fig. 4.34). Should the fetus have emerged from the amniotic sac into a secondary space between the placental membranes, then the amniotic sac may persist as a frill around the cord insertion, although occasionally a small amniotic sac may be identified.

Table 4.6. Types of anomaly seen in amnion rupture sequence

Time of rupture	Craniofacial	Trunk	Limbs	Placenta
<4 weeks	Anencephaly Inappropriate facial cleft Proboscis, eye defects Encephalocoele		Absent limb	Adherence of head to chorion
<6 weeks	Cleft lip	Thoracic wall defect Abdominal wall defect Severe scoliosis	Syndactyly Limb reduction	Abdominal wall attached to chorion Short or absent umbilical cord
<12 weeks	Cleft palate Ear deformity Craniostenosis	Omphalocoele	Amputation of digits/part limb Limb hypoplasia Asymmetrical limb size	Short umbilical cord Amnion "strings" or bands
>12 weeks			Compression deformities	Oligohydramnios

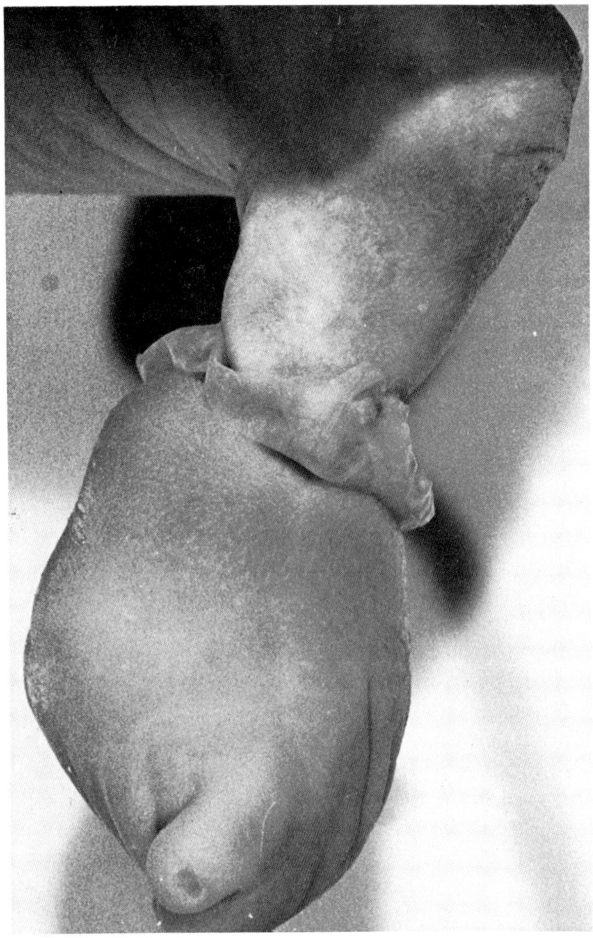

a

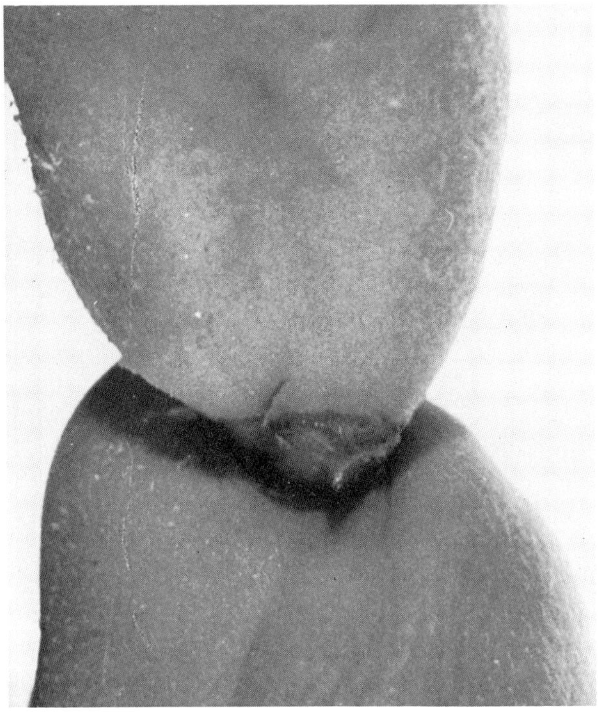

b

Fig. 4.34a,b. Amnion rupture sequence. **a** Frill of placental membrane surrounds the fetal leg; the foot is very oedematous. **b** Membrane has been cut away to display a deep groove in soft tissues.

References

American Journal of Medical Genetics (1990) 35: 157–218

Arulkumaran S, Rodeck CH (1990) Invasive prenatal diagnostic techniques. Fetal Med Review 2: 171–185

Aitken DA, May HM, Ferguson-Smith MA (1984) Amniotic band disruption syndrome associated with elevated amniotic AFP and normal acetylcholinesterase gel test. Prenat Diagn 4: 443–446

Balfour RO, Laurence KM (1980) Raised serum AFP levels and fetal renal agenesis. Lancet I: 317

Ballantyne JW (1902) Manual of antenatal pathology and hygiene. Green, Edinburgh, pp 272–277

Barson AJ, Donnai P, Ferguson A, Donnai D, Read AP (1980) Haemangioma of the cord: further cause of raised maternal serum and liquor alphafetoprotein. Br Med J 281: 1252

Batcup G, Clarke JP, Purdie DW (1988) Disposal arrangements for fetuses lost in the second trimester. Br J Obstet Gynaecol 95: 547–550

Benirschke K, Lowry RB, Opitz JM, Schwarzacher HG, Spranger JW (1979) Developmental terms—some proposals: first report of an international working group. Am J Med Genet 3: 297

Bieber FR, Petres RE, Bieber JMcN, Nance WE (1979) Prenatal detection of a familial nuchal bleb simulating encephalocoele. Birth Defects XV (5A): 51–61

Bogart MH, Paradian MR, Jones VW (1987) Abnormal maternal serum chorionic gonadotrophin levels in pregnancies with fetal chromosome abnormalities. Prenat Diagn 7: 623–630

Boulot P, Hedon B, Deschamps F et al. (1990) Anencephaly-like malformation in surviving twin after embryonic reduction. Lancet 335: 1155–1156

Boyd PA, Keeling JW, Lindenbaum RH (1988) Fraser syndrome (cryptophthalmos-syndactyly syndrome: a review of eleven cases with postmortem findings. Am J Med Genet 31: 159–168

Boyd PA, Keeling JW, Selinger M, MacKenzie IZ (1990) Limb reduction and chorion villus sampling. Prenat Diagn 10: 437–441

Boyd PA (1992) Why might maternal serum AFP be high in pregnancies in which the fetus is normally formed? Br J Obstet Gynaecol 99: 93–95

Brock DJH, Sutcliffe RG (1972) Alpha-fetoprotein in the antenatal diagnosis of anencephaly and spina bifida. Lancet II: 197–199

Brock DJH, Barron L, Bedgood D, Hawward C (1985) Prospective prenatal diagnosis of cystic fibrosis. Lancet I: 1175–1178

Canadian Collaborative CVS-amniocentesis Clinical Trial Group (1989) Multicentre randomised clinical trial of chorionic villus sampling and amniocentesis. Lancet I: 1–6

Canadian Medical Research Council (1977) Diagnosis of genetic disease by amniocentesis during the second trimester of pregnancy. A Canadian study. Report No 5. Supply Services, Ottawa, Canada

Canick JA, Knight GJ, Palomaki GE, Haddow JE, Cuckle HS, Wald NJ (1988) Low second trimester maternal serum unconjugated oestriol in pregnancies with Down's syndrome. Br J Obstet Gynaecol 95: 330–333

Carter CO (1963) The genetics of common malformation. In: Proceedings, II international conference on congenital malformations. The Medical Congress Ltd, New York, pp 306–313

Carter CO (1969) Genetics of common disorders. Br Med Bull 25: 52–57

Chemke J, Miskin A, Rav-acha Z, Porath A, Sagiv M, Katz Z (1977) Prenatal diagnosis of Meckel syndrome: alphafetoprotein and betatrace protein in amniotic fluid. Clin Genet 11: 285–289

Chitayat D, Kalousek DK, Bamforth JS (1989) Lymphatic abnormalities in fetuses with posterior cervical cystic hygroma. Am J Med Genet 33: 352–356

Clayton-Smith J, Farndon PA, McKeown C, Donnai D (1990) Examination of fetuses after induced abortion for fetal abnormality. Br Med J 300: 295–297

Colten HR (1990) Screening for cystic fibrosis. N Engl J Med 322: 328–329

Cowchock FS, Wapner RJ, Kurtz A, Chatzkel S, Barnhart JS Jr, Lesnick DC (1982) Brief clinical report: not all cystic hygromas occur in the Ullrich–Turner syndrome. Am J Med Genet 12: 327–331

Cuckle HS, Wald NJ, Goodburn SF, Sneddon J, Amess JAL, Carlson Dunn S (1990) Measurement of activity of urea resistant neutrophil alkaline phosphatase as an antenatal screening test for Down's syndrome. Br Med J 301: 1024–1026

Daffos F, Capella-Pavlovsky M, Forestier F (1983) Fetal blood sampling via the umbilical cord using a needle guided by ultrasound. Prenat Diagn 3: 271–274

Elder SH, Laurence KM (1991) The impact of supportine intervention after second trimester termination of pregnancy for fetal abnormality. Prenat Diagn 11: 47–54

Elejalde BR, Elejalde MM, Acuna JM et al. (1990) Prospective study of amniocentesis performed between weeks 9 and 16 of gestation: its feasibility, risks, complications and use in early genetic prenatal diagnosis. Am J Med Genet 35: 188–196

Emery AEH, Rimoin DL (eds) (1990) Principles and practice of medical genetics. Churchill Livingstone, Edinburgh, Chapters 18 and 19

Eydoux P, Choiset A, le Porrier N et al. (1989) Chromosomal prenatal diagnosis: study of 936 cases of intrauterine abnormalities after ultrasound assessment. Prenat Diagn 9: 255–268

Ferguson-Smith MA (1983) The reduction of anencephalic and spina bifida births by maternal serum alpha-fetoprotein screening. Br Med Bull 39: 365–372

Firth HV, Boyd PA, Chamberlain P, Mackenzie IZ, Lindenbaum RH, Huson SM (1991) Severe limb abnormalities after chorion villus sampling at 56–66 days gestation. Lancet 337: 762–763

Fitzsimons JS, Filshie GM, Hill AS, Kime R (1976) Antenatal diagnosis of trisomy 13 with unexpected increase in alpha-fetoprotein. J Med Genet 13: 400–412

Fu YH, Kuhl DPA, Pizzutr A et al. (1991) Variation of the CGG repeat at the fragile X site results in genetic stability: resolution of the Sherman paradox. Cell 67: 1047–1058

Gardner RJM, Sutherland GR (1989) Chromosome abnormalities and genetic counselling. Oxford Monographs on Medical Genetics No 17. Oxford University Press

Gau GS, Napier K, Bhundia J (1991) Use of a tissue adhesive to repair fetal bodies after dissection. J Clin Pathol 44: 759–760

Gitlin D (1975) Normal biology of alpha-fetoprotein. Ann NY Acad Sci 259: 7–16

Graham J, Smith D (1981) Dominantly inherited pterygium colli. J Pediatr 98: 664–665

Graham JM, Edwards MJ, Lipson AH, Webster NS (1988) Gestational hyperthermia as a cause for Moebius' syndrome. Teratology 37: 461–462

Hall JG (1990) Genomic imprinting: review and relevance to human diseases. Am J Hum Genet 46: 857–873

Hall JG, Pauli RM, Wilson KM (1980) Maternal and fetal sequelae of anticoagulation during pregnancy. Am J Med 68: 122–140

Harrod MJE, Friedman JM, Santos-Ramos R, Rutledge J, Weinberg A (1984) Etiologic heterogeneity of fetal hydrocephalus diagnosed by ultrasound. Am J Obstet Gynecol 150: 38–40

Hauge M, Bugge M, Nielsen J (1983) Early prenatal diagnosis of omphalocoele constitutes indication for amniocentesis. Lancet II: 507

Higginbottom MC, Jones KL, Hall BD, Smith DW (1979) The amniotic band disruption complex: timing of amniotic rupture and variable spectra of consequent defects. J Pediatr 95: 544–549

Hoagland MH, Frank KA, Hutchins GM (1988) Prune-belly syndrome with prostatic hypoplasia, bladder wall rupture, and massive ascites in a fetus with trisomy 18. Arch Pathol Lab Med 112: 1126–1128

Hobbins JC, Grannum PAT, Berkowitz RL, Silverman R, Mahoney MJ (1979) Ultrasound in the diagnosis of congenital anomalies. Am J Obstet Gynecol 134: 331–345

Hook EB (1990) Chromosome abnormalities in older women by maternal age. Am J Med Genet 35: 184–187

Jacobs PA, Szulman AE, Funkhouser J, Matsuura JS, Wilson CC (1982) Human triploidy: relationship between parental origin of the additional haploid complement and development of partial hydatiform mole. Ann Hum Genet 46: 223–231

Jones KL (1988) Smith's recognizable patterns of human malformation, 4th edn. Saunders, Philadelphia

Jones KL, Smith DW, Ulleland N, Streissguth AP (1973) Pattern of malformation in offspring of chronic alcoholic mothers. Lancet 1: 1267–1271

Kalousek DK, Barrett I, McGillivray BC (1989) Placental mosaicism and intrauterine survival of trisomies 13 and 18. Am J Hum Genet 44: 338–343

Kalousek DK, Fitch N, Paradice BA (1990) Pathology of the human embryo and previable fetus. An atlas. Springer-Verlag, New York

Keeling JW, Manning N, Chamberlain P (1990) Accuracy of fetal anomaly scanning. Pediatr Pathol 10: 653
Kerem B, Rommens JM, Buchanan JA et al. (1989) Identification of the cystic fibrosis gene: genetic analysis. Science 245: 1073–1080
Kjessler B, Johansson SGO, Sherman M, Gustavson KH, Hultqvist G (1975) Alphafetoprotein in antenatal diagnosis of congenital nephrosis. Lancet I: 432–433
Knowles SAS (1986) Examination of products of conception terminated after prenatal investigation. J Clin Pathol 39: 1049–1065
Koontz WL, Seeds JW, Adams NJ, Johnson AM, Cefato RC (1983) Elevated maternal serum alpha-fetoprotein, second-trimester oligohydramnios and pregnancy outcome. Obstet Gynecol 62: 301–304
Lamb MP (1975) Gangrene of a fetal limb due to amniocentesis. Br J Obstet Gynaecol 82: 829–830
Lammer EJ, Chen DT, Hoar RM et al. (1985) Retinoic acid embryopathy. N Engl J Med 313: 837–841
Lancet (1991) Editorial. Imprinting makes an impression. Lancet 338: 413–414
Laurence KM (1982) Antenatal detection of neural tube defects. In: Barson AJ (ed) Fetal and neonatal pathology. Praeger, New York, p 87
Laurence KM, Martin D (1959) A technique for obtaining undistorted specimens of the central nervous system. J Clin Pathol 12: 188–190
Lilford RJ (1991) Editorial. The rise and fall of chorion villus sampling. Br Med J 303: 936–937
Macken MB, Grantmyre EB, Vincer MJ (1989) An ultrasonic view of the developing fetus. Obstet Gynecol Surv 38: 375–398
Manchester DK, Pretorius DH, Avery C et al. (1988) Accuracy of ultrasound diagnoses in pregnancies complicated by suspected fetal anomalies. Prenat Diagn 8: 109–117
Mann L, Alroomi L, McNay M, Ferguson-Smith MA (1983) Placental haemangioma. Case report. Br J Obstet Gynaecol 90: 983–986
Mann L, Ferguson-Smith MA, Desai M, Gibson AAM, Raine PAM (1984) Prenatal assessment of anterior abdominal wall defects and their prognosis. Prenat Diagn 4: 427–435
Manning FA, Harman CR, Lange IR et al. (1983) Antepartum chronic fetal vesico-amniotic shunts for obstructive uropathy: a report of two cases. Am J Obstet Gynecol 145: 819
Marchese C, Savin E, Dragone E et al. (1985) Cystic hygroma: prenatal diagnosis and genetic counselling. Prenat Diagn 5: 221–227
Markowski B, Lawler SD (1977) Use of early fetal tissues obtained from suction termination of pregnancy. Lancet I: 186–188
Martinez-Frias M-L (1991) Valproic acid and spina bifida. Lancet 338: 196–197
McKusick VA (1990) Mendelian inheritance in man. Catalogs of autosomal dominant, autosomal recessive and X-linked phenotypes, 8th edn. John Hopkins, Baltimore
Medical Research Council (1978) An assessment of the hazards of amniocentesis. Br J Obstet Gynaecol 85 (suppl 2): 1–41
Medical Research Council (1991a) European trial of chorion villus sampling. Lancet 337: 1491–1499
Medical Research Council (1991b) Prevention of neural tube defects: results of the Medical Research Council vitamin study. Lancet 338: 131–137
Merkatz IR, Nitowsky HM, Macri JN, Johnson WE (1984) An association between low maternal serum alphafetoprotein and fetal chromosome abnormalities. Am J Obstet Gynecol 148: 886–894
Nevin NC, Nevin J, Thompson W, O'Hara MD (1983) Cystic hygroma simulating encephalocele. Prenat Diagn 3: 249–252
NICHD National Registry for Amniocentesis Study Group (1976) Midtrimester amniocentesis for prenatal diagnosis. Safety and accuracy. JAMA 236: 1471–1476
Nicolaides KH, Rodeck CH, Gosden GM (1986) Rapid karyotyping in non-lethal fetal malformations. Lancet I: 283–287
Norgaard-Pedersen B, Bagger P, Bang J et al. (1985) Maternal serum alphafetoprotein screening for fetal malformations in 28 062 pregnancies. A four-year experience from a low-risk area. Acta Obstet Gynecol Scand 64: 511–514
Oberlé I, Rousseau F, Heitz D et al. (1991) Instability of a 550 bp DNA segment and abnormal methylation in fragile X syndrome. Science 252: 1097–1102
Ornoy A (1991) The effects of pharmacological agents on the human fetus. Pediatr Pathol 11: 807–812
Ossipoff V, Hall D (1977) Etiologic factors in the amniotic band syndrome: a study of 24 patients. Birth Defects XIII (3D): 117–132
Pagon RA, Stephens TD, McGillivray BC et al. (1979) Body wall defects with reduction limb anomalies: a report of fifteen cases. Birth Defects XV (5A): 171–185
Quintero RA, Romero R, Mahoney MJ, Vecchio M, Holden J, Hobbins JC (1992) Fetal haemorrhagic lesions after chorionic villus sampling (letter). Lancet 339: 193
Reeders ST, Breuning MH, Davies KE et al. (1985) A highly polymorphic DNA marker linked to adult polycystic kidney disease on chromosome 16. Nature 317: 542–544
Rehder H (1978) Fetal limb deformities due to amniotic constrictions (a possible consequence of preceding amniocentesis). Pathol Res Pract 162: 316–326
Rehder H, Weitzel H (1978) Intrauterine amputations after amniocentesis. Lancet I: 382
Riordan JR, Rommens JM, Kerem B et al. (1989) Identification of the cystic fibrosis gene: cloning and characterisation of complementary DNA. Science 245: 1066–1073
Rommens JM, Ianuzzi MC, Kerem B et al. (1989) Identification of the cystic fibrosis gene: chromosome walking and jumping. Science 245: 1059–1065
Rushton DI (1981) Examination of products of conception from previable human pregnancies. J Clin Pathol 34: 819–835
Rutledge JC, Weinberg AG, Friedman JM, Harrod MJ, Santos-Ramos R (1986) Anatomic correlates of ultrasonographic prenatal diagnosis. Prenat Diagn 6: 51–61
Schinzel A (1984) Catalogue of unbalanced chromosome aberrations in man. Walter de Gruyter, Berlin, New York
Seeds JW, Cefalo RC, Herbert WNP (1982) Amniotic band syndrome. Am J Obstet Gynecol 144: 243–248
Seller MJ, Creasy MR, Alberman ED (1974) Alphafetoprotein levels in amniotic fluids from spontaneous abortions. Br Med J II: 524–525
Seller MJ, Dumon JE, Vanderheyden JS (1977) Amniotic fluid in multiple pregnancy. Br Med J I: 1600
Seppala M (1973) Increased alphafetoprotein in amniotic fluid associated with a congenital oesophageal atresia of the fetus. Obstet Gynecol 42: 623–624
Shen-Schwartz S, Neish C, Hill LM (1989) Antenatal ultrasound for fetal anomalies: importance of perinatal autopsy. Pediatr Pathol 9: 1–10
Singer N, Gersen S, Warburton D (1987) The value of chromosome analysis in cases of neural tube defects: a case of anencephaly associated with fetal dup(2)(p24 → pter). Prenat Diagn 7: 567–571

Smith DW (1982) Recognizable patterns of human malformation. (Major problems in clinical pediatrics, vol VII), Saunders, London

Spranger J, Benirschke K, Hall JG et al. (1982) Errors of morphogenesis: concepts and terms. Recommendations of an International Working Group. J Pediatr 100: 160–165

Stirrat GM, Gough JD, Bullock S, Wald NJ, Cuckle HS (1981) Raised maternal serum AFP, oligohydramnios and poor fetal outcome. Br J Obstet Gynaecol 88:231–235

Swift PGF, Driscoll IB, Vawles KDJ (1979) Neonatal small bowel obstruction associated with amniocentesis. Br Med J I: 720

Szulman AE, Surti U (1982) The clinicopathologic profile of the partial hydatidiform mole. Obstet Gynecol 59: 597–602

Tabor A, Philip J, Marsden M, Bary J, Obel FB, Morgaard-Pedersen B (1986) Randomised controlled trial of genetic amniocentesis in 4606 low-risk women. Lancet I: 1287–1293

Terry GM, Ho-Terry L, Warren RC et al. (1986) First trimester prenatal diagnosis of congenital rubella: a laboratory investigation. Br Med J 292: 930–932

Therkensen AJ, Rehder H (1981) Intestinal atresia caused by second trimester amniocentesis. Br J Obstet Gynaecol 88: 559–562

Thom H, Johnstone FD, Gibson JI, Scott GB, Noble DW (1977) Fetal proteinuria in diagnosis of congenital nephrosis detected by raised alpha-fetoprotein in maternal serum. Br Med J I: 16–18

Torfs C, Curry C, Roeper P (1990) Gastroschisis. J Pediatr 116: 1–6

van de Kaa CA (1991) Interphase cytogenetics in paraffin sections of routinely processed hydatidiform moles and hydropic abortions. J Pathol 165: 281–287

van der Putte SCJ (1977) Lymphatic malformation in human fetuses: a study of fetuses with Turner's syndrome or Status Bonnevie-Ullrich. Virchows Arch (A) 376: 233–246

Vinson PC, Goldenberg RL, Davis RO et al. (1977) Fetal bladder neck obstruction and elevated amniotic fluid alphafetoprotein. New Engl J Med 297: 1351

Wald NJ, Cuckle H, Stirrat GM, Turnbull AC (1978) Maternal serum alphafetoprotein and birth weight in twin pregnancies. Br J Obstet Gynaecol 85: 582–584

Wald NJ, Cuckle HS, Densem JW et al. (1988) Maternal serum screening for Down's syndrome in early pregnancy. Br Med J 297: 883–887

Warburton D, Byrne J, Canki N (1991) Chromosome anomalies and prenatal development: an atlas. Oxford University Press

Weatherall DJ (1991) The new genetics and clinical practice, 3rd edn. Oxford University Press

Weidemann H-R, Grosse K-R, Dibbern H (1985) An atlas of characteristic syndromes. A visual aid to diagnosis. Wolfe Medical, London

Weinberg AG, Milunsky A, Harrod MJ (1975) Elevated amniotic fluid alphafetoprotein and duodenal atresia. Lancet II: 496

Wisniewski L, Skrgydlewski Z, Orciuch J (1974) Alphafetroprotein in amniotic fluid in early normal pregnancy and intrauterine fetal death. Br Med J III: 742

Young ID, Lindenbaum RH, Thompson EM, Pembrey ME (1985) Amniotic bands in connective tissue disorders. Arch Dis Child 60: 1061–1063

Youroukos S, Papadelis F, Matsaniotis N (1980) Porencephalic cysts after amniocentesis. Arch Dis Child 55: 814–815

Yu S, Kremer E, Pritchard M et al. (1991) The fragile X gene type is characterised by an unstable region of DNA. Science 252: 1179–1181

Chapter 5

Genetic Metabolic Disease

Geoffrey A. Machin

Introduction

Genetic metabolic diseases (GMD; inborn errors of metabolism), are of considerable importance in paediatric pathology. Many individual diseases have been described, and detailed knowledge is required to encompass the field of GMD (reviewed by Benson and Fensom 1985). Historically, the understanding of GMD has evolved in several stages. First came recognition of the "inborn errors of small molecules", as envisaged by Garrod, e.g. phenylketonuria, galactosaemia. Then it was confirmed that abnormal enzyme function (absence or reduction) was responsible for abnormalities in metabolic pathways. Workers at that time recognised that GMD could be studied at the level of the gene product, i.e. enzymes and structural and functional proteins such as haemoglobin, factor VIII, alpha-1-antitrypsin and collagen. During the same period, the peptide sequences of several human polypeptides were worked out. Finally, the genetic code was elucidated, and the mechanisms of transcription and translation of genetic information were partially understood (Fig. 5.1).

Progress in the analysis of the whole human genome will ultimately allow the assignment of gene products and genes to all genetic diseases, including those in which the place and mode of action of the gene product is at present unknown. The recent delineation of the genes and gene products for Duchenne muscular dystrophy and cystic fibrosis are early examples of this trend.

There are two common types of mutation in genetic disease:

1. Point mutation (i.e. base substitution) in a codon results in two possibilities; there may be substitution of one amino acid residue by another in such a way as to alter significantly the three-dimensional structure and function of the polypeptide gene product. Point mutation may also convert a triplet from coding for an amino acid to coding for STOP (a nonsense mutation). The resulting gene product may thus lack a large proportion of its original length.

In about 5%–10% of point mutations, the change in the triplet alters the ability of the codon to participate in a restriction fragment site. The classic example is the mutation causing the sickle globin gene; there is a cleavage site at position 6 of the normal β-globin gene, but this is abolished by the mutation to β-S GAG to GTG (Fig. 5.2).

2. Deletions of varying lengths of DNA are also common forms of mutation. They may involve a short segment of DNA, such as a triplet (as in the most common form of cystic fibrosis), or very long segments, as in the gene for Duchenne muscular dystrophy.

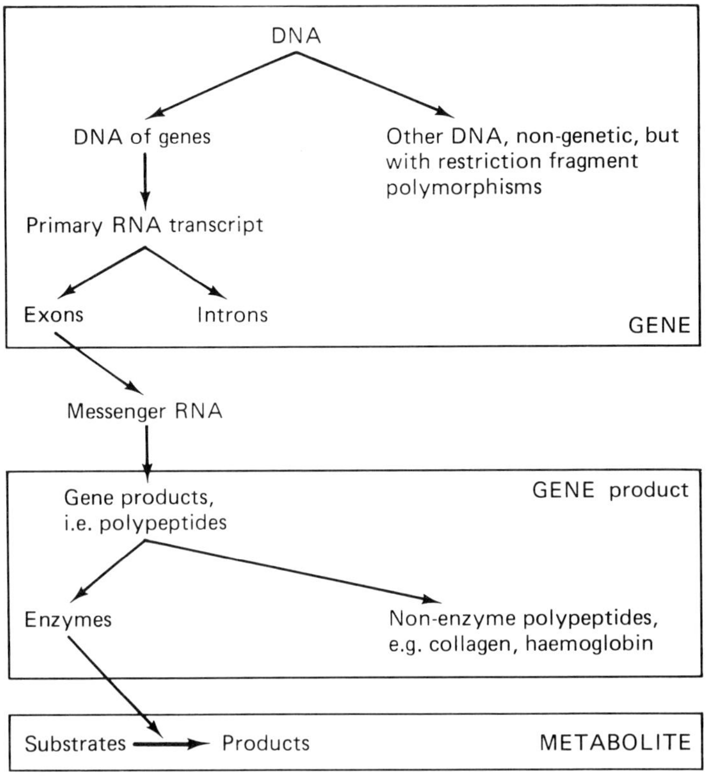

Fig. 5.1. The flow of information in normal and abnormal metabolism is from gene to gene product and metabolite; historically, the GMDs were understood first at the level of metabolites and only latterly at the level of the genes. (Genetic diseases include all diseases in which there are abnormal gene products, i.e. polypeptides).

Restriction fragment length polymorphism (RFLP) methodology is used for the detection of RFLP sites that are close to genes but not in them. An example is shown in Fig. 5.3.

There has been considerable expansion of prenatal diagnosis of GMD. Amniocentesis is now routine in prenatal diagnosis of many congenital anomalies, including GMD. Fetal blood sampling, liver and skin biopsy, and chorionic villus biopsy are now carried out in many centres.

Classic anatomical pathology has played a major role in the diagnosis of GMD, and will continue to play a part. The emphasis will be to coordinate studies on tissues obtained at biopsy, necropsy and termination of pregnancy. These studies will include histological and ultrastructural examination, tissue culture and biochemical techniques, including DNA analyses. The pathologist will also be involved in the assessment of results of treatment of GMDs, including transplantation.

The objectives of this chapter are to examine current horizons in the prenatal diagnosis of GMD, to describe the clinical presentation of GMD in the fetus and neonate, and to consider principles and practice of neonatal screening for GMD and some selective methods used at necropsy and biopsy.

As the underlying DNA defects in genetic disease become apparent, the distinction becomes blurred between genetic metabolic diseases and other genetic diseases. It is not always clear whether the haemoglobinopathies, osteogenesis imperfecta, haemophilia, cystic fibrosis and Duchenne muscular dystrophy, for example, should be considered as GMDs. All genetic diseases with Mendelian inheritance are caused by mutations in the DNA code and, hence, have their pathogenesis in abnormal gene products. It is rather arbitrary to separate GMDs as a distinct group, and there are disease entities that are hard to categorise as GMD or other genetic disease, e.g. haemoglobinopathies, chronic granulomatous disease, haemophilia. For general purposes, GMDs fall into two main categories: (1) diseases of small molecules which, in the

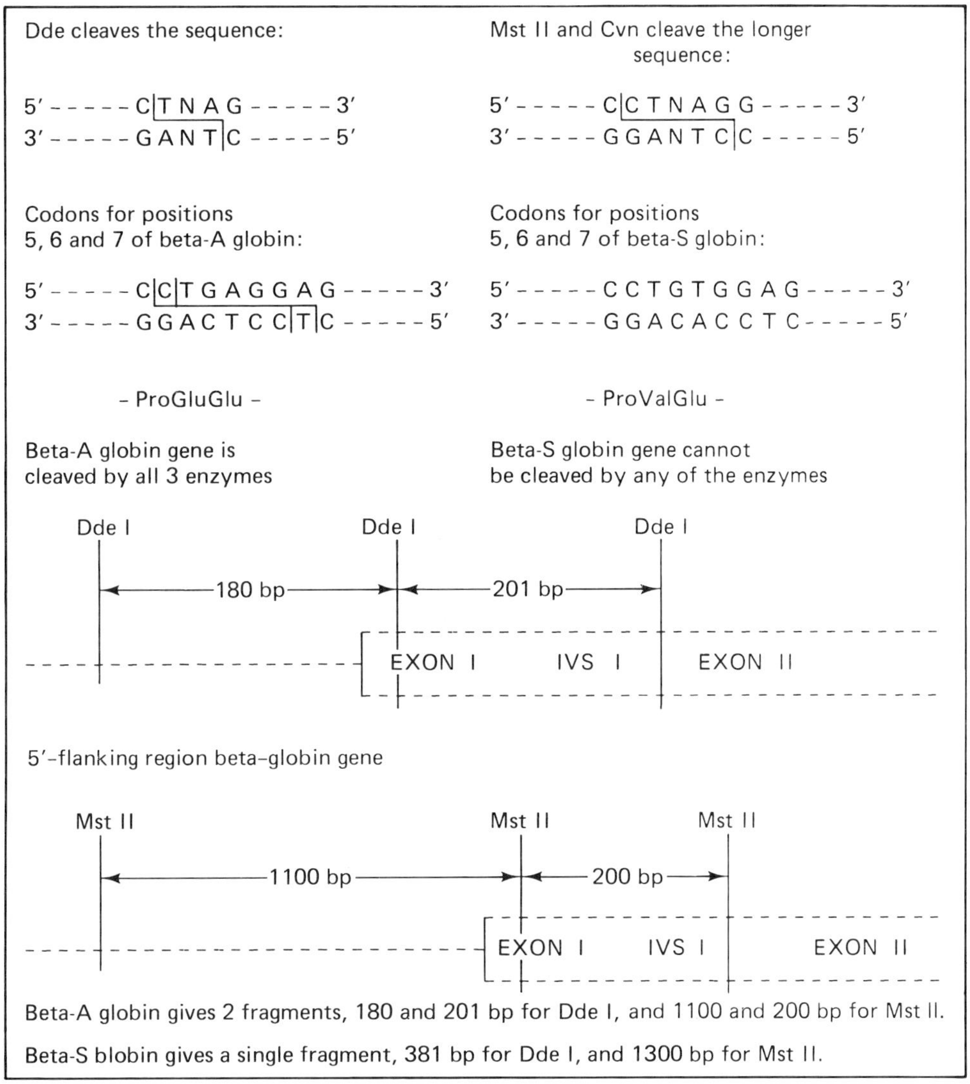

Fig. 5.2. The restriction endonucleases Dde I, Mst II and Cvn I have a cleavage site involving position 6 of the normal beta-globin gene.

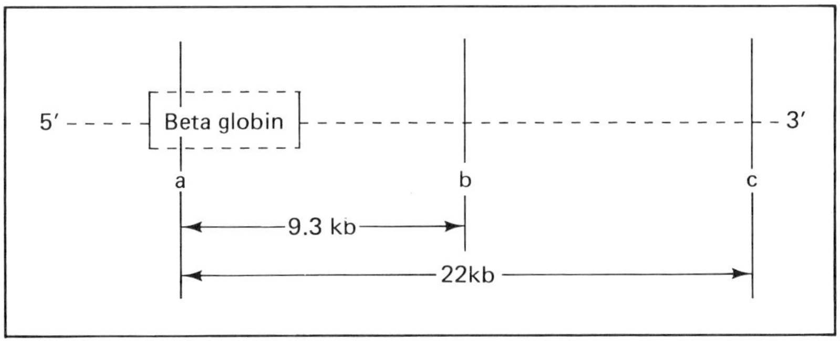

Fig. 5.3. An RFLP site is cleaved by Bam HI, and is closely linked with the beta0-thalassaemia gene. In Sardinians and Chinese, the 22 kb fragment is not found in individuals with homozygous beta0-thalassaemia, i.e. the cleavage site at point b is linked with the gene for beta0-thalassaemia.

neonatal period, cause neurological distress or energy deficiency (with lactic acidosis) and, (2) diseases of large molecules that result from failure of catabolic conversion of large molecules (e.g. cell and organelle wall constituents) to small components, i.e. the storage disorders. Disorders of small molecules do not often cause specific histopathological changes in the fetus and neonate. The storage disorders often produce striking structural pathology but rarely cause disease in the fetus and newborn.

Prenatal Diagnosis

The standard method of prenatal diagnosis in the fetus at risk of most GMDs is assay of the appropriate enzyme in cultured fibroblast-like cells obtained by amniocentesis at about 16 weeks' gestation. At-risk pregnancies are recognised because of affected siblings or the known carrier status of the mother (X-linked GMD), or of both parents (autosomal-recessive GMD). Prenatal diagnosis of GMD by amniocentesis and enzyme assay is a great step forward, but has two disadvantages. These are time constraint and the degree of expression of genes in cultured amniocytes. For most enzyme assays, large numbers of cultivated cells are needed; thus the assay is done close to the legal limit for selective termination as amniocentesis is difficult before 16 weeks' gestation. Although the cultured amniocyte is an undifferentiated cell, it does not express all the genes. Notable exceptions are tissue-specific polypeptides such as those synthesised by the liver (e.g. phenylalanine hydroxylase and ornithine transcarbamylase) and by mature red cells (haemoglobins). The diversity of methods of prenatal diagnosis now available represents a response to these disadvantages:

1. For most enzyme assays, several million cells are required. Microtechniques have been developed in some centres, so that enzyme assays can be carried out on small numbers of cells after shorter periods of culture.

2. The use of fetal blood and tissue biopsies (liver, skin) for organ-specific diseases such as the haemoglobinopathies, immunodeficiency disorders, liver enzymopathies and genodermatoses allows direct detection of GMD in the organ system concerned. Fetal blood leucocytes can be used for enzyme assays in GMDs that could be assayed in amniocytes, when there is some urgency, e.g. late maternal presentation for prenatal diagnosis or failure of amniocyte culture (Rodeck et al. 1983). However, these invasive methods are not without risk to the fetus.

3. The problem of lack of expression of certain polypeptides in amniocytes is also being overcome by the use of the new DNA methodologies which can detect the gene for the polypeptide whether or not transcription and translation to the gene product actually occur. These techniques may obviate fetal blood and tissue biopsy, and will probably become the most frequently used methods in the next few years.

4. Chorionic villus biopsy in the first trimester yields fetal tissue samples in early pregnancy. This has been used for chromosome analysis, and increasing numbers of GMDs are being diagnosed by this method. Sufficient material is obtained to allow direct analysis by enzyme assay, without the necessity for tissue culture. Sampling is done at 8–11 weeks' gestation. Light and electron microscopy are occasionally used. DNA methodology has been applied to chorionic villus biopsies, extending diagnostic possibilities to include the full range of GMDs. Metabolites can also be measured directly, e.g. in Zellweger syndrome and cystinosis.

5. In the interests of speed, uncultured amniotic cells have sometimes been used for diagnosis of GMD. Many centres regard this method as unreliable, and it is likely to be superseded by use of chorionic villus biopsy. Uncultured cells can be used for some restriction endonuclease methods and also for electron microscope studies.

6. In some renal tubular transport disorders and certain amino acid and organic acid disorders, significant amounts of abnormal small molecular metabolites may be found in the amniotic fluid. Certain organic acidurias can be diagnosed reliably by examination of supernatant amniotic fluid, such as tyrosinaemia (Gagné et al. 1982), glutaric aciduria (Boué et al. 1984), methyl malonic aciduria, and citrullinaemia (Kleijer et al. 1984). Elevated levels of glycosaminoglycans are found in amniotic fluid in certain of the mucopolysaccharidoses (MPSs). Congenital nephrosis can be diagnosed by elevated alpha-fetoprotein in amniotic fluid supernatant. Attempts at

Table 5.1. Classification of levels of understanding of mechanisms which may produce GMD

Level	Mechanism	Example
Level I:	*Altered DNA structure (mutation)*	
	1. Point mutations (mis-sense)	Sickle cell disease
	(nonsense)	One type of beta0-thalassaemia
	2. Deletion mutation	Alpha-thalassaemia
	3. Frame-shift mutation	Hgb Wayne
	4. Gene duplication	Hgb Grady
Level II:	*Altered polypeptide enzyme function*	
	1. Absent activity (enzyme may or may not be detectable antigenically)	Galactosaemia
	2. Reduced activity;	
	decreased substrate affinity	
	decreased cofactor affinity	
	unstable enzyme structure	G-6-PD deficiency
	Altered non-enzyme polypeptides	
	1. Defective post-translational modification	Alpha-1-antitrypsin ZZ status
	2. Tendency to aggregate or polymerise	Sickle cell disease
	3. Defective ligand binding	Testicular feminisation
Level III:	*Effects on whole cell or organ*	
	1. Altered flow through metabolic pathways	
	Accumulation of toxic precursor	PKU, lysosomal storage diseases
	Deficiency of product (synthetic)	Familial goitre
	2. Altered feedback regulation of metabolic pathways	
	Overproduction of endproduct because of ineffective feedback regulator	Familial hypercholesterolaemia
	3. Disordered membrane function	
	Deficient transmembrane transport	Cystinuria
	Deficient receptor-mediated endocytosis	Familial hypercholesterolaemia (some types)
	4. Disordered intracellular compartmentation	
	Accumulation of unprocessed protein	Alpha-1-antitrypsin ZZ status
	Mislocation of protein	I-cell disease
	5. Distorted cell, tissue or organ shape	
	Altered cell shape	Sickle cell disease
	Altered organelle structure	Kartagener syndrome
	Altered extracellular matrix	Ehlers–Danlos type III

Abbreviations: G-6-PD, glucose-6-phosphate dehydrogenase; PKU, phenylketonuria

prenatal diagnosis of cystic fibrosis indicate that levels of some enzymes may be elevated in amniotic fluids of affected fetuses.

7. In particular circumstances, the analysis of maternal serum permits the diagnosis of a fetus affected by GMD. This is uncommon, but has recently been reported in a case of fetal I-cell disease (Hug et al. 1984b).

Application of these newer methodologies to replace amniocentesis and amniocyte culture has been swift. All methods are aimed at earlier diagnosis using less invasive methods.

Pathogenesis and Classification

GMD can be classified according to the specificity of current understanding of the defect, at any level of the cascade from DNA through metabolite to whole cell (Table 5.1). In some cases, the defect is understood at many levels, including that of the causative mutation (e.g. sickle cell disease). In others, only the clinically obvious syndrome is recognised, but little is known of its causes and effects at the level of metabolite, polypeptide or gene (e.g. cystic fibrosis). Ultimately, all genetic diseases result from altered DNA structure, and the aim of human molecular genetics is to understand all these diseases at that level of the cascade. A classification of GMD by biochemical type is shown in Table 5.2.

Few of these disorders cause mortality or major morbidity in the third trimester and newborn period, but the pathologist needs to be familiar with the gamut of disorders that can be diagnosed prenatally, so that the morphological equivalents can be documented in affected fetuses when pregnancy is selectively

Table 5.2. Biochemical types of GMD

Group	Example
1. Carbohydrate disorders	Galactosaemia, glycogenoses
2. Amino acids	Hyperphenylalaninaemia, alkaptonuria
3. Urea cycle disorders	Citrullinaemia
4. Organic acidaemias	Methylmalonic acidaemia
5. Lipoprotein & lipid metabolism	Abetalipoproteinaemia; familial hypercholesterolaemia
6. Lysosomal enzyme disorders	Mucopolysaccharidoses; I-cell disease; oligosaccharidoses; Niemann–Pick disease; gangliosidoses
7. Steroid metabolism	Congenital adrenal hyperplasia Primary gout; Lesch–Nyhan syndrome;
8. Purine metabolism	adenine deaminase deficiency
9. Metal metabolism	Wilson's disease; Menke's disease; idiopathic haemochromatosis
10. Porphyrin & haem metabolism	Porphyrias; Gilbert's syndrome
11. Collagen disorders	Ehlers–Danlos syndrome; osteogenesis imperfecta; Marfan syndrome; recessive epidermolysis bullosa
12. Muscle disorders	Myotonic dystrophy; Duchenne muscular dystrophy
13. Disorders of blood & blood-forming tissues	Spherocytosis; glucose-6-phosphate dehydrogenase deficiency; haemoglobinopathies; thalassaemias
14. Disorders of transport	Intestinal lactase deficiency; vitamin-D-dependent rickets; cystinuria; cystic fibrosis
15. Immune system disorders	X-linked hypogammaglobulinaemia; complement system abnormalities; chronic granulomatous disease

terminated. The clinical expression of GMD in the stillborn fetus and the sick neonate can be unusual, subtle and non-specific, and the possibility of GMD needs to be considered in the differential diagnosis in a number of clinical situations.

Clinical Presentation

In the interests of time and economy, there must be selection of necropsy and biopsy cases for full investigation for GMD. On the other hand, inappropriate parental counselling can result from failure to suspect and diagnose GMD. It is preferable to err on the side of initiating full studies, including biochemical analyses, and to be prepared to cancel these at the earliest moment should it become apparent that the clinical picture is adequately explained by disease other than GMD. Rapid processing of histological findings, including frozen section during necropsy or biopsy, and use of the "scrimp" (scrape and imprint) technique may be useful in confirming the presence of a GMD, so that appropriate steps are taken to collect and process blood and tissues for biochemical and ultrastructural studies. A suggested protocol for handling of tissues is given later in this chapter (see p. 160).

GMDs have three main presentations in the fetus and neonate: acute neonatal disease, dysmorphism with intrauterine growth retardation, and insidious neonatal disorders.

Acute Neonatal Disease

Most GMDs that produce acute symptoms in the first few weeks of life are defects of small molecules, which become symptomatic when the newborn infant is challenged with dietary oligosaccharides and amino acids and no longer has the protection of the placenta and maternal metabolism. Symptoms and signs suggestive of GMD include acute and severe unexplained jaundice, persistent hypoglycaemia, vomiting, diarrhoea, unexplained acidosis, electrolyte disturbances, seizures, coma, unusual body odour and abnormal hair. The clinical features are reviewed by Aleck and Shapiro (1978) and Burton (1987) and laboratory investigation summarised by Applegarth et al. (1983).

In general, histological findings in acute GMD of small molecules are not specific but suggest the possibility of GMD. If liver enzymes are deficient, there may be cirrhosis, cholestasis, fatty change or non-specific necrosis of hepatocytes. Metabolic causes of cirrhosis in infancy and early childhood are reviewed by Hardwick and Dimmick (1976). GMDs that affect the central nervous system directly or indirectly usually result in non-specific features such as neuronal necrosis or disturbed myelination.

GMDs of small molecules that may present in the newborn period are listed below:

1. *The urea cycle disorders*, with ammonia intoxication causing lethargy, irritability, tachypnoea, seizure, coma and death in untreated cases. In these disorders, enzyme activity is analysed in liver and/or cultured fibroblasts.

2. *Glycogenosis type I* (glucose-6-phophatase deficiency) with hypoglycaemia, hyperuricaemia, hyperlacticacidaemia and hepatomegaly. Fresh liver tissue is required for the enzyme analysis. The liver cells are distended with intracytoplasmic glycogen particles. The appearances of glycogenosis type IB have recently been reported in two neonates (Buchino et al. 1983).

3. *Galactosaemia* presents with irritability, vomiting, diarrhoea, hypoglycaemia, jaundice and hepatomegaly. The picture may be complicated by bacterial sepsis. Diagnosis depends on assay of red cell galactose-1-phosphate uridyl transferase activity. Galactosaemia is one of the GMDs that causes neonatal cirrhosis.

4. *Hereditary fructose intolerance* has many clinical features in common with galactosaemia and requires liver tissue for assay or fructose-1-phosphate aldolase activity.

5. Of the many *aminoacidopathies*, only maple syrup urine disease (MSUD) and phenylketonuria are relevant to the neonatal period. MSUD causes a rapidly downhill course of hyperglycaemia, vomiting, flaccidity, seizures, apnoea and death. The enzyme deficiency can be assayed from leucocytes or fibroblasts (Cox et al. 1978). The clinical signs of phenylketonuria are subtle and evasive. Untreated cases should not be seen by pathologists in this era of neonatal metabolic screening.

6. *Organic acidaemias* present with ketoacidosis, vomiting, lethargy, seizures and hypotonia. Leucocytes and fibroblasts can be used for the enzyme assays.

Some macromolecular disorders may present with fetal hydrops, which may be identified prenatally or constitute a neonatal emergency. Lysosomal storage disorders are cited as a cause of fetal hydrops by several authors. In 1414 cases of hydrops fetalis 20 (1.4%) had a GMD (Machin 1989). The diagnoses in these 20 cases were: Gaucher disease (5 cases), G_{M1}-gangliosidosis (2 cases), sialidosis (6 cases), MPS VII (3 cases), idiopathic neonatal iron storage (1 case), I-cell disease (1 case), MPS IVa (2 cases). Placental villi often show evidence of storage in trophoblastic cells and stromal Hoffbauer cells. Homozygous alpha-thalassaemia (Fig. 5.4), glucose-6-phosphate dehydrogenase deficiency and osteogenesis imperfecta may present clinically with hydrops fetalis.

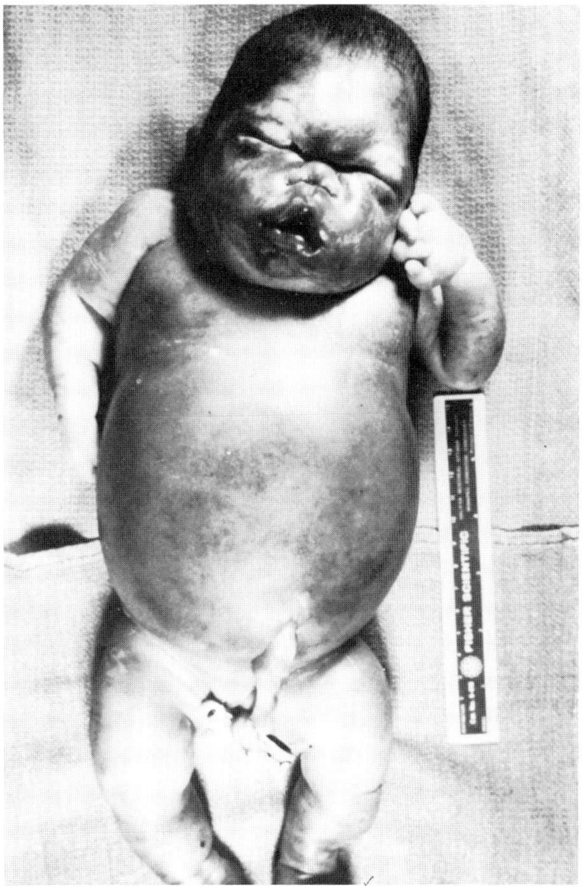

Fig. 5.4. Hydrops fetalis, a baby with homozygous alpha-thalassaemia.

A second acute presentation of macromolecular GMD is as fetal, congenital or neonatal ascites without hydrops. Several mechanisms may be involved including portal hypertension with severe degrees of liver infiltration by storage cells, and accumulation of stored material in endothelial cells, resulting in abnormal peritoneal, capillary or venular permeability. Fifty-six infants with lysosomal storage disease presenting as congenital ascites (Daneman et al. 1983; Gillan et al. 1984) included cases of sialidosis, Salla disease, G_{M1}-gangliosidosis and Gaucher's disease. Alpha-1-

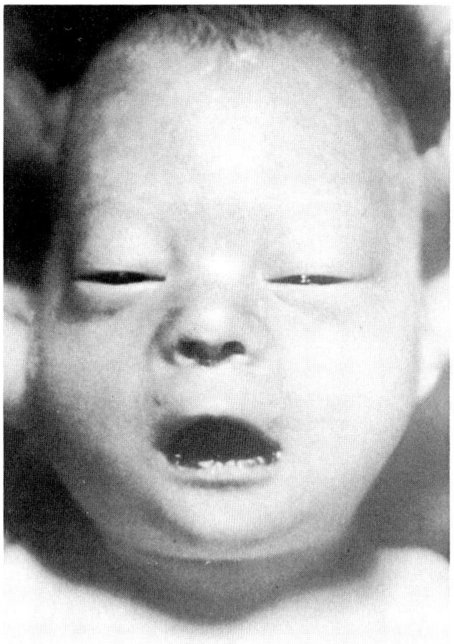

Fig. 5.5. Typical facies of cerebrohepatorenal (Zellweger) syndrome.

antitrypsin deficiency can also present as neonatal ascites (Ghishan et al. 1983).

Dysmorphism and Intrauterine Growth Retardation

It is becoming clear that some selected GMDs of small molecules produce fetal growth retardation and malformations as well as metabolic disturbances. In cerebrohepatorenal (Zellweger) syndrome, features include micropolygyria, hepatic dysgenesis leading to cirrhosis, multiple renal cortical cysts and facial anomalies such as Brushfield spots, epicanthic folds, shallow supraorbital ridges and micrognathia (Fig. 5.5; Kelley 1983). The biochemical basis of Zellweger syndrome is known to be a deficiency of a peroxisomal enzyme, and absence of peroxisomes has been shown ultrastructurally. Glutaric aciduria type II has dysmorphic manifestations with hydrocephalus, dysmorphism of the face and ears, ventricular septal defect and renal enlargement with cortical cysts (see Fig. 4.25, p. 137; Sweetman et al. 1980). Another GMD with dysmorphisms involves a defect in valine metabolism. In one reported case the infant had facial anomalies, tetralogy of Fallot and agenesis of the corpus callosum (Brown et al. 1982).

In all of these examples the clinical course is typical of acute or subacute GMD of small molecules, but malformations appear to be genuine components of the disease. It is postulated that these malformations are "automalformations", imposed on the developing fetus by disturbed metabolism of its own cells, so that the findings of structural malformations do not exclude a GMD.

Insidious Neonatal Disorders

When macromolecular GMDs present in the neonatal period, the symptoms are often insidious, but they often have characteristic histopathology.

Alpha-1-antitrypsin Deficiency

Alpha-1-antitrypsin deficiency can present in the newborn with jaundice and cirrhosis. The diagnosis is made by electrophoresis of serum samples (Fig. 5.6) and the use of immunoperoxidase techniques to show the presence of excessive alpha-1-antitrypsin in hepatocytes.

Lysosomal Storage Disorders

Lysosomal storage disorders (LSDs) present at various ages from the prenatal period to adulthood. The majority become apparent in early childhood, but several cause symptomatology in the fetus and newborn. Frequent findings are neurological deficit, hepatosplenomegaly and dysostosis multiplex congenita. The histopathologist may be involved in the diagnosis in the fetus (including selectively aborted fetuses), during neonatal necropsy or in the biopsy investigation of neonates for suspected LSD.

The acid hydrolases within lysosomes catalyse the breakdown of high molecular weight complex molecules that have a limited life span as components of the walls of cells or cell organelles, or have entered into the cytoplasm by endocytosis. Lysosomes are particularly abundant in phagocytic cells, but are also present in all other cell types. Many different hydrolases are involved in the stepwise degradation of macromolecules, and absence of any one of them may result in significant accumulation of partially degraded

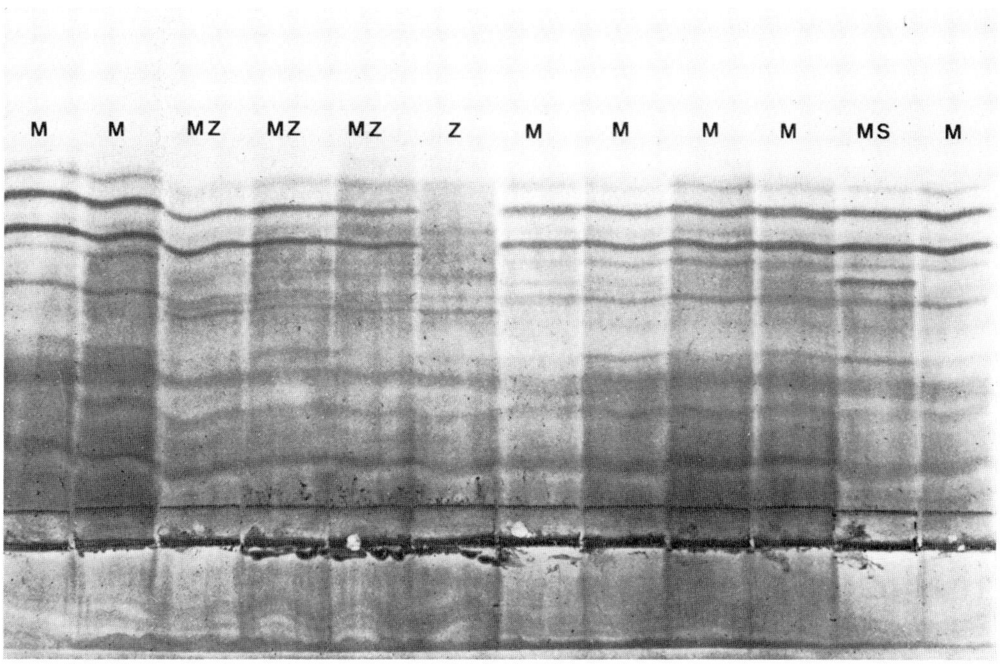

Fig. 5.6. Isoelectric focusing of sera from families with alpha-1-antitrypsin deficiency. The ZZ genotype is of the propositus, with neonatal cirrhosis; sera from his heterozygous carrier parents were run in lanes 4 and 5 (from the *left*).

cell membrane material in lysosomes, to the extent that such "storage disorders" are readily visible by light and electron microscopy. The greatly enlarged lysosomes distort the cell and interfere with normal metabolic functions. There are differences in organ and tissue involvement and in histological detail within this group of disorders (O'Brien 1982). Typical inclusions are illustrated in Fig. 5.7.

Diagnosis. Although diagnosis is best made by biochemical means, there are occasions when fetal material is not suitable, or intra-uterine death occurs prior to termination. In these cases, confirmation depends on histo-pathological assessment. Even when bio-chemical investigations are undertaken it is desirable to undertake histological and electron microscopy examination in order that the gestational age at which significant storage is seen is reliably known.

Tissue biopsy and blood samples can be used in the investigation of suspected LSD, and the pathologist may occasionally interpret findings as compatible with storage disease in the newborn period. Brunning (1970) summarises the appearances of peripheral blood cells by standard haematological stains in a number

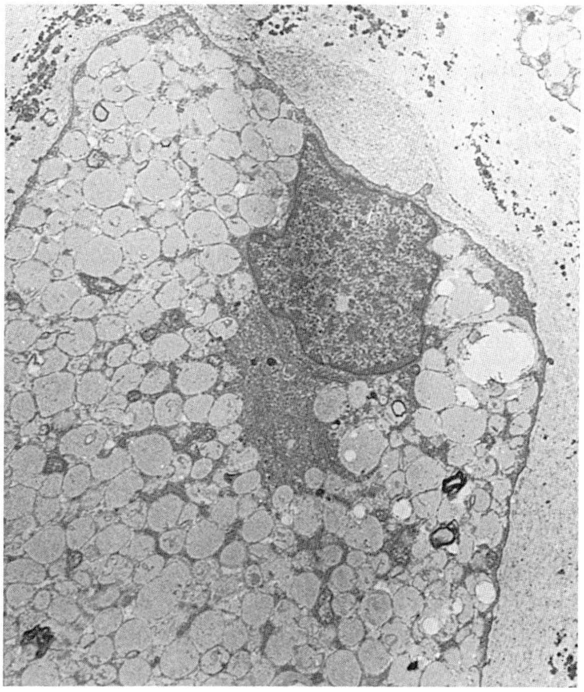

Fig. 5.7. Iliac crest resting chondrocyte in a case of MPS. (×1000 approx.)

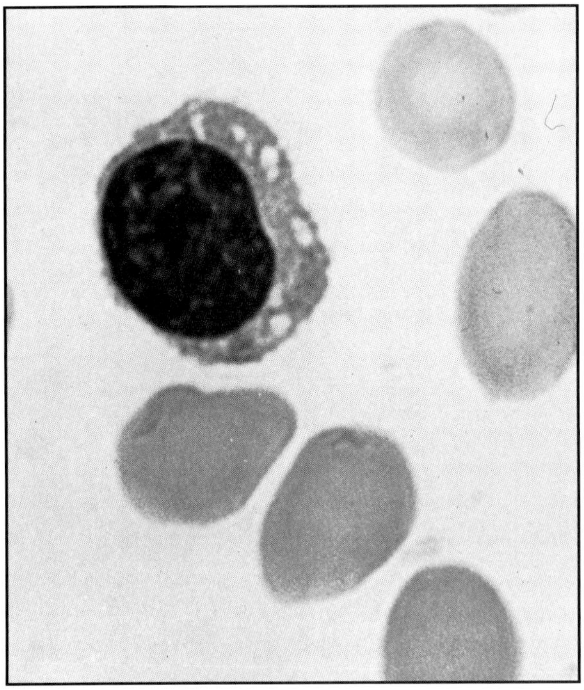

Fig. 5.8. Vacuolated peripheral blood lymphocyte in case of Niemann-Pick disease (Wright stain, ×800 approx.)

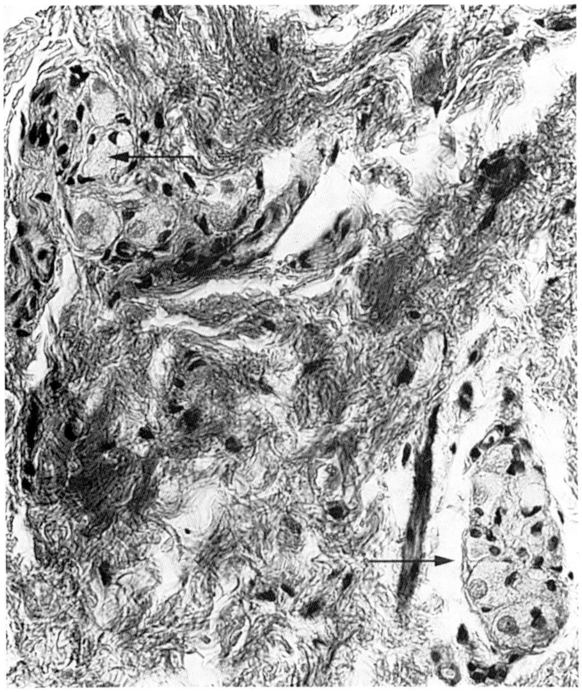

Fig. 5.9. Distended ganglion cells (*arrows*) in the myenteric plexus of a full-thickness rectal biopsy from a case of Niemann-Pick disease (PAS stain, ×265 approx.)

of genetic diseases, including the storage disorders (Fig. 5.8). The ultrastructure of leucocytes in a range of LSDs has also been examined (Ikeda et al. 1982). Leucocytes are abnormal in all the mucopolysaccharidoses (MPSs) and in G_{M1}-gangliosidosis, but are not affected in metachromatic leucodystrophy, Gaucher's disease or mucolipidosis (ML) type III. The appearance of leucocytes in MPSs has been reported in detail by Markesberry et al. (1980), and the typical features of bone marrow histiocytes in storage disorders are described by Savage (1984).

Conjunctival biopsies can be used for light microscopy, ultrastructure and tissue culture for the diagnosis of LSD. Kenyon (1982) reviewed more than 1000 cases, and all MPSs showed abnormalities caused by storage in fibroblasts, histiocytes, epithelial cells, endothelial cells and Schwann cells. Similar changes are described in the limited number of sphingolipidoses tested, in I-cell disease and ML type IV. It is not clear whether gangliosidoses also show storage changes in the conjunctiva.

The histological changes in MPSs also have been described in iliac crest chondrocytes (Silberberg et al. 1972; see Fig. 5.7). Abnormalities in skin biopsies are present in the majority of LSDs, with the exception of Gaucher's and Krabbe's disease (O'Brien et al. 1975; Carpenter 1987). Skin and conjunctival biopsies have largely replaced rectal biopsies that contain enteric plexus used to indicate the involvement of the central nervous system (Fig. 5.9). A large series and literature review of light microscopic appearances (Brett and Berry 1967) has been extended by an ultrastructural review (Yamano et al. 1982). Mucosal macrophages may be affected in other disorders, where ganglion cells are not, e.g. ceroid lipofuscinosis (Rapola et al. 1984). Detailed reviews of the pathological appearances of individual LSDs have also been published: ML type IV (Livni and Merin 1978); fucosidosis (Landing et al. 1976).

Lysosomal disorders that regularly cause clinical problems in the neonate are listed below:

1. *G_{M1}-gangliosidosis, type I (infantile).* These patients have coarse facial features, motor and mental deterioration, poor weight gain, ineffective swallowing, aspiration pneumonia and radiological evidence of dystosis multiplex (widened metacarpal diaphyses, oval-shaped vertebrae and spatulate ribs). Foam cells are

present in biopsies of bone marrow and liver. At necropsy, there is widespread visceral storage, largely in vacuolated histiocytes, storage in renal gomerular epithelial cells, and neuronal lipidosis. Definitive diagnosis is by assay of ganglioside beta-galactosidase activity in leucocytes and cultured fibroblasts.

2. *MPSs* generally show normal development in the first year of life, followed by progressive skeletal deterioration. MPS type VII is an exception, presenting in infancy (Sheets Lee et al. 1985). These patients have beta-glucuronidase deficiency, which can be measured in leucocytes and cultured fibroblasts. Clinical features include coarse facies, hepatosplenomegaly and thoracolumbar gibbus. The bone marrow contains vacuolated granulocytes, and storage can also be seen in peripheral blood. Cases of MPS type VII have recently been described in which the clinical onset is prenatal and presentation is as non-immune hydrops fetalis (see Chap. 11, p. 258).

3. *I-cell disease (ML type II)* has clinical features similar to MPS, but with a severe and early onset.Vacuolated histiocytes and fibroblasts are present in subcutaneous connective tissue, Schwann cells and axons. The renal glomerular and tubular epithelium is markedly affected; the placenta is also involved (Aula et al. 1975; Martin et al. 1975).

4. *Other disorders of glycoprotein degradation* include mannosidosis, fucosidosis, sialidoses and aspartylglycosaminuria. Of these, the severe infantile form of mannosidosis may present in the newborn period with rapidly progressive mental retardation, hepatosplenomegaly and dysostosis multiplex. Vacuolated circulating lymphocytes are present, and findings at necropsy include neuronal lipidosis, with vacuolated hepatocytes and Kupffer cells (Dickersin et al. 1980). Sialidosis type II is another LSD that can present with hydrops fetalis (Stevenson et al. 1983). The pathology of this disease is reviewed by Lowden and O'Brien (1979).

5. *Wolman's disease (acid lipase deficiency)* presents with forceful vomiting, marked abdominal distension and persistent, low-grade fever in early infancy. Vacuolated lymphocytes and bone marrow storage cells are consistent features. A particular feature of diagnostic importance is calcification of the adrenals. Necropsy findings are vacuolation of hepatic parenchymal cells, foamy histiocytes, calcification of the inner cortex of symmetrically enlarged adrenals, storage cells in the lamina propria of the bowel mucosa, splenic storage and storage in oligodendrocytes (Lowden et al. 1970).

6. A severe infantile form of *Farber's disease (ceramidase deficiency)* presents with painful swollen joints with palpable nodules. Foamy macrophages accumulate in subcutaneous tissues and many viscera.

7. *Gaucher's disease type 2* is an acute neuropathic form, of which a subgroup may present with hydrops fetalis. Gaucher cells are distributed in the splenic red pulp, lymph nodes, alveolar capillaries, bone marrow and perivascular spaces of the brain, including the Virchow–Robin spaces. Diagnosis is made by bone marrow examination, raised serum levels of non-tartrate-inhibitable acid phosphatase, and the demonstration of decreased glucocerebrosidase activity in leucocytes or cultured fibroblasts.

The pathologist may be involved in the biochemical and histopathological confirmation of storage disorders in proven biochemically affected fetuses that are selectively aborted. Fetal and placental tissues should be studied by light microscopy and ultrastructurally. In general, those storage disorders that present clinically in the perinatal period will also cause early structural changes in placenta and fetal tissues. For diseases that have a later onset, minimal or questionable structural changes are seen in early gestation, and biochemical confirmation is the reliable method (Martin and Centerick, 1988).

Screening

The objectives of population screening are the ascertainment of the prevalence of the disease, the identification of adult carriers at risk of having affected children and, most importantly, the detection and early treatment of affected neonates. Neonatal screening of total, unselected populations is undertaken to identify individuals with certain GMDs that have serious consequences, usually on intellectual function, that do not have obvious clinical signs at birth and which can be effectively treated. Some advocate screening also for diseases that cannot be treated, since clinical presentation in the propositus may be sufficiently delayed that further affected siblings may be born without benefit of prenatal diagnosis.

Screening for phenylketonuria was the first neonatal test to be introduced, and many other diseases can now be detected. These include hypothyroidism (1 in 6000 liveborn), cystinuria (1 in 7000), alpha-1-antitrypsin deficiency (1 in 8000), histidinaemia (1 in 17000), hyperprolinaemia (1 in 40000), galactosaemia (1 in 57000), MSUD (1 in 200000) and homocystinuria (1 in 200000). There are some important disorders for which neonatal screening is not currently available, e.g. hereditary fructose intolerance, hyperuricacidaemias, hyperlipoproteinaemias, Wilson's disease, adrenogenital syndrome, or is of doubtful specificity (cystic fibrosis).

These tests are made on heel prick blood taken at the age of 2–4 days, after the neonates have been exposed to significant dietary intake of amino acids and saccharides. Screening tests have to be cheap, permit no false negatives and few false positives. Several studies have shown adequate cost-effectiveness of screening at least for the more common GMDs, and present discussions concern how many GMDs should be screened. The following are screened in most centres: phenylketonuria, galactosaemia, hypothyroidism, homocystinuria and MSUD. If sickle cell disease is added to this battery, the incidence of GMD can be expected at 1 in 3000 births.

Screening for haemoglobin abnormalities, sickle cell disease and thalassaemias has not always been well received (Grover et al. 1978), but it seems that awareness of the diagnosis of sickle cell disease reduces mortality from sepsis in infancy (Nussbaum et al. 1984). In the UK, screening has been carried out in limited geographical areas where there is a high-risk population (Henthorn et al. 1984); 7% of screened neonates had haemoglobinopathies. Southeast Asians and blacks are selected populations in which alpha- and beta-thalassaemia trait, haemoglobin S, haemoglobin C and haemoglobin Lepore may be found; in a recent study almost 40% of those screened had a haemoglobinopathy (Stein et al. 1984).

Early attempts at screening for GMD by use of neonatal urine were largely discredited because of non-specificity. Some centres have continued to screen for GMDs that have a rather low prevalence in the population (Jones 1984). The number of cases of GMD picked up by this simple methodology is impressive (Levy et al. 1980). The major programmes have been carried out in Massachusetts, New South Wales and Quebec. Approximately 1 in 3000 newborns have a detectable GMD in urine, but none of these GMDs has a clinical impact comparable with hypothyroidism or phenylketonuria.

Because of the high prevalence of cystic fibrosis in Caucasian populations (1 in 2000), much effort has been spent on development of screening programmes, although it is not proven that early diagnosis leads to a better prognosis and life expectancy. The metabolic basis of cystic fibrosis has not yet been elucidated, and methods of diagnosis are indirect. The sweat test is cumbersome, and cannot be applied as a screening test. Several methods for neonatal screening have been proposed in the last 15 years which depend on assessment of pancreatic function, although this is not always impaired in cystic fibrosis. Two methods are used: one demonstrates increased albumin in meconium (attributable to reduced pancreatic tryptic activity), and the other depends on increased serum immunoreactive trypsin (attributable to pancreatic duct obstruction; Wilcken et al. 1983). Evaluation of these tests, alone or in combination, continues, and opinion is divided about the use of immunoreactive trypsin for screening for cystic fibrosis in the newborn (Brock 1984; Holtzman 1984). The identification of the most common deletion mutation (ΔF508) in Caucasians with cystic fibrosis raises the possibility of screening for heterozygotes (Lemna et al. 1990).

Screening in selected populations at high risk for certain GMDs that segregate in ethnic subgroups may be useful. Sickle cell disease, alpha- and beta-thalassaemia, Tay–Sachs disease and glucose-6-phosphate dehydrogenase deficiency are typical examples. Real effects on prevalence in the newborn have been shown as the result of screening and prenatal diagnosis of beta-thalassaemia in Cypriots in the UK (Modell et al. 1984). It can be anticipated that newborn screening for GMD will increase greatly in the future.

Necropsy and Biopsy Investigation

There is no standard method for necropsy of the aborted fetus or neonate with GMD, since the sampling and handling of tissues must be tailored to the type of GMD and its anatomical distribution. Procedures must be undertaken as soon as necropsy permission is obtained, even when this involves out-of-hours work. Much valuable information will be lost if there is a delay of even a few hours.

The objective of necropsy is precise diagnosis. The type of sample that may be needed are as follows:

1. Enzyme studies can only be done on cultured cells. Gonad or fascia lata are recommended for tissue culture and can be obtained in sterile fashion. Skin is not used if deeper, uncontaminated tissues are obtainable. Amniotic membrane or chorionic plate are also useful, particularly if there is fetal autolysis. Samples should be placed in tissue culture medium after being cut into small pieces, about 2–3-mm cubes. They should be kept at 4°C, but not frozen, prior to being sent to a reference laboratory. A method of frozen storage of tissue for later thaw and culture is described by Fowler (1984). DNA can be extracted from gram quantities of any tissue, and is often well preserved even in autolysed material.

2. Samples of unfixed organs, such as placenta, muscle, brain, liver, spleen and kidney should be snap frozen in liquid nitrogen or dry ice for biochemical analysis. They are individually wrapped in airtight material, e.g. aluminium foil, and stored at −70°C prior to transportation. About 50–100 g of tissue is a useful size. When there is major neurological disease, the brain can be cut sagittally; one half can then be frozen and the other half fixed for morphological study. Biochemical and topographical correlations can then be made of different regions of the brain. These tissues can be used for enzyme analysis and for analysis of stored or other abnormal metabolites.

3. Plasma, urine and CSF can be studied for evidence of small molecule GMDs. Some of the specimen should be deproteinised immediately. All samples should be stored at −70°C. Blood may be used for haemoglobin electrophoresis of red cell haemolysates.

4. Most organs should be sampled for histological examination, since the distribution of abnormalities in tissues may give clues to the likely diagnosis. Standard histological methods, "scrimp" technique, special stains and ultrastructure can all be used, and it is better to sample too many organs than too few. Bowel, skin, bone marrow, muscle, spinal cord, eye, fibrous connective tissue and placenta may be informative. Standard glutaraldehyde fixation is required for ultrastructural studies.

There are few reports on the morphology of GMDs in aborted fetuses. Lowden et al. (1973) showed the findings in G_{M1}-gangliosidosis, and Kleijer et al. (1983) reported on MPSs. Whilst LSDs can be identified by the deposition of stored material, even in the second trimester fetus, GMDs of small molecules do not produce histological abnormality in the fetus.

Methods of fetal examination are those of Perry (1981) and Keeling (1984).

Biopsy samples are generally processed for morphological study, including ultrastructure, and may also be used for enzyme analysis and tissue culture. Circumstances will dictate the number of procedures for which GMD biopsies are used, but there will often be multiple uses.

Reference Laboratories for Investigation of Metabolic Disorders

Information can be obtained from:

Prenatal Diagnosis Group (UK),
Dr. A. McDermot,
SW Regional Cytogenetics Centre,
Southmead Hospital,
Bristol BS10 5NB,
UK.

Inventory of Genetic Consultation Centres,
The Liaison Section of the Public Health
Committee (PA),
Council of Europe,
The Danish National Health Service,
1 Store Kongensgade,
DK–1264 Copenhagen K,
Denmark.

Cell Repositories,
Institute for Medical Research,
Camden,
New Jersey,
USA.

A list of 352 medical genetic centres in 45 countries is available from March of Dimes Genetic Services, International Directory,

March of Dimes Birth Defects Foundation, White Plains, New York, USA.

References

Aleck KA, Shapiro LJ (1978) Genetic-metabolic considerations in the sick neonate. Pediatr Clin North Am 25: 431–451

Applegarth DA, Toone JR, Macleod PM (1983) Laboratory diagnosis of inborn errors of metabolism in children. Pediatr Pathol 1: 107–130

Aula P, Rapola J, Autio S, Raivio K, Karjalainen O (1975) Prenatal diagnosis and fetal pathology of I-cell disease (mucolipidosis type II). J Pediatr 87: 221–226

Benson PF, Fensom AH (1985) Genetic biochemical disorders. Oxford University Press, Oxford

Boué J, Chalmers RA, Tracey BM et al. (1984) Prenatal diagnosis of dysmorphic neonatal-lethal type II glutaricaciduria. Lancet I: 846–847

Brett EM, Berry CL (1967) Value of rectal biopsy in paediatric neurology: report of 165 biopsies. Br Med J 3: 400–403

Brock DJ (1984) Cystic fibrosis. In: Wald NJ (ed) Antenatal and neonatal screening. Oxford University Press, Oxford, pp 192–220

Brown KG, Hunt SM, Scholem R et al. (1982) Beta-hydroxyisobutyryl coenzyme A decyclase deficiency: a defect of valine metabolism associated with physical malformations. Pediatrics 70: 532–538

Brunning RD (1970) Morphologic alterations in nucleated blood and marrow cells in genetic disorders. Hum Pathol 1: 99–124

Buchino JJ, Brown BI, Volk DM (1983) Glycogen storage disease type IB. Arch Pathol Lab Med 107: 283–285

Burton BK (1987) Inborn errors of metabolism: the clinical diagnosis in early infancy. Pediatrics 79: 359–369

Carpenter S (1987) Skin biopsy for diagnosis of hereditary metabolic disease. Arch Dermatol 123: 1618–1621

Cox RP, Hutzler J, Dancis (1978) Antenatal diagnosis of maplesyrup-urine disease. Lancet II: 212

Daneman A, Stringer D, Reilly BJ (1983) Neonatal ascites due to lysosomal storage disease. Radiology 149: 463–467

Dickersin GR, Lott IT, Kolodny EH, Dvorak AM (1980) A light and electron microscopic study of mannosidosis. Hum Pathol 11: 245–256

Fowler KJ (1984) Storage of skin biopsies at −70°C for future fibroblast culture. J Clin Pathol 37: 1191–1193

Gagné R, Lescault A, Grenier A, Laberge C, Melancon SB, Dallaire L (1982) Prenatal diagnosis of hereditary tyrosinemia: measurement of succinylacetone in amniotic fluid. Prenat Diagn 2: 185–188

Ghishan FK, Gray GF, Greene HL (1983) Alpha-1-antitrypsin deficiency presenting with ascites and cirrhosis in the neonatal period. Gastroenterology 85: 435–438

Gillan JE, Lowden JA, Gaskin K, Cutz E (1984) Congenital ascites as a presenting sign of lysosomal storage disease. J Pediatr 104: 225–231

Grover R, Wethers D, Shahidi S, Grossi M, Goldberg D, Davidow B (1978) Evaluation of the expanded newborn screening program in New York City. Pediatrics 61: 740–748

Hardwick DF, Dimmick JE (1976) Metabolic cirrhosis of infancy and early childhood. Perspect Pediatr Pathol 3: 103–144

Henthorn J, Anionwu E, Brozovic M (1984) Screening cord blood for sickle haemoglobinopathies in Brent. Br Med J 289: 479–480

Holtzman NA (1984) Routine screening of newborns for cystic fibrosis: not yet. Pediatrics 73: 98–99

Hug G, Bove KE, Soukup S et al. (1984) Increased serum hexosaminidase in a woman pregnant with a fetus affected by mucolipidosis II (I-cell disease). N Engl J Med 311: 988–989

Ikeda K, Goebel HH, Burck U, Kohlschutter A (1982) Ultrastructural pathology of human lymphocytes in lysosomal disorders: a contribution to their morphological diagnosis. Eur J Pediatr 138: 179–185

Jones JD (1984) Screening tests for inherited metabolic diseases. Mayo Clin Proc 59: 347–349

Keeling JW (1984) Postmortem examination of the fetus. In: Rodeck CH, Nicolaides KH (eds) Prenatal diagnosis. Proceedings of the eleventh study group of the Royal College of Obstetricians and Gynaecologists. Wiley, Chichester, pp 347–371

Kelley RI (1983) Review: the cerebrohepatorenal syndrome of Zellweger, morphologic and metabolic aspects. Am J Med Genet 16: 503–517

Kenyon KR (1982) Conjunctival biopsy for diagnosis of lysosomal disorders. Prog Clin Biol Res 82: 103–122

Kleijer WJ, Thompson EJ, Niermeijer MF (1983) Prenatal diagnosis of the Hurler syndrome: report on 40 pregnancies at risk. Prenat Diagn 3: 179–186

Kleijer WJ, Blom W, Huijmans JGM, Mooyman MCT, Berger R, Niermeijer MF (1984) Prenatal diagnosis of citrullinemia: elevated levels of citrulline in the amniotic fluid in the three affected pregnancies. Prenat Diagn 4: 113–118

Landing BH, Donnell GN, Alfi OS et al. (1976) Fucosidosis: clinical, pathologic and biochemical studies of five patients. In: Volk BW, Schnecke L (eds) Current trends in sphingolipidoses and allied disorders. Plenum, New York, pp 147–165

Lemna WK, Feldman GL, Kerem BS et al. (1990) Mutation analysis for heterozygote detection and the prenatal diagnosis of cystic fibrosis. N Engl J Med 322: 291–296

Levy HL, Coulombe HT, Shih JT (1980) Newborn urine screening. In: Bickel H, Guthrie R, Hammerson G (eds) Neonatal screening for in born errors of metabolism. Springer, Berlin Heidelberg New York, pp 89–103

Livni, N, Merin S (1978) Mucolipidosis IV. Ultrastructural diagnosis of a recently defined genetic disorder. Arch Pathol Lab Med 102: 600–604

Lowden JA, O'Brien JS (1979) Sialidosis: a review of human neuraminidase deficiency. Am J Hum Genet 31: 1–18

Lowden JA, Barson AJ, Wentworth P (1970) Wolman's disease: a microscopic and biochemical study showing accumulation of ceroid and esterified cholesterol. Can Med Assoc J 102: 402–405

Lowden JA, Cutz E, Conen PE, Rudd N, Doran TA (1973) Prenatal diagnosis of GM1-gangliosidosis. N Engl Med 288: 225–228

Machin GA (1989) Hydrops revisited: literature review of 1414 cases published in the 1980s. Am J Med Genet 34: 366–390

Markesbery WR, Robinson RO, Falace PV, Frye MD (1980) Mucopolysaccharidoses: ultrastructure of leucocyte inclusions. Ann Neurol 8: 332–336

Martin JJ, Leroy JG, Farriaux JP, Fontaine G, Desnick RJ, Cabello A (1975) I-cell disease (mucolipidosis II). A report on its pathology. Acta Neuropathol 33: 285–305

Martin JJ, Centerick C (1988) The contribution of pathology

to the study of storage disorders. Path Res Pract 183: 375–385

Modell B, Petrou M, Ward RHT et al. (1984) Effect of fetal diagnostic testing on birth-rate of thalassaemia major in Britain. Lancet II: 1383–1386

Nussbaum RL, Powell C, Graham HL, Caskey CT, Fernbach DJ (1984) Newborn screening for sickling hemoglobinopathies. Am J Dis Child 138: 44–48

O'Brien JF (1982) Laboratory report: the lysosomal storage diseases. Mayo Clin Proc 57: 192–197

O'Brien JS, Bernett J, Veath ML, Paa D (1975) Lysosomal storage disorders. Diagnosis by ultrastructural examination of skin biopsy specimens. Arch Neurol 32: 592–599

Perry TL (1981) Autopsy investigation of disorders of amino acid metabolism. In: Barson AJ (ed) Laboratory investigation of fetal disease. Wright, Bristol, pp 429–451

Rapola J, Satavuori P, Savilahti E (1984) Suction biopsy of rectal mucosa in the diagnosis of infantile and juvenile types of neuronal ceroid lipofuscinoses. Hum Pathol 15: 352–360

Rodeck CH, Tansley LR, Benson PF, Fensom AH, Ellis M (1983) Prenatal exclusion of Hurler's disease by leucocyte alpha-L-iduronate assay. Prenat Diagn 3: 61–63

Savage RA (1984) Specific and not-so-specific histiocytes in bone marrow. Lab Med 15: 467–471

Sheets Lee JE, Falk RE, Ng WG, Donnell GN (1985) Beta-glucuronidase deficiency. A heterogeneous mucopolysaccaridosis. Am J Dis Child 139: 57–59

Silberberg R, Rimoin DL, Rosenthal RE, Hasler MB (1972) Ultrastructure of cartilage in the Hurler and Sanfillipo syndromes. Arch Pathol Lab Med 94: 500–510

Stein J, Berg C, Jones JA, Detter JC (1984) A new screening protocol for a prenatal population at risk for inherited hemoglobin disorders: results of its application to a group of Southeast Asians and blacks. Am J Obstet Gynecol 150: 333–341

Stevenson RE, Lubinsky M, Taylor HA, Wenger DA, Schroer RJ, Olmstead PM (1983) Sialic acid storage disease with sialuria: clinical and biochemical features in the severe infantile type. Pediatrics 72: 441–448

Sweetman L, Nyhan WL, Trauner DA, Merritt TA, Singh M (1980) Glutaric aciduria type II. J Pediatr 96: 1020–1026

Wilcken B, Brown ARD, Urwin R, Brown DA (1983) Cystic fibrosis screening by dried blood spot trypsin assay: results in 75000 newborn infants. J Pediatr 102: 383–387

Yamano T, Shimada M, Okada S, Yutaka T, Kato T, Yabauuchi H (1982) Ultrastructural study of biopsy specimens of rectal mucosa. Arch Pathol Lab Med 106: 673–677

Chapter 6

Epidemiology of Fetal and Neonatal Death

Jean Golding

Introduction

The study of perinatal mortality rates has become increasingly popular. The results are quoted variously by politicians, sociologists and clinicians according to the point which they wish to make. Government spokesmen quote a fall in the perinatal mortality rate as vindication of their policies. Politicians in opposition and clinicians quote high national rates in comparison with selected other countries and claim that the government is not spending enough on maternity or neonatal services. Sociologists point to the differential mortality between advantaged and disadvantaged social groups and claim that better housing, or increased minimum wages, or decreased levels of unemployment would result in an improvement in perinatal mortality rates.

Are any of these claims justified? In order to interpret any data successfully, whether they relate to a small area or a large country, it is essential to understand the difficulties inherent in statistics. On the face of it, there should be no difficulty in ascertaining the perinatal mortality of a particular population. The only items of information necessary are the absolute numbers of total births and perinatal deaths. However, there are two major problems: first, that of definition and, second, that of recording.

Accuracy of Perinatal Death Statistics

Definition Problems

There are no problems in identifying as livebirths, infants who are born alive and survive well into the first week of life. However, there has been inconsistency in defining those livebirths who survive for only a short time. To this end, therefore, the World Health Organisation (1976, 1977) defined a livebirth as: "the complete expulsion or extraction from its mother of a product of conception, irrespective of the duration of pregnancy, which after such separation, breathes and shows any evidence of life such as beating of the heart, pulsation of the umbilical cord of definite movement of voluntary muscles, whether or not the umbilical cord has been cut, or the placenta is attached: each product of such a birth is considered liveborn". Since some very early abortions show such signs, the identification of some livebirths depends on the assiduousness with which the attending clinician observes and records.

A definition of a fetal death is consequently as difficult as that of livebirth in an infant showing marginal signs of life. Perhaps more importantly, there is a difference between and within countries concerning which fetal deaths should be registered as such. Thus, in Japan, all fetal deaths occurring after 13 weeks' gestation are registered (Kamimura 1976), whereas, in the UK, only those occurring at or after 28 weeks are recorded (Macfarlane and Mugford 1984). Even within such wide limits there is still some confusion concerning the distinction between neonatal death and late fetal death (stillbirth). In some countries a livebirth that dies before registration as liveborn is registered as a fetal death.

Within countries, particular factors may also influence whether a death is registered as a late fetal death or a neonatal death. These include the laws governing the entitlement to a maternity grant.

Finally, assuming that fetal deaths, livebirths and neonatal deaths have been registered, what should the definition of a perinatal death be? The World Health Organisation (1977) recommends that for *national* statistics, the term "perinatal death" should include all early neonatal deaths together with those fetal deaths that weigh 500 g or more (or, if weight is unknown, of gestation 22 weeks or more, or crown–heel length of 25 cm or more). For *international* statistics they recommend including only those fetal deaths of weight 1000 g or more (or, if weight is unknown, of gestation 28 weeks or more, or crown–heel length of 35 cm or more). There has been much discussion concerning the bias generated by taking a definition for international comparison that is based on birthweight rather than gestation (Goldstein and Butler 1977; Meyer 1977). Nevertheless, because gestation is often unknown it is felt that a criterion based on weight will give more comparable figures than would have pertained had gestation been used.

Personal Variation in Interpretation of Definitions

In Belgium and the Netherlands an elegant study was carried out by Keirse (1984). To specialist and trainee obstetricians in the two countries he sent a questionnaire purporting to be concerned with the management of preterm labour. Amongst the material were three case histories and the respondent was asked whether he would or would not register the deaths. The three deaths had the following characteristics; (1) normally formed, 23 weeks, 590 g, livebirth, died aged 4 min; (2) anencephalic, 24 weeks, 600 g, died after a few minutes; (3) anencephalic, 24 weeks, 600 g, stillborn. In both countries, by law, cases 1 and 2 should have been registered and 3 should not. Only 6% of obstetricians would have registered all three correctly! No similar studies have been carried out in other countries, but studies of this nature are an essential prerequisite in order to assess the validity of published perinatal mortality data.

Registration Failure

Clinicians may fail to recognise when a perinatal death should be registered; however, even when they fill in the forms appropriately, these may not reach the registrar. A prime example of this type of error was found in the American state of Georgia. Interest was aroused by a peculiar pattern of birthweight-specific mortality rates. A study was carried out to ascertain how many of the registered livebirths of low birthweight had indeed survived. It was found that a large proportion (21%) of neonatal deaths had never been registered as such. Their inclusion in the mortality rates would have raised the overall neonatal mortality rate by 25% (Alley and Terry 1979; McCarthy et al. 1980). As a result of this study all hospitals in Georgia now notify those deaths which have occurred and if registration forms are not received, steps are taken to obtain them. For fetal deaths it has been reported from Wisconsin that 18% were not registered, the shortfall being particularly those of shortest gestation (Greb et al. 1987).

Elsewhere it has been shown that there are similar problems. For example, in Enschede in the Netherlands, Smits (1981) found that 31% of perinatal deaths had not been registered. In Amsterdam hospitals Doornbos and Nordbeck (1985) found that 15% of deaths were not registered, but they were not able to estimate what the rate of home deaths might be. In Northern Ireland, Scott and colleagues (1981) suggested that there was a 10% shortfall. In the Greek National Birth Survey (Tzoumaka-Bakoula 1987), 31% of the perinatal deaths had not been registered and in the Jamaican Perinatal Mortality Survey the proportion was over 90% (McCaw-Binns 1991).

It is essential that each study of perinatal deaths starts by ascertaining the defects in the data. In local hospital-based studies, for example, one would need to be aware of transfers to other hospitals (or home) and the outcome of each before publishing a neonatal or perinatal mortality rate. Within the UK, national birth surveys have, to a certain extent, provided information that enables us to state that a large majority of perinatal deaths are, in fact, registered as such (Butler and Alberman 1969; Chamberlain et al. 1975).

Epidemiological Analyses

Given all the problems of definition outlined above, together with the unknown extent of the inaccuracies that are present, is there any point in analysing data concerning perinatal mortality? In effect, one can only satisfactorily analyse perinatal data if one has a clear idea of what one may and may not be measuring, if the comparison is of like with like, and if the conclusions take account of the limitations of the data.

It is essential to remember that statistics are a useful tool to be used in describing patterns, but they can rarely be used to prove a causal hypothesis. Medical literature gives copious examples of unwarranted conclusions being reached from valid statistics. One of the examples that used to be quoted compared the annual number of newly registered mentally handicapped persons with the number of television sets bought. A positive correlation does not prove that watching television results in mental handicap.

Place of Birth

Closer to the subject of this book, Tew has repeatedly published data (1978, 1980, 1985, 1990) that purport to show that delivery in a consultant unit results in more perinatal deaths than delivery at home, with the conclusion that home delivery is safest for the baby. Here the statistics are not wrong, and control for high-risk factors does not totally eliminate the association. The defect in her studies is that she is not comparing like with like.

In order to make the point clearer, suppose that instead of observational data she had been able to set up a randomised controlled trial in which mothers were allocated n_1 to home and n_2 to hospital delivery. Out of the n_1 randomised to deliver at home, x_1 will develop some complication that will necessitate their transfer to hospital care (e.g. rising blood pressure, placenta praevia, proteinuria, abruptio placenta, suspected growth retardation, reduction in fetal movements, suspected fetal death, prolonged labour with failure to progress ect). Of the n_2 originally in the group for hospital care, x_2 will also develop these abnormalities.

There are now, at the point of delivery:

$n_1 - x_1$ at home

$n_2 + x_1$ in hospital

The only valid comparison is either between the $(n_1 - x_1)$ at home and the $(n_2 - x_2)$ in hospital that did not develop complications, or between the original n_1 *intended* to deliver at home and the n_2 *intended* to deliver in hospital. When the latter strategy has been attempted on observational studies (Hobbs and Acheson 1966; Fedrick and Butler 1972), the data have shown that *intention* to deliver at home carries a higher mortality than *intention* to deliver in a consultant unit. This point has been discussed in more detail by Golding and Peters (1988).

Time Trends

Other examples where data are difficult to interpret are found in examining time trends. So many different factors vary over time, from the social and geographical composition of the sample to features of obstetric practice. Therefore, it is not valid to observe, for example, the increasing use of fetal monitoring techniques and the falling perinatal mortality rate and claim that one has caused the other. A first step in an analysis in time trends would be to document the basic changes in the population (including maternal age, parity, marital status, ethnic group, maternal smoking, prevalence of severe pre-eclampsia, birthweight and gestation distributions). If a hospital population is being used, then it is vital to ascertain the numbers of mothers referred from outside the normal catchment area (these should be excluded) and those inside the area that have delivered elsewhere (these should be included).

Studies of Perinatal Mortality

Given that one knows the biases inherent in case definition and ascertainment, there are four possible ways in which studies may be mounted. All have their advantages and disadvantages.

1. *National statistics*
Advantages: Large numbers.
Disadvantages: Limited amount of information. Cause of death data meaningless. Possible under-ascertainment of deaths. Lack of quality control on information.

2. *National surveys*, using data specially collected over a defined period of time, e.g. Greek National Survey (Tzoumaka-Bakoula 1987); British National Surveys (Butler and Bonham 1963; Chamberlain et al. 1975); Jamaican National Survey (Ashley et al. 1988).
Advantages: Improved quality of data. Ability to classify deaths in a standard way. Large amount of information available for analysis.
Disadvantages: Relatively small numbers of deaths unless the sample is extended, as in the First British Perinatal Mortality Survey (Butler and Bonham 1963) or the Jamaican study (Ashley et al. 1988).

3. *Ongoing area-based maternity information*
Advantages: Quality control is possible, especially if organised so that research clerks abstract the information using well-formulated rules, with referral to consultant obstetricians in cases of difficulty (e.g. Cardiff Birth Survey and Aberdeen Survey).
Disadvantages: Relatively small numbers of deaths in any one year. Difficulty in accomodating within the system new obstetric and neonatal procedures introduced during the course of the study.

4. *Hospital-based statistics*
Advantages: As above.
Disadvantages: As above. In addition, the data are epidemiologically uninterpretable unless the hospital serves the whole of a geographical population. Otherwise it is essential to ascertain the outcome of pregnancy in all women resident in the referral area but delivered outside the hospital.

5. *Prospective studies*
Advantages: Surveys starting in pregnancy or even before have the benefit of greater accuracy in determining features relating to the mother and the pregnancy prior to the death occurring.
Disadvantages: High cost; relatively small numbers.

When studies have been carried out on valid populations a number of consistent and striking associations have been found for perinatal mortality in general. These are described below.

Causes of Perinatal Death

In order to identify ways in which perinatal deaths may be prevented, one needs a valid system of classification.

Interpretation of the causes of death that appear on the perinatal death certificate is extremely difficult. Frequently, for example, the causes of death are written down by junior medical staff often before the results of any post-mortem examination are known. Occasionally, the registered causes of death are given after necropsy, but even then a histological examination is unlikely to have been made, and the results of bacteriological and chromosome examinations or other tests will rarely be available.

A number of studies have now been carried out comparing registered causes of stillbirth or neonatal death with post-mortem findings (Fedrick and Butler 1972; Edouard 1982; Duley 1986), each showing poor correlation. Not surprisingly, overt congenital malformations are most likely to have been identified, but even for anencephalus, only 90% of cases had such a term on the death certificate (Fedrick and Butler 1972). At the other end of the spectrum, for a third of neonatal deaths ascribed to hyaline membrane disease there was no evidence at necropsy to support this (Duley 1986).

Much of the confusion in assigning causes to perinatal deaths lies in the multiplicity of contributing factors. For example, consider the following case:

> The mother was unmarried and aged 17. She was smoking 30 cigarettes a day and had not booked until the third trimester of pregnancy when she was found to have fulminating pre-eclampsia. Her membranes ruptured spontaneously and she went into labour at 35 weeks. A retroplacental haemorrhage was found and the female infant was severely growth retarded. She was severely asphyxiated at birth but recovered rapidly after ventilation; nevertheless after 4 hours she developed signs of respiratory distress and was treated appropriately but her condition rapidly deteriorated and she died 2 hours later. Necropsy showed resolving hyaline-membrane disease, a small ventricular septal defect and an intraventricular haemorrhage.

Among other terms that might have been recorded on the death certificate are the following: "maternal pre-eclampsia"; "maternal abruptio placentae"; "premature rupture of membranes"; "unmarried mother"; "heavy maternal smoking"; "preterm delivery"; "growth retardation"; "low birthweight"; "placental insufficiency"; "birth asphyxia";

"respiratory distress syndrome", "intraventricular haemorrhage"; and "congenital heart disease".

The International Classification of Diseases would have assigned each of these terms to a different code. One suggestion on methods of coping with multiple causes of death is that up to five different causes should be coded for each death. Even so, it is difficult to know which of the 13 terms listed above would be most relevant; there are few published data to suggest which the underlying cause of death should be. The answer is clearly that we do not yet know. Certainly, the *risk* of perinatal death is greater if the mother is unmarried, a teenager, a smoker, or if she develops pre-eclampsia, but that does not mean that *in this particular case* any of these factors contributed at all to this death. Unlike deaths in adults, where there is often an identifiable disease process and hence an underlying cause of death which would be recognised as such by many workers, in the perinatal field this rarely occurs.

This has prompted many authors to develop their own systems of classification. These really depend on either a combination of clinical and pathological findings (Baird et al. 1954; Hovatta et al. 1983), the pathological lesions found at necropsy (Claireaux 1962; Autio-Harmainen et al. 1983), placental and fetal pathology (Naeye 1977), or clinical features of the perinate (Wigglesworth 1980). The classification systems used are described below:

Aberdeen Clinicopathological Classification

The Aberdeen clincopathological classification was first described by Baird et al. in 1954 and has been used extensively since then (McIlwaine et al. 1979). In the earlier paper the authors stated that necropsy findings usually indicate only the immediate cause of death and have little relevance from the point of view of aetiology. As an example, they cited the infant weighing 1.36 kg (3 lb) delivered by caesarean section, after placenta praevia had been identified. Post-mortem examination showed a tentorial tear, but the authors considered that *placenta praevia* was a more meaningful cause of death than either prematurity or birth trauma. They developed very detailed rules for classification of perinatal deaths, almost entirely based on clinical information, and defined eight categories as follows:

1. *Premature, cause unknown*:
a) Baby weighs ≤2500 g, but otherwise normal apart from possible maceration. Pregnancy and labour normal even though onset of labour may have been preterm.
b) If lesions (such as intracranial haemorrhage or infection) are found at necropsy but baby weighs <1800 g. and there have been no serious abnormalities of pregnancy.

2. *Mature, cause unknown*: Pregnancy clinically normal, labour normal, baby weighing 2501 g+.

3. *Mechanical*: All deaths without major malformations 1801 g+ with breech or shoulder presentation, or with obstruction of the cord. In vertex deliveries, the degree of moulding and characteristics of labour are taken into account. Diagnosis of trauma may be made in the absence of necropsy evidence of birth injury.

4. *Toxaemia*: Intrauterine or neonatal death caused by prematurity or anoxia when eclampsia or severe or moderate pre-eclampsia have been present. When antepartum haemorrhage has also occurred, cases are classified as toxaemia.

5. *Antepartum haemorrhage*: All cases with placenta praevia, accidental haemorrhage or antepartum haemorrhage of uncertain origin.

6. *Maternal disease*: "Cases in which the mother has suffered during pregnancy from an incidental medical or surgical condition such as diabetes, pneumonia, syphilis, or appendicitis, apparently leading to intrauterine death or to the expulsion of a feeble, toxic (usually premature) baby which dies in the first week."

7. *Deformity*: Malformations incompatible with life or likely to have been the prime factor contributing to death.

8. *Other causes*: Includes cases in which mother had rhesus antibodies and cases in which infants, healthy at birth, died of infection, haemorrhagic disease etc. Subsequently this class was divided into two groups: blood group incompatibility, which took precedence over all other causes except deformity, and the remainder.

This classification has been used in a number of studies of perinatal death; thus it is interesting to compare the results (Table 6.1). As expected, the proportion of deaths "caused by" trauma and blood group incompatibility has fallen dramatically, whereas the proportion associated with malformation and prematurity (cause unknown) has risen.

Table 6.1. Distribution of perinatal deaths according to the Aberdeen clinicopathological classification

Clinical classification	Aberdeen[a] 1938–1952	Great Britain[b] 1958	Scotland[c] 1977	Northern Region[d] 1981–1982
Premature, cause unknown	19.7%	17.4%	29.8%	31.9%
Mature, cause unknown	13.7%	15.1%	10.5%	12.4%
Trauma	18.8%	13.1%	4.9%	2.7%
Toxaemia	10.0%	13.1%	8.8%	7.1%
Antepartum haemorrhage	10.9%	13.1%	12.5%	15.0%
Malformation	15.6%	18.0%	26.2%	21.2%
Maternal disease	6.0%	2.4%	4.4%	4.4%
Other		2.4%	1.3%	3.5%
—incompatibility	5.3%	4.8%	1.6%	0.9%
Number of deaths (= 100%)	1008	2210	1012	988

[a] Cases booked at Aberdeen Maternity Hospital (Baird et al. 1954).
[b] First National Perinatal Mortality Survey (Baird and Thomson 1969).
[c] The Scottish Perinatal Mortality Survey (McIlwaine et al. 1979).
[d] The Northern Regional Health Authority Coordinating Group (1984).

Within the last few years there have been two attempts to update and rationalise the classification. On the one hand Cole et al. (1986) suggested a number of subdivisions within each group but Whitfield et al. (1986) recommended more substantial changes to identify 12 subgroups as shown in Table 6.2.

Table 6.2. Modification of the Aberdeen classification of perinatal deaths

Aberdeen classification[a]	Whitfield classification[b]
1. Premature unknown	→ spontaneous preterm intrauterine growth retardation unexplained IUD
2. Mature unknown	→ intrapartum asphyxia ↗
3. Mechanical	→ trauma
4. Toxaemia	→ hypertension
5. Maternal disease	→ maternal disease
6. Antepartum haemorrhage	→ antepartum haemorrhage
7. Deformity	→ fetal abnormality
8a. Blood group incompatibility	→ haemolytic disease
8b. Other	→ infection ↘ other

[a] Baird et al. (1954).
[b] Whitficed et al. (1986).

British Necropsy Classification

For the 1958 British Perinatal Mortality Survey (BPMS), Claireaux (1962) developed a classification based on post-mortem findings. His results are compared in Table 6.3 with those from the perinatal mortality survey in Cuba (Rajas Ochoa 1981) and from Machin's (1975) study in London: as in other systems hierarchical decisions had to be made. For example, an infant with evidence of both intrauterine asphyxia and cerebral birth trauma was always classified as trauma; an infant with pneumonia and another major lesion was always grouped with the other lesion.

Table 6.3. Distribution of deaths according to British necropsy classification

Classification of primary anatomical lesion	BMPS[a] 1958	London[b] 1970–1973	Cuba[c] 1973
Congenital malformation	15.1%	23.8%	12.3%
Blood group incompatability	4.0%	3.3%	2.6%
Antepartum asphyxia	13.4%	21.3%	14.9%
Intrapartum asphyxia	20.8%	20.9%	22.7%
Intracranial birth trauma	8.9%	4.0%	4.2%
Intraventricular haemorrhage	2.4%	10.6%	3.7%
Hyaline membranes	5.8%	6.2%	11.4%
Massive pulmonary haemorrhage	2.7%	1.2%	2.1%
Pneumonia	4.1%	5.0%	6.9%
Extrapulmonary infection	0.3%	1.2%	2.9%
Other lesion	1.1%	4.9%	1.9%
Resorption atelectasis (no HM)	3.3%	0.6% (combined)	14.2% (combined)
No anatomical lesion found	18.1%		
Number of deaths (= 100%)	2368	721	1400

Abbreviation: HM, hyaline membranes
[a] Claireaux (1962) (population based).
[b] Machin (1975) (hospital based).
[c] Rojas Ochoa (1981) (population based).

That there were disadvantages in assuming that one lesion was the most important rapidly became apparent both to the team analysing the BPMS data and to Valdes-Dapena and Arey (1970) in the USA. Later analyses of the BPMS deaths examined all deaths with a particular pathological abnormality and looked at the interactions with other lesions, as well as with clinical factors (Fedrick and Butler 1970a,b, 1971a,b,c,d).

An attempt to address the problems inherent in multiple causes has been attempted by Hey et al. (1986). They suggest dividing the congenital malformations category into six groups (Chromosomal, inborn error of metabolism, neural tube defect, congenital heart disease, renal abnormality, other malformation), the hyaline membrane disease (HMD) group into three classes (HMD, HMD + intraventricular haemorrhage (IVH), HMD + infection), the two infection groups into four (necrotising enterocolitis, antepartum infection, intrapartum infection, postpartum infection). They suggest there should be further categories for "other intracranial bleeding", "cot death", "unattended delivery" and "undocumented or unclassified".

Placental and Fetal Pathology Classification

Naeye (1977) Classified causes of perinatal death according to placental and fetal pathology, as follows:

1. *Acute amniotic fluid infection syndrome*: Acute congenital pneumonia associated with acute inflammation of extraplacental membranes, acute funisitis, acute inflammation of the chorionic plate of the placenta. Membranes had to have been intact at start of labour
2. *Abruptio placentae*: Clinical evidence of abruption and retroplacental clot + evidence of fetal hypoxia, e.g. aspirated squamae and petechiae on surface of visceral organs
3. *Premature rupture of membranes*: If <37 weeks gestation: membranes rupture prior to onset of labour; if ≥37 weeks, membranes rupture at least 20 h prior to onset of labour
4. *Congenital anomalies*: Severe and incompatible with survival
5. *Large placental infarcts*: At least 25% of placenta involved by one or more infarcts over 3 cm in diameter; no other known explanation for death
6. *Intervillous thrombi of placenta*: If more than 3 cm in diameter and involving at least 25% of placenta
7. *Umbilical cord compression*: Breech delivery with cord compressed by head, or cord prolapse, or cord tightly round neck
8. *Cord knots*: If knots were tight, no other explanation for death
9. *Placental growth retardation*: Placenta 40% below weight for gestation and no other explanation for death
10. *Placenta praevia*: Placenta encroached on the cervical os and death caused by blood loss or consequences of premature delivery
11. *Rhesus erythroblastosis*
12. *Birth trauma*: (not defined by Naeye, but 91% of his group of cases had subdural haematomas)
13. *Polyhydramnios*: Excess amniotic fluid initiated preterm labour and infant died from consequences of immaturity
14. *Caesarean section*: Gestational age overestimated and infant died from consequences of immaturity
15. *Marginal sinus rupture*: A marginal tear in the placenta which appeared responsible for antepartum haemorrhage and fetal hypoxia
16. *Severe fetal undernutrition*: Gross and microscopic characteristics (undefined) of undernutrition without any known causes except maternal weight loss or poor weight gain
17. *Uterine rupture*
18. *Postmaturity*: Gestation <44 weeks, gross and microscopic evidence of undernutrition and no other explanation for death
19. *Congenital syphilis*: Spirochaetes in the infant's tissues
20. *Other disorders*

The figures in Table 6.4 indicate the proportion of stillbirths and neonatal deaths which were placed in each category using deaths from the USA, South Africa and Ethiopia. It will be noted that categories 6, 8, 11, 13–18 have been replaced by fetal hypoxia, obstructed labour, other acute infections or amalgamated into the "other" category.

Wigglesworth Classification

The classification proposed by Wigglesworth (1980) is an attempt to produce a simple system

Table 6.4. Mortality rates (per 1000) attributable to placental/fetal pathology

Naeye's classification	Durban South Africa	Addis Ababa Ethiopia	USA
Amniotic fluid infection	14.2	17.5	5.9
Abruptio placentae	8.1	4.5	3.8
Premature rupture of membranes	1.1	1.1	3.5
Congenital anomalies	2.7	2.4	3.2
Large placental infarcts	0.9	1.5	2.1
Umbilical cord compression	2.2	3.4	1.2
Placental growth retardation	0.5	0.2	0.9
Placenta praevia	1.0	1.6	0.7
Birth trauma	3.9	0.9	0.5
Congenital syphilis	3.2	4.3	0.1
Fetal hypoxia	6.5	3.6	2.6
Obstructed labour	3.3	8.4	—
Other acute infections	0.9	0.3	0.4
Other disorders	4.8	3.5	3.9
Diagnosis unknown	0.8	0.2	4.6
Total	54.6	53.4	33.4

Data abstracted from Ross et al. 1982.

for classifying perinatal deaths and purports to be relatively accurate whether or not post-mortem examination is carried out. The five categories are:

1. Normally formed antepartum fetal death
2. Congenital malformation
3. Conditions associated with immaturity
4. Asphyxial conditions developing in labour
5. Specific conditions other than the above

The five categories seem to be fairly straightforward, but problems arise in a minority of cases. For example, should one really put a macerated stillbirth with a minor isolated defect (e.g. polydactyly, cleft palate) in category 2, rather than category 1? How does one classify the neonatal death of an infant of weight 3500 g and 41 weeks' gestation who died with an intraventricular haemorrhage? The cause of death is certainly one that is usually associated with immaturity even though the index infant was mature.

An attempt to address such ambiguities was made by Barson and his colleagues (1984), who ruled that a malformation which could be lethal if found in isolation took precedence over all other causes and that preterm infants would be placed in category 4 if there was profound hypoxia at birth unresponsive to resuscitation. They included neonatal necrotising enterocolitis and meningitis in category 5 but placed preterm infants with pneumonia in category 3. Nevertheless, these modifications still leave a number of unanswered questions which were addressed by Keeling et al. (1989) who set out clearer rules in order to clarify ambiguities.

Comparison of various studies using the Wigglesworth classification is shown in Table 6.5. It can be seen that the proportion of normally formed macerated stillbirths has increased, but those associated with asphyxia and other conditions (mainly rhesus disease and infection) have decreased. There is increasing evidence of the validity of using this classification. An important study (Lumley and Tzoumaka-Bakoula 1992) has, for example, compared perinatal mortality in Greece with that to Greeks living in Australia. They showed that the reduced perinatal mortality rate in Australia was entirely due to a reduction in the intrapartum asphyxia group.

The classification has been found to be particularly useful in developing countries. In Jamaica the major cateogry was intrapartum asphyxia, accounting for 44% of perinatal deaths. Analysis of the data showed that the mortality rate associated with intrapartum asphyxia was reduced in areas with access to specialist obstetric and neonatal facilities (Samms-Vaughan and Golding 1992).

Table 6.5. Distribution of perinatal deaths deaths according to Wigglesworth classification

Wigglesworth classification	BPMS[b] 1958	Manchester[a] 1976–1981	Northern Region[b] 1981–1982	Hammersmith Hospital[c] 1978–1979
Macerated	20.8%	28.9%	40.7%	24.3%
Malformation	19.3%	24.8%	22.1%	13.5%
Immaturity	12.3%	24.3%	15.0%	41.9%
Asphyxia	32.2%	16.4%	16.8%	16.2%
Other	15.4%	5.7%	5.4%	4.1%
Number of deaths (=100%)	2368	440	988	74

[a] Barson et al. (1984).
[b] Northern Regional Health Authority Coordinating Group (1984).
[c] Wigglesworth (1980).

Finnish Pathological Classifications

Neonatal Deaths

In the classification proposed by Autio-Harmainen et al. (1983), the immediate cause of death was used if considered more serious than the underlying cause, but the underlying cause was taken when it alone would have been sufficient to cause death. When cerebral haemorrhage occurred in association with hyaline membranes or infection, haemorrhage was taken as the primary cause of death. Infection was considered as primary cause only when no other potentially lethal lesions were present. "Immaturity" was taken as the cause when both the clinical and pathological findings supported this and there was no other abnormality. The distribution of the six categories among 1020 neonatal deaths was:

Cerebral haemorrhage 20.2%
Hyaline membrane disease 21.6%
Infection 10.9%
Malformation 35.3%
Immaturity 3.5%
Miscellaneous 8.5%

Stillbirths

For stillbirths, Hovatta et al. (1983) produced both a necropsy classification and a clinicopathological assessment and showed the ways in which 243 stillbirths would be distributed in each.

Necropsy classification
- *Asphyxia* 38.3% (including meconium aspiration, petechiae on serous membranes, intracerebral haemorrhage)
- *Major malformations* 16.9%
- *Severe erythroblastosis* 0.8%
- *Maceration only* 42.8%
- *No cause found* 1.2% (non-macerated fetus with no pathological findings)

Clinicopathological classification
- *Abruptio placentae* 14.4%
- *Large placental infarcts* 10.7%
- *Cord complication* 11.9% (includes prolapse, velamentous insertion, strangulation, single umbilical artery)
- *Other placental failure* 25.4% (includes severe pre-eclampsia, cholestasis of pregnancy, twin pregnancy, immature birth, uterine anomaly etc.)
- *Unexplained asphyxia* 3.3%
- *Maternal isoimmunisation* 3.3%
- *Fetal bleeding* 2.9%
- *Severe chorioamnionitis* 2.1%
- *Major malformations* 16.9%
- *Unexplained* 9.1%

Avoidability of Death

Given so many different classifications of perinatal death, and so many factors that influence the risk of death, the person assessing each death is likely to bring his own experience, expertise and biases into play. To get over this problem there has been a move to institute "Confidential Enquiries" using a committee approach (Chalmers 1985). This requires a subjective decision to be made about possible avoidability of death.

The aetiology of perinatal deaths is extraordinarily complex. I agree with Baird (1980), who said "I think it is a mistake to talk about avoidability of perinatal deaths. Who can tell whether a perinatal death could have been avoided? What one can do is describe the circumstances in which the death occurred and the type of death".

Nevertheless, a number of regions have undertaken such studies. If the criterion of "avoidable death" was meaningful, and local efforts were made to remedy any faults in obstetric or neonatal practice that might have been identified, then it is reasonable to postulate that subsequent mortality might be reduced. One study (Thomas et al. 1985) claims that it has, but Elbourne and Mutch (1984) compared the improvements in mortality rates in all those British regions that had ongoing Confidential Enquiries with the areas that had no such monitoring system. The fall in mortality was similar in each group, thus suggesting that, although of interest locally, it was unlikely that such enquiries would actually prevent many deaths.

Cause or Association

Baird et al. (1954) produced a logical argument to support the largely clinical classification they advocated, as opposed to a classification based on necropsy findings, on the basis that the clinical abnormalities usually resulted in the lesions that led to the death of the fetus. Yet, even 30 years on from their original publication are we actually able to say that the death of an infant born to a mother with moderate pre-eclampsia is the result of that maternal disease? Perusal of the statistics shows that perinatal deaths are 30% and 130% more likely if the mother has either moderate or severe pre-eclampsia. This means that out of every 130 deaths to mothers with moderate pre-eclampsia, 100 would have been expected to occur anyway and thus only 30 would actually be associated with the pre-eclampsia. Are we yet in a position to assert positively that we are able, either from clinical history or post-mortem examination, to distinguish the 100 from the 30? Until we can do this it would surely be wrong to use only the clinical classification.

What then should be used? The answer must surely depend on the use to which the system is put. Not unexpectedly, obstetricians have found the Aberdeen clinical classification of most use, and only pathologists appear to have used the mainly anatomical classifications (Machin 1975; Naeye 1979a). Consequently, epidemiological analyses of factors associated with specific causes of death are difficult to compare with one another.

The need for a simple system of use to all who are interested in perinatal deaths may be answered by the Wigglesworth classification. This has been shown to have validity and repeatability regardless of the experience of the classifier and the extent of post-mortem examination (Keeling et al. 1989). It is being increasingly found to be of great value in the monitoring of trends in perinatal mortality and comparison of different populations. If this is not feasible, the best option may well be to follow the guidelines of the FIGO Standing Committee on Perinatal Mortality and Morbidity (1982) and compare perinatal deaths of birthweight 1000 g+, both including and excluding lethal malformations. This procedure has proved helpful in local studies (Mutch et al. 1981), but, nevertheless, still requires complete ascertainment of perinatal deaths.

Maternal and Environmental Factors Associated with Perinatal Death

When studies have been carried out on valid populations a number of consistent and striking associations have been found for perinatal mortality in general. These are described below.

Maternal Age

There is generally a U-shaped variation with the risk of perinatal death, very young and older mothers having the highest rates (Cahalane et al. 1965; Naeye and Tafari 1983; Pharaoh and Alberman 1988). However there are differences in pattern according to time of death, with the stillbirth rate increasing with maternal age and a shallow U-shape for neonatal deaths (Golding 1990a). Only in Jamaica has there been an analysis to look at the specific mechanisms involved. The authors showed that the relationship between advanced maternal age and stillbirths was mainly associated with antepartum fetal deaths, and was explained by the increased rates of hypertension, bleeding and syphilis in the older mothers. The same survey demonstrated a marked increase in risk of Wigglesworth group 3—neonatal deaths associated with immaturity—among the births to teenagers which could not be explained by specific complications of pregnancy (Ashley et al. 1993).

Parity

Parity is measured as number of previous pregnancies resulting in live- or stillbirth. The parities with least risk of perinatal death are parities 1 and 2 (i.e. second and third pregnancies). Thereafter, in general, the risk rises with increasing parity. There is some evidence that the difference in risk between parities 0 and 1 has decreased over time (Golding 1990a), but it is still apparent in most countries (Golding 1990b).

Past Obstetric History

History tends to repeat itself. Sometimes the repetition is due to similar combinations of genes in the conceptuses, but more often to a continuing biological abnormality or environmental hazard in the mother. Whatever the reason, the most important factor in predicting the risk to the current pregnancy is the outcome of previous pregnancies of the same mother. In Britain, a history of previous miscarriage results in a 68% increase in perinatal death, but the increase is 200% if there has been previous perinatal death (Fedrick and Adelstein 1977). In Jamaica, the risk was increased by 33% when there had been one but by 129% when there had been two or more previous miscarriages, by 190% in the presence of a previous stillbirth and by 130% if there had been a prior early neonatal death. The risk to the current pregnancy was always increased further if the previous loss had occurred in the immediately preceding pregnancy. There was also support to suggest that the type of death using the Wigglesworth classification tended to be repeated (Ashley et al. 1993). Another feature of the past obstetric history that was shown to be predictive of perinatal death was previous antepartum haemorrhage (mainly associated with Wigglesworth group 3).

Interpregnancy Interval

There is much confusion in analysis of interpregnancy interval. It is essential that this is measured as the length of time from the preceding delivery to the last menstrual period of the index pregnancy. This becomes problematic in mothers with unknown LMP, or who conceived again prior to menstruating; however, these problems can be overcome with clinical or necropsy estimation of gestation. Women with preceding miscarriage or perinatal loss tend to have very short interpregnancy intervals. Thus, analysis must always take account of the past obstetric history. There is now reliable evidence from Britain and Norway that a prolonged interval between pregnancies carries an increased risk of stillbirth, but that a short interval (i.e. less than 6 months from preceding delivery to current conception) carries an increased risk of neonatal death (Bakketeig et al. 1984; Fedrick and Adelstein 1973).

Ethnic Group

In the USA, perinatal mortality rates among the black population are greater than among whites; in Australia the aborigines have a higher mortality rate than the white settlers; in Israel, the Arabs have a higher mortality than the Jews; in Sweden and the UK, immigrants have a higher mortality than the indigenous population. Reasons for the differences are multiple and vary from country to country. In the UK, immigrants from India/Bangladesh/Pakistan have the highest rates (Gillies et al. 1984), much of the excess being associated with congenital malformations. Some of the differences may be due to inbreeding (consanguinity rates in these groups are very high), to dietary differences, especially the vitamin D deficiency which develops following arrival in the UK, or to socioeconomic factors.

Social Class

In the UK, the classification of social disadvantage that most clearly reflects differing risks in perinatal mortality is based on a classification of the father's occupation into I (higher professionals such as doctors, ministers of religion, barristers); II (other professionals and managers, including teachers, nurses, company directors); IIIN (skilled non-manual such as salesmen, clerks, draughtsmen); IIIM (skilled manual, e.g. plumbers, carpenters, lorry drivers); IV (semi-skilled, such as caretakers, machine minders, postmen); V (unskilled, including cleaners and labourers). Single mothers are not included in this classification. In general, the perinatal mortality rate in social class V is almost twice that in social class I (Pharaoh and Alberman, 1985).

Other classifications have used parental education categories, and shown that whether in the industrial or the third world, there is a strong trend with highest perinatal mortality rate when the parent has received the lowest level of education (Golding 1990a). Nevertheless, in Greece a U-shaped variation has been found; women with lowest and highest education levels had the highest mortality rates (Tzoumaka-Bakoula et al. 1989).

Single Parents

In countries and times when the unmarried state was relatively unusual, there was a marked increase in mortality rates (Golding 1990a), but in countries where unmarried deliveries were not unusual there is still an excess in perinatal death (Golding 1990c; Skjaerven and Irgens 1988; Tzoumaka-Bakoula et al. 1989). It has been shown that there is an increase of about 40% in the risk to the fetus of an unmarried mother in Britain, over and above that related to her age and parity (Golding et al. 1986). From Jamaica there is evidence that unmarried mothers living in a stable relationship with the father of the child are also at increased risk, but the group who are living apart from the father of the child are at much greater risk (Ashley et al. 1993).

Maternal Size

Pre-pregnant maternal weight has rarely been studied. In the US, the risk increased with increasing weight (Naeye 1979b) but in Brazil, the relationship was found for stillbirths but not for neonatal deaths (Barros et al. 1987). In general both studies have shown an increase in risk with low maternal weight gain, but this finding is uninterpretable, being confounded by the fact that women who deliver preterm are bound not to have put on as much weight during pregnancy as women going to term. In the US mothers who put on excessive weight were at increased risk, but this was not true of mothers in Brazil.

Maternal height was considered important when the British Perinatal Mortality Survey showed an increased risk in short mothers (Butler and Bonham 1963), but this was not found in the USA (Naeye and Tafari 1983). In Brazil there was no relationship with stillbirth, but for neonatal deaths there was increasing risk with decreasing maternal height (Barros et al. 1987).

Season

Conceptions at times of peak fertility are at least risk of perinatal death. For the UK, therefore, conceptions in midsummer with expected date of delivery the following spring have the lowest risk (Golding and Sunderland 1990).

Smoking

Risk of perinatal death is elevated in mothers who smoke, although there is not a clear dose–response effect. The increased mortality is partly due to the fact that the infants of smoking mothers are more likely to be delivered preterm and also to be growth retarded. Nevertheless, one of the most important relationships is with antepartum fetal death (Golding et al. 1992).

Alcohol Consumption

Although possibly implicated in spontaneous abortion (Kline et al. 1980), there is no clear evidence that mild or moderate alcohol consumption has an adverse effect on the fetus. Indeed in Jamaica mothers who drank some alcohol had a slightly reduced risk of losing their baby (Ashley et al. 1993). In contrast, the fetus of the alcoholic mother is certainly at risk of growth retardation and dysmorphism, but it is not clear whether perinatal mortality rates are elevated.

Diet

Although it is often assumed that maternal diet has a major impact on perinatal mortality, the evidence for this is lacking. Supplement studies are rarely large enough to show any effect on perinatal mortality, and studies that have looked at general aspects of the diet have very rarely taken account of other features that may be contributing to perinatal mortality (Golding 1990a).

Of the supplement studies that have been carried out, a calorie protein supplement compared with placebo resulted in a reduction in perinatal mortality in Germany, which was just statistically significant (Mora et al. 1978). In America a randomised control trial of high-protein supplements resulted in a higher neonatal death rate when compared with controls receiving a placebo (Rush et al. 1986). In general, it is now considered that there may be a reduction in fetal death of the order of 2 per 1000 with appropriate dietary intervention in populations with poor diet in general (Rush et al. 1988).

Pre-eclampsia

Although severe maternal pre-eclampsia is associated with a much increased risk of mortality in the infant, mild pre-eclampsia (defined as a rise to maximum diastolic of 90–99 mm in the third trimester) carries no increase in risk at all. It is therefore essential to determine the degree of pre-eclampsia before ascribing it as a contributory cause of death.

Bleeding

A history of bleeding in pregnancy is associated with elevated risk of perinatal death. Most attention is paid to pregnancies with placenta praevia or where accidental haemorrhage has developed. Certainly, they both have high associated mortality rates (Huisjes et al. 1979; Naeye 1978; Naeye et al. 1977; Record and McKeown 1956). Nevertheless, numerically more deaths are actually associated with unspecified antepartum haemorrhage or even bleeding in the first two trimesters (Ashley et al. 1993; Butler and Bonham 1963).

Other Maternal Disorders

Data from the US Collaborative Study have indicated that perinatal mortality rates are elevated in the presence of maternal heart disease, asthma, epilepsy, urinary infection within 15 days of delivery, glomerulonephritis and, of course, diabetes (Naeye and Tafari 1983). From the major Jamaican study there was no relationship with urinary infection but marked associations with maternal anaemia and syphilis (Ashley et al. 1993).

Other Factors

There is no firm evidence that housing conditions or employment result in higher mortality rates in the developed world. In Bangladesh, however, there are reported associations with type of latrine and crowding within the household (Rahman et al. 1985).

There is some prospective evidence that stressful life events in pregnancy may result in the onset of preterm labour (Newton et al. 1979) and hence an increased risk of neonatal death. There is also prospective evidence that if the mother had, at the start of pregnancy, a negative attitude to pregnancy there is an increased risk of perinatal death (Laukaran and van der Berg 1980).

Characteristics of the Infant

Sex of Fetus

Stillbirth rates do not vary markedly with the sex of the fetus, but neonatal death rates are higher in males. This is largely due to the fact that boys are more likely than girls to be delivered prematurely (Karlberg et al. 1990).

Birthweight

In all countries a distinctive pattern is found when perinatal mortality rates are plotted against birthweight. There is a marked reduction in risk with increasing birthweight up to 3500 g, and then an upturn, with heavier infants being slightly more likely to die.

Low birthweight, however, is made up of three major components: multiple births, growth retardation and preterm delivery.

Twins. The perinatal mortality rate in twins is at least four times that of singletons (Golding 1990d). In addition, the second twin is at 35% greater risk of neonatal death than the first twin. Mortality of twins weighing under 1500 g is similar to that of singletons of the same weight; mortality of twins weighing 1500–2500 g is less than that of singletons of the same weight; mortality of twins weighing 2500 g or more is higher than that of singletons of similar weight (Golding 1990d).

Growth retardation. Whether measured in terms of percentiles or standard deviations from the mean, the infants at the mean or median have the lowest risk of perinatal death and those at the lowest extreme (i.e. with marked growth retardation) have the highest risk.

Preterm delivery. The gestation with the lowest perinatal mortality rate is in the period 39–41 weeks. From there, the lower the gestation the higher the risk, but there is also an increased risk among the postmature.

Preterm delivery and growth retardation. It is important to remember that, in spite of the patterns above, for a given birthweight the growth-retarded fetus has a lower mortality than the normally grown, but that the growth-accelerated fetus has a higher perinatal mortality rate than normally grown fetuses of the same weight.

Genetics

Although there is a recurrence effect, in that mothers who have had one perinatal death are at increased risk of further perinatal deaths, this does not necessarily imply a genetic effect. It could equally apply to continuing environmental conditions or medical problems in the mother. Nevertheless, one particular cause of perinatal deaths was certainly associated with a specific gene in the past. This occurred when rhesus-negative mothers were exposed to rhesus-positive fathers in one pregnancy and then reacted against any subsequent pregnancy that was rhesus positive. This cause of perinatal mortality has fallen rapidly in association with primary preventive methods involving the administration of anti-D after delivery (Clarke et al. 1985).

As to whether consanguineous mating results in increased risk of perinatal mortality, over and above that associated with congenital malformations, there has been conflicting evidence. The best data are probably those collected by Stevenson and his colleagues (1966). Their international study found a relative risk of perinatal death among consanguineous matings of 1.73 in comparison with unrelated parents. Nevertheless, no analysis was done to assess whether this was an artefact; it is conceivable that consanguineous mating may be more prevalent in the lower social groups or in religious groups that have particular habits that are harmful to the fetus.

Conclusions

In this chapter we have shown the way in which perinatal mortality rates vary with the different definitions used, and that registration of perinatal deaths is rarely, if ever, strictly accurate.

The cause of death classification varies from centre to centre, but in general the Wigglesworth classification appears to be simpler and more repeatable than many others. It has the added advantage of being interpretable by both clinicians and lay personnel.

The factors contributing towards perinatal mortality are varied, and point mostly to environmental factors. Nevertheless, the mechanism of these relationships has rarely been identified. Further progress into the understanding of perinatal deaths should involve studies of geographically defined populations with accurate data collection on both deaths and the background control population. The epidemiological method can assess ways in which perinatal mortality rates are higher than expected, and can give pointers to appropriate preventive strategies.

References

Alley J, Terry J (1979) Under-reporting of neonatal deaths—Georgia 1974–77. CDC Morbidity and Mortality Weekly Report 28: 253–254

Ashley D, McCaw-Binns A, Foster-Williams K (1988) The perinatal morbidity and mortality survey of Jamaica. Paediatr Perinat Epidemiol 2: 138–147

Ashley D, Golding J, Keeling J (1993) Perinatal mortality in Jamaica. University of the West Indies Press

Autio-Harmainen H, Rapola J, Hoppu K, Osterlund K (1983) Causes of death in a paediatric hospital neonatal unit. Acta Paediatr Scand 72: 333–337

Baird D (1980) Mortality equiries: discussion. In: Chalmers I, McIlwaine G (eds) Perinatal audit and surveillance. Royal College of Obstetricians and Gynaecologists, London, p 164
Baird D, Thomson AM (1969) The effects of obstetric and environmental factors on perinatal mortality by clinicopathological causes. In: Butler NR, Alberman ED (eds) Perinatal problems. Livingstone, Edinburgh, pp 211–226
Baird D, Walker J, Thomson AM (1954) The causes and prevention of stillbirths and first week deaths. Part III. A classification of deaths by clinical cause. J Obstet Gynaecol Br Emp 61: 433–448
Bakketeig LS, Hoffman HJ, Oakley ART (1984) Perinatal mortality. In: Bracken MB (ed) Perinatal epidemiology. Oxford University Press, New York, pp 99–151
Barros FC, Victoria CG, Vaughan JP, Estanislau HJ (1987) Perinatal mortality in southern Brazil: a population-based study of 7392 births. Bull WHO 65: 95–104
Barson AJ, Tasker M, Lieberman BA, Hillier VF (1984) Impact of improved perinatal care on the causes of death. Arch Dis Child 59: 199–207
Butler NR, Alberman ED (1969) Perinatal problems: the second report of the British National Perinatal Mortality Survey. Livingstone, Edinburgh
Butler NR, Bonham DG (1963) Perinatal mortality: the first report of the 1958 British Perinatal Mortality Survey. Livingstone, Edinburgh
Cahalane SF, Kennedy JD, McNicholl B, O'Dwyer E (1965) Perinatal mortality survey for County Galway, 18 months, October 1958 through March 1960. J Ir Med Assoc 57: 135–141
Chalmers I (1985) Enquiry into perinatal death. Br J Obstet Gynaecol 92: 545–549
Chamberlain R, Chamberlain G, Howlett B, Claireaux A (1975) British births 1970, volume I. Heinemann Medical, London
Claireaux AE (1962) Perinated mortality in the United Kingdom. In: Keller RJ (ed) Modern trends in obstetrics 3. Butterworths, London, pp 191–211
Clarke CA, Mollison PL, Whitfield AGW (1985) Deaths from Rhesus haemolytic disease in England and Wales in 1982 and 1983. Br Med J 291: 17–19
Cole SK, Hey EN, Thomson AM (1986) Classifying perinatal death: an obstetric approach. Br J Obstet Gynaecol 93: 1204–1212
Doornbos JPR, Nordbeck HJ (1985) Perinatal mortality. Obstetric factors in a community of mixed ethnic origin in Amsterdam. ICG Printing, Dordrecht
Duley LMM (1986) A validation of underlying cause of death, as recorded by clinicians on stillbirth and neonatal death certificates. Br J Obstet Gynaecol 93: 1223–1235
Edouard L (1982) Validation of the registered underlying causes of stillbirth. J Epidemiol Community Health 36: 231–234
Elbourne D, Mutch L (1984) Do locally-based enquiries into perinatal mortality reduce the risk of perinatal death? In: Smith A (ed) Recent advances in community medicine, vol 3. Churchill-Livingstone, London, pp 221–229
Fedrick J, Adelstein P (1973) The influence of pregnancy spacing on outcome of pregnancy. Br Med J 4: 753–756
Fedrick J, Adelstein P (1977) Preceding pregnancy loss as an index of risk of stillbirth or neonatal death in the present pregnancy. Biol Neonate 31: 84–93
Fedrick J, Butler NR (1970a) Certain causes of neonatal death: I Hyaline membranes. Biol Neonate 15: 229–255
Fedrick J, Butler NR (1970b) Certain causes of neonatal death: II Intraventricular haemorrhage. Biol Neonate 15: 257–290
Fedrick J, Butler NR (1971a) Certain causes of neonatal death: III Pulmonary infection (a) Clinical factors. Biol Neonate 17: 458–471
Fedrick J, Butler NR (1971b) Certain causes of neonatal death: III Pulmonary infection (b) Pregnancy and delivery. Biol Neonate 18: 45–57
Fedrick J, Butler NR (1971c) Certain causes of neonatal death: IV Massive pulmonary haemorrhage. Biol Neonate 18: 243–262
Fedrick J, Butler NR (1971d) Certain causes of neonatal death: V Cerebral birth trauma. Biol Neonate 18: 321–329
Fedrick J, Butler NR (1972) Accuracy of registered causes of neonatal deaths. Br J Prev Soc Med 26: 101–105
Fedrick J, Butler NR (1978) Intended place of delivery and perinatal outcome. Br Med J i: 763–765
FIGO Standing Committee on Perinatal Mortality and Morbidity (1982) Report of the Committee following a workshop on Monitoring and Reporting Perinatal Mortality and Morbidity. Chameleon, London
Gillies DRN, Lealman GT, Lumb KM, Congdon P (1984) Analysis of ethnic influence on stillbirths and infant mortality in Bradford 1975–81. J Epidemiol Community Health 38: 214–217
Golding J (1990a) The epidemiology of perinatal death. In: Kiely M (ed) Reproductive and perinatal epidemiology. CRC Press, Boston, pp 401–436
Golding J (1990b) Maternal age and parity. In: Golding J (ed) Social and biological effects on perinatal mortality, vol III. Perinatal analyses. University of Bristol, Bristol, pp 183–218
Golding J (1990c) Other factors related to perinatal mortality statistics. In: Golding J (ed) Social and biological effects on perinatal mortality, vol III. Perinatal analyses. University of Bristol, Bristol, pp 299–332
Golding J (1990d) The outcome of twin pregnancy. In: Golding J (ed) Social and biological effects on perinatal mortality, vol. III Perinatal analyses. University of Bristol, Bristol, pp 67–104
Golding J, Peters TJ (1988) Are hospital confinements really more dangerous for the fetus? Early Hum Dev 17: 29–36
Golding J, Sunderland R (1990) Month and day of delivery. In: Golding J (ed) The third report of the WHO study of social and biological effects on perinatal mortality. University of Bristol, Bristol
Golding J, Henriques J, Thomas P (1986) Unmarried at delivery. II Perinatal morbidity and mortality. Early Hum Dev 14: 217–228
Golding J et al. (1992) Factors associated with antepartum fetal death in two continents (in preparation)
Goldstein H, Butler NR (1977) Definition of perinatal mortality. Lancet I: 1254
Greb AE, Pauli RM, Kirby RS (1987) Accuracy of fetal death reports: comparison with data from an independent stillbirth assessment program. Am J Public Health 77: 1202–1206
Hey EN, Lloyd DJ, Wigglesworth JS (1986) Classifying perinatal death: fetal and neonatal factors. Br J Obstet Gynaecol 93: 1213–1223
Hobbs MST, Acheson ED (1966) Obstetric care in the first pregnancy. Lancet i: 761–764
Hovatta O, Lipasti A, Rapola J, Karjalainen O (1983) Causes of stillbirth: a clinicopathological study of 243 patients. Br J Obstet Gynaecol 90: 691–696
Huisjes HJ, Touwen BCL, Van Doorm JM (1979) Perinatal mortality and late sequelae in children born after abruptio placentae. Eur J Obstet Gynaecol Reprod Biol 9: 45–49
James WH (1974) Parental age differences. J Biosoc Sci 6: 93–106

Kamimura K (1976) Epidemiology of twin births from a climatic point of view. Br J Prev Soc Med 30: 175–179
Karlberg P, Golding J, Bolander A–M (1990) Sex differences. In: Golding J (ed) The third report of the WHO study of social and biological effects on perinatal mortality. University of Bristol, Bristol
Keeling JW, MacGillivray I, Golding J, Wigglesworth J, Berry J, Dunn PM (1989) Classification of perinatal death. Arch Dis Child 64: 1345–1351
Keirse MJNC (1984) Perinatal mortality rates do contain what they purport to contain. Lancet i: 1166–1169
Kline J, Shrout P, Stein Z, Susser M, Warburton D (1980) Drinking during pregnancy and spontaneous abortion. Lancet ii: 176–180
Laukaran VH, van den Berg BJ (1980) The relationship of maternal attitude to pregnancy outcomes and obstetric complications: a cohort study of unwanted pregnancy. Am J Obstet Gynecol 136: 374–379
Lumley J, Bakoula C (1992) Perinatal mortality in Greece and to Greek-born women in Australia. What does a "natural experience" suggest? Europ J Obstet Gynaecol Reprod Biol (in press)
Macfarlane A, Mugford M (1984) Birth counts: statistics of pregnancy and childbirth. HMSO, London
Machin GA (1975) A perinatal mortality survey in South East London 1970–73: the pathological findings in 726 necropsies. J Clin Pathol 28: 428–434
McCarthy BJ, Terry J, Rochat RW, Quave S, Tyler CW Jr (1980) The underregistration of neonatal deaths: Georgia 1974–77. Am J Public Health 70: 977–982
McCaw-Binns A (1991) Does antenatal care make a difference? An examination of antenatal care in Jamaica and its impact on pregnancy outcome. PhD thesis, University of Bristol, Bristol
McIlwaine G, Howat RCL, Dunn F, MacNaughton MC (1979) The Scottish Perinatal Mortality Survey. Br Med J 2: 1103–1106
Meyer MB (1977) Definition of perinatal mortality. Lancet ii: 246–247
Mora JO, Clement J, Christiansen N, Suescun J, Wagner M, Herrera MG (1987) Nutritional supplementiation and outcome of pregnancy, III. Perinatal and neonatal mortality. Nutr Rep Int 18: 167
Mutch LMM, Brown NJ, Speidel BD, Dunn PM (1981) Perinatal mortality and neonatal survival in Avon. Br Med J 282: 119–122
Naeye RL (1977) Causes of perinatal mortality in the US Collaborative Perinatal Project. JAMA 238: 228–229
Naeye RL (1978) Placenta praevia: predisposing factors and effects on the fetus and surviving infants. Obstet Gynecol 52: 521–525
Naeye RL (1979a) Causes of fetal and neonatal mortality by race in a selected US population. Am J Public Health 69: 857–861
Naeye RL (1979b) Weight gain and the outcome of pregnancy. Am J Obstet Gynecol 135: 3–9
Naeye RL, Tafari N (1983) Risk factors in pregnancy and diseases of the fetus and newborn. Williams and Wilkins, Baltimore
Naeye RL, Harkness WL, Utts J (1977) Abruptio placentae and perinatal death: a prospective study. Am J Obstet Gynecol 128: 740–746
Newton RW, Webster PAC, Binu PS, Maskrey N, Phillips AB (1979) Psychosocial stress in pregnancy and its relation to the onset of premature labour. Br Med J ii: 411–413
Northern Regional Health Authority Coordinating Group (1984) Perinatal mortality: a continuing collaborative regional survey. Br Med J 288: 1717–1720
Pharoah POD, Alberman ED (1988) Annual statistical review. Arch Dis Child 63: 1511–1515
Rahman M, Mujibur Rahaman M, Wojtyniak B, Aziz KMS (1985) Impact of environmental sanitation and crowding on infant mortality in rural Bangladesh. Lancet ii: 28–31
Record RG, McKeown T (1956) Investigation of foetal mortality associated with placenta praevia. Br J Prev Soc Med 10: 25–31
Rojas Ochoa, FR (1981) Investigacion perinatal by Instituto de Desarrollo de la Salud. Editorial Cientifico-Tecnica, La Habana, Cuba
Ross SM, MacPherson TA, Naeye RL, Khatree MHD, Wallace JA (1982) Causes of fetal and neonatal mortality in a South African black community. S Afr Med J 12: 905–908
Rush D (1986) Nutrition in preparation for pregnancy. In: Pregnancy care: a manual for practice. Chamberlain G, Lumley J (eds). Wiley, London 113–139
Rush D, Alvir JM, Kenny DA, Johnson SS, Horvitz DG (1988) Historical study of pregnancy outcomes. Am J Clin Nutr 48: 412–428
Samms-Vaughan ME, Golding J (1992) Area variation in perinatal mortality in Jamaica: Association with type of hospital services available. In: Perinatal problems of islands in relation to the prevention of handicap. INSERM, Paris, pp 90–98
Scott MJ, Ritchie JW, McClure BG, Reid MM, Halliday HL (1981) Perinatal death recording: time for a change? Br Med J 282: 707–710
Skjaervan R, Irgens LM (1988) Perinatal mortality and mother's marital status at birth in subsequent siblings. Early Hum Dev 18: 199–212
Smits F (1981) De doeltreffendheid van het selectiessysteem binnen de verloskundige zorg. MD Thesis, Nijmegen, p 66
Stevenson AC, Johnston HA, Stewart MIP, Golding DR (1966) Congenital malformations: a report of a study of a series of consecutive births in 24 centres. Bull WHO vol 34 (supplement)
Tew M (1978) The case against hospital deliveries: the statistical evidence. In: Kitzinger S, Davies JA (eds) The place of birth. Oxford University Press, Oxford, pp 55–65
Tew M (1980) Facts not assertions of belief. Health Soc Serv J LXXXX (4710): 1194–1197
Tew M (1985) Place of birth and perinatal mortality. J Coll Gen Pract 35: 390–394
Tew M (1990) Safer childbirth? A critical history of maternity care. Chapman and Hall, London
Thomas J, Edwards J, Bowen-Simpkins P et al. (1985) Use of refined perinatal mortality rate trends to evaluate the effect of a confidential enquiry. Lancet II: 197–199
Tzoumaka-Bakoula C (1987) The Greek national perinatal survey: I: Design, methodology, case ascertainment. Paediatr Perinat Epidemiol 1: 43–55
Tzoumaka-Bakoula C (1990) Assessment of the incidence of perinatal deaths in Greece using two separate sources. In: Golding J (ed) The third report of the WHO study of social and biological effects on perinatal mortality. University of Bristol, Bristol, pp 389–390
Tzoumaka-Bakoula C, Lekea-Karanika V, Matsaniotis NS, Golding J (1989) The Greek national perinatal survey. II: Socioeconomic factors and perinatal mortality in Greece. Paediatr Perinat Epidemiol 3: 43–54
Valdes-Dapena MA, Arey JB (1970) The causes of neonatal mortality: an analysis of 501 autopsies on newborn infants. J Pediatr 77: 366–375
Whitfield CR, Smith NC, Cockburn F, Gibson AAM (1986) Perinatally related wastage—a proposed classification of

primary obstetric factors. Br J Obstet Gynaecol 93: 694–703
Wigglesworth J (1980) Monitoring perinatal mortality: a pathophysiological approach. Lancet ii: 684–686
World Health Organisation (1967) Manual of the international statistical classification of diseases, injuries and causes of death, 8th rev, vol 1. WHO, Geneva
World Health Organisation (1977) Manual of the international statistical classification of diseases, injuries and causes of death, 9th rev, vol 1. WHO, Geneva
Yerushalmy J, Palmer CE, Kramer M (1940) Age and parity as factors in puerperal fatality. Public Health Rep 55: 1195

Chapter 7

Macerated Stillbirth

Isabella E. Moore

Introduction

Despite the increasing accuracy of prenatal detection of birth defects and genetic disorders, necropsy still provides the final diagnosis in many cases and serves as an "ultimate audit". In Berger's view (1978) "Any single autopsy may not have dramatic import for progress in medicine, but it may have profound and life-long implications for helping the dead child's family". Necropsy results are of great importance to the parents of stillborn infants. However, the task of autopsy on a macerated stillbirth is too often delegated to the least experienced junior trainee pathologist.

In recent years, a fall in intrapartum deaths has been observed as part of the decline in overall perinatal mortality rates in developed countries (Georgsdottir et al. 1989). Thus a larger proportion of perinatal deaths is now attributable to antepartum causes. Antepartum stillbirths may comprise more than one-third of perinatal deaths (Keeling 1987). In order to achieve even lower perinatal mortality rates, efforts should be focused primarily on the investigation of antepartum deaths.

The importance of adequate pathological examination of both fetus and placenta has been emphasised by Naeye (1983). The examination of a macerated fetus should not be looked upon as a low priority excercise. The necropsy of a macerated baby may not provide an exact cause of death but it can produce valuable information concerning the time of death, details of fetal growth and development and identify unsuspected malformations. All this information will assist the obstetrician in counselling distressed parents who often experienced the death of their child without any warning, during the course of an apparently normal pregnancy.

Even in the absence of parental consent for post-mortem examination, weight and external measurements, whole body X-ray, photographs, placental examination or even ultrasound scan can be usefully performed.

Changes Associated with Maceration

Maceration (Latin *macerare*—to soften by soaking) describes the softening effect of soaking on solid tissues and is applied to the degenerative changes occurring in a fetus retained in utero after death. Autolysis, due to endogenous proteolytic enzymes, contributes to softening of the tissues and should not be confused with maceration. The earliest signs of maceration are seen in the skin in the form of skin slipping (Strachan 1922), approximately 6 h and certainly 12 h after intrauterine death (IUD). The epidermis can be easily separated from the dermis by applying oblique stress (Fig. 7.1). Loss of the epidermis exposes a red, shiny,

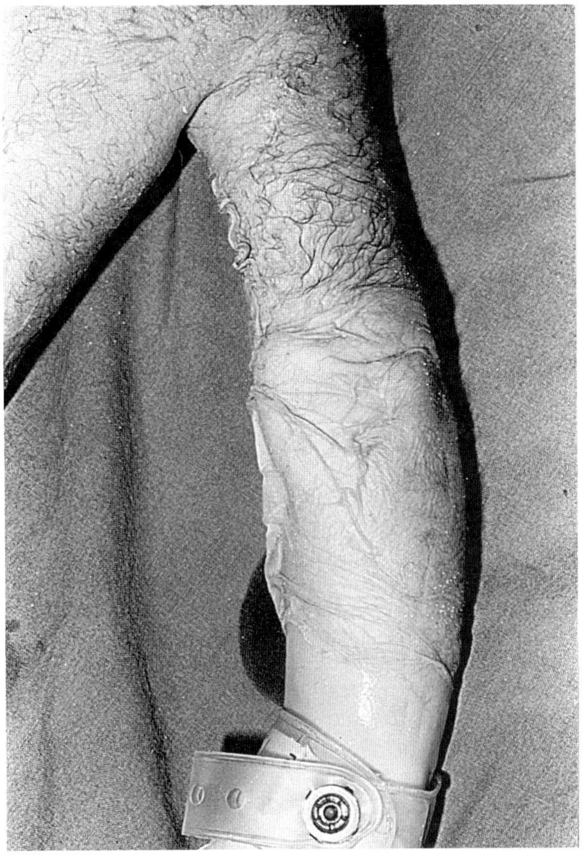

Fig. 7.1. The earliest sign of maceration is skin slipping following obliquely applied pressure, revealing a shiny, moist dermal surface.

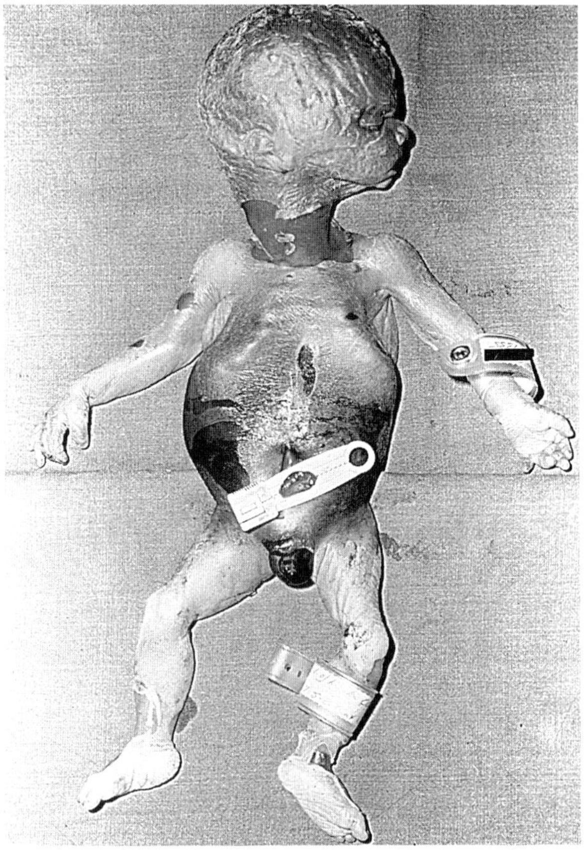

Fig. 7.2. Severely macerated stillborn fetus: the exposed dermis shows dark red discoloration (neck, right flank, external genitalia). There is post-mortem abdominal distension.

moist dermal surface. This is particularly noticeable over bony prominences. Approximately 24 h after IUD fluid-filled bullae are formed between dermis and epidermis. Fetal epidermis loses its integrity completely within the first 3–4 days and scalp oedema can be seen on the ultrasound scan (halo sign). Up to 5 mm of subcutaneous oedema may be present by the 5th day after IUD (Hill et al. 1989). Longstanding IUD may occasionally mimic hydrops fetalis and unusual sonographic appearances associated with IUD should be distinguished from true pathological abnormalities. For example, fluid accumulation at the nape of the neck related to advanced maceration should not be mistaken for a cystic hygroma or occipital encephalocoele.

Approximately 48 h after death, the internal fetal organs and connective tissue show increasing purple discoloration due to haemolysis and breakdown of red cells. Dark, red-stained fluid accumulates in the serous cavities. This should be distinguished from serous effusions acquired antemortem. Proteolytic digestion by kallikrein contributes to increased vascular permeability in a macerated fetus (Singer and Macpherson 1990).

Similar colour changes are observed in the amniotic fluid which shows deep, dark red colour ("tobacco juice") or in the event of passage of meconium, a thick brown ("pea soup") appearance. The volume of the amniotic fluid diminishes following fetal death and the level of alpha-fetoprotein in it may be raised because of a concentration effect and increased fetal skin permeability.

Autolysis of connective tissue contributes to laxity of joints and lack of definition of cut surface margins of the solid organs. The abdominal organs may show green discoloration due to leakage of bile pigments from the gall bladder. In an IUD occurring not less than a week previously, meconium may be released into the abdominal cavity through the dissolving bowel wall. Occasionally, the protruding autolysed liver mass can produce an abnormal ultrasonographic appearance which could be mistaken for omphalocoele (Hill et al. 1989) (Fig. 7.2). Dystrophic calcification may develop in the autolysed liver tissue.

After 4–5 days, the cranial vault bones become separated from the dura and periosteum. Overlapping of the bones produces the characteristic Spalding sign on ultrasound examination. Maceration may permit distortion of the skull during vaginal delivery and may lead to an erroneous diagnosis of hydrocephalus. Squeezing of the autolysed brain tissue into the spinal cord and along the spinal nerve roots into the retropleural and retroperitoneal areas may produce tumorous masses of neural tissue which should not be mistaken for a neurogenic neoplasm (Kalousek et al. 1988) (Fig. 7.3).

When the fetus is retained in utero for 7–10 days, further changes in colour occur, from purple to brown discoloration. During retention of the fetus for several weeks, a fading of colour to yellow-grey will occur. Progressive loss of fluid from the fetus will eventually result in the formation of "fetus papyraceus". Dehydration results in shrinkage and compaction of tissues and organs. Very occasionally an extrauterine pregnancy may be retained for years forming so-called lithopedion (Greek *lithos*—stone, *paidion*–small child), a calcified fetus retained in the abdominal cavity (Mathieu 1939).

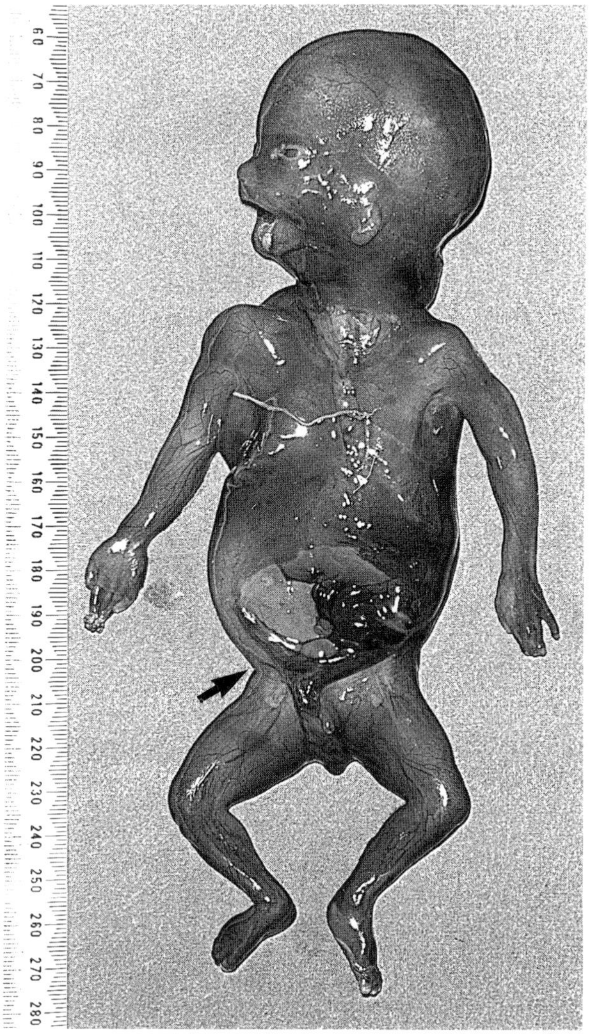

Fig. 7.3. Macerated and autolysed fetus with inguinal masses (*arrow*) of autolysed cerebral tissue; and the cranial vault is collapsed.

Limitations of Examination

Even in the presence of advanced maceration as full and detailed a necropsy as possible should be performed. Some measurements and weights may be altered by the process of maceration, nevertheless, when used together, they may help in evaluation of fetal growth.

Body weight and external measurements should be recorded irrespective of the degree of maceration. Connective tissue autolysis may allow stretching and elevate both crown–rump and crown–heel lengths. In this situation, the foot length still remains the least altered parameter and supplies a reliable marker for gestational assessment.

Overlapping of the cranial vault bones may invalidate the head circumference measurement but if taken with care and used in conjunction with foot length, it may add extra information to the assessment of fetal growth.

In a longstanding IUD, body and organ weights will not be accurate. Organ weight ratios rather than absolute values should be used.

Softening of tissues may produce difficulties in the dissection of the internal organs, particularly when a congenital malformation is suspected as, for example, congenital heart defect.

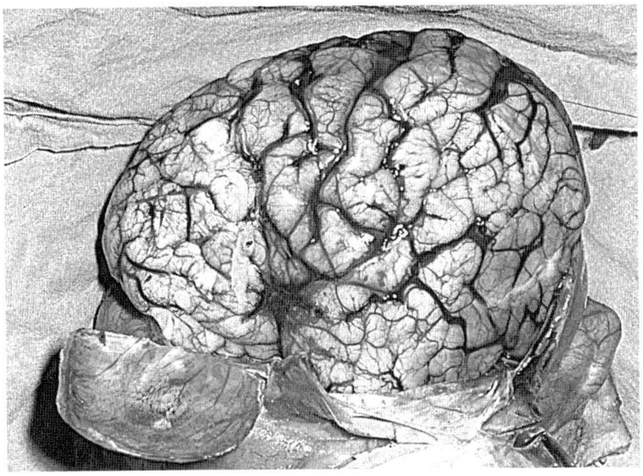

Fig. 7.4. Macerated stillbirth: the skull has been opened to expose the surface of the cerebral hemispheres. The complexity of the gyral pattern can aid assessment of gestational age (consistent with 38 weeks' gestation; death occurred 24–48 h previously).

Brief formalin fixation (for 24–48 h) will produce some hardening of the tissue and permit adequate dissection and demonstration of structural abnormality.

Organs most severely affected by autolysis in macerated stillbirths are usually those from the abdominal cavity (pancreas, liver, spleen, adrenal glands) and brain. The presence of proteolytic enzymes, abundant in liver tissue, accounts for their rapid and extensive autolysis.

Fetal brain with its high water content is very soft and friable even in normal conditions. In the presence of maceration and advanced autolysis, the removal of the brain may be very difficult. Despite the rapid softening of the tissue, the gyral pattern on the surface of the cerebral hemispheres is retained and careful inspection of the gyri after opening of the skull and dura may help in assessment of gestational age, particularly important when there is intrauterine growth retardation (Fig. 7.4).

Removal of the brain into a formalin-filled container has been advocated to minimise trauma associated with handling. A soft cloth can also be used to transport and suspend the brain in a suitable container for fixation with good structural preservation (Fig. 7.5).

Histological Examination

Even in cases of severe maceration, histological sampling of all internal organs should be undertaken. Histological examination can help in the assessment of gestational age at the time of death, the mode of death (sudden or associated with prolonged stress), presence of viral infection or maternal diabetes.

Routine haematoxylin and eosin stain is frequently not very helpful as, with progressive autolysis, there is increased loss of nuclear

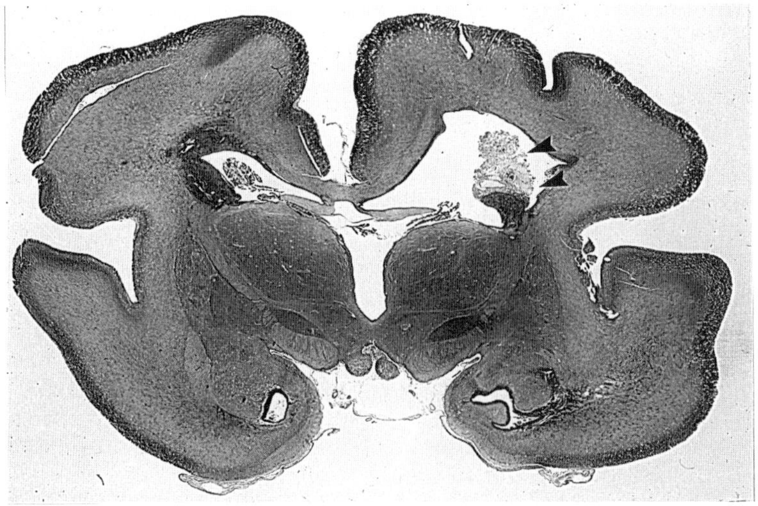

Fig. 7.5. Macerated stillbirth at 27 weeks of gestation. The brain was suspended and fixed in formalin for 4 weeks prior to dissection. This coronal section at the level of the foramen of Monro reveals old intraventricular haemorrhage (*arrow*) (H&E, ×1.4)

detail. However, connective tissue stains (trichrome or reticulin stain) may outline the architectural detail and may enable assessment of organ development and identification of pathological abnormalities. In the abdominal cavity the histological detail of the liver and spleen is lost quickly but kidneys and adrenal glands retain their details for longer. A frozen section of the adrenal gland allows the assessment of the distribution of the intracellular lipid and supplies information about the mode of death (Becker and Becker 1976).

Additional Investigations

Microbiological Studies

There is conflicting evidence about the significance and frequency of infection in cases of IUD. Infection is probably less frequent in macerated stillbirths compared to fresh stillbirths and neonatal deaths (Keeling 1987).

"Amniotic fluid infection" is listed as one of the common causes of fetal death in the US collaborative perinatal project (Naeye 1977). A recent study by Lessing et al. (1989) described a variety of positive bacterial cultures in 28 out of 57 fetuses delivered after IUD. The most commonly isolated organisms were *E. coli* and *Proteus mirabilis*. These findings were not confirmed by histological examination of the membranes and fetal organs and could be of questionable significance.

Genital mycoplasmas are present in 8.3% of stillbirths and neonatal deaths, significantly more often associated with acute chorioamnionitis and funisitis (Madan et al. 1988). However, isolation of genital mycoplasmas from fetal tissues is not associated with increased incidence of IUDs.

In macerated stillbirths routine bacteriological and viral cultures are not justified in every case but should be performed in cases where clinical information and pathological findings are suggestive of infection. These would include not only cases with obvious signs of infection (opacity and necrosis of the placental membranes) but also severe intrauterine growth retardation and non-immune hydrops. In the last two conditions intrauterine viral infection should be considered. Congenital echovirus infection (echovirus type 33 and 27) might be suspected in the fetus with marked haemorrhagic necrosis, particularly in the peripheral muscles, and viral cultures should be undertaken in such cases (Garcia et al. 1990).

Chromosomal Analysis

Chromosomal studies in macerated stillbirths are fraught with difficulties but chromosomal analysis should be attempted in cases with congenital defects, severe intrauterine growth retardation or non-immune hydrops (Pitkin 1987).

Although 30%–35% of stillbirths may have notable congenital defects (Mueller et al. 1983), only 5%–11% of macerated stillbirths may be expected to have chromosomal abnormalities (Carey 1987; Magani et al. 1990). Chromosomal abnormalities found in macerated stillbirths were of the same type as those present in neonatal deaths but were twice as common (11.5% compared to 5.6%) in a study by Alberman and Creasy (1977).

In slightly macerated stillbirths lung and diaphragm cultures should be attempted, but very often the only viable tissue left is that of the placenta. A small sample of amnion (1–2 cm^2) should be removed with a sterile forceps, placed in a sterile container with or without a culture medium, and transported immediately at room temperature. Success in cell cultures from such material varies considerably between different laboratories and published data on abnormal karyotypes should therefore be interpreted with caution. Sutherland and Carter (1983) obtained successful chromosomal analyses from 54% of macerated stillbirths and detected abnormalities in 19% of these.

Radiographic Examination

Radiographic appearances of the fetus are not affected by maceration. In fact, the laxity of joints enables easy alignment of the upper and lower limbs. Radiography may contribute to assessment of gestational age and provides an accurate record of any suspected skeletal abnormalities.

The usefulness of radiological investigation is well documented (Winter et al. 1984). In cases of hydrocephalus, craniolacunae may be identified on radiological examination of the head. Out of 400 fetuses examined in the study by Kalifa et al. (1989), additional information was

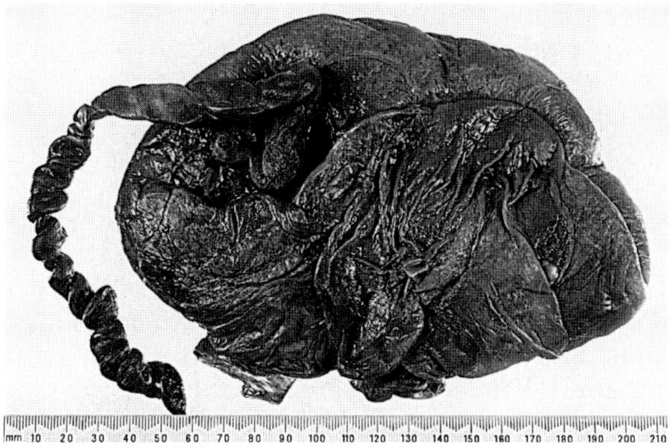

Fig. 7.6. Dark-red discoloration and excessive twisting of the cord in a macerated stillbirth.

obtained from post-mortem radiographic examination in 34.5% of cases.

Ultrasound

In cases where parents are unwilling to consent to a full necropsy, permission may be obtained for ultrasound scanning examination, or ultrasound-guided needle biopsy in cases of suspected metabolic disorders (Furness et al. 1989).

Examination of the Placenta

Placental examination should be considered as an integral part of the autopsy on a macerated stillborn infant. After death in utero the placenta still remains a viable organ and undergoes progressive morphological changes which commence 24 h after fetal death and are fully established 5 or 6 days later (Fox 1978).

Macroscopically recognisable changes associated with IUD include maternal floor infarction (Benirschke and Driscoll 1967). In cases of IUD of a few weeks' duration the placental tissue becomes firm and whitish in colour with progressive reduction of the placental volume.

Extensive subchorial thrombus formation or so-called Breus' mole may be apparent following IUD, possibly related to sudden slowing of the blood flow through the intervillous space.

Following the cessation of fetal circulation, several characteristic post-mortem changes are observed on histological examination of the placental villi. The villi show an increased number of syncytial knots. The number of cytotrophoblastic cells is increased and thickening of the basement membrane is observed. The basement membrane of the trophoblast may become mineralised in the first 5 days after death in utero (Wigglesworth 1984). Many of the villi show prominent stromal fibrosis, capillary collapse and fibromuscular sclerosis of the fetal stem arteries with narrowing and full obliteration of their lumen.

Occasionally, villous oedema may be seen and aggregates of placental dystrophic calcification observed. Calcification is as common in fresh stillbirths as in liveborn infants but, in longstanding IUD, there is a progressive loss of calcium from the placenta rather than excessive accumulation (Fox 1978).

Several post-mortem changes are also observed in the umbilical cord. Oedema and dull-red discoloration, particularly at the fetal end of the cord, are frequently seen in macerated stillbirths. Excessive twisting of the cord has been described in relation to increased fetal flotational movements after IUD (Edmonds 1954) (Fig. 7.6). Usually, it is more prominent at the fetal end of the cord and it should be distinguished from antemortem twisting which remains permanent after the separation of the fetus and placenta (Browne 1925). Histological examination will show congestion, thrombosis and oedema at the site of antemortem coiling and these features are absent in cases of post-mortem twisting. Edmonds (1954) suggested that a cord stricture is another post-mortem artefact due to maceration of the cord close to the fetal end. The majority of such strictures have been described in stillborn infants and probably do not antedate fetal death in utero (Gilbert and Zugibe 1974; Weber 1963).

The presence of true tight knots should be clearly distinguished from "false-knots" represented by local dilatation of umbilical vessels or focal thickening of Wharton's jelly. A previously loose knot might become tightened during delivery. Any cord with a tight knot should be carefully examined for the presence of marked and permanent grooving on the surface of the cord at the site of the knot, loss of Wharton's jelly and constriction of the vessels. The presence of thrombus in the lumen of the vessels and iron-laden macrophages in the Wharton's jelly would support the observation of antemortem formation of the knot. Very rarely a tight cord knot may contribute to intrauterine demise particularly in association with excessive length of the cord (greater than 90 cm) (Keeling 1987). The significance of knots in the cord was disputed by Browne (1925).

Cord and placental complications have been suggested as chief contributory factors in 10%–20% of IUDs (Pitkin et al. 1987) and placental abnormalities as a major contributing factor in 58% of stillbirths (Magani et al. 1990).

Significant pathological abnormalities identified on macroscopic examination of the placenta include retroplacental haemorrhage, placental infarction and opacity of the placental membranes indicating infection. However, retroplacental haemorrhage and infection are not as frequent in macerated stillbirths as they are in the placentae from fresh stillborn infants. The margination of maternal neutrophils in the subchorionic tissue of the placental disc in response to a dead fetus, should be distinguished from chorioamnionitis due to ascending infection. Infarcts occupying more than 10% of the placental cross-section area should be considered as an indication of compromised uteroplacental blood flow (Fox 1978) (Fig. 7.7). Massive areas of infarction may be observed in placentas from mothers with lupus anticoagulant and anticardiolipin antibodies.

Placentas from hydropic stillborn infants are usually heavy, pale and oedematous. Microscopically, numerous nucleated red cells may be detected in the fetal blood vessels indicating severe anaemia.

Haemorrhagic endovaculitis with thrombosis of the chorionic vessels, extravasation and fragmentation of red blood cells were found in 17% of the placentas from stillborn fetuses in the study by Sander and Stevens (1984). The significance of this lesion is uncertain.

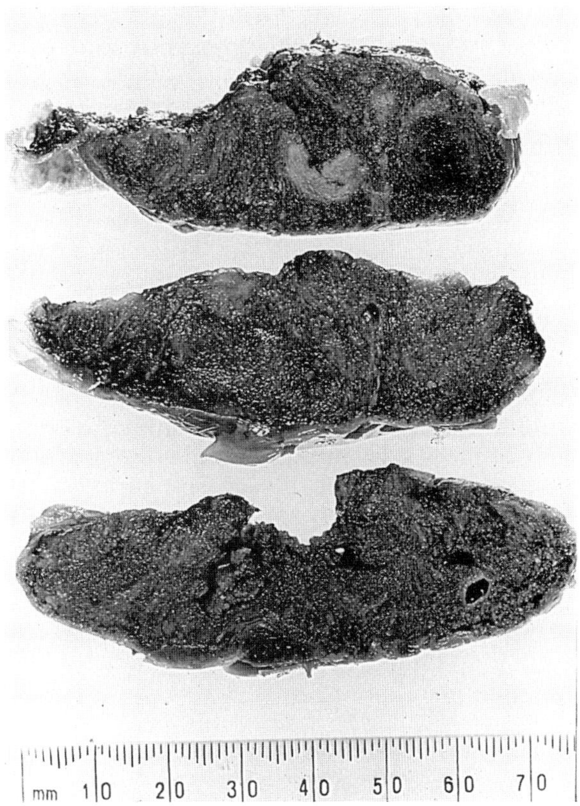

Fig. 7.7. Slices of the placenta from a stillbirth showing numerous areas of infarction of different duration.

Pathological Findings in Macerated Stillbirths

Incidence

Approximately 1% of pregnancies are complicated by death of a fetus after 20 weeks (Pitkin 1987). The incidence of pathological abnormalities in macerated stillbirths is difficult to ascertain as frequently only broad categories are described and only selected findings are quoted. The search for aetiological factors may overshadow other pathological findings which may be considered as of no particular significance.

A direct cause of death is found in only 50% of stillbirths. Slightly higher figures were quoted by Brandt and Holmskov (1990) in whose study the diagnosis was established in 78% of prenatal deaths. Studies by Hovatta et al. (1983) and Magani et al. (1989) quoted anoxic changes as the most common finding in stillbirths but did not distinguish between antepartum and intrapartum deaths. Histological examination was not performed in all of their cases.

Mode of Death

Acute and chronic modes of death can be established in stillbirths by careful evaluation of external appearances of the organs, their weights, the weight ratios and from the histological examination.

In acute mode of death (death occurring within 24 h from the initial incident), asphyxial petechial haemorrhages are detected on the surface of the thoracic organs (Fig. 7.8). Abdominal organs are very congested but with normal weight ratios.

Examination of the adrenal gland plays a crucial role in the assessment of mode of death (Becker and Becker 1976). Frozen sections stained with Oil Red O or Sudan Black demonstrate the pattern of lipid distribution in this organ. In the acute mode of death of a previously uncompromised fetus, there is absence of lipid in the fetal cortex with preservation of lipid in the definitive cortex. A similar distribution of fat is seen in the normal adrenal gland. In chronic IUD, with the disease process lasting for at least 3 weeks, the fetal zone of the adrenal gland demonstrates accumulation of lipid and in such cases placental pathology frequently suggests chronic fetal hypoxia.

Delprado and Baird (1984) reported a very similar pattern of lipid deposition in the adrenal gland and suggested that any lipid deposition in the fetal cortex was a marker of chronic fetal hypoxia. Similar changes were observed by Claireaux (1950) in the adrenal glands of hydropic infants from rhesus-incompatible pregnancies.

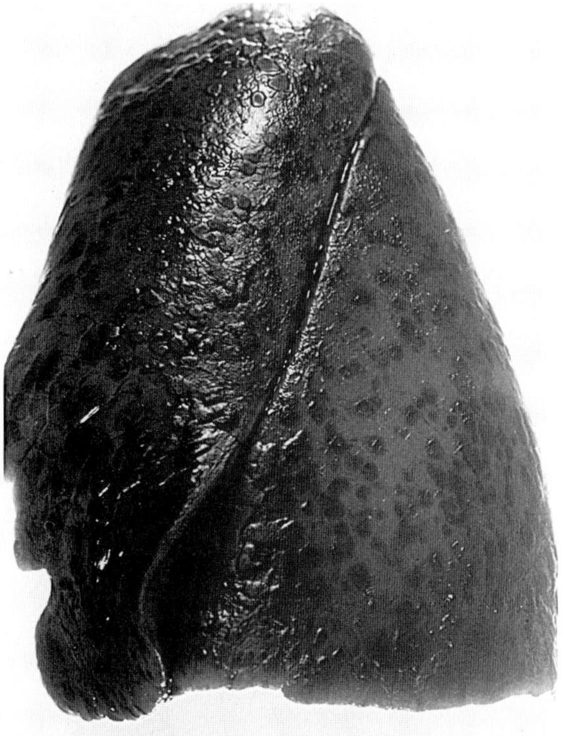

Fig. 7.8. Lungs from a stillbirth: many petechial haemorrhages are present in the visceral pleura. This was accompanied by marked congestion of the abdominal organs.

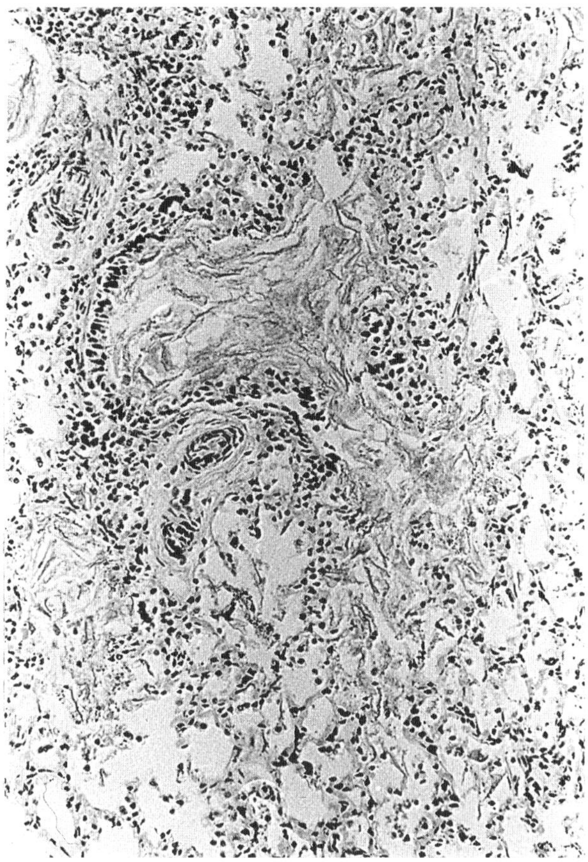

Fig. 7.9. Section from the lungs revealing large amount of squamous debris filling the terminal airways, consistent with meconium aspiration in an asphyxial episode in utero. (H&E, ×40)

Asphyxia

In a study from Scotland, half of fetal deaths were attributed to asphyxia (Whitfield et al. 1986). Pathological signs of asphyxia include thoracic visceral and parietal serosal petechial haemorrhages, squamous debris aspirated into the distal airways, splanchnic haemorrhagic necroses in liver, spleen, kidneys, adrenals and cerebral subependymal/intraventricular haemorrhages (Figs. 7.9, 7.10, 7.11). In a fetus retained after death in utero for longer than 3

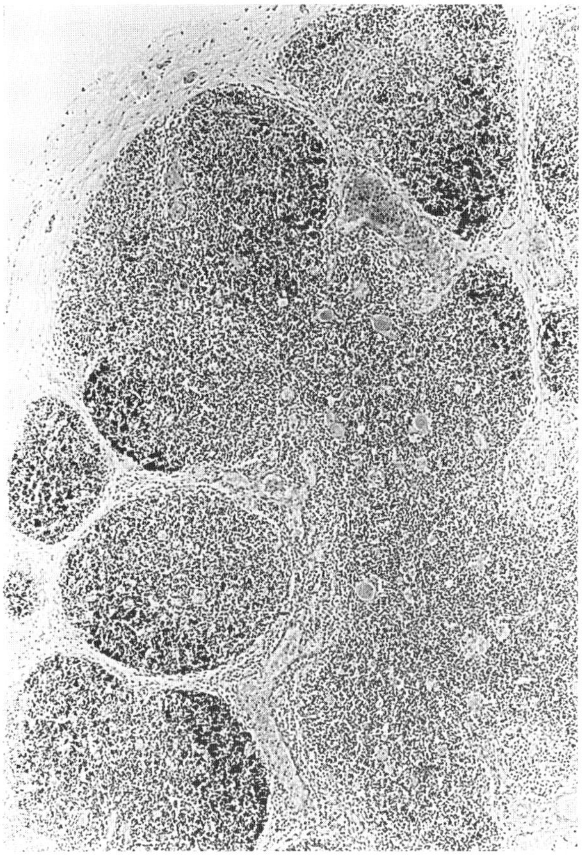

Fig. 7.10. Thymus displaying loss of lymphocytes from poorly developed cortex with exaggerated separation of thymic lobules in a case of prolonged intrauterine stress finally presenting as a stillbirth. (H&E, ×16)

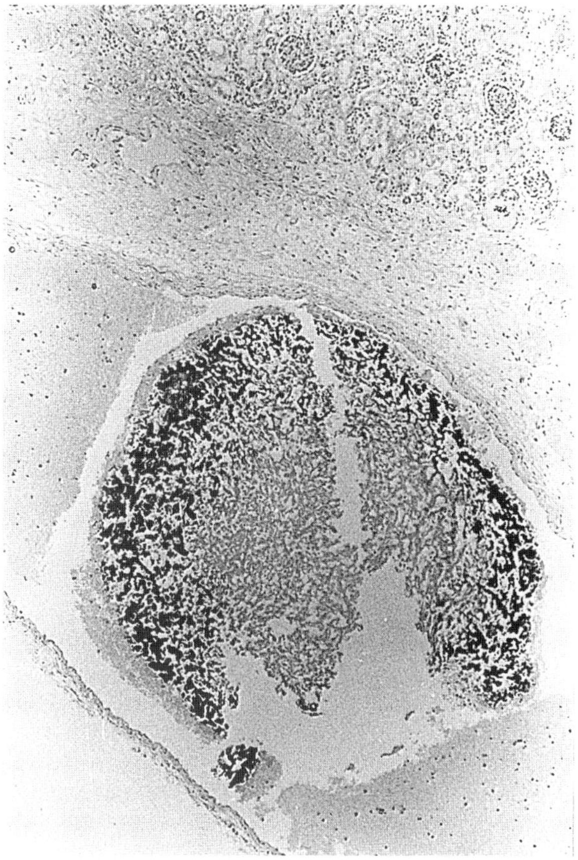

Fig. 7.11. Kidney from a macerated stillborn infant. There is calcified antemortem thrombus in a renal vein. (H&E, ×40)

days, petechial haemorrhages gradually fade away.

Abruptio placentae is one of the commonest causes of asphyxia and contributes to up to one-third of fetal deaths (Kochenour 1987). Polyhydramnios, trauma and short umbilical cord are traditionally thought to be associated with abruptio placentae. This event occurs more commonly in hypertensive mothers (Abdella et al. 1984).

Antepartum haemorrhage due to placenta praevia is not a very common finding in macerated stillbirths. Naeye reported its presence in 11 stillbirths out of 53 518 pregnancies (Naeye 1978).

Cord accidents (true knots, cord prolapse and cord around the neck) accounted for 48% of fetal asphyxia in Morrison and Olsen's study (1985), while a recent account by Magani et al. (1990) supports the view that mechanical factors, including cord accidents are not very common in stillbirths (12% overall incidence).

Cerebral pathology

Ischaemic lesions in the brain, including intraventricular haemorrhage (IVH) and periventricular leucomalacia (PVL) have been documented in fetuses dying in utero before the onset of labour (Bose 1978; Taylor and Roessmann 1984). Approximately 6% of stillbirths are noted to have IVH at autopsy (Harcke 1972). Detailed histological examination of brains from stillbirths shows features of ischaemia and prenatal damage much more often than initially anticipated. Sims et al. (1985) demonstrated IVH and gliosis in 25 out of 433 consecutively

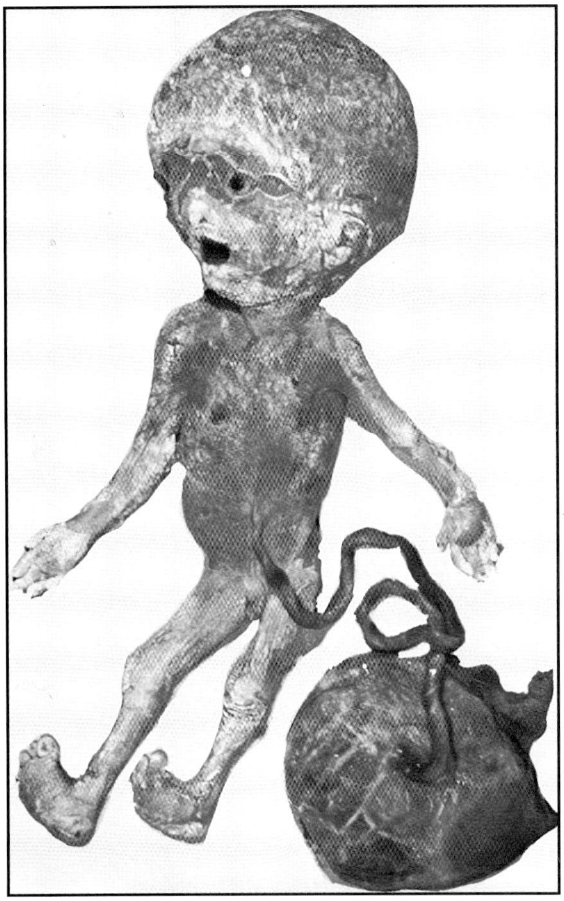

Fig. 7.12. Macerated stillbirth with disproportion of head and trunk and talipes. Culture of placental amnion revealed triploid karyotype.

examined stillbirths. 36% of cases with cerebral pathology were associated with presence of chorioamnionitis.

A recent study from Oxford (Squier and Keeling, 1991) describes the presence of ischaemic and haemorrhagic brain damage in 40% of stillborn infants. The most frequent lesion found in this study was diffuse white matter ischaemia, seen in 26% of cases. This abnormality was only detected in brains of fetuses of more than 27 weeks' gestation.

Pontosubicular neuronal necrosis, comprising neuronal necrosis with karyorrhexis in pontine nuclei and in the subicular segment of the Ammon's horn has been observed in 40% of brains from stillbirths by Skullerud and Skjaeraasen (1988). This lesion was associated with maternal diabetes and intrauterine growth retardation.

Malformations

Major congenital defects are not seen as frequently in stillbirths as they are in neonatal deaths. Machin (1975) described lethal malformations in 11% of 185 antepartum deaths and a 10% rate was quoted by Hovatta et al. (1983). In a study of 253 macerated stillbirths examined in Oxford, malformations were found in 13% of stillbirths (Table 7.1). Many of these cases showed malformations in several systems and, in many, prolonged extrauterine existence would not have been possible without surgical intervention. The most common major congenital anomalies include CNS anomalies, congenital heart defects and major renal anomalies.

The recognition of a combination of defects commonly associated with fetal mortality may provide an accurate cause of death e.g. holoprosencephaly, congenital heart defect and facial anomalies in trisomy 13, or dysmorphism and growth retardation in triploidy (Fig. 7.12). However, the presence of minor anomalies with their overall frequency of 1%–3%, may not by itself indicate a malformation syndrome or provide a cause of death, but may lead to a diagnosis of a common disorder such as trisomy 21. The rate of minor abnormalities is increased in stillbirths compared with the general population. Single umbilical artery has been documented in 3.1% of stillbirths while in the general population it is of the order of 0.5% (Heifetz 1983).

The association of malformations and intrauterine growth retardation is well known. They are seen in 5%–15% of growth retarded infants (Chiswick 1985). The Oxford study documented an increased number of malformations in infants of low birthweight amongst 253 macerated stillbirths (Table 7.2).

Stillbirths with congenital malformations have a higher frequency of chromosomal abnormalities (5%–10%). The most common of these include trisomies (21,18,13) and monosomy X. Stillbirths with these chromosomal disorders may show hydrops fetalis—particularly common are monosomy X and trisomy 21.

Placental Abnormalities

Infarction is one of the commoner placental abnormalities detected on macroscopic examination. It was shown in 15% of placentas from stillbirths (Hovatta et al. 1983). These are usually multiple small areas of infarction,

Table 7.1. Malformations amongst 253 macerated stillbirths (Keeling 1987)

System affected	Details of malformation	Number of cases
CNS	Hydrocephalus; exomphalos; tracheo-oesophageal fistula; oesophageal atresia. Hydrocephalus; meningomyelocoele; VSD. Hydrocephalus; periventricular calcification. Hydrocephalus; exomphalos; renal agenesis; sirenomyelia. Hydrocephalus; exomphalos. Hydrocephalus; ambiguous genitalia. Hydrocephalus. Anencephalus.	8
Cardiac	Cardiac rhabdomyomas; hydrops fetalis. Cardiac rhabdomyomas. Atrioventricular canal defect; asplenia syndrome; hydrops fetalis. Atrioventricular canal defect. Hypoplastic left heart; gross ascites. Interrupted aortic arch; aortopulmonary window; Klippel–Feil anomaly. TGA; VSD; exomphalos; cleft palate. TGA; VSD; cleft lip and palate; minor anomalies. TGA; polydactyly; flexion deformities. Cardiac conduction system anomaly; hydrops fetalis. VSD (3). Sinus venosus atrial septal defect.	14
Renal	Renal hypoplasia; hydrops fetalis. Renal agenesis (3). Bilateral polycystic kidneys.	5
Gastrointestinal	Exomphalos; volvulus; intestinal infarction. Oesophageal atresia; tracheo-oesophageal fistula. L. diaphragmatic hernia; hydrops fetalis.	3
Skeletal	Thanatophoric dysplasia. Absent radii and thumbs; flexion deformities.	2
Respiratory	Adenomatoid malformation lung; hydrops fetalis.	1
		TOTAL 33

Abbreviations: TGA, transposition of great arteries; VSD, ventricular septal defect

Table 7.2. 253 macerated stillbirths grouped by necropsy weight and form (Keeling 1987)

	<1000 g	<1500 g	<2000 g	<2500 g	<3000 g	>3000 g	Total
Malformed	11	11	3	6	0	2	33
Normally formed:	38	37	48	32	31	34	220
Signs of asphyxia	13	14	20	18	19	24	108
No asphyxia	25	23	28	14	12	10	112
Total	49	48	51	38	31	36	253

sometimes mixed with larger and recently acquired infarcts.

Table 7.3 shows the pathological abnormalities identified in fetus and placenta in 220 normally formed macerated stillbirths (Keeling 1987). Placental abnormalities, including retroplacental haemorrhage, infarction and tight umbilical cord knots, were twice as common in stillbirths with signs of asphyxia as in those without such signs. Although not all the placental abnormalities present in this table could be causally related to IUD, retroplacental haemorrhages, infarction and tight knots in the cord were considered as likely causes of death.

Table 7.3. Pathological abnormalities in 220 normally formed macerated stillbirths (Keeling 1987)

	Signs of asphyxia $n = 108$	No asphyxia $n = 112$	Total
Fetus:			
Intrauterine growth retardation	26	7	33
Hydrops with ascites	4	6	10
Renal vein thrombosis	5	1	6
Renal artery thrombosis	1	—	1
Renal cortical necrosis	1	—	1
Inflammatory infiltration of myocardium and calcification	2	2	4
Calcification of myocardium	1	—	1
Inflammation in several organs	—	1	1
Hepatosplenomegaly	—	1	1
Thyroid enlargement	—	1	1
Cardiac teratoma	—	1	1
Neuroblastoma in situ	1	—	1
Flexion deformities	2	1	3
Mild hydronephrosis and hydroureter	—	1	1
Uterus unicornis	1	—	1
Dysmorphic features	2	—	2
Single umbilical artery	—	1	1
	46 (43%)	23 (21%)	69 (32%)
Placenta and cord:			
Retroplacental haemorrhage	20	11	31
Haemorrhage and infarction	33	20	53
Hydrops	2	4	6
Chorionamnionitis	6	2	8
Funisitis	2	—	2
Circummarginate placenta	2	—	2
Tight cord knots	3	1	4
Cord enlargement	6	1	6
Placental artery aneurysm	1	—	1
Iatrogenic vasculitis and thrombosis	—	1	1
	75 (68%)	39 (37%)	114 (52%)

Maternal Disorders Associated with Stillbirth

One of the major factors influencing the increased risk of stillbirth is a history of chronic maternal disease such as hypertension or diabetes. Nevertheless, even increased maternal age (women in their 30s) or a very young maternal age (women less than 20 years of age) are associated with higher risk of stillbirths (Brans et al. 1984; Naeye 1983a).

Maternal hypertension is a major cause of perinatal mortality (Lin et al. 1982) with a higher risk of fetal death when eclampsia is superimposed (Sibai et al. 1984). Abruptio placentae is often seen in hypertension and extensive placental infarcts have been reported by Strachan (1922).

Maternal diabetes is another important cause of perinatal mortality, also contributing to increased incidence of congenital malformations (Ballard et al. 1984). It has been shown that the placental blood flow in pregnancy complicated by diabetes is decreased by 35%–45% (Nylund et al. 1982). Mimouni et al. (1989) suggested that the increased risk of perinatal hypoxia in insulin-dependent diabetic mothers might reflect a "left shift" of the blood–oxygen dissociation curve caused by increased concentrations of glycosylated haemoglobin, in effect producing a decreased availability of the oxygen to the fetus.

Connective tissue disorders in the mother are associated with a high risk of fetal death and recurrent spontaneous abortion in the first and second trimesters. Nilsson et al. (1975) documented a very high incidence of pregnancy loss in women with lupus anticoagulant. Lupus anticoagulant is an antiphospholipid antibody interfering with coagulation pathways and leading to thrombotic events and vasculopathy involving the placental decidual vessels and resulting in infarction. It has recently been suggested that lupus anticoagulant and raised levels of anticardiolipin antibodies are each independently associated with fetal loss and they should be sought even in apparently healthy mothers following fetal loss (Creagh et al. 1991).

In fetal deaths associated with antiphospholipid antibodies, demise appears to be a consequence of the uteroplacental vascular damage. Another mechanism which contributes to a small proportion of fetal deaths to mothers with connective tissue disorders is development of complete heart block in the fetus. There is a strong association between a complete congenital heart block and maternal connective tissue disease. It is present or subsequently develops in 30% of mothers of affected infants. Extensive endocardial damage with fibrosis in the region of the atrioventricular node has been shown in such cases (Steier et al. 1987).

Massive fetomaternal haemorrhage is rare, demonstrated in 0.04% of all births (Laube and Schauberger 1982) but it is probably an underestimated cause of fetal death, particularly amongst macerated stillbirths. Small fetomaternal haemorrhages occur in up to 39% of otherwise normal pregnancies but these haemorrhages are of no significance. Clinically significant haemorrhage occurs when 20% of fetal blood volume is lost (Owen et al. 1989). Even with significant fetomaternal haemorrhage, much in excess of the calculated fetal blood volume, post-mortem findings may not be very striking (Fay 1983). Occasionally, distinctive pallor of skin and mucous membranes may be observed when the fetus is delivered shortly after the incident.

Certain maternal occupations carry a higher risk of stillbirth. Maternal work in the rubber, plastics and textile industries, as well as lead exposure, increases the risk of stillbirth, preterm delivery and small-for-gestational age infants (Savitz et al. 1989).

Maternal smoking is a well-recognised risk factor for fetal death. It is estimated that if all pregnant women stopped smoking, the number of fetal and infant deaths would be reduced by 10% (Kleinmann et al. 1988). Naeye (1980) described an increased incidence of abruptio placentae and placenta praevia in smoking mothers.

Stillbirth and Multiple Gestation

The incidence of multiple births in England and Wales decreased constantly from the early 1950s. This trend was reversed in the 1980s, when introduction of fertility drugs which induce ovulation and, more recently, in vitro fertilisation techniques have contributed to increased multiple births. Mortality in multiple births is about five times higher than for singletons (Botting et al. 1987). Twins were three times as common amongst macerated stillbirths (18 out of 253) examined in Oxford (Keeling 1987).

Intrauterine death of one of twins may not be recognised for some time, although this is less likely with ready access to ultrasonography. Cerebral and renal cortical necroses have been described in a surviving twin after death of the co-twin (Moore et al. 1969). The most common cerebral lesion found in the longer-surviving twin is widespread periventricular leucomalacia. The hazards of multiple pregnancy are discussed further in Chapter 9.

Conclusions

Although there are still pathologists and obstetricians who regard necropsy on a macerated stillbirth as an unnecessary procedure, one study has shown clinically important differences between clinical and pathological diagnoses present in 36% of stillbirths (54 out of 150 cases) (Porter and Keeling 1987).

The necropsy on a macerated stillbirth may be aesthetically unpleasant but this should not deter one from as full and as diligent an examination as possible. This should include histological examination, radiology and cytogenetic studies, and microbiology in some cases: clinical diagnosis was reached after histological examination of the tissues in 20% of stillbirths (Porter and Keeling 1987).

During post-mortem examination of macerated stillbirths, abnormalities which are not causally related to IUD will be detected; these may have clinical importance. Even negative findings after carefully performed necropsy are useful in future parental counselling.

Pathological investigation of stillbirths plays an important role as improvement in the quality of information obtained from necropsies is an essential component of any strategies aiming at reduction of perinatal mortality (Chalmers 1989).

References

Abdella TN, Sabai BM, Hays JM, Anderson GD (1984) Relationship of hypertensive disease to abruptio placentae. Obstet Gynecol 63: 365–370

Alberman ED, Creasy MR (1977) Frequency of chromosomal abnormalities in miscarriages and perinatal deaths. J Med Genet 14: 313–315

Ballard JL, Holroyde J, Tsang RC, Chan G, Sutherland JM, Knowles HC (1984) High malformation rates and de-

creased mortality in infants of diabetic mothers managed after the first trimester of pregnancy (1956–1978). Am J Obstet Gynecol 148: 1111–1118
Becker MJ, Becker AE (1976) Fat distribution in the adrenal cortex as an indication of the mode of intrauterine death. Hum Pathol 7: 495–504
Benirschke K, Driscoll SG (1967) The pathology of the human placenta. Springer, Berlin Heidelberg New York
Berger LR (1978) Requesting the autopsy. A pediatric perspective. Clin Pediatr 17: 445–452
Bose C (1978) Hydrops fetalis and in utero intracranial hemorrhage. J Pediatr 93: 1023–1024
Botting BJ, Macdonald Davies I, Macfarlane AJ (1987) Recent trends in the incidence of multiple births and associated mortality. Arch Dis Child 62: 941–950
Brandt CA, Holmskov A (1990) The prevalence of prenatal death in the community of Viborg, Denmark. Acta Obstet Gynecol Scand 69: 7–10
Brans YN, Escobedo MB, Hayashi RH, Huff RW, Kagan-Hallet KS, Ramamurthy RS (1984) Perinatal mortality in a large perinatal centre: five-year review of 31 000 births. Am J Obstet Gynecol 148: 284–289
Browne FJ (1925) On the abnormalities of the umbilical cord which may cause antenatal deaths. J Obstet Gynaecol Br Emp 32: 17–48
Carey JC (1987) Diagnostic evaluation of the stillborn infant. Clin Obstet Gynecol 30: 342–351
Chalmers I (1989) Inquiry into stillbirths and infant deaths. Br Med J 299: 339–340
Chiswick M (1985) Intrauterine growth retardation. Br Med J 291: 845–848
Claireaux AE (1950) Haemolytic disease of the newborn. 1. A clinicopathologial study of 157 cases. Arch Dis Child 25: 61–70
Creagh MD, Malia RG, Cooper SM, Smith AR, Duncan SLB, Greaves M (1991) Screening for lupus anticoagulant and anticardiolipin antibodies in women with fetal loss. J Clin Pathol 44: 45–47
Delprado WJ, Baird PJ (1984) The fetal adrenal gland: lipid distribution with associated intrauterine hypoxia. Pathology 16: 25–29
Edmonds HW (1954) The spiral twist of the normal umbilical cord in twins and in singletons. Am J Obstet Gynecol 67: 102–120
Fay RA (1983) Fetomaternal haemorrhage as a cause of fetal morbidity and mortality. Br J Obstet Gynaecol 90: 443–446
Fox H (1978) Pathology of the placenta. Saunders, London
Furness ME, Weckert RC, Parker SA, Knowles S (1989) Ultrasound in perinatal necropsy. J Med Genet 26: 368–372
Garcia AGP, Basso NGDS, Fonseca MEF, Outani HN (1990) Congenital Echovirus infection—morphological and virological study of fetal and placental tissue. J Pathol 160: 123–127
Georgsdottir I, Geirsson RT, Johannsson JH, Biering G, Snaedal G (1989) Classification of perinatal and late neonatal deaths in Iceland. Acta Obstet Gynecol Scand 68: 101–108
Gilbert ER, Zugibe FT (1974) Torsion and constriction of the umbilical cord. A cause of fetal death. Arch Pathol 97: 58–59
Harcke HT, Naeye RL, Storch A, Blanc WA (1972) Perinatal cerebral intrauterine haemorrhage. J Pediatr 80: 37–42
Heifetz S (1983) Single umbilical artery: a statistical analysis of 237 autopsy cases. Lab Invest 48: 6p
Hill LM, Macpherson T, Belfar HL, Kislak S (1989) Role of the perinatal autopsy in evaluating unusual sonographic findings of intrauterine fetal death. Am J Perinatol 6: 331–333
Hovatta O, Lipasti A, Rapola J, Karjalainen O (1983) Causes of stillbirth: a clinicopathological study of 243 patients. Br J Obstet Gynaecol 90: 691–696
Kalifa G, Barbet JP, Labbe F, Houette A, Sellier N (1989) Value of systematic post-mortem radiographic examinations of fetuses—400 cases. Pediatr Radiol 19: 111–113
Kalousek DK, Pantzar T, Craver R (1988) So-called primitive neuroectodermal tumor in aborted previable fetuses. Pediatr Pathol 8: 503–511
Keeling JW (1987) Macerated stillbirth. In: Keeling JW (ed) Fetal and neonatal pathology. Springer-Verlag, London, pp 167–177
Kleinman JC, Pierre MB Jr, Madans JH, Land GH, Schramm WF (1988) The effects of maternal smoking on fetal and infant mortality. Am J Epidemiol 127: 274–282
Kochenour NK (1987) Other causes of fetal death. Clin Obstet Gynecol 30: 312–321
Laube DW, Schauberger CW (1982) Fetomaternal bleeding as a cause for "unexplained" fetal death. Obstet Gynecol 60: 649–651
Lessing JB, Amster R, Berger SA, Peyser MR (1989) Bacterial infection and human fetal wastage. J Reprod Med 34: 975–976
Lin CH, Lindheimer MD, River P, Moawad AH (1982) Fetal outcome in hypertensive disorders of pregnancy. Am J Obstet Gynecol 142: 255–260
Machin GA (1975) A perinatal mortality survey in south-east London 1970–73: the pathological findings in 726 necropsies. J Clin Pathol 28: 428–434
Madan E, Meyer MP, Amortegui AJ (1988) Isolation of genital mycoplasmas and *Chlamydia trachomatis* in stillborn and neonatal autopsy material. Arch Pathol Lab Med 112: 749–751
Magani IM, Rafla NH, Mortimer G, Meehan FP (1990) Stillbirths: a clinicopathological survey (1972–1982) Pediatr Pathol 10: 363–374
Mathieu A (1939) Lithopedion developed from extrauterine gestation in intrauterine and extrauterine pregnancy. Am J Obstet Gynecol 37: 297–302
Mimouni F, Miodovnik M, Siddiqi T, Khoury J, Tsang RC (1988) Perinatal asphyxia in infants of insulin-dependent diabetic mothers. J Pediatr 113: 345–353
Moore CM, McAdams AJ, Sutherland J (1969) Intrauterine disseminated intravascular coagulation: a syndrome of multiple pregnancy with a dead twin fetus. J Pediatr 74: 523–528
Morrison I, Olsen J (1985) Weight-specific stillbirths and associated causes of death: an analysis of 765 stillbirths. Am J Obstet Gynecol 152: 975–980
Mueller RF, Sybert VP, Johnson J, Brown ZA, Chen WJ (1983) Evaluation of a protocol for post-mortem examination of stillbirths. N Engl J Med 309: 586–590
Naeye RL (1977) Causes of perinatal mortality in the US collaborative perinatal project. JAMA 238: 228–229
Naeye RL (1978) Placenta previa. Predisposing factors and effects on the fetus and surviving infants. Obstet Gynecol 52: 521–525
Naeye RL (1980) Abruptio placentae and placenta praevia. Frequency, perinatal mortality and cigarette smoking. Obstet Gynecol 55: 701–704
Naeye RL (1983a) Maternal age, obstetric complications and the outcome of pregnancy. Obstet Gynecol 61: 210–216
Naeye RL (1983b) The investigation of perinatal deaths. N Engl J Med 309: 611–612
Nilsson IM, Astedt B, Hedner U, Berezin D (1975) Intrauterine death and circulating anticoagulant ("anti-

thromboplastin"). Acta Med Scand 197: 153–159
Nylund L, Lunell N-O, Lewander R, Persson B, Sarby B (1982) Uteroplacental blood flow in diabetic pregnancy: measurements with indium 113 m and a computer-linked gamma camera. Am J Obstet Gynecol 144: 298–302
Owen J, Stedman CHM, Tucker TL (1989) Comparison of predelivery versus postdelivery Kleihauer-Betke stains in cases of fetal death. Am J Obstet Gynecol 161: 663–666
Pitkin RM (1987) Fetal death: diagnosis and management. Am J Obstet Gynecol 157: 583–589
Porter HJ, Keeling JW (1987) Value of perinatal necropsy examination. J Clin Pathol 40: 180–184
Sander CH, Stevens NG (1984) Hemorrhagic endovasculitis of the placenta: an in depth morphologic appraisal with initial epidemiological observations. Pathol Annu 19: 37–79
Savitz DA, Whelan EA, Kleckner RC (1989) Effects of parents' occupational exposures on risk of stillbirth, preterm delivery and small-for-gestational age infants. Am J Epidemiol 129: 1201–1218
Sibai BM, Spinnato JA, Watson DL, Hill GA, Anderson GD (1984) Pregnancy outcome in 303 cases with severe preeclampsia. Obstet Gynecol 64: 319–325
Sims ME, Beckwitt Turkel S, Halterman G, Paul RH (1985) Brain injury and intrauterine death. Am J Obstet Gynecol 151: 721–723
Singer DB, Macpherson T (1991) Fetal death and the macerated stillborn fetus. In: Wigglesworth JS, Singer DB (eds) Textbook of fetal and perinatal pathology. Blackwell Scientific Publications, Oxford, pp 263–283
Skullerud K, Skjaeraasen J (1988) Clinicopathological study of germinal matrix hemorrhage, pontosubicular necrosis, and periventricular leukomalacia in stillborn. Childs Nerv Syst 4: 88–91
Squier W, Keeling JW (1991) The incidence of prenatal brain injury. Neuropathol Appl Neurobiol 17: 29–38
Steier JA, Akslen LA, Flesland O, Askvik K (1987) Fetal heart block, anti-SSA and anti-SSB antibodies. Association with intrauterine growth retardation, fetal death and lupus anticoagulant. Acta Obstet Gynecol Scand 66: 737–739
Strachan GI (1922) The pathology of foetal maceration. A study of 24 cases. Br Med J ii: 80–82
Sutherland GR, Carter RF (1983) Cytogenetic studies: an essential part of the paediatric necropsy. J Clin Pathol 36: 140–142
Taylor SR, Roessmann U (1984) Hypotensive brain stem necrosis in a stillborn. Acta Neuropathol (Berl) 65: 166–167
Weber J (1963) Constriction of the umbilical cord as a cause of foetal death. Acta Obstet Gynecol Scand 42: 259–268
Whitfield CR, Smith NC, Cockburn F, Gibson AAM (1986) Perinatally related wastage—a proposed classification of primary obstetric factors. Br J Obstet Gynaecol 93: 694–703
Wigglesworth J (1984) Perinatal pathology, Saunders, London
Winter RM, Sandin BM, Mitchell RA, Price AB (1984) The radiology of stillbirths and neonatal deaths. Br J Obstet Gynaecol 91: 762–765

Chapter 8

Prematurity

Gillian Batcup

Introduction and Definitions

The aim of every obstetrician is to achieve safe delivery of a baby whose development has reached such a stage as to enable him or her to be ready for extrauterine life. It has long been recognised that some babies have not acquired this degree of maturity at birth, and are, in the widest sense of the word, "premature". These infants are at risk of increased morbidity and mortality; they are usually small, and many, but not all, have had a shortened gestational period.

Historically, "prematurity" was defined as that state associated with a birthweight below 2500 g, but refinement of this concept has led to the introduction of new terms with more exact meanings. Some small babies have grown normally in utero but are born at an abnormally early gestational age; these infants, who will show signs of organ immaturity and are particularly liable to suffer respiratory distress, are designated "preterm", defined by the Working Party of the Second European Congress of Perinatal Medicine (Neligan 1970) as having a gestation period of less than 37 weeks. Other babies, however, may be either term or preterm, but are abnormally low in weight for their gestational age, usually as a result of poor blood flow to the placental bed, or of chronic intrauterine infection or chromosomal anomaly. These infants are described as "light-for-dates" and show the features of intrauterine growth retardation, described fully in Chapter 1. This chapter is chiefly concerned with the pathology of the preterm infant whose weight is appropriate for the gestational age. This pathology is related to lack of maturity, and especially so in a relatively new group of neonates, the "very low birthweight" (VLBW) infants of less than 1500 g at delivery, who now survive because of expert neonatal intensive care.

The importance of immaturity as a cause of death is illustrated in Fig. 8.1, where birthweight has been taken as a crude measure of maturity. This histogram, derived from the Office of Population Censuses and Surveys returns for 1987, shows that infants within the weight range 3000–3499 g accounted for 38% of livebirths, but only 11% of neonatal deaths. By contrast, infants weighing less than 1500 g, although accounting for only 0.95% of the births, were responsible for 49% of neonatal deaths. The last decade, however, has seen an encouraging decrease in mortality as the result of increasing clinical skills and improved bioengineering in neonatal intensive care units. Table 8.1 shows the neonatal death rates from 1978 to 1986 in VLBW infants and in those weighing 3000–3499 g. In the latter group the rate, which was already low, showed a slight but steady improvement, whereas in the former group the improvement has been dramatic, and there is every reason to suppose that this trend will continue. These national figures are mirrored by reports such as that of Thompson and Khot (1985) who found

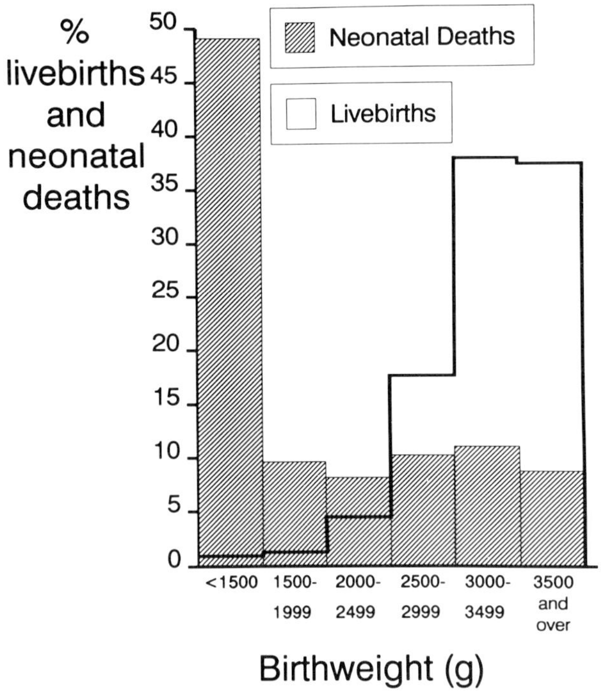

Fig. 8.1. Percentage of total livebirths and neonatal deaths by birthweight, England and Wales, 1987. (Returns for neonatal deaths which did not include birthweight details are omitted.)

Table 8.1. Neonatal mortality rates in two birthweight groups. 1978–1986, England and Wales

Year	<1500 g	3000–3499 g
1978	449	3
1979	455.4	2.5
1980	395.8	2.4
1981	312.7	1.9
1982	293	2.0
1983	295.5	1.7
1984	278.9	1.7
1985	262.4	1.6
1986	262.3	1.6

a decreased mortality rate within their unit in infants less than 33 weeks' gestation and in VLBW infants from 1978 to 1982; they attributed this improvement to the introduction of effective respiratory support at the beginning of this period.

Predisposing Factors

The precise aetiology of preterm labour is largely unknown, but some of the major recognised causes or predisposing factors are listed in Table 8.2. Depending on the obstetric policies of the hospital concerned, one-third to two-fifths of preterm deliveries will occur electively; the proportion of such deliveries has increased in recent years with the knowledge that the preterm infant survival rate has improved so dramatically. The remaining preterm labours occur spontaneously, and it is estimated that in over half no cause can be found (Chamberlain 1984).

Induction of Labour as a Cause of Preterm Delivery

Preterm delivery becomes an obstetric necessity where prolongation of the pregnancy would seriously jeopardise the wellbeing of either the mother or the fetus. If induction is contemplated, knowledge of the exact gestational age of the fetus is all-important, since the danger of prolonging the pregnancy has to be weighed against the degree of fetal immaturity. The accepted use of ultrasound to measure the fetal biparietal diameter in early pregnancy (from 14 to 20 weeks' gestation, when assessment of gestational age is most accurate) has, in recent years, greatly increased obstetric confidence in planning the time of delivery.

Pre-eclampsia

Pre-eclamptic toxaemia is usually manifest in the last weeks of pregnancy, but may present at any time after 20 weeks' gestation. Fulminant pre-eclampsia is an indication for immediate delivery in order to preserve the mother's health. Less severe forms of the disease, although not so dangerous to the mother, will still reduce uterine blood flow to the placenta, resulting in fetal growth retardation. Early elective delivery is then undertaken to avoid the further complication of intrauterine fetal death, with or without placental abruption.

Essential Hypertension

Essential hypertension and the other non-gestational causes of raised blood pressure are usually already evident in the first half of pregnancy. Pre-eclamptic toxaemia often supervenes, and the clinical problems are as described above.

Table 8.2. Aetiology of preterm delivery

Induction (planned preterm delivery)	Spontaneous (accidental or unintended preterm delivery)
Pre-eclamptic toxaemia (Chamberlain 1984)	Premature rupture of membranes (Romero and Mazor 1988)
Essential hypertension (Chamberlain 1984)	Cervical incompetence (Parisi 1988)
Intrauterine growth retardation (Jones and Roberton 1984)	Polyhydramnios (Naeye and Peters 1978)
	Multiple pregnancy (Papiernik 1984)
Placenta praevia (Chamberlain 1984)	Maternal infections (Papiernik 1984)
Rhesus disease (Tovey et al. 1983)	Congenital uterine abnormalities (Myerscough 1982)
Diabetes (Lavin et al. 1983)	Abruptio placentae (Chamberlain 1984)
	Pre-eclampsia (Naeye 1989)
	First and second trimester uterine bleeding (Papiernik 1984)
	Medical and social factors (Papiernik 1984):
	low socioeconomic status
	maternal age (<18 years or >35 years)
	excessive maternal activity
	multiparity (4 or more children)
	previous preterm birth
	maternal cigarette smoking
	Other causes, including early initiation of labour (Huszar and Naftolin 1984)

Intrauterine Growth Retardation

Many cases of intrauterine growth retardation are due to a compromised blood flow within the uterine placental bed and are commonly associated with maternal pre-eclampsia. When fetal growth is poor and maternal urinary oestriol levels begin to fall away from their expected values, the fetus is in danger and delivery will be expedited. The clinical attendants must bear in mind, however, that there are other causes of fetal growth retardation, particularly fetal viral infections and certain chromosomal anomalies, where no benefit to the fetus will be gained by an early delivery.

Placenta Praevia

Bleeding from a placenta praevia usually occurs in the early part of the third trimester, especially at around 32 weeks, when the lower segment of the uterus is beginning to form. Except for the most minor degree of placenta praevia, delivery must be by caesarean section, often before 37 weeks. The risk of placenta praevia in a subsequent pregnancy is 10 times that expected in the population as a whole (Chamberlain 1984).

Rhesus Disease

The incidence of elective preterm delivery for infants affected by rhesus disease has fallen dramatically since the advent of anti-D immunoglobulin prophylaxis. Immunoglobulin is given routinely to rhesus negative mothers within 72 h of the delivery of a rhesus positive infant. The protection so afforded has been increased in recent years by giving immunoglobulin antenatally as well as after delivery. In a trial of antenatal anti-D immunoglobulin administration at 28 and 34 weeks in primigravidae (Tovey et al. 1983), it was found that treatment reduced the incidence of rhesus sensitisation by a factor of 8, compared with the routine postnatal regimen. Protection, although high, was not complete; it was postulated that some failures may be due to fetomaternal haemorrhage in early pregnancy. It is unlikely that rhesus disease will disappear entirely in the near future.

Maternal Diabetes

The fetus of a diabetic mother is at risk of intrauterine death, particularly in the last few weeks of pregnancy. Until recently many diabetic pregnancies ended in induction of labour or caesarean section, usually at around 38–39 weeks but sometimes earlier, particularly if the diabetes was poorly controlled or severe pre-eclampsia supervened. Lavin and his colleagues (1983) reported their experience with 107 diabetic pregnancies. The perinatal mortality rates were 0, 16.1 and 9.3/1000 births respectively among their Class A (diet only), insulin-requiring and total diabetic populations. These rates compared favourably with that of the general population at that time; the improvement in survival was attributed to better care and biochemical monitoring of the mother during pregnancy. Preterm delivery occurred in 7% of the Class A and 19% of the insulin-requiring patients; caesarean section rate was 66% in the latter group.

At the present time, diabetic mothers are usually managed jointly by an obstetrician and a physician specialising in diabetes. Biochemical monitoring includes both blood glucose measurements and estimates of glycosylated haemoglobin levels, which provide an "averaged" measure of recent blood sugar control. However, despite meticulous care, the diabetes may become uncontrollable and severe maternal retinopathy or nephropathy may suddenly appear. Early delivery is now undertaken primarily for maternal wellbeing; perinatal mortality attributable to diabetes has fallen to zero over the last decade.

Spontaneous Preterm Delivery

Preterm Premature Rupture of Membranes and Chorioamnionitis

Preterm premature rupture of membranes (PPROM) is defined as spontaneous rupture of the fetal membranes prior to the onset of preterm labour, and is a common and important antecedent of spontaneous preterm delivery. Over an 8-month period in Oxford more than one-third of all preterm births were associated with PPROM (Zaaijman et al. 1982). Harger et al. (1990) have quoted an incidence range of 15% to 40% in preterm births. PPROM occurs particularly in the late second and early third trimesters and is often associated with an infection of the fetal membranes (chorioamnionitis). There is thus a temporal relationship between preterm labour, PPROM and infection of the fetal membranes, and it is likely that infection may act as a precipitating agent, both for labour and for the membrane rupture.

The importance of membrane infection as an aetiological factor in preterm labour is being recognised with increasing frequency (Charles and Hurry 1983; Drife 1989; Naeye 1988; Romero and Mazor 1988). Chorioamnionitis is best considered in terms of inflammation of the placental membranes, and the histological appearances are described in Chapter 2. The inflammatory infiltrate usually denotes an acute infection, but a more chronic reaction is occasionally encountered. Clinically, chorioamnionitis is suspected in the presence of maternal fever, uterine tenderness, leucocytosis, positive blood culture and purulent vaginal discharge, but such signs are late or inconstant manifestations, and undoubtedly give an underestimate of the incidence of infection. Bacteria from the placental membranes frequently invade the amniotic fluid, and the third mode of diagnosis is by culture after amniocentesis, either by a transabdominal approach, or by means of a transcervical catheter following membrane rupture; the latter method is subject to contamination by vaginal flora.

Chorioamnionitis usually originates in the membranes adjacent to the cervical os, as an ascending infection caused by vaginal organisms, although occasionally transabdominal diagnostic or therapeutic procedures are responsible. The organisms identified have included aerobic and anaerobic bacteria, mycoplasmas, *Chlamydia trachomatis* and yeasts. Naeye (1988) was able to recover bacteria or mycoplasmas from over 70% of placentas and extraplacental membranes that showed histological evidence of chorioamnionitis. The organisms may arise from the indigenous vaginal population, or may be introduced by the male partner. Naeye and Ross (1982), in a study of urban black mothers in South Africa, noted that premature delivery was four times more frequent following recent coitus and in the presence of histological chorioamnionitis, than when either factor was absent, and Toth et al. (1988) found a correlation between premature rupture of the membranes and a history of multiple sexual partners. The organisms responsible for chorioamnionitis may be cultured in the usual way, but more rapid though less specific markers of acute infection have been measured recently. These include serum estimations of C-reactive protein (Fisk et al. 1987) and amniotic fluid assays for interleukins and other cytokines (Romero and Mazor 1988; Romero et al. 1990).

The incidence of histological chorioamnionitis increases with decreasing gestational age at the time of labour. Naeye and Peters (1980), investigating preterm labour before membrane rupture, found 23% of patients at 20–28 weeks' gestation to have chorioamnionitis, as opposed to 11% at 33–37 weeks. This change in incidence is due, in part, to variations in the bactericidal and bacteriostatic activity of the amniotic fluid. Bratlid and Lindback (1978) found that amniotic fluid bacteriolytic activity was increased threefold from the 25th gestational week to term, after which a slight reduction was found.

It was postulated that the lytic activity was due to lysozyme, either alone or with other factors. Other investigators have found that at term a zinc-peptide complex plays an important part (Blanco et al. 1982; Tafari et al. 1977). Tafari et al. (1977) found amniotic infection to be responsible for nearly one-third of perinatal deaths in Addis Ababa, Ethiopia. Of 53 term amniotic fluid specimens which they collected, one was bactericidal, 12 were bacteriostatic and 40 were non-inhibitory to bacterial growth. Higher bacterial titres and lower amniotic fluid zinc concentrations were related to maternal undernourishment.

The mechanism whereby infection of the placental membranes induces labour is not fully understood, but appears to be related to an increase in prostaglandin activity. The factors thought to be responsible for term labour are outlined on p. 205, although preterm labour may not be initiated in an identical manner. Lamont et al. (1985) found that when cultured cells from the amnion were exposed to bacterial products from *Escherichia coli* and *Streptococcus faecalis*, their prostaglandin E output rose considerably. Romero et al. (1986) measured the levels of prostaglandin E2 and $F_{2\alpha}$ in amniocentesis speciments from 18 patients with premature rupture of membranes and positive amniotic fluid cultures, and found a significantly higher level of both substances, when compared to matched patients of the same gestational length whose amniotic fluid was sterile. An evaluation of prostaglandin production by fetal membranes obtained at various gestational ages was undertaken by López Bernal et al. (1989), who found that inflamed amnion and choriodecidua from spontaneous preterm deliveries were capable of generating large quantities of prostaglandin E following short-term incubation. It has been observed that some pathogenic bacteria possess phospholipase activity, and are thus able to initiate the chain of events leading to uterine contraction.

The consequences of PPROM and membrane infection are overwhelmingly those of prematurity (Zaaijman et al. 1982), but once the infection reaches the amniotic cavity, the fetus may be contaminated through the acts of respiration and swallowing, and develop a septicaemia within a few hours of birth.

Cervical Incompetence, Polyhydramnios and Multiple Pregnancy

Cervical incompetence, polyhydramnios (for whatever cause) and multiple pregnancy are all known associations of preterm delivery. McDonald (1980) has estimated that approximately one in five midtrimester spontaneous deliveries is due to an incompetent cervix, and Papiernik (1984) found that preterm labour occurred in 35%–40% of twin pregnancies. These three conditions may act in the same way, as they all tend to increase the amount of membrane exposed at the cervical os, rendering infection of the membrane more probable (Charles and Hurry 1983).

Cervical incompetence may occur spontaneously, but in many cases there is a history of previous midtrimester spontaneous abortion, termination of pregnancy accompanied by dilatation and curettage, or trauma to the cervix (McDonald 1980). Women exposed to diethylstilboestrol in utero also have an increased incidence of cervical incompetence (Parisi 1988). Naeye and Peters (1978) noted a high perinatal mortality rate caused by amniotic fluid infections in association with previous incompetence of the cervix and with polyhydramnios. Paradoxically, cervical cerclage, designed to prevent preterm labour and infection, may actually increase their incidence, either by stitch abscess formation (McDonald 1980), the release of cervical prostaglandins which stimulate myometrial contraction (Charles and Hurry 1983), or by the preservation of an area of membrane already infected as a result of early cervical dilatation (Charles and Edwards 1981). These last authors found that the optimum time in pregnancy to perform cerclage was between the 14th and 18th weeks; the incidence of clinical and bacteriological chorioamnionitis was increased 2.6 times where the operation was delayed until later in the second trimester.

Maternal Infections

The extrauterine maternal infections linked with preterm labour are in general those which are sited within the abdominal cavity. These include appendicitis, acute pyelonephritis and acute cholecystitis (Papiernik 1984). Inflammatory conditions such as Crohn's disease and ulcerative colitis have also been associated with an increased risk of preterm delivery (Sandler et al. 1990).

Congenital Uterine Abnormalities

Congenital uterine abnormalities are a rare cause of preterm birth (Chamberlain 1984), but include abnormalities of fusion of the Müllerian ducts where the uterine cavity is abnormal in shape or restricted in size (Myerscough 1982).

Abruptio Placentae

Only about one-third of placental abruptions occur before 37 weeks' gestation (Chamberlain 1984). Delivery often occurs spontaneously following the haemorrhage, but caesarean section may be necessary to save a viable fetus when haemorrhage is severe.

First and Second Trimester Uterine Bleeding

Uterine bleeding during the first and second trimesters has a high predictive value for preterm birth in that pregnancy. Papiernik (1984) showed that 75% of bleeding episodes occurred before 18 weeks' gestation; these haemorrhages were observed in 34% of mothers who delivered before 35 weeks.

Pre-eclampsia

Naeye (1989) has found an association between spontaneous preterm delivery and both pre-eclampsia and normal blood pressure with placental histological evidence of low utero-placental blood flow (placental infarcts and excessive numbers of syncytial knots). These two conditions were linked with 26% of the 5414 preterm births in his study.

Medical and Social Factors

Some of the more important medical and social factors are listed in Table 8.2; they are not independent variables and many are interrelated.

Several studies have correlated parental low socioeconomic status with increased incidence of preterm birth. Papiernik (1984) quotes the results of a large study in Paris which showed that delivery at less than 33 weeks' gestation was 3.3 times higher in the lowest compared with the highest social class. This may be related to inadequate diet, poor hygiene and to increased physical activity, both at home and at work. In a study of the relationship between occupational fatigue and preterm birth rates, Mamelle and Laumon (1984) found preterm births to increase with the number of hours worked per week. Special risk factors included a standing posture for more than 3 h a day, work involving strenuous effort or the carrying of heavy loads, work at boring or routine tasks, and work in a noisy, cold or very wet environment. A more recent study, however, has related the incidence of preterm birth to occupation, rather than to working conditions (Saurel-Cubizolles et al. 1991).

A history of a previous preterm delivery is a useful indicator of the likelihood of recurrence. Carr-Hill and Hall (1985) evaluated 6572 reproductive careers of certain gestational length, after exclusion of stillbirths, multiple pregnancies and liveborn inductions. They found the risk of preterm birth tripled after one previous preterm birth and increased sixfold after two previous preterm births.

A multicentre case-control study by Harger et al. (1990) identified three independent risk factors for PPROM: antepartum vaginal bleeding in more than one trimester, current cigarette smoking, and previous preterm delivery. The authors noted that nicotine could cause arteriolar constriction and thus decidual necrosis and chronic placental abruption, and they postulated a causal link between smoking and antepartum vaginal bleeding.

Other Causes

A small number of preterm deliveries occurring shortly before 37 weeks' gestation represent the lower limit of the normal distribution curve of pregnancy duration. These babies (about 1 in 5000 of all deliveries) are likely to be functionally mature and cause no anxiety to their attendants.

The remaining preterm deliveries are grouped together and reflect present ignorance of their causation. This group is large, accounting for about half of all spontaneous preterm labours.

There may be a biochemical trigger which initiates labour at an earlier stage than usual. Even the initiation of normal term labour is incompletely understood, and preterm labour may be a quite different phenomenon (Turnbull 1977).

Current knowledge of the biochemical and physiological changes occurring within the myometrium and uterine cervix in preparation for labour has been reviewed in depth by Huszar and Naftolin (1984). Normal term labour clearly represents a complex sequence of interrelated chemical and ultrastructural events designed to promote rhythmical contraction of the uterine smooth muscle following maturation of the cervix. The number of gap junctions joining myometrial smooth muscle cells increases prior to labour, as does the number of oxytocin receptor sites. Oxytocin and prostaglandin inhibit the intracellular sequestration of calcium in storage vesicles and increase the amount of free cytoplasmic calcium, which acts on the enzyme myosin light-chain kinase to promote phosphorylation of myosin and contraction through the subsequent formation of actomyosin. Changes in steroid concentrations result in instability of the lysosomal membranes, and an increase in phospholipase activity. Within placental membranes, this enzyme catalyses the hydrolysis of glycerophospholipids to form arachidonic acid, which is subsequently converted into prostaglandins. Diffusion of these substances into the myometrium causes uterine contractions (Lamont et al. 1985). Maturation of the cervix also involves complex changes, the most important of which are fragmentation of collagen fibres and increased hyaluronic acid and water content.

These events are thought to be under fetal control through the secretion of adrenal cortisol (Turnbull 1977). Most of our knowledge has been gained from studies of ovine parturition. In sheep, cortisol acts on the placenta to stimulate production of androgens from progesterone. Since androgens are rapidly converted to oestrogens, the oestrogen/progesterone ratio rises, and this, together with a rise in prostaglandin levels, triggers uterine and cervical changes in preparation for labour.

How preterm labour may be viewed in relation to the process of normal labour is still a matter for speculation. For example, the fetal adrenal may discharge its cortisol at an inappropriately early stage, as a response to "stress". Alternatively, fetal adrenal discharge may be bypassed and labour initiated by a trigger further down the chain of events, for example increased local production of prostaglandin by the cervix or placental membranes. The elucidation of the many biochemical pathways involved is an important first step in the formulation of rational preventative measures and treatment of preterm labour.

Pathology of the Preterm Infant

The main problems for the preterm infant are those of organ and system immaturity and of iatrogenic complications which are often inseparable from the intensive treatment necessary to maintain life. The more important problems are discussed below; Fig. 8.2 illustrates their temporal relationships. A comprehensive list of complications is given by Gibson (1982), and iatrogenic disorders are discussed in detail in Chapter 14.

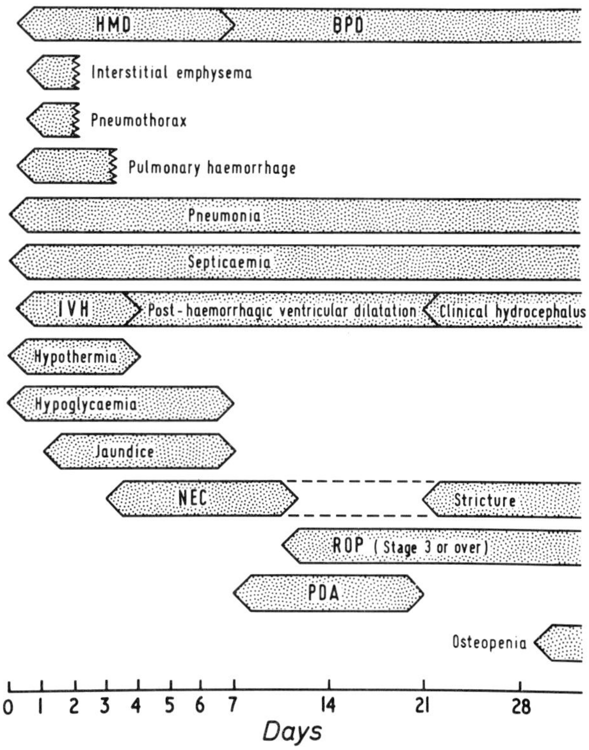

Fig. 8.2. Some important complications of prematurity with approximate time of onset and duration. HMD, hyaline membrane disease; BPD, bronchopulmonary dysplasia; IVH, intraventricular haemorrhage; NEC, necrotising enterocolitis; ROP, retinopathy of prematurity; PDA, patent ductus arteriosus.

Respiratory problems

Hyaline Membrane Disease

There are three essential requirements for the establishment of effective respiration in the newborn infant. First, a sufficient number of pulmonary blood–air barriers must develop in order to allow gaseous exchange to occur; second, sufficient surfactant should be generated and released; and, third, the airways must be cleared of fluid and the pulmonary vascular resistance must fall.

The anatomical development of the lung has been summarised by Whittle (1984), and a brief résumé is given here. At about 6 weeks after fertilisation the trachea and the main and subsidiary bronchi have developed. In the pseudoglandular phase (7–17 weeks) there is further extensive branching of the respiratory tree with cartilage formation. The most peripheral branches are lined by glandular epithelium with clear cytoplasm, which secretes fluid into the lumen. The glands are separated by mesenchyme and not intimately related to the developing pulmonary vascular system. During the canalicular phase (18–24 weeks) the walls of the terminal bronchioles become thinner as the result of a decrease in height of the lining cells. A capillary plexus develops around the terminal bronchioles. The terminal sac phase (24 weeks to term) is characterised by subdivision into respiratory bronchioles and terminal saccules. Effective gaseous exchange is possible via rudimentary blood–air barriers in some infants born as early as 24–26 weeks, but true alveoli do not appear until near term. Alveolar development continues after birth for up to 8 years and size of alveoli increases until maturity (Hislop and Reid 1974).

Surfactant is a complex of proteins, salts, neutral lipids and phospholipids, of which the most important are phosphatidylcholine and phosphatidylglycerol. It is manufactured by type II pneumocytes in terminal air passages. Although these cells produce characteristic osmiophilic granules as early as 20–24 weeks of gestation, surfactant is not made in large quantities until about 34 weeks. It has three major functions. It lowers the surface tension of peripheral airways, thus preventing their collapse on expiration and allowing respiratory movements to be accomplished with less effort. It seems to protect the delicate lung tissue against the effects of oxygen, either at atmospheric or increased tensions. Surfactant also helps to clear the lungs of fluid following the first breath. Adrenaline is elevated in the fetus during labour and promotes both surfactant release and lung fluid absorption; it is more effective at term than during preterm labour.

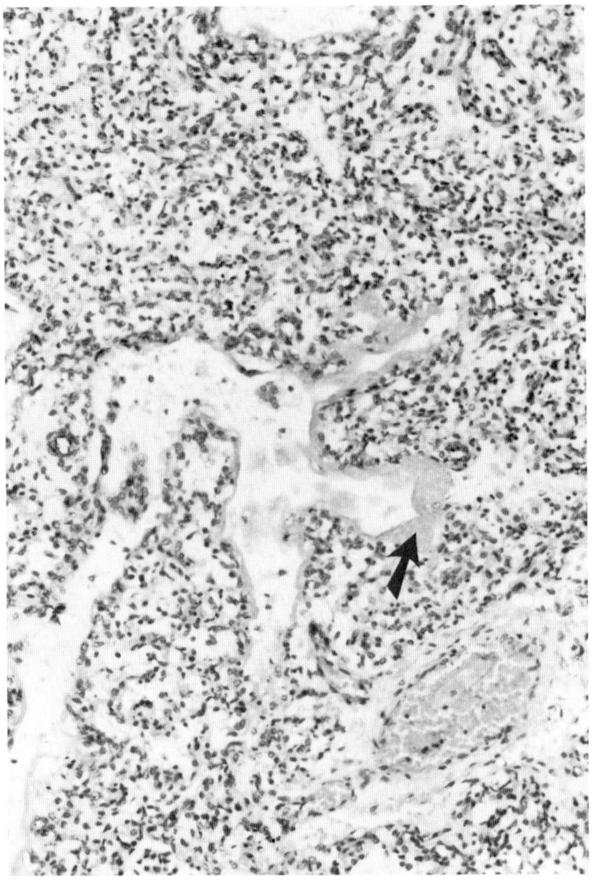

Fig. 8.3. Hyaline membrane disease. The bronchioles and terminal bronchioles are patent, but their epithelium has been partially replaced by a hyaline membrane (*arrow*). The surrounding air saccules are collapsed. (H&E, ×130)

An infant born much before term is likely to be deficient in both surfactant and alveoli. Damage to peripheral airways epithelium ensues and results, within a few hours, in *hyaline membrane disease* (HMD). This is characterised by progressive tachypnoea and inspiratory indrawing of a mechanically unstable chest wall; however, other respiratory disorders, notably pulmonary infection or diffuse haemorrhage, may produce a similar clinical picture. Babies dying in the early stages of HMD, or "idiopathic" respiratory distress syndrome, have plum-coloured, poorly aerated lungs, which microscopically show collapse of air saccules caused by insufficient surfactant production. Peripheral airways supplying the saccules (bronchioles and terminal bronchioles), being cylindrical rather than spherical and having a more robust connective tissue support, remain open and may become distended. These aerated peripheral airways are damaged by air in the absence of surfactant and after a few hours membranes composed of extravasated plasma proteins and necrotic epithelium are apparent (Fig. 8.3). The majority of babies with HMD are now mechanically ventilated to improve tissue oxygenation, but this procedure has its own dangers. The fragile airways may be overdistended and finally rupture, causing interstitial emphysema; this is sometimes so marked as to result in macroscopic lung "cysts", causing compression of vessels and airways (Fig. 8.4). Subsequent rupture of the pleural surface will result in a pneumothorax, which bears a temporal relationship with intraventricular haemorrhage (see Fig. 8.2); air may also find its way into the pericardial or peritoneal cavities or even the systemic circulation. Drainage of a pneumothorax may result in the relatively rigid tube piercing and entering the lung itself (Fig. 8.5).

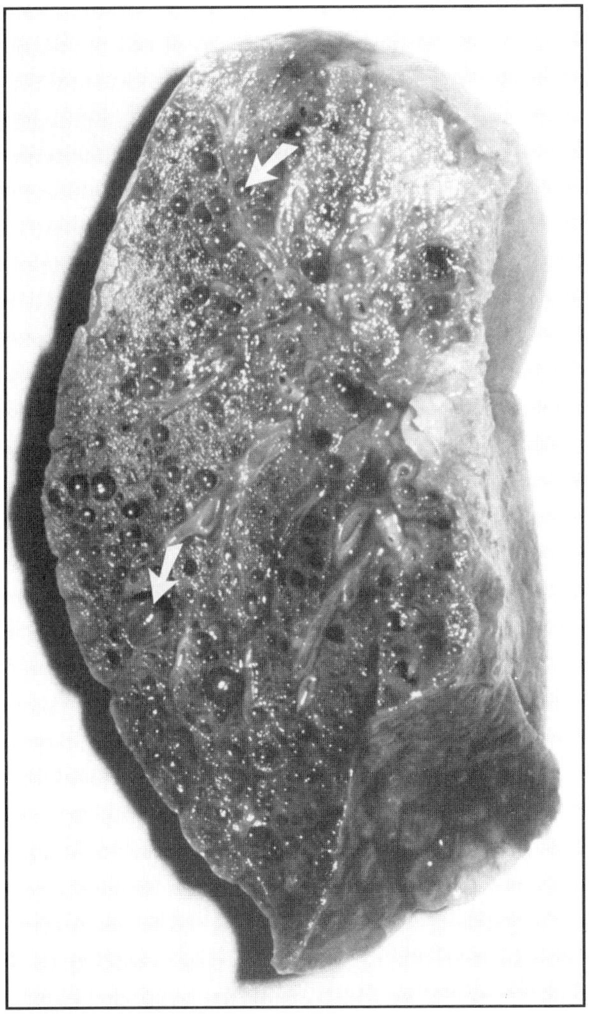

Fig. 8.4. Pulmonary interstitial empysema. When severe, the emphysema produces macroscopic "cysts" (*arrows*), which must be distinguished from congenital cystic disorders of the lung.

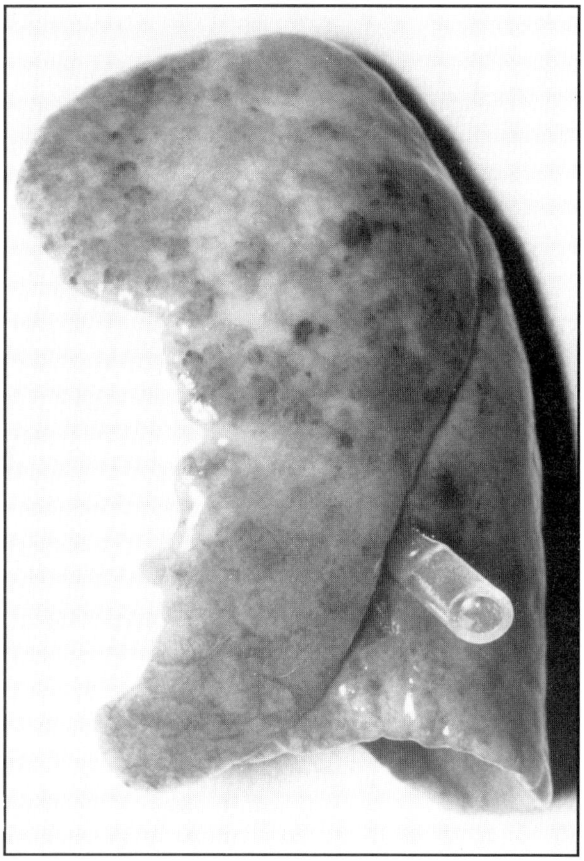

Fig. 8.5. The rigid catheter inserted into the pleural cavity to drain a pneumothorax has pierced the visceral pleura and entered the lung substance.

Bronchopulmonary Dysplasia

In the majority of infants with HMD the abnormalities resolve and ventilator treatment

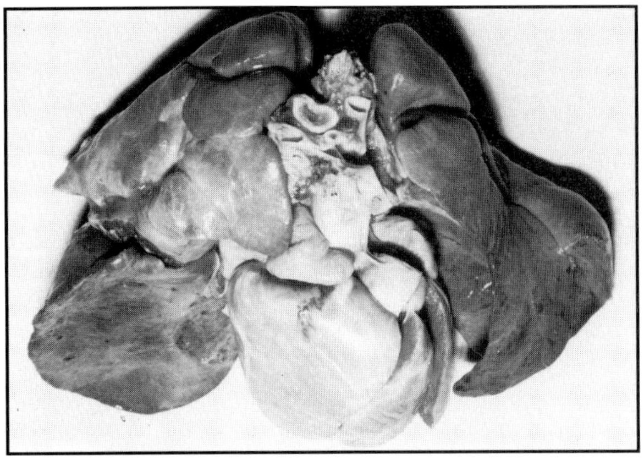

Fig. 8.6. Bronchopulmonary dysplasia. The lungs are voluminous and show a random distribution of collapsed and overinflated areas. The heart is enlarged because of right ventricular hypertrophy.

can be discontinued after a few days. However, a few babies require prolonged ventilation for weeks or even months, and develop *bronchopulmonary dysplasia* (BPD), characterised by pulmonary repair and regeneration. These changes were not infrequent 20–25 years ago when mechanical ventilation was introduced into neonatal units; for a description of the severe changes then encountered see Taghizadeh and Reynolds (1976). These authors drew attention to a correlation between severe BPD at necropsy and high peak airways pressure during ventilation; other causative factors are discussed in Chapter 14 (see p. 332).

The lungs of infants with BPD are voluminous and have randomly distributed areas of collapse and overinflation (Fig. 8.6). The heart is invariably enlarged as the result of hypertrophy of the right ventricle, and the ductus arteriosus remains patent. Microscopically, in severe BPD there is interstitial fibrosis (Fig. 8.7a); fibroblasts extend into terminal airways and produce focal persistent collapse of the peripheral lung. There is epithelial regeneration in bronchi with squamous metaplasia, which may be so exuberant as to contribute to airways obstruction. Lobular arteries show medial hypertrophy, and those infants dying later exhibit diminished alveolar formation. Changes of this severity are a rarity now; despite the occurrence of clinical respiratory distress and macroscopic pulmonary abnormality, the microscopic changes are more subtle. In the non-emphysematous areas the amount of interstitial tissue is usually increased by young fibrous tissue which cannot generally be demonstrated by conventional collagen stains. In addition, there are scattered eosinophilic "membranes" containing elastic fibres and elongated nuclei which line some of the distorted peripheral airways (Fig. 8.7b). It is possible that these may contribute to the loss of blood–air barriers; they may perhaps represent organisation of hyaline membranes. Obliterative and epithelial proliferative changes are now rare.

Pulmonary Haemorrhage

Petechial haemorrhages within the interstitial tissue and lumen of the airways are common in neonates of all gestational ages, particularly if there has been an episode of hypoxia. Massive pulmonary haemorrhage, which is, in fact, haemorrhagic oedema, can be difficult to distinguish clinically from HMD. It is also associated with perinatal asphyxia. The preterm baby, with an increased liability to infection, may develop a consumptive coagulopathy and, because of hepatic immaturity, may be deficient in many clotting factors, the levels of which cannot be raised by administration of vitamin K.

Apnoea

Apnoea is defined as a respiratory pause of 20 s or longer (Rigatto 1982). Its frequent occurrence in preterm infants—90% at 28 weeks' gestation—has resulted in a policy of elective ventilation from birth for many very small babies. Apnoea in VLBW infants is thought to be due to immaturity of the central control of respiration. Ventilatory sensitivity and response to inhaled CO_2 is less in preterm than in term infants. Prolonged apnoea is a serious occurrence, leading to a lowered arterial oxygen tension, bradycardia and ultimate brain damage.

Many of the established complications of prematurity are likely to produce episodes of apnoea. Even mild hypoxia can result in apnoea, the initial stimulation of ventilatory rate being followed by respiratory depression. Furthermore, worsening hypoxia diminishes sensitivity to increasing CO_2 levels. Severe HMD and patent ductus arteriosus with its associated pulmonary oedema are often complicated by apnoeic spells. Pneumonia and other infections give rise to apnoea both by a

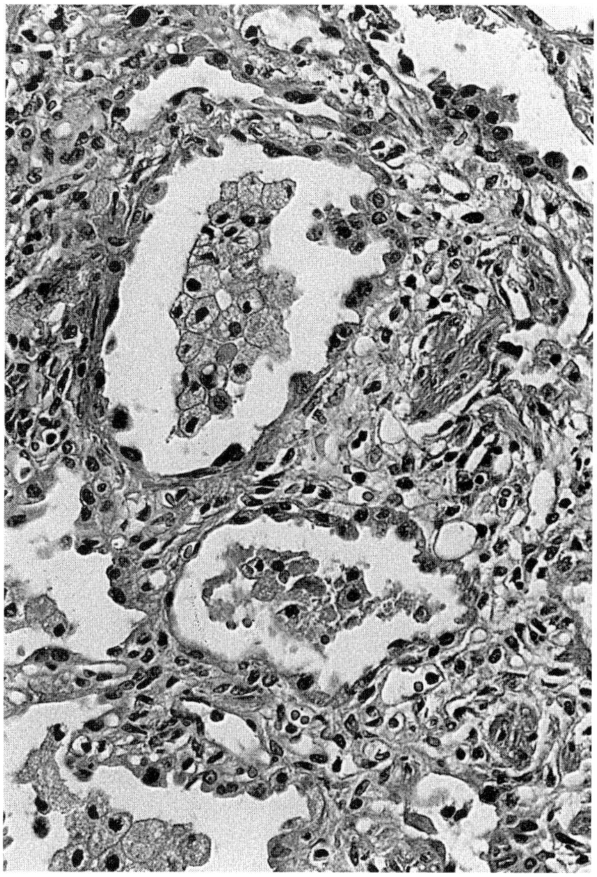

a

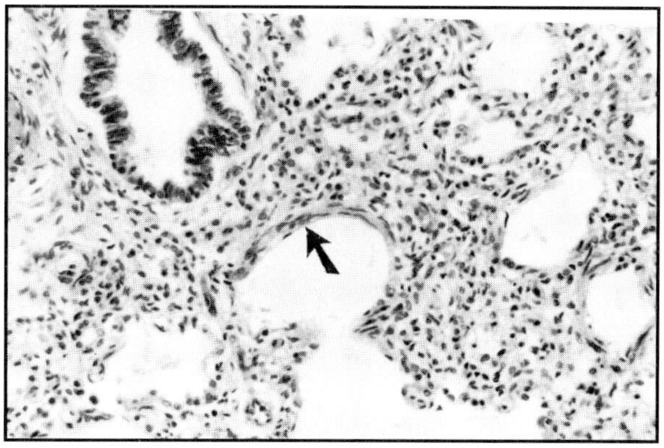

b

Fig. 8.7. **a** Interstitial fibrosis in the lung of a 4-month old male infant, born at 35 weeks' gestation with severe birth asphyxia. There is marked hypertrophy and desquamation of the alveolar lining cells. (H&E, ×294). **b** Bronchopulmonary dysplasia. The interstitial tissue is increased in thickness. Nucleated "membranes" (*arrow*) line some of the peripheral airways. (H&E, ×140)

peripheral action on the lungs and a central depressive effect on the respiratory centre.

Other causes of apnoea include birth asphyxia, cerebral birth trauma, intraventricular haemorrhage, hypothermia, hypoglycaemia and hypocalcaemia. Oversedation of the mother before delivery may also depress the infant's respiratory drive.

Problems of the Central Nervous System

Intraventricular Haemorrhage

Germinal layer haemorrhage (GLH) and intraventricular haemorrhage (IVH) are common neurological events in the preterm infant and are directly related to the development of HMD and other causes of respiratory difficulty. The haemorrhage originates within the periventricular germinal matrix layer, which is packed with small cells from which are derived glial cells and the migrating neuroblasts destined for the cerebral cortex. The germinal matrix layer is prominent in the early stages of development up to at least 24 weeks' gestation. By 31–32 weeks, however, the width of the layer is reduced by half and only remnants can be identified at 36 weeks (Szymonowicz et al. 1984). GLH can spread into the lateral ventricle or the adjacent parenchyma (Fig. 8.8). If ventricular involvement is substantial, blood tracks downwards through the ventricular system to reach the subarachnoid space and accumulates particularly over the lower brain stem and inferior surfaces of the cerebellar hemispheres (Fig. 8.9). Blood is sometimes also present in the subdural space, without evidence of a dural tear or injury to the vein of Galen, and in such cases is probably secondary to dural haemorrhages of hypoxic origin.

Parenchymal extension of a GLH is not the only cause of haemorrhages near the angle of the lateral ventricle, and the differential diagnosis must include bleeding into an area of periventricular leucomalacia and localised venous infarction. In GLH, sudden extension of haemorrhage is usually fatal, and the picture is that of white matter torn apart by the bleeding. A more restricted area of haemorrhage with infarction may be due to local venous compression caused by the ventricular dilatation, and the lesion is closely apposed to the ependymal lining. In periventricular leucomalacia the primary pathology is of infarction in a watershed zone, and at the edge of the haemorrhage one can distinguish necrotic tissue with reactive microglia; the infarct is often separated

a

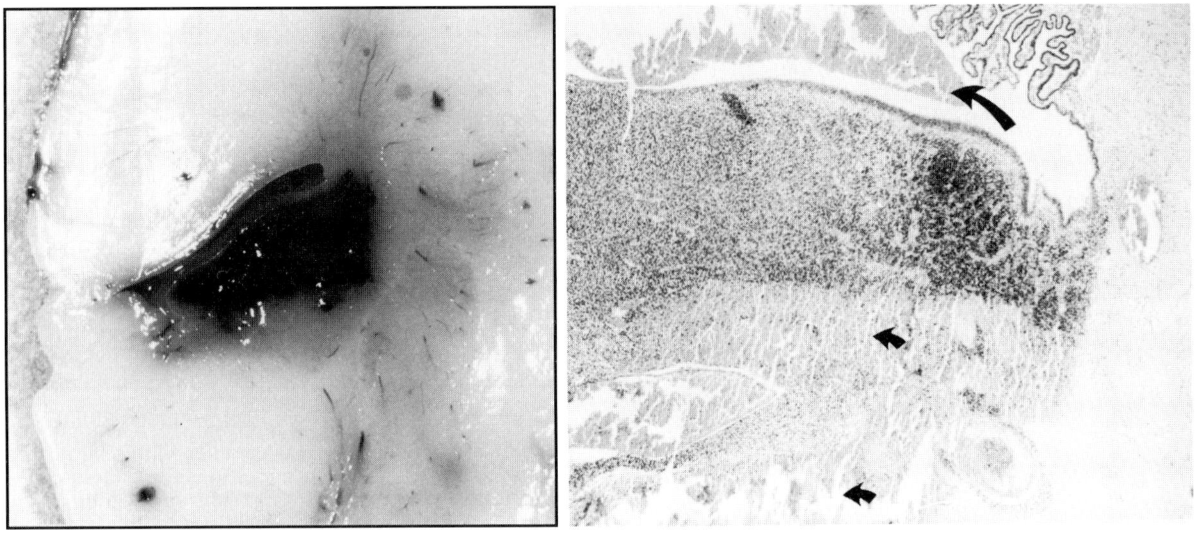

b

Fig. 8.8. **a** Germinal layer haemorrhage with minimal extension into the parenchyma. **b** Haemorrhage within the deeper parts of the germinal matrix layer (*short arrows*) has at some other point burst through the ependyma to form an intraventricular haemorrhage (*long arrow*). (H&E, ×30)

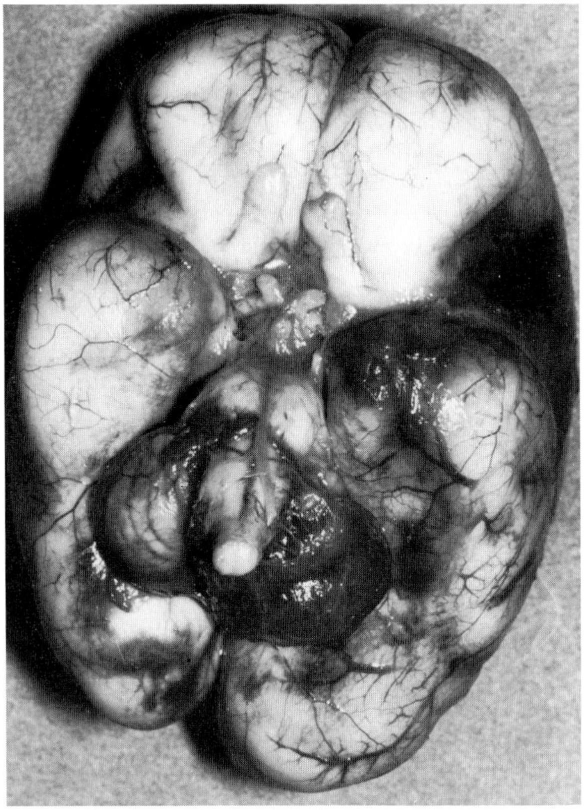

Fig. 8.9. A large intaventricular haemorrhage has tracked down through the ventricular system to reach the subarachnoid space. The blood accumulates within the Sylvian fissures and covers the inferior surface of the cerebellar hemispheres.

from the ventricular cavity by a narrow strip of normal brain. As a further complication, periventricular leucomalacia and GLH may coexist.

GLH and IVH were previously considered terminal, catastrophic events, but the advent of CT scans and, more recently, ultrasound examination in neonatal units has revealed that only about one-half of these haemorrhages are correctly predicted on the basis of clinical criteria (Tarby and Volpe 1982). The incidence of GLH is related to gestational age. Szymonowicz et al. (1984) found that progressive involution of the germinal matrix layer with increasing gestational age was parallelled by a reduction in the incidence of GLH. At 23–24 weeks' gestation the incidence of GLH was 80%, dropping to 32% at 31–32 weeks and zero at 35–36 weeks.

The pathogenesis of GLH is complex, but elucidation of these problems has been greatly stimulated by Wigglesworth and Pape (1978), who stressed that the vascular anatomy of the developing brain changes from a predominantly basal ganglia-orientated pattern at 24 weeks to a cortically orientated pattern at 34 weeks, and that autoregulation of the cerebral circulation may break down in the sick, hypoxic neonate. At 24 weeks' gestation the basal ganglia and adjacent germinal matrix tissue have a well-developed arterial supply, particularly via Heubner's artery; thus it was postulated that blood flow must normally be increased in this area at this stage of gestation.

Pasternak et al. (1982), using the unanaesthetised newborn beagle pup as a model for IVH, studied regional cerebral blood flow by means of a labelled blood flow indicator and subsequent quantitative autoradiography of brain slices. Germinal matrix blood flow was low, with a mean value one-eighth and one-sixth of that calculated for the cerebral cortex and caudate nucleus respectively. This low flow seems at first to be at variance with the presence of dilated vessels in the germinal matrix in the brains of preterm infants dying with IVH. However, it appears that cerebral blood flow control is lost once a neonate becomes hypoxic. In the human adult, blood flow is controlled within a physiological range of blood pressure by changes in cerebrovascular resistance, largely independent of autonomic stimuli and dependent rather on local metabolic activity (Wigglesworth and Pape 1978). In the infant with respiratory distress, arterial hypoxia and hypercarbia dilate the cerebral vessels and autoregulation of flow is lost. Lou et al. (1979), using the ^{133}Xe clearance technique in hypoxic infants, showed that cerebral blood flow became dependent upon blood pressure (pressure passive cerebral blood flow). Continuous arterial blood pressure recordings via umbilical catheters are now routine in neonatal intensive care units, and the tracings show that wide swings of blood pressure can accompany apnoeic episodes, fits, therapeutic or diagnostic procedures, and spontaneous pneumothorax.

Hill et al. (1981) have investigated the relationship between pneumothorax and IVH in preterm infants. Using a Doppler technique, they measured blood flow velocity in the anterior cerebral arteries and found that the mean diastolic amplitude of flow was increased following spontaneous pneumothorax, and that this was reflected in an increase in systemic mean and diastolic blood pressure; all nine infants with tension pneumothorax developed an IVH soon afterwards. The sequence of events is thought to be as follows: pneumothorax increases intrathoracic pressure, which by decreasing venous return to the heart decreases cardiac output. There is then a reflex rise in systemic peripheral vascular resistance with an increase in mean and diastolic blood pressure, which is mirrored in increased cerebral diastolic flow velocity.

However, pressure and flow changes in vessels of the germinal matrix are only part of the answer. The vessels themselves are thin walled and poorly supported. Preterm babies are vitamin E-deficient compared with mature infants; vitamin E administration to a group of babies under 32 weeks' gestation reduced the incidence of IVH from 56.3% in controls to 18.8% in supplemented babies (Chiswick et al. 1983). It was suggested initially that vitamin E, an antioxidant, might protect the integrity of endothelial cell membranes; if so, a reduction in the incidence of haemorrhage confined to the germinal layer might be expected, but none has been demonstrated (Law et al. 1990). The germinal matrix itself may play a role in the development of GLH, since it is known to be rich in fibrinolytic factors; prophylactic administration of fresh frozen plasma to infants in neonatal intensive care units appears to reduce substantially the incidence of GLH and IVH (Beverley et al. 1985).

Post-haemorrhagic Hydrocephalus

In many of those infants who survive IVH, the blood will disperse, leaving little to show apart from distortion of the ventricular outline and one or more small cysts in the region of the germinal matrix layer when haemorrhage there has been extensive (Fig. 8.10a,b). These cysts have a lining of neuroglial tissue and are often traversed by small blood vessels; they may contain haemosiderin aggregates, but frequently do not. In a few infants, blood or tissue debris may block the ventricular pathway, or else cause obstruction to the flow of cerebrospinal fluid by means of an obliterative arachnoiditis, especially over the caudal aspects of the posterior fossa structures. At first the ventricular system will enlarge without an increase in head circumference (post-haemorrhagic ventricular dilatation), but later clinical hydrocephalus becomes apparent; drainage of cerebrospinal fluid by means of a ventriculoperitoneal shunt is often required (Fig. 8.11).

Periventricular Leucomalacia

Periventricular leucomalacia (PVL) is the term given to areas of cerebral necrosis caused by a fall in systemic blood pressure in the hypoxic newborn infant with pressure passive cerebral blood flow (Wigglesworth and Pape 1978). The region involved, an area of white matter peripheral to the lateral ventricles, is a watershed zone between the centripetal and centrifugal

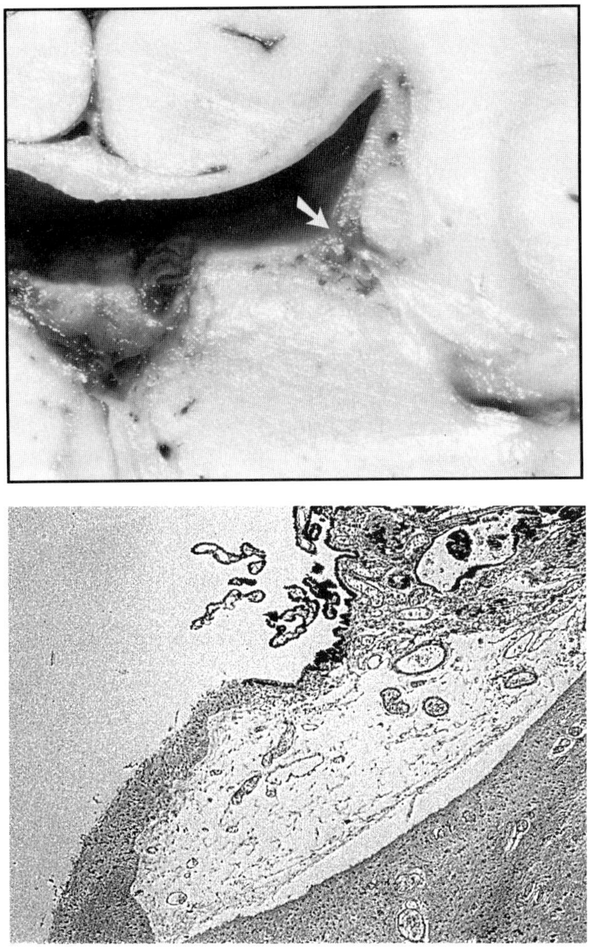

Fig. 8.10. Germinal layer haemorrhage, late appearances. **a** In this coronal section of the cerebral hemispheres the ventricles are dilated. At the *arrow*, the ventricular outline is angulated and small poorly defined cysts are visible in the adjacent tissue. An infant born at 29 weeks' gestation developed bilateral intraventricular haemorrhages and subsequent hydrocephalus. He died at a postnatal age of 3 weeks. **b** The cyst has a lining of neuroglial tissue and is traversed by small blood vessels. Haemosiderin is deposited near the choroid plexus. (H&E, ×34)

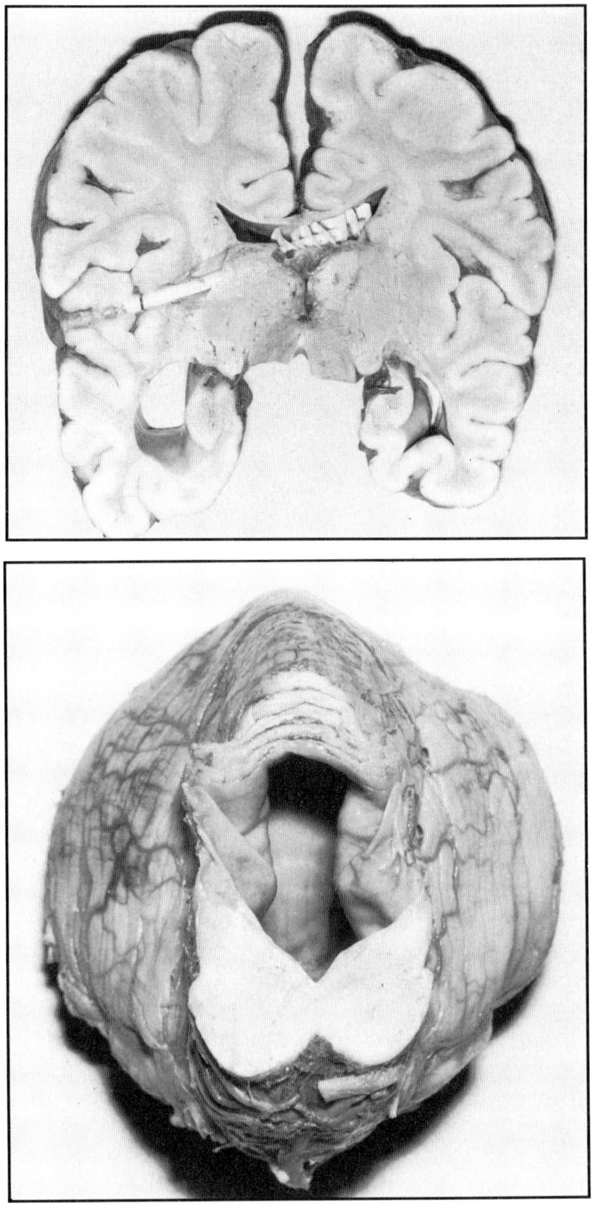

Fig. 8.11. Post-haemorrhagic hydrocephalus. Same case as illustrated in Fig. 8.10. **a** The hydrocephalus has been drained by means of a ventriculoperitoneal shunt. **b** Superior view of the brain stem and cerebellum to show the marked enlargment of the fourth ventricle.

arteries of the cerebral hemispheres (Fig. 8.12). The lesions of PVL are not usually haemorrhagic, but may be so if extensive (Fig. 8.13). PVL is not confined to preterm infants and is seen in term infants subjected to severe birth asphyxia (see Chap. 24, p. 582). It is probably the major cause of mental handicap in surviving babies.

Jaundice and Kernicterus

Unconjugated hyperbilirubinaemia is common in preterm infants because of hepatic immaturity. The maximum bilirubin level may not be reached until the end of the first week of life and some preterm infants may have elevated levels up to the 14th day. Breast milk jaundice is rare in premature infants, and rhesus haemolytic disease, a major contributory factor in the past, is now far less common. Very high levels of unconjugated bilirubin ($\geqslant$340 µmol/l)

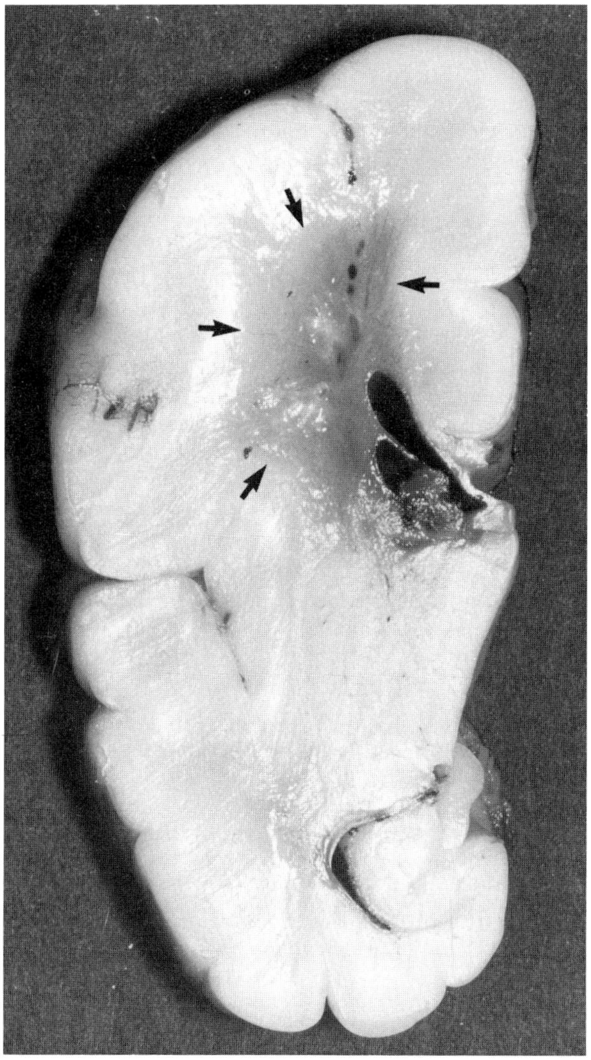

Fig. 8.12. Periventricular leucomalacia. The area of necrosis is outlined by the *arrows*. A germinal layer haemorrhage is also present.

predispose to development of kernicterus (bilirubin staining of the basal ganglia, pons and cerebellum), but may occur in preterm infants with hypoxia or neonatal sepsis at lower serum levels. This heightened susceptibility may be due both to a relative increase in unbound bilirubin because of low serum albumin levels and to increased entry of albumin-bound bilirubin into a brain damaged by hypoxia. Kernicterus is seen at necropsy in 3%–10% of low birthweight infants (<2500 g; Cashore and Stern 1982), but its incidence is dependent on the handling of the brain. Affected brains which are fixed in formalin for a week or two in order to demonstrate haemorrhagic or necrotic lesions are likely to lose some of their bilirubin content, and the staining will fade once exposed to air. If kernicterus is suspected, it is best to cut the brain fresh and photograph it immediately.

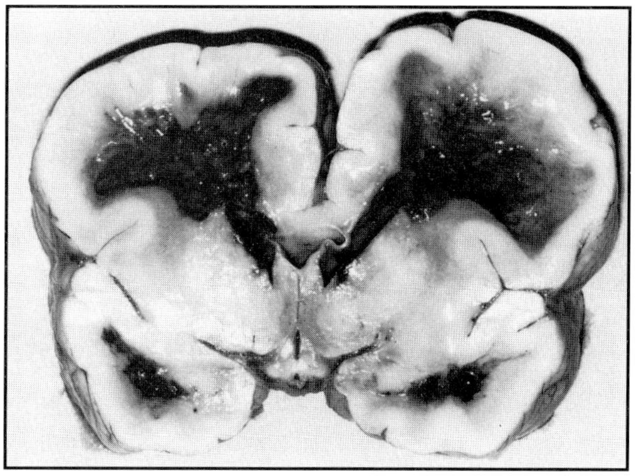

Fig. 8.13. Extensive haemorrhagic periventricular leucomalacia. A zone of necrotic brain tissue can be identified at the periphery of the haemorrhagic areas.

Conjugated hyperbilirubinaemia in preterm infants can be a complication of prolonged parenteral nutrition and appears to be related to the composition of amino acids in intravenous infusions, and to the lack of hormones acting on the biliary excretory system when enteral feeding is withheld.

Problems of the Alimentary System

Intestinal Motility

Premature babies may develop a Hirschsprung-like syndrome, caused by functional immaturity of their ganglion cells. Rectal biopsy is usually normal.

Necrotising Enterocolitis

Necrotising enterocolitis (NEC) is a serious condition largely confined to preterm infants; only about 10% of affected infants are of more than 37 weeks' gestation (Kliegman and Fanaroff 1984). The disease is particularly prevalent in the very premature; overall incidence in neonatal units is about 2% but rises to 13.3% in VLBW babies (Yu et al. 1984). NEC has a mortality of 20%–40%.

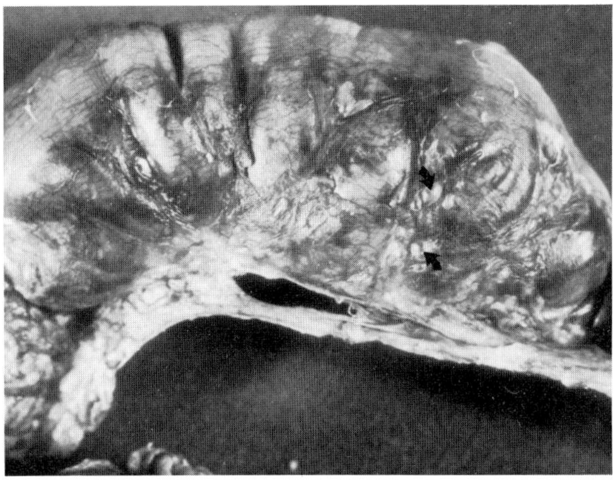

Fig. 8.14. Necrotising enterocolitis. The bowel wall is necrotic and small blebs of gas are present beneath the serosa (*arrows*).

Clinical manifestations, which start to appear about 4 days after birth, include retained gastric contents, blood-streaked or loose stools, abdominal distension and signs of shock, including recurrent apnoea, pallor and temperature instability. Radiographs show gaseous distension of the small and large bowel; there may be intramural gas (Fig. 8.14) which can permeate the portal venous system. Peritonitis and pneumoperitoneum are acute complications and are indications for surgery.

Most infants who survive NEC, with or without surgery, regain normal intestinal function. Intestinal strictures, usually in the colon, occur in 10% of cases and require surgical resection. When only mucosal damage has occurred, regeneration, perhaps with distortion of glandular pattern and Paneth cell metaplasia, is usual. When submucosa and muscle coats are damaged, the bowel can only heal by granulation and a fibrous scar will result. Loss of muscular continuity and myenteric plexus injury add a functional element to the anatomical obstruction. Strictures usually take several months to develop.

The pathogenesis of NEC is still uncertain, although ischaemia of the intestine plays an important part (Brown and Sweet 1982). The ischaemia is thought to result from an overzealous reflex diversion of blood from intestines and other abdominal organs to the heart and brain, and is considered to be analogous to the diving reflex which protects the vital organs of aquatic mammals from hypoxia during prolonged submersion. The initiating factors may include a poor cardiac output for any cause, a decrease in blood volume or hyperviscosity of the blood. Polycythaemia with a haematocrit of over 60% is known to increase the viscosity of the blood and has been demonstrated as a significant factor in the pathogenesis of severe NEC (Yu et al. 1984). Undoubtedly the introduction of milk feeds is another contributing factor, since the disease rarely develops in infants who have never been fed. Brown and Sweet (1982) suggest that fluid passes from the vascular compartment into the intestinal lumen to make its contents iso-osmolar, and causes reduction of the circulating blood volume. NEC is known to be associated with hyperosmolarity of both formula feeds and oral drugs. Oral feeding has a second important effect: it introduces large numbers of bacteria into the intestine, where they proliferate and can invade mucosa which has already suffered ischaemic injury. Gas cysts in the bowel wall and portal vessels are almost certainly of bacterial origin. In some cases, bacteria and endotoxins will pass into the systemic circulation and produce intravascular coagulation and other manifestations of toxic shock.

Associated clinical factors are birth asphyxia, respiratory distress syndrome, apnoea and thermal instability, but most of these are also related to prematurity. Yu et al. (1984) investigated perinatal risk factors for NEC in 50 VLBW infants, taking a large number of unaffected VLBW infants as controls. The only adverse factors were hypothermia (less than 35.5°C) on admission to hospital and a higher incidence of polycythaemia in severely affected infants. Much remains to be learnt of this engimatic condition. Iatrogenic factors related to NEC are discussed in Chapter 14 (see p. 340).

Retinopathy of Prematurity (Retrolental Fibroplasia)

The term "retinopathy of prematurity" (ROP) describes a vasoproliferative and fibroblastic reaction in the developing retina to various metabolic insults, especially abnormalities of arterial oxygen tension. Most instances of ROP are associated with prematurity, only a very small number of cases occurring in term infants. At its most severe (Fig. 8.15) it is a major cause of blindness, particularly affecting babies weighing less than 1000 g at birth (Anon 1991). Lucey and Dangman (1984) estimated

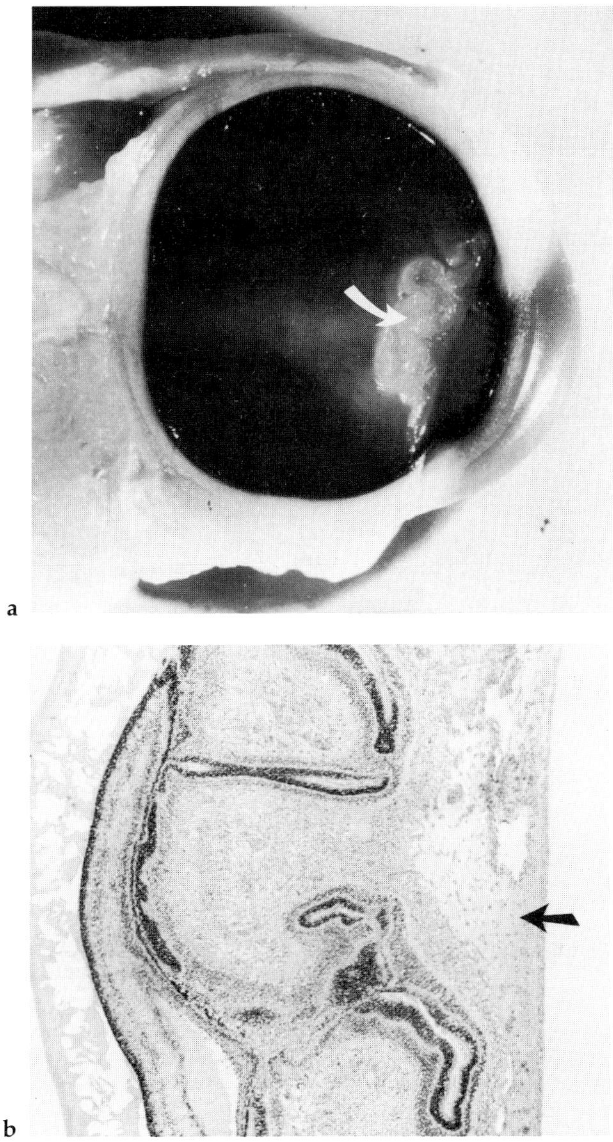

Fig. 8.15. Retrolental fibroplasia (Stage 5). **a** The retina is totally detached and lies in a folded mass (*arrow*) just behind the anterior chamber. (The lens is not included in plane of section.) (Case of Dr. R.W. Blewitt.) **b** The retina is folded and bound anteriorly by fibrovascular tissue (*arrow*). (H&E, ×30)

that ROP now occurs in approximately 7% of infants with a birthweight between 1001 and 1500 g, but increases to 42% or more among survivors weighing 500–750 g at birth.

About 20 years ago, it was thought that high levels of inspired oxygen, administered over several weeks, were responsible for the development of ROP, and clearly hyperoxia did play a major part at that time, since the incidence of ROP fell with better control of oxygen use. It has become clear, however, that ROP can occur in preterm infants who have never received oxygen therapy. Preterm infants may be hyperoxaemic for many hours and yet not develop ROP. Hyperoxaemia is not the only aetiological factor; it seems likely that low oxygen tensions and hypotension also matter.

ROP is assigned ophthalmoscopically to one of five stages (Keith et al. 1981). Fortunately, the majority of cases of ROP fall into stages I and II, which are reversible, but more advanced disease may lead to blindness. A proportion of less severely affected infants become myopic, although the pathogenesis of this complication is not fully understood. ROP is described in Chapter 28 (p. 679).

Osteopenia

Placental transfer of calcium from mother to fetus increases dramatically in the last trimester, and the calcium requirements of preterm babies are therefore substantial (more than 130 mg/kg/day). The placenta is far more efficient at supplying calcium to the fetus than is the intestine of the preterm infant; the mean calcium intake in such babies is of the order of 90 mg/kg/day and cannot be increased much more without rendering the feed hyperosmolar. Infants of less than 32 weeks' gestational age, whose bone mineral content can be measured in life, do not achieve adequate mineralisation when they have reached an age equivalent to term gestation and the deficit is particularly severe in infants with a birthweight of 1000 g or less (Horsman et al. 1989). Clinical rickets may become evident at about 5 months after birth. Vitamin D-metabolising enzymes are thought to function in the preterm infant, with deficiency of calcium and phosphate as the major aetiologial factor (Brooke and Lucas 1985).

Rickets is evident as bone fractures with abundant callus, especially in the ribs (Fig. 8.16a). Costochondral junctions are also expanded and have a bizarre, irregular growth pattern, with poor alignment of the cartilage columns, virtual loss of a linear cartilage/bone junction and poor calcification of the matrix (Fig. 8.16b).

Miscellaneous Problems

Some of the complications listed below are evident to the pathologist at necropsy. Others, of

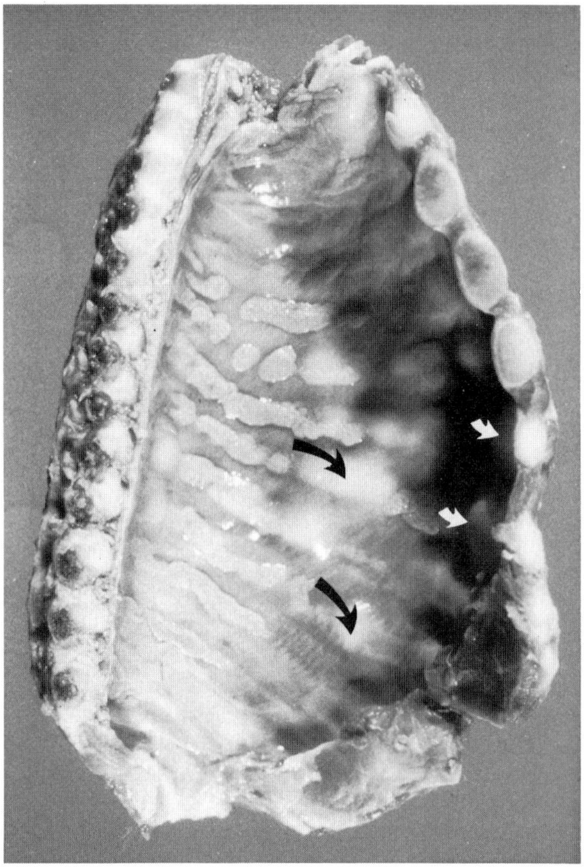
a

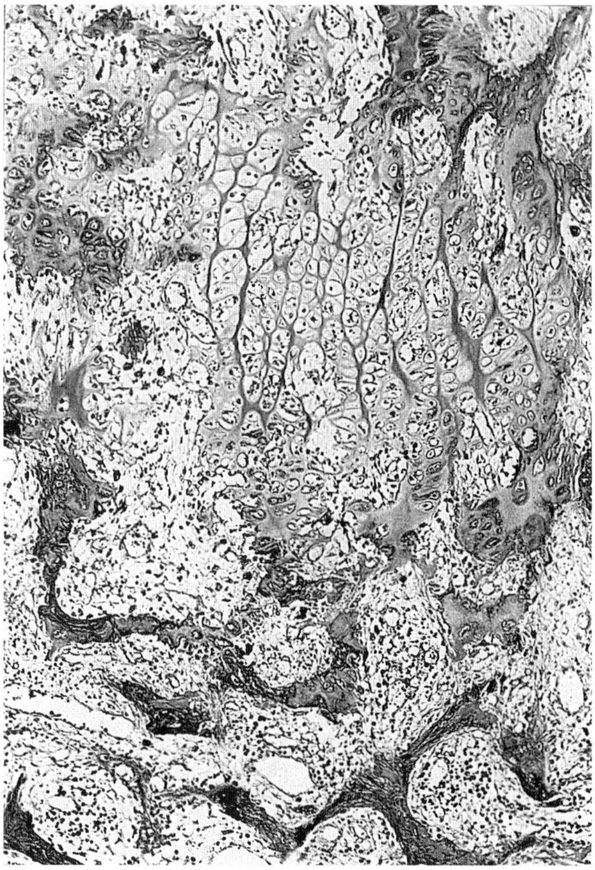
b

Fig. 8.16. **a** Rickets. The rib fractures have healed with abundant callus formation (*long arrows*). Expansion of the costochondral junctions is just visible (*short arrows*). **b** Rickets. The costochondral junction shows an irregular growth pattern with loss of the linear transition from cartilage to bone. (Masson trichrome, ×69).

a metabolic or functional nature, are difficult or impossible to demonstrate after death, but, nevertheless, may have had an adverse effect on the baby's progress.

Hyperkalaemia

Hyperkalaemia is a condition found not uncommonly in VLBW babies. Potassium is well tolerated by preterm infants, and hyperkalaemia in this context is defined as a serum potassium level in excess of 8.5 mmol/l. These very high levels are associated with post-haemorrhagic haemolysis complicating bruising, IVH and pulmonary haemorrhage. Hyperkalaemia causes supraventricular tachycardias, ventricular fibrillation and asystole.

Hypoglycaemia

The metabolic needs of the normal term newborn infant are high, and storage of glycogen in preparation for these needs is a necessary feature of intrauterine development. Shelley and Neligan (1966) have demonstrated that carbohydrate storage within the liver increases sharply from 36 weeks' gestation to term, and thus that preterm babies have relatively low levels of liver carbohydrate, which are exhausted rapidly after birth. Preterm infants also have smaller fat reserves and even greater metabolic needs than term babies. It is not surprising, therefore, that they may become hypoglycaemic. Symptoms are non-specific and include apnoeic attacks, reluctance to feed, jittery movements and fits, and can be cured instantaneously by glucose administration. Promptly treated episodes will leave no recognisable pathology, but prolonged hypoglycaemia, refractory to treatment, will cause brain damage, with scattered areas of necrosis in the white matter of the cerebral cortex.

Hypoglycaemia is not a condition unique to prematurity, and has been recognised for many years as a particular problem in the light-for-dates baby. The mechanism here is poor placental nutrition, reflected in the lower liver-to-brain-weight ratio and low liver carbohydrate stores even at term. Other rare causes of hypoglycaemia are various inborn errors of metabolism (especially those concerned with glycogen storage and release) and functional abnormalities of the pancreas, with inappropriate insulin secretion.

Patent Ductus Arteriosus

Every normally formed infant is, of course, born with a widely patent ductus arteriosus, which has shunted most of the blood away from the lungs during fetal life. The patency of the ductus is maintained by endogenous prostaglandin production for which hypoxaemia is a major stimulating factor. When respiratory function is adequate after birth, the blood oxygen tension rises, depressing the production of prostaglandin and causing a functional closure of the ductus within the first 10–15 h (see Chap. 18, p. 455). The ductus may open and close sporadically during the first few days, but thereafter undergoes progressive anatomical closure, which is usually complete at about 10 days of age.

Preterm infants, especially those below 32 weeks' gestational age, show poor ductal development of both media and intimal cushions, and because of their respiratory immaturity are very likely to become hypoxaemic. Iatrogenic fluid overload for any reason will cause pulmonary oedema, with a further deterioration in blood oxygen tensions. All these factors combine to maintain the patency of the ductus. The pulmonary arterial pressure is normally high immediately after birth, but within the first few days falls so that the systemic arterial pressure becomes the greater. If the ductus is still widely patent at this time, a left-to-right shunt occurs with pulmonary hyperperfusion and left heart strain. Bounding pulses and a heart murmur complete the clinical presentation, which is usually apparent by the end of the first week. Treatment centres on restriction of fluid, adequate oxygenation, administration of a prostaglandin antagonist (usually indomethacin), and sometimes surgical ligation of the ductus.

Hypothermia

Very premature infants have decreased amounts of both brown fat and insulating subcutaneous fat and have difficulty in maintaining their core temperature. Infants allowed to become hypothermic expend extra energy to raise their temperature and require more oxygen. Thus, the respiratory problems already present are compounded. In addition, hypothermic premature infants are more susceptible to other complications, including disseminated intravascular coagulation and necrotising enterocolitis. For this reason, thermal regulation in these babies is a major concern.

Infection

The increased susceptibility to infection of preterm infants over their term counterparts is due to the relative immaturity of their immune system and to the hostile microbiological environment which many of them encounter. Immunological immaturity affects both humoral and cellular systems. IgG in the neonate is largely of maternal origin and is transferred via the placenta in the last trimester. Thus very premature infants would be expected to have low IgG levels. Conway et al. (1985) confirmed this low level and failed to detect any endogenous IgG generation during the first 15 weeks of life. Most babies had no detectable serum IgA at birth. Initial IgM concentrations were variable and were not related to gestational age. Other investigators have noted that even in term infants serum complement activity is low and that both number and function of phagocytic cells are depressed.

Infections are acquired by different routes during fetal and neonatal development. Congenital infection of the fetus is usually transplacental, and the well-known agents include cytomegalovirus, rubella, *Treponema pallidum, Listeria monocytogenes* and *Toxoplasma gondii.* These agents may cause fetal death or premature delivery, but are also likely to result in an infant of term gestation who is light-for-dates.

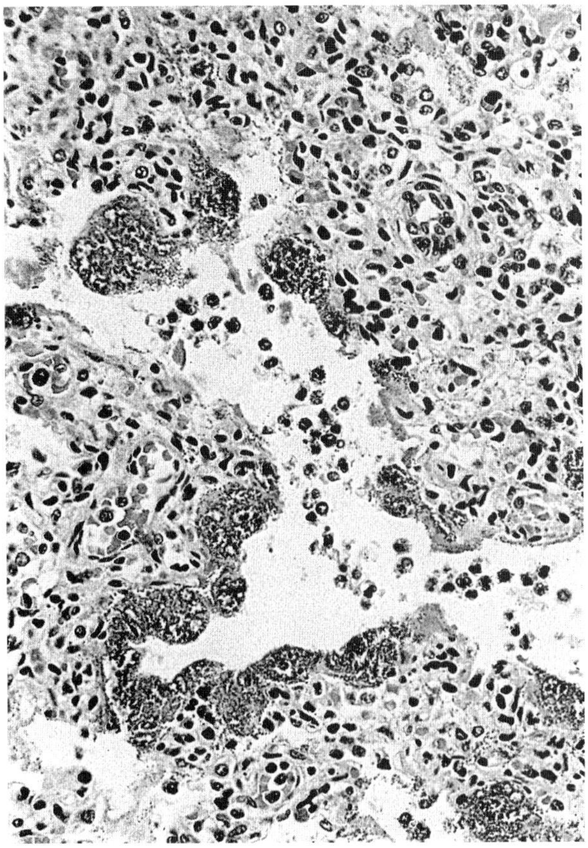

Fig. 8.17. Pneumonia. This infant was born at 31 weeks' gestation, following rupture of the membranes for 2 weeks. β-haemolytic streptococci were grown from the placenta and from the baby's blood and pleural fluid. Polymorphs fill the airways, and the hyaline membranes are colonised by bacteria. (H&E, ×266).

Bacteria and viruses make their next onslaught at the time of delivery, when the infant comes in contact with the organisms of the maternal birth canal. As discussed above (p. 202), preterm premature rupture of membranes is associated with premature delivery. The organisms may colonise the infant's skin and be inhaled or swallowed with the remaining amniotic fluid; only a small percentage of colonised babies develop clinical infection.

The immediate environment of the neonate forms the final source of infection in the first days after birth. The preterm infant is at particular risk here because of the invasive techniques commonly employed, including the use of arterial and venous catheters, chest drains and endotracheal tubes.

Serious infections in the newborn characteristically show one of two clinical patterns which are related to onset. Early-onset disease occurs in the first week of life and may be obvious within hours of birth. Symptoms are non-specific and may be indistinguishable from those of HMD. The two conditions may indeed coexist, and if organisms have previously been inhaled from an infected amniotic fluid or source of infection from the upper respiratory tract, a pneumonia will become established (Fig. 8.17), bacterial clusters sometimes colonising the hyaline membranes. The resulting septicaemia is manifest clinically by sudden deterioration, with apnoea attacks, bradycardia and hypotension. Late-onset disease, occurring after the first week of life, is a more insidious process, presenting clinically with low-grade fever, irritability and feeding difficulties. Meningitis occurs more frequently in this form of infection than in the early-onset disease.

Septicaemia and meningitis are still important causes of mortality in the newborn, and Hurley (1983) has emphasised the vulnerability of low birthweight babies. She recorded an overall mortality rate of 40.1% for septicaemia, rising to 62.5% in those of a birthweight less than 1000 g. Where meningitis supervened, the mortality rate rose to 83%.

The organisms responsible for neonatal infection are many and varied, reflecting the many types present in the mother's birth canal and in the ward environment. Group B streptococci and *Escherichia coli*, however, are still dangerous pathogens at this age, responsible for both early- and late-onset disease. Group B streptococci in particular can be responsible for a fulminant septicaemia over which antibiotics have no control. Other pathogenic organisms include streptococci of other Lancefield groups, *Pseudomonas aeruginosa*, *Klebsiella aerogenes*, *Proteus* species, *Staphylococcus aureus* and *Listeria monocytogenes*. Pseudomonas septicaemia can be suspected clinically and at necropsy by its propensity to cause haemorrhagic ulcerated lesions on the skin and mucous membranes (Fig. 8.18). Histologically, infected organs contain obvious clusters of bacteria with virtually no polymorph response.

Very premature babies may be infected with organisms which are less pathogenic to term infants. *Staphylococcus epidermidis* is frequently isolated from blood cultures and can be a cause of clinical disease. Candida infections of the placental membranes are not infrequent even at term (Fig. 8.19); in premature babies the

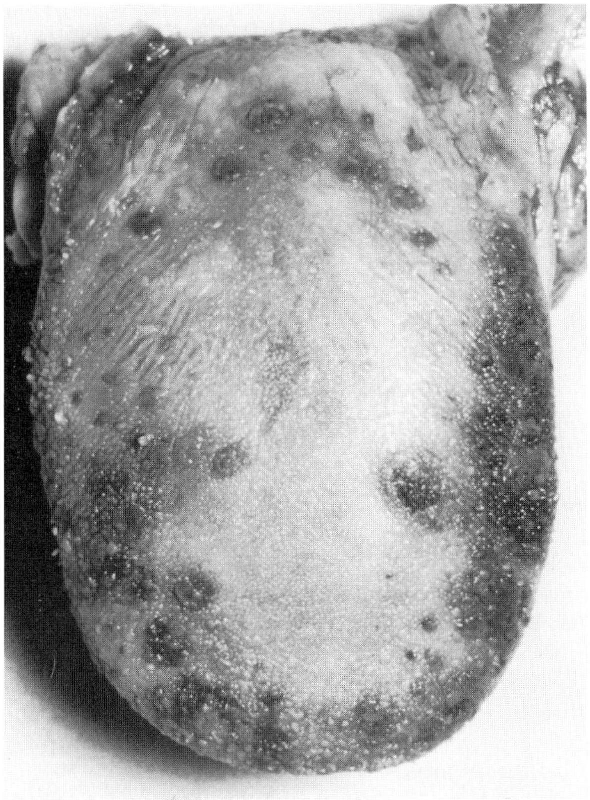

Fig. 8.18. Tongue. Pseudomonas septicaemia causes haemorrhagic and ulcerated lesions on the skin and mucous membranes.

fungi may colonise the lungs (Fig. 8.20) or may in the neonatal period contaminate fluids administered intravenously. Smith and Congdon (1985) reported ten cases of systemic candidiasis in preterm babies, eight of which were 28 weeks' gestation or less. All had received prolonged ventilation, multiple courses of broad-spectrum antibiotics and intravenous hyperalimentation. The yeasts showed a predilection for the urinary tract, forming fungal abscesses, and could be cultured from suprapubic urine specimens.

Late Complications of Prematurity

Very premature babies may require prolonged treatment and observation in neonatal intensive care units. A small number never recover completely because of damage to the central nervous system or, more rarely, develop chronic lung problems secondary to bronchopulmonary dysplasia. A proportion of infants

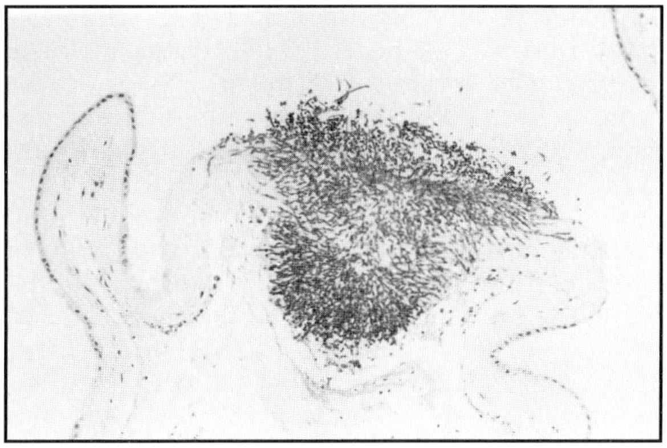

Fig. 8.19. Candida infection of the placental membranes. (PAS, ×100)

appear to become functionally mature and are discharged from hospital, only to die shortly thereafter suddenly and unexpectedly.

Sudden Infant Death Syndrome

Postneonatal infant mortality in infants admitted to a neonatal intensive care unit was

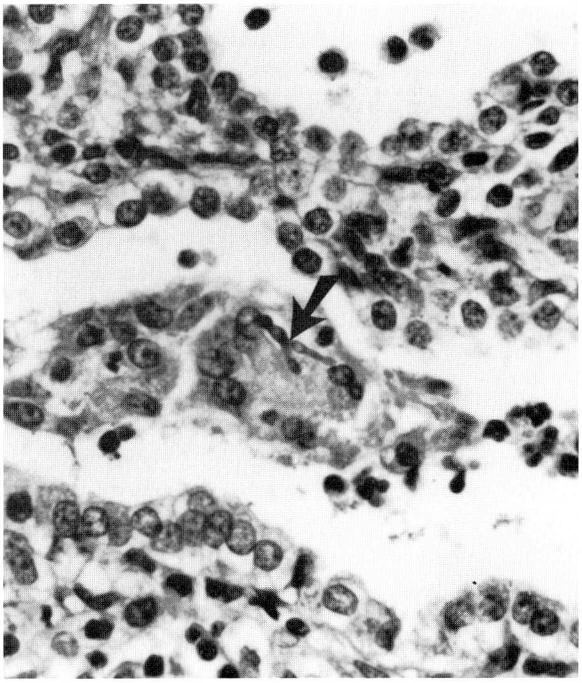

Fig. 8.20. Candida pneumonia in a very premature infant. A peripheral airway contains inflammatory cells including a multinucleate giant cell which has phagocytosed fungal elements (*arrow*). (PAS, ×640)

investigated by Kulkarni et al. (1978). The mortality rate was 44 per 1000 live births in those surviving to an age of 28 days; 79% of deaths were associated with major congenital defects, brain damage or other serious disease and were not unexpected. Of the remaining 21% about half were ascribed to sudden infant death syndrome (SIDS), although only three of these eight infants had necropsy examinations. Thus the mortality rate for SIDS was calculated as 4.5 per 1000 live births, a figure two or three times that of the general population. Six of the eight deaths were in babies who had been preterm with birthweights ranging from 900 to 2489 g. Besides low infant birthweight, poor socioeconomic status of the parents was also confirmed as a contributory factor.

Neurodevelopmental Handicap

Critics of the first neonatal intensive care units predicted that the rescue of very small infants would lead to an increased incidence of serious neurological handicap. Assessment within the field is necessarily slow, since many years are required for full developmental potential to be realised.

Major handicap presents clinically as cerebral palsy, mental retardation, hearing loss, visual defect or hydrocephalus. More subtle handicaps may be revealed with continued assessment, and these include impairment of reasoning, comprehension, articulation and motor coordination, with poor ability to read or calculate (Taylor 1984). A comprehensive analysis of 111 studies reporting morbidity among surviving VLBW infants born since 1960 (Escobar et al. 1991) has found the median incidence of cerebral palsy to be 7.7%, with little variation over the last 20 years, and the relative risk of cerebral palsy in this group was calculated to be 38 times that in the general population. The incidence of disability of all types, including pulmonary disorders, was around 25%, and the studies which followed children up for longer periods tended to report higher disability rates. Outcome may be improved for infants whose parents have a higher educational attainment (McCormick 1989).

Attention is now being directed towards extremely low birthweight infants (birthweight less than 1000 g). Kitchen et al. (1987) assessed 50 such infants at 5.5 years; 5 had severe sensorineural or intellectual impairments, 5 had mild to moderate impairments, 10 had minor neurobehavioural abnormalities, and 30 appeared unimpaired. As this cohort of children attains school age, the more sophisticated assessment techniques then available will allow a more reliable evaluation of outcome.

Some of the major handicaps have a specific pathological counterpart, which allows some speculation as to their aetiology. Cerebral palsy is generally the late complication of periventricular leucomalacia, itself a consequence of cerebral hypoperfusion. Where the infarcted area includes the descending corticospinal fibres, the corresponding paralysis of legs (spastic diplegia) or all four limbs (spastic quadriplegia) will result. Periventricular haemorrhage with extension into the parenchyma is also cited as a cause of cerebral palsy, but it seems unlikely that this is a major aetiological factor.

Hydrocephalus can occur when an intraventricular haemorrhage which has tracked down to the cisterna magna undergoes organisation, rather than clearance by the phagocytic mechanisms, thus blocking cerebrospinal fluid flow; meningitis in which exudate at the cisterna magna fails to resolve may also produce hydrocephalus.

Significant hypothermia (below 34°C) has been associated with subsequent spastic diplegia, and great care is now taken to prevent loss of body heat, especially during transfer of small infants from one treatment centre to another.

Prolonged and recurrent hypoglycaemia is also well known to cause neurological handicap. It may be recognised at necropsy by the presence of small scattered necrotic foci in white matter.

Hyperbilirubinaemia of more than 255 μmol/l increases the risk of handicap, but the threshold falls in the presence of perinatal hypoxia. The unbound bilirubin penetrates the brain and may damage the basal ganglia and cranial nuclei. Late clinical manifestations include fits, involuntary movements, mental deficiency, partial hearing loss and abnormalities of eye movement.

Conclusion

Mortality rates in preterm infants show evidence of a substantial decrease since the introduction of neonatal intensive care units and of improved obstetric practice, and the incidence of severe neurological handicap appears to remain steady. However, room for further improvement still exists. The role of the pathologist is to record accurately all abnormalities present in those infants and children coming to necropsy and to search for adverse effects of treatment. The clinical, investigative and pathological findings must all be correlated if a true assessment of disease and its treatment is to be made.

References

Anon (1991) Retinopathy of prematurity. Lancet 337: 83–84

Bratlid D, Lindback T (1978) Bacteriolytic activity of amniotic fluid. Obstet Gynecol 51: 63–66

Beverley DW, Pitts-Tucker T, Arthur RJ, Congdon PJ, Tate G (1985) Prevention of intraventricular haemorrhage by fresh frozen plasma. Arch Dis Child 60: 710–713

Blanco JD, Gibbs RS, Krebs LF, Castaneda YS (1982) The association between the absence of amniotic fluid bacterial inhibitory activity and intra-amniotic infection. Am J Obstet Gynecol 143: 749–755

Bobitt JR, Ledger WJ (1978) Amniotic fluid analysis. Its role in maternal and neonatal infection. Obstet Gynecol 51: 56–62

Brooke OG, Lucas A (1985) Metabolic bone disease in preterm infants. Arch Dis Child 60: 682–685

Brown EG, Sweet AY (1982) Neonatal necrotising enterocolitis. Pediatr Clin North Am 29: 1149–1170

Carr-Hill RA, Hall MH (1985) The repetition of spontaneous preterm labour. Br J Obstet Gynaecol 92: 921–928

Cashore WJ, Stern L (1982) Neonatal hyperbilirubinemia. Pediatr Clin North Am 29: 1191–1203

Cashore WJ, Stern L (1984) Neonatal problems of the preterm baby. Clin Obstet Gynaecol 11: 391–413

Chamberlain G (1984) Epidemiology and aetiology of the preterm baby. Clin Obstet Gynaecol 11: 297–314

Charles D, Edwards WR (1981) Infectious complications of cervical cerclage. Am J Obstet Gynecol 141: 1065–1071

Charles D, Hurry DJ (1983) Chorioamnionitis. Clin Obstet Gynaecol 10: 123–148

Chiswick ML, Johnson M, Woodhall C et al. (1983) Protective effect of vitamin E (DL-alpha-tocopherol) against intraventricular haemorrhage in premature babies. Br Med J II: 81–84

Conway SP, Dear PRF, Smith I (1985) Immunoglobulin profile of the preterm baby. Arch Dis Child 60: 208–212

Drife J (1989) Infection and preterm birth. Br J Obstet Gynaecol 96: 1128–1132

Escobar GJ, Littenberg B, Petitti DB (1991) Outcome among surviving very low birthweight infants: a meta-analysis. Arch Dis Child 66: 204–211

Fisk NM, Fysh J, Child AG, Gatenby PA, Jeffery H, Bradfield AH (1987) Is C-reactive protein really useful in preterm premature rupture of the membranes? Br J Obstet Gynaecol 94: 1159–1164

Gibson AAM (1982) Prematurity. In: Barson AJ (ed) Fetal and neonatal pathology. Praeger, Eastbourne, pp 205–211

Hargar JH, Hsing AW, Tuomala RE et al. (1990) Risk factors for preterm premature rupture of fetal membranes: A multicenter case-control study. Am J Obstet Gynecol 163: 130–137

Hill A, Perlman JM, Volpe JJ (1982) Relationship of pneumothorax to occurrence of intraventricular haemorrhage in the premature newborn. Pediatrics 69: 144–149

Hislop A, Reid L (1974) Growth and development of the respiratory system–anatomical development. In: Davis JA, Dobbing J (eds) Scientific foundations of paediatrics. Heinemann, London, pp 214–254

Horsman A, Ryan SW, Congdon PJ, Truscott JG, James JR (1989) Osteopenia in extremely low birthweight infants. Arch Dis Child 64: 485–488

Hurley R (1983) Serious infections in the newborn. Clin Obstet Gynaecol 10: 65–91

Huszar G, Naftolin F (1984) The myometrium and uterine cervix in normal and preterm labor. N Engl J Med 311: 571–481

Jones RAK, Roberton NRC (1984) Problems of the small-for-dates baby. Clin Obstet Gynaecol 11: 499–524

Keith CG, Smith ST, Lansdell BJ (1981) Retrolental fibroplasia. A study of the incidence and aetiological factors 1977–1979. Med J Aust 2: 589–592

Kitchen WH, Ford GW, Rickards AL, Lissenden JV, Ryan MM (1987) Children of birth weight <1000 g: changing outcome between ages 2 and 5 years. J Pediatr 110: 283–288

Kliegman RM, Fanaroff AA (1984) Necrotising enterocolitis. N Engl Med 310: 1093–1103

Kulkarni P, Hall RT, Rhodes PG, Sheehan MB (1978) Postneonatal infant mortality in infants admitted to a neonatal intensive care unit. Pediatrics 62: 178–183

Lamont RF, Rose M, Elder MG (1985) Effect of bacterial products on prostaglandin E production by amnion cells. Lancet ii: 1331–1333

Lavin JP, Lovelace DR, Miodovnik M, Knowles HC, Barden TP (1983) Clinical experience with one hundred seven diabetic pregnancies. Am J Obstet Gynecol 147: 742–752

Law MR, Wijewardene K, Wald NJ (1990) Is routine vitamin E administration justified in very low-birthweight infants? Dev Med Child Neurol 32: 442–450

López Bernal A, Hansell DJ, Khong TY, Keeling JW, Turnbull AC (1989) Prostaglandin E production by the fetal membranes in unexplained preterm labour and preterm labour associated with chorioamnionitis. Br J Obstet Gynaecol 96: 1133–1139

Lou HC, Lassen NA, Friis-Hansen B (1979) Impaired autoregulation of cerebral blood flow in the distressed newborn infant. J Pediatr 94: 118–121

Lucey JF, Dangman B (1984) A reexamination of the role of oxygen in retrolental fibroplasia. Pediatrics 73: 82–96

Mamelle N, Laumon B (1984) Occupational fatigue and preterm birth. In: Chamberlain G (ed). Pregnant women at work. Royal Society of Medicine and Macmillan, London, pp 105–115

McCormick MC (1989) Long-term follow-up of infants discharged from neonatal intensive care units. JAMA 261: 1767–1772

McDonald IA (1980) Cervical cerclage. Clin Obstet Gynaecol 7: 461–479

Myerscough PR (1982) Dystocia associated with malformations of the uterus and vagina. In: Munro Kerr's operative obstetrics, 10th edn. Baillière Tindall, London, pp 187–202

Naeye RL (1988) Acute bacterial chorioamnionitis. Prog Clin Biol Res 281: 73–86

Naeye RL (1989) Pregnancy hypertension, placental evi-

dences of low uteroplacental blood flow, and spontaneous premature delivery. Hum Pathol 20: 441–444
Naeye RL, Peters EC (1978) Amniotic fluid infections with intact membranes leading to perinatal death: a prospective study. Pediatrics 61: 171–177
Naeye RL, Peters EC (1980) Causes and consequences of premature rupture of fetal membranes. Lancet i: 192–194
Naeye RL, Ross S (1982) Coitus and chorioamnionitis: a prospective study. Early Hum Dev 6: 91–97
Neligan GA (1970) Working party to discuss nomenclature based on gestational age and birthweight. Arch Dis Child 45: 730
Papiernik E (1984) Prediction of the preterm baby. Clin Obstet Gynaecol 11: 315–336
Parisi VM (1988) Cervical incompetence and preterm labor. Clin Obstet Gynecol 31: 585–598
Pasternak JF, Groothuis DR, Fischer JM, Fisher DP (1982) Regional cerebral blood flow in the newborn beagle pup: the germinal matrix is a "low-flow" structure. Pediatr Res 16: 499–503
Rigatto H (1982) Apnea. Pediatr Clin North Am 29: 1105–1116
Romero R, Mazor M (1988) Infection and preterm labor. Clin Obstet Gynecol 31: 553–584
Romero R, Emamian M, Quintero R, Wan M, Hobbins JC, Mitchell MD (1986) Amniotic fluid prostaglandin levels and intra-amniotic infections. Lancet i: 1380
Romero R, Avila C, Santhanam U, Sehgal PB (1990) Amniotic fluid interleukin 6 in preterm labor. Association with infection. J Clin Invest 85: 1392–1400
Sandler RS, Baird DD, Narendranathan M (1990) Reproductive outcomes in women with inflammatory bowel disease. Gastroenterology 98: A202
Saurel-Cubizolles MJ, Subtil D, Kaminski M (1991) Is preterm delivery still related to physical working conditions in pregnancy? J Epidemiol Community Health 45: 29–34
Shelley HJ, Neligan GA (1966) Neonatal hypoglycaemia. Br Med Bull 22: 34–39
Smith H, Congdon P (1985) Neonatal systemic candidiasis. Arch Dis Child 60: 365–369
Szymonowciz W, Schafler K, Cussen LJ, Yu VYH (1984) Ultrasound and necropsy study of periventricular haemorrhage in preterm infants. Arch Dis Child 59: 637–642
Tafari N, Ross SM, Naeye RL, Galask RP, Zaar B (1977) Failure of bacterial growth inhibition by amniotic fluid. Am J Obstet Gynecol 128: 187–189
Taghizadeh A, Reynolds EOR (1976) Pathogenesis of bronchopulmonary dysplasia following hyaline membrane disease. Am J Pathol 82: 241–258
Tarby TJ, Volpe JJ (1982) Intraventricular hemorrhage in the premature infant. Pediatr Clin North Am 29: 1077–1104
Taylor D (1984) Low birthweight and neurodevelopmental handicap. Clin Obstet Gynaecol 11: 525–542
Thompson MH, Khot AS (1985) Impact of neonatal intensive care. Arch Dis Child 60: 213–214
Toth M, Witkin SS, Ledger W, Thaler H (1988) The role of infection in the etiology of preterm birth. Obstet Gynecol 71: 723–726
Tovey LAD, Stevenson BJ, Townley A, Taverner J (1983) The Yorkshire antenatal anti-D immunoglobulin trial in primigravidae. Lancet ii: 244–246
Turnbull AC (1977) Aetiology of pre-term labour. In: Anderson A, Beard R, Brudenell JM, Dunn PM (eds) Preterm labour. Proceedings of the Fifth Study Group of the Royal College of Obstetricians and Gynaecologists. RCOG, London, pp 56–78
Whittle MJ (1984) Lung maturation. Clin Obstet Gynaecol 11: 353–372
Wigglesworth JS, Pape KE (1978) An integrated model for haemorrhagic and ischaemic lesions in the newborn brain. Early Hum Dev 2: 179–199
Yu VYH, Joseph R, Bajuk B, Orgill A, Astbury J (1984) Perinatal risk factors for necrotising entercolitis. Arch Dis Child 59: 430–434
Zaaijman J du T, Wilkinson AR, Keeling JW, Mitchell RG, Turnbull AC (1982) Spontaneous premature rupture of the membranes: bacteriology, histology and neonatal outcome. J Obstet Gynaecol 2: 155–160

Chapter 9

Pathology of Twinning

Geoffrey A. Machin

Introduction

As other causes of perinatal morbidity and mortality are reduced by improving standards of prenatal and perinatal care, stubborn problems remain. The continuing problem of lethal congenital anomalies is well recognised. Multiple pregnancy is a "hidden" but endemic risk which is not usually thus categorised, but contributes an excess of perinatal deaths, compared to singletons within the categories antepartum fetal death, prematurity and congenital anomalies. Twinning is also common among spontaneous abortuses, although exact statistics are not available. In the era of ovulation induction and in vitro fertilisation, higher-order multiple pregnancies are becoming more common. However, it is the monochorionic (MC) multiple pregnancies which carry particularly high perinatal risks that warrant classification as a primary cause of perinatal death.

Prevalence, Types and Causes of Multiple Births

Spontaneous multiple pregnancies occur in 1 in 80 deliveries in the western world, but twinning rates are geographically quite variable worldwide. One in 40 births is from a multiple pregnancy, and the great majority of these births are twins. Induced higher-order multiple pregnancies are increasing, often followed by selective reduction from very high order to twins and triplets (Berkowitz et al. 1988; Wapner et al. 1990). Monozygotic (MZ) twins are excessively represented in these induced multiple pregnancies (Derom et al. 1987).

Among Caucasians, roughly 70% of twins are dizygotic (DZ), resulting from simultaneous ovulation of two ova, most frequently from two ovaries, possibly from two follicles in the same ovary, or even from one follicle. These two ova are usually fertilised by two sperm from the same ejaculate, perhaps from two ejaculates of the same father and, rarely, by different fathers. Evidence is lacking in humans for twins from fertilisation of ova from successive cycles. DZ twinning can occur in families, is thought to result from increased levels of follicle-stimulating hormone, and shows secular variation. DZ twinning is excessive in Nigeria and uncommon in Japan. DZ twins have dichoronic (DC) placentation, either separate or fused. Interfetal vascular anastomoses have been reported infrequently in DC, DZ placentas. There may be marked growth discrepancy between DZ twins despite the absence of anastomoses.

MZ twin pairs originate from single zygotes; the fission of the twins occurs at different times after fertilisation, as reflected in the four different types of placentation found in MZ twins (Fig. 9.1). Early fission of the twins, prior

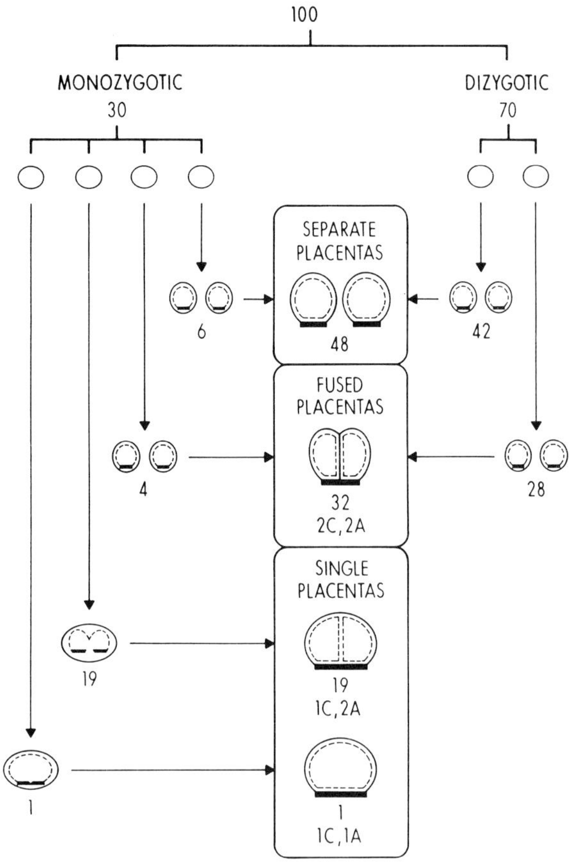

Fig. 9.1. Twin zygosity and types of placentation in Caucasians. Unlike-sex twins are DZ (unless they are heterokaryotypic MZ twins). MC twins are MZ but MZ twins can have all four types of placentation. No DZ twins are MC (Benirschke and Kim 1973).

to the development of the blastocyst, results in DC placentation, whereas fission after the blastocyst stage yields MC diamniotic (DA) twins. Rarely, fission is delayed until after the development of the amniotic sac, when MC monoamniotic (MA) placentation results. Most conjoined twins (caused by incomplete fission of the zygote) have MC,MA placentas. Roughly two-thirds of MZ twins have MC placentas, with a resulting high rate of complications caused by interfetal placental vascular anastomoses. The causes of MZ twinning are not known; prevalence varies with maternal age, but there is no other significant association and MZ twinning rates are quite similar throughout the world. There is an excess of females among MZ twins compared with singletons and DZ twins (Table 9.1); this has led to the proposal that the process of X-chromosome inactivation (which probably occurs in humans at about the same time as MC twin fission) may cause "cloning" of the two cell lines, one each with predominantly the paternally or maternally derived X chromosome inactivated (Burn et al. 1986; Richards et al. 1990; Nance 1990). There is conflicting evidence about the prevalence of congenital anomalies in DZ and MZ twins, but it seems likely that there is an excess of midline-type malformations in MZ twins; this may reflect abnormal cell division/migration/adhesion causally linking the MZ twinning process with midline malformations.

Table 9.1. Sex ratios in twins by zygosity and chorionicity

	Derom et al. (1988)	James (1980)	Gedda et al. (1981)
Singletons (control)	0.518	0.514	
All twins			0.499
All DZ	0.518	0.514	0.516
All MZ (DC and MC)	0.487	0.496	0.472
All MC	0.484		
MC, DA	0.493		
MC, MA	0.231	0.420	
Conjoined		0.250	

A third type of twinning may arise from simultaneous ovulation of two oocytes derived from the same oogonium; such twins might have a genetic status somewhere between MZ and DZ; as recombination occurs prior to first meiotic division, mono-oogonial oocytes would be genetically distinct. Only one pair of possible mono-oogonial human twins has been reported so far (Bieber et al. 1981), but the concept is important, because it implies that at least some DZ twins might arise from abnormal cell division and be susceptible to midline anomalies.

Methods of Zygosity Determination

Morphological phenotype is reliable for zygosity determination in older twins, but is not reliable in like-sexed newborns or infants. Classic genetic methods include analysis of blood groups, enzymes, HLA-typing and placental status. It is generally accepted that unlike-sex twins are DZ and that twins with MC placentas are MZ; DC placentas may be DZ or MZ.

DNA "fingerprinting", using high- or low-stringency restriction fragment polymorphism, is the definitive method for determining zygosity (Derom et al. 1985; Hill and Jeffreys 1985; Azuma et al. 1989). It can be used on cord blood, amniotic fluid, fetal tissues, including placenta, and can give good results from small or autolysed fetuses from whom blood cannot be obtained (Derom et al. 1989).

Accurate zygosity determination is necessary for twin research when its purpose is to distinguish between genetic and environmental causations of human characteristics. MZ twin pairs reared apart show remarkably similar physical and mental characteristics (Bouchard T.J. et al. 1990) and response to overfeeding (Bouchard C et al. 1990).

Prenatal Detection of Twin Pregnancy

Since MC twins carry high prenatal and perinatal risks, prenatal identification of MC,MZ twins is desirable, and can be achieved with reasonable accuracy. The DC septum is a robust and relatively thick structure that is easily seen by ultrasound (Barss et al. 1985; Hertzberg et al. 1987; Townsend et al. 1988; D'Alton and Dudley 1989; Winn et al. 1989); MC,DA twin septa contain two layers of amnion, seen as tenuous "hair-like" membranes by obstetric ultrasound; there is no septum in MC,MA pregnancies. Since MC,MA twinning may be complicated by mutual intertwining of the umbilical cords, braided cords may be detected by ultrasound (Townsend and Filly 1988). Conjoined twins appear in constant relationship to each other on ultrasound examination.

Complications of Monochorionic Twinning

Prenatal and perinatal complications are higher in MC than DC twins, regardless of the zygosity of DC twins. This is largely because of the presence of interfetal vascular anastomoses (IFVA) in most MC placentas; IFVA can result in the development of twin transfusion syndrome (TTS) and twin reversed arterial perfusion (TRAP). The MC placenta is truly single rather than fused, and, during placental angiogenesis, perfusion zones for each embryo are not necessarily equal in size. A small minority of MC placentas do not have any IFVA. These twins are usually born at or near term after uncomplicated pregnancies, although they may be growth-discrepant. The majority of MC placentas do have IVFA; anastomotic arrangement is unique to each placenta, although certain patterns and perinatal outcomes are common.

Twin Transfusion Syndrome

IFVA are of three types; any combination of these types can occur in MC placentas (Arts and Lohman 1971; Benirschke 1961; Strong and Corney 1967; Yoshida and Soma 1984). The combinations and complexities of types of IFVA are responsible for differences in severity and onset of TTS and TRAP. The functioning of the IFVA almost certainly varies during gestation. The three types of IFVA are:

Arteriovenous anastomoses (AVA). These are small vessel anastomoses within the placental parenchyma, usually close to the equatorial zones. AVA may be single or multiple, and multiple AVA may be unidirectional or bidirectional. Net transfusion of blood occurs in TTS from the donor on the arterial side to the recipient on the venous side of the AVA. If there is significant and uncompensated AV transfusion, death of both twins usually occurs in the second trimester. AVA are not malformations, but rather result from the monochorionicity of the placenta itself. AVA can also be regarded as representing a disproportion between zones of arterial perfusion and venous return in MC placentas (Bendon and Siddiqi 1989); thus, if arterial perfusion zones are roughly equal, but venous drainage is predominantly to one twin, AV flow will occur from the twin with the smaller venous drainage zone to the twin with the larger venous zone. This causes severe early TTS if not compensated by other IFVA.

Arterio-arterial anastomoses (AAA). These run above the chorionic plate. AAA are common in MC placentas, but it is unlikely that they can account for TTS; rather, they act as routes for compensatory return of blood from recipient to donor in TTS. AAA are the anatomic basis for the development of TRAP (see below). They may be single or multiple.

Venovenous anastomoses (VVA). These also run above the chorionic plate. VVA are uncommon, and, like AAA, may function as return vessels that moderate the effects of net AVA transfusion. They may also alleviate the effects of unequal venous perfusion zones. Ischaemic/necrotic organ lesions are found in some MC twin survivors with fetal death of the co-twins; it has been proposed that these lesions result from the liberation of thromboplastins released by necrotic tissue in the dead co-twin; VVA could be paths for diffusion of such thromboplastins. VVA are usually present in TRAP twins.

There is current interest in the criteria for the prenatal diagnosis of TTS (Blickstein 1990; Danskin and Neilson 1989). Prenatal interventions are being developed to reduce or reverse the worst consequences of TTS, polyhydramnios, fetal congestive cardiac failure, hydrops, preterm delivery and fetal death. Classic features of TTS seen postnatally are: MC placenta with AVA and often other IFVA, significant intertwin growth discrepancy, (>15% of the weight of the larger twin) and significant intertwin discrepancy of haemoglobin values (>5 g/l) (Galea et al. 1982; Strong and Corney 1967). These criteria are somewhat arbitrary. Because of perinatal reversed TTS (see below) the criteria are not always met postnatally and they are of limited use prenatally. The problem with prenatal TTS is that fetal physiology is already disturbed when lesions are large enough to be detectable by ultrasound. Prenatal signs of TTS include polyhydramnios/oligohydramnios and hydrops (Brennan et al. 1982; Elejalde et al. 1983; Wittman et al. 1981). There may be growth discrepancy; however, growth discrepancy also occurs in DC twins, and in MC twins with unequal venous zones who do not have TTS. The usefulness of Doppler umbilical artery velocimetry in TTS is unclear since some changes may be due to growth discrepancy rather than TTS per se (Erskine et al. 1986; Giles et al. 1985; Pretorius et al. 1988).

For the pathologist, the diagnosable substrate for TTS is the presence in MC placentas of IFVA that can cause TTS, i.e. AVA. In any MC twin death, TTS should be suspected unless placental anastomoses are absent. Clinical data on birthweights and initial haemoglobin values of survivors should be obtained in cases where only one twin dies.

Perinatal death in MC twins may relate directly to TTS and TRAP, or only indirectly, because of preterm delivery. Uncompensated TTS via AVA results in hyperperfused cardiovascular systems in the recipients, and chronic anaemia and undernourishment in the donors; donors or recipients may die in utero. Net transfusion of whole blood into the recipient causes increased fetal micturition, possibly mediated by atriopeptin (Nageotte et al. 1989); in turn, this causes polyhydramnios of the sac of the recipient, who nevertheless develops progressively raised haematocrit values as more blood is transfused; hyperviscosity probably causes circulatory failure and hydrops, followed by fetal death if unrelieved. Polyhydramnios is probably the single most important factor in preterm delivery of TTS twins (Kirshon 1989), because of uterine distention and/or premature ruptured membranes. A further possible effect of high-pressure polyhydramnios (Nicolini et al. 1989) is reduced blood flow in the superficial IFVA, which may previously have functioned to compensate for transfusion via AVA.

Chronic loss of transfused blood from the donor twin stimulates erythropoiesis (Schwartz et al. 1984), so that donors are not severely anaemic. If increased donor erythropoiesis is hormonally mediated, the recipient is similarly stimulated, via IFVA, thus exacerbating the plethora. Donor twins usually show growth lag. It is not clear whether the oligohydramnios of the donor twin sac is a component of intrauterine growth retardation or whether it is passively compressed by the overdistended recipient sac. The donor lies in a small sac and may become a "stuck" twin (Hashimoto et al. 1986; Mahony et al. 1985). There may be amnion nodosum, and the stuck twin may show positional deformities at birth. Donor twins sometimes develop hydrops.

TTS is usually progressive, and prenatal diagnosis in the second trimester presents dilemmas in management. However, there are rare reports of apparently spontaneous resolution of severe TTS (Lubinsky and Rapoport 1983; Montan et al. 1985); placental details are lacking, but AVA may thrombose, or AAA and VVA open up to relieve the effects of partially compensated TTS. Detailed prenatal Doppler studies of flow in surface IFVA may clarify these issues.

Fetal death from TTS can adversely affect surviving co-twins; four principal patterns are described, depending on the timing of fetal death:

Vanishing twin (Landy et al. 1982; Landy et al. 1986; Levi 1976). It has been documented repeatedly by ultrasound that multifetal pregnancies may spontaneously reduce to singleton pregnancies; many of these instances are probably MC,MZ twin pregnancies with complications of IFVA. Diligent search for remnants of the vanished twin may be successful (Sulak and Dodson 1986; Yoshida and Soma 1986; Jauniaux et al. 1988), but absolute anatomical and histological criterial have not been established.

Spontaneous abortion of both twins is noted in some reports. The prevalence of twins among spontaneous abortuses is greater than twin prevalence at birth, ranging from 1 in 35 (Livingstone and Poland 1980) to 1 in 44 (Uchida et al. 1983) conceptuses. Criteria for zygosity and chorionicity were not rigidly applied, but there appears to be an excess of MC twins (Uchida 1990), including conjoined twins and cases of early severe TTS (Fig. 9.2).

Early death and retention of one twin, with the development of fetus papyraceus, can result in aplasia cutis congenita and/or multiple bowel atresias in survivors (Mannino et al. 1977; Yoshida and Soma 1986; Wagner et al. 1990) (Fig. 9.3). Arterial blood supply to mesodermal structures and skin are closely related in early gestation.

Second or third trimester death of one twin results in a pattern of organ infarction involving brain, lungs, kidney and liver in the survivor (Szymonowicz et al. 1986; Fisher and Siongco 1989; Bulla et al. 1987). Thrombi and/or thromboemboli have been reported in the lungs of affected infants (Moore et al. 1969; Wagner et al. 1990). It is commonly thought that thromboplastins are liberated from the tissues of the dead twin, and reach the surviving co-twin via IFVA or across the interfetal septum from the amniotic fluid; however, it is also possible that abnormal flow in IFVA after intrauterine death of the fetus may result in episodes of hypotension and shock in the survivor (Dimmick et al. 1971).

Follow-up studies show an excess of neurological and developmental delay in MC twins, probably resulting from vascular events in utero (Durkin et al. 1976); detailed examination of the placenta should be carried out on all twin pregnancies in order to document zygosity, membrane disposition and IFVA status for correlation with clinical follow-up.

The most common picture in TTS is that of MC,MZ twins who are growth discrepant, with the larger recipient twin being plethoric and the smaller donor having normal or reduced haemoglobin level. The donor may be positionally deformed by the effects of polyhydramnios/oligohydramnios. Either twin may be hydropic. Visceral infarction in the survivor may complicate fetal death of one twin.

Less commonly, reversed twin transfusion may supervene during delivery (Bendon and Siddiqi 1989). If the chronic recipient is delivered first, IFVA may drain placental blood into the second-born donor, who may then appear as plethoric as the recipient twin.

Rupture of vasa praevia may cause anaemia in the first-born recipient. Rarely, the second twin may also exsanguinate via IFVA when vasa praevia of the first twin are torn (Antoine et al. 1982).

Spontaneous resolution of prenatally documented TTS may result in no residual abnormality or there may be ill-defined right ventricular pathology and continuing myocardial failure.

In addition to the macroscopic lesions of organ infarction that may complicate fetal death of one twin, changes may occur at tissue and cellular level, including aganglionosis and neuromuscular abnormalities (Hall et al. 1983; Siplovich et al. 1983).

Exceptions to the expected pattern of TTS should prompt careful placental examination in an attempt to correlate the clinical status of the twins with their placental anatomy. There are also rare reports of IFVA and actual TTS occurring in DC (and also DZ) twins (Robertson and Neer 1983; Lage et al. 1989).

Twin Reversed Arterial Perfusion

One of the most severe human congenital anomalies is holoacardius acephalus, which is found in MC twins who have major AAA and VVA as the associated placental anatomy (Moore et al. 1990; Van Allen et al. 1983). It has been shown by prenatal Doppler flow studies that the intact "pump" twin perfuses the acardiac twin retrogradely via the umbilical artery of the latter (Kirkinen et al. 1989), with arterial flow being reversed in the major portion

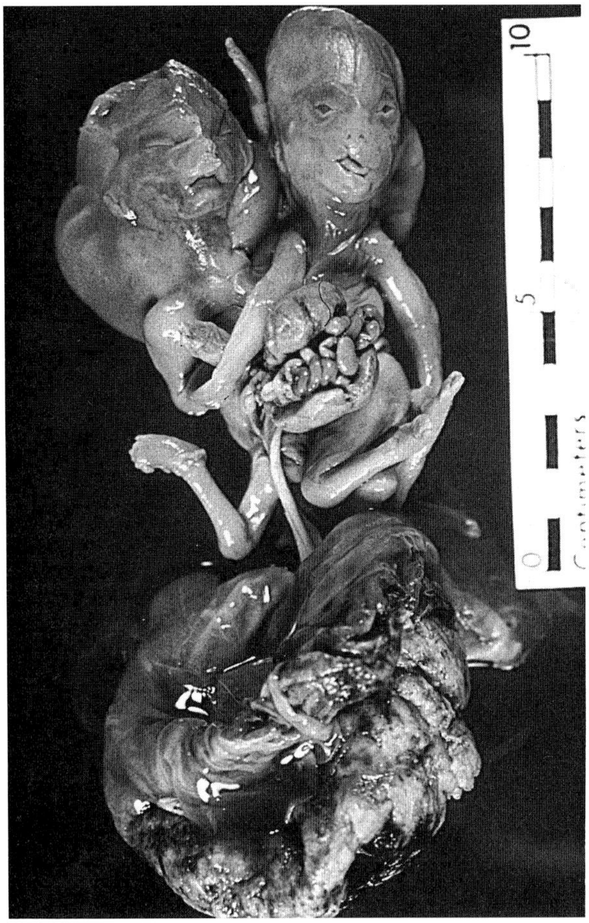

a

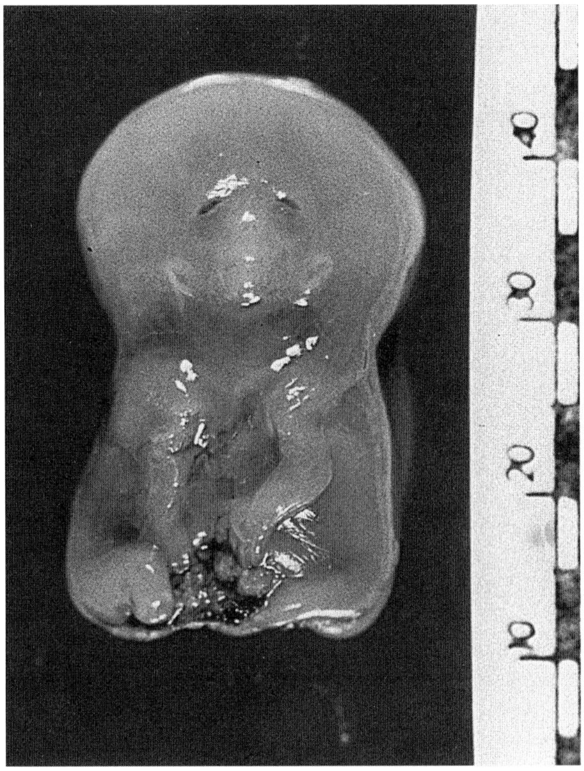

c

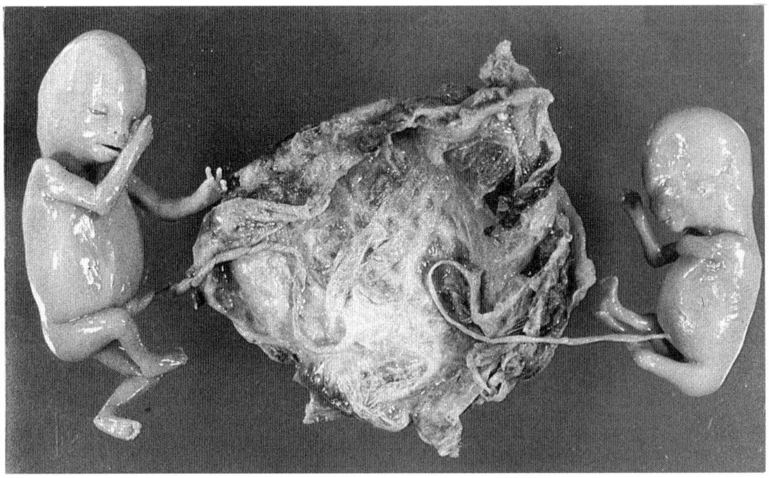

b

Fig. 9.2. MZ twins among spontaneously aborted conceptuses: **a** Conjoined thoracopagus female twins with cystic hygromas, probably representing 45X chromosome constitution (Turner's syndrome). **b** Spontaneous abortion of MC twins at 8 weeks of gestation, with evidence of TTS. There is growth retardation of the right twin, which has a flexed attitude. **c** Cephalothoracopagus conjoined twins, spontaneously aborted at 11 weeks of gestation.

Continued

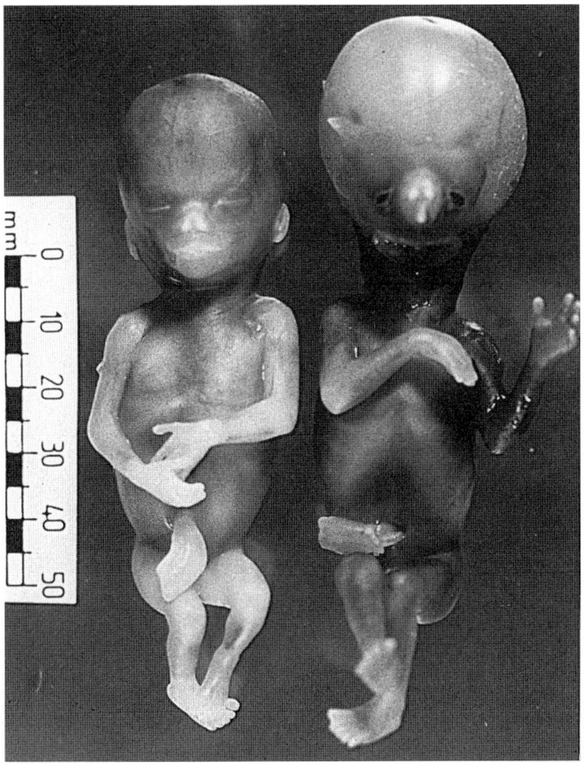

d

Fig. 9.2(*continued*). **d** Spontaneous abortion of MC twins at 13 weeks that are discordant for holoprosencephaly. Twin on left is normal; twin on right has holoprosencephaly/synotia.

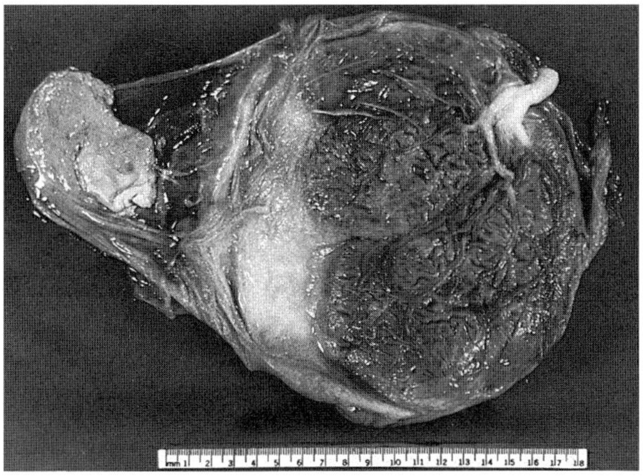

Fig. 9.3. Fetus papyraceus in MC twin pregnancy. The co-twin survived intact.

of the aorta; a proportion of the arterial blood of the pump twin, destined for the placenta, crosses instead in large AAA to reach the common iliac arteries of the acardiac. Thus, structures in the lower half of the body often survive better than those further from the portal of entry of arterial blood. A further consideration is the metabolic requirements of various organ systems, notably the brain, which usually does not survive the abnormal haemodynamics.

Serial ultrasound examinations show that initially apparently nearly normal acardiacs can undergo progressive deterioration in the interval before delivery. The pathology of the acardiac probably depends largely on the interval between the onset of regression and the time of delivery (Fig. 9.4).

Two mechanisms are proposed for the development of TRAP. One regards TRAP as an unusual outcome of TTS in which the particular anatomical arrangement of IFVA allows the surviving twin to perfuse a fetal co-twin who has died from complications of severe, early TTS. The other posits that the acardiac twin is malformed from the outset in such a fashion that there is circulatory failure in early fetal life. This would result in spontaneous abortion in a singleton, but the fetus is passively perfused by the co-twin. It is possible that both of these mechanisms can occur; only circumstantial evidence of cause is available. A proportion of acardiac fetuses appear to have true malformations in addition to the disruptive lesions caused by TRAP (Van Allen et al. 1983; Stocker et al. 1987; Luebke et al. 1990), and some acardiacs are chromosomally abnormal, while their co-twins are chromosomally normal (heterokaryotypia) (Deacon et al. 1980). These observations support the idea that at least some acardiac fetuses have major or multiple malformations that result in cardiac failure, with the pump twin assuming the function of the circulation, albeit in an anatomically unusual way.

Pump twins have a high morbidity and mortality, largely connected with preterm delivery (Moore et al. 1990; Van Allen et al. 1983). Many of these pregnancies are complicated by polyhydramnios, which is reported to occur only in those cases where the acardiac fetus has kidneys (Mack et al. 1982). It is not clear how many pump twins have organ infarction as a result of the circulatory failure of the regressing acardiac co-twin. The diagnosis of TRAP can be made prenatally (Billah et al. 1981; Gibson et al. 1986; Lindahl et al. 1984);

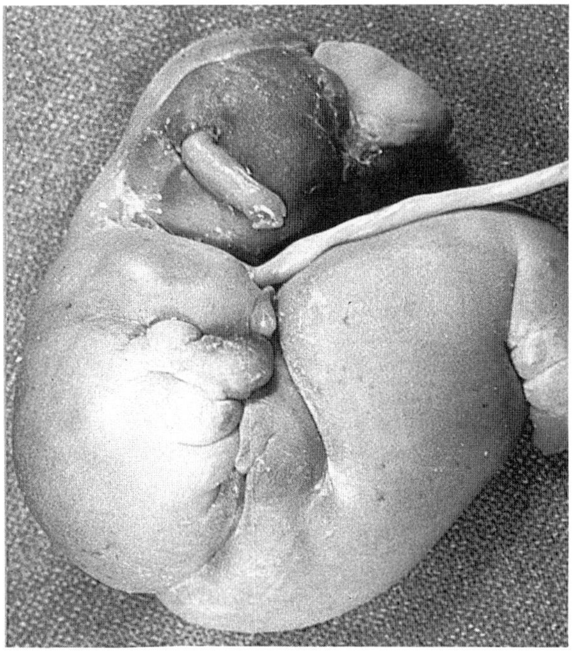
a

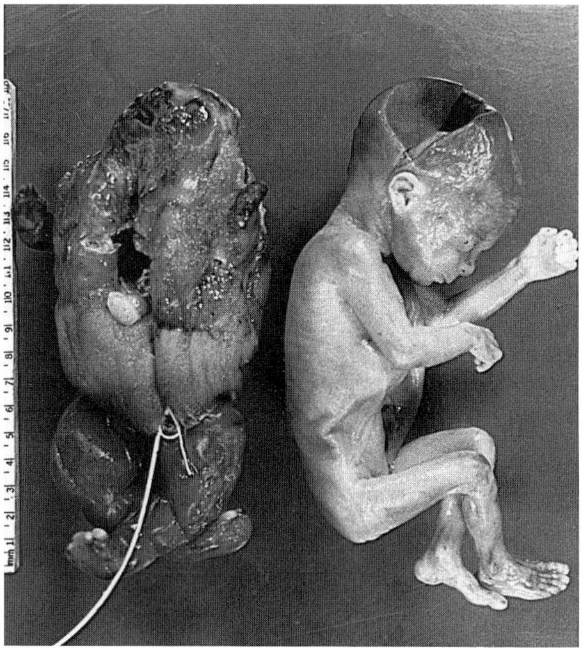
b

Fig. 9.4. TRAP syndrome: **a** Death relatively soon after onset of regression, with mummified head and upper limb still evident. **b** Facial features and four limbs can be delineated.

monitoring the wellbeing of the pump twin seems warranted. If kidneys are detected in the acardiac, premature delivery might be anticipated and treated by reducing the degree of polyhydramnios.

Complications of Monoamniotic Twinning

In addition to the risks posed by IFVA, monoamniotic (MA) twins have further problems because of the possibility of cord complications. These are of three types:

Cord/cord entanglement is likely to occur during early fetal life as the twins move freely in a common amniotic cavity; this can be detected prenatally (Halfar 1987; Townsend and Filly 1988). Prevalence of cord braiding is not known, but approaches 25%. Both twins usually die when knotting is extensive, but single twin survival is also known (Fig. 9.5).

Cord/twin entanglement may occur when the cord of one MA twin becomes entwined around the body of the co-twin. In the event of vaginal delivery of MA twins, a nuchal cord of the first-born twin may actually belong to the second twin; division of the cord will cause asphyxia of the second twin (Kassam and Tompkins 1980; McLeod and McCoy 1981).

Cord prolapse of the second cord may occur prior to delivery of the first MA twin (Lumme and Saarikoski 1986).

Cord complications, in addition to IFVA, cause MA twins to have the highest mortality of all twins, approaching 50% (Benirschke and Kim 1973; Carr et al. 1990).

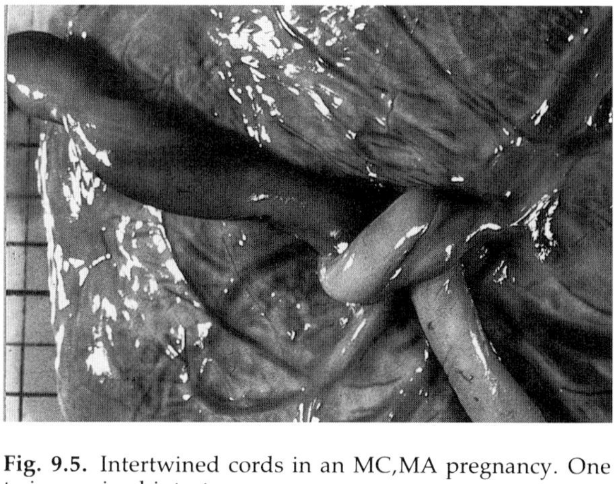

Fig. 9.5. Intertwined cords in an MC,MA pregnancy. One twin survived intact.

Congenital Anomalies in Twins

Many studies of congenital anomalies in twins are marred by inadequate documentation of chorionicity and zygosity; the present situation is confused. Anomalies resulting from monochorionicity (e.g. "stuck" twins, conjoined twins, TRAP and vascular complications of fetal death of the co-twin) must be excluded from any consideration of the prevalence of malformations of other aetiology. Some of the classic studies are based on like-sexed twins (Schinzel et al. 1979), assumed to be MZ, but do not consider chorionicity. These studies have been justly criticised (Boklage 1987). There is as yet no confirmation of a causal link between the process of MZ twinning and the genesis of midline malformations. Further, it is not clear whether MC,MZ twins are at greater risk for malformation than DC,MZ twins, and whether anomalies in DC,MZ twins may result from disruptional events, such as forcible rupture of the zona pellucidum. If the so-called "third twin" (mono-oogonial twin) is confirmed in humans, it remains to be seen whether malformation is more common in this category than in other DZ twins.

Most studies confirm that anomalies are more common in twins than singletons, and the suspicion remains that midline malformations are more common in MZ than DZ twins. Further documentation of anomalies in twins, analysed by zygosity and chorionicity, should clarify these problems.

Active Management of Vascular Sequelae in Monochorionic Twins

TTS may be progressive, leading to double fetal death, hydrops or severe sequelae of single fetal death. Since the disease is readily diagnosed and monitored, it is reasonable to attempt intervention when the prognosis appears poor. If maturity is not a consideration, delivery may be expedited; more commonly, TTS presents with severe complications in the second trimester. The aims of treatment are to reduce polyhydramnios, reduce the risk of markedly preterm delivery, and retard or reverse the transfusion process itself. Pathologists should expect to see fetuses and newborn infants with partially treated TTS, and need to assess the effects of treatment on the anatomy of IFVA. Similar considerations apply to TRAP pregnancies. The types of interventions and their rationales are listed in Table 9.2.

Table 9.2. Interventions in twin pregnancies with IFVA; methods and outcomes

Intervention	Outcome	Reference
Maternal digitalis therapy (Case no. 2)	100% mortality	Pretorius et al. (1988)
Maternal digitalis therapy	Both survived	DeLia et al. (1985)
Amniocentesis (Case no. 1, no. 2)	50% perinatal mortality with embolism, organ infarction	Feingold et al. (1986)
Amniocentesis	50% perinatal mortality, donor hydropic	Brennan et al. (1982)
Amniocentesis (Case no. 2)	100% perinatal mortality	Chescheir and Seeds (1988)
Amniocentesis (Case no. 1, no. 2)	50% perinatal mortality	Montan et al. (1985)
Amniocentesis, 8 pairs	31% perinatal mortality	Mahony et al. (1990)
Amniocentesis, 17 pairs	31% perinatal mortality	Elliott et al. (1991)
Selective feticide (Case no. 4)	Other twin died neonatally	Chescheir and Seeds (1988)
Selective feticide	Intact survival of TTS recipient	Wittmann et al. (1986)
Selective feticide (Case no. 2)	Intracardiac KCl to donor. Both died	Baldwin and Wittmann (1990)
Hysterectomy for TRAP	Pump twin died of antepartum haemorrhage	Golbus et al. (1988)
Hysterectomy and cord ligation of acardiac fetus	Pump twin survived intact	Robie et al. (1989)
Occlusive coil in umbilical artery of acardiac fetus	Pump twin survived intact	Porreco et al. (1991)
Laser coagulation of IFVA, 3 pairs	4 of 6 twins survived	DeLia et al. (1990)

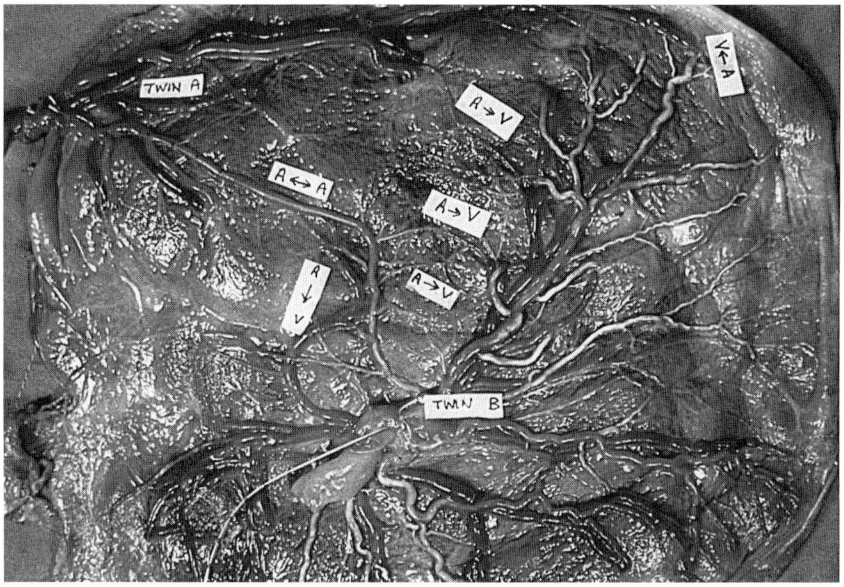

a

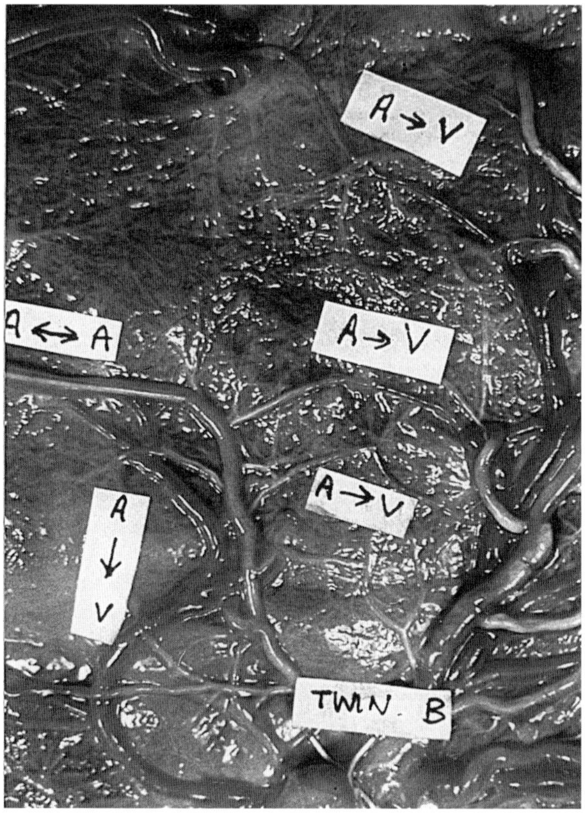

b

Fig. 9.6. **a** Perfusion study of MC,DA placenta. This case is more complex than usual, with one AAA and multiple, bidirectional AVA. **b** Close-up view of areas of potential AVA.

Practical Twin Pathology

The Placenta

The placenta should not be subject to examination on the labour ward but transferred to the pathology laboratory intact and with umbilical cords identified. Describe and classify as DC, separate or fused, MC,DA or MC,MA. Note identity of cords for each twin, and cord insertions, especially velamentous.

In MC placenta, document IFVA. This may require perfusion studies (Fig. 9.6a,b). When cords are identified and TTS is clinically suspected, it is best to perfuse an umbilical artery of the donor and an umbilical vein of the recipient. Half-strength barium gives good outlines and also shows well in the histological sections. AAA and VVA are easily seen. It is usually difficult to cause adequate perfusion through AVA, and sufficient evidence for presumed presence of AVA is furnished by the anatomical arrangement of artery and vein connecting to different cords from a single perfusion zone.

In addition to IFVA, it is useful to document the relative areas of venous perfusion by the twins, as this could account for growth discrepancy in the absence of other features of TTS. Perfusion studies should also be done in TRAP and in cases with FP.

The thickness of the septum, when present, gives immediate diagnosis of chorionicity. It is best to make membrane rolls of septum, and also T-junction preparations, so that chorionicity is permanently archived and recorded by microscopy (Fig. 9.7a,b).

Gross evidence of chorionamnionitis or oligohydramnios (amnion nodosum) should be noted. There may be histological differences in the placental parenchyma (Fig. 9.8a,b). Cord blood or placental tissue can be used to confirm zygosity by any method, such as RFLP, should this be clinically important.

It is good practice to photograph the gross appearances of all twin placentas.

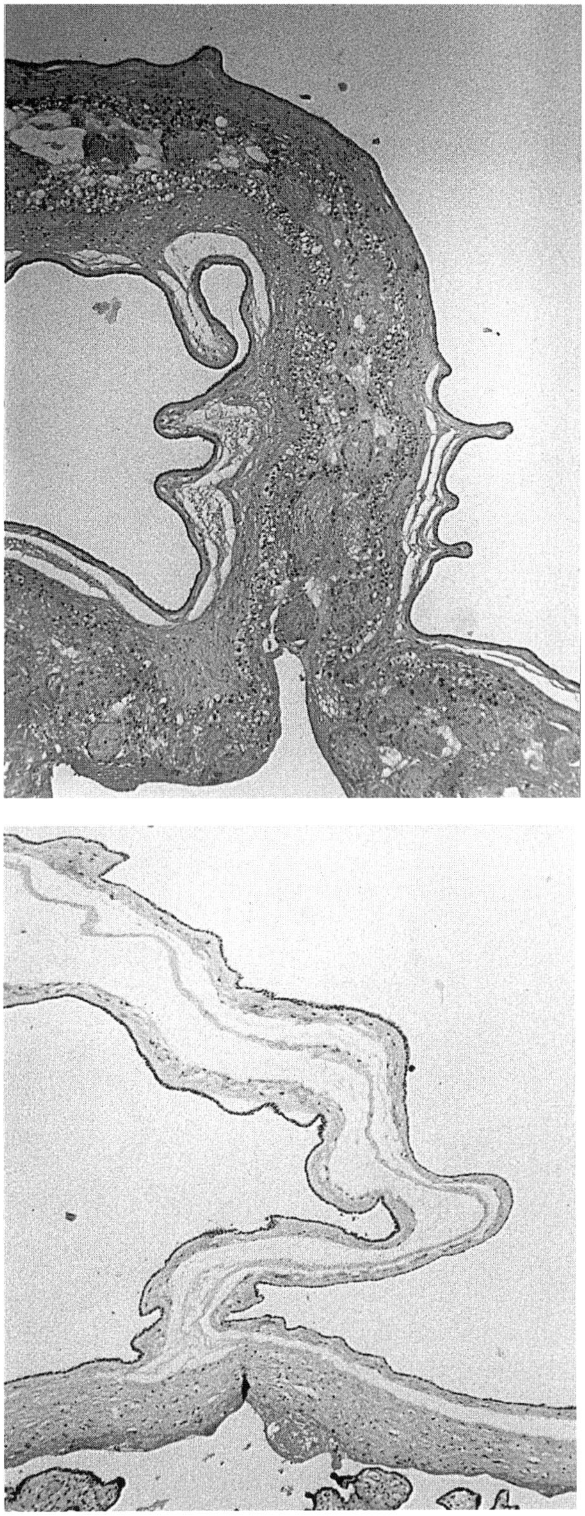

a

b

Fig. 9.7. **a** T-junction of DC,MA twin placenta. **b** T-junction of MC,DA twin placenta.

Necropsy of Twins

When only one twin dies, it is best to gather full clinical information about the survivor, and to compare birthweights and initial haemoglobin values in MC twins. While it is not always the case that deaths in MC twins are

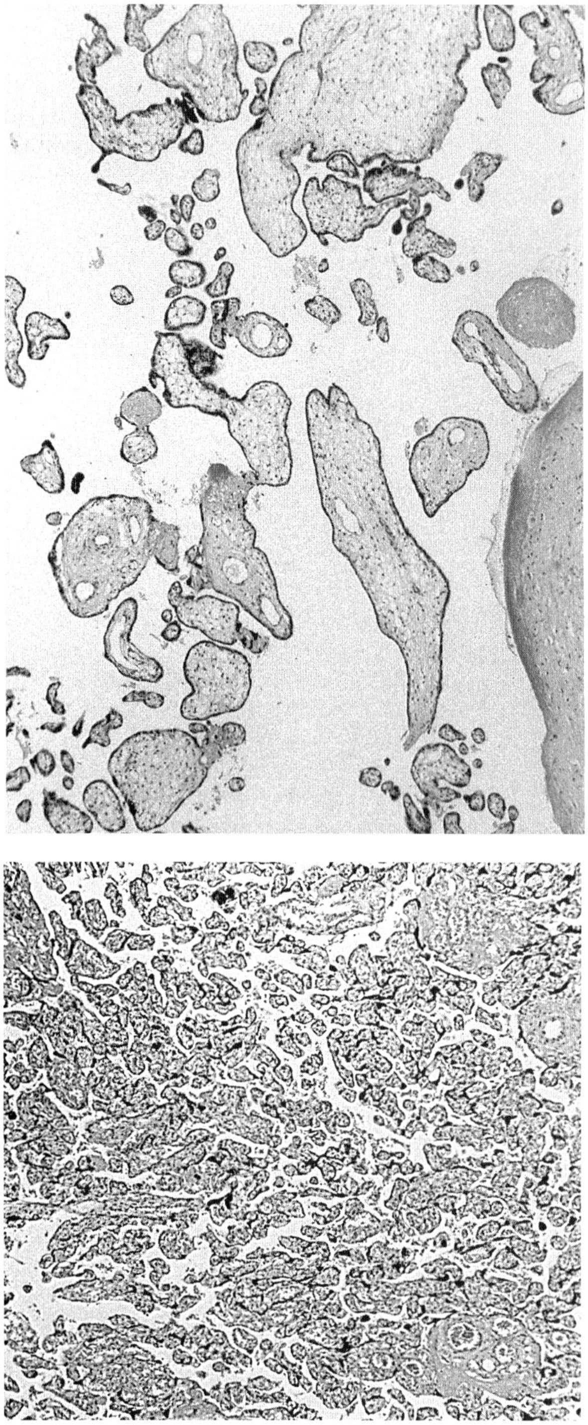

a

b

Fig. 9.8. **a** Chorionic villi of recipient, with stromal oedema. **b** Chorionic villi of donor, with perivillar fibrin deposition and accelerated maturation.

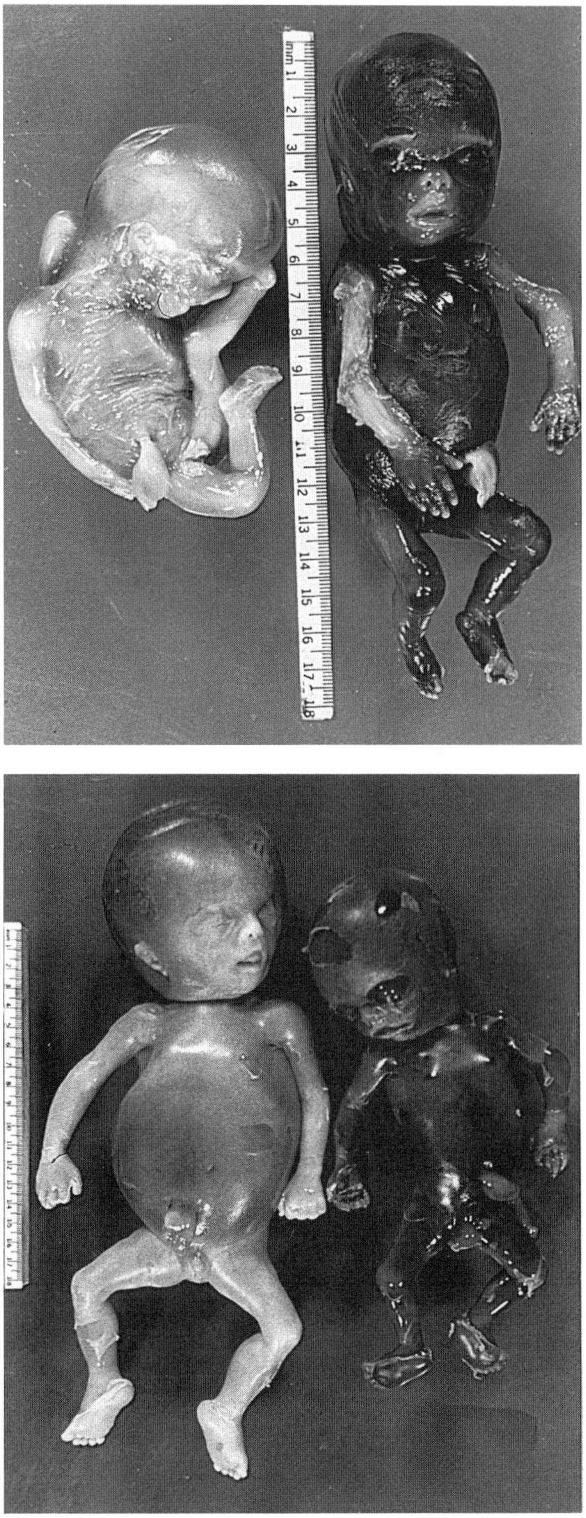

a

b

Fig. 9.9. **a** Typical acute, second trimester TTS, with small, flexed, "stuck" twin and larger, plethoric recipient twin. **b** Acute perinatal TTS, in which the chronic donor (*right*) has been acutely transfused in reverse by the chronic recipient (*left*).

directly or indirectly due to monochorionicity, it is highly likely.

When both twins are examined, they should be photographed together (Fig. 9.9a,b) and, if necessary, during dissection, in order to document growth discrepancy, plethora and anaemia, organ infarction and malformation.

Careful documentation of congenital anomalies is important, so as to distinguish between mechanical deformities and true malformations. "Stuck" twins usually show positional effects of oligohydramnios.

References

Antoine C, Young BK, Silverman F, Greco MA, Alvarez SP (1982) Sinusoidal fetal heart rate pattern with vasa previa in twin pregnancy. J Reprod Med 27: 295–330
Arts NFT, Lohman AHM (1971) The vascular anatomy of monochorionic diamniotic twin placentas and the transfusion syndrome. Eur J Obstet Gynaecol Reprod Biol 1: 85–93
Azuma C, Kamiura S, Nobunaga T, Negoro T, Saji F, Tanizawa O (1989) Zygosity determination of multiple pregnancy by deoxyribonucleic acid fingerprints. Am J Obstet Gynecol 160: 734–736
Baldwin VJ, Wittmann BK (1990) Pathology of intragestational intervention in twin-to-twin transfusion syndrome. Pediatr Pathol 10: 79–93
Barss VA, Benacerraf BR, Frigoletto FD (1985) Ultrasonographic determination of chorion type in twin gestation. Obstet Gynecol 66: 779–783
Bendon RW, Siddiqi T (1989) Clinical pathology conference: acute twin-to-twin transfusion. Pediatr Pathol 9: 591–598
Benirschke K (1961) Twin placenta in perinatal mortality. NY State J Med 61: 1499–1508
Benirschke K, Kim CK (1973) Multiple pregnancy. N Engl J Med 288: 1276–1284, 1329–1336
Berkowitz RL, Lynch L, Chitkara U, Wilkins IA, Mehalek KE, Alvarez E (1988) Selective reduction of multifetal pregnancies in the first trimester. N Engl J Med 318: 1043–1047
Bieber FR, Nance WE, Morton CC, Brown JA, Redwine FO (1981) Genetic studies of an acardiac monster: evidence of polar body twinning in man. Science 213: 775–777
Billah KL, Shah K, Odwin C (1984) Ultrasonic diagnosis and management of acardius anencephalic twin pregnancy. Med Ultrasound 8: 108–109
Blickstein I (1990) The twin-twin transfusion syndrome. Obstet Gynecol 76: 714–722
Boklage CE (1987) Invited editorial essay. Twinning, nonrighthandedness, and fusion malformations: evidence for heritable causal elements held in common. Am J Med Genet 28: 67–84
Bouchard C, Tremblay A, Despres J-P et al. (1990) The response to long-term overfeeding in identical twins. N Engl J Med 322: 1477–1487
Bouchard TJ, Lykken DT, McGur M, Segal NL, Tellegen A (1990) Sources of human psychological differences: The Minnesota study of twins reared apart. Science 250: 223–228
Brennan JN, Diwan RV, Rosen MG, Bellon EM (1982) Fetofetal transfusion syndrome: prenatal ultrasonographic diagnosis. Radiology 143: 535–536
Bulla M, von Lilien T, Goecke H, Roth B, Ortmann M, Heising J (1987) Renal and cerebral necrosis in survivor after in utero death of co-twin. Arch Gynecol 240: 119–124
Burn J, Povey S, Boyd Y et al. (1986) Duchenne muscular dystrophy in one of monozygotic twin girls. J Med Genet 23: 494–500
Carr SR, Aronson MP, Coustan CR (1990) Survival rates of monoamniotic twins do not decrease after 30 weeks' gestation. Am J Obstet Gynecol 163: 719–722
Chescheir NC, Seeds JW (1988) Polyhydramnios and oligohydramnios in twin gestations. Obstet Gynecol 71: 882–884
D'Alton ME, Dudley DK (1989) The ultrasonographhic prediction of chorionicity in twin gestation. Am J Obstet Gynecol 160: 557–561
Danskin FH, Neilson JP (1989) Twin-to-twin transfusion syndrome: What are appropriate diagnostic criteria? Am J Obstet Gynecol 161: 365–369
Deacon JS, Machin GA, Martin JME, Nicholson S, Nwankwo DC, Wintemute R (1980) Investigation of acephalus. Am J Med Genet 5: 85–99
DeLia JE, Emery MG, Sheafor SA, Jennison TA (1985) Twin transfusion syndrome: successful in utero treatment. Int J Gynaecol Obstet 23: 197–201
DeLia JE, Cruikshank DP, Keye WR (1990) Fetoscopic neodymium: YAG laser occlusion of placental vessel in severe twin-twin transfusion syndrome. Obstet Gynecol 75: 1046–1053
Derom C, Bakker E, Vlietinck R et al. (1985) Zygosity determination in newborn twins using DNA variants. J Med Genet 22: 279–282
Derom C, Vlietinck R, Derom R, Van den Berghe H, Thiery M (1987) Increased monozygotic twinning rate after ovulation induction. Lancet i: 1236–1238
Derom C, Vlietinck R, Derom R, Van den Berghe H, Thiery M (1988) Population-based study of sex proportion in monoamniotic twins. N Engl J Med 319: 119–120
Derom C, Vlietinck R, Derom R, Thiery M, Van den Berghe H (1989) Genotyping macerated stillborn twin fetuses. In: Proceedings of the 6th international congress on twin studies, Rome
Dimmick J, Hardwick D, Ho-Yuen B (1971) A case of renal necrosis and fibrosis in the immediate newborn period. Association with twin-to-twin transfusion syndrome. Am J Dis Child 122: 345–247
Durkin MV, Kaveggia EG, Pendleton E, Neuhauser G, Opitz JM (1976) Analysis of etiologic factors in cerebral palsy with severe mental retardation. Eur J Pediatr 123: 67–81
Elejalde BR, de Elejalde MM, Wagner AM, Lebel RR (1983) Diagnosis of twin transfusion syndrome at 18 weeks of gestation. J Clin Ultrasound 11: 442–446
Elliot JP, Urig MA, Clewell WH (1991) Aggressive therapeutic amniocentesis for treatment of twin-twin transfusion syndrome. Obstet Gynecol 77: 537–540
Erskine RLA, Ritchie JWK, Murnaghan GA (1986) Antenatal diagnosis of placental anastomosis in a twin pregnancy using Doppler ultrasound. Br J Obstet Gynaecol 93: 955–959
Feingold M, Cetrulo CL, Newton ER, Weiss J, Shakr C, Schmoys S (1986) Serial amniocentesis in the treatment of twin to twin transfusion complicated with acute hydramnios. Acta Genet Med Gemellol 35: 107–113

Fisher JE, Siongco A (1989) Complications from in utero death of a monozygous co-twin. Pediatr Pathol 9: 765–771
Galea P, Scott JM, Goel KM (1982) Feto-fetal transfusion syndrome. Arch Dis Child 57: 781–794
Gedda L, Lun MT, Carrega R, Roselli E (1981) Parental age, sibship's size, and sibship's sex ratio in twins. A progress report. In: Gedda L, Parisi P, Nance WE (eds) Twin research 3: twin biology and multiple pregnancy. Liss, New York, pp 75–80
Gibson JY, D'Cruz CA, Patel RB, Palmer SM (1986) Acardiac anomaly: review of the subject with case report and emphasis on practical sonography. J Clin Ultrasound 14: 541–545
Giles WB, Trudinger BJ, Cook CM (1985) Umbilical waveforms in twin pregnancy. Acta Genet Med Gemellol 43: 233–237
Golbus MS, Cunningham N, Goldberg JD, Anderson R, Filly R, Callen P (1988) Selective termination of multiple gestations. Am J Med Genet 31: 339–348
Halfar MM (1987) Collaborative management of twins. Two case studies. J Nurse-Midwifery 32: 140–148
Hall JG, Reed SD, McGillivray BC et al. (1983) Part II. Amyoplasia: twinning in amyoplasia—a specific type of arthrogryposis with an apparent excess in discordantly affected identical twins. Am J Med Genet 15: 591–599
Hashimoto B, Callen PW, Filly RA, Laros R (1986) Ultrasound evaluation of polyhydramnios and twin pregnancy. Am J Obstet Gynecol 154: 1069–1072
Hertzberg BS, Kurtz AB, Choi HY et al. (1987) Significance of membrane thickness in the sonographic evaluation of twin gestations. AJR 148: 151–153
Hill AVS, Jeffreys AJ (1985) Use of minisatellite DNA probes for determination of twin zygosity at birth. Lancet ii: 1394–1395
James WH (1980) Sex ratio and placentation in twins. Ann Hum Biol 7: 273–276
Jauniaux E, Elkhazen N, LeRoy F, Wilkin P, Hustin J (1988) Clinical and morphologic aspects of the vanishing twin phenomenon. Obstet Gynecol 72: 577–581
Kassam SH, Tompkins MG (1980) Monoamniotic twin pregnancy and modern obstetrics. Report of a case with a peculiar cord complication. Diagn Gynecol Obstet 2: 213–220
Kirkinen P, Herva R, Rasanen J, Airaksinen J, Ikaheimo M (1989) Documentation of paradoxical umbilical blood supply of an acardiac twin in the antepartum state. J Perinat Med 17: 63–65
Kirshon B (1989) Fetal urine output in hydramnios. Obstet Gynecol 73: 240–242
Lage JM, Vanmarter LJ, Mikhail E (1989) Vascular anastomoses in fused, dichorionic twin placentas resulting in twin transfusion syndrome. Placenta 10: 55–59
Landy HJ, Keith L, Keith D (1982) The vanishing twin. Acta Genet Med Gemellol 31: 179–194
Landy HJ, Weiner S, Corson SL, Batzer FR, Bolognese RJ (1986) The "vanishing twin": Ultrasonographic assessment of fetal disappearance in the first trimester. Am J Obstet Gynecol 155: 14–19
Levi S (1976) Ultrasonic assessment of the high rate of human multiple pregnancy in the first trimester. J Clin Ultrasound 4: 3–5
Lindahl SA, Baldwin V, Wakeford J, Wittmann BK (1984) Early diagnosis of an acardiac acephalus twin by ultrasound. Med Ultrasound 8: 105–107
Livingstone JE, Poland BJ (1980) A study of spontaneously aborted twins. Teratology 21: 139–148
Lubinsky M, Rapoport P (1983) Transient fetal hydrops and "prune belly" in one identical female twin. N Engl J Med 308: 256–257
Luebke HJ, Reiser CA, Pauli RM (1990) Fetal disruptions: assessment of frequency, heterogeneity and embryologic mechanisms in a population referred to a community-based stillbirth assessment program. Am J Med Genet 36: 56–72
Lumme RH, Saarikoski SV (1986) Monoamniotic twin pregnancy. Acta Genet Med Gemellol 35: 99–105
Mack LA, Gravett MG, Rumack CM et al. (1982) Antenatal ultrasonic evaluation of acardiac monsters. J Ultrasound Med 1: 13–18
Mahony BS, Petty CN, Nyberg DA et al (1990) The "stuck twin" phenomenon: ultrasonographic findings, pregnancy outcome and management with serial amniocentesis. Am J Obstet Gynecol 163: 1513–1522
Mahony BS, Filly RA, Callen PW (1985) Amnionicity and chorionicity in twin pregnancies: prediction using ultrasound. Radiology 155: 205–209
Mannino FL, Jones KL, Benirschke K (1977) Congenital skin defects and fetus papyraceus. J Pediatr 91: 559–564
McLeod FN, McCoy DR (1981) Monoamniotic twins with an unusual cord complication. Case report. Br J Obstet Gynaecol 88: 774–775
Montan S, Jorgensen C, Sjoberg NO (1985) Amniocentesis in treatment of acute polyhydramnios in twin pregnancies. Acta Obstet Gynecol Scand 64: 537–539
Moore CM, McAdams AJ, Sutherland J (1969) Intrauterine disseminated intravascular coagulation: a syndrome of multiple pregnancy with a dead twin fetus. J Pediatr 74: 523–528
Moore TR, Gale S, Benirschke K (1990) Perinatal outcome of 49 pregnancies complicated by acardiac twinning. Am J Obstet Gyneol 163: 907–912
Nageotte MP, Hurwitz SR, Kaupke CJ, Vaziri ND, Pandian MR (1989) Atriopeptin in the twin transfusion syndrome. Obstet Gynecol 73: 867–870
Nance WE (1990) Invited editorial: Do twin Lyons have larger spots? Am J Hum Genet 46: 646–648
Nicolini U, Fisk NM, Talbert G et al. (1989) Intrauterine manometry: technique and applications to fetal pathology. Prenat Diagn 9: 243–254
Porreco RP, Barton SM, Haverkamp AD (1991) Occlusion of umbilical artery in acardiac, acephalic twin. Lancet 337: 326–327
Pretorius DH, Manchester D, Barkin S, Parker S, Nelson TR (1988) Doppler ultrasound in twin transfusion syndrome. J Ultrasound Med 7: 117–124
Richards CS, Watkins SC, Hoffman EP et al. (1990) Skewed X inactivation in a female MZ twin results in Duchenne muscular dystrophy. Am J Hum Genet 46: 672–681
Robertson EG, Neer KJ (1983) Placental injection studies in twin gestation. Am J Obstet Gynecol 147: 170–174
Robie GF, Payne GG, Morgan MA (1989) Selective delivery of an acardiac, acephalic twin. N Engl J Med 320: 512–513
Schinzel AAGL, Smith DW, Miller JR (1979) Monozygotic twinning and structural defects. J Pediatr 95: 921–930
Schwartz JL, Maniscalco WM, Lane AT, Currao WJ (1984) Twin transfusion syndrome causing cutaneous erythropioesis. Pediatrics 74: 527–529
Siplovich L, Carmi R, Bar-Ziv J, Karplus M, Mares AJ (1983) Discordant Hirschsprung's disease in monozygotic twins. J Pediatr Surg 18: 639–640
Stocker JT, Heifetz SA (1987) Sirenomelia. A morphological study of 33 cases and review of the literature. Perspect Pediatr Pathol 10: 7–50
Strong SJ, Corney G (1967) The placenta in twin preg-

nancy. Pergamon, Oxford

Sulak LE, Dodson MG (1986) The vanishing twin: pathologic confirmation of an ultrasonographic phenomenon. Obstet Gynecol 68: 811–815

Szymonowicz W, Preston H, Yu VYH (1986) The surviving monozygotic twin. Arch Dis Child 61: 454–458

Townsend RR, Filly RA (1988) Sonography of nonconjoined monoamniotic twin pregnancies. J Ultrasound Med 7: 665–670

Townsend RR, Simpson GF, Filly RA (1988) Membrane thickness in ultrasound prediction of chorionicity of twin gestations. J Ultrasound Med 7: 413–416

Uchida I (1990) Twinning in spontaneous abortions and developmental abnormalities. In: Kalter H (ed) Issues and reviews in teratology, vol 5: Plenum, New York, pp 155–180

Uchida IA, Freeman VCP, Gedeon M, Goldmaker J (1983) Twinning rate in spontaneous abortions. Am J Hum Genet 35: 987–993

Van Allen MI, Smith DW, Shepard TH (1983) Twin reversed arterial perfusion (TRAP) sequence: a study of 14 twin pregnancies with acardius. Semin Perinatol 7: 285–293

Wagner DS, Klein RL, Robinson HP, Novak RW (1990) Placental emboli from a fetus papyraceus. J Pediatr Surg 25: 538–542

Wapner RJ, Davis GH, Johnson A et al. (1990) Selective reduction of multifetal pregnancies. Lancet 335: 90–93

Winn HN, Gabrielli S, Reece EA, Roberts JA, Salafia C, Hobbins JC (1989) Ultrasonographic criteria for the prenatal diagnosis of placental chorionicity in twin gestations. Am J Obstet Gynecol 161: 1540–1542

Wittman BK, Baldwin VJ, Nichol B (1981) Antenatal diagnosis of twin transfusion syndrome by ultrasound. Obstet Gynecol 58: 123–127

Wittmann BK, Farquharson DF, Thomas WDS, Baldwin VJ, Wadsworth LD (1986) The role of feticide in the management of severe twin transfusion syndrome. Am J Obstet Gynecol 155: 1023–1026

Yoshida K, Soma H (1984) A study of twin placentation in Tokyo. Acta Genet Med Gemellol 33: 115–120

Yoshida K, Soma H (1986) Outcome of surviving cotwin of a fetus papyraceus or a dead twin fetus. Acta Genet Med Gemellol 35: 91–98

Chapter 10

Intrapartum Asphyxia and Birth Trauma

Jean W. Keeling

Introduction

There has been a commendable reduction in intrapartum and neonatal deaths associated with birth trauma and asphyxia during the last 40 years. Any death related to intrapartum insult deserves attention. Necropsy and clinical management should be carefully reviewed to identify any avoidable factors. It is particularly important that a good obstetric and neonatal history is available in these cases before necropsy is begun, so that evidence of asphyxia or trauma is not overlooked. A history of intrapartum death or a description of intrapartum difficulties will not be found in all cases. The pathologist should be aware that pallor, shock, hypotonia and difficulty in initiating or maintaining respiration at birth may be the result of intrapartum asphyxia or trauma. These signs do not specifically imply intrapartum insult and may be the presenting features of some major malformations, particularly those accompanied by pulmonary hypoplasia (see Table 17.1, p. 415), congenital heart disease or infection.

Better antenatal care means that in most pregnancies both mother and baby are in good condition at the onset of labour; this improved standard of care, together with more reliable intrapartum monitoring techniques, has led to better anticipation of problems which might arise during labour enabling appropriate delivery to be planned. The availability of facilities for caesarean section has improved the outcome for those emergencies that do occur. It is appropriate to consider birth asphyxia and trauma together as there is usually an asphyxial contribution to deaths where major trauma is identified. More frequently, the observed physical injury is unlikely to be fatal and is an indication of intrapartum difficulty. It should alert the pathologist to the probability of cerebral compression sufficient to induce fetal shock with bradycardia and reduced cardiac output, so that ischaemia will exacerbate any hypoxic stress.

The effect of intrapartum asphyxia is probably underestimated amongst babies delivered prematurely, when prematurity-associated pathology commands attention both in the nursery and the post-mortem room (Barson et al. 1984). Asphyxia alone may be sufficient to induce certain physical changes; some are immediately apparent, e.g. visceral petechial haemorrhages or haemorrhage into muscles, or become manifest following degenerative sequelae of the initial insult, as is the case with some forms of hypoxic cerebral or myocardial injury.

Fetal Response to Asphyxia

A dictionary definition of asphyxia as "suspended animation due to lack of oxygen in blood" describes the physiological effects of the combination of hypoxaemia, hypercapnia and acidosis. The fetal response to hypoxaemia is a redistribution of the circulation to maintain oxygenation of vital organs and to conserve oxygen (Dawes 1968). Cohn et al. (1974) have shown in fetal lambs that, in the short term, hypoxaemia results in increased blood flow to the brain, heart and adrenals, whilst the flow to kidney and spleen fall and that to other organs, including the placenta, remains unchanged. Cardiac output and blood pressure are maintained by means of a fall in heart rate and increase in stroke volume.

In the human fetus, hypoxaemia depresses breathing movements; thus tachycardia, which accompanies the tachypnoeic response to hypoxia in adults, is abolished. Bradycardia, which is the primary cardiovascular response to hypoxia, is therefore the observed fetal response to hypoxia. In the face of hypoxaemia, the fetus can use lactate as an energy source and engage in anaerobic metabolism, which extends its ability to endure asphyxial insults.

Fetal asphyxia in labour is recognised by abnormalities of heart rate in relation to uterine contractions and depression of blood pH. Now that more sophisticated monitoring equipment is available, additional parameters can be used. Abnormalities of fetal electrocardiograph or electroencephalographic recordings and reduction in fetal breathing movements, particularly if gasping efforts are observed, are recognised as responses to asphyxial stress.

Fetal Response to Labour

Our understanding of the fetal reponse to labour is far from complete, but continuous recording of fetal heart rate during labour and its relationship to blood gas measurements in fetal scalp and cord blood samples and to fetal condition at birth in both complicated and uncomplicated labour has contributed to our understanding of fetal wellbeing or the lack of it during labour (Low et al. 1981). A normal fetal electrocardiograph has a baseline rate between 120 and 160 beats per minute (bpm) with a variability between 5 and 15 bpm. Reactivity, i.e. accelerations associated with fetal movement, is normal up to 15 bpm, as are decelerations synchronous with contractions of less than 15 bpm (early decelerations, Type I dips; Steer 1985). Late decelerations (Type II dips) indicate fetal hypoxia, and loss of baseline variability is seen when there is fetal metabolic acidosis. An increase in baseline fetal heart rate is observed up to delivery in both normal and abnormal labours but is more common in the latter (Low et al. 1981) and may be the first sign of hypoxic stress. It is also seen when there is maternal pyrexia, infection or anxiety. Tachycardia is a physiological response in the preterm fetus.

Fetal wellbeing during labour is dependent on the complex relationship between uterine muscular activity, the shape and distensibility of the birth canal and the size, position and configuration of the fetus, and on the continuing function of the placenta. During labour the fetus is dependent on adequate placental perfusion for survival. In late pregnancy and in labour, uterine perfusion may be adversely affected by compression of the aorta and vena cava by the gravid uterus when the mother is supine. Crawford et al. (1972) documented the association of birth asphyxia and caval compression during caesarean section. The same group (Atkins et al. 1981) demonstrated rapid circulatory compensation for large vessel compression in the normal parturient woman but stressed the hazard that changes in utero-placental vascular dynamics pose for the human fetus.

Placental perfusion is interrupted by uterine contractions and there must be an adequate recovery phase between contractions to permit reperfusion and oxygenation of fetal tissues. Even in normal labour, the normal, optimally positioned fetus will experience a fall in capillary pH during both first and second stages of labour (Beard et al. 1967). Such acidosis indicates the inefficiency of placental transfer and obligatory anaerobic metabolism provoked by the interruption to placental exchange by uterine contractions. The fetus may experience stress during vaginal delivery as a result of compression of the head and trunk, resulting in elevated levels of circulating noradrenalin and adrenalin when compared with babies delivered by elective caesarean section (Jones and Greiss 1982). Amniotomy in early labour produces transient changes in fetal heart rate patterns (Smis and Thiery 1980), presumably as a result of increased pressure to the fetal head. Svenningsen et al. (1988) measured fetal head compression during spontaneous labour. They recorded large differences in maximum compression pressure during maternal bearing down. There was no relationship between maximum pressure and presence of retinal haemorrhage and concluded that the fetus could withstand marked head compression for short periods with no ill effect.

The normal fetus may be subject to abnormal stresses during labour in several circumstances. It may be stressed because labour is prolonged. Excessive uterine contraction, either naturally occurring or because of the use of oxytoxic drugs (Schwarcz et al. 1974), may adversely affect the fetus. Increased pressure to the fetal head may occur because the abnormal shape or resistance of the birth canal impedes fetal passage (Stewart and Philpott 1980). This problem may be aggravated by maternal bearing down efforts, which can impair uterine circulation by interference with both arterial perfusion and venous drainage, by compression of the aorta and vena cava respectively by the gravid uterus (Bassell et al. 1980). The fetus which is abnormal as a result of intrauterine growth retardation, infection, malformation or injury may be unable to withstand the amount of physical stress engendered by a normal labour (Steer 1985).

Incidence

Intrapartum death of normally formed babies as the result of fetal asphyxia, trauma or a combination of the two accounted for 40.3% of stillbirths and 19.6% of neonatal deaths in the 1958 British Perinatal Mortality Survey (Butler and Bonham 1963), a rate of 10.2 per 1000 births. In one area of the UK 13 years later, intrapartum problems amongst stillbirths had fallen to 31%, but the proportion of neonatal deaths related to intrapartum events was virtually unchanged, although the mortality rate from these conditions had fallen to 5.2 per 1000 births (Machin 1975). In the US Collaborative Perinatal Study, there were 76 intrapartum deaths at term, comprising 32% of the normally formed stillbirths in that study (Lilien 1970). The deaths of 97 normally formed babies occurred during labour in Scotland in 1976, (McIlwaine et al. 1979). This comprised 13% of perinatal deaths or 24% of normally formed stillbirths in that year. By 1989, this had fallen to 19 (0.2/1000) with an additional 32 early neonatal deaths resulting from hypoxia/birth trauma (Scottish Stillbirth and Neonatal Death Report 1990). Two small hospital-based European studies showed a much lower incidence of intrapartum deaths: they accounted for 9.1% of stillbirths in Helsinki (Hovatta et al. 1983) and 8.3% of stillbirths in Malmö (Löfgren and Polberger 1983). The incidence of intrapartum problems is a good indicator of the provision of facilities for delivery. Brans et al. (1984) found one-third of stillbirths occurred intrapartum, a stillbirth rate of 9.2 per 1000 births in one disadvantaged area of the US. In Jamaica 61% of perinatal deaths in 1986–87 were fresh stillbirths or first day deaths to mature babies (Coard et al. 1991). The perinatal mortality rate was 38 per 1000 births. More detailed analysis of factors related to adverse intrapartum events showed an association between both intrapartum asphyxia and maternal mortality and the type of hospital facilities in the mother's parish of residence (Samms-Vaughan and Golding 1992).

Placental Factors During Labour

Any pathological condition of the placenta which affects maternoplacental gas exchange, such as hydrops, widespread villitis and infarction of more than 10% of parenchymal volume, will increase the risk of asphyxial insult to the fetus during labour.

Some causes of birth asphyxia are unpredictable and constitute obstetric emergencies. Placental abruption is the commonest of these. Its association with toxaemia of pregnancy has long been recognised, and although ultrasound examination has led to earlier, more certain recognition of the problem and thus to better management, our lack of understanding of its aetiology offers little prospect for more precise anticipation.

Placenta praevia as a cause of birth asphyxia is more often associated with preterm than term labour. This is in part because the lower uterine segment extends as pregnancy advances so that the placenta appears to "move away" from the internal os and also because premature separation of the placenta from the lower segment may result in retroplacental haemorrhage, overt vaginal bleeding and uterine contractions. There is often premonitory minor haemorrhage, and increased use of ultrasound examination in the third trimester and during labour is identifying an increasing proportion of cases.

Velamentous insertion of the cord (see p. 63) prediposes to birth asphyxia because of circulatory obstruction resulting from direct pressure by the presenting fetal part on the poorly supported vessels in their intramembranous course. If there is vasa praevia then vessel rupture may occur and asphyxia be compounded by hypovolaemia.

Cord obstruction during labour may result from cord prolapse complicating non-engagement of the presenting part from any cause such as multiparity, multiple pregnancy or compound presentation. Tightening of cord knots during fetal descent and an unduly short or very long umbilical cord are all associated with intrapartum asphyxia (see pp. 63, 64).

Maternal Factors in Labour

Fetuses of women with certain medical disorders such as diabetes mellitus, renal disease, hypertension and malnutrition are at increased risk of intrapartum stress. Maternal anaemia from any cause enhances intrapartum asphyxial insult and should be sought and treated before labour commences. In pre-eclamptic toxaemia, failure in adaptation of decidual vessels (see Chap. 2, p. 68) causes chronic uteroplacental ischaemia resulting in fetal growth retardation. This accentuates placental ischaemia produced by uterine contraction. The fetus does not seem to be at increased risk of asphyxial stress when chorioamnionitis is diagnosed during labour (Maberry et al. 1990) and operative delivery is not justified when labour is progressing at a normal rate.

Maternal pelvic pathology, such as uterine fibroids, ovarian cysts and abnormalities of pelvic shape, may predispose to breech presentation or interfere with descent of the presenting fetal part. Poor uterine tone in the grande multipara is associated with breech or compound presentation.

Asphyxia as a result of long labour because of cephalopelvic disproportion or poor uterine action is uncommon in developed countries, where these problems are likely to be recognised and delivery expedited. They are still a serious cause of fetal and maternal morbidity and mortality in countries where specialist maternity services are not available to a large part of the population.

Instrumental delivery can produce some forms of cranial trauma, particularly when rotation of the fetal head has been attempted. However, it is important to distinguish between abnormalities related to the reason for which instrumental delivery was undertaken and those related to the mode of delivery itself. Documentation of increased fetal mortality and morbidity (Friedman and Sachtleben 1971; Chiswick and James 1979) and fear of litigation increased the number of operative deliveries for occipitoposterior position, deep transverse arrest and delayed second stage. More recent studies (Healey et al. 1982; Cardozo et al. 1983) suggest that, provided there is observation of clearly defined criteria for selection for forceps delivery and adherence to documented instrumental technique, instrumental delivery offers no increased risk to the baby compared with caesarean section. They also found that risks to the mother in current and subsequent pregnancies were lower when instrumental delivery rather than caesarean section had been undertaken.

Drugs administered to the mother which can result in fetal hypoxia because of maternal hypotension and reduced uteroplacental perfusion include those drugs used to treat hypertension as well as spinal, epidural and general anaesthetic agents. Maternal anaesthesia is thus a further hazard to the fetus when instrumental or operative delivery is required. Narcotic analgesics administered to the mother can depress the fetal respiratory centre. This provokes neonatal rather than intrapartum problems for the baby.

Fetal Factors in Labour

Fetal size is an important determinant of the successful outcome of labour. The large baby is at risk of both asphyxia and physical injury related to its size (Fedrick 1969). Manipulation to overcome shoulder dystocia may lead to excessive neck stretching and injury to the brachial plexus or cervical cord. Cephalopelvic disproportion inclines towards delay in descent of the presenting part, and signs of asphyxia may precipitate instrumental delivery and risk of injury to the face and head.

The small baby, whether preterm or growth retarded, is at risk of asphyxia and abnormal presentation. When the baby is growth retarded these problems may be compounded by the underlying causes of poor growth such as uteroplacental ischaemia and placental infarction (Fox 1967) or infection.

The fully flexed fetus with the vertex presenting and occiput anterior is in the optimal position for delivery as the smallest diameter of the fetal head is accommodated by the birth canal. Incomplete neck flexion results in a larger cranial diameter and predisposes to failure of rotation of the fetal head to the occipitoanterior position during its descent through the pelvis. Incomplete flexion of the head is encouraged by poor uterine contractions, an excess of liquor amnii and abnormalities of pelvic shape. Fetal abnormality, such as Klippel–Feil anomaly of the cervical spine or cervical tumour, may also prevent full head flexion.

Breech presentation is associated with higher perinatal mortality and morbidity than vertex presentation, but much of the excess appears to be related to the underlying cause (Faber-Nijholt et al. 1983). Prematurity is the commonest of these. In the second trimester when there is a relatively large amount of liquor, fetal position changes frequently; by 34 weeks' gestation the head is usually the presenting part. Conditions which impede fetal movement such as oligohydramnios, multiple pregnancy and fetal neuromuscular abnormality are associated with breech presentation. Situations which permit excess fetal movement such as polyhydramnios and multiparity also encourage abnormal presentation. Factors which impede engagement of the fetal head such as placenta praevia, lower segment uterine fibroids and hydrocephalus predispose to breech presentation, and antepartum recognition of these problems influences management of delivery.

Even when the adverse effects of aetiological factors of breech presentation are acknowledged, there are hazards related to vaginal delivery of the fetus presenting by the breech. Prolapsed cord or descent of the breech through an incompletely dilated cervix with subsequent delay to delivery of the head result in asphyxia. Manoeuvres undertaken to deliver the head, with or without forceps, may result in cervical cord injury or occipital osteodiastasis. Decreased muscle tone because of asphyxia increases the risk of some traumatic injuries. The baby presenting by the breech is thus susceptible to fractures of long bones inflicted when there is difficulty in bringing down the limbs. Cervical and visceral injuries occur following manipulation of the neck and trunk and are more likely in the presence of asphyxia. Haemorrhage into leg and gluteal muscles resulting from hypoxia and congestion of the dependent part may be sufficient to cause significant hypovolaemia or neonatal jaundice.

Some pathological conditions of the fetus substantially increase the risk of birth trauma in otherwise propitious circumstances. The most easily recognised of these is type II osteogenesis imperfecta, where the skull is poorly mineralised and easily deformed so that intracranial trauma is readily inflicted. These babies develop multiple fractures of long bones and ribs in utero and, although healing with callous formation takes place, the limbs are often deformed. Manipulation of the deformed limbs increases still further the likelihood of additional fractures of the very brittle bones in this condition.

Babies with neuromuscular disorders which are apparent at birth, such as severe forms of Werdnig–Hoffmann disease, dystrophia myotonia congenita or hydrocephalus, are at increased risk of birth injury. Their reduced muscular activity in utero increases the proportion of babies presenting by the breech, and restriction of the range of movement at joints makes manipulation of fetal parts more difficult. Fetal deformity or limitation of joint movement is also seen as a result of oligohydramnios (Fig. 10.1). The reduced level of muscle traction can affect the configuration

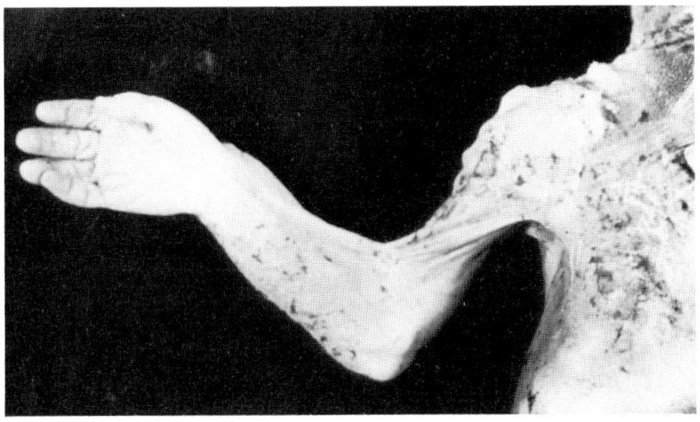

Fig. 10.1. Limitation of movement and webbing at shoulder and elbow joints in a preterm infant born following leakage of liquor amnii for 8 weeks.

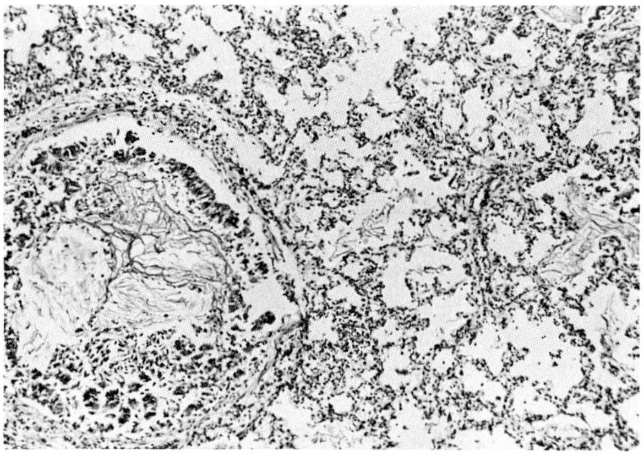

Fig. 10.2. Lung of a mature baby subject to birth asphyxia. Plugs of squamous material are present within the bronchial lumen and terminal airways.

of long bones, which are unduly slender and fragile and liable to fracture.

Some fetal conditions are associated with undue fragility of connective tissue. This may relate to abnormalities of collagen, such as those seen in osteogenesis imperfecta and dystrophia myotonica, or result from changes which accompany other disorders, such as those which result in fetal hydrops.

Congenital tumours and tumour-like conditions, such as teratoma or vascular malformations of the liver, achieve a large size by term and can obstruct delivery or be themselves subject to trauma, when serious haemorrhage may occur.

Intrapartum Asphyxial Insult

The extent of asphyxial damage to vital organs is difficult to ascertain in the fetus who dies intrapartum or shortly after birth. The manifestations of asphyxial injury appear trivial in these babies. The full extent of the insult may take several days to develop and be seen only in those babies who have been maintained on life-support systems.

Cutaneous Petechial Haemorrhages

Cutaneous petechial haemorrhages which are delivery-related are usually restricted to an anatomical region which has been subjected to increased capillary pressure as well as asphyxial stress. They might be restricted to the legs and lower trunk in breech delivery or a single arm which has prolapsed through the cervix. Petechiae are restricted to the head when the cord is tightly around the neck during vertex vaginal delivery. The restricted distribution of delivery-related petechiae is usually sufficient to allow distinction from the generalised petechial rash which accompanies intrauterine infection (see Fig. 13.1, p. 297) or platelet abnormalities.

Other Asphyxial Insults

Meconium staining of the skin is often apparent in the mature fetus subject to asphyxial stress either before or during labour. The pathologist should examine skin creases and ears for residual staining as even a stillborn fetus may have been washed before being shown to the parents and despatched to the mortuary.

Petechial haemorrhages in thoracic viscera are often apparent on gross examination beneath both visceral and parietal pleura, along the course of coronary arteries and within the thymus.

Violent inspiratory efforts in response to hypoxic stress result in the aspiration of amniotic fluid (Fig. 10.2). Should a mature fetus have recently passed meconium into the amniotic fluid, then this may be seen within the trachea and main bronchi and sometimes in the stomach. The histological appearances of the lung in hypoxia are described in Chapter 17 (see p. 421).

The most serious hypoxic injuries are those inflicted on brain, heart, kidneys and adrenals. When facilities for ventilation are available, the factor which limits survival is the presence and extent of ischaemic damage to the myocardium. The role of myocardial injury in perinatal mortality caused by birth asphyxia has been seriously under-rated until recently. This relates to the paucity of histological changes in the myocardium in babies dying within 24 h of birth and the failure to undertake routine histological examination of all organs in the investigation of perinatal death. Clinicians drew attention to the need to examine the heart with more care by demonstrating ECG abnormalities and poor myocardial contractility on ultrasound examination. Ischaemic injury is frequently restricted to the inner third of the myocardium and papillary muscle. Histological

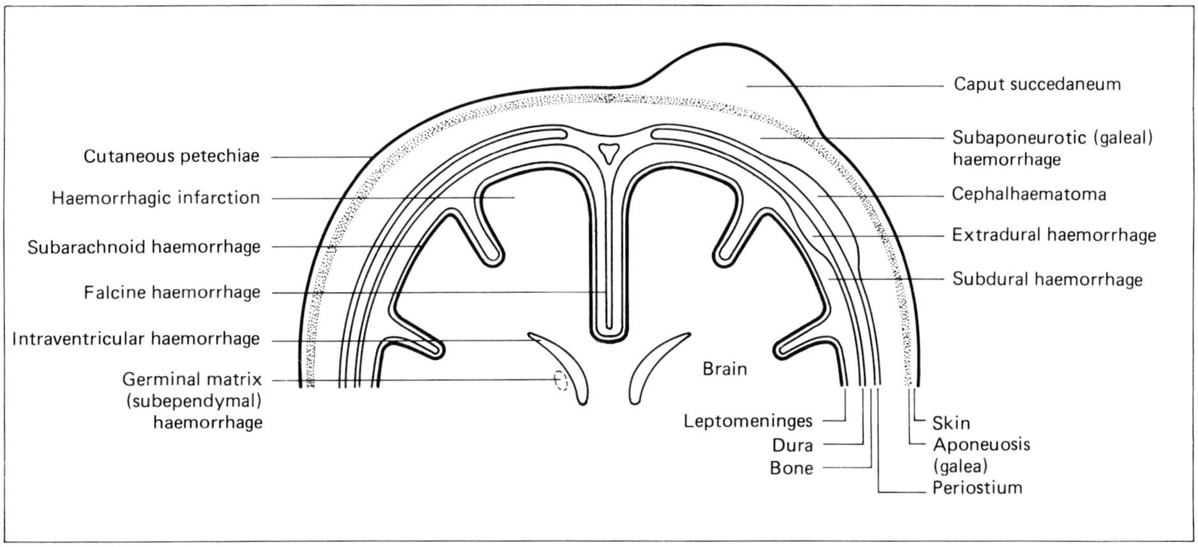

Fig. 10.3. Sites of asphyxial (*left side*) and traumatic (*right side*) pericranial and intracranial haemorrhage.

abnormalities are related to the time of the insult and the length of survival (see Chap. 18, p. 450).

The importance of hypoxic cerebral injury is not only its contribution to perinatal and infant mortality but its relationship to serious morbidity in survivors (Stanley 1984). Sites of pericranial and intracranial haemorrhage are illustrated diagrammatically in Fig. 10.3. Those which are the result of asphyxia are listed on the left of the figure; individual lesions are described in Chapter 24. Ischaemic cerebral injury in neonates is underestimated for two reasons: it is often difficult to identify in babies who die shortly after the insult has occurred or it may produce such extensive cerebral disruption after a few days have elapsed that ischaemic injury may be discounted as artefact or the result of poor fixation (see Chap. 24, p. 576). Infarction is more easily identified (Fig. 10.4). The end result of hypoxic damage is cystic degeneration, which may affect the whole of the cerebral white matter and takes 4–6 weeks to develop (Fig. 10.5).

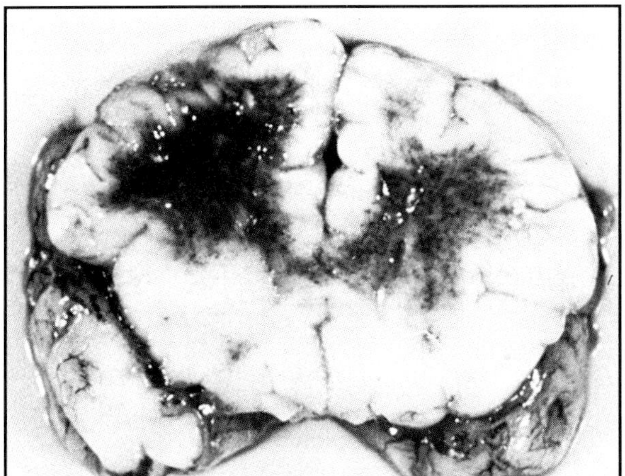

Fig. 10.4. Bilateral cerebral infarction in a preterm baby who died aged 3 days.

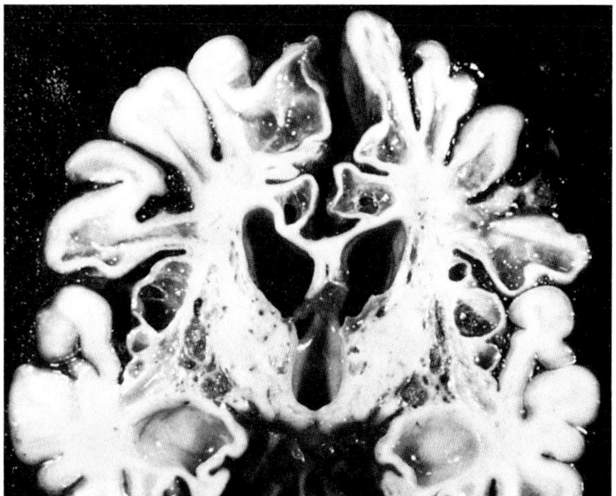

Fig. 10.5. Extensive cystic degeneration involving cortical white matter in a term infant subject to severe birth asphyxia who died at 37 days of age.

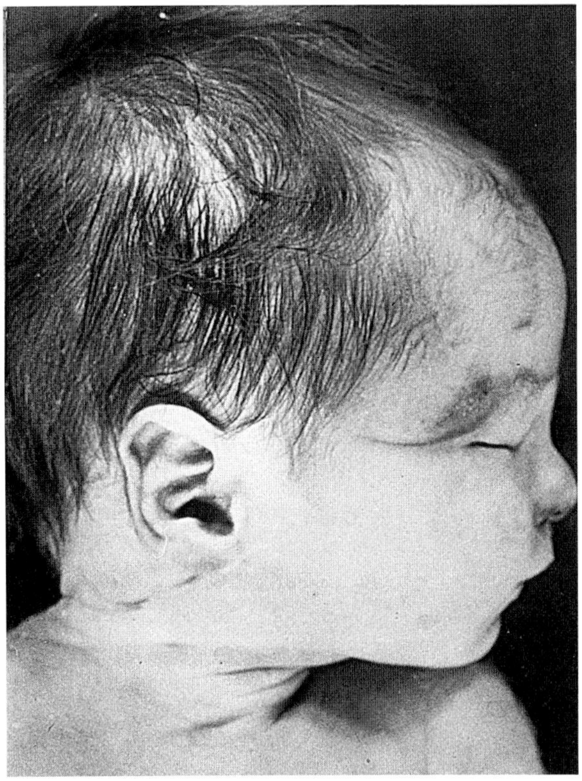

Fig. 10.6. Bruising at the lateral margin of the orbit following rotational forceps delivery. The margin of the forceps blade is clearly seen.

Traumatic Birth Injury

Birth injury can involve almost any organ. Some forms of injury are very common and readily recognised; others, though uncommon, may be life threatening or fatal. Some are easily missed by a necropsy examination using only techniques appropriate to the post-mortem examination of adults. A review of birth trauma by Walker (1985) details clinical associations and findings and describes those abnormalities which are unlikely to be encountered by the pathologist and are therefore omitted here.

Bruises

Bruises involving skin, subcutaneous tissue and muscles are common injuries, particularly, but not exclusively, following instrumental delivery. Bruising of the face and head is frequent following forceps delivery, particularly if rotation of the head has been undertaken (Fig. 10.6). Bruises following the application of forceps follow the outline of the instrument. Serious sequelae may follow the application of a blade directly over the eye or the course of the facial nerve.

Bleeding into gluteal muscles and the muscles of thighs and legs is often very extensive following breech delivery, particularly when the baby is delivered prematurely. The severity of muscle haemorrhage is often belied by the trivial extent of subcutaneous bruising (Fig. 10.7). Genital bruising and excoriation is found in male infants following breech delivery (Tiwary 1989).

Laceration

Cutaneous laceration occasionally occurs during emergency caesarean section. Such injury is usually of a trivial nature.

Pericranial Injury

A variety of soft tissue injuries to the fetal head are described. Whilst they are more common following instrumental delivery, they can occur during spontaneous delivery or even caesarean section. The sites of traumatic pericranial haemorrhage are illustrated on the right in Fig. 10.3.

Caput Succedaneum

Caput succedaneum is a superficial soft tissue swelling of the fetal presenting part where it overlies the internal os and is thus unsupported. A caput develops best over the head because of the better fit of the smooth curve of the cranium to the margin of the os. Stewart and Philpott (1980) have graded the extent of caput formation and used it as an index of cephalopelvic disproportion.

Congestion and petechial haemorrhage can be seen within the skin. Subcutaneous tissues are oedematous and congested. Local haemorrhage may occur and is of no consequence. Rapid resolution without sequelae is usual.

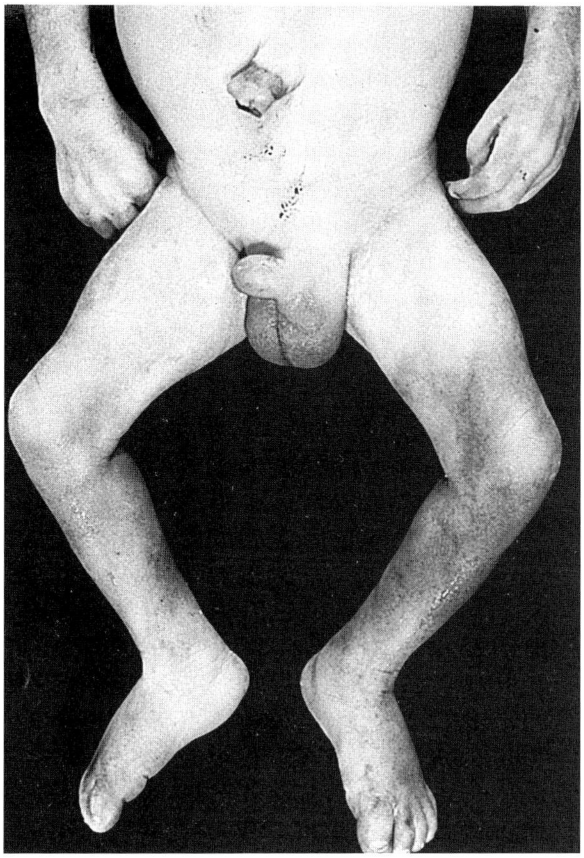

Fig. 10.7. Bruising of the lower thighs and legs in a preterm infant who presented by the breech.

Chinon

Circumscribed soft tissue oedema with localised haemorrhage may follow the use of a vacuum extractor to expedite delivery. Excoriation of the overlying skin is common and usually heals without scarring but occasionally this is more serious and permanent baldness results.

Subaponeurotic Haemorrhage

Subaponeurotic haemorrhage is a serious form of pericranial injury. Haemorrhage occurs into the loose connective tissue beneath the dense layer of the scalp aponeurosis (galea). The plane of haemorrhage is superficial to the periosteum, and haemorrhage may extend to cover the whole of the cranium (Fig. 10.8). The scalp is diffusely boggy to touch. It is important to recognise subaponeurotic haema-

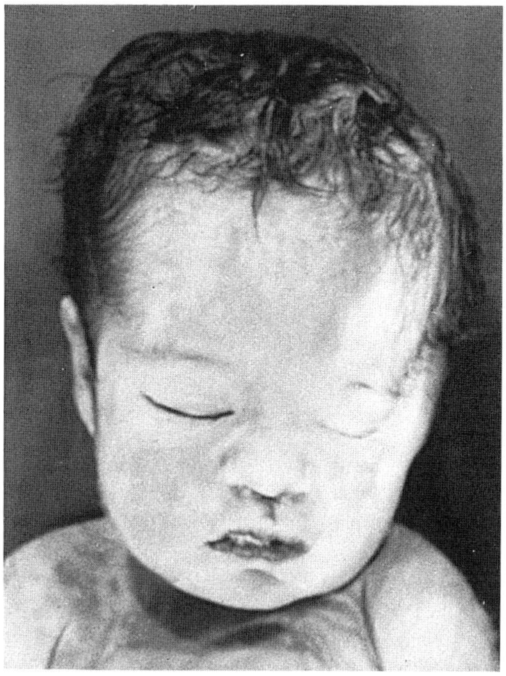

a

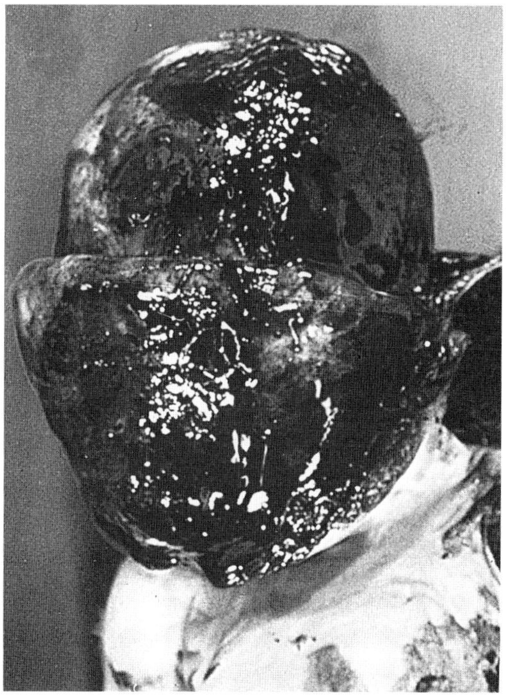

b

Fig. 10.8. **a** Asymmetric scalp swelling following forceps delivery. **b** Reflection of the scalp reveals the extent of subaponeurotic haemorrhage.

toma, as a significant volume of blood may be lost and require urgent replacement. Plauché (1980) found fatal outcome in 22.8% of cases in a review of reported experience.

This type of haemorrhage typically complicates rotational forceps delivery but has been described following the use of a vacuum extractor in a small proportion (0.13%) of cases (Plauché 1979) and is occasionally seen after spontaneous delivery.

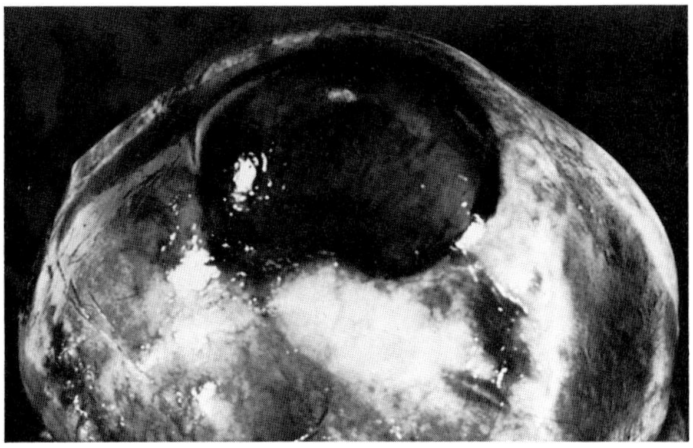

Fig. 10.9. Subperiosteal haematoma (cephalhaematoma) overlying the right parietal bone.

Subperiosteal Haematoma

Bleeding beneath the periosteum of a single skull bone (cephalhaematoma), usually the parietal bone, is a common and trivial birth injury. Haemorrhage is limited by firm attachment of the periosteum around the margin of the bone (Fig. 10.9), and the periosteum is elevated by the accumulated blood. Bone is laid down beneath the elevated periosteum producing a hard lump on the baby's head within which the haematoma resorbs (Fig. 10.10). Remodelling of the bone takes place slowly and the original contour is restored. The bony lump may give rise to considerable parental anxiety and occasionally provoke suspicion of non-accidental injury.

Cephalhaematoma may complicate instrumental delivery, but most occur after spontaneous uncomplicated delivery. A few are accompanied by fracture of the underlying bone.

Extradural Haemorrhage

Bleeding on the outer side of the dura mater is an uncommon birth injury and almost always accompanies fracture of a skull bone. The extent of haemorrhage is usually small.

Subdural Haemorrhage

Haemorrhage into the subdural space is usually the result of tearing of one or more bridging veins running unsupported from the surface of the brain to their insertion in the dural membranes. This occurs because of rapid or excessive deformity of the skull during birth. It may be the result of rapid passage through the birth canal during spontaneous delivery or vacuum extraction (Hanigan et al. 1990). More commonly it complicates instrumental manipulation. The premature infant is at particular risk of subdural haemorrhage. Tears of the tentorium are often seen when there is subdural haemorrhage but are only causally related when the tear extends into a dural sinus.

Injury to the vein of Galen and its tributaries is an uncommon cause of massive subdural haemorrhage during instrumental delivery; venous congestion is a contributory factor. Laceration into the sigmoid sinus following occipital osteodiastesis can result in serious,

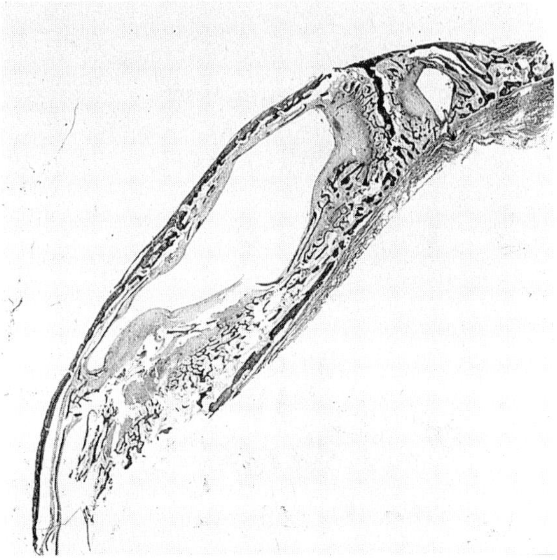

Fig. 10.10. Section through an organising subperiosteal haematoma. New bone is present beneath the periosteum. The outer table of the parietal bone forms the inferior margin of the cavity.

often fatal, subdural haemorrhage in the posterior fossa.

Tears of Falx and Tentorium

Tears of the membranous supports of the brain are the result of excessive distortion of the infant skull during delivery. Tears of the tentorium, often superficial (Fig. 10.11), at its junction with the falx are the most commonly encountered injuries. They frequently accompany subdural haemorrhage as bridging veins are likely to be disrupted by the same distorting force.

Tears of the falx and tentorium are only the cause of subdural haemorrhage when they extend into a sinus and are more usually merely evidence that excessive skull deformity has occurred. Tears in the falx are much less common than those in the tentorium and are the result of forceful distortion.

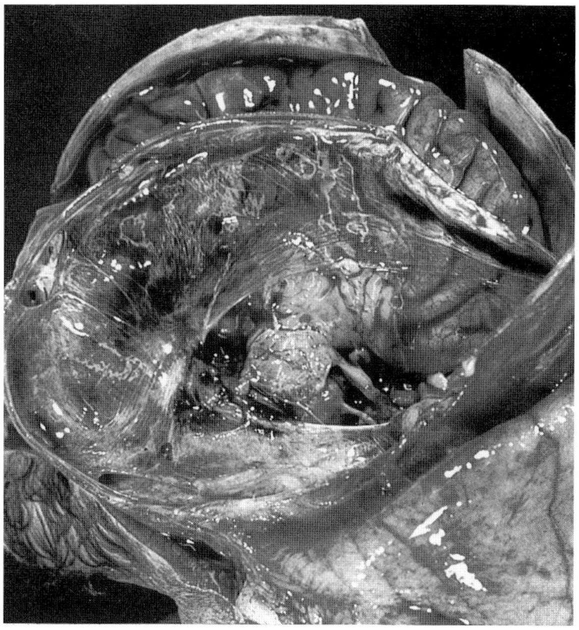

Fig. 10.11. Tear at the angle of the right tentorium cerebelli and falx. The smooth margin of the tentorium is lost. There is a "V" shaped defect as the tear is stretched open.

Skull Fracture

The commonest skull fracture is a linear fracture in the parietal bone running into the bone from the midpoint of its medial border (Fig. 10.12). Most fractures go unrecognised and are likely to be seen by the pathologist when they accompany other forms of traumatic or hypoxic birth injury. They usually complicate instrumental delivery. Irregular, multiple fractures of skull bones are occasionally seen and may even complicate emergency caesarean section when delivery of the head (Fig. 10.13) has been particularly difficult.

Occipital Osteodiastesis

Inward displacement of the inferior margin of the squamous part of the occipital bone in respect of its lateral portions is usually a complication of breech delivery, when dislocation of the inferior part of the bone is the result of pressure from the internal aspect of maternal pubic bones during delivery of the head (Wigglesworth and Husemeyer 1977). It is occasionally seen following instrumental vertex delivery.

Dislocation may directly injure the cerebellum or cause subdural haemorrhage when an overlying venous sinus is torn. It is important to reflect the posterior scalp flap down to the level of the foramen magnum during necropsy examination so that the whole of the occipital bone can be seen, otherwise this injury is easily missed.

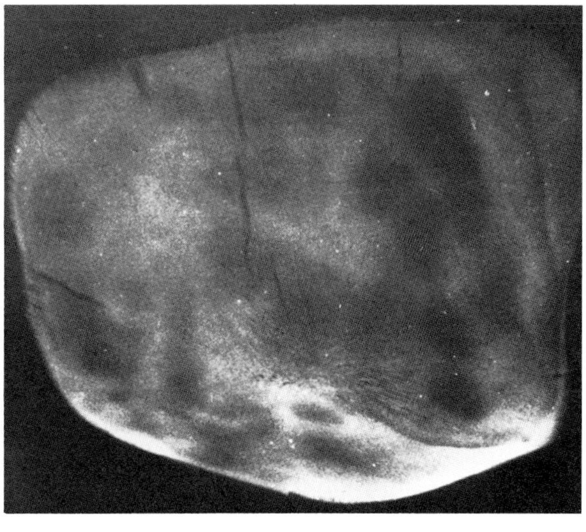

Fig. 10.12. Radiograph of excised parietal bone. Undisplaced linear fractures run into the bone from its medial and posterior borders.

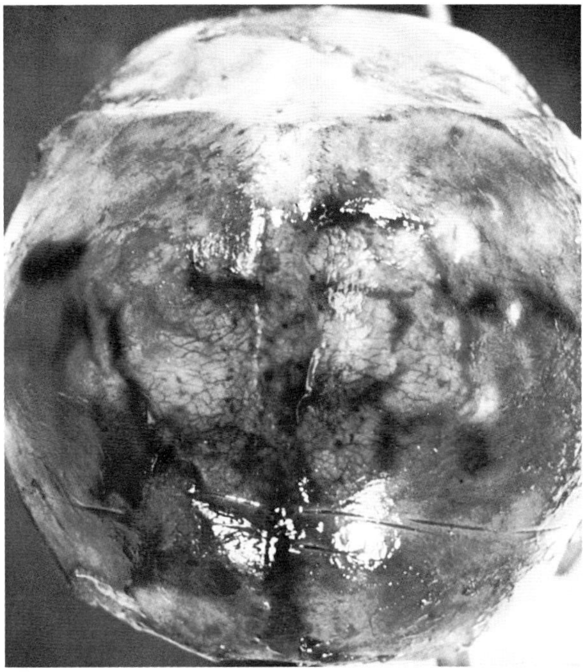

Fig. 10.13. Irregular fractures of both parietal bones following emergency caesarean section for failure to progress.

Spinal Cord Injury

Damage to the spinal cord is a manifestation of birth trauma which is easily missed by both clinician and pathologist (Gresham 1975). Imaging techniques such as ultrasound (Babyn et al. 1988) and magnetic resonance imaging (Lanska et al. 1990) can demonstrate spinal cord injury very clearly. Their use causes little disturbance to the infant and their increasing use will give a more realistic idea of the incidence of cord trauma. Such injuries result from traction and may complicate vaginal delivery with either cephalic or breech presentation. The injury is more likely when traction is accompanied by neck flexion or torsional stress.

The clinical picture of shock and hypotonia is common to other forms of traumatic or hypoxic injury and neuromuscular disorders. Cord injury is often missed by the pathologist because examination of the spinal cord is often not routine. Even when the possibility of spinal injury is raised, the full extent of injury may be missed when the cervical spinal cord is divided during removal of the brain. High cervical cord contusion and laceration is the type of injury seen following difficult delivery with cephalic presentation but it may be discounted as the result of poor dissection technique. Following breech delivery, damage is likely to be found in the lower part of the cervical cord. It is in this situation that removal of the cord within an intact spinal canal (see Chap. 1, p. 26) will reveal the full extent of injury to the cord, nerve roots and vertebral arteries.

Nerve Injuries

Nerve injuries are a rare form of birth trauma except amongst large babies and are unlikely to be encountered by the pathologist. They result from traction on nerve roots, shoulder dislocation (Dunkerton 1989), or pressure on a superficial nerve. The large baby is particularly vulnerable, especially if there is shoulder dystocia (Walker 1985; Sjöberg et al. 1988; Wikström et al. 1988).

Long Bone Fractures

The clavicle is the commonest site of birth-related fracture. Oppenheim et al. (1990) found 58 fractured clavicles during a 5-year period (2.7/1000 births). Three babies had Erb's palsy. It is most commonly seen in big babies, associated with shoulder dystocia and midcavity forceps delivery. It is seen at necropsy in association with more serious injuries, or occasionally as a fortuitous finding.

Long Bone Fractures

Femoral fractures are usually the result of manipulations to bring down the legs during breech delivery (Fig. 10.14). Loss of protective muscle tone because of hypoxia, and in some cases failure to develop mechanical strength because of inappropriate intrauterine muscular activity, probably contribute to the ease of fracture in some cases. Fracture of the femur is not a common birth injury but can result in serious shock and haemorrhage.

Fractures of the humerus are seen more commonly than femoral fractures. They are similarly associated with obstetric manipulations when there is shoulder dystocia (Wikström et al. 1988).

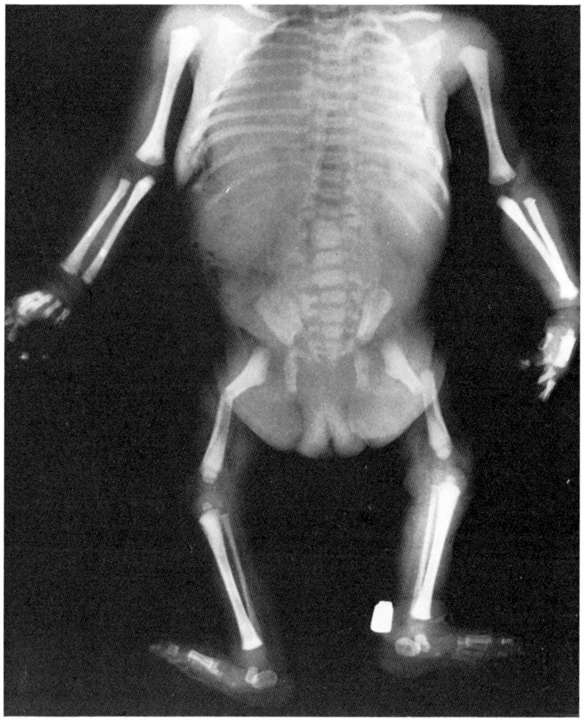

Fig. 10.14. Bilateral femoral fractures following vaginal breech delivery. There is apparent shortening and lateral rotation of the lower limbs.

Hepatic Injury

Injury to the liver is the most common visceral birth injury. This is usually a subcapsular haematoma, but occasionally a parenchymal rupture is seen (see Fig. 16.20, p. 391). The usual victim is the premature infant presenting by the breech (Shankaran et al. 1991). Hypoxic hypotonia often plays a part in this type of injury. It is usually seen on the anterior aspect of the right hepatic lobe in relation to the costal margin (see Fig. 16.21, p. 391). Significant blood loss usually follows traumatic rupture of Glisson's capsule. When the capsule remains intact, blood loss is limited by increased pressure within the haematoma. Jaundice accompanies organisation of large haematomas. Hepatomegaly for any reason such as heart failure, excessive haemopoesis or angioma increases the likelihood of traumatic injury.

Abdominal Visceral Injury

Abdominal visceral injury outwith the liver is very uncommon. Splenic injury occasionally occurs and splenomegaly is a predisposing factor. Perirenal haematoma is reported following avulsion of the renal pedicle during precipitate delivery (Newman and Smith 1987). Injury to the gastrointestinal tract is very rare in the neonate; those injuries which do occur are more likley to be postnatally acquired during energetic resuscitation than acquired intrapartum.

References

Atkins AJF, Watt JM, Milan P, Davies P, Crawford S (1981) The influence of posture upon cardiovascular dynamics throughout pregnancy. Eur J Obstet Gynecol Reprod Biol 12: 357–372

Babyn PS, Chuang SH, Daneman A, Davidson GS (1988) Sonographic evaluation of spinal cord birth trauma with pathologic correlation. Am J Roentgenol 151: 763–766

Barson AJ, Tasker M, Lieberman BA, Hillier VF (1984) Impact of improved perinatal care on the causes of death. Arch Dis Child 59: 199–207

Bassell GM, Humayun SG, Marx GF (1980) Maternal bearing down efforts—another fetal risk? Obstet Gynecol 56: 39–41

Beard RW, Morris ED, Clayton SG (1967) pH of foetal capillary blood as an indicator of the condition of the foetus. J Obstet Gynaecol Br Cmwlth 74: 812–822

Brans YW, Escobedo MB, Hayashi RH, Huff RW, Kagan-Hallet KS, Ramamurthy RS (1984) Perinatal mortality in a large perinatal center: five-year review of 31 000 births. Am J Obstet Gynecol 148: 284–289

Butler NR, Bonham DG (1963) Perinatal mortality. The first report of the 1958 British Perinatal Mortality Survey under the auspices of The National Birthday Trust Fund. Livingstone, Edinburgh.

Cardozo LD, Gibb DMF, Studd JWW, Cooper DJ (1983) Should we abandon Kielland's forceps? Br Med J 287: 315–317

Chiswick ML, James DK (1979) Kielland's forceps: association with neonatal morbidity and mortality. Br Med J 1: 7–9

Coard K, Codrington G, Escoffrey C, Keeling JW, Ashley D, Golding J (1991) Perinatal mortality in Jamaica 1986–1987. Acta Paediatr Scand 80: 581–587

Cohn HE, Sacks EJ, Heymann MA, Rudolph AM (1974) Cardiovascular responses to hypoxemia and acidemia in fetal lambs. Am J Obstet Gynecol 120: 817–824

Crawford JS, Burton M, Davies P (1972) Time and lateral tilt at Caesarean section. Br J Anaesth 44: 477–484

Dawes GS (1968) Fetal and neonatal physiology. Year Book Medical Publishers, Chicago, p 97

Dunkerton MC (1989) Posterior dislocation of the shoulder associated with obstetric brachial plexus palsy. J Bone Joint Surg 71: 764–766

Faber-Nijholt R, Huisjes HJ, Touwen BCL, Fidler VJ (1983) Neurological follow-up of 281 children born in breech presentation: a controlled study. Br Med J 286: 9–12

Fedrick J (1969) Comparison of birth weight/gestation distribution in cases of stillbirth and neonatal death according to lesions found at necropsy. Br Med J 3: 745–748

Fox H (1967) The significance of placental infarction in perinatal morbidity and mortality. Biol Neonate 11: 87–105

Friedman EA, Sachtleben MR (1971) High risk labour. J Reprod Med 7: 28–32

Gresham EL (1975) Birth trauma. Pediatr Clin North Am 22: 317–328

Hanigan WC, Morgan AM, Stahlberg LK, Hiller JL (1990) Tentorial hemorrhage associated with vacuum extraction. Pediatrics 85: 534–539

Healey DL, Quinn MA, Pepperall RJ (1982) Rotational delivery of the fetus: Keilland's forceps and two other methods compared. Br J Obstet Gynaecol 89: 501–506

Hovatta O, Lipasti A, Rapola J, Karjalainen O (1983) Causes of stillbirth: a clinicopathological study of 243 patients. Br J Obstet Gynaecol 90: 691–696

Jones CM, Greiss FC (1982) The effect of labor on maternal and fetal circulating catecholamines. Am J Obstet Gynecol 144: 149–153

Lanska MJ, Roessmann U, Wiznitzer M (1990) Magnetic resonance imaging in cervical cord birth injury. Pediatrics 85: 760–764

Lilien AA (1970) Term intrapartum fetal death. Am J Obstet Gynecol 107: 595–603

Löfgren O, Polberger S (1983) Perinatal mortality: changes in the diagnostic panorama 1974–1980. Acta Paediatr Scand 72: 327–332

Low JA, Cox MJ, Karchmar EJ, McGrath MJ, Pancham SR, Piercy WN (1981) The effect of maternal, labor, and fetal factors upon fetal heart rate during the intrapartum period. Am J Obstet Gynecol 139: 306–310

Maberry MC, Ramin SM, Gilstrap LC, Leveno KJ, Dax JS (1990) Intrapartum asphyxia in pregnancies complicated by intra-amniotic infection. Obstet Gynecol 76: 351–354

Machin GA (1975) A perinatal mortality survey in south-east London 1970–73: the pathological findings in 726 necropsies. J Clin Pathol 28: 428–434

McIlwaine GM, Howat RCL, Dunn F, Macnaughton MC (1979) The Scottish Perinatal Mortality Survey. Br Med J II: 1103–1106

Newman B, Smith S (1987) Unusual renal renal mass in a newborn infant. Radiology 163: 193–194

Oppenheim WL, Davis A, Growdon WA, Dorey FJ, Davlin LB (1990) Clavicle fractures in the newborn. Clin Orthop 250: 176–180

Plauché WC (1979) Fetal cranial injuries related to delivery with the Malstrom vacuum extractor. Obstet Gynecol 53: 750–757

Plauché WC (1980) Subgaleal hematoma. A complication of instrumental delivery. JAMA 244: 1597–1598

Samms-Vaughan ME, Golding J (1992) Area variation in perinatal mortality in Jamaica: Association with type of hospital services available. In: Perinatal problems of islands in relation to prevention of handicap. INSERM, Paris, pp 90–98

Schwarcz RL, Belizan JM, Cifuentes JR, Cuadro JC, Marques MB, Caldeyro-Barcia R (1974) Fetal and maternal monitoring in spontaneous labors and in elective inductions. A comparative study. Am J Obstet Gynecol 120: 356–362

Scottish Stillbirth and Neonatal Death Report 1989 (1990) Common Serivces Agency for the Scottish Health Service, Edinburgh

Shankaran S, Elias E, Ilagan N (1991) Subcapsular haemorrhage of the liver in the very low birth weight neonate. Acta Paediatr Scand 80: 616–619

Sjöberg I, Erichs K, Bjerre I (1988) Cause and effect of obstetric (neonatal) brachial plexus palsy. Acta Paediatr Scand 77: 357–364

Smis B, Thiery M (1980) Fetal heart rate pattern before, during and after amniotomy. Eur J Obstet Gynecol Reprod Biol 11: 163–171

Stanley F (1984) Perinatal risk factors in the aetiology of the cerebral palsies. In: Stanley F, Alberman ED (eds) The epidemiology of the cerebral palsies. Clinics in developmental medicine No 87, SIMP, Blackwell, Oxford, pp 98–115

Steer PJ (1985) Fetal distress. In: Crawford JW (ed) Risks of labour. Wiley, Chichester, pp 11–13

Stewart KS, Philpott PH (1980) Fetal response to cephalopelvic disproportion. Br J Obstet Gynaecol 87: 641–649

Svenningsen L, Lindemann R, Eidal K (1988) Measurements of fetal head compression pressure during bearing down and their relationship to the condition of the newborn. Acta Obstet Gynecol Scand 67: 129–133

Tiwary CM (1989) Testicular injury in breech delivery: possible implications. Urology 34: 210–212

Walker CHM (1985) Birth trauma. In: Crawford JW (ed) Risks of labour. Wiley, Chichester, pp 71–93

Wigglesworth JS, Husemeyer RO (1977) Birth trauma in vaginal breech delivery. Br Med J I: 320–321

Wikström I, Axelsson O, Bergström R, Meirik O (1988) Traumatic injury in large-for-date infants. Acta Obstet Gynecol Scand 67: 259–264

Chapter 11

Fetal Hydrops

Jean W. Keeling

Introduction

Fetal hydrops is a general increase in interstitial fluid occurring prenatally, manifest as oedema, with abnormal fluid distribution in body compartments. There is usually an increase in total body water. Severe degrees of oedema are accompanied by effusions in body cavities. Fetal hydrops may be accompanied by oedema of the placenta and umbilical cord. Oedema of the placenta is not universal and when present may not be uniformly distributed through the organ; to a certain extent, its presence reflects the underlying cause of the hydropic state. Hydrops may be observed at any gestation from first trimester to term.

The clinical presentation of fetal hydrops is gestation-related. In the first trimester of pregnancy hydrops is observed coincidentally in spontaneous abortions. It is recognised during routine ultrasound scanning as well as during scans prior to chorion villus sampling. Those women whose pregnancy is complicated by fetal hydrops in the second trimester often present with signs and symptoms related to intrauterine death of the fetus. An increasing proportion of mid-trimester fetal hydrops is being recognised when ultrasound examination is undertaken, either for estimation of fetal size and gestation or prior to amniocentesis (Boyd and Keeling 1992). The majority of cases which present in the third trimester are discovered during the investigation of women who are large for dates. Many of these women have clinically apparent polyhydramnios or rapid-onset pre-eclampsia (Keeling et al. 1983). In the third trimester fetal hydrops often gives rise to premature onset of labour and third-stage complications, particularly postpartum haemorrhage and manual removal of the placenta (Hutchison et al. 1982; Gough et al. 1986).

The underlying cause of hydrops is more likely to be discovered in those cases where it is observed whilst the fetus is still alive. This enables a much wider range of investigations to be undertaken. The increasing use of ultrasound examination has resulted in a marked reduction in the number of cases designated "unexplained" (Fleischer et al. 1981; Gough et al. 1986; Boyd and Keeling 1992) when compared with earlier studies where ultrasound examination was not routine (Macafee et al. 1970; Hutchison et al. 1982). Serial ultrasound examination has documented the spontaneous resolution of even severe degrees of fetal hydrops (Platt et al. 1978; Iliff et al. 1983).

The incidence of generalised oedema of the fetus is difficult to quantify. Minor fetal hydrops is very common, particularly amongst preterm neonates, and is often unexplained (Cartlidge and Rutter 1986). Major or severe fetal hydrops, defined as generalised oedema of >5 mm subcutaneous oedema in a third trimester fetus and accompanied by an effusion in at least one body cavity, was identified in

1:1400 pregnancies when cases caused by rhesus incompatability had been excluded (Iliff et al. 1983).

Mild subcutaneous oedema is often observed when intrauterine death has occurred and its significance is dubious. The intraperitoneal accumulation of fluid post mortem may be distinguished from significant ascites by its colour, which is usually dark red, and the site and appearance of viscera. In the presence of longstanding ascites the intestines are compressed into the central posterior part of the peritoneal cavity, and pleural effusions not only cause some degree of pulmonary hypoplasia but also affect lobar contour, with loss of concavity of the inferior surface of the lower lobes and the acute angle of the inferior border.

Distribution and Control of Fetal Fluid

Water is the major constituent of the human body. Its contribution to body mass changes with maturity, comprising 88% of fetal mass at 18–20 weeks' gestation and 73% at term (Friis-Hansen 1971). Water may be intracellular or extracellular, the latter comprising both the intravascular compartment and the interstitial space. The volume of the intracellular compartment depends on the relationship between osmotic forces both within and outwith the cell, and on a functioning sodium pump within cell membranes.

The distribution of extracellular water between interstitial and intravascular compartments is dependent on a variety of mechanisms. Its control is clearly more complex than that postulated by Starling. Mayerson et al. (1960) suggest that bulk flow of water accompanies protein molecules across capillaries in the lung and liver, which have capillary pores large enough to permit the passage of protein molecules. In other sites, water escapes from the intravascular compartment by simple diffusion through intercellular clefts in the capillary wall.

The stability of the relationship between interstitial and intravascular fluid depends on the structure and components of the interstitial space. This comprises a gel of mucopolysaccharide molecules (largely hyaluronic acid) lying in the spaces of a collagen network. The gel contains protein and salts, particularly sodium ions, and is only partially saturated with water. Normally no free fluid is present within the interstitial space. Water is attracted into it by the partially saturated gel, and removed by the small, negative hydrostatic force exerted by the pumping action of lymphatics.

Small changes in water content produce large changes in interstitial fluid pressure until saturation of the gel occurs. At this point, a large increase in water content has little effect on interstitial fluid pressure (Guyton 1963) but should more water enter the interstitial space, pooling of free fluid and, consequently, oedema, occurs. This fluid can move under the influence of gravity.

Amniotic fluid volume increases as pregnancy progresses, although not at a constant rate. Its chemical composition alters as the fetus matures. The relationship between fetal size, weight and amniotic fluid volume also changes with increasing fetal maturity.

During embryogenesis, amniotic fluid volume is greatly in excess of fetal volume. A fluid-filled amniotic cavity is recognisable around the time of implantation, before the embryo is distinguishable (Boyd and Hamilton 1970). Amniotic fluid is not dependent on the embryo, it continues to accumulate both when the fetus fails to develop or is resorbed. It is thought to be secreted by the amnion.

In the early fetal period, amniotic fluid volume is closely related to fetal size (Abramovich 1968; Lind et al. 1972). It increases from 25 ml at 10 weeks' gestation to around 400 ml, at 20 weeks; its composition closely resembles fetal plasma. There is rapid diffusion of water between fetus and amniotic fluid estimated at 400–500 ml per hour. This is grossly in excess of the net increase in amniotic fluid volume (about 0.5 ml per hour, assuming a steady increase of about 100 ml per week). In the first half of pregnancy, fetal skin and umbilical cord amnion are freely permeable to water and solutes (Page et al. 1978). In the rhesus monkey, amniotic fluid volume may change in order to maintain the tonicity of fetal extracellular fluid (Schruefer et al. 1972). Before mid-pregnancy, it is unlikely that fetal swallowing or micturition exert any influence on either composition or volume of amniotic fluid.

In the second half of pregnancy, the relationship between fetal size and amniotic fluid volume is no longer linear. Whilst there is around 800 ml of fluid at term, its rate of increase is outstripped by that of fetal size and weight. Keratinisation of fetal skin begins at 19–20 weeks' gestation and is well developed by 25 weeks. Free diffusion of water and solutes through the skin is then no longer possible. The amniotic fluid loses its function both as a physiological buffer and as an extension of the fetal extracellular compartment. It becomes an externalised fluid affording physical protection. Its volume is increased continually by voiding of fetal urine; a similar volume is removed by fetal swallowing.

There is exchange of fluid across the respiratory tract during the third trimester. It has been largely ignored and its contribution to amniotic fluid volume not determined.

During the last trimester of pregnancy, fetal anomalies that interfere with swallowing are often accompanied by polyhydramnios and those which result in reduced voiding of urine with oligohydramnios. It is known that water can cross both umbilical cord amnion and the chorionic plate of the placenta close to term (Abramovich and Page 1973). However, there is no evidence to suggest that fluid exchange at either site modifies amniotic fluid volume in the presence of a healthy fetus; such routes might be important when this is not the case.

The volume of amniotic fluid falls rapidly after 40 weeks' gestation to around 400 ml at 42 weeks and then to 200 ml at 44 weeks (Queenan et al. 1972). The reason for this has not been determined.

Mechanisms of Fetal Hydrops

Consideration of the types of pathological abnormality in published series of fetal hydrops reveals common features from which causal mechanisms may be inferred (Keeling et al. 1983). The three most important failures of fetal homeostasis which are associated with hydrops are severe chronic anaemia, e.g. rhesus incompatability (Whitfield 1981) and alpha-thalassaemia (Thumasathit et al. 1968); hypoproteinaemia, e.g. congenital nephrotic syndrome (Worthen et al. 1959); and intrauterine heart failure, e.g. high-output failure through arteriovenous anastomoses (Knoth et al. 1976) or cardiac arrhythmias (Fleischer et al. 1981). Whilst any one of these three mechanisms may be the initiating factor, complications arise as fluid balance deteriorates. Eventually all three mechanisms may contribute to worsening of the hydropic state. Phibbs et al. (1974) found that the severity of the hydrops in severe rhesus disease correlated better with serum albumin level than with red cell volume, and Gordon et al. (1966) found that they could not reverse rhesus hydrops when adequate haemoglobin levels were achieved and maintained by intrauterine transfusion, suggesting that irreversible capillary damage had already occurred.

In addition to the three mechanisms outlined above, there is little doubt that a variety of structural abnormalities which primarily interfere with the fetoplacental circulation, usually obstructing venous return from the placenta, are causally related to fetal hydrops. It seems that obstruction to venous return from the placenta initiates a series of events where increased venous pressure → placental oedema → impaired gas exchange → fetal hypoxia → fetal capillary damage → loss of plasma proteins → fetal hydrops. Examples of this situation include premature closure of the ductus arteriosus (Kohler 1978), right-sided diaphragmatic hernia (Keeling et al. 1983) and abdominal tumours (Moerman 1982).

Oedema of the placenta interferes with maternofetal transfer (Bryan 1977), and this may contribute to the worsening of the fetal condition in two ways: poor protein transport may contribute to a decrease in fetal plasma protein levels, and less efficient oxygenation may produce hypoxic damage to fetal capillaries and loss of plasma proteins into the interstitial space.

It is likely that the time of onset and rate of change of a particular initiating abnormality matters as much as its ultimate abnormal value. The rarity of hydrops in analbuminaemia and erythrogenesis imperfecta, where levels of serum albumin and haemoglobin respectively are extremely low throughout pregnancy, lends support to this suggestion (Barnes et al. 1977).

Causes and Associations of Fetal Hydrops

Until recently, the problem of fetal hydrops in Europe, North America and Australia was dominated by the effects of rhesus incompatability (Anderson et al. 1983). Following the introduction of effective management and prevention of rhesus disease (Whitfield 1981), other causes, taken together, are now numerically more important (Keeling et al. 1983; Machin 1989).

Worldwide, alpha-thalassaemia is the commonest cause of fetal hydrops (Thumasathit et al. 1968). Fetal hydrops is an uncommon but serious manifestation of intrauterine infection in the UK, whilst syphilis is still a numerically important cause of hydrops in parts of south-east Asia (Bryan and Nicholson 1981). A spectrum of fetal malformations has been described in association with fetal hydrops (Keeling et al. 1983; Machin 1989; Boyd and Keeling 1992). Many associated anomalies are likely to precipitate intrauterine heart failure in various ways, such as shunting through vascular malformations and cardiac abnormalities which are likely to be accompanied by arrhythmias. Fetal cardiac arrhythmias have been documented in both anatomically normal and malformed hearts (Kleinman et al. 1982) in association with hydrops.

Many major malformations which have been described in association with fetal hydrops have concomitant pulmonary hypoplasia affecting one or both lungs as an additional finding. Larroche (1982) poses the fundamental question, "Should the presence of the commonly associated finding [of fetal hydrops] of pleural effusion, be considered a cause or a consequence of pulmonary hypoplasia?" but does not answer it. She draws attention to the more common association of pulmonary hypoplasia and oligohydramnios and to the role of pulmonary secretions in the production and composition of amniotic fluid. Observation of many of the associated anomalies suggests that their relationship to lung hypoplasia and hydrops is that they produce the former because they reduce the thoracic volume and subsequently initiate hydrops because high intrathoracic pressure impedes venous return from the placenta. The rôle of lung hypoplasia is probably that of innocent bystander.

During the last decade, many more hydropic fetuses have been identified during life, improving the likelihood of determining all associations or underlying cause. Furthermore, changes in the associations of fetal hydrops have been observed as a result of the increasing proportion of cases identified in the second trimester (Hansmann et al. 1989; Boyd and Keeling 1992). There is a higher proportion of chromosomally abnormal fetuses and of those with dysmorphic features suggestive of chromosome anomaly where tissue culture failed because of intrauterine death (Boyd and Keeling 1992). It is likely that formerly, these fetuses were delivered some time after intrauterine death and not submitted for pathological examination.

A very large number of associations of fetal hydrops have accumulated. They are listed in Tables 11.1, 11.2 and 11.3.

Table 11.1. Cardiothoracic disorders associated with fetal hydrops

Structural cardiac anomalies
Complex with ambiguous cardiac situs (Kleinman et al 1982; Keeling et al. 1983)
Transposition of great arteries (Keeling et al. 1983; Holzgreve et al. 1984)
Tetralogy of Fallot (Kleinman et al. 1982)
Truncus arteriosus (Im et al. 1984; Holzgreve et al. 1984)
Atrial septal defect (Holzgreve et al. 1984)
Atrioventricular canal defect (Kleinman et al. 1982; Allan et al. 1986)
Large ventricular septal defect (Etches and Lemons 1979; Holzgreve et al. 1984)
Single ventricle (Holzgreve et al. 1984)
Aortic valve atresia (Moller et al. 1966)
Aortic valve stenosis (Moerman et al. 1982; Allan et al. 1986)
Hypoplastic left heart syndrome (Hutchison et al. 1982; Holzgreve et al. 1984)
Mitral atresia + EFE (Wilkin and Parmentier 1961)
Pulmonary valve atresia (Ito et al. 1961; Allan et al. 1986)
Absent pulmonary valve + EFE (Moller et al. 1966; Kleinman et al. 1982)
Tricuspid valve atresia (Keeling et al. 1983; Holzgreve et al. 1984)
Tricuspid valve atresia and ectopia cordis (Allan et al. 1986)
Ebstein's anomaly (Moller et al. 1966; Allan et al. 1986)
Acardia (twin pregnancy) (Kleinman et al. 1982; Boyd and Keeling 1991)
Other cardiac pathology
Myocarditis (Keeling et al. 1983; Mostoufi-Zadeh et al. 1985)
Myocardial infarction (coronary artery embolus) (Kleinman et al. 1982)
Cardiomyopathy (Holzgreve et al. 1984; Allan et al. 1986)
Premature closure of foramen ovale (Naeye and Blanc 1964; Pesonen et al. 1983)
Premature closure of ductus arteriosus (Becker et al. 1977; Kohler 1978)
EFE ± hepatitis (Spahr et al. 1980; Keeling et al. 1983)
Cardiac tumours
Rhabdomyoma (Kleinman et al. 1982; Keeling et al. 1983)
Rhabdomyoma and tuberous sclerosis (Ostor and Fortune 1978)
Cardiac teratoma (Mahony et al. 1984)
Atrial angioma (Platt et al. 1981)

Table 11.1. *Continued*

Cardiac arrhythmias
Paroxysmal atrial tachycardia (Radford et al. 1976; Im et al. 1984)
Supraventricular tachycardia (Radford et al. 1976; Kleinman et al. 1982)
Bundle branch block (Cowan et al. 1975)
Complete heart block (Etches and Lemons 1979; Holzgreve et al. 1984)
Complete heart block and maternal connective tissue disease (McCue et al. 1977; Hardy et al. 1979)
Arrhythmia + EFE (Hull et al. 1966)
Arrhythmia and conduction system anomaly (Esscher and Scott 1979; Ho et al. 1985)
Familial heart block (Cooke et al. 1980)
Bradycardia (Im et al. 1984)
Wolff–Parkinson–White syndrome (Lauener et al. 1985)

Intrathoracic abnormalities
Adenomatoid malformation (Kleinman et al. 1982; Keeling et al. 1983)
Pulmonary sequestration (Etches and Lemons 1979; Kleinman et al. 1982)
Tracheal atresia (Keeling et al. 1983; Mostoufi-Zadeh et al. 1985)
Pulmonary agenesis (Engellenner et al. 1989)
Tracheobronchomalacia (Phillips et al. 1985)
Diaphragmatic hernia (Kleinman et al. 1982; Keeling et al. 1983)
Mesenchymal hamartoma (Khong and Keeling 1990)
Oesophageal atresia (Larroche 1982)

Vascular abnormalities
Haemangioma
fetus (Larroche 1977; Keeling et al. 1983)
fetus multiple (Shturman-Ellstein et al. 1978)
placenta (Jones et al. 1973; Keeling et al. 1983)
Atrial angioma (Platt et al. 1981)
Meningeal angiomatosis (Boyd and Keeling 1992)
Calcific arteriopathy (Ivemark et al. 1962; Keeling et al. 1983)
Pulmonary lymphangiectasia (Hutchison et al. 1982)
Diffuse lymphangiectasia (Laurence 1955; Windebank et al. 1987)
Cystic hygroma (Etches and Lemons 1979; Keeling et al. 1983)
Acardiac monozygous twin pregnancy (Kleinman et al. 1982; Boyd and Keeling 1992)
Venacaval thrombus (Rudolph and Levin 1977)
Coronary artery embolus (Kleinman et al. 1982)
Fetal entanglement with umbilical cord (Keeling et al. 1983)

Table 11.2. Other systemic fetal disorders associated with fetal hydrops

Intra-abdominal
Gastrointestinal
Jejunal atresia (Spahr et al. 1980)
Small intestinal volvulus (Seward and Zusman 1978)
Meconium ileus ± peritonitis (Etches and Lemons 1979; Hutchison et al. 1982)
Intestinal infarction (Holzgreve et al. 1984)
Intestinal obstruction (Mahony et al. 1984)
Hepatitis (Hutchison et al. 1982; Keeling et al. 1983)
Hepatic necrosis (Hutchison et al. 1982)
Cirrhosis (Spahr et al. 1980; Keeling et al. 1983)

Tumours
Neuroblastoma (Anders et al. 1973; Moerman et al. 1982)
Hepatoblastoma (Kazzi et al. 1989)
Glioblastoma multiforme (Sabet 1982)
Primitive neuroectodermal tumour (Boyd and Keeling 1992)
Teratoma
sacrococcygeal (Kohler 1976; Hutchison et al. 1982)
mediastinal (Beischer et al. 1971; Fleischer et al. 1981)
intrapericardial (Holzgreve et al. 1984; Mahony et al. 1984)
Mesoblastic nephroma (Larroche 1977; Gray 1989)
Cardiac rhabdomyoma (Ostor and Fortune 1978; Keeling et al. 1983)

Urogenital abnormalities
Cystic renal dysplasia (Larroche 1982)
Renal hypoplasia (Etches and Lemons 1979; Keeling et al. 1983)
Urethral obstruction
valves (Holzgreve et al. 1984)
atresia (Keeling et al. 1983)
Congenital nephrotic syndrome (Worthen et al. 1959; Mostoufi-Zadeh et al. 1985)
Meckel's syndrome (Boyd and Keeling 1992)
Fraser's syndrome (Potter 1943; Keeling et al. 1983)
Vaginal atresia, hydrometrocolopos syndrome (Hutchison et al. 1982; Moerman et al. 1982)
Mesoblastic nephroma (Larroche 1977; Gray 1989)

Musculoskeletal
Achondrogenesis I (Mostoufi-Zadeh et al. 1985)
Achondrogenesis II (Golbus et al. 1977; Moerman et al. 1982)
Chondroectodermal dysplasia (Mahony et al. 1984)
Saldino–Noonan syndrome (Richardson et al. 1977)
Osteogenesis imperfecta (Hutchison et al. 1982; Mostoufi-Zadeh et al. 1985)
Jeune's asphyxiating thoracic dystrophy (Hutchison et al. 1982)
Thanatophoric dysplasia (Fleischer et al. 1981)
Multiple pterygium syndrome (Holzgreve et al. 1984)
Popliteal pterygium syndrome (Mahony et al. 1984)
Neu–Laxova syndrome (Holzgreve et al. 1984)
Pena Shokeir I syndrome (Holzgreve et al. 1984)
Myotonic dystrophy (Mahony et al. 1984)
Hydrocephaly, arthrogryposis (Holzgreve et al. 1984)
Holoprosencephaly (Mostoufi-Zadeh et al. 1985)
Amniotic bands (Holzgreve et al. 1984)

Table 11.3. Other associations of fetal hydrops

Genetic metabolic disease
Infantile Gaucher (Im et al. 1984; Mostoufi-Zadeh et al. 1985)
Mucopolysaccharidosis (Mahony et al. 1984)
Sialidosis (Johnson et al. 1980; Beck et al. 1984)
Neimann–Pick (Rossier et al. 1958)
? GM_1 gangliosidosis (Etches and Lemons 1979)
Hypoalbuminaemia (Turski et al. 1978)
Carnitine deficiency (Steenhout et al. 1990)

Chromosome anomalies
45XO (Kleinman et al. 1982; Mahony et al. 1984)
Trisomy 21 (Moerman et al. 1982; Holzgreve et al. 1984)
Trisomy 18 (Macafee et al. 1970; Keeling et al. 1983)
Trisomy 13 (Sahn et al. 1982; Mahony et al. 1984)
Trisomy 15 (Kuller and Laifer 1991)
Triploidy (Hutchison et al. 1982)
Cystic hygroma and hypoplastic aortic arch (Keeling et al. 1983)

Haematological disorders
Inherited
Diamond–Blackfan syndrome (Scimeca et al. 1988)
Dyserythropoietic anaemia (Carter et al. 1989)
Rhesus incompatibility (Whitfield 1981)
ABO incompatibility (McCue et al. 1977; Huchet and Soulié 1979)
Kell incompatibility (Miser et al. 1975; Scanton and Muirhead 1976)
Alpha-thalassaemia (Thumasathit et al. 1968; Holzgreve et al. 1984)
Haemoglobin Bart's (Weatherall et al. 1970; Boer and Anido 1979)
Glucose-6-phosphate dehydrogenase deficiency (Perkins 1971; Mentzer and Collier 1975)
Pyruvate kinase deficiency (Hennekam et al. 1990)
Haemoglobin Bart's + H (Lie and Lie 1961)
Haemophilia A (Mahony et al. 1984)

Acquired
Chronic fetomaternal haemorrhage (Debelle et al. 1977; Mostoufi-Zadeh et al. 1985)
Fetofetal haemorrhage (twin-transfusion syndrome) (Keeling et al. 1983; Mahony et al. 1984)
Haemorrhage into fetal organs
  intracranial associated with ischaemia (Bose 1978; Etches and Lemons 1979)
  intracranial associated with tumour (Boyd and Keeling 1992)
  intra-abdominal (Seward and Zusman 1978)

Infection
CMV (Hutchison et al. 1982; Holzgreve et al. 1984)
Herpes virus 1 (Im et al. 1984)
Rubella virus (Spahr et al. 1980)
Toxoplasmosis (Bain et al. 1956; Spahr et al. 1980)
Syphilis (Bulova et al. 1972; Bryan and Nicholson 1981)
Coxsackie virus (Bates 1970)
Myocarditis NOS (Keeling et al. 1983; Mostoufi-Zadeh et al. 1985)
Parvovirus (Burton 1986; Porter et al. 1988; Morey et al. 1992)

Table 11.3. *Continued*

Maternal disorders
Connective tissue disorders (Altenberger et al. 1977; Hardy et al. 1979)
Diabetes mellitus (Graves and Baskett 1984)
Maternal anaemia with two hydropic pregnancies (Macafee et al. 1970; Larroche 1982)
Choriocarcinoma (Zarafu et al. 1978)

To get an idea of the importance of particular associations Keeling (1991) surveyed 17 reported series of 10 or more cases totalling 594 cases. A summary of this updated survey, now 1097 cases, is presented in Table 11.4. Twenty-three per cent had cardiovascular pathology, particularly congenital heart disease; 17% had extracardiac anomalies and 13% were chromosomally abnormal. Machin (1989) approached the problem in a different way. He surveyed non-selected series (804 cases) and individual case reports (610 cases) published between 1981 and 1988. His findings were similar, but he found a bigger proportion of cardiovascular anomalies (26%); 12% had chromosome anomalies or suggestive dysmorphology and 12% had extracardiac anomalies.

Table 11.4. Associations of non-immunological fetal hydrops compiled from 22 published series of 10 or more cases

	No. of associations	% association
Cardiac malformations	159	23.2
Arrhythmias	34	
Other cardiac	44	
Arterial pathology	17	
Non-cardiovascular anomalies	183	16.7
Pulmonary malformation	30	
Diaphragmatic hernia	32	
Renal anomaly	29	
Skeletal anomaly	72	
Other malformation	20	
Chromosome anomaly	111	13.4
Cystic hygroma	36	
Monochorionic twin pregnancy	79	7.2
Infection	71	6.5
Anaemia	28	2.6
Tumours	19	1.7
Gastrointestinal pathology	22	2.0
Genetic metabolic disease	6	0.5
Obstructed venous return NOS	2	0.2
Unexplained	286	26.0
TOTAL	1097	100%

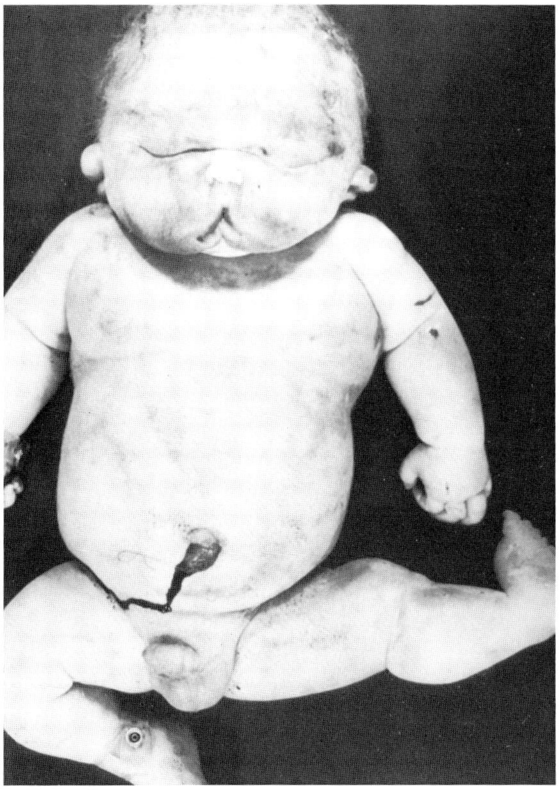

Fig. 11.1 Gross hydrops involving head, trunk and limbs. Severe oedema introduces facial deformity.

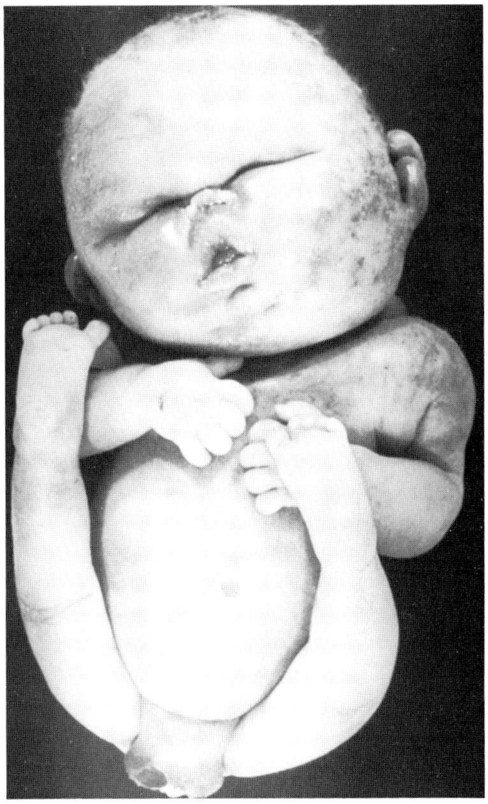

Fig. 11.2 Hydropic stillbirth with large angioma involving the left side of the face, head and shoulder. Head and trunk are grossly hydropic, limbs relatively spared.

Pathological Findings

External

The affected fetus is pale and usually preterm. The amount and distribution of soft tissue oedema is variable, the head and face are often markedly affected whilst the limbs are sometimes spared. When oedema is gross (Fig. 11.1), the deforming effect, particularly of the head, both obliterates dysmorphic features, such as the facies associated with some chromosome anomalies, and produces changes which may be wrongly interpreted as specific dysmorphic features. Gross external abnormalities, e.g. skeletal dysplasia (see Fig. 26.3 and Fig. 26.8) or extensive angiomata (Fig. 11.2) are not obliterated and should be observed carefully as they may be causally related to the hydropic state. The distribution of oedema may itself suggest a diagnosis, such as the disproportionate amount of postnuchal fluid seen in monosomy X (Fig. 11.3) although it is not specific for this condition and may occur with other chromosome abnormalities (Fig. 11.4) or with normal chromosomes. The abdomen is often distended because of ascites (Fig. 11.5) or hepatomegaly (Fig. 11.6).

Internal

Serous effusions are often present and are always found when hydrops is severe. It is usual to find an excess of fluid in all body cavities, although not usually to the same degree. Sometimes, there is disproportionate ascites and it is likely that in some, if not many of these babies, ascites accumulates first and hydrops follows because elevated intra-abdominal pressure distorts the umbilical vein and impedes venous return from the placenta. In a review of fetal ascites, Machin (1985) found that many of the associations of fetal ascites were also associated with generalised

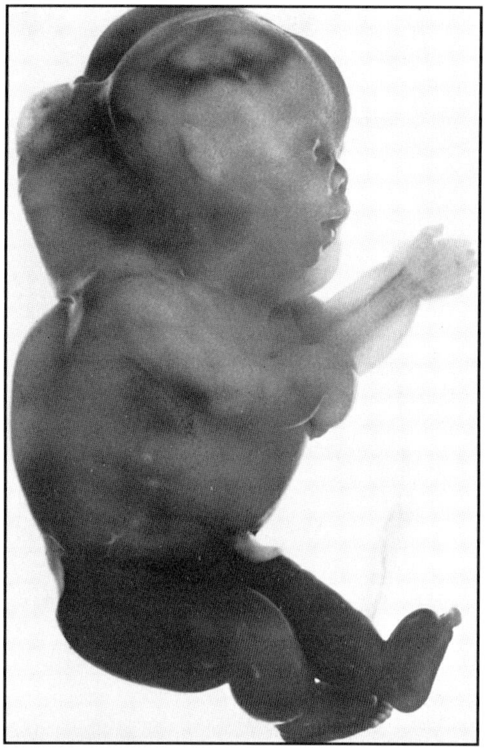

Fig. 11.3

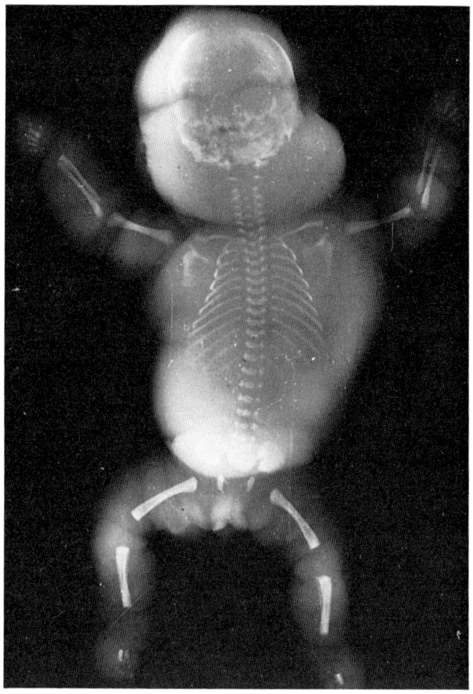

Fig. 11.4

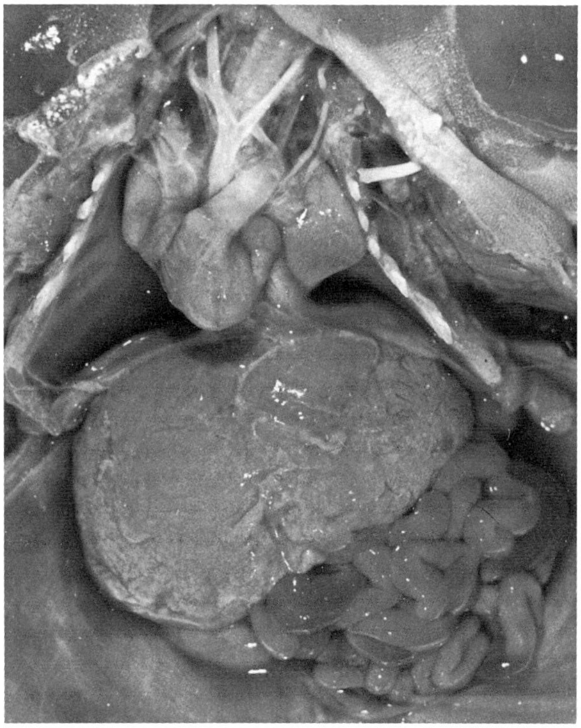

Fig. 11.5

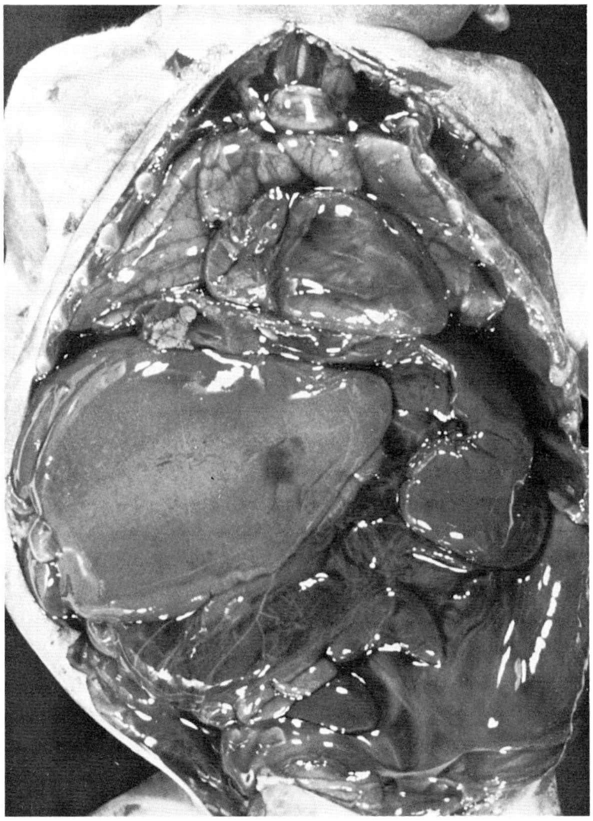

Fig. 11.6

Fig. 11.3 Fetus with generalised hydrops and marked postnuchal fluid accumulation: karyotype was 45XO. Termination of pregnancy for fetal anomaly.

Fig. 11.4 Radiograph of 19 weeks' gestation fetus with generalised hydrops and disproportionate postnuchal fluid accumulation. Karyotype was 47 + 21 (Keeling et al. 1983).

Fig. 11.5 Hydropic fetus was 45XO karyotype. The pulmonary trunk is larger than the ascending aorta and the distal part of the aortic arch is very narrow. The peritoneal cavity is very large and intestines compressed because of ascites.

Fig. 11.6 Fetal hydrops due to severe rhesus incompatibility. Massive hepatosplenomegaly is the result of increased erythropoiesis.

hydrops, although there was an excess of intra-abdominal abnormalities such as urinary tract obstruction and gastrointestinal or hepatic abnormalities.

The heart and liver are often enlarged even in the absence of specific abnormality in these organs (Fig. 11.7). This is particularly likely when hydrops is due to heart failure. In rhesus disease and chronic anaemia from other causes, including infection such as toxoplasmosis, hepatosplenomegaly is usual because of increased, persistent haemopoesis (Fig. 11.6). The liver is often much enlarged in the osteochondrodysplasias as it is the main organ of erythropoesis because of reduced bone marrow volume.

Complex congenital heart disease, pulmonary malformations (Figs. 11.8, 11.9) and intrathoracic masses (Figs. 11.10, 11.11, 11.12) are amongst the commonest associations of fetal hydrops (Table 11.1, 11.4) and should always be sought. Intra-abdominal causes

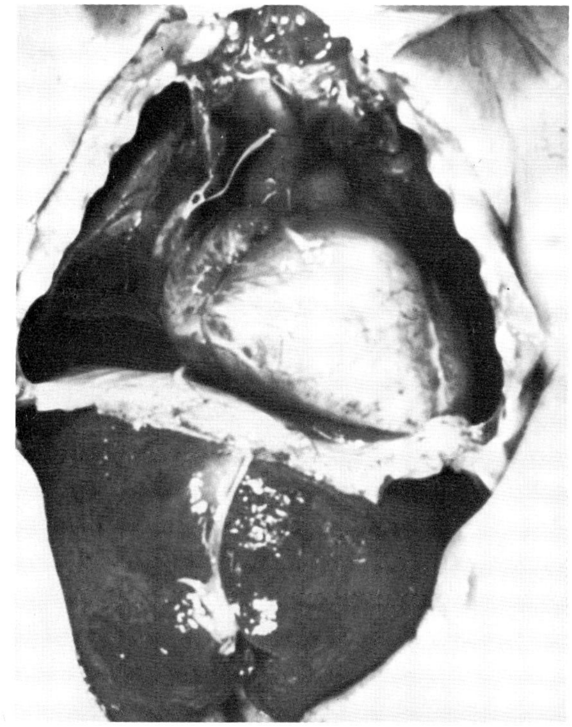

Fig. 11.7 Cardiomegaly with biventricular hypertrophy and hepatomegaly in a stillborn infant with diffuse arterial calcification (Keeling et al. 1983).

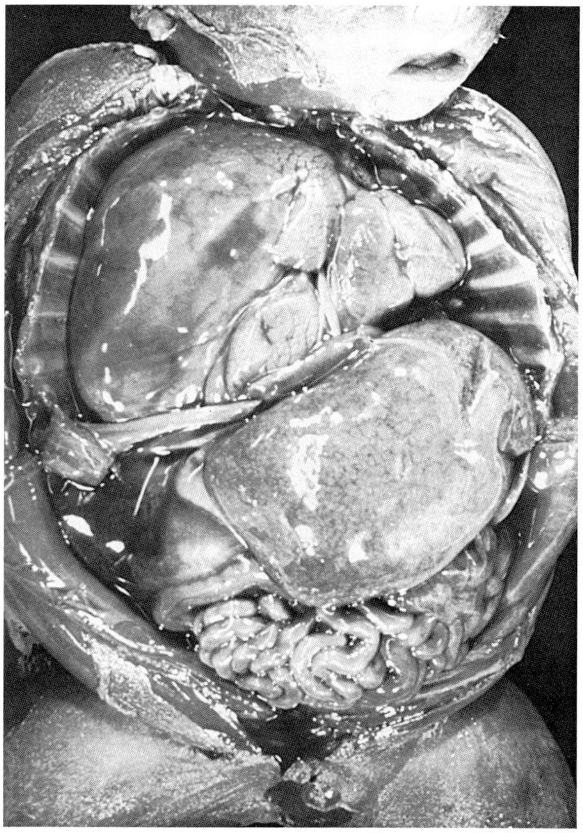

Fig. 11.8 Hydropic stillbirth: adenomatoid malformation of right upper lobe of lung. There is mediastinal shift and displacement of the liver by the depressed right hemidiaphragm. (Keeling et al. 1983).

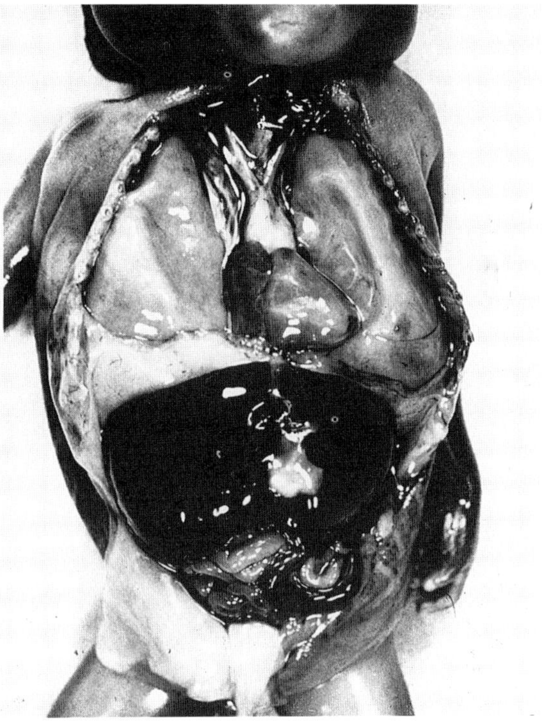

Fig. 11.9 Fetus of 20 weeks' gestation. There is massive distension of both lungs producing depression of the diaphragm, ascites and hydrops. There was severe laryngeal stenosis obstructing pulmonary drainage.

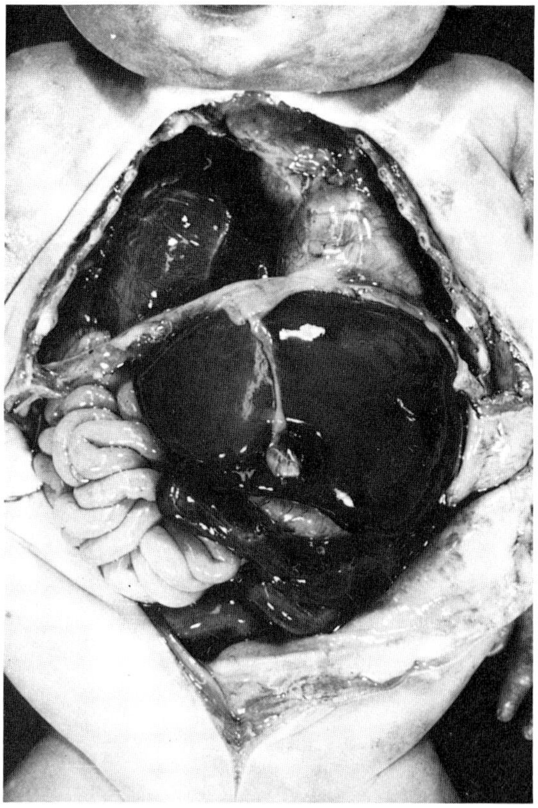

Fig. 11.10 Right-side diaphragmatic hernia associated with fetal hydrops and polyhydramnios. The heart and lungs are displaced to the left by the right lobe of the liver (Keeling et al. 1983).

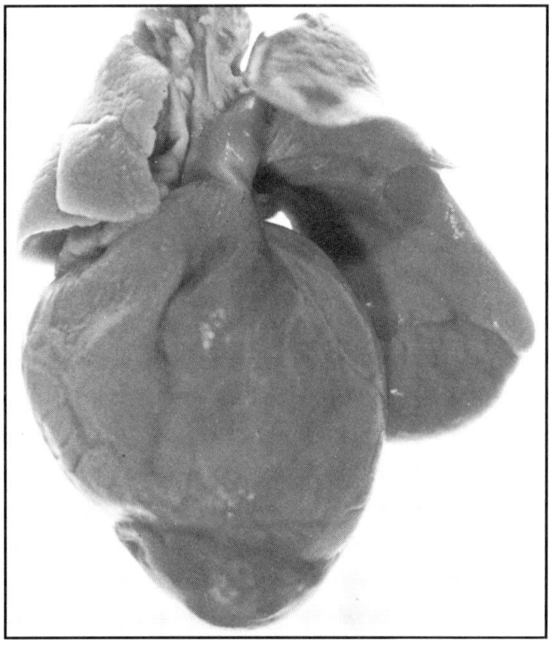

Fig. 11.11 Fetal hydrops with cardiomegaly: a mass arises within the ventricular myocardium and is apparent at the apex. (×2)

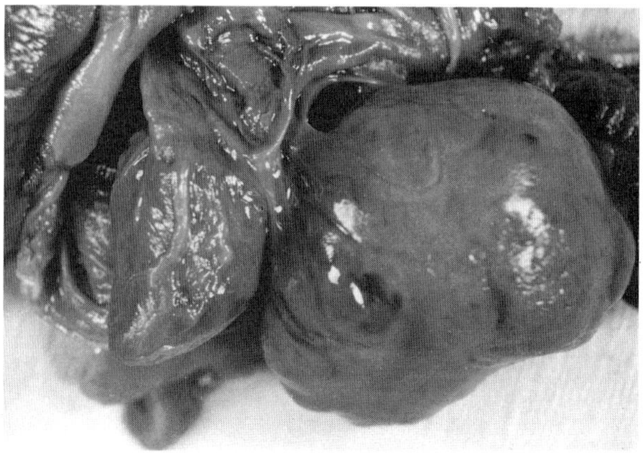

Fig. 11.12 Hydrops at 25 weeks' gestation. A teratoma arises from the right atrium/great artery origins. A large pericardial effusion was present.

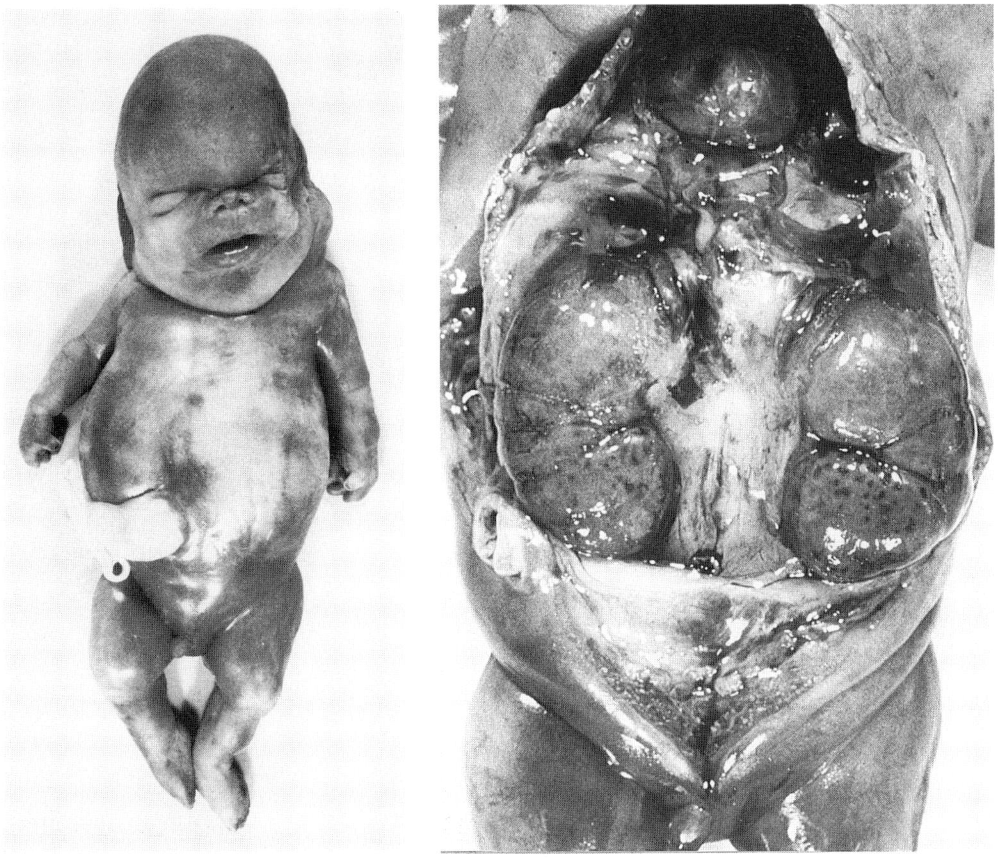

a b

Fig. 11.13 Meckel's syndrome. Hydropic fetus at 22 weeks' gestation **a** Massive ascites, shortening of all limbs and abdominal distension. **b** Massive renomegaly (Keeling 1991).

include tumours, cystic kidneys (Fig. 11.13), lower genitourinary obstruction and intestinal pathology with haemorrhage or infarction (Table 11.2).

Intracranial pathology includes necrosis and calcification resulting from infection, tumours and vascular abnormalities (Table 11.3), cerebral haemorrhage may be present.

Histological Examination

Routine sampling of organs for histological examination should be undertaken (see Chap. 1) even when a gross abnormality thought to be causally related to the hydrops has been identified. Histological appearances of the heart and lungs may be particularly useful. The heart should be sampled initially in such a manner that the conductive system is undisturbed as subsequent systematic detailed conductive examination may be necessary. Histology will distinguish between different pulmonary hamartomata and the types of cystic kidneys (see Chap. 19). In the heart, infection, infarction or rhabdomyomata may be found. The nature of vascular pathology can be established (Fig. 11.14). Useful information about the nature of fetal infection can be obtained either from the histological appearances or from more specific investigations including immunohistochemistry or in situ hybridisation (Fig. 11.15).

The Placenta

The placenta is often extremely thick and may weigh more than 1000 g. It is pale and friable and there is usually marked oedema of the umbilical cord. Placental appearance is related to the underlying cause of hydrops and is hydropic when there is severe anaemia and when there is obstruction to venous return

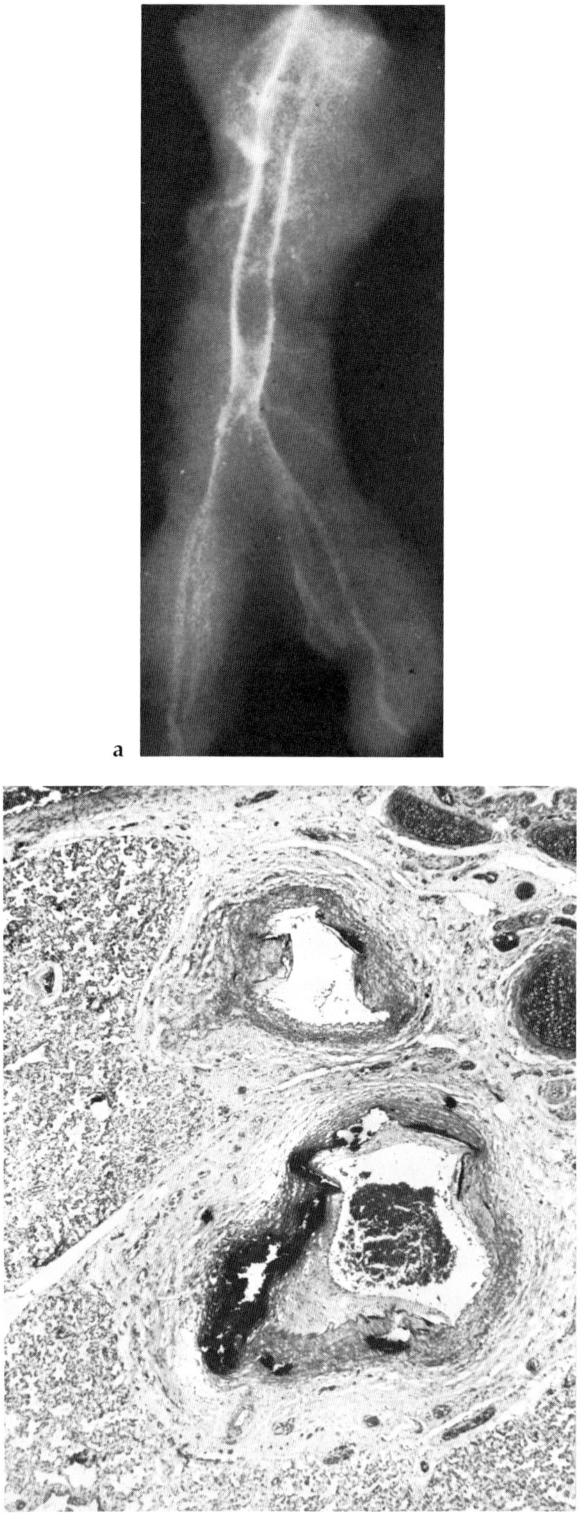

Fig. 11.14 Same case as in Figs. 11.1 and 11.7. **a** Radiograph of the aorta and iliac vessels demonstrates extensive calcification. **b** Calcification in the media of a pulmonary artery with overlying intimal proliferation (Keeling et al. 1983).

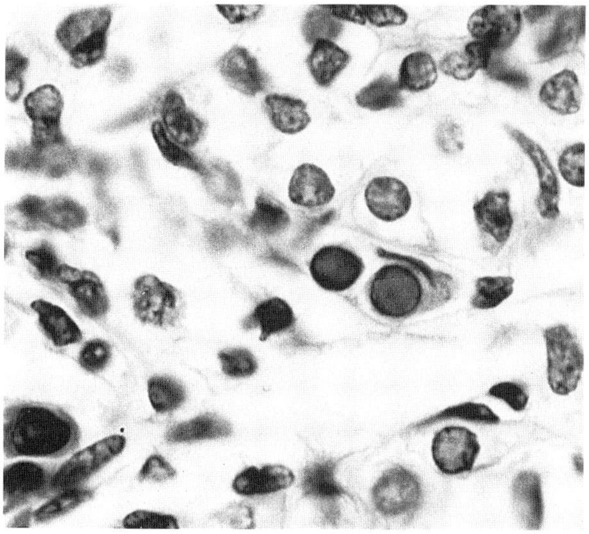

Fig. 11.15 Parvovirus infection. Intranuclear inclusions are present in cells in pulmonary capillaries.

from the placenta. In congenital nephrotic syndrome, placental oedema is gross even when the fetus is only mildly affected. The placenta may appear grossly normal even when the fetus is severely hydropic due to high-output heart failure or some chromosome anomalies.

Placental abnormalities causally related to fetal hydrops are large angiomata (Fig. 11.16) and monochorionic, diamniotic twin pregnancy. When there is significant twin transfusion (Fig. 11.17), there is usually a marked difference in appearance between the parts of the placenta related to each baby. The donor part is pale, friable and often thicker

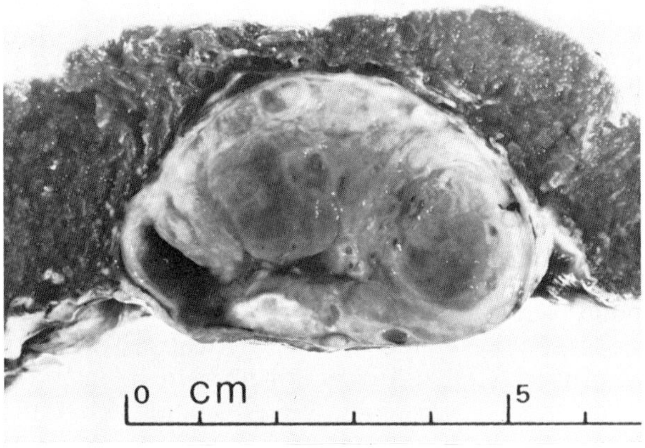

Fig. 11.16 Slice of placenta with large angioma from a pregnancy complicated by third trimester fetal hydrops and polyhydramnios.

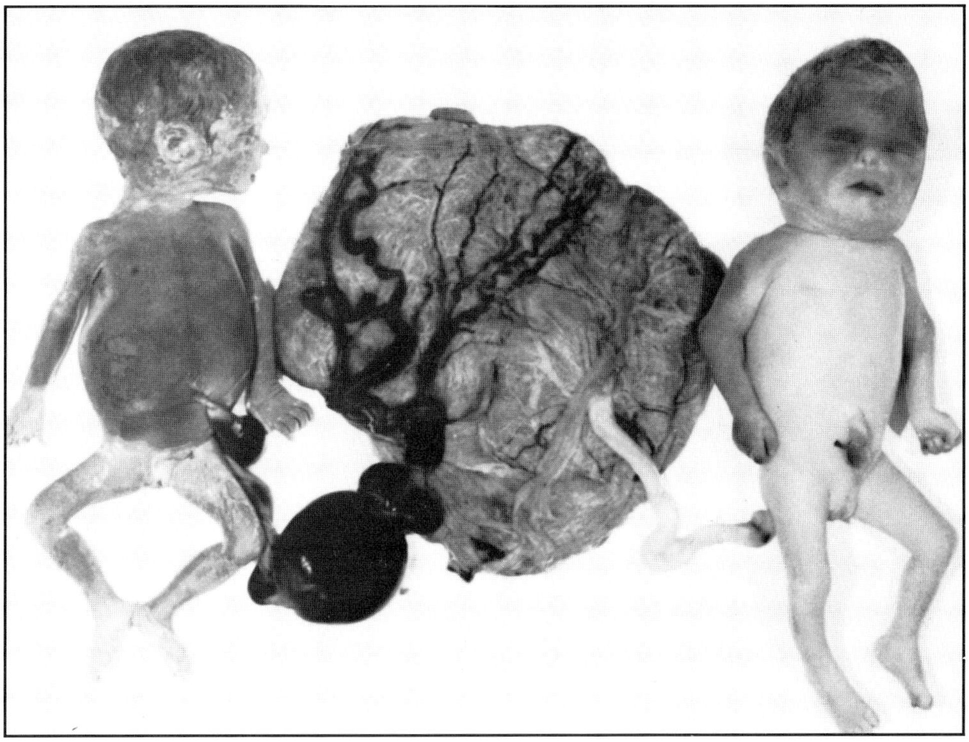

Fig. 11.17 Twin transfusion syndrome. The donor twin (*right*) is hydropic and pale. The recipient is plethoric, and placental vascular congestion is marked.

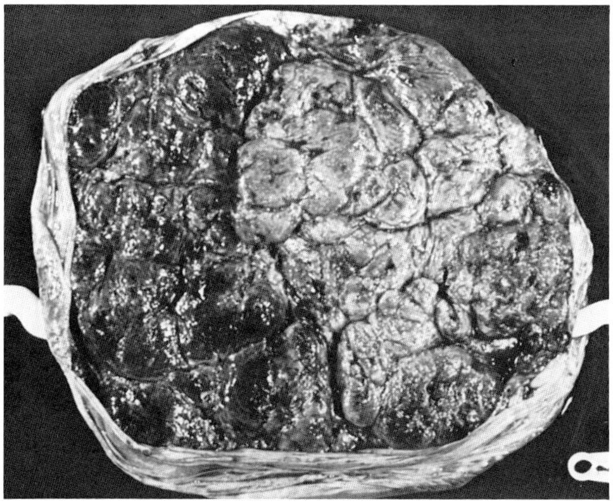

Fig. 11.18 Twin transfusion syndrome. The right side of the placenta is pale, bulky and hydropic (donor), the left side very congested (recipient).

than that related to the recipient, which is intensely congested (Fig. 11.18). Vascular communications between the two circulations can be readily demonstrated in chorionic plate vessels and within the placental parenchyma. Monochorionic, monoamniotic twins rarely exhibit signs of twin transfusion.

Histological examination of the placenta of a hydropic fetus reflects, to some extent, the gross appearance. When the placenta is hydropic, the villi may be uniformly oedematous, e.g. congenital nephrotic syndrome, and Hofbauer cells are readily seen. In rhesus disease, villous hydrops is not usually gross and is patchy in distribution; many villi are of normal size. There is persistence of cytotrophoblast so that villi appear immature. Careful examination of the non-hydropic villi shows plugging of villous capillaries by clumps of erythropoetic cells (Fig. 11.19). In the fetus with neuroblastoma, similar capillary plugging by clumps of tumour cells is seen (Fig. 11.20). Prominence or increased size of trophoblast cells with cytoplasmic vacuolation is present in some fetuses of genetic metabolic disease such as the lysosomal disorder sialidosis (Fig. 11.21).

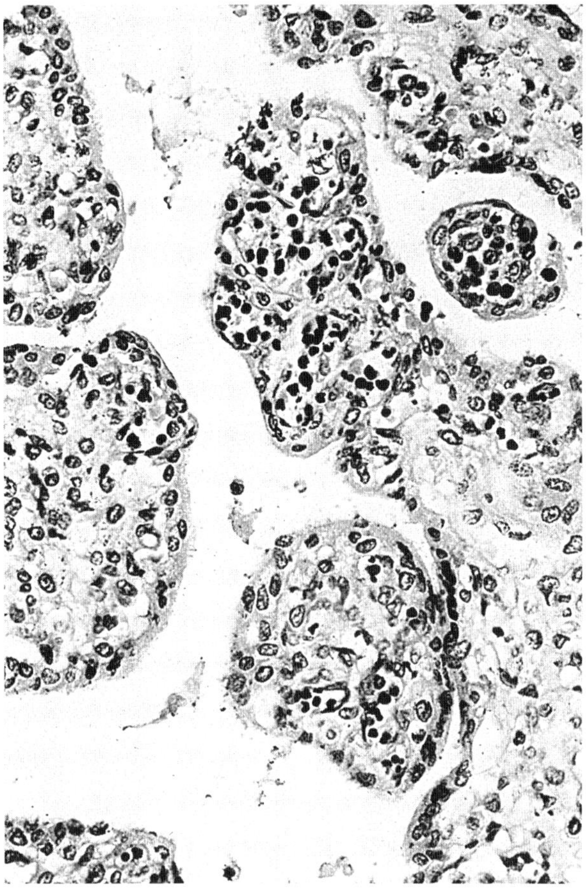

Fig. 11.19 The placenta in Rhesus hydrops. Hydropic change is non-uniform. Capillaries of non-hydropic villi are plugged by erythropoietic foci.

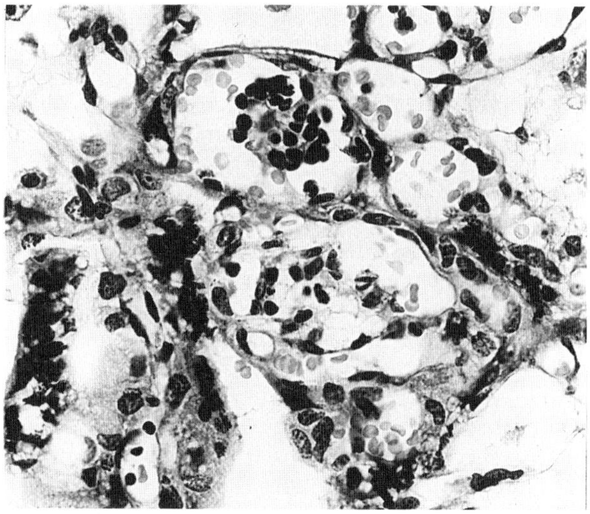

Fig. 11.20 Hydropic fetus with neuroblastoma. Tumour emboli are present within villous capillaries in the placenta (Keeling 1991).

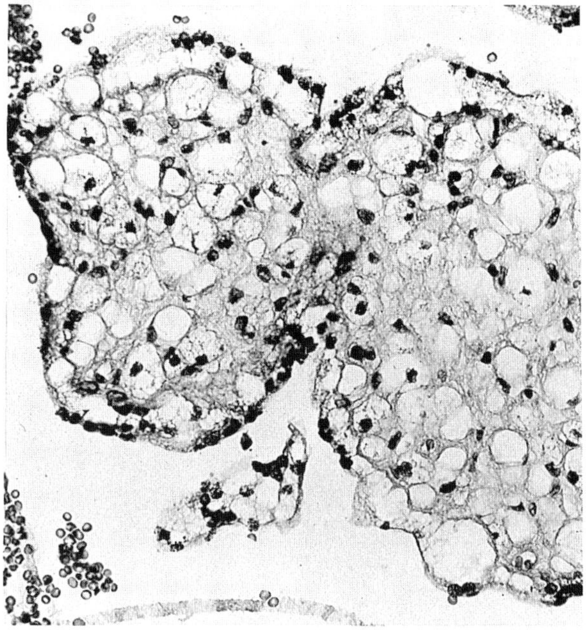

Fig. 11.21 Placenta at 25 weeks' gestation; prominent, vacuolated trophoblast and villous hydrops; sialidosis.

Significance of Pathological Abnormalities

When assessing the relationship between fetal hydrops and any pathological abnormalities present, it is important that a causal relationship is not immediately implied and that thorough, systematic investigations are undertaken.

Careful thought must be given to all the findings, clinical and pathological, so that the sequence of events culminating in fetal hydrops might be better understood. This is particularly important as particular clinical skills are developed and effective fetal therapy to alleviate the hydropic state is introduced.

McFadden and Taylor (1989) question an association with congenital heart disease and prenatal closure of the foramen ovale. They found no difference in the type of malformations in hydropic and non-hydropic babies subjected to necropsy examination. Looking at the types of cardiac malformation in series of 10 or more cases of hydrops (Keeling 1991), there seems to be an excess of complex cardiac anomalies such as those with ambiguous cardiac situs, where structural abnormalities of the cardiac conduction system and arrhythmias are common (Fleischer et al. 1981; Kleinman et al. 1982; Keeling et al. 1983).

Intracranial ischaemia (Kobori and Urich 1986; Squier and Keeling 1991) and intracranial haemorrhage (Bose 1978) require careful evaluation. Ischaemic cerebral injury seems to be a consequence of the underlying cause of hydrops; Squier and Keeling (1991) found these changes in both the hydropic and non-hydropic twin of twin-transfusion pairs. One of these babies had an intracerebral haemorrhage which occurred in an area with pre-existing ischaemic change.

Newbold et al. (1991) investigated the relationship between endocardial fibroelastosis (EFE) (Fig. 11.22) and hydrops in both the presence and absence of rhesus disease. They concluded that EFE was secondary to congestive cardiac failure. I endorse their conclusion that EFE is a response to insult rather than a primary disorder but find it difficult to ascribe the changes to congestive cardiac failure. It seems more likely that the common factor amongst its various antecedents is hypoxia. The presence of mature elastic and collagen fibres beneath the endothelium and the lack of cytological evidence of myohypertrophy suggests to me that in many cases congestive cardiac failure is a response to increased work in overcoming the impedance of EFE to normal contractility.

It is evident that careful consideration must be given to all pathological findings in the examination of the hydropic fetus. Assessment of histological changes may permit observations in respect of the chronology of changes present and contribute to our understanding of the mechanisms of fetal hydrops.

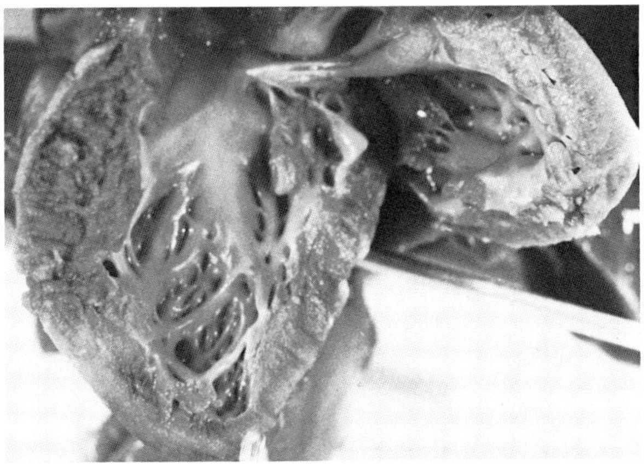

a

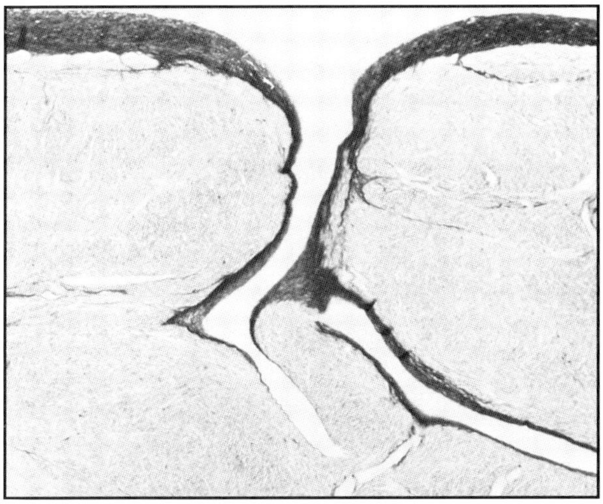

b

Fig. 11.22 a Endocardial fibroelastosis accentuates the trabecular pattern of the ventricular myocardium. **b** Irregular deposition of fibroelastic tissue beneath the endocardium. (Weigert's elastic—Van Geison's method).

Investigation of Fetal Hydrops

The aims of investigations following the discovery of fetal hydrops are to ascertain the underlying cause or association and to document the severity of fetal oedema, the presence or absence of effusions in body cavities, the degree of polyhydramnios and the extent of placental involvement so that rational decisions can be made about patient management and estimates of risk of recurrence given (Holzgreve et al. 1984).

Some urge immediate delivery when a diagnosis of fetal hydrops is made in the third trimester, arguing that pulmonary hypoplasia secondary to pleural effusions constitutes the major risk to the fetus (Anderson et al. 1983). Others (Fleischer et al. 1981; Kleinman et al. 1982) advocate careful ultrasound examination to identify the fetus with major malformation. Mahony et al. (1984) found that they were unable to predict outcome on the basis of ultrasonographic examination alone.

Immediate investigation with selective delivery, medical management in some cases and careful repeated observation was advocated by Gough et al. (1986), because of the high incidence of major malformations, which have a poor outcome even in the most favoured circumstances, the difficulties encountered during resuscitation of the hydropic infant and the impact of caesarean section on the mother's reproductive career. Spontaneous resolution of fetal hydrops has been observed with favourable outcome for both mother and fetus (Platt et al. 1978; Keeling et al. 1983).

A number of different types of ultrauterine therapy for fetal hydrops have been tried, with some success. This underlines the need for rapid and specific diagnosis of the underlying problem. The earliest specific therapy was digoxin or beta blockers administered to the mother (Rees et al. 1980; Fleischer et al. 1981; Iliff et al. 1983). Subsequently these drugs have been given to the fetus directly to counteract poor or unpredictable placental transfer (Hansmann et al. 1989). Blood transfusion (Soothill 1990) and albumin infusion (Shimokawa et al. 1988) have been used in different circumstances. Drainage of pleural effusions to encourage lung growth and of ascites and the urinary bladder to reduce intra-abdominal pressure have also been undertaken.

Table 11.5. Investigations to be undertaken when fetal hydrops is diagnosed prenatally

Investigation of the mother	Ultrasonography
Haemoglobin, Kleihauer	Severity of hydrops
ABO and rhesus group	Severity of polyhydramnios
Serum alpha-fetoprotein	Multiple pregnancy
Haemolysins, haemaglutinins	Fetal heart rate/rhythm
Minor blood group antigens	Fetal anomaly:
Antinuclear factor	heart
Autoantibodies	other
Serological tests for syphilis	Placenta:
Glucose tolerance test	thickness
Placental biopsy/amniocentesis:	other abnormality
chromosomes	
virus culture	

When the diagnosis of fetal hydrops is made, the investigations listed in Table 11.5. should be undertaken as a matter of urgency. All the investigations should be undertaken, even though results might have been normal earlier in pregnancy. The investigations identify that small group of cases where immediate delivery or active antenatal management may be life saving. These conditions include minor blood group abnormalities (anti e, b or c or Kell), fetal cardiac arrhythmias, placental chorioangioma, twin–twin transfusion syndrome, fetomaternal haemorrhage, maternal anaemia or diabetes mellitus.

Amniocentesis with controlled removal of fluid may contribute to maternal comfort, decrease the likelihood of spontaneous premature onset of labour and yield samples for microbiological culture and biochemical examination, which may assist management.

When a hydropic fetus is born alive and the underlying cause of hydrops is not apparent, the investigations listed in Table 11.6 should be contemplated. Essential post-mortem investigations are also indicated in this Table.

Table 11.6. Investigation of the hydropic neonate

At birth:	
Full blood count	Echocardiogram
Blood group and antibodies	Radiological examination
Clotting screen	Cardiac catheterisation
Liver function tests	Effusions:
Viral antibodies	culture
WR, karyotype	biochemical analysis
Necropsy:	
Photographic record	Histological examination
Weight and measurements	Virus culture and antibodies
Malformation:	Blood group and antibodies
cardiac	Effusions:
other	culture
Lung weight	biochemical analysis

Abbreviation: WR, Wassermann reaction

References

Abramovich DR (1968) The volume of amniotic fluid in early pregnancy. J Obstet Gynaecol Br Cmwlth 75: 728–731

Abramovich DR, Page KR (1973) Pathways of water transfer between liquor amnii and the fetoplacental unit at term. Eur J Obstet Gynecol Reprod Biol 3: 155–158

Allan LD, Crawford DC, Sheridan R, Chapman MG (1986) Aetiology of nonimmune hydrops: the value of echocardiography. Br J Obstet Gynaecol 93: 223–225

Altenberger KM, Jedziniak M, Roper WL, Hernandez J (1977) Congenital complete heart block associated with hydrops fetalis. J Pediatr 91: 618–620

Anders D, Kindermann G, Pfeifer U (1973) Metastasising fetal neuroblastoma with involvement of the placenta simulating fetal erythroblastosis. J Pediatr 82: 50–53

Andersen HM, Drew JH, Beischer NA, Hutchison AA, Fortune DW (1983) Non-immune hydrops fetalis: changing contribution to perinatal mortality. Br J Obstet Gynaecol 90: 636–639

Bagozzi DC, Tagliabue P, Salmoiraghi MG, Tischer MC, Marini A, Flauto U (1988) Neonatal evaluation of non immunologic hydrops fetalis. Report of 31 cases. Pathologica 80: 677–686

Bain AD, Bowie JH, Flint WF, Beverley JKA, Beattie CP (1956) Congenital toxoplasmosis simulating haemolytic disease of the newborn. J Obstet Gynaecol Br Cmwlth 63: 826–832
Barnes E, Bryan EM, Harris DA, Baum JD (1977) Oedema in the newborn. Mol Aspects Med 1: 187–282
Bates HR (1970) Coxsackie virus B3 calcific pancarditis and hydrops fetalis. Am J Obstet Gynecol 106: 629–630
Beck AM, Bender SW, Reither H-L, Otto W, Bassler R, Dancygier H, Gehler J (1984) Neuraminidase deficiency presenting as nonimmune hydrops fetalis. Eur J Pediatr 43: 135–139
Becker AE, Becker MJ, Wagenvoort CA (1977) Premature contraction of the ductus arteriosus: a cause of fetal death. J Pathol 121: 187–191
Beischer NA, Fortune DW, Macafee J (1971) Non-immunologic hydrops fetalis and congenital abnormalities. Obstet Gynecol 38: 86–95
Boer HR, Anido G (1979) Hydrops fetalis caused by Bart's haemoglobin. South Med J 72: 1623–1624
Bose C (1978) Hydrops fetalis and in utero intracranial haemorrhage. J Pediatr 93: 1023–1024
Boyd JD, Hamilton WJ (1970) The human placenta. Heffer, Cambridge, p 22
Boyd PA, Keeling JW (1992) Fetal hydrops. J Clin Genet 29: 91–97
Bryan EM (1977) IgG deficiency in association with placental oedema. Early Hum Devel 1/2: 133–143
Bryan EM, Nicholson E (1981) Hydrops fetalis in South Korea. Ann Trop Paediatr 1: 181–187
Bulova SI, Schwartz E, Harrer WV (1972) Hydrops fetalis and congenital syphilis. Pediatrics 49: 285–287
Burton PA (1986) Intranuclear inclusions in marrow of hydropic fetus due to parvovirus infection. Lancet ii: 1155
Carlson DE, Platt LD, Medearis AL, Horenstein J (1990) Prognostic indicators of the resolution of nonimmune hydrops fetalis and survival of the fetus. Am J Obstet Gynecol 163: 1785–1787
Carter C, Darbyshire PJ, Wickramasinghe SN (1989) A congenital dyserythropoietic anaemia variant presenting as hydrops fetalis. Br J Haematol 72: 289–290
Cartlidge PHT, Rutter N (1986) Serum albumin concentrations and oedema in the newborn. Arch Dis Child 61: 657–660
Cooke RWJ, Mettau JW, van Coppelle AW, de Villeneuve VH (1980) Familial congenital heart block and hydrops fetalis. Arch Dis Child 55: 479–480
Cowan RH, Waldo HB, Harris G et al. (1975) Neonatal paroxysmal supraventricular tachycardia with hydrops. Pediatrics 55: 248–230
Debelle GD, Gillam GL, Tauro GP (1977) A case of hydrops fetalis due to maternal haemorrhage. Aust Pediatr J 13: 131–133
Engellenner W, Kaplan C, van de Vegte GL (1989) Pulmonary agenesis association with nonimmune hydrops. Pediatr Pathol 9: 725–730
Esscher E, Scott JS (1979) Congenital heart block and maternal systemic lupus erythematosus. Br Med J i: 1235–1238
Etches PC, Lemons JA (1979) Nonimmune hydrops fetalis: report of 22 cases including three siblings. Pediatrics 64: 326–332
Fleischer AC, Killam AP, Boehm FH et al. (1981) Hydrops fetalis: sonographic evaluation and clinical implications. Radiology 141: 163–168
Friis-Hansen B (1971) Body composition during growth. In vivo measurements and biochemical data correlated to differential anatomical growth. Pediatrics 47(2): 264–274
Golbus MS, Hall BD, Filly RA, Poskaizer LR (1977) Prenatal diagnosis of achondrogenesis. J Pediatr 91: 464–466
Gordon H, Grausz JP, Raphael M, McClure Browne JC (1966) Experience with intraperitoneal transfusion. J Obstet Gynaecol Br Cmwlth 73: 917–922
Gough JD, Keeling JW, Castle B, Iliff PJ (1986) The obstetric management of non-immunological hydrops. Br J Obstet Gynaecol 93: 111–119
Graves GR, Baskett TF (1984) Nonimmune hydrops fetalis: antenatal diagnosis and management. Am J Obstet Gynecol 148: 563–565
Gray ES (1989) Mesoblastic nephroma and non-immunological hydrops fetalis (letter). Pediatr Pathol 9: 607–609
Guyton AC (1963) A concept of negative interstitial pressure based on pressures in implanted perforated capsule. Circ Res 12: 399–414
Hansmann M, Gembruch U, Bald R (1989) New therapeutic aspects in nonimmune hydrops fetalis based on 402 prenatally diagnosed cases. Fetal Therapy 4: 29–36
Hardy JD, Solomon S, Banwell GS, Beach R, Wright V, Howard FM (1979) Congenital complete heart block in the newborn associated with maternal systemic lupus erythematosus and other connective tissue disorders. Arch Dis Child 54: 7–13
Hennekam RC, Beemer FA, Cats BP, Jansen G, Staal GE (1990) Hydrops fetalis associated with red cell pyruvate kinase deficiency. Genet Couns 1: 75–79
Ho SY, Mortimer G, Anderson RH, Pomerance A, Keeling JW (1985) Conduction system defects in three perinatal patients with arrhythmia. Br Heart J 53: 158–163
Holzgreve W, Curry CJR, Golbus MS, Callen PW, Filly RA, Smith JC (1984) Investigation of nonimmune hydrops fetalis. Am J Obstet Gynecol 150: 805–812
Huchet J, Soulié JC (1979) Anasarque fœto-placentaire et incompatibilité ABO. Rev Fr Transfus Immuno-hémat 22: 191–193
Hull D, Binns BAO, Joyce D (1966) Congenital heart block and widespread fibrosis due to maternal lupus erythematosus. Arch Dis Child 41: 688–690
Hutchison AA, Drew JH, Yu VYH, Williams ML, Fortune DW, Beischer NA (1982) Nonimmunologic hydrops fetalis: a review of 61 cases. Obstet Gynecol 59: 347–352
Iliff P, Nicholls JM, Keeling JW, Gough JD (1983) Nonimmunologic hydrops fetalis: a review of 27 cases. Arch Dis Child 58: 979–982
Im SS, Rizos N, Joutsi P, Shime J, Benzie RJ (1984) Nonimmunologic hydrops fetalis. Am J Obstet Gynecol 148: 566–569
Ito T, Engle MA, Holswade GR (1961) Congenital insufficiency of the pulmonic valve. Pediatrics 28: 712–718
Ivemark B, Lagergren C, Ljungqvist A (1962) Generalised arterial calcification associated with hydramnios in two stillborn infants. Acta Paediatr Scand [Suppl] 135: 103–110
Johnson WG, Thomas GH, Miranda AF et al. (1980) Congenital sialidosis: biochemical studies, clinical spectrum in four sibs; two successful prenatal diagnoses. Am J Hum Genet 32: 43A
Jones CE, Rivers RP, Chir B, Taghizadeh A (1973) Disseminated intravascular coagulation and fetal hydrops in a newborn infant in association with a chorioangioma of placenta. Pediatrics 50: 901–907
Kazzi NJ, Chang CH, Roberts EC, Shankaran S (1989) Fetal hepatoblastoma presenting as nonimmune hydrops. Am J Perinatol 6: 278–280

Keeling JW (1991) Hydrops fetalis and other forms of excess fluid collection in the fetus. In: Wigglesworth JS, Singer DB (eds) Textbook of fetal and perinatal pathology. Blackwell Scientific, Oxford, pp 429–454
Keeling JW, Gough DJ, Iliff P (1983) The pathology of non-rhesus hydrops. Diagn Histopathol 6: 89–111
Khong TY, Keeling JW (1990) Massive congenital mesenchymal malformation of the lung: another cause of non-immune hydrops. Histopathology 16: 609–611
Kleinman CS, Donnerstein RL, de Vore GR et al. (1982) Fetal echocardiography for evaluation of in utero congestive heart failure: a technique for study of nonimmune fetal hydrops. N Engl J Med 306: 568–575
Knoth M, Rygaard J, Hesseldahl H (1976) Chorioangioma with hydramnios and intrauterine fetal death. Acta Obset Gynecol Scand 55: 279–281
Kobori JA, Urich H (1986) Intrauterine anoxic brain damage in nonimmune hydrops fetalis. Biol Neonate 49: 311–317
Kohler H (1976) Sacrococcygeal teratoma and "nonimmunological" hydrops fetalis. Br Med J ii: 422–423
Kohler HG (1978) Premature closure of the ductus arteriosus (PCDA): a possible cause of intrauterine circulatory failure. Early Hum Devel 2(1): 15–23
Kuller JA, Laifer SA (1991) Trisomy 15 associated with nonimmune hydrops. Am J Perinatol 8: 39–40
Larroche J-Cl (1977) Nonimmunologic hydrops fetalis. Developmental pathology of the neonate. Excerpta Medica, Amsterdam, pp 179–181
Larroche J-Cl (1982) Anasarque foeto-placentaire (hydrops) sans immunisation. Med Hyg 40: 2061–2073
Lauener P-A, Payot M, Micheli J-L (1985) Congenital hydrops and WPW Syndrome. Pediatr Cardiol 6: 113–116
Laurence KM (1955) Congenital pulmonary cystic lymphangiectasis. J Pathol Bacteriol 70: 325–333
Lie ILE, Lie HG (1961) Abnormal haemoglobin production as a probable cause of erythroblastosis and hydrops foetalis in uniovular twins. Acta Hematol 25: 192–199
Lind T, Kendall A, Hytten FE (1972) The role of the fetus in the formation of amniotic fluid. J Obstet Gynaecol Br Cmwlth 79: 289–298
Macafee CAJ, Fortune DW, Beischer NA (1970) Non-immunological hydrops fetalis. J Obstet Gynaecol Br Cmwlth 77: 226–237
McCue CM, Mantakes ME, Tingelstad JB, Ruddy S (1977) Congenital heart block in newborns of mothers with connective tissue disease. Circulation 56: 82–90
McFadden DE, Taylor GP (1989) Cardiac abnormalities and nonimmune hydrops fetalis: coincidental, not causal, relationship. Pediatr Pathol 9: 11–17
Machin GA (1981) Differential diagnosis of hydrops fetalis. Am J Med Genet 19: 341–350
Machin GA (1985) Diseases causing fetal and neonatal ascites. Pediatr Pathol 4: 195–211
Machin GA (1989) Hydrops revisited: literature review of 1414 cases published in the 1980s. Am J Med Genet 34: 366–390
Mahony BS, Filly RA, Callen PW, Chinn DH, Golbus MS (1984) Severe nonimmune hydrops fetalis: sonographic evaluation. Radiology 151: 757–761
Mayerson HS, Wolfram CG, Shirley HH Jr, Wasserman K (1960) Regional differences in capillary permeability. Am J Physiol 198: 155–160
Mentzer WC, Collier E (1975) Hydrops fetalis associated with erythrocyte G-6-PD deficiency and maternal ingestion of fava beans and ascorbic acid. J Pediatr 86: 565–569
Miser A, Geraci TK, Wennberg RP (1975) Fetal erythroblastosis fetalis due to anti-Kell isoimmune disease. J Pediatr 86: 567–569
Moerman P, Fryns J-P, Goddeeris P, Lauweryns JM (1982) Nonimmunological hydrops fetalis. A study of ten cases. Arch Path Lab Med 106: 635–640
Moller JH, Lynch RP, Edwards JE (1966) Fetal cardiac failure resulting from congenital anomalies of the heart. J Pediatr 68: 699–703
Morey AL, Keeling JW, Porter HJ, Fleming KA (1992) Clinical and histopathological features of parvovirus B_{19} infection in the human fetus. Br J Obstet Gynecol 99: 566–574
Mostoufi-Zadeh M, Weiss LM, Driscoll SG (1985) Nonimmune hydrops fetalis: a challenge in perinatal pathology. Hum Pathol 16: 785–789
Naeye RL, Blanc WA (1964) Prenatal narrowing or closure of the foramen ovale. Circulation 30: 736–742
Nakamura Y, Komatsu Y, Yano H et al. (1987) Nonimmunologic hydrops fetalis: a clinico-pathological study of 50 autopsy cases. Pediatr Pathol 7: 19–30
Newbould MJ, Armstrong GR, Barson AJ (1991) Endocardial fibroelastosis in infants with hydrops fetalis. J Clin Pathol 44: 576–579
Ostor AG, Fortune DW (1978) Tuberous sclerosis initially seen as hydrops fetalis: report of a case and review of the literature. Arch Path Lab Med 102: 34–39
Page KR, Abramovich DR, Garden AS, Jandial L (1978) Solute levels in uterine fluids of patients with normal values of amniotic fluid and with hydramnios. Eur J Obstet Gynecol Reprod Biol 8(5): 287–293
Perkins RP (1971) Hydrops fetalis and stillbirth in a male glucose-6-phosphate dehydrogenase deficient fetus possibly due to maternal ingestion of sulfisoxazole. Am J Obstet Gynecol 111: 379–381
Pesonen E, Haavistu H, Anumala P, Teramu IC (1983) Intrauterine hydrops caused by premature closure of the foramen ovale. Arch Dis Child 58: 1015–1016
Phibbs RH, Johnson P, Tooley WH (1974) Cardiorespiratory status of erythroblastotic newborn infants: II. Blood volume, hematocrit, and serum albumin concentration in relation to hydrops fetalis. Pediatrics 53: 13–23
Phillips RR, Batcup G, Vinall PS (1985) Non-immunologic hydrops fetalis. Arch Dis Child 60: 84
Platt LD, Collea JV, Joseph DM (1978) Transitory fetal ascites: an ultrasound diagnosis. Am J Obstet Gynecol 132: 906–908
Platt LD, Geirmann CA, Turkel SB, Young G, Keegan KA (1981) Atrial hemangioma and hydrops fetalis. Am J Obstet Gynecol 141: 107–109
Porter HJ, Khong TY, Evans MF, Chan VT-W, Fleming KA (1988) Parvovirus as a cause of hydrops fetalis: detection by in situ hybridisation. J Clin Pathol 41: 381–383
Potter EL (1943) Universal edema of the fetus unassociated with erythroblastosis. Am J Obstet Gynecol 46: 130–134
Queenan JT, Thompson W, Whitfield CR, Shah SI (1972) Amniotic fluid volumes in normal pregnancies. Am J Obstet Gynecol 114: 34–38
Radford DJ, Izukawa T, Rowe RD (1976) Congenital paroxysmal atrial tachycardia. Arch Dis Child 51: 613–617
Rees L, Vlies PR, Adams J (1980) Hydrops fetalis, an unusual cause, presentation and method of diagnosis. Br J Obstet Gynaecol 87: 1169–1170
Richardson MM, Wagner ML, Malini S, Rosenberg HS, Lucci JA (1977) Prenatal diagnosis of recurrence of Saldino-Noonan dwarfism. J Pediatr 91: 467–471
Rossier A, Caldera R, Sarrut S (1958) Sur un cas de maladie

de Niemann–Pick chez un nouveau-né. Presse Med 66: 535–537

Rudolph N, Levin EJ (1977) Hydrops fetalis with venae cavae thrombosis in utero. NY State J Med 3: 421–423

Ruiz-Villaespesa A, Suarez Mier MP, Lopez Ferrer P, Alvarez Baleriola I, Rodriguez Gonzalez JI (1990) Nonimmunologic hydrops fetalis: an etiopathogenetic approach through the postmortem study of 59 patients. Am J Med Genet 35: 274–279

Sabet LM (1982) Congenital glioblastoma multiforme associated with congestive heart failure. Arch Path Lab Med 106: 31–34

Sahn DJ, Shenker L, Reed KL, Valdes-Cruz LM, Sobonya R, Anderson C (1982) Prenatal ultrasound diagnosis of hypoplastic left heart syndrome in utero associated with hydrops fetalis. Am Heart J 104: 1368–1372

Scanton JW, Muirhead DM (1976) Hydrops fetalis due to anti-Kell isoimmune disease: survival with optimal long-term outcome. J Pediatr 88: 484–485

Schruefer JJ, Seeds AE, Behrman RE, Hellegers AE, Bruns PD (1972) Changes in amniotic fluid volume and total solute concentration in the rhesus monkey following replacement with distilled water. Am J Obstet Gynecol 112: 807–815

Scimeca PG, Weinblatt ME, Slepowitz G, Harper RG, Kohen JA (1988) Diamond–Blackfan syndrome: an unusual cause of hydrops fetalis. Am J Pediatr Hematol Oncol 10: 241–243

Seward JF, Zusman J (1978) Hydrops fetalis associated with small bowel volvulus. Lancet ii: 52–53

Shimokawa H, Hara K, Maeda H, Miyamoto S, Koyanagi T, Nakano H (1988) Intrauterine treatment of idiopathic hydrops fetalis. J Perinat Med 16: 133–138

Shturman-Ellstein R, Greco MA, Myrie C, Goldman EK (1978) Hydrops fetalis, hydramnios and hepatic vascular malformation associated with cutaneous haemangioma and chorioangioma. Acta Paed Scand 67: 239–243

Soothill P (1990) Intrauterine blood transfusion for non-immune hydrops fetalis due to parvovirus B19 infection. Lancet 336: 121 (letter)

Spahr RC, Botti JJ, MacDonald HM, Holzman IR (1980) Nonimmunologic hydrops fetalis: a review of 19 cases. Int J Gynaecol Obstet 18: 303–307

Squier MV, Keeling JW (1991) The incidence of prenatal brain injury. Neuropathol Appl Neurobiol 17: 29–38

Steenhout P, Elmer C, Clercx A et al. (1990) Carnitine deficiency with cardiomyopathy presenting as neonatal hydrops: successful response to carnitine therapy. J Inherited Metab Dis 13: 69–75

Thumasathit B, Nondasuta A, Silpisornkosol S, Lousuebsakul B, Unchalipongse P, Mangkornkanok M (1968) Hydrops fetalis associated with Bart's haemoglobin in Northern Thailand. J Pediatr 73: 132–138

Turski DM, Shahidi N, Viseskul C, Gilbert E (1978) Nonimmunologic hydrops fetalis. Am J Obstet Gynecol 131: 586–587

Weatherall DJ, Clegg JB, Wong HB (1970) The haemoglobin constitution of infants with the haemoglobin Bart's hydrops fetalis syndrome. Br J Haematol 18: 357–367

Whitfield CR (1981) Prediction of Rhesus haemolytic disease. In: Barson AJ (ed) Laboratory investigation of fetal disease. Wright, Bristol pp 299–319

Wilkin P, Parmentier R (1961) Hydrops foeto-placentaire et fibroelastose sousendocardique. Bull Soc R Belge Gynec Obstet 31: 35–44

Windebank KP, Bridges NA, Ostman-Smith I, Stevens JE (1987) Hydrops fetalis due to abnormal lymphatics. Arch Dis Child 62: 198–200

Worthen HG, Vernier RL, Good RA (1959) Infantile nephrosis. Am J Dis Child 98: 731–748

Zarafu IW, Tseng PI, Chuachingco J (1978) Hydrops fetalis, fetal maternal transfusion and choriocarcinoma of the placenta. Pediatr Res 12: 537

Chapter 12

Congenital Tumours

P. Jeremy Berry

Introduction

Tumours presenting in the newborn period are rare, although not as rare as the published literature suggests (Gale et al. 1982; Isaacs 1985; Campbell et al. 1987; Davis et al. 1988; Crom et al. 1989). Any pathologist working near a busy obstetric or neonatal unit can expect to see occasional cases. Many of these tumours are peculiar to infants, or behave differently from their counterparts in older children. Unfamiliarity with neonatal tumours may lead to unnecessarily aggressive therapy or well-intentioned neglect.

Although many tumours of early infancy are unique to that age group, virtually all childhood neoplasms have been described at some time or another in the perinatal period. (For a comprehensive review see Dehner 1981.) This chapter will concentrate on the special characteristics of neonatal tumours which influence their diagnosis and management, and outline some areas where study of neonatal tumours has clarified our understanding of neoplasia in general.

A congenital tumour is one that is present at birth, but it is reasonable to suppose that any tumour presenting in the first 3 months of life was congenital. Although there is no clear difference between the types of tumours presenting at birth and those of early infancy some distinction is worth preserving. Tumours may be diagnosed in utero by ultrasound scanning and pose difficult management problems (Kurjak et al. 1989). A fetal tumour may be influenced in utero by placental and maternal hormones or maternal immunoglobulins. The fetal circulation may be responsible for the pattern of metastases seen at birth. Large tumours can rupture or obstruct delivery. Poor drug tolerance may complicate chemotherapy in the newborn (Gale et al. 1982).

Many of the tumours seen in the newborn are not neoplasms but hamartomas, e.g. haemangiomas and melanocytic naevi. Such lesions may be symptomatic and occasionally fatal. Others are not easily classifiable, e.g. the congenital fibromatoses and phakomatoses. The difficulty of deciding which are true neoplasms is reflected in terminology such as "congenital fibrosarcoma-like fibromatosis", which some regard as fibrosarcoma and others as a fibromatosis. The term "tumour" will be used here in its literal sense to mean a mass or swelling.

Some of the true neoplasms of childhood are collectively referred to as blastomas, embryomas, or embryonic tumours. With few exceptions they are confined to childhood, and include nephroblastoma (Wilms' tumour), neuroblastoma, hepatoblastoma and medulloblastoma. These tumours recapitulate the embryonic tissues of the organ in which they arise, and are thought to result from neoplastic change in fetal and embryonic tissue. This would explain their restricted age range and unique histology. A conceptual flaw in this argument is that most of these tumours do not arise until the child is several years old, long after the supposed tissue of origin has disappeared. Study of the fetus and neonate has shown that such immature tissues occasionally persist and may develop into tumours later in childhood. These premalignant lesions exemplified by in situ neuroblastoma and nephroblastomatosis (Shanklin and Sotelo-Avila 1969) will be discussed with their respective tumours.

Incidence

Benign tumours of the newborn are so common that they are difficult to enumerate. Vascular naevi and haemangiomas are present in 6%–25% of the paediatric population, most being present from birth. Melanocytic naevi are found in 3% of newborn white infants and 16% of blacks.

Malignant tumours are uncommon. Wells (1940) reported four congenital tumours, all neuroblastomas, in a necropsy series of 3000 newborn infants, and reviewed a further 255 congenital tumours of all types reported in the literature up to that time. More recent studies (Barson 1978; Las Heras and Isaacs 1980) derived from pathology records probably underestimate the incidence of congenital leukaemia, which may not be adequately represented in such data (Table 12.1). With that exception these figures are essentially similar to data from the United Kingdom Children's Cancer Study Group and the Oxford Childhood Cancer Research Group registry (Broadbent 1986).

Table 12.1. Benign and malignant tumours in newborn children and infants. Percentage by tumour type

Tumour	Neonates (Barson 1980)[a]	Neonates (Las Heras and Isaacs 1980)	Infants up to 1 year (Isaacs 1983)
Teratoma	24%	40%	18%
Neuroblastoma	23%	12%	13%
Mesenchymal	8%	9%	23%
Renal	7%	5%	7%
CNS	6%	2%	9%
Leukaemia	6%	12%	6%
Number of cases	286	42	265

[a] Tumours accounting for less than 5% of the total in Barson's series are not shown.

Amongst solid tumours, benign and malignant germ cell tumours are the most common, followed by neuroblastoma, mesenchymal tumours of various types, renal tumours and brain tumours. Less common conditions seen in the neonatal period include histiocytosis X, hepatoblastoma and retinoblastoma. Lymphoma is notable for its extreme rarity in very young infants.

The Third US National Cancer Survey (1969–1971) estimated the incidence of malignant neoplasms in infants less than 29 days of age as 36.5 per million live births per year (Bader and Miller 1979). Mortality was approximately one-fifth of the incidence, reflecting the relatively benign course of several histologically malignant tumours in this age group. Pathologists must be aware that standard histological criteria of malignancy do not always indicate malignant behaviour in congenital tumours.

Aetiology

Congenital tumours appear to offer a system in which to study oncogenesis free from the multiple environmental influences which complicate such studies in adults. However, embryo and fetus are exposed to many chemical, physical and infective agents in utero. Despite this, considerable insight has been gained in recent years into the pathogenesis of neoplasms in infants and young children, and some are beginning to be understood at the molecular level (Gilbert 1984; Littlefield 1984; Knudson 1989). Genetic, chromosomal, syndromic and environmental associations that have been recognised in childhood cancer will be discussed here as they apply to perinatal pathology.

Some childhood tumours are inherited. For example, 40% of retinoblastomas and a proportion of Wilms' tumours are familial (Knudson and Strong 1972); 9% of retinoblastomas are present at birth and these are almost always heritable (Gaitan-Yanguas 1978). Sibships affected by neuroblastoma, teratoma, hepatoblastoma and congenital fibromatoses have been reported. Many inherited syndromes predispose to tumour development, although such tumours are not usually present at birth (Bolande 1984; Table 12.2).

Hereditary tumours only account for a small proportion (2.2%) of childhood cancers (Bader et al. 1980). Neurofibromatosis, heritable

Table 12.2. Some inherited syndromes associated with childhood cancer

Inherited syndrome	Childhood cancer
Phakomatoses and hamartoses	
Neurofibromatosis	Brain tumours; sarcomas; leukaemia
Tuberous sclerosis	Brain tumours
Basal cell naevus syndrome	Medulloblastoma; basal cell carcinoma
Turcot's syndrome	Medulloblastoma
Multiple mucosal neuroma syndrome	Medullary thyroid carcinoma; phaeochromocytoma
Metabolic disorders	
Glycogenosis Type I	Hepatocellular carcinoma
Hereditary tyrosinaemia	Hepatocellular carcinoma
Alpha-1-antitrypsin deficiency	Hepatocellular carcinoma
Chromosome breakage and repair defects	
Bloom's syndrome	Leukaemia; gastrointestinal tumours
Ataxia telangiectasia	Leukaemia; lymphoma
Fanconi's anaemia	Leukaemia; hepatoma
Xeroderma pigmentosum	Skin cancers; melanoma
Immune deficiency disorders	
Wiscott–Aldrich syndrome	Leukaemia; lymphoma (often in CNS)
Sex-linked lymphoproliferative syndrome	B-cell lymphoma
Severe combined immunodeficiency	Leukaemia; lymphoma
Bruton's agammaglobulinaemia	Leukaemia; lymphoma

retinoblastoma and familial Wilms' tumour were the commonest in this study. A further group of patients had constitutional aneuploidy, mainly trisomy 21.

The association of constitutional karyotypic abnormalities and childhood cancer further emphasises the importance of the genome in oncogenesis (Table 12.3). These associations are highly specific for certain tumour types,

Table 12.3. Constitutional chromosomal anomalies predisposing to childhood cancer

Chromosomal anomaly	Childhood cancer
Down's syndrome (trisomy 21)	Acute leukaemia
Turner's syndrome (45 XO)	Neurogenic tumours
13q-syndrome	Retinoblastoma
11p-syndrome	Nephroblastoma
Monosomy 7	Preleukaemia and non-lymphoblastic leukaemia
XY gonadal dysgenesis	Gonadoblastoma
Trisomy 18	Nephroblastoma
Klinefelter syndrome	Leukaemia; teratoma; breast carcinoma

and give important clues to the location of the genes responsible. For example the retinoblastoma gene has now been mapped to the long arm of chromosome 13 and characterised as a nuclear phosphoprotein (Gallie et al. 1990) and at least two genes involved in Wilms' tumour are located on the short arm of chromosome 11 (Rose et al. 1990; Dunlop 1991). The most frequent associations seen in the perinatal period are nephroblastomatosis and trisomy 18, and a congenital leukaemia-like syndrome in trisomy 21.

Several sporadic dysmorphic syndromes and malformations carry a significant risk of childhood cancer (Bolande 1976; Table 12.4), particularly hemihypertrophy and Beckwith–Wiedemann syndrome. Up to 10% of children with Beckwith's syndrome develop malignant neoplasms (Sotelo-Avila and Gooch 1976; Tank and Kay 1980). The occasional occurrence of neuroblastoma in children with Hirschsprung's disease and Ondine's curse suggests that it may sometimes be part of a generalised disorder of neural crest development.

Table 12.4. Congenital anomalies associated with childhood cancer

Congenital anomaly	Childhood cancer
Hemihypertrophy and Beckwith's syndrome	Nephroblastoma; adrenal cortical carcinoma; hepatoblastoma
Sporadic aniridia	Wilms' tumour
Poland's syndrome	Leukaemia
Hirschsprung's disease	Neuroblastoma

The association of malformations in general and childhood tumours is less clear. Some authors describe an increased incidence of congenital malformations in children with cancer (Kobayashi et al. 1968), but methods of ascertainment and inclusion of minor malformations invalidate comparison with national incidence rates. A retrospective review of the case records of nearly 400 children with embryonic tumours showed no excess of major malformations when those discovered because of the tumour or possibly attributable to it were discounted (Berry et al. 1970). Nevertheless, associations between Wilms' tumour and genitourinary abnormalities, and sacrococcygeal teratoma with hindgut, sacral and genitourinary malformations are firmly entrenched in the literature. It is possible that both tumour and malformation result from disordered development. More recent reports describe malformations in children with rhabdomyosarcoma (Ruymann et al. 1988), histiocytosis X (Sheils and Dover 1989) and other childhood malignancies (Nakissa et al. 1985).

There is good experimental evidence that teratogenesis and oncogenesis are closely linked (Bolande 1976; Einhorn 1983). The embryo is resistant to carcinogens. However, agents which induce tumours in the fetus produce malformations when given earlier in gestation. Ionising radiation shows a similar gestation-related response (Einhorn 1983).

There are many examples of exogenous teratogens in man (Berry 1989), but evidence that intrauterine exposure produces tumours is scanty. Children exposed in utero to atomic bomb radiation at Hiroshima had an increased incidence of congenital malformations but not of cancers, whilst those exposed after birth developed more tumours (Jablon and Kato 1970). Conflicting reports of prenatal irradiation and childhood cancer are reviewed by MacMahon (1981), who concluded that the question is still largely unresolved. However, it is now accepted that prenatal radiation predisposes to childhood leukaemia (Butturini and Gale 1989; Roman and Beral 1991).

Apart from the well-known association of maternal ingestion of diethylstilboestrol during pregnancy with genital tract malformations and clear-cell adenocarcinoma of the vagina and cervix in their daughters (Herbst 1981), evidence that intrauterine exposure to chemical agents induces tumours in man is anecdotal (Bove et al. 1979; Seeler et al. 1979; Tuman et al. 1980; Chadduck et al. 1987).

A number of reports have linked maternal virus infections with subsequent development of cancer in the offspring (Fine et al. 1985). Viruses implicated include varicella, cytomegalovirus, influenza and possibly rubella. Leukaemia has occurred in the infants of leukaemic mothers, although there is no evidence for vertical transmission. Paternal occupational exposure to hydrocarbons has been implicated in Wilms' tumour, and maternal use of neurotropic drugs, alcohol and hair dyes during pregnancy in neuroblastoma (Terracini et al. 1983; Kramer et al. 1987).

In 1971, Knudson proposed a two-hit theory of carcinogenesis which was later extended by others to build a conceptual framework uniting the bewildering array of observations outlined above into a manageable whole (Bolande 1984). From studies of retinoblastoma Knudson (1971) postulated that two separate random genetic events or "hits" are required to transform a cell and produce a tumour. In patients with hereditary retinoblastoma the first "hit" has already affected the genome, thus explaining the predisposition of these children to develop retinoblastomas which often arise early and may be multifocal. Knudson has more recently included Wilms' tumour and neuroblastoma in his two-hit hypothesis (Knudson and Strong 1972; Knudson and Meadows 1976). Although the theory does not explain all the observed facts and alternative models have been proposed, it has had a profound effect on theoretical oncology (Bolande and Vekemans 1983).

The various dysmorphic syndromes, focal tissue abnormalities, chromosomal anomalies and inherited disorders predisposing to childhood cancers are all evidence that the "first hit" has already occurred, and that the child is vulnerable to any subsequent "hit" or oncogenic event. In retinoblastoma evidence of the first hit may be a positive family history or the 13q- phenotype. For Wilms' tumour the visible evidence may be nephroblastomatosis, hemihypertrophy, the Beckwith–Wiedemann syndrome or a deletion of chromosome 11 with aniridia. The development of both retinoblastoma and nephroblastoma is associated with further genetic events resulting in homozygosity for deletions in regions of chromosome 13 and 11 respectively. These regions contain genes involved in control of normal growth and development of the retina and kidney. Although it is not their usual function these genes have been called "tumour suppressor genes" because their homozygous loss or mutation results in tumours (Paul 1988; Haber and Housman 1991). Similar genetic events are involved in sporadic retinoblastoma and Wilms' tumour.

We are ignorant of the molecular mechanisms responsible for the phenotype of most malformations and dysmorphic syndromes. Recent work on the Beckwith-Wiedemann syndrome promises to throw light on the relationship between dysmorphic syndromes and cancer. Patients with Beckwith's syndrome were thought to have a normal karyotype, but high-resolution banding techniques show that at least some individuals are trisomic for part of the short arm of chromosome 11 (Turleau et al. 1984). The segment involved, 11p15, is close to the genes coding for insulin, insulin-like growth factor II and the c-Ha-*ras* 1 oncogene offering a possible explanation for the abnormalities of growth, carbohydrate metabolism and tumour susceptibility seen in this syndrome (Olshan 1986). Genes linked to the major histocompatibility complex may be involved in both abnormal development and carcinogenesis (Gill 1984).

Investigation of Congenital Tumours

In stillbirths it is important to establish whether the baby was normal apart from his tumour, or whether the tumour was part of a syndrome with genetic implications for subsequent pregnancies. This requires a full perinatal necropsy (see Chap. 1, p. 9).

When the child is liveborn it is important to provide an accurate diagnosis and prognosis to direct further management. In addition to preparing paraffin-embedded sections it is necessary to snap-freeze fresh tissue for immunohistochemistry and preserve a sample in glutaraldehyde for electron microscopy. The karyotype of both the tumour and any normal tissue included in the biopsy may be informative.

Tissue markers with important implications, such as adrenal cytomegaly, pancreatic islet-cell hyperplasia and nephroblastomatosis should be sought in both post-mortem and surgical material. In both liveborn and stillborn babies the placenta should be examined for metastases.

Many histologically malignant tumours behave in a relatively benign way in neonates (Bolande 1976; Table 12.5). The pathologist must base his advice on knowledge of the behaviour of the tumour in children of the same age. Advances in neonatal surgery and oncology mean that many babies are cured and grow up to lead normal lives.

Table 12.5. Some tumours of early life showing benign tendencies (after Bolande 1984)

Infantile congeners of Wilms' tumour
Neuroblastoma:
- in situ neuroblastoma
- stage IV-S neuroblastoma
- neuroblastoma under 1 year of age

Congenital myeloproliferative disorder in trisomy 21
Congenital fibromatosis (myofibromatosis)
Congenital fibrosarcoma
Yolk sac tumour of testis under 2 years of age
Hereditary retinoblastoma (retinomas)

Teratomas

Teratomas are the commonest congenital tumours and have been the subject of several excellent reviews (Berry et al. 1969; Grosfield et al. 1976; Marsden et al. 1981; Gonzalez Crussi 1982; Dehner 1983; Tapper and Lack 1983). The sites of teratomas in children are shown in Table 12.6. In infancy, sacrococcygeal teratomas outnumber all others.

Table 12.6. Percentage of childhood teratomas by site; 578 cases pooled from 9 series (after Gonzalez-Crussi 1982)

Sacrococcygeal	44.8%
Ovary[a]	29.7%
Mediastinum	7.0%
Testis	5.8%
Neck	3.4%
Retroperitoneum	3.4%
CNS	2.7%
Head (extracranial)	1.7%
Abdomen	0.69%
Perineum	0.34%

[a] The proportion of ovarian tumours in much less in neonates

The origin of teratomas is controversial, and it is likely that not all arise in the same way. Studies of chromosome markers show that sacrococcygeal teratomas arise from totipotent somatic cells and are always of the host sex (Linder 1983).

The majority of congenital teratomas fulfil the usual diagnostic criteria and contain tissues from all three germ layers, although about one-quarter do not. Highly differentiated teratomas with limbs and organoid development may be confused with a parasitic twin or fetus in fetu. Teratomas differ from these conditions because they lack a notochordal or vertebral axis and have an inherent tendency towards progressive uncoordinated growth. Teratoma and fetus in fetu have been reported occurring together (Du Plessis et al. 1974) and the distinction between these two entities may not be as clearcut as often suggested.

The most important prognostic factors in teratomas of the newborn period, apart from age, are the presence or absence of yolk sac tumour, site, and completeness of excision. Immature elements should be related to the maturity of the host. Immature neural elements are not an adverse factor in neonates; teratomas with a high degree of fetiformity occasionally recur.

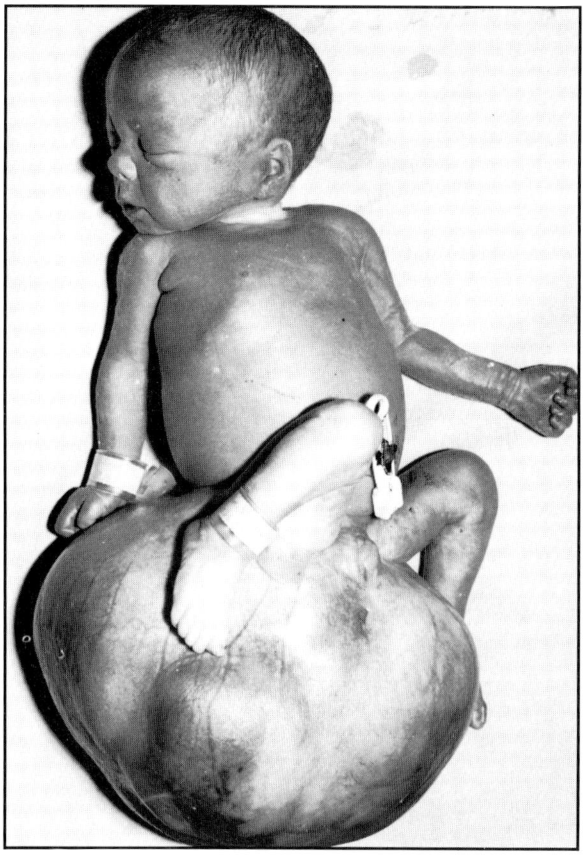

Fig. 12.1. Congenital sacrococcygeal teratoma. The anus is displaced anteriorly by a tumour between the sacrum and rectum. Obstructed labour necessitated caesarean section. The tumour was histologically benign. (Courtesy of the publishers of *Hospital Update*)

Sacrococcygeal Teratomas

Sacrococcygeal teratomas occur in 1:30 000–1:170 000 live births, with a male to female ratio of 1:3. A strong family history of twinning is described. Associated malformations of the hindgut, caudal spinal cord and distal genitourinary tract are sometimes present. Whilst these malformations may be due to local effects of the tumour on growth and development, the same disorder of differentiation may be responsible for both. Lemire and Beckwith (1982) and Bale (1984) described an extraordinary variety of developmental abnormalities and tumour-like conditions of the sacrococcygeal region in children and related them to the complex embryology of this area.

Most sacrococcygeal teratomas are sporadic, but familial cases occur with sacral defects. In addition to the sacral anomaly there may be rectal stenosis, retrorectal abscesses and a postcoccygeal dimple. Inheritance in these cases is autosomal dominant (Hunt et al. 1977).

Most tumours are apparent at birth (Fig. 12.1). Sacrococcygeal teratomas have been visualised by ultrasound as early as the second trimester and are one cause of a raised maternal serum alpha-fetoprotein level (see Table 4.1, p. 118) and amniotic fluid acetylcholinesterase. The outcome is often favourable, and so appropriate management may include repeated aspirations of large cysts, and planned delivery by caesarean section in a centre with expert paediatric surgery. Unfavourable factors are rapid tumour growth and the development of fetal hydrops or placentomegaly. Extensively cystic tumours are usually benign, but a predominantly solid tumour raises the question of malignancy (Flake et al. 1986; Holzgreve et al. 1987; Gross et al. 1987; Kurjak et al. 1989). The tumour may be so large that obstructed labour, maternal injury or intrapartum rupture occur. The overlying skin is sometimes ulcerated and occasionally bears a rudimentary tail or digit. Some tumours are vascular and telangiectases in the overlying skin should warn of the risk of haemorrhage into the tumour or high-output heart failure. Sometimes the tumour is inconspicuous, marked externally only by a skin tag, dimple or tuft of hair.

Sacrococcygeal teratomas may be entirely postsacral (external), presacral (internal), or dumbbell shaped (Altman et al. 1974). The risk of malignancy is increased both when the tumour is internal and when diagnosis is delayed beyond the newborn period. These factors may be related. Benign tumours are usually well defined with a solid or cystic cut surface. Some tumours are highly differentiated with well-formed bronchial or intestinal cysts. Neuroglia, with or without choroid plexus, is seen in most cases and may predominate. Occasionally, adrenal cortical tissue may produce secondary effects as a result of secretion of steroid hormones.

The main objectives of pathological examination are to assess the completeness of excision and offer a guide to prognosis. Experience has shown that failure to remove the coccyx results in an increased risk of recurrence, so it is important to identify this structure in the surgical specimen (occasional patients have coccygeal aplasia). The tumour must be adequately sampled, taking at least one block per centimetre of diameter and sampling areas of haemorrhage and necrosis which may indicate

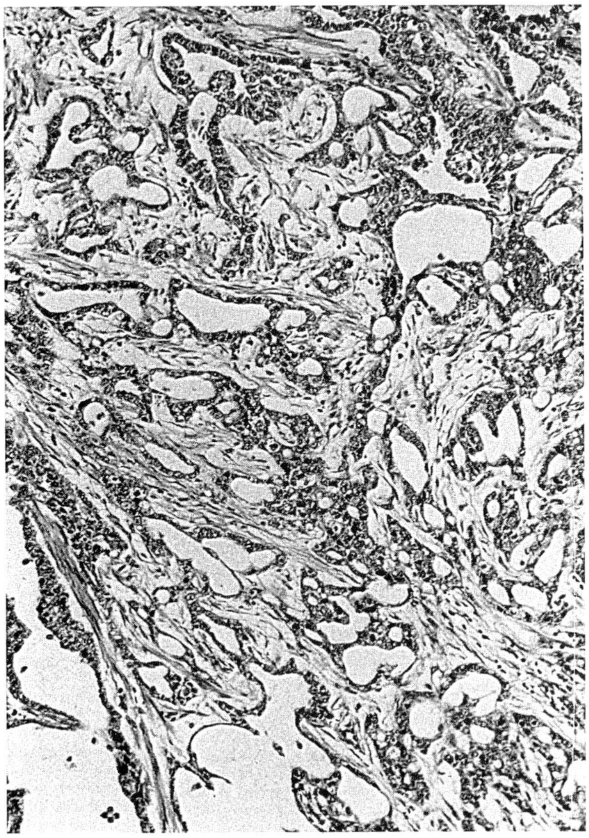

Fig. 12.2. Yolk sac tumour (polyvesicular pattern) in a malignant sacrococcygeal teratoma. Alpha-fetoprotein was demonstrated by an immunoperoxidase technique (H&E, ×94)

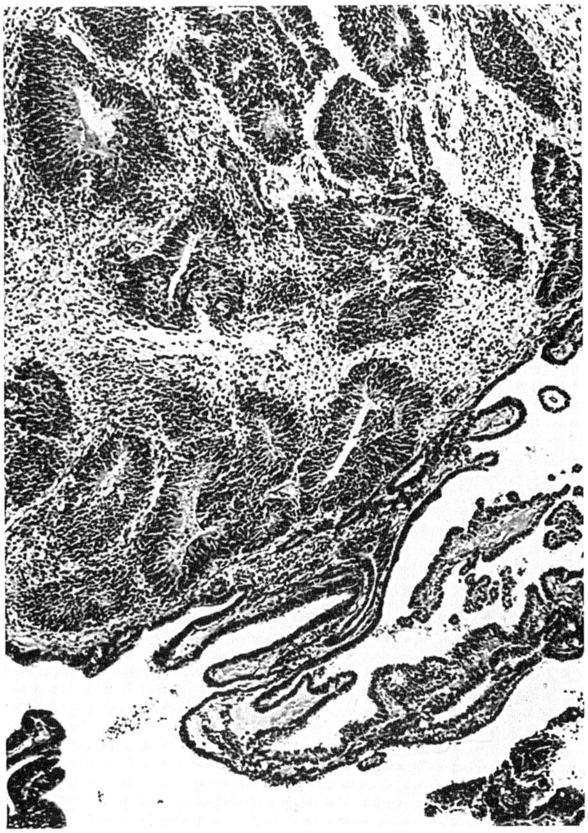

Fig. 12.3. Immature neural tissue resembling developing neural tube in a sacrococcygeal teratoma. This tissue does not indicate malignancy in neonates. Choroid plexus is also present in this field. (H&E, ×65)

malignancy. About 10% of sacrococcygeal teratomas presenting in the newborn period are malignant, including all those with yolk sac elements or embryonal carcinoma (Berry et al. 1969; Fig. 12.2). Choriocarcinoma and germinoma have not been reported in neonatal sacrococcygeal teratomas. About 20% of otherwise histologically benign sacrococcygeal teratomas contain immature elements; the commonest of these is neural tissue resembling neuroblastoma or the developing neural tube (Fig. 12.3) and does not indicate malignancy in this context (Bale 1984). Neural elements may recur as local implants (dermal-subcutaneous gliomatosis) without ominous significance (Dehner 1983). However, despite the good outcome of most immature sacrococcygeal teratomas it is important to recognise that occasional tumours without frankly malignant elements at presentation recur as malignant tumour and cause death (Hawkins et al. 1986); follow-up for at least 2 years is recommended regardless of histological type.

Teratomas in Other Sites

Other teratomas that characteristically affect the newborn include orbital, intrapericardial, facial and cervical tumours.

Mediastinal tumours may be congenital, but may not present until adolescence. In the neonatal period they may present with hydrops fetalis or respiratory obstruction caused by compression of adjacent structures. Carter et al. (1982) emphasised the benign behaviour of mediastinal teratomas in infants, even when histologically immature.

Intrapericardial tumours present in infancy with cardiomegaly, muffled heart sounds and cardiac tamponade caused by a pericardial effusion. Of 48 cases reported by Torres-Aybar et al. (1975), 24 were in infants less than 3 months old. They arise close to the root of the great vessels, often on the right side, and may be fatal because of their location.

Teratomas involving the pharynx and base of the skull arise from pluripotent cells around Rathke's pouch and the oral membrane at the point of contact of the buccopharyngeal membrane and the rostral notocord (Gonzales-Cruzzi 1982). They frequently prevent fusion of the palatal processes, resulting in clefting. Large tumours project from the mouth (epignathus) and cause polyhydramnios by preventing fetal swallowing. Tumour site often precludes complete excision, and death occurs from asphyxia (Fig. 12.4), or from meningitis if the base of the skull is involved.

A related lesion peculiar to infancy is the hairy polyp of the nasopharynx. The tumour-like lesion consists of a mass of fibroadipose tissue covered by hair-bearing skin projecting into the mouth or pharynx. This entity is best regarded as a hamartoma.

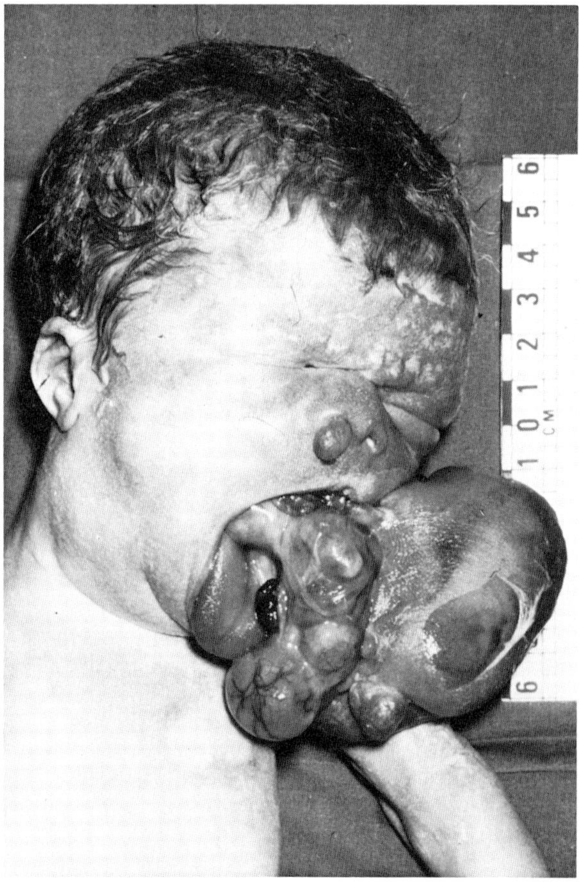

Fig. 12.4. Congenital pharyngeal teratoma. Death was due to respiratory obstruction. The tumour was histologically benign.

Orbital teratomas are peculiar to the neonate and have often reached a large size by the time of birth. There is exophthalmos of striking proportions; the extrinsic muscles of the eye are stretched over a retrobulbar mass which may have an intracranial extension. Differential diagnosis includes haemangioma, lymphangioma, epidermal inclusion cyst and metastatic neuroblastoma.

Cervical teratomas account for 3%–4% of childhood teratomas and are usually evident as a large mass at birth. Their size and location may prevent swallowing and cause polyhydramnios, and are responsible for their high mortality (Rosenfeld et al. 1979); 17% of affected babies are stillborn and 35% die before surgery. Many tumours are intimately related to the thyroid. Although extracranial germ cell tumours of the head and neck in early infancy are usually benign, yolk sac tumours can occur (Dehner et al. 1990).

Congenital Neuroblastoma

Neuroblastoma has been diagnosed antenatally by ultrasound scanning (Kurjak et al. 1989; Holzgreve et al. 1991) and may produce symptoms in the mother due to secretion of catecholamines. It is the commonest malignant solid tumour presenting in the neonatal period. Its microscopic appearance does not differ significantly from that in older children but its behaviour and metastatic pattern are distinctive. The majority have an abdominal primary site either in the adrenal gland or retroperitoneum (Schneider et al. 1965). Rare cases are familial (Mancini et al. 1982), associated with Beckwith's syndrome (Emery et al. 1983), or part of a disorder of neural crest such as Von Recklinghausen's neurofibromatosis, Hirschsprung's disease (Chatten and Witzleben 1975), Ondine's curse (Bower and Adkins 1980) or nesidioblastosis (Grotting et al. 1979). There may be placental involvement with widespread plugging of villous capillaries (Fig. 12.5) resulting in hydrops fetalis (see Chap. 11, p. 255). Metastasis to the skin is common in neonates. Hepatic involvement, often massive, was present in 65% of the neonatal cases reviewed by Schneider et al. (1965; Fig. 12.6). The terms

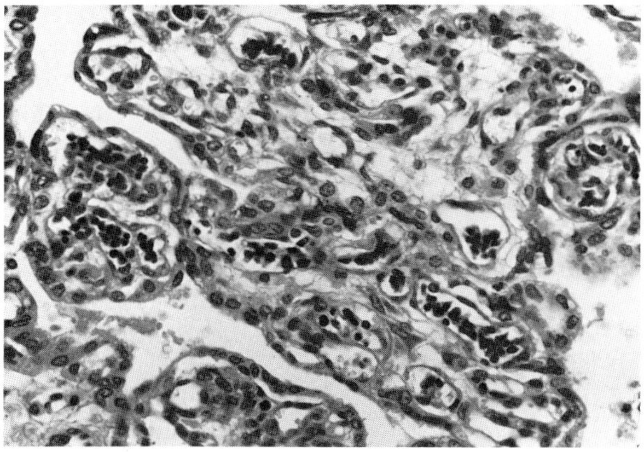

Fig. 12.5. Congenital neuroblastoma with placental involvement. Villous capillaries are plugged by darkly staining neuroblasts. (H&E, ×165)

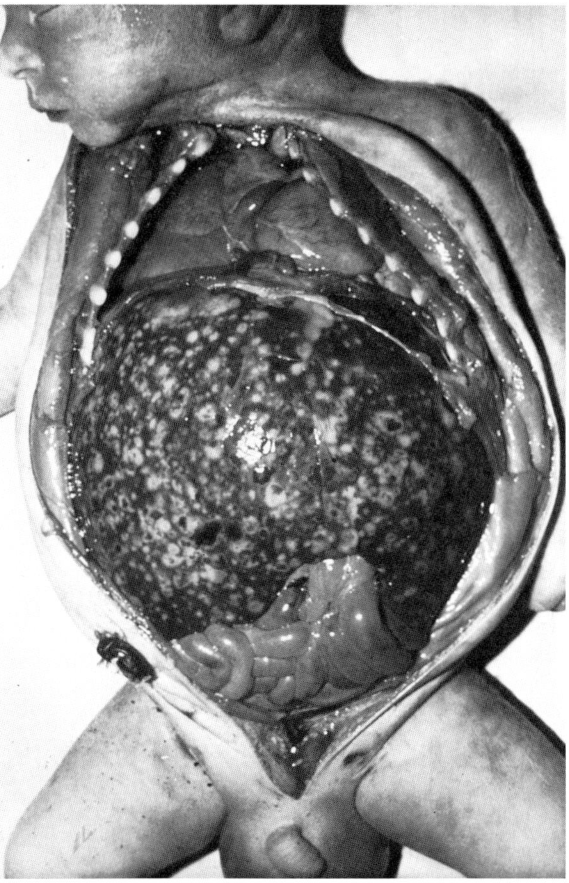

Fig. 12.6. Congenital neuroblastoma with massive liver involvement (Pepper's syndrome).

"Pepper's syndrome" and "Hutchinson's syndrome" are no longer fashionable; the former described massive liver involvement by adrenal neuroblastoma which is virtually confined to young infants. It has been suggested that the liver may be reseeded from the placenta via the umbilical vein whilst the lungs are spared by diversion of blood through the foramen ovale and ductus arteriosus (Wieberdink 1982).

Congenital neuroblastoma undergoes spontaneous regression more commonly than any other tumour. This is usually the result of necrobiosis, but maturation to ganglioneuroma may occur. This remarkable phenomenon has been well documented and accounts in part for the relatively good prognosis of neuroblastoma in young children (Table 12.7).

Table 12.7. Age and survival in neuroblastoma (after Bolande 1976)

Age of onset	2-year survival
Neonatal or congenital	62%–70%
Before 1 year	35%
Second year	19%
After second year	5%

About 10% of children and at least 30% of neonates have a special pattern of metastasis, termed Stage IV-S neuroblastoma, which has a particularly favourable outlook. It comprises patients with small primary tumours and dissemination to liver, skin and bone marrow, but without bone lesions (D'Angio et al. 1971; Evans et al. 1981); survival is much better in babies with skin metastases (93%) compared with 32% survival when these are absent (Stephenson et al. 1986). Ordinary Stage IV disseminated disease occurs rarely in neonates and has a poor prognosis.

Various explanations have been advanced for the relatively benign behaviour of neuroblastoma in neonates. Recent work has shown that malignant neuroblastoma contains extra non-banding chromosomal material which may be absent in Stage IV-S disease (Balaban and Gilbert 1983). This appears to be made up of repeated gene sequences and contains many extra copies of the N-*myc* oncogene believed to be responsible for malignant neuroblastoma. Thus Stage IV-S neuroblastoma may lack the gene structure necessary for fully malignant behaviour.

The histological appearance of neuroblastoma in neonates is the same as that in older chil-

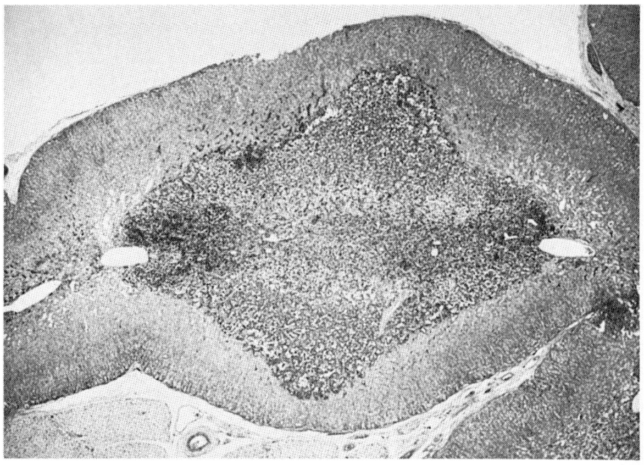

Fig. 12.7. In situ neuroblastoma. A nodule of immature neuroblasts is present in the adrenal gland of a neonate with a lethal congenital heart defect. Note the permeation of cortical sinusoids by darkly staining neuroblasts. (H&E, ×15)

dren and presents similar diagnostic problems. Grading systems which correlate with prognosis have been proposed by Beckwith and Martin (1968) and Shimada et al. (1984). Favourable prognosis correlates with low N-*myc* copy number, aneuploidy, and no loss of heterozygosity of chromosome 1p (Look et al. 1984; Brodeur et al. 1986; Kaneko et al. 1987). Diagnostic aids such as the measurement of catecholamines and their metabolites in body fluids (Graham-Pole et al. 1983), immunohistochemistry for neural antigens including neuron-specific enolase, catecholamine autofluorescence and electron microscopy may be helpful (Triche and Askin 1983).

Small nodules of neuroblasts up to 400 μm in diameter with a modal size of 60 μm are seen in the adrenal glands of all fetuses (Turkel and Itabashi 1974). They become less frequent after 20 weeks of gestation and are uncommon at birth. "In situ neuroblastoma" refers to larger nodules of undifferentiated neuroblasts a few millimetres in diameter situated in the adrenal medulla (Beckwith and Perrin 1963; Fig. 12.7). Some are visible to the naked eye (Guin et al. 1969). Systematic search shows in situ neuroblastoma in 1%–2% of routine perinatal necropsies.

The natural history of in situ neuroblastoma is unknown, but it is not found after 3 months of age. In situ neuroblastoma is seen in malformed infants, often with cardiovascular anomalies, and it has been argued that it is part of a generalised dysontogenic process. If present in the normal population with the same high frequency as in the necropsied population, then the majority of in situ neuroblastomas must regress spontaneously, very few becoming malignant tumours. The favourable prognosis of neuroblastoma in infancy has stimulated screening programmes based on catecholamine metabolites in urine to detect the tumour before it is clinically manifest (Huddart and Mann 1991). Although the effectiveness of these programmes in preventing death is still in question, it is clear that a majority of neuroblastomas are detectable by 6 months and so many may in fact be congenital. Carlsen (1988) argues on theoretical grounds that almost all childhood neuroblastomas arise in utero.

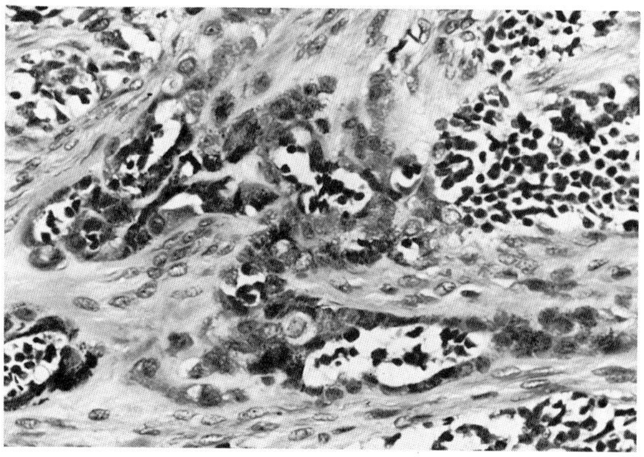

Fig. 12.8. Pigmented neuroectodermal tumour of infancy. Nests of neuroblasts are surrounded by cuboidal cells containing granular melanin pigment. (H&E, ×190)

Melanotic Neuroectodermal Tumour of Infancy

Another tumour of neuroectodermal origin virtually confined to infancy and with a good prognosis is the melanotic progonoma, or melanotic neuroectodermal tumour of infancy. Over 90% occur in the head and neck region and characteristically involve the maxilla. Other sites include the epididymis, mediastinum and thigh. The histological appearance is striking, with nests of neuroblast-like cells surrounded by cuboidal cells containing melanin in a connective tissue stroma (Fig. 12.8). Although the local recurrence rate is 15%, metastasis is rare and most cases follow a benign course (Johnson et al. 1983).

Renal Tumours

Between 5% and 7% of congenital tumours arise in the kidney. Although in the past most were called Wilms' tumours, it is now recognised that classic Wilms' tumour is extremely rare in neonates and only 2.4% occur in the first 6 months of life (Lemerle et al. 1976). The description of mesoblastic nephroma by Bolande et al. (1967) led to the recognition of a group of tumours and tumour-like conditions, collectively known as infantile congeners of Wilms' tumour, which occur in very young children and have a generally favourable prognosis (Table 12.8). Clear cell sarcoma of kidney and malignant rhabdoid tumour may occasionally occur in neonates (Ugarte et al. 1981; Schmidt et al. 1982).

Table 12.8. Infantile congeners of Wilms' tumour

Congenital mesoblastic nephroma
The nephroblastomatosis complex
Variants of Wilms' tumour:
cystic, partially differentiated nephroblastoma
monomorphic epithelial Wilms' tumour
fetal rhabdomyomatous nephroblastoma

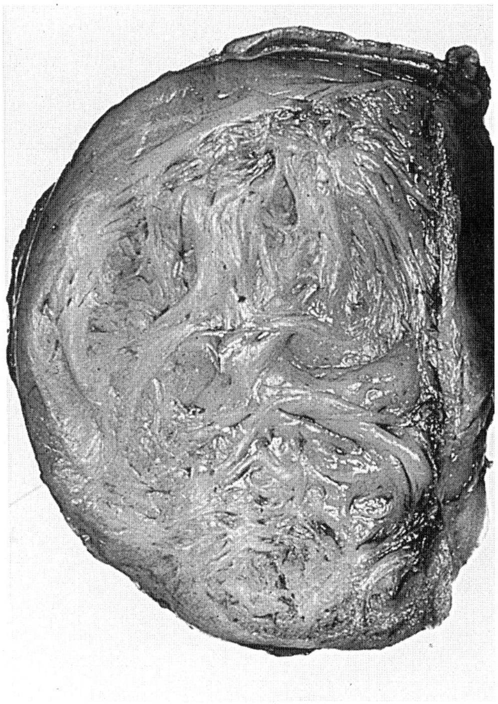

Fig. 12.9. Congenital mesoblastic nephroma. Bisected kidney with adrenal (*above*) and normal kidney (*bottom centre*). The fibroid-like cut surface and ill-defined junction with normal kidney are typical of this tumour. (Courtesy of Dr. A. King, Cambridge)

Congenital Mesoblastic Nephroma

Congenital mesoblastic nephroma (fetal renal hamartoma) is the commonest neonatal renal tumour (Bolande 1973). Pregnancy may be complicated by polyhydramnios. Mesoblastic nephroma may also be associated with a salt-losing state or hypertension, both of which resolve rapidly on removal of the tumour. Renin can be demonstrated by immunohistochemistry (Cook et al. 1988). The tumour is usually found on routine examination in the neonatal period and is unusual beyond 3–6 months of age. Macroscopically the kidney is enormously enlarged by an intrarenal mass whose cut surface resembles a uterine fibroid (Fig. 12.9). It is described in Chapter 19 (see p. 477). Simple nephrectomy with complete removal of the tumour is adequate therapy in neonates.

It was thought that all neonatal mesenchymal renal tumours were benign, but rare recurrence and metastasis of otherwise apparently typical examples of congenital mesoblastic nephroma are described (Yazaki et al. 1982; Steinfeld et al. 1984). Mesoblastic nephroma with increased cellularity and mitotic activity reported as cellular variants (Snyder et al. 1981) or atypical mesoblastic nephroma (Marsden and Lawler 1983) did not metastasise or recur after simple nephrectomy. Although the great majority of mesoblastic nephromas are adequately treated by nephrectomy alone with careful removal of any extrarenal extension, tumours showing dense cellularity, necrosis and abundant mitotic activity in children over 3 months of age may occasionally recur (Joshi et al. 1986). It is suggested by some that infants over 6 months of age with the cellular variant of congenital mesoblastic nephroma should receive adjuvant chemotherapy, whilst infants under 3 months of age are adequately treated by complete excision alone. A conservative approach is advocated by others (Beckwith and Weeks 1986). These cellular or atypical tumours may be aneuploid, but this has not been shown to predict adverse outcome (Barrantes et al. 1991).

In the study of Gormley et al. (1989) positive surgical margins was the only significant variable predicting recurrent disease, while all infants with cellular mesoblastic nephroma

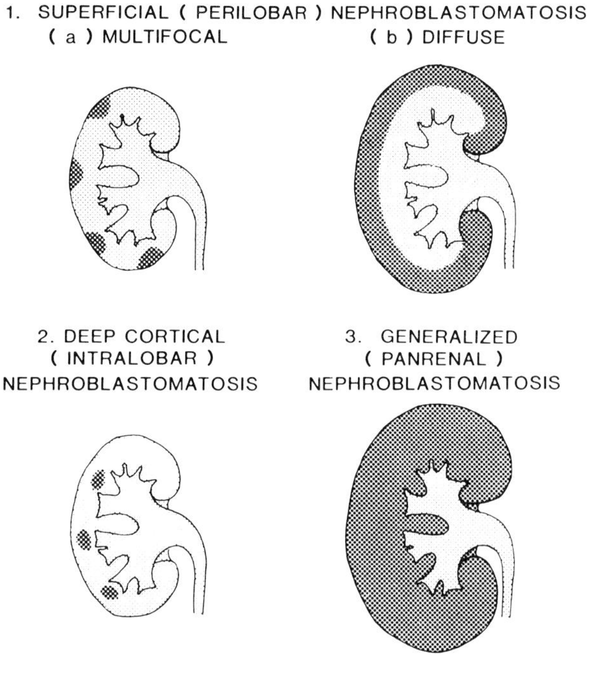

Fig. 12.10. Nephroblastomatosis. Diagrammatic representation of the location of the different types of nephroblastomatosis. (Based on Bove and McAdams 1976; Machin 1980, 1984. Courtesy of Churchill Livingstone)

and clear pathological margins were cured by surgery alone.

Nephroblastomatosis and Nephrogenic Rests

Nephroblastomatosis has been defined as the persistence of renal metanephric blastema beyond 36 weeks' gestation when nephrogenesis ceases, or in an inappropriate location or amount before that time (Machin 1980). It is of great interest as a putative precursor of Wilms' tumour, being present in less than 1% of neonatal necropsies but in 20%–40% of kidneys with Wilms' tumour. In the neonatal period it presents in two ways, either as a rare cause of bilateral renal enlargement, or as an incidental macroscopic or microscopic postmortem finding, when it should alert the pathologist to the possibility of associated syndromes. In older children it is seen in kidneys removed for Wilms tumour, and occasionally in association with cystic renal dysplasia (Dimmick et al. 1989). The classification of nephroblastomatosis is complex because different terms have been used to describe similar lesions (Fig. 12.10). This complexity is compounded by transition of one type to another, sometimes as a result of chemotherapy (Kulkarni and Bailie 1980).

Commonly, nephroblastomatosis involves the periphery of the renal lobe in a subcapsular position or along the columns of Bertin. Microscopic nests of embryonal renal epithelial cells with minor tubular differentiation and no embryonal stromal component situated beneath the renal capsule, sometimes surrounded by immature glomeruli, are termed "persistent nodular renal blastema" (Fig. 12.11). Bove and McAdams (1976) describe differentiation or maturation into other types with the formation of tubules (metanephric hamartoma) and a prominent collagenous stroma (sclerosing metanephric hamartoma). Hyperplastic lesions arise within these nodules with progression from adenoma to incipient Wilms' tumour to Wilms' tumourlet. The last is defined as a neoplastic nodule of embryonal renal elements from 1.0 to 3.5 cm in diameter composed of monomorphous embryonal epithelium indistinguishable from that of a nephroblastoma. Wilms' tumourlets may be multiple and have limited capacity for metastasis.

Occasionally, persistent blastema forms a continuous layer around each renal lobe resulting in considerable renal enlargement. There may be tubule formation, but no stromal elements. This superficial diffuse type of nephroblastomatosis is rare, and may be related to the nodular types described above (Fig. 12.12). Data on nine cases are reviewed by Machin (1980), several of which presented in early infancy.

Superficial nephroblastomatosis is seen in patients with Beckwith–Wiedemann syndrome, hemihypertrophy, pseudohermaphroditism, trisomy 18 and some familial cases of Wilms' tumour. The nephroblastomas that develop in this form of nephroblastomatosis tend to show epithelial or blastemal predominance, with scanty stroma and rare heterotopic tissues such as striated muscle.

A more recently recognised deep cortical form of nephroblastomatosis involving the juxtamedullary cortex is associated with aniridia and the development of nephroblastoma with a predominant striated muscle component (fetal rhabdomyomatous nephroblastoma; (Wigger 1976; Machin and McCaughey 1984). Here the teratological insult may occur earlier in organogenesis when the metanephric blastema is committed to stromagenesis. This would

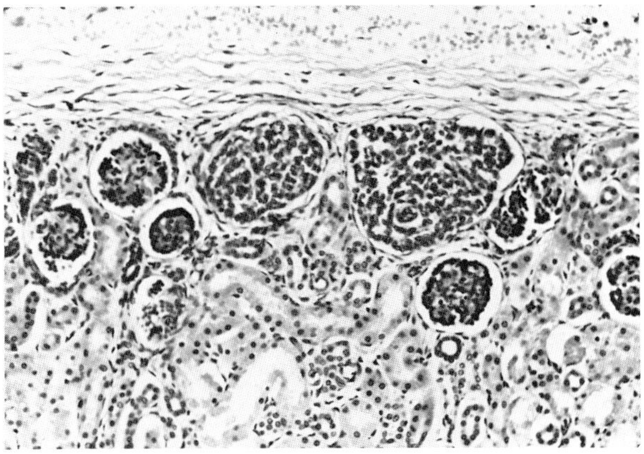

Fig. 12.11. Nephroblastomatosis. Persistent nodular renal blastema. Incidental finding in a 3-month old cot death. (H&E, ×110.) Compare with Fig. 19.1, p. 466.

explain both the deep location of the precursor lesion and the predominant stromal component of this tumour.

Finally, both the cortex and the medulla may be diffusely affected, resulting in marked nephromegaly. This very rare form (generalised or panrenal nephroblastomatosis) is probably incompatible with life. Its relationship to the other types of nephroblastomatosis and to Wilms' tumour is unknown. Machin (1980) cites only the original case of Hou and Holman (1961).

In 1990 Beckwith et al. proposed a new and unifying classification preferring the term nephrogenic rest for a single focus of persistent nephrogenic cells, and restricting the use of nephroblastomatosis to cases with multiple or diffuse nephrogenic rests. Nephrogenic rests are divided according to their location (intralobar or perilobar) and subclassified by gross and microscopic appearance (dormant, maturing, hyperplastic or neoplastic). Nephroblastomatosis may be perilobar, intralobar, combined or universal. This authoritative scheme is comprehensible, biologically relevant and clinically meaningful and so is likely to be adopted. The reader is referred to this key reference for further dicussion beyond the scope of this chapter.

Although multiple nephrogenic rests in the perinatal period are usually diagnosed at necropsy, nephroblastomatosis is occasionally found following biopsy of an enlarged kidney in infancy. The microscopic appearances of nephrogenic rests and nephroblastoma can be indistinguishable in a biopsy, and so the macroscopic pattern of the lesion is critical (Beckwith et al. 1990). The precise risk of developing Wilms' tumour in each type of nephroblastomatosis is unknown but most nephrogenic rests probably do not become neoplastic, particularly those found incidentally. Nephroblastomatosis must be presumed to be bilateral, and so renal tissue should be conserved. Nephroblastomatosis is not malignant, and so it is reasonable to follow most patients by regular imaging of both kidneys. If there is progression then chemotherapy is effective and probably reduces the malignant potential of nephroblastomatosis. Nephroblastomatosis in-

a 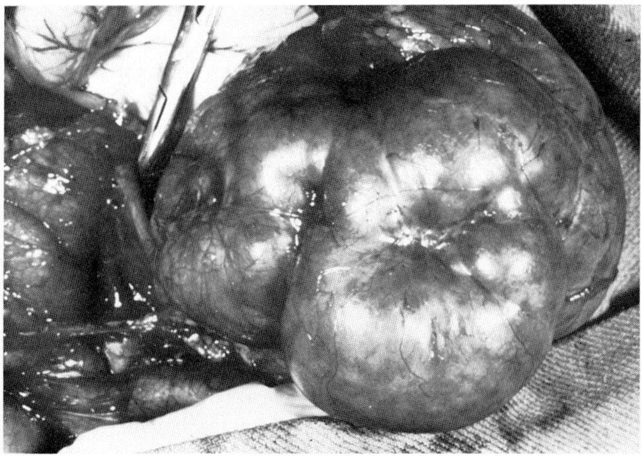 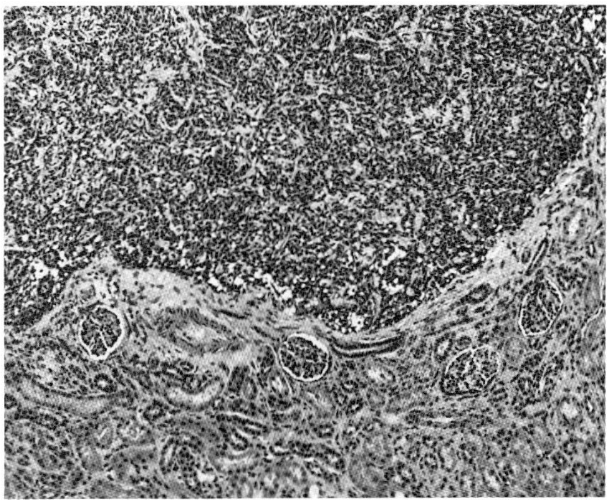 b

Fig. 12.12. Nephroblastomatosis. **a** Extensive almost confluent superficial nephroblastomatosis at exploratory laparotomy for bilateral renal enlargement. **b** Subcapsular blastema forms a rind beneath the renal capsule. (H&E, ×54.) This patient subsequently developed Wilms' tumour.

dicates the possibility of bilateral Wilms' tumours but does not affect the prognosis.

Nephroblastoma

Classic triphasic Wilms' tumour is very rare in the neonatal period. Some of the earlier reported cases were probably not nephroblastomas at all, and some would now be classified as malignant rhabdoid tumour (Kalousek et al. 1977). Of the 30 renal tumours seen by Marsden and Lawler (1983) in the first year of life, 15 were classic Wilms' tumours, and 1 of these might be considered congenital.

Variants of nephroblastoma with a favourable prognosis are more common in the first year of life (Ugarte et al. 1981). Fetal rhabdomyomatous nephroblastoma describes tumours in which the major component is differentiating striated muscle (Wigger 1976). Wilms' tumours composed exclusively of epithelial tubules also have a relatively favourable outlook (Chatten 1976). Cystic, partially differentiated nephroblastoma is a distinct entity composed of epithelium-lined cysts with immature metanephric tissue in their walls (Joshi 1979; Andrews et al. 1983). It is adequately treated by complete excision.

Two highly malignant renal tumours, clear cell sarcoma and malignant rhabdoid tumour, are unrelated to Wilms' tumour and are occasionally seen in the first few months of life. Clear cell sarcoma or bone metastasising tumour (Marsden and Lawler 1980) is easily confused with a cellular congenital mesoblastic nephroma. Malignant rhabdoid tumour is recognised by the presence of filamentous cytoplasmic inclusions and large single nucleoli in characteristic rhabdoid cells. It is associated with separate primary brain tumours in some cases (Weeks et al. 1989).

A rare and apparently benign tumour described in neonates is the ossifying renal tumour of infancy (Jerkins and Callihan 1986).

Liver Tumours

Liver tumours in the newborn are uncommon. Vascular tumours, hepatoblastoma and mesenchymal hamartoma are the only lesions seen with any frequency (Dehner 1981; Weinberg and Finegold 1983).

Vascular Tumours

Vascular tumours of the liver may be encountered as incidental necropsy findings. Large tumours present with high-output heart failure, an abdominal mass, hepatic failure or intra-abdominal haemorrhage following rupture during delivery. Occasionally, sequestration of platelets causes a bleeding diathesis (Kasabach–Merritt syndrome). Forty per cent of patients also have cutaneous haemangiomas.

Spontaneous regression is less common in visceral than in cutaneous haemangiomas, but occurs in approximately 60% of cases. The prognosis of hepatic vascular tumours is good in the absence of clinical complications.

Hepatoblastoma

Hepatoblastoma is the commonest malignant liver tumour of infancy (Weinberg and Finegold 1983). It occurs in children with hemihypertrophy and the Beckwith–Weidemann syndrome. It has also rarely been reported in siblings, in conjunction with nephroblastoma, in association with maternal use of oral contraceptives, and in the fetal alcohol syndrome (Lack et al. 1982). Serum alpha-fetoprotein is usually markedly elevated.

The histological pattern of hepatoblastoma has prognostic significance. Survival is commoner in children with predominantly fetal tumours than in those with conspicuous embryonal or mesenchymal components (Haas et al. 1989). Two special variants with a particularly unfavourable prognosis are the anaplastic type (Kasai and Watanabe 1970), and the macrotrabecular pattern recognised by Gonzalez-Crussi et al. (1982). Surgical excision is a prerequisite for survival and is possible in 75% of patients with hepatoblastoma. It results in cure in 30%–50% of cases.

Mesenchymal Hamartoma

Mesenchymal hamartoma is a tumour of infants and young children. Of 30 cases reported by Stocker and Ishak (1983), 7 patients were less than 3 months old. A few patients had adrenal cytomegaly and pancreatic islet hyperplasia.

Most growth after birth occurs by enlargement of cystic spaces within the lesion and may promote suspicion of malignancy. Surgical excision is curative.

Congenital Mesenchymal Tumours

Mesenchymal lesions comprise about 10% of neonatal tumours. Kauffman and Stout (1965) reported 125 congenital mesenchymal tumours of soft tissue. Fibromatoses, mesenchymomas rhabdomyosarcomas, smooth muscle tumours and haemangiopericytomas were the commonest types in their series. Since that time a number of new entities have been described which might necessitate reclassification of some of their cases. However, their conclusion that congenital mesenchymal tumours seldom behave in a malignant way and differ biologically from those in adults is still valid.

Fibromatoses

The fibrous proliferations of infancy and childhood include a number of distinctive lesions unique to this age group which are recognisable as much by their clinical presentation as by their histology. All have in common the proliferation of spindle cells resembling fibroblasts, which are locally invasive, but lack the capacity to metastasise. Fibromatoses seen in infancy are usually more cellular than the adult type, although the latter do occur in childhood. Discussion will be restricted to the fibrous proliferations that are seen in neonates and young infants (Table 12.9; Enzinger and Weiss 1988).

Table 12.9. Fibrous proliferations of infancy and childhood

Congenital fibromatosis (myofibromatosis):
solitary
multicentric
Infantile desmoid-type fibromatosis
Fibromatosis colli (sternomastoid tumour)
Infantile digital fibromatosis (recurring digital fibroma)
Fibrous hamartoma of infancy
Calcifying aponeurotic fibroma
Juvenile hyaline fibromatosis
Gingival fibromatosis
Giant cell

Congenital Fibromatosis (Solitary and Multicentric)

A rare distinctive lesion of neonates has been described under a variety of synonyms, including congenital diffuse fibromatosis, congenital generalised fibromatosis and infantile myofibromatosis (Chung and Enzinger 1981; Wiswell et al. 1988). This fibromatosis may be solitary, usually involving the soft tissues of the head, neck and trunk. Multicentric involvement of the skin, bones and viscera is less common; 60% of lesions are congenital. Macroscopically they are well demarcated, often vascular nodules up to several centimetres in diameter. Microscopically they are cellular with plump spindle cells showing mitotic activity. The centre of the lesion characteristically has a haemangiopericytomatous pattern. Necrosis and intravascular growth are seen and are not of adverse significance (Fig. 12.13). Although solitary lesions sometimes recur they do not metastasise, and the outlook is excellent. The prognosis is less good for patients with multicentric lesions, particularly if the lungs are involved (Rosenberg et al. 1978). Death results from extensive organ infiltration or obstruction of hollow viscera. New lesions may continue to appear after birth. Spontaneous regression can occur even in patients with multiple lesions. Both autosomal-recessive and dominant modes of inheritance have been suggested in some

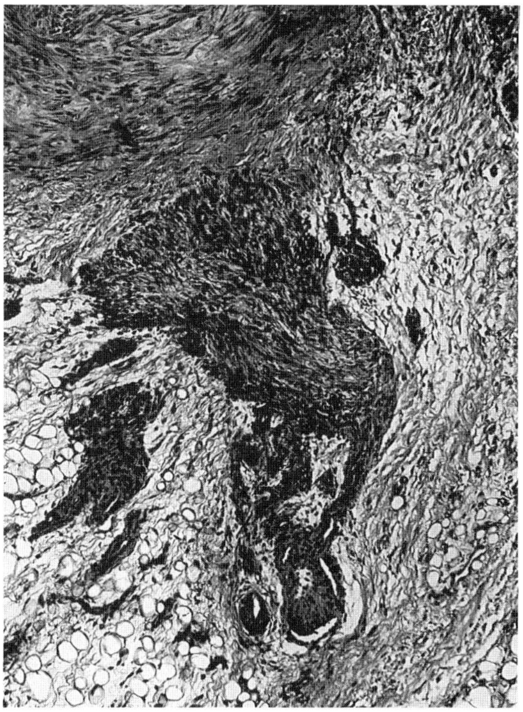

Fig. 12.13. Solitary congenital fibromatosis. At the edge of the lesion fingers of myofibroblast extend into vessels in adjacent adipose tissue. This feature should not lead to a diagnosis of malignancy. (H&E, ×66)

cases (Jennings et al. 1984). The histogenesis is believed to be from myofibroblasts or even smooth muscle (Fletcher et al. 1987).

Infantile Desmoid-type Fibromatosis

Infantile desmoid-type fibromatosis corresponds to the musculoaponeurotic fibroma (desmoid tumour) of adults. It arises in muscle, aponeurosis or fascia. Muscles of the head and neck, shoulder, upper arm and thigh are favoured sites. The macroscopic appearance is of an ill-defined mass of grey-white tissue which consists of spindle cells infiltrating surrounding tissues at the periphery. The histological appearance varies. Some resemble the adult desmoid tumour, but more cellular examples are indistinguishable from infantile fibrosarcoma. Another pattern seen in very young infants is of immature cells, intermediate between primitive mesenchymal cells and fibroblasts, scattered in a myxoid background and surrounded by abundant reticulin. This appearance may be confused with other myxoid tumours such as a lipoblastoma or rhabdomyosarcoma.

Infantile desmoid-type fibromatosis tends to recur and infiltrate locally, but does not metastasise. Local excision is the treatment of choice but may be difficult because of the involvement of vital structures.

Fibromatosis Colli

Fibromatosis colli (sternomastoid tumour) typically occurs as a horizontally mobile mass in the sternomastoid muscle of an infant between the second and fourth weeks of life. After a period of growth it becomes stationary and may regress, to be followed by shortening of the sternomastoid muscle resulting in torticollis. In 50% of cases there is a history of complicated delivery. Occasional cases occur in families.

Microscopy shows proliferating fibroblasts surrounding degenerating residual striated muscle cells (Fig. 12.14). This lesion never behaves aggressively.

Infantile Digital Fibromatosis

Another lesion unique to young children is the infantile digital fibromatosis (recurring digital fibroma). It appears as a dome-shaped swelling on the sides or dorsum of the middle and distal interphalangeal joints of the fingers and toes. Sometimes more than one lesion is present. Most patients are less than 1 year of age, and in one-third of cases infantile digital fibromatosis is congenital. Microscopic examination shows a uniform proliferation of spindle cells, which have been shown by electron microscopy to be myofibroblasts (Mortimer and Gibson 1982). A characteristic feature seen in no other fibromatosis is the presence of a variable number of eosinophilic cytoplasmic inclusions with a filamentous ultrastructure. A histologically identical lesion has recently been described in an extradigital location in a $2\frac{1}{2}$-year-old child (Purdy and Colby 1984).

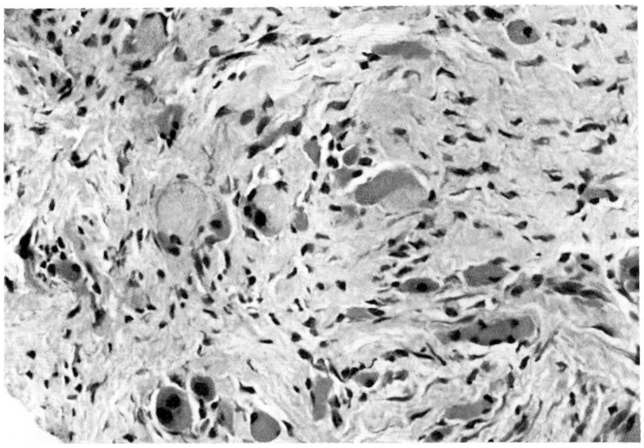

Fig. 12.14. Fibromatosis colli. Degenerating striated muscle cells are surrounded by dense fibrous tissue. (H&E, ×115)

Spontaneous regression may occur, and surgery is only required for diagnosis or if function is affected (Enzinger and Weiss 1988). As the name implies, there is a tendency to local recurrence after excision.

Fibrous Hamartoma of Infancy

Fibrous hamartoma of infancy occurs in the lower dermis and subcutaneous tissue as a soft mass which also rarely involves the superficial aspect of underlying muscle. About 20% of cases are congenital. Favoured sites are around the shoulder and upper arm, particularly the axillary folds, thigh and inguinal region. Grossly it appears as an ill-defined fibrofatty lump. Microscopically it is made up of three components: trabeculae of fibrous tissue, mature fat, and areas of immature mesenchy-

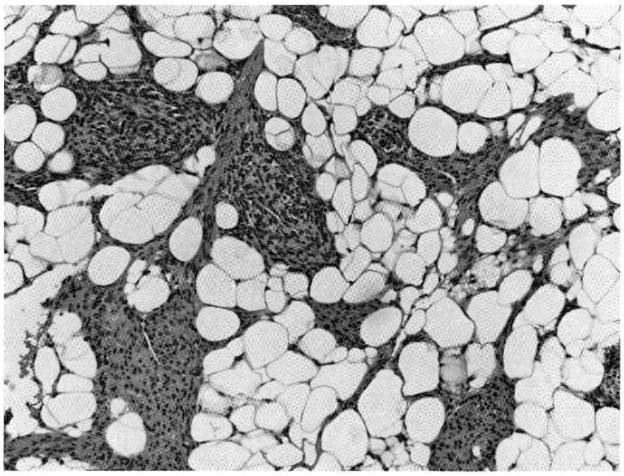

Fig. 12.15. Fibrous hamartoma of infancy. Lump from the axilla of a young infant. The typical organoid pattern composed of islands of immature mesenchymal cells, fibrous trabeculae and adipose tissue is clearly shown. (H&E, ×45)

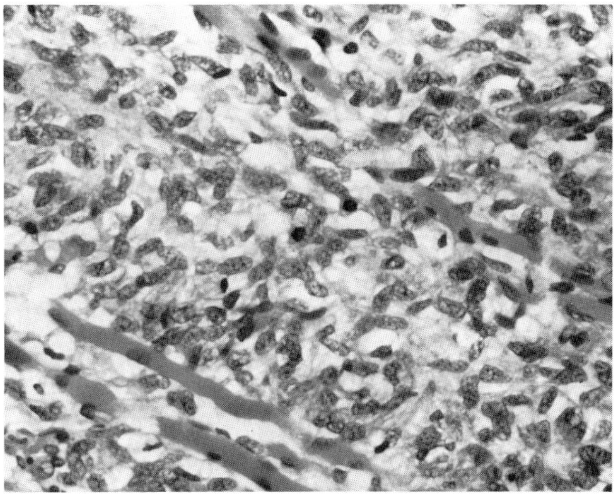

Fig. 12.17. Congenital fibrosarcoma. The tumour is composed of undifferentiated spindle cells with frequent mitoses invading striated muscle. (H&E, ×200)

mal cells often arranged in nests (Fig. 12.15). This lesion is benign but may rarely recur locally (Enzinger and Weiss 1988).

Congenital Fibrosarcoma

About half the cases of infantile fibrosarcoma described by Chung and Enzinger (1976) were present at birth and occurred preferentially in the extremities. Some lesions are very large (Fig. 12.16). The microscopic appearance may vary from that of an adult-type fibrosarcoma to a tumour composed of immature spindle cells with little evidence of fibroblastic differentiation (Fig. 12.17). The electron microscopic appearance is distinctive (Gonzalez-Crussi 1970). Metastases occur in 10% of cases; the

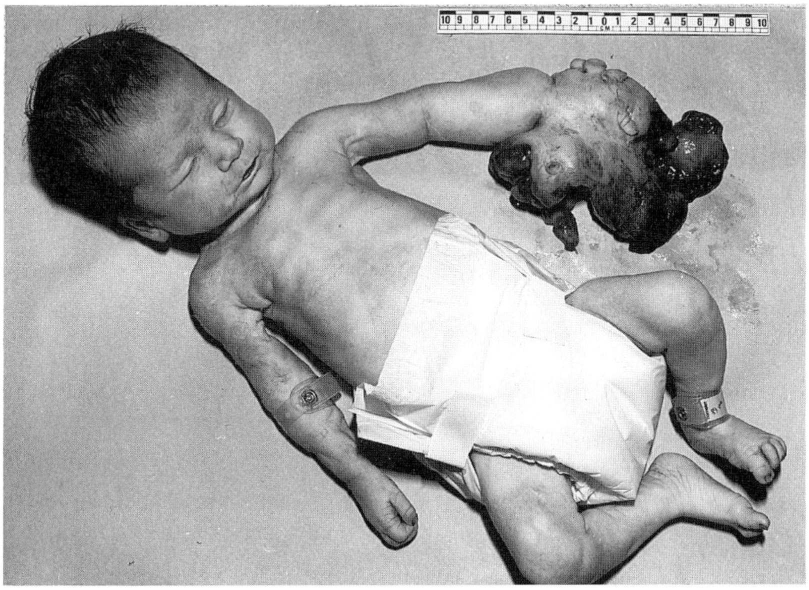

Fig. 12.16. Congenital fibrosarcoma involving the left hand and forearm. The tumour ruptured during delivery causing exsanguination.

5-year survival rate is 84% (Chung and Enzinger 1976). Congenital fibrosarcoma has been reviewed by Blocker et al. (1987).

Other Mesenchymal Tumours of Infancy

Rhabdomyosarcoma of the head, neck or urogenital tract can present in the neonatal period (Ragab et al. 1986; Hayashi et al. 1988). It is usually of the botryoid type and behaves as in older children. It is important to distinguish this tumour from fetal rhabdomyoma, which resembles fetal muscle and is benign (Di Sant' Agnese and Knowles 1980).

Congenital Leukaemia

Congenital leukaemia is rare but is a major cause of cancer deaths in the first month of life. It differs from leukaemia in older children in that most cases are non-lymphoid, and half have skin involvement. Leukaemia must be distinguished from florid leukaemoid reactions seen in neonates. Three diagnostic criteria must be fulfilled: proliferation of immature cells of the myeloid or lymphoid series; infiltration of non-haemopoietic tissues; and absence of other diseases that might cause diagnostic confusion such as erythroblastosis fetalis, congenital syphilis, and viral and bacterial infections (Engle et al. 1983). The diagnosis must be backed up by cytochemical, immunological and chromosome studies (Warrier et al. 1983; Gray et al. 1986). Congenital leukaemia is seen in Down's syndrome, Bloom's syndrome, Turner's syndrome, trisomy 13, Fanconi's anaemia and the Ellis–van Creveld syndrome. The outlook in neonatal leukaemia is very poor.

A syndrome closely mimicking congenital myeloblastic leukaemia is seen in trisomy 21 and commonly remits spontaneously. A similar syndrome is seen in children with trisomy 21 mosaicism, the leukaemoid reaction being confined to trisomic cells (Stockman 1982). The myeloproliferative disorder in trisomy 21 may be managed expectantly unless there is life-threatening progression. Older children with Down's syndrome have a 20 times increased risk of acute leukaemia, which does not regress spontaneously. Both the transient leukaemia-like syndrome and acute leukaemia in trisomy 21 may show megakaryoblastic differentiation (Hayashi et al. 1988).

Tumours of the Central Nervous System

Congenital tumours of the brain and spinal cord are rare and amount to only 5% of all congenital tumours. Up to a quarter of brain tumours diagnosed in the first year of life are evident at birth (Gerlach et al. 1982). The commonest presentation, regardless of tumour type, is enlargement of the head because of hydrocephalus or the tumour mass. The ability of the neonatal skull to expand enables some of these tumours to grow very large indeed. One in four cases is stillborn, and decompression of the skull may be required to effect vaginal delivery. Occasionally, a haemorrhagic glioma mimics intracerebral haemorrhage. This possibility should be considered in term infants with intracerebral bleeding. In children less than 1 year of age the majority of intracerebral tumours are supratentorial.

The commonest congenital brain tumours are teratomas (Takaku et al. 1978; Gerlach et al. 1982; Buetow et al. 1990). These usually arise either in the pineal region or in continuity with a pharyngeal teratoma. They are often very large but, with few exceptions, histologically benign. The other common types are gliomas, craniopharyngiomas and choroid plexus papillomas. The latter produce hydrocephalus by hypersecretion of cerebrospinal fluid.

Maternal Malignant Disease in Pregnancy

Cancer in pregnant women is probably commoner than primary malignant tumours in their offspring. Figures for maternal cancer range from 1 per 1000 pregnancies (Potter and Schoeneman 1970) to 1 per 6000 livebirths (Haas 1984). The coexistence of pregnancy and maternal malignancy imposes difficult therapeutic dilemmas which are beyond the scope of this chapter (Donegan 1983; Rosenstock 1983). Management may be influenced by the supposed risk of metastatic spread of the maternal tumour to the fetus. Available evidence shows that this concern is largely unjustified and confined to cases where tumour is already widely disseminated. Of the 35 cases of fetal and placental metastasis reported in the 106 years prior to 1973, only 11 involved the fetus (Rothman et al. 1973). Although a wide range of tumour types metastasised to the placenta, leukaemia, lymphoma and melanoma accounted for 10 of the 11 affected fetuses. There was a single case of transplacental metastasis of hepatocellular carcinoma. The placenta is probably always affected if there are metastases in the fetus (see Chap. 2, p. 70).

The placenta may act as a physical barrier to maternal tumours, and the fetus may be able to recognise and reject foreign maternal antigens expressed by the tumour. Maternal malignant melanoma metastatic to the fetus has regressed spontaneously (Rothman et al. 1973).

Witzleben and Bruninga (1968) have drawn attention to a rare but characteristic syndrome of infantile choriocarcinoma caused by metastatic placental choriocarcinoma. The young infant develops anaemia, hepatomegaly, bleeding and endocrine abnormalities such as breast enlargement, with signs of disseminated tumour. Evidence of choriocarcinoma in the mother may precede or follow its appearance in the child (Tsukamoto et al. 1986).

References

Altman RP, Randolph JG, Lilly JR (1974) Sacrococcygeal teratoma: American Academy of Pediatrics Surgical Section Survey—1973. Pediatr Surg 9: 389–398

Andrews MJ, Askin FB, Fried FA, McMillan CW, Mandell J (1983) Cystic partially differentiated nephroblastoma and polycystic Wilms' tumor. A spectrum of related clinical and pathologic entities. J Urol 129: 557–580

Bader JL, Miller RW (1979) US cancer incidence and mortality in the first year of life. Am J Dis Child 133: 157–159

Bader JL, Meadows AT, Lemerle J et al. (1980) Neurofibromatosis and other genetic defects associated with childhood cancer. Am J Hum Genet 32: 97A

Balaban G, Gilbert F (1983) Neuroblastoma IV-S: chromosome analysis. N Engl J Med 309: 989

Bale PM (1984) Sacrococcygeal developmental abnormalities and tumors in children. Perspect Paediatr Pathol 1: 9–56

Barrantes JC, Toyn C, Muir KR et al. (1991) Congenital mesoblastic nephroma: possible prognostic and management value of assessing DNA content. J Clin Pathol 44: 317–320

Barson AJ (1978) Congenital neoplasia; the Society's experience. Arch Dis Child 53: 436

Beckwith JB (1983) Wilms' tumor and other renal tumors of childhood. Hum Pathol 14: 481–492

Beckwith JB, Martin RF (1968) Observations on the histopathology of neuroblastomas. J Pediatr Surg 3: 106–110

Beckwith JB, Perrin EV (1963) In situ neuroblastomas. Am J Pathol 43: 1089–1104

Beckwith JB, Weeks DA (1986) Congenital mesoblastic nephroma. When should we worry? Arch Pathol Lab Med 110: 98–99

Beckwith JB, Kiviat NB, Bonadio JF (1990) Nephrogenic rests, nephroblastomatosis, and the pathogenesis of Wilms' tumour. Pediatr Pathol 10: 1–36

Berry CL (1989) Congenital malformations. In: Berry CL (ed) Paediatric pathology. Springer, Berlin Heidelberg New York, pp 41–62

Berry CL, Keeling J, Hilton C (1969) Teratoma in infancy and childhood. A review of 91 cases. J Pathol 98: 241–252

Berry CL, Keeling J, Hilton C (1970) Coincidence of congenital malformation and embryonic tumours of childhood. Arch Dis Child 45: 229–231

Blocker S, Koenig J, Ternberg J (1987) Congenital fibrosarcoma. J Pediatr Surg 22: 665–670

Bolande RP (1973) Congenital mesoblastic nephroma of infancy. In: Rosenberg HS, Bolande RP (eds) Perspectives in pediatric pathology, vol 1. Year Book Medical Publishers, Chicago, pp 227–250

Bolande RP (1976) Neoplasia of early life and its relationship to teratogenesis. In: Rosenberg HS, Bolande RP (eds) Perspectives in pediatric pathology, vol 3. Year Book Medical Publishers, Chicago, pp 145–183

Bolande RP (1984) Models and concepts derived from human teratogenesis and oncogenesis in early life. J Histochem Cytochem 32: 874–884

Bolande RP, Vekemans MJ-J (1983) Genetic models of carcinogenesis. Hum Pathol 14: 658–662

Bolande RP, Brough AJ, Izant RJ (1967) Congenital mesoblastic nephroma of infancy. A report of eight cases and the relationship to Wilms' tumor. Pediatrics 40: 272–278

Bove KE, McAdams AJ (1976) The nephroblastomatosis complex and its relationship to Wilms' tumor. A clinicopathologic treatise. In: Rosenberg HS, Bolande RP (eds) Perspectives in pediatric pathology, vol 3. Year Book Medical Publishers, Chicago, pp 185–223

Bove KE, Bhathena D, Wyatt RJ, Lucas BA, Holland NH (1979) Diffuse metanephric adenoma after in utero aspirin intoxication. Arch Pathol Lab Med 103: 187–190

Bower RJ, Adkins JC (1980) Ondine's curse and neurocristopathy. Clin Pediatr 19: 655–668

Broadbent VA (1986) Malignant disease in the neonate. In: Roberton NRC (ed) Textbook of neonatology. Churchill Living-stone, Edinburgh, pp 689–695

Brodeur GM, Seeger R, Sather H et al. (1986) Clinical implications of oncogene activation in human neuroblastomas. Cancer 58: 541–545

Buetow PC, Smirniotopoulos JG, Done S (1990) Congenital brain tumors: a review of 45 cases. AJNR 11: 793–799

Butturini A, Gale RP (1989) Age of onset and type of leukaemia. Lancet ii: 789–791

Campbell AN, Chan HSL, O'Brien A, Smith CR, Becker LE (1987) Malignant tumours in the neonate. Arch Dis Child 62: 19–23

Carlsen NLT (1988) Why age has independent prognostic significance in neuroblastomas. Evidence for intrauterine development, and implications for treatment of the disease. Anticancer Res 8: 255–262

Carter D, Bibro MC, Touloukian RJ (1982) Benign clinical behaviour of immature mediastinal teratoma in infancy and childhood. Cancer 49: 398–402

Chadduck WA, Gollin SM, Gray BA, Norris JS, Araoz CA, Tryka AF (1987) Gliosarcoma with chromosome abnormalities in a neonate exposed to heptachlor. Neurosurgery 21: 557–559

Chatten J (1976) Epithelial differentiation in Wilms' tumor: a clinocopathologic appraisal. In: Rosenberg HS, Bolande RP (eds) Perspectives in pediatric pathology, vol 3. Year Book Medical Publishers, Chicago, pp 225–254
Chatten J, Witzleben CL (1975) Neuroblastoma and Hirschsprung's disease. Am J Pathol 78: 2a
Chung EB, Enzinger FM (1976) Infantile fibrosarcoma. Cancer 38: 729–739
Chung EB, Enzinger FM (1981) Infantile myofibromatosis. Cancer 48: 1807–1818
Cook HT, Taylor GM, Malone P, Risdon RA (1988) Renin in mesoblastic nephroma: an immunohistochemical study. Hum Pathol 19: 1347–1351
Crom DB, Williams JA, Green AA, Pratt CB, Jenkins JJ, Behm FG (1989) Malignancy in the neonate. Med Pediatr Oncol 17: 101–104
D'Angio GJ, Evans AE, Koop CE (1971) Special pattern of widespread neuroblastoma with a favourable prognosis. Lancet I: 1046–1049
Davis CF, Carachi R, Young DG (1988) Neonatal tumours: Glasgow 1955–86. Arch Dis Child 63: 1075–1078
Dehner LP (1981) Neoplasms of the fetus and neonate. In: Naeye RL, Kissane JM, Kaufman N (eds) Perinatal diseases. Williams and Wilkins, Baltimore, pp 286–345
Dehner LP (1983) Gonadal and extragonadal germ cell neoplasia of childhood. Hum Pathol 14: 493–511
Dehner LP, Mills A, Talerman A, Billman GF, Krous HF, Platz CE (1990) Germ cell neoplasms of head and neck soft tissues: a pathological spectrum of teratomatous and endodermal sinus tumours. Hum Pathol 21: 309–318
Dimmick JE, Johnson HW, Coleman GU, Carter M (1989) Wilms' tumorlet, nodular renal blastema and multicystic renal dysplasia. J Urol 142: 484–485
Di Sant'Agnese PA, Knowles DM (1980) Extracardiac rhabdomyoma: a clincopathologic study and review of the literature. Cancer 46: 780–789
Donegan WL (1983) Cancer and pregnancy. CA 33: 194–214
Dunlop MG (1991) Allele loss and onco-suppressor genes. J Pathol 163: 1–5
Du Plessis JPG, Winship WS, Kirstein JDL (1974) Fetus in fetu and teratoma: a case report and review. S Afr Med J 48: 2119–2122
Einhorn L (1983) Are there factors preventing cancer development during embryonic life? Oncodevel Biol Med 4: 219–229
Emery LG, Shields M, Shah NR, Garbes A (1983) Neuroblastoma associated with Beckwith–Weidemann syndrome. Cancer 52: 176–179
Engle WA, Schreiner RL, Baehner RL (1983) Neonatal white blood cell disorders. Semin Perinatol 7: 184–200
Enzinger FM, Weiss SW (1988) Soft tissue tumors, 2nd edn. Mosby, St Louis
Evans AE, Baum E, Chard R (1981) Do infants with Stage IV-S neuroblastomas need treatment? Arch Dis Child 56: 271–274
Fine PE, Adelstein AM, Snowman J, Clarkson JA, Evans SM (1985) Long term effects of exposure to viral infections in utero. Br Med J 290: 509–511
Flake AW, Harrison MR, Adzick NS, Laberge J-M, Warsof SL (1986) Fetal sacrococcygeal teratoma. J Pediatr Surg 21: 563–566
Fletcher CDM, Achu P, Van Norden S, McKee PH (1987) Infantile myofibromatosis: a light microscopic, histochemical and immunohistochemical study suggesting true smooth muscle differentiation. Histopathology 11: 245–258
Gaitan-Yanguas M (1978) Retinoblastoma: analysis of 235 cases. Int J Radiat Oncol Biol Phys 4: 359–365.
Gale GB, D'Angio GJ, Uri A, Chatten J, Koop CE (1982) Cancer in neonates: the experience at the Children's Hospital of Philadelphia. Pediatrics 70: 409–413
Gallie LB, Squire JA, Goddard A et al. (1990) Mechanism of oncogenesis in retinoblastoma. Lab Invest 62: 394–406
Gerlach H, Janisch W, Schreiber D (1982) Intracranial and spinal tumours in newborns and infants. In: Voth D, Gutjahr P, Langmaid C (eds) Tumours of the central nervous system in infancy and childhood. Springer, Berlin Heidelberg New York, pp 51–57
Gilbert F (1984) Solid tumors of children: chromosome abnormalities and the development of cancer. J Cell Physiol [Suppl] 3: 165–170
Gill TJ (1984) The borderland of embryogenesis and carcinogenesis. Major histocompatibility complex-linked genes affecting development and their possible relationship to the development of cancer. Biochim Biophys Acta 738: 93–102
Golbus MS (1987) Experience with 8 cases of prenatally diagnosed sacrococcygeal teratomas. Fetal Ther 2: 88–94
Gonzalez-Grussi F (1970) Ultrastructure of congenital fibrosarcoma. Cancer 26: 1289–1299
Gonzalez-Crussi F (1982) Extragonadal teratomas. In: Hartman WH (ed) Fascicle 18: Atlas of tumor pathology. Armed Forces Institute of Pathology, Washington DC
Gonzalez-Crussi F, Sotelo-Avila C, Kidd JM (1981) Mesenchymal renal tumors in infancy: a reappraisal. Hum Pathol 12: 78–85
Gonzalez-Crussi F, Upton MP, Maurer HS (1982) Hepatoblastoma. Attempt at characterization of histologic subtypes. Am J Surg Pathol 6: 599–612
Gormley TS, Skoog SJ, Jones RV, Maybee D (1989) Cellular congenital mesoblastic nephroma: what are the options. J Urol 142: 479–483
Graham-Pole J, Salmi T, Anton AH, Abramovsky C, Gross S (1983) Tumor and urine catecholamines in neurogenic tumors. Cancer 51: 834–839
Gray ES, Balch NJ, Kohler H, Thompson WD, Simpson JG (1986) Congenital leukaemia: an unusual cause of stillbirth. Arch Dis Child 61: 1001–1006
Grosfield JL, Ballantine TVN, Lowe D, Baehner RL (1976) Benign and malignant teratomas in children: analysis of 85 patients. Surgery 80: 297–305
Gross SJ, Benzie RJ, Sermer M, Skidmore MB, Wilson SR (1987) Sacrococcygeal teratoma: prenatal diagnosis and management. Am J Obstet Gynecol 156: 393–396
Grotting JC, Kassel S, Dehner LP (1979) Nesidioblastosis and congenital neuroblastoma. Arch Pathol Lab Med 103: 642–646
Guin GH, Gilbert EF, Jones B (1969) Incidental neuroblastoma in infants. Am J Clin Pathol 51: 126–136
Haas JF (1984) Pregnancy in association with a newly diagnosed cancer: a population based epidemiologic assessment. Int J Cancer 34: 229–235
Haas JE, Muczinski KA, Krailo M et al. (1989) Histopathology and prognosis in childhood hepatoblastoma and hepatocarcinoma. Cancer 64: 1082–1095
Haber DA, Housman DE (1991) Rate-limiting steps: the genetics of pediatric cancers. Cell 64: 5–8
Hawkins EP, Finegold MJ, Hawkins HK, Krischer JP, Starling KA, Weinberg A (1986) Nongerminomatous malignant germ cell tumors in children. A review of 89 cases from the Pediatric Oncology Group, 1971–1984
Hayashi K, Ohtsuki Y, Takahashi K et al. (1988) Congenital alveolar rhabdomyosarcoma with multiple skin metastases. Acta Pathol Jpn 38: 241–248
Hayashi Y, Eguchi M, Sugita K et al. (1988) Cytogenetic

findings and clinical features in acute leukemia and transient myeloproliferative disorder in Down's syndrome. Blood 72: 15–23

Herbst AL (1981) Clear cell adenocarcinoma and the current status of DES-exposed females. Cancer 48: 484–488

Holzgreve W, Miny P, Anderson R et al. (1991) Neuroblastoma diagnosed antenatally: a treatment dilemma. In: Proceedings of the 2nd international symposium on neuroblastoma screening. University of Minnesota, Minneapolis, p 18

Hou LT, Holman RL (1961) Bilateral nephroblastomatosis in a premature infant. J Pathol Bacteriol 82: 249–255

Huddart SN, Mann JR (1991) Screening for neuroblastoma. Arch Dis Child 66: 1272–1273

Hunt PT, Davidson KC, Ashcraft KW, Holder TM (1977) Radiography of hereditary presacral teratoma. Radiology 122: 187–191

Isaacs H (1983) Neoplasms in infants: a report of 265 cases. Pathology Annu 18(2): 165–214

Isaacs H (1985) Perinatal (congenital and neonatal neoplasms): a report of 110 cases. Pediatr Pathol 3: 165–216

Jablon S, Kato H (1970) Childhood cancer in relation to prenatal exposure to atomic-bomb radiation. Lancet II: 1000–1003

Jennings TA, Duray PH, Collins FS, Sabetta J, Enzinger FM (1984) Infantile myofibromatosis; evidence for an autosomal dominant disorder. Am J Surg Pathol 8: 529–538

Jerkins GR, Callihan TR (1986) Ossifying renal tumor of infancy. J Urol 135: 120–121

Johnson RE, Scheithauer BW, Dahlin DC (1983) Melanotic neuroectodermal tumor of infancy. A review of seven cases. Cancer 52: 661–666

Joshi VV (1979) Cystic partially differentiated nephroblastoma: an entity in the spectrum of infantile renal neoplasia. In: Rosenberg HS, Bolande RP (eds) Perspectives in pediatric pathology, vol 5. Masson, New York, pp 217–235

Joshi VV, Kasznica J, Walters TR (1986) Atypical mesoblastic nephroma. Pathological characterization of a potentially aggressive variant of conventional congenital mesoblastic nephroma. Arch Pathol Lab Med 110: 100–106

Kalousek DK, De Chadarevian JP, Mackie GG, Bolande RP (1977) Metastatic infantile Wilms' tumor and hydrocephalus. A case report with a review of the literature. Cancer 39: 1312–1316

Kaneko Y, Kanda N, Maseki N et al. (1987) Different karyotypic patterns in early and advanced stage neuroblastomas. Cancer Res 47: 311–318

Kasai M, Watanabe I (1970) Histological classification of liver-cell carcinoma in infancy and childhood and its clinical evaluation. A study of 70 cases collected in Japan. Cancer 25: 551–563

Kauffman SL, Stout AP (1965) Congenital mesenchymal tumors. Cancer 18: 460–476

Knudson AG (1971) Mutation and cancer: statistical study of retinoblastoma. Proc Natl Acad Sci USA 68: 820–823

Knudson AG (1989) Hereditary cancers: clues to the mechanisms of carcinogenesis. Br J Cancer 59: 661–666

Knudson AG, Meadows AT (1976) Developmental genetics of neuroblastoma. JNCI 57: 675–682

Knudson AG, Strong LC (1972) Mutation and cancer. A model for Wilms' tumor of the kidney. JNCI 48: 313–324

Kobayashi N, Furukawa T, Takatsu T (1968) Congenital anomalies in children with cancer. Pediatr Univ Tokyo 16: 31

Koppersmith DL, Powers JM, Hennigar GR (1980) Angiomatoid neuroblastoma with cytoplasmic glycogen. Cancer 45: 553–560

Kramer S, Ward E, Meadows AT, Malone K (1987) Medical and drug risk factors associated with neuroblastoma: a case-control study. J Nat Cancer Inst 78: 797–804

Kulkarni R, Bailie MD, Bernstein J, Newton B (1980) Progression of nephroblastomatosis to Wilms' tumor. J Pediatr 96: 178

Kurjak A, Zalud I, Jurkovic D, Alfirevic Z, Tomic K (1989) Ultrasound diagnosis and evaluation of fetal tumors. J Perinat Med 17: 173–193

Lack EL, Neave C, Vawter GF (1982) Hepatoblastoma. A clinical and pathologic study of 54 cases. Am J Surg Pathol 6: 693–705

Las Heras J, Isaacs H (1980) Congenital and neonatal tumors: a 15-year experience, Lab Invest 42: 175

Lemerle J, Tournade MF, Gerard-Marchant R et al. (1976) Wilms' tumor; natural history and prognostic factors. A retrospective study of 248 cases. Cancer 37: 2557–2566

Lemire RJ, Beckwith JB (1982) Pathogenesis of congenital tumors and malformations of the sacrococcygeal region. Teratology 25: 201–213

Linder D (1983) The origin of teratomas. In: Damjanov I, Knowles BB, Solter D (eds) The human teratomas, experimental and clinical biology. Humana, Clifton, NJ, pp 68–80

Littlefield JW (1984) Genes, chromosomes and cancer. J Pediatr 104: 489–494

Look AT, Hayes A, Nitschke R, McWilliams NB, Green AA (1984) Cellular DNA content as a predictor of response to chemotherapy in infants with unresectable neuroblastoma. N Engl J Med 311: 231–235

Machin GA (1980) Persistent renal blastema (nephroblastomatosis) as a frequent precursor of Wilms' tumor; a pathological and clinical review Parts 1–3. Am J Pediatr Haematol Oncol 2: Part 1 165–172; Part 2 253–261; Part 3 353–362

Machin GA, McCaughey WTE (1984) A new precursor lesion of Wilms' tumor (nephroblastoma): intralobar multifocal nephroblastomatosis. Histopathology 8: 35–53

MacMahon B (1981) Childhood cancer and prenatal irradiation. In: Burchenal JH, Oettgen HF (eds). Cancer achievements, challenges and prospects for the 1980s, vol 1. Grune and Stratton, New York, pp 223–228

Mancini AF, Rosito P, Faldella G, Serra L, Vallicelli R, Vecchi V, Vivarelli F, Paolucci G (1982) Neuroblastoma in a pair of identical twins. Med Pediatr Oncol 10: 45–51

Marsden HB, Lawler W (1980) Bone metastasising renal tumour of childhood. Histopathological and clinical review of 38 cases. Virchows Arch [A] 387: 341–251

Marsden HB, Lawler W (1983) Primary renal tumours in the first year of life. Virchows Arch [A] 399: 1–9

Marsden HB, Birch JM, Swindell R (1981) Germ cell tumours of childhood: a review of 137 cases. J Clin Pathol 34: 879–883

Mortimer G, Gibson A (1982) Recurring digital fibroma. J Clin Pathol 35: 849–854

Nakissa N, Constine LS, Rubin P, Strohl R (1985) Birth defects in three common pediatric malignancies; Wilms' tumor, neuroblastoma and Ewing's sarcoma. Oncology 42: 358–363

Olshan A (1986) Wilms' tumor, overgrowth, and fetal growth factors: a hypothesis. Cancer Genet Cytogenet 21: 303–307

Paul J (1989) Tumour suppressor genes: oncogenesis update. Histopathology 15: 1–9

Platt MS, Agamanolis DP, Krill CE, Boeckman C, Potter JL, Robinson H, Lloyd J (1983) Occult hepatic sinusoid tumor of infancy simulating neuroblastoma. Cancer 52:

1183–1189
Potter JF, Schoeneman M (1970) Metastasis of maternal cancer to the placenta and fetus. Cancer 25: 380–388
Purdy JL, Colby TV (1984) Infantile digital fibromatosis occurring outside the digit. Am J Surg Pathol 8: 787–790
Ragab AH, Heyn R, Tefft M, Hays D, Newton WA, Beltangady M (1986) Infants younger than 1 year with rhabdomyosarcoma. Cancer 58: 2606–2610
Roman E, Beral V (1991) Possible aetiological factors in childhood leukaemia. Arch Dis Child 66: 179–180
Rose EA, Glaser T, Jones C et al. (1990) Complete physical map of the WAGR region of 11p13 localises a candidate Wilms' tumor gene. Cell 60: 495–508
Rosenberg HS, Stenback WA, Spjut HJ (1978) The fibromatoses of infancy and childhood. In: Rosenberg HS, Bolande RP (eds) Perspectives in pediatric pathology. vol 4. Year Book Medical Publishers, Chicago, pp 269–348
Rosenfeld CR, Coln CD, Duenhoelter JH (1979) Fetal cervical teratoma as a cause of polyhydramnios. Pediatrics 64: 176–179
Rosenstock JG (1983) Neoplasia: the mother and the neonate. Semin Perinatol 7: 226–235
Rothman LA, Cohen CJ, Astarloa J (1973) Placental and fetal involvement by maternal malignancy: a report of rectal carcinoma and review of the literature. Am J Obstet Gynecol 116: 1023–1034
Ruymann FB, Maddux HR, Ragab A et al. (1988) Congenital abnormalities associated with rhabdomyosarcoma: an autopsy study of 115 cases. A report from the Intergroup Rhabdomyosarcoma Study committee (representing the Children's Cancer Study Group, the United Kingdom Children's Cancer Study Group, the Pediatric Oncology Group, and the Pediatric Intergroup Statistical Centre). Med Pediat Oncol 16: 33–39
Schmidt D, Harms D, Zieger G (1982) Malignant rhabdoid tumour of the kidney. Histopathology, ultrastructure and comments on differential diagnosis. Virchows Arch [A] 398: 101–108
Schneider KM, Becker JM, Krasna IH (1965) Neonatal neuroblastoma. Pediatrics 36: 359–366
Seeler RA, Israel JN, Royal JE, Kaye CI, Raos S, Abulaben M (1979) Ganglioneuroblastoma and fetal hydantoin-alcohol syndromes. Pediatrics 63: 524–527
Shanklin DR, Sotelo-Avila C (1969) In situ tumors in fetuses, newborns and young infants. Biol Neonate 14: 286–316
Sheils C, Dover GJ (1989) Frequency of congenital anomalies in patients with histiocytosis X. Am J Hematol 31: 91–95
Shimada H, Chatten J, Newton WA, Sachs N, Hamoudi AB, Chiba T, Marsden HB, Misugi K (1984) Histopathologic prognostic factors in neuroblastic tumors. JNCI 73: 405–416
Snyder HM, Lack EE, Chatty-Backtavizian A, Bauer SB, Colodny AH, Retik AB (1981) Congenital mesoblastic nephroma: relationship to other renal tumors of infancy. J Urol 126: 513–516
Solomon E (1984) Recessive mutation in aetiology of Wilms' tumour. Nature 309. 111–112
Sotelo-Avila C, Gooch WM (1976) Neoplasms associated with the Beckwith–Wiedemann syndrome. In: Rosenberg HS, Bolande RP (eds) Perspectives in pediatric pathology, vol 3. Year Book Medical Publishers, Chicago, pp 255–272
Steinfeld AD, Crowley CA, O'Shea PA, Tefft M (1984) Recurrent and metastatic mesoblastic nephroma in infancy. J Clin Oncol 2: 956–960
Stephenson SR, Cook BA, Mease AD, Ruymann FB (1986) The prognostic significance of age and pattern of metastases in Stage IV-S neuroblastoma. Cancer 58: 372–375
Stocker JT, Ishak KG (1978) Undifferentiated (embryonal) sarcoma of the liver. Report of 31 cases. Cancer 42: 336–348
Stocker JT, Ishak KG (1983) Mesenchymal hamartoma of the liver: report of 30 cases and review of the literature. Pediatr Pathol 1: 245–267
Stockman JA (1982) Disorders of leukocytes. In: Oski FA, Naiman JL (eds) Hematologic problems in the newborn. Saunders, Philadelphia, pp 223–244
Takaku A, Kodama N, Ohara H, Hori S (1978) Brain tumor in newborn babies. Childs Brain 4: 365–375
Tank ES, Kay R (1980) Neoplasms associated with Beckwith's syndrome, hemihypertrophy and aniridia. J Urol 124: 266–268
Tapper D, Lack EE (1983) Teratomas in infancy and childhood. A 54 year experience at the Children's Hospital Medical Centre. Ann Surg 198: 398–410
Terracini B, Pastore G, Segnan N (1983) Association of father's occupation and cancer in children. Biol Res Pregnancy Perinatol 4: 40–45
Torres-Aybar FG, Basora G, Lopez-Busquets RH et al. (1975) Intrapericardial teratomas. Bol Asoc Med PR 67: 366–368
Triche TJ, Askin FB (1983) Neuroblastoma and the differential diagnosis of small-, round-, blue-cell tumors. Hum Pathol 14: 569–595
Tsukamoto N, Matsumura M, Matsukuma K, Kamura T, Baba K (1986) Choriocarcinoma in mother and fetus. Gynecol Oncol 24: 113–119
Tuman KJ, Chilcote RR, Berkow RI, Moohr JW (1980) Mesothelioma in a child with prenatal exposure to isoniazid. Lancet II: 362
Turleau C, de Grouchy J, Chavin-Colin F, Martelli H, Voyer M, Charlas R (1984) Trisomy 11p15 and Beckwith–Wiedemann syndrome. A report of two cases. Hum Genet 67: 219–221
Turkel SB, Itabashi HH (1974) The natural history of neuroblastic cells in the fetal adrenal gland. Am J Pathol 76: 225–244
Ugarte N, Gonzalez-Crussi F, Hsueh W (1981) Wilms' tumor: its morphology in patients under one year of age. Cancer 48: 346–353
Warrier RP, Ravindranath Y, Inoue S, Kaplan J, Emami A (1983) Congenital leukaemia: two transient regressions without treatment in one patient. Pediatrics 72: 916–917
Weeks DA, Beckwith JB, Mierau GW, Lucky DW (1989) Rhabdoid tumor of kidney. A report of 111 cases from the National Wilms' Tumor Study Pathology Center. Am J Surg Pathol 13: 439–458
Wells HG (1940) Occurrence and significance of congenital malignant neoplasms. Arch Pathol 30: 535–601
Weinberg AG, Finegold MJ (1983) Primary hepatic tumours of childhood. Hum Pathol 14: 512–537
Wieberdink J (1982) Metastasis in neonatal neuroblastoma. In: Pochedly C (ed) Neuroblastoma, clinical and biological manifestations. Elsevier, New York, pp 13–21
Wigger HJ (1976) Fetal rhabdomyomatous nephroblastoma—a variant of Wilms' tumor. Hum Pathol 7: 613–623
Wiswell TE, Davis J, Cunningham BE, Solenberger R, Thomas PJ (1988) Infantile myofibromatosis: the most common fibrous tumor of infancy. J Pediatr Surg 23: 314–318
Wiztleben CL, Bruninga G (1968) Infantile choriocarcinoma: a characteristic syndrome. J Pediatr 73: 374–378
Yazaki T, Akimota M, Tsuboi N, Kawai H, Miyamato M, Suzuki T (1982) Congenital mesoblastic nephroma. Urology 20: 446–450

Chapter 13

Infection in Pregnancy and the Neonatal Period

Helen Holzel

Adverse Effects of Infection During Pregnancy

Introduction

Precise information on the frequency of infection in pregnancy is not available. Specific diseases are easily documented but non-specific or asymptomatic infection is less likely to be investigated or diagnosed. Much of our information stems from large prospective studies carried out in the 1960s and 70s. Amongst 30 000 pregnancies, Sever and White (1968) showed that 5.2% were complicated by at least one clinically recognisable illness. Influenza or influenza-like illness was identified most frequently. Another study, looking at pregnancy outcome following recognised viral illness, found clear-cut evidence of fetal damage only after rubella infection: 6%–8% of affected neonates had major defects (Manson et al. 1960). Congenital infection accounts for only a small proportion of infectious disease of the newborn. Many congenital infections show national differences in incidence. Group B streptococcal infection is more common in the USA than in the UK and toxoplasmosis is more common in France and Austria than in the UK. Within countries, infection rates may be social class and race related. An estimate of the prevalence of congenital infections in the UK in the 1980s was 3.4 per 1000 births (Rudd and Peckham 1988).

Estimates of the frequency of bacterial infection of the fetus and gestation sac are particularly difficult. Maternal symptoms are often non-specific and there may be problems in acquiring appropriate samples for culture and in interpretation of results. Viral infection is more amenable to study although several studies of viral infection in abortion have failed to identify common viruses (Boué and Loffredo 1970; Catalano and Sever 1971).

Viral Infection

Rubella

Rubella infection is worldwide in distribution. In the UK it has an epidemic pattern with four-year cycles; its incidence has declined since 1986. Selective immunisation of schoolgirls and susceptible adult women, begun in the UK in 1970, was augmented in 1988 by mass vaccination of all children with combined measles, mumps and rubella vaccine. The aim is to eliminate endemic rubella virus.

Spontaneous abortion due to rubella infection in pregnancy is unusual, affecting about 4% of infected women (Miller et al. 1982). The total impact of rubella as a cause of fetal wastage includes those therapeutic abortions performed because of disease, contact or inadvertent immunisation (Table 13.1). Of women in the UK with first trimester rubella infection, 94% underwent therapeutic abortion (Miller et al. 1982). The role of rubella as a cause of congenital abnormalities has been well documented since its association with congenital cataract (Gregg 1941). In contrast to the mild, self-limiting postnatal disease, prenatal infection is often widespread and persistent (Alford et al. 1964). Disseminated disease does not always occur: in some cases a single organ is involved or infection is avoided. Clinical manifestations and pathology are reviewed by Hanshaw et al. (1985).

Table 13.1. Rubella-associated terminations of pregnancy

	Disease or contact		Vaccination
Year	Number	Rate per 100 000 pregnancies*	Number
1971	1018	115	43
1972	738	88	38
1973	816	103	23
1974	633	84	31
1975	504	70	27
1976	213	31	40
1977	184	27	37
1978	830	116	66
1979	575	75	156
1980	200	25	101
1981	134	17	63
1982	180	24	46
1983	231	30	72
1984	141	18	93
1985	65	8	41
1986	110	14	30
1987	73	9	31
1988	44	5	11
1989	18	2	17

*includes all live and still births and terminations of pregnancy in residents, England and Wales. (Miller et al. 1991)

The risk of congenital rubella depends on the prevalence of infection in the community, the immune status of the mother and the stage of pregnancy at which infection occurs. Immunisation programmes have greatly reduced the number of cases worldwide although clusters of congenital infection have occurred in countries where overall uptake of immunisation is high (Lamprecht et al. 1982). During 1990, reports from US health departments showed a major increase in congenital rubella syndrome (CRS) (Morbidity and Mortality Weekly Report 1991).

In the UK between 1971 and 1990 when large and moderate rubella epidemic years were interspersed with non-epidemic years, the number of confirmed or suspected cases reported to the National Congenital Rubella Surveillance Programme showed corresponding fluctuation but an overall reduction from 60 cases in 1970 to 7 in 1990 (Miller et al. 1991).

Fetal infection results from primary maternal infection. Reinfection was thought not to be a risk (Boué et al. 1971). Isolated reports of fetal infection and malformation following maternal reinfection have occurred (Morgan-Capner 1986). Seven cases of maternal reinfection resulting in five cases of CRS and virus isolation from two therapeutic abortions have been reported (Best et al. 1989; Das et al. 1989). The actual risk of fetal damage following maternal reinfection is not yet clear but is likely to be rare (Best et al. 1989) and is being investigated prospectively by Miller (1990).

Prospective studies of the risk of fetal injury and timing of maternal infection have been undertaken in many countries. In Sweden, the risk of major defects following first trimester maternal infection was 10% (Lundstrom 1962) and in the UK was 15.8% with 2% in controls (Manson et al. 1960). The most recent study followed 1000 women who contracted infection at different stages of pregnancy (Miller et al. 1982). Forty per cent of pregnancies continued and offspring were followed for 2 years. Congenital infection followed more than 80% of first trimester infections, 54% of infections at 13–14 weeks' gestation and 25% of infections at the end of the second trimester. An unexpected and unexplained increase in infection rate occurred during the last trimester. Malformations related to the timing of infection are detailed in Table 13.2. No defects attributable to rubella were found in 63 children infected after 16 weeks' gestation. Sequelae of rubella infection have presented as late as 8 years of age (Menser and Forest 1974).

Cytomegalovirus

Cytomegalovirus (CMV) is a typical herpes virus possessing the property of latency.

Table 13.2. Rubella defects found at follow-up in infants infected at successive stages of pregnancy (Miller et al. 1982)

Stage of pregnancy (weeks)	Seropositive infants				Overall risk[a] of rubella defect (%)
	No. followed up	Heart and other defect	Deafness alone	Percentage with defect	
<11	9	5	4	100	90
11–12	4	0	2	50	33
13–14	12	0	2	17	11
15–16	14	0	7	50	24
17–18	10	0	0	—	—
>18	53	0	0	—	—
Total	102	5	15	20	—

[a] Estimated from congenital infection rate following symptomatic rubella at different stages of pregnancy (table II; Miller et al. 1982). Overall risk = percentage seropositive with defects × percentage of infants infected.

CMV infection is endemic worldwide with no seasonal variation; most infections are asymptomatic. It is the most frequent cause of congenital infection (Fig. 13.1), affecting 1800 infants in England and Wales and 35 000 in the USA each year (Rudd and Peckham 1988; Stagno 1990).

Antibody positivity amongst women of childbearing age is related to national, racial and socioeconomic factors (Stagno 1990). Primary infection during pregnancy shows similar variation, 0.7%–4% of pregnant women become infected (Alford et al. 1990). In the UK primary infection in pregnancy occurs in 1% of susceptible women with fetal infection in 30%–40% of cases (Griffiths and Baboonian 1984). Fetal infection follows both primary and recurrent maternal infection (Peckham et al. 1983; Griffiths and Baboonian 1984; Stagno et al. 1986; Griffiths et al. 1991). Griffiths and Baboonian (1984) found virus transmission was 20% in the first trimester but did not occur in the second trimester, although in 40% of third trimester infections transmission was demonstrated. Subsequent studies show no gestational age effect on CMV transmission. The risk of neonatal disease, with attendant sequelae, appears to be higher when infection occurs in the first half of pregnancy (Stagno and Whitley 1985a; Stagno et al. 1986).

Primary maternal infection resulting in excess fetal loss has been noted by some workers (Griffiths and Baboonian 1984) but not others (Stagno et al. 1986). The majority of neonates with congenital CMV infection (90%) are asymptomatic at birth. Of the remainder,

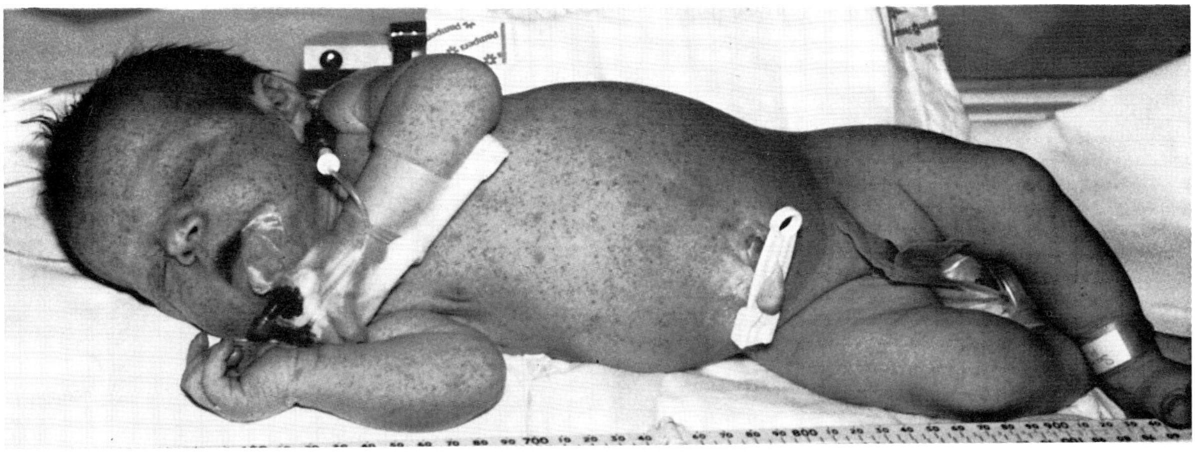

Fig. 13.1. Congenital CMV infection: generalised petechial rash. Hepatosplenomegaly was present. (Courtesy of Dr. A. Wilkinson, Oxford)

5% suffer an acute illness whose clinical manifestations are shown in Table 13.3. The rest have mild (Fig. 13.1) or atypical disease. Mortality may reach 30% amongst those severely affected (Pass et al. 1980). Most deaths are neonatal and due to multiorgan disease with severe hepatic dysfunction, disseminated intravascular coagulation and secondary bacterial infection. Psychomotor retardation, neurological dysfunction and hearing loss are frequent late complications. There are few normal survivors amongst symptomatic infants (Stagno 1990).

Table 13.3. Manifestations of congenital cytomegalic inclusion disease (Peckham and Marshall 1983)

Low birthweight	Hypotonia
Hepatosplenomegaly	Encephalitis
Hepatitis: jaundice	Chorioretinitis
Hyperbilirubinaemia	Cerebral calcification
Thrombocytopenic purpura	Microcephaly
Haemolytic anaemia	Mental retardation
Pneumonitis[a]	

[a] in less than 1% (Stagno 1990)

Ahlfors et al. (1981) described the first case of congenital disease following recurrent maternal infection. Since then further cases have been documented (Rutter et al. 1985; Griffiths et al. 1991). The risk of disease is significantly greater for infants born after primary maternal infection than after reinfection (Stagno 1990).

Herpes Simplex

Herpes simplex virus (HSV) in pregnancy may be disseminated or localised, primary or recurrent. Disseminated maternal infection is rare with high maternal mortality and fetal mortality greater than 50% (Stagno and Whitley 1985b). Localised genital infection is much more common and prospective studies found it in 1% of women at any time during gestation (Nahmias et al. 1983). Most infections are recurrent. Maternal primary infection prior to 20 weeks' gestation may be complicated by spontaneous abortion (Nahmias et al. 1971). Later infection does not predispose to pregnancy loss (Harger et al. 1983). Recurrent infection during pregnancy is more common and fetal transmission is related to viral shedding at delivery. It has been estimated that viral excretion at delivery ranges from 0.01%–0.39% of all women (Nahmias et al. 1983). Cervical virus shedding is lower in recurrent genital infection (Corey 1982; Corey et al. 1983) so that the type of maternal infection can influence neonatal acquisition of HSV as does transplacental acquisition of maternal neutralising antibodies (Prober et al. 1987).

Neonatal HSV infection is common in the USA where rates between 1 in 1500 and 1 in 5000 deliveries are observed (Whitley 1990). This results in infection of some 1500–2200 newborns annually (Whitley et al. 1991). In contrast, notifications to the British Paediatric Surveillance Unit (BPSU) between July 1986 and December 1990 identified 112 cases of suspected neonatal HSV infection of which only 62 were later confirmed (approximately 1 in 50 000 livebirths).

Neonatal HSV infection results from intrauterine, intrapartum or postnatal transmission. The majority (85%–90%) are acquired intrapartum from contact with infected maternal genital secretions (Whitley 1990). Intrauterine infection is uncommon by either the transplacental or the ascending route. Following intrauterine transmission, severe infection may be apparent at birth with skin vesicles and scarring, eye disease, microcephaly or hydranencephaly (South et al. 1969; Florman et al. 1973; Hutto et al. 1987). Unlike rubella, severe disease may follow infection at any stage of gestation.

Intrapartum or postnatal disease may be (1) localised to skin, eye and mouth, (2) encephalitis with or without skin involvement, (3) disseminated infection involving many organs including the central nervous system (Whitley 1990). In the BPSU study 27% of infants died within 1 month of birth. HSV 1 infections were as common as type 2 and fatality rates were similar. Maternal genital infection occurred in less than one-third of women and in most cases infection was diagnosed retrospectively. In 11 cases a postnatal source of infection was identified. In 24% of infants no skin lesions were present. Nine of these 15 died, and in 6 the diagnosis was made post mortem.

Varicella

Varicella is primarily a disease of young children and infection in pregnancy is uncommon. Two American studies found attack rates of 0.8 and 5.0 per 10 000 pregnancies (Siegal and Fuerst 1966; Sever and White 1968). Gershon

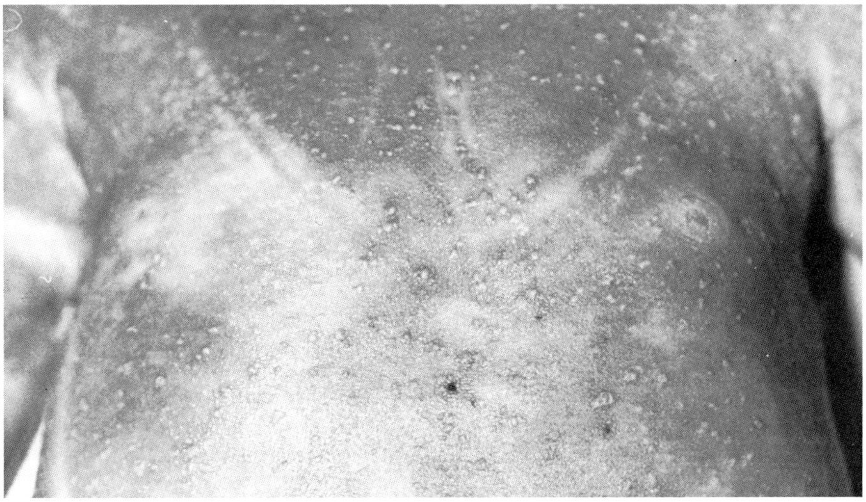

Fig. 13.2. Congenital varicella with diffuse vesicular rash; death from pneumonitis.

(1990) reviewed maternal mortality associated with gestational varicella in 118 women. Eleven deaths occurred, all amongst the 24 women (20%) who had pneumonia. He concluded that in the absence of pneumonia, chickenpox is not more serious in pregnant females than in adults in general.

There is no increase in abortion, fetal death, low birthweight, prematurity or congenital defects following varicella in pregnancy (Siegal and Fuerst 1966; Siegal et al. 1966; Parjani and Arvin 1986). There are 37 reports of similar abnormalities occurring in babies following varicella in early pregnancy. These include cicatricial skin lesions, limb hypoplasia, chorioretinitis, microphthalmia and cerebral cortical atrophy. In all but one of these cases onset of maternal infection was before the 20th week of gestation. The incidence of fetal damage following maternal varicella zoster infection is 2.3% (Preblud et al. 1986).

The outcome of varicella in late pregnancy is influenced by the onset of maternal illness in relation to delivery. The severity of neonatal disease seems to be modified by transfer of maternal antibody (Brunell 1967). Gershon (1975) found that when maternal rash appeared within 4 days of delivery and onset of infant disease was between 5 and 10 days of age, then 9 of 23 babies were seriously ill and 7 died (Fig. 13.2). When maternal infection occurred 5 or more days before delivery and the infant's rash appeared between birth and 4 days of age, all survived.

Influenza

The effect of influenza in pregnancy varies with the virulence of the infecting strain. During the pandemic of 1918–1920 when illness was complicated by pneumonia, maternal mortality was over 50% and abortion or preterm labour was common. Harris (1919) found the risk of abortion or preterm labour to be 39% following first trimester infection, 21% following second trimester illness and 25% in the third trimester. When maternal pneumonia occurred, corresponding figures were 64%, 43% and 56%. Despite high fetal losses no congenital defects were reported. Viraemia is not a feature of influenza-like infection (Monif et al. 1972)—adverse effects on the fetus must be indirect. A causal relationship between congenital defects and maternal influenza has been suggested (Coffey and Jessop 1959; Pleydell 1960; Griffiths et al. 1980). Doll et al. (1960) found no fetal effect even when illness occurred in early pregnancy. Leck's review (1963) concluded that a causal relationship between influenza and congenital malformation was unclear, particularly as defects found were common in the population. As influenza and influenza-like illness are the commonest infections in pregnancy it is surprising that if a causal relationship exists it has not been firmly established.

Symptomatic influenzal infection may be prevented during the first months of life if maternal antibodies are transferred transplacentally (Puck et al. 1980; Reumen et al. 1987).

Measles

Measles infection in adults is rare and occurs less frequently during pregnancy than chickenpox or mumps (Siegal and Fuerst 1966); preterm labour may occur. Outbreaks sometimes occur in isolated communities when first trimester infection leads to heavy fetal losses (Jesperson et al. 1977). An outbreak in Israel resulted in five preterm deliveries of low birthweight babies; none developed measles (Gazala et al. 1985). No teratogenic effect is described.

Mumps

The incidence of mumps in pregnancy in the pre-vaccine era ranged between 0.8 and 10 cases per 10 000 pregnancies (Sever and White 1968). Today it is unknown. When mumps occurs in pregnant women, illness is generally benign. First trimester disease may provoke abortion (Gershon 1990). Kurtz et al. (1982) isolated mumps virus from a 10-week spontaneous abortus after maternal infection. There is no association between gestational mumps and low birthweight (Siegal and Fuerst 1966) or malformation (Manson et al. 1960; Siegal 1973). No relationship between gestational mumps and subendocardial fibroelastosis has been convincingly demonstrated (Finland 1973).

Enteroviruses

Although transplacental passage of Coxsackie virus has been documented at term (Kibrick and Benirschke 1956; Brightman et al. 1966; Cherry et al. 1968), transmission during first and second trimesters is less clear and is documented by some workers (Burch et al. 1968) but not by others (Plager et al. 1962). Transplacentally acquired echovirus has been noted throughout pregnancy (Berkovich and Smithwick 1968; Jones et al. 1980) and transmission of poliovirus has frequently been observed late in gestation (Shelakov and Weinstein 1951; Blattner 1963) although there is little evidence for this early in pregnancy (Schaeffer et al. 1954). There is no good evidence of an association of abortion and maternal Coxsackie virus infection (Cherry 1990) or echovirus infection (Rantasalo et al. 1960; Landsman et al. 1964). Polio virus can give rise to abortion; Kaye et al. (1953) noted 19 abortions in 101 women with poliomyelitis in pregnancy. Polio virus does not appear to be teratogenic (Bates 1955; Siegal and Greenberg 1956; Horn 1955), nor does echovirus (Cherry 1990). Suggestions of a teratogenic effect of Coxsackie virus were poorly supported (Brown and Karunas 1972) but another study suggests that severe central nervous system defects may be produced (Gauntt et al. 1985).

Stillbirth may follow late Coxsackie viral (Burch et al. 1968), echoviral (Freedman 1979) and polio viral infection (Cherry 1990). The last can provoke preterm labour.

Hepatitis A Virus

Age of acquisition of antibody to hepatitis A virus (HAV) varies considerably and prevalence of antibody in young adults ranges from 3.5% in Scandinavia to 15% in the UK and 80%–90% in Italy and Spain (Mortimer 1980).

Following illness late in pregnancy, the common complication of presumed HAV infection is onset of labour (Siegal and Fuerst 1966). Several studies have provided no evidence that HAV infection in pregnancy poses a risk for either mother or fetus (Heiber et al. 1977; Schwer and Moosa 1978; Tong et al. 1981). Claims of an association between HAV infection and Down's syndrome (Stoller and Collman 1965; Pantelakis et al. 1970) have not been supported by other studies (Kucera 1970; Dietzman et al. 1972).

Hepatitis B Virus

The frequency of hepatitis B virus (HBV) infection in pregnancy is related to local prevalence. Primary infection is rare, transmission of infection during the first two trimesters is low (10%) but following acute illness in the third trimester or early postpartum period transmission of virus is high (76%) and risk of neonatal hepatitis is 50% (Schweitzer et al. 1973; Cossart 1974). Irrespective of antigen status of the neonate, a high incidence of prematurity and low birthweight occurs following acute maternal HBV infection (Schweitzer et al. 1973). Infection of the neonate occurs during parturition (Merrill 1972; Cossart 1974) and so results from exposure to antigen in utero or ingestion of blood-contaminated fluid and not from small amounts of hepatitis B surface antigen (HBsAg) in breast milk (Derso et al. 1978). Transmission of HBV from asymptomatic carrier mothers is rare in western industrialised countries but common in Taiwan and Japan (Zeldis and Crumpacker 1990). The importance of e antigen in intrapartum transmission has been confirmed by several workers (Okada et al. 1976; Lee et al. 1978). HBV may be transmitted in consecutive pregnancies and this has been associated with fatal hepatitis (Fawaz et al. 1975). The majority of infants who become HBsAg positive remain clinically healthy but are likely to be chronic carriers and may show persistently elevated alanine transferase (ALT) and histological evidence of chronic hepatitis (Zeldis and Crumpacker 1990). Although neonatal hepatitis is usually benign there are three reports of severe fatal neonatal hepatitis (Kattamis et al. 1974; Dupuy et al. 1975; Fawaz et al. 1975). Prevention of neonatal HBsAg positive hepatitis involves prompt immunisation of infants of carrier mothers with HBsAg vaccine plus high titre hepatitis B immunoglobin at birth (Maupas et al. 1981; Zeldis and Crumpacker 1990).

Hepatitis C Virus

Vertical transmission of hepatitis C virus (HCV) from infected mothers to their children has been documented. Using a PCR technique HCV RNA was found in 8 neonates delivered by seropositive mothers. Antibody persisted for 2–19 months. In 7 infants antibody cleared by 9 months of age and then remained undetectable. Serum ALT was raised in 3 infants (Thaler et al. 1991).

Hepatitis D and E

Hepatitis D virus is a defective agent which requires coinfection with HBV before it can replicate. It has a worldwide distribution and has been shown to have been in existence for some 60 years (Buitrago et al. 1986). Incidence of transmission and clinical consequences of infection in the newborn are currently being determined (Zeldis and Crumpacker 1990).

Hepatitis E is the main cause of enterically transmitted, non-A non-B hepatitis, occurring in both epidemic and sporadic forms, and generally associated with sewage-contaminated drinking water. Outbreaks have affected mainly young and middle-aged adults with a very high mortality (20%–39%) in infected pregnant women (Zuckerman 1990).

Parvovirus

Adverse effects of parvovirus B19 in pregnancy were first noted by Brown et al. (1984) and Knott et al. (1984). Since then some 20–30 fetal deaths have been documented where fetal tissue contained B19 DNA (Centre for Disease Control 1989; Morey et al. 1992). An aborted fetus with eye abnormalities was reported (Weiland et al. 1987) but its relationship to parvoviral infection was tenuous. The virus replicates in erythroid progenitor cells (Caul et al. 1988), inhibiting maturation, and the resulting anaemia produces heart failure, hydrops and death (Anderson 1990). Virus has been demonstrated in fetal myocardial cells (Porter et al. 1988) and circulating leucocytes (Kurtzman et al. 1988) by in situ hybridisation. A Public Health Laboratory Service (PHLS) working party on Fifth Disease serologically documented B19 infection in 190 pregnant women of whom 168 (91%) had a rash. Fifty per cent had arthralgia or arthritis, upper respiratory tract symptoms or general malaise. Half of the 16 women with no rash experienced joint and respiratory symptoms, 6 were asymptomatic (PHLS 1990). Of these women 168 elected to continue pregnancy and 156 (84%) delivered a normal baby. Follow-up of 114 infants to 1 year of age showed no abnormalities although serological evidence of intrauterine infection was present in 27. Total fetal loss rate was 16%, similar to that in an uninfected antenatal sample, but there was a marked excess of second trimester fetal loss in infected women. Risk of fetal death from parvovirus infection was 9% and transplacental transmission of virus 30%. Therapeutic termination of pregnancy following maternal infection is not indicated (PHLS 1990).

Human Immunodeficiency Virus

Human immunodeficiency virus (HIV_1) infection in infants and children is relatively recent and the natural history of HIV-related disease in children is still evolving. Maternal risk factors include origin from high incidence areas, history of intravenous drug use, consort with known risk factors, multiple partners or multiple blood transfusions (Falloon and Pizzo 1990). In the UK, anonymous HIV testing of pregnant women showed the prevalence to be 1:515 in inner London, 1:1440 in the remaining Thames regions, and 1:16000 in another NHS region (PHLS 1991).

Early reports suggested that HIV may be transmitted from mother to offspring by transplacental passage, intrapartum exposure to infected blood or secretions or postnatal exposure to breast milk (Cowan et al. 1984; Lapointe et al. 1985; Jovaisas et al. 1985). The mode of vertical transmission is still unknown but early onset of clinical and immunological abnormalities in 80%–90% of infected children suggests that intrauterine transmission is likely (European Collaborative Study (ECS) 1991). However rapid onset of HIV-related illness has also been reported in children infected by transfusion at birth (Saulsbury 1987). The ECS reports a vertical transmission rate of 12.9%. This is lower than that found in other studies, which varied from 27% in France to 39% in Zambia.

Scott et al. (1985) showed that preterm delivery and maternal symptoms in pregnancy were common. Infectivity is persistent with transmission of infection to later-born infants. Two African studies have suggested that babies of women with AIDS or symptomless HIV infection are of lower birthweight than those of seronegative mothers (Hira et al. 1989; Ryder et al. 1989). This has not been confirmed (Johnstone et al. 1988; Selwyn et al. 1989) and it is likely that low birthweights reflect differences in maternal health or socioeconomic status rather than intrauterine infection.

In the ECS, clinical findings in the perinatal period did not discriminate between infected and uninfected infants. There was no excess of congenital abnormalities and HIV dysmorphic syndrome was not seen, unlike other studies (Marion et al. 1986, 1987). In the European study HIV-related signs and symptoms were oral candidiasis or any two of lymphadenopathy, hepatomegaly or splenomegaly, concurrent and persisting for more than 2 months. Signs and symptoms associated with HIV infection are shown in Table 13.4. Encephalopathy and other neurological abnormalities were uncommon in children in the pre-AIDS period (ECS 1991). Sixty-four per cent of the 64 antibody-positive children showed some features of HIV by 3 months of age, increasing to 83% by 6 months, and 90% by 12 months of age. Thirty per cent developed AIDS within 6 months. AIDS-related infections appeared at 2–3 months of age in 6 of 17 children who developed AIDS or died of HIV-related illness in the first 12 months of life.

Parasitic Infection

Toxoplasma Gondii

Acquisition of *T. gondii* follows consumption of infected undercooked meat or exposure to oocysts in cat excreta or infected soil. Most infections are asymptomatic or result in a mild influenza-like illness. Antibody studies in different populations show marked differences in antibody status in pregnant women. In Paris prevalence of toxoplasma antibody rose from 80% in the 15–19 year age group to 95% at 30–34 years. Corresponding differences in New York were from 16%–40% and in London from 15%–34% (Desmonts and Couvreur 1974). Data collected in 1985 in an EEC Co-operative Study showed a prevalence of 21% in women of western origin in London, similar to that found previously, whilst in Paris the prevalence had dropped to 72%. The prevalence in Stuttgart and Padua was 36% and 56% respectively (Remington and Desmonts 1990). The decrease in France may result from changes in eating habits or to differences in animal husbandry.

Infection during pregnancy accompanied by parasitaemia can lead to placental infection. Transmission to the fetus occurs in 45% of affected pregnancies (Desmonts and Couvreur 1979). Infection in early pregnancy can cause abortion. Its status as a cause of recurrent abortion was reviewed by Remington (1973) who found it possible in chronically infected women but considered it was not a significant cause of abortion or perinatal loss. Prospective studies in France indicate that the risk to the fetus is greatest when maternal infection occurs in the third trimester, with 59% transmission compared with 14% and 29% for infection in the first and second trimesters (Desmonts and Couvreur 1974). Severe neonatal manifestations are not usually seen with third trimester infection but occur in 80% of infants following first trimester disease and 30% of second

Table 13.4. Signs and symptoms associated with HIV infection (European Collaborative Study 1991)

Sign/symptom	Infected pre-AIDS	Presumed uninfected	Rate ratio	p
Oral candidosis*	13	2	51.5	<0.001
Parotitis	7	2	28.0	<0.001
Petechiae	2	1	15.1	0.02
Eczcma	12	33	2.9	0.002
Unexplained fever	9	11	6.5	<0.001
Diarrhoea†	20	47	4.0	<0.001
Bronchitis/bronchiolitis	3	28	0.8	0.6
Gram-negative septicaemia/ septicaemia > 1 month's duration	7	0		<0.001
Gram-negative pneumonia	4	2	15.4	0.001
Other pneumonia	13	21	5.3	<0.001
Chronic otitis media	6	18	2.5	0.03
Chronic purulent rhinitis	10	44	1.8	0.06
Encephalopathy	1	0		0.1
Other abnormal neurology*‡	2	5	3.0	0.2
Failure to thrive§	2	3	4.9	0.08
Lymphadenopathy*¶	33	44	9.6	<0.001
Hepatomegaly*	37	54	9.5	<0.001
Splenomegaly*	27	16	17.4	<0.001
Hyper IgG‖	40	8	90.8	<0.001
Hyper IgA‖	16	5	35.0	<0.001
Hyper IgM‖	10	5	20.5	<0.001
Low T4/T8**	32	15	22.0	<0.001
No. of children	64	343		
No. of years of observation	102.5	753.1		
No. of examinations	441	2566		

No. of children with at least one episode for each sign and symptom.

* On 2 consecutive examinations at least 2 months apart.

† Persisting > 21 days.

‡ Abnormal reflexes or gait, seizures, paresis.

§ Fall of >1.0 in weight for age SD score to <−2.5, or >0.5 to <−3.0.

¶ On at least 2 sites, bilaterally.

‖ >125% of upper reference level for age; in 2 consecutive samples at least 1 month apart.

** In 2 consecutive samples at least 1 month apart; below reference level R—R = 1.2 − A/100 if $0 < A < 20$, and R = 1.0 if $A \geqslant 20$ where A is age in months.

trimester infections (Desmonts and Couvreur 1974). The incidence of congenital toxoplasmosis is uncertain; it has been estimated at 1–2 per 1000 births in the USA (Stagno 1980), 1 in 2000 in France (Desmonts and Couvreur 1979) and 1 in 5–10 000 births in the UK (Fleck 1979). A survey of congenital toxoplasmosis in the UK between 1975 and 1980 (Hall 1983) suggests a lower incidence; infection was confirmed in only 13 of 91 babies and a further 20 infections were postnatally acquired. Prevalence data for congenital toxoplasmosis in the UK are poor. Discrepancy exists between the 13 annual cases reported to the Communicable Disease Surveillance Centre (CDSC) and the prediction of 40–50 damaged infants derived from extrapolation of French data (PHLS 1990). There are probably 300 infected but asymptomatic babies each year who later develop chorioretinitis. Recent results from Swansea and Scotland give a primary infection rate of 2 per 1000 pregnant women (Joynson and Payne 1988).

The majority of newborns are asymptomatic. Overt disease at birth is recognised in only 10%–20% (Alford et al. 1974; Desmonts and Couvreur 1979). Severe neonatal manifestations are low birthweight, jaundice, hepatomegaly, thrombocytopenia, meningoencephalitis and hydrocephalus. Hydrocephalus, intracranial calcification and chorioretinitis constitute the "classic triad" of congenital toxoplasmosis. Although asymptomatic at birth, many have CSF abnormalities. Careful follow-up of these infants is required as damage to eyes, ears or brain may develop (Stagno and Whitley 1977b). Long-term assessment revealed that 85% of infected newborns developed late sequelae (Wilson et al. 1980).

Malaria

Prenatally acquired malaria is rare among the indigenous population of malarial areas despite heavy infestation of the placenta (Ransome-Kuti 1972). It is found more frequently in infants of non-immune women who contract malaria during pregnancy (Covell 1950). Occasional reports from non-malarial countries involve travellers or immigrants (Hindi and Azimi 1980; Quinn et al. 1982). Loss of anti-malarial immunity during pregnancy, particularly in primipara, has been suggested (Wyler 1983). The incidence of abortion is inversely proportional to the degree of maternal immunity (Ransome-Kuti 1972). Placental infection is often associated with severe maternal anaemia, an increased risk of preterm labour, fetal growth retardation and low birthweight (Reinhardt 1980). A malarial eradication scheme in the British Solomon Islands resulted in a fall in the proportion of infants less than 2500 g birthweight (MacGregor and Avery 1974). Symptoms of congenital infection, fever, anaemia and splenomegaly are present in more than 80% of cases. Reticulocytosis is common, jaundice and hyperbilirubinaemia are seen in one-third of cases, hepatomegaly is less frequent (Arvin et al. 1990).

Mycoplasma and Chlamydia

Mycoplasmas have been linked with spontaneous abortion for 20 years but their adverse role in pregnancy is still unclear (Kundsin and Driscoll 1970). They are recovered with equal frequency from both pregnant and non-pregnant women (Eschenbach 1977). In a prospective study, *Mycoplasma hominis* was isolated most frequently from women who experienced threatened abortion whilst the prevalence of other micro-organisms was similar in all groups (Munday et al. 1984). In high-risk pregnancies compared with normal pregnancies, isolation of *M. hominis* was significantly higher where prolonged membrane rupture, spontaneous abortion, stillbirth or early neonatal death occurred (Embree et al. 1980). This study recovered *Ureaplasma urealyticum* but not *M. hominis* in the high-risk group. It was associated with intrauterine growth retardation, prematurity and low birthweight. Some studies found maternal colonisation was associated with lower infant birthweight (Klein et al. 1969; Foy et al. 1970; Dimusto et al. 1973). This was not supported by Naessens et al. (1983). Both *M. hominis* and *U. urealyticum* have been isolated more frequently from couples with pregnancy loss than from those with successful outcome (Quinn et al. 1983). Detailed serological investigations suggested that certain ureaplasma serotypes may be more pathogenic than others.

Chlamydia trachomatis is a common sexually transmitted pathogen. Cervical colonisation in pregnant women varies with race and social class; rates between 2% and 47% have been found in the USA and Sweden (Rettig 1988). UK studies found marked variation in infection, from 7% in pregnant women in urban Liverpool (Wood et al. 1984) to zero amongst higher social class women (Ross et al. 1981). No relationship was found between the isolation of *C. trachomatis* and abortion (Munday et al. 1984). It may be related to preterm delivery and perinatal death (Martin et al. 1982) particularly when IgM antibody is present (Harrison et al. 1983). Association between maternal colonisation and infection in the neonate is well established. Risk has been summarised by Rettig (1988). Schachter et al. (1986) found 4.7% of pregnant women to be chlamydia positive and 60% of their infants showed serological evidence of infection: chlamydiae were isolated from 36%. Culture-positive pneumonia was diagnosed in 16% and conjunctivitis found in 18%.

Bacterial Infection

Bacterial infection of mother and baby is the most frequent type of infection. Acquisition of organisms is usually from the genital tract via the ascending route, particularly following prolonged rupture of membranes. Transplacental transfer occurs during haematogenous infection. Bacteria gain access during vaginal delivery or as a result of direct innoculation into the gestation sac during amniocentesis or intrauterine transfusion.

Ascending Bacterial Infection

Ascending bacterial infection is far more common than infection via other routes. The organisms involved are commensal flora of the vagina and intestine. Although a common association of midtrimester abortion, prolonged rupture of membrane, preterm labour and neonatal infection, there is little population-based information about the incidence of ascending infection. Epidemiological studies are hampered by ethical considerations, lack of specific serological markers and contamination of samples for culture (Blanc 1981). Ascending bacterial infection is responsible, directly or indirectly, for much perinatal mortality (Naeye 1979).

Maternal Bacteriuria and Pyelonephritis

Bacteriuria complicates 2%–5% of pregnancies (Savage et al. 1967). Variation occurs with age and social class (Norden and Kass 1968) and rates in pregnant women are similar to those in non-pregnant women of similar age. Kass (1960) found that birthweight less than 2500 g fell from 24% in women with asymptomatic bacteriuria to 10% after eradication of infection. In London and Birmingham, prematurity was 12.9% in untreated bacteriuric patients but in treated women was 6.7% (Williams et al. 1978). An American study (Sever et al. 1978) showed that symptomatic bacterial pyelonephritis in pregnancy was strongly associated with preterm delivery and high infant mortality. In 1982, Kass found that women with symptomatic bacteriuria experienced high rates of symptomatic pyelonephritis as well as increased low birthweight and perinatal mortality. These infections are preventable by screening and treatment during pregnancy.

Syphilis and Gonorrhoea

Treponema pallidum readily crosses the placenta. Antenatal screening has dramatically reduced the number of cases of congenital syphilis. In the UK only 17 cases below the age of 2 years were notified in Special Clinic Returns over 4 years to 1986.

In the US the incidence of congenital syphilis has steadily increased during the past decade, now 1 in 10 000 liveborn infants is affected (Centre for Disease Control 1988). They are usually the offspring of deprived women with no prenatal care and, in some, substance abuse is a significant factor (Ricci et al. 1989). Syphilitic infection of the fetus can occur at any stage of pregnancy. Formerly it was thought rare in early pregnancy but organisms have been demonstrated in first trimester villi by immunofluorescence (Epstein and King 1985). Abortion is uncommon but a Florida study found that 34% of infants with congenital syphilis were stillborn. Preterm labour and premature rupture of membranes were more common in infected pregnancies. Twenty-one per cent of infants were growth retarded (Ricci et al. 1989). Prenatal haematogenous spread results in disseminated disease. In the perinatal period the earliest signs of syphilis are rhinitis, snuffles, skin and vascular lesions (Ingall et al. 1990). Osteochondritis and perichondritis are often widespread. Hepatomegaly, thrombocytopenia and jaundice are common. If untreated, survivors develop interstitial keratitis, neurosyphilis and nerve deafness (Fiumara and Lessell 1970).

Figures for the incidence of *Neisseria gonorrhoea* infection in the UK are not available: about half of infected women are asymptomatic. Untreated pregnancies are complicated by preterm delivery (13%–67%), fetal distress (5%–10%), perinatal death (2%–11%) (Gutman and Holmes 1990).

After birth, ophthalmia neonatorum presents at 2–5 days of age. Twenty to 40 cases per annum are reported to the CDSC; this has remained constant since 1975.

Listeria Monocytogenes

Listeria is widely distributed in animals and the environment. Most cases of listeriosis are sporadic but in the 1980s, community outbreaks occurred in Canada, USA and Europe (Gill 1988) and were food related. The organism is often carried asymptomatically; up to 70% of the population are short-term carriers (Kampelmacher and Van Noorle Jansen 1972). In Scotland *L. monocytogenes* was isolated from the faeces of only 1 in 54 pregnant women and 1 in 60 non-pregnant women (Lamont and Postlethwaite 1986). In the UK between 1983 and 1986 laboratories reported 115–149 cases. In 1988 this increased to 291 (5.8 per million population) and pregnancy-related cases were 14 per 100 000 total births. A similar rate was detected in the US in 1986 by active surveillance in five states (Schuchat et al. 1991). In 1990 in England and Wales the rate fell to 2.3 per million and pregnancy-related disease was 3.6 per 100 000 total births (Newton et al. 1990); fluctuation involved pregnancy-associated disease and serotype 4 infection. Maternal listerial bacteraemia may be asymptomatic or produce a flu-like illness. Abortion occurs and it is suggested that up to 6% of abortions in East Germany and France are caused by listeriosis (Seeliger and Finger 1983). Neonatal listeriosis may be of early or late onset. Early onset disease presents as stillbirth, generalised sepsis at or shortly after birth, and results from transplacental spread (PHLS 1990). Late-onset disease typically presents at 3–7 days of life and meningitis is common (Spencer 1987). Infection is acquired from the mother intrapartum or postpartum or by nosocomial spread in the nursery (McLaughlin et al. 1986).

Infection in the Neonate

Introduction

Risk of infection in the neonatal period is greater than at any other time of life. A minority of infections result from sepsis acquired in utero. More frequently, neonatal infection results from exposure to microbes during passage through the birth canal or from attendants during the first weeks of life. The usual route of acquisition of a range of organisms is shown in Table 13.5. Congenital infection may give rise to classic signs and symptoms which are immediately apparent at birth. Usually, clinical signs are non-specific such as growth retardation, prolonged jaundice or failure to thrive. Occasionally, the baby appears normal. Neonatal sepsis may develop during the first few hours or days of life. Early infection is usually caused by maternally derived organisms; late-onset disease comes from attendants, other babies or the environment. Neonates requiring intensive care are at risk of nosocomial infection from invasive monitoring procedures or therapy.

The normal fetus is sterile until shortly before birth, as long as the placental membranes remain intact. After birth the neonate rapidly acquires commensal bacteria which colonise the skin, mucous membranes and the gastrointestinal tract. Rotimi and Duerden (1981) studied the acquisition of bacterial flora in neonates and found that *streptococcus viridans* and *Streptococcus salivarius* were present in the mouth from 8 h after birth and that *Staphylococcus aureus* was the predominant species isolated from the umbilicus (21.7% on day 1, rising to 87% by day 6). These authors provided valuable data on the acquisition of bowel flora, demonstrating that the predominant organisms by the end of the first week were anaerobes. Clostridia were isolated in 78.3% of cases by day 6. They isolated Enterobacteriaceae in 52% of neonates on the second day of life, in 70% by day 3 and in 83% by day 6. The sequence of acquisition of faecal flora in the neonate is shown in Table 13.6.

Table 13.5. Routes of transmission of some organisms known to cause fetal and neonatal infection

Infection	Transplacental	Ascending	Intrapartum	Postpartum
Rubella	+			
CMV	+		±	±
Herpes simplex	$\pm\!\!\!\!-$	±	+	±
Toxoplasma	+			
Syphilis	+		±	
Listeria	+		+	+
Group B streptococcus		+	+	±

+, usual mode; ±, occasional mode; $\pm\!\!\!\!-$, rare.

Table 13.6. Development of neonatal faecal flora during the first 6 days of life in 23 neonates (Rotimi and Duerden 1981)

Bacterial group	Number of neonates colonised by the given bacteria on			
	day 1	day 2	day 3	day 6
Enterobacteria	0	12	16	19
Enterococci	1	21	23	23
Pseudomonads	0	0	0	1
Streptococci	2	4	4	8
Staphylococci	6	17	17	11
Non-sporing anaerobes				
Gram-negative rods	0	7	14	18
Gram-positive rods	0	17	22	23
Clostridia	0	6	16	18
Anaerobic cocci	0	3	8	12

Bacterial colonisation of the neonate must be distinguished from infection but colonisation may proceed to invasion of both superficial and deep sites.

Congenital Infection

Neonates with congenital infection usually have non-specific signs or symptoms, failure to thrive or intrauterine growth retardation. Occasionally, findings are so specific that they suggest the nature of the infection. Clinical features commonly associated with rubella and toxoplasma infections are detailed in Tables 13.7 and 13.8. Those associated with congenital CMV infection are shown in Table 13.4. Diagnosis of congenital infection during life is usually made using a combination of serological tests on both maternal and infant sera; specific IgM antibodies are sought in the neonate after maternal serum screening (Holliman 1990), although in toxoplasmosis, up to 30% of affected infants lack a demonstrable IgM response (Desmonts et al. 1981).

Viruses may be cultured from samples of saliva, nasopharyngeal aspirate or urine obtained during life, but may take several weeks for a positive result to be obtained. HSV and varicella can be demonstrated rapidly in the vesicle fluid by electron microscopy.

Demonstration of cytopathic effects of organisms causing congenital infection has been made much easier and more reliable with the advent of molecular biological techniques and immunohistochemistry. They enable large or multiple samples to be screened rapidly. This is important when relatively few cells have characteristic inclusions, which is the case when initial infection occurred weeks or months previously.

Necropsy examination may reveal features which are typical or suggestive of a particular infection but routine sampling of all organs for histological examination may be diagnostic

Table 13.7. Clinical aspects of congenital rubella (Hanshaw et al. 1985a)

General
Intrauterine growth retardation; spontaneous abortion; stillbirth; small for gestational age; failure to thrive; increase in neonatal and infant mortality; slow development in infancy and early childhood

Ocular
Cataracts; pigmentary retinopathy; microphthalmus; glaucoma; cloudy cornea; macular degeneration of the retina; iris hypoplasia; strabismus

Cardiovascular lesions
Persistent ductus arteriosus (PDA); PDA and pulmonary arterial lesions; pulmonary arterial lesions: (1) hypoplasia of artery, (2) supravalvular stenosis, (3) valvular stenosis, (4) peripheral branch stenosis; renal artery stenosis; ? cerebrovascular stenosis; aortic stenosis; ventricular septal defects and tetralogy of Fallot; myocardial damage; neonatal myocarditis

Auditory
Sensorineural deafness; central auditory imperception; deafness with speech defects, with or without mental retardation; ? delayed speech with normal hearing and intelligence

Central nervous system
Microcephaly; full anterior fontanelle; meningoencephalitis; mental retardation; lethargy; hypotonia; irritability; unreactive, hypotonic infant; late onset of irritability and hypotonia; late onset of convulsions and "meningitis"; progressive panencephalitis; autism

Visceral
Hepatosplenomegaly; hepatitis and jaundice

Haematological
Neonatal thrombocytopenic purpura; anaemia; haemolytic anaemia

Osseous
Osteopathy; lack of calcification of osteoid

Pulmonary
Interstitial pneumonitis

Immunological
Chronic rubelliform rash; thymic hypoplasia; dysgammaglobulinaemia; circulating immune complexes

Miscellaneous
Adenopathy; thymic hypoplasia; hypogammaglobulinaemia; recurrent or persistent infections; chronic diarrhoea; growth hormone deficiency; diabetes mellitus; dermatoglyphic abnormalities; hypothyroidism

Table 13.8. Signs and symptoms observed in the newborn period in a prospective study of 108 infants born to women who acquired toxoplasmosis during pregnancy (adapted from Remington and Desmonts 1983)

Finding	No. examined	Percentage positive
Prematurity	108	10.2
Intrauterine growth retardation	108	2.7
Postmaturity	108	8.3
Jaundice	107	11.2
Hepatosplenomegaly	108	4.6
Thrombocytopenic purpura	108	1.8
Abnormal blood count	105	4.8
Microcephaly	108	8.3
Hydrocephalus	108	3.7
Hypotonia	108	6.5
Convulsions	108	4.6
Psychomotor retardation	108	4.6
Intracranial calcifications	108	15.5
Abnormal EEG	95	8.4
Abnormal CSF	94	68.0
Microphthalmia	108	3.7
Strabismus	108	8.3
Chorioretinitis	108	24.9

when congenital infection was previously unsuspected. Immunohistochemistry or in situ hybridisation is particularly helpful here; although CMV inclusions are usually readily apparent other viral inclusions are not so striking and can easily be missed.

Syphilis in the Fetus and Newborn

Congenital syphilis presents as fetal hydrops (see Chap. 11), unexplained stillbirth or neonatal hepatosplenomegaly with or without jaundice. The differential diagnosis includes the TORCH agents. The stillborn syphilitic infant is often macerated with a protuberant abdomen. Any dermal bullous or vesicular lesions contain large numbers of treponemes. Hepatomegaly with fibrosis and persistent extramedullary haemopoiesis is present. Wright and Berry (1974) used silver stains to demonstrate large numbers of treponemes even in histologically normal liver. The spleen may also be enlarged. Obliterative pulmonary fibrosis is rare whilst pancreatitis is often severe. In the kidney, glomerular injury caused by immune complex deposition may be present. Meningeal involvement is commonly found around the brain stem and optic chiasma. Syphilitic endocarditis may be present. Widespread skeletal involvement is characteristic with osteochrondritis, periostitis and osteomyelitis of long bones or ribs. Anaemia is common and severe when the fetus is hydropic.

Diagnosis is by demonstration of treponemes by dark-ground microscopy of fluid from cutaneous lesions, or specific silver staining of tissue sections. Fetal and maternal serological investigations should include a quantitative cardiolipin test (Venereal Disease Research Laboratory (VDRL)) with confirmation of positive results by a fluorescent treponemal antibody (FTA) test. In infants the VDRL is normally less than or equal to that in maternal serum. An infant's VDRL titre more than four times higher than the maternal level is strongly suggestive of congenital disease. Presence of FTA IgG may reflect passive maternal transfer of antibody but the presence of FTA IgM in infant serum is consistent with congenital infection. The test for specific IgM in serum is useful but can give false positive cross-reactions with other IgM and false negatives if maternal IgG is very high (PHLS 1990).

Bacterial Infection

Two distinct patterns of disease occur in neonatal septicaemia and meningitis. Early onset infection presents in the first 4 days of life and is likely when the infecting organism is either virulent or present in large numbers. Obstetric complications, prematurity and low birthweight are common. Organisms are acquired from the birth canal during delivery and mortality is high (15%–50%) (Klein and Marcy 1990). Sepsis may be apparent at birth or appear within a few hours. Clinical signs are non-specific and include tachycardia or bradycardia, tachypnoea, apnoea and poor peripheral perfusion. Pneumonia is frequent (Davies and Gothefors 1984).

Late-onset disease may present as early as 5 days of life but is more commonly recognised after 7 days. Infecting organisms may be maternal in origin or derived from the neonate's own flora, altered by frequent handling, exposure to antibiotics and invasive neonatal care.

Between 1977 and 1987 laboratory reports of neonatal bacteraemia made to the CDSC increased threefold.

Table 13.9. Neonatal septicaemia: Gram-negative organisms. Reports to the CDSC 1988–1990

Year	Bacteraemia (annual total)	*E. coli*		*Klebsiella/ Enterobacter*		*Pseudomonas ae*/ species*		*Salmonella/* other coliforms	
		n	%	*n*	%	*n*	%	*n*	%
1988	720	101	(14)	37	(5)	15/14	(4)	3/12	(2)
1989	1102	134	(12)	84	(7)	20/13	(3)	4/28	(2)
1990	1082	159	(15)	59	(5)	15/11	(2)	4/20	(2)

n, number of cases per annum. *ae* aeruginosa*
( ) % of total annual neonatal septicaemia.
Other included: *Acinetobacter* sp., *Citrobacter, Achromobacter, Alkaligenes, Agrobacter-Radiobacter, Flavobacter* sp. (Total Gram-negative rods = 25%–26% of all episodes.)

Neonatal Septicaemia

Gram-negative Aerobic Bacteria

During a 3-year period 1988–1990, Gram-negative bacteria were isolated in one-quarter of cases of neonatal septicaemia reported to CDSC. *Escherichia coli* was the most frequent isolate (Table 13.9). Pseudomonas sepsis was detected in 2%–4% of bacteraemia; 39%–48% of these strains were of environmental origin.

About 36% of strains of *E. coli* isolated from neonates with septicaemia and 75% of strains causing neonatal meningitis carry the K_1 capsular antigen (McCracken et al. 1974; Robbins et al. 1974). Mortality in infants with meningitis caused by K_1 strains was higher than that caused by non-K_1 strains. Severity of disease was directly related to presence, amount and persistence of K_1 antigen in the CSF (Mulder et al. 1984). Colonisation with K_1 strains occurs in pregnancy and most are maternal in origin (Sarff et al. 1975).

Assisted ventilation and antibiotics in sick neonates favours colonisation with resistant Gram-negative flora and superinfection. In our neonatal surgical unit, Gram-negative organisms accounted for 16% of 75 septicaemic episodes over 33 months. *E. coli* was the most common pathogen followed by organisms of the *Klebsiella, Enterobacter* and *Citrobacter* groups.

Gram-positive Aerobic Bacteria

Maternal group B streptococcal colonisation is a risk factor for neonatal disease (Ancona et al. 1980). Anorectal and genital carriage of group B streptococci in pregnant women is about 25% in the UK (Easmon and Hastings 1985). Ethnic differences exist: carriage rates are lower among Asians and higher among women of Afro-Caribbean origin. In early-onset group B streptococcal disease, septicaemia and pneumonia occur in about 40% of cases and meningitis in 30%. Respiratory distress is frequent whether pneumonia is present or not and may be clinically and radiologically indistinguishable from hyaline membrane disease (Baker and Edwards 1990). Early-onset disease has a case fatality rate between 20% and 50%. Early infection may affect mature babies but tends to involve low birthweight preterm infants. Heavy maternal vaginal colonisation with the organism (Ancona et al. 1980), prolonged rupture of membranes and absence of protective IgG antibody (Boyer et al. 1984) are common. The same bacterial strains are isolated from the maternal genital tract and from infant nose and skin (Stringer et al. 1981).

Late-onset disease (5 days to 3 months) is not associated with prematurity or obstetric factors. Septicaemia is accompanied by meningitis, the presenting sign in 85% of cases. Infection is predominantly associated with serotype III organisms and low levels of type III antibody are found in both infants and mothers (Baker et al. 1981). Mortality is lower than in early-onset disease.

A review of isolates from cases of neonatal bacteraemia in the UK reported to the CDSC between 1988 and 1990 showed that group B streptococci were commonest (Tables 13.9, 13.10, 13.11).

Listeria monocytogenes is a less frequent cause of septicaemia (Table 13.10); 84 cases were reported from 1988 to 1990. Early-onset disease contributes about 80% of cases. Fulminating listeriosis may be present at birth, a skin rash with vesicles (focal granulomata) may be present. These are also found in the pharynx. Meningitis, meningoencephalitis or brain abscess all occur. Gram-positive organisms

Table 13.10. Neonatal septicaemia: Group B streptococcus and *Listeria monocytogenes*. Reports to the CDSC 1988–90

Year	Bacteraemia (annual total)	Group B Streptococcus *n*	%	*L. monocytogenes* *n*	%
1988	720	131	(18)	26	(4)
1989	1102	219	(20)	46	(4)
1990	1082	221	(20)	12	(1)

n, number of cases per annum.

are demonstrable within granulomata. *Staphylococcus aureus* and *Staph. epidermidis* caused acute bacteraemia in 11%–13% and 14%–18% of cases of neonatal sepsis between 1988 and 1990 (Table 13.11). Systemic *Staph. aureus* infection or toxin-mediated skin disease may follow umbilical sepsis. Skin sepsis is seen, from pustules and paronychia to mastitis or postoperative wound infection. If not treated promptly, *Staph. aureus* bacteraemia can result in septic arthritis, osteomyelitis, endocarditis, meningitis and cerebral abscess. *Staph. epidermidis* is now the second most frequently isolated organism in neonatal bacteraemia reported to the CDSC and is almost always associated with colonisation and vascular cannulation in infants in intensive care.

Table 13.11. Neonatal septicaemia: *Staphylococcus aureus* and coagulase-negative staphylococci. Reports to the CDSC 1988–1990

Year	Bacteraemia (annual total)	*Staph. aureus* *n*	%	Coagulase negatives *n*	%
1988	720	95	(13)	132	(18)
1989	1102	119	(11)	155	(14)
1990	1082	123	(11)	180	(17)

n, number of cases per annum.

Anaerobic Septicaemia

Anaerobic septicaemia is uncommon in newborns in the UK and usually follows gastrointestinal surgery. From 1988 to 1990, these organisms caused 2%–3% of cases of neonatal septicaemia. *Bacteroides* species (predominantly *B. fragilis*) and *Clostridium* species were most frequently isolated.

Infection with β haemolytic streptococci (Groups A, C, G) is uncommon in the newborn period (8–13 cases per annum).

Other Organisms

There was only one case of *Neisseria meningitidis* infection noted during the 3-year period 1988–1990 whilst 20–40 cases of *Streptococcus pneumoniae* were noted and 10–20 cases of *Haemophilus influenzae* were reported each year, accounting for 5%–6% of neonatal septicaemia. During this 3-year period between 5 and 30 cases of fungal sepsis were reported (0.8%–3% of septicaemia). Isolates were predominantly *Candida albicans*. This is likely to be a serious underestimate of neonatal fungal infection which is often unsuspected and becomes apparent at necropsy. Fungal sepsis nearly always occurs following protracted antibiotic therapy in sick, preterm infants. Multiple breaches of mucocutaneous surfaces by venous, arterial and bladder catheters are contributory factors. If not promptly treated, candidaemia produces multiple abscesses and occasionally endocarditis (Figs. 13.3, 13.4).

Neonatal Meningitis

Meningitis in neonates is a life-threatening condition with a high mortality. It complicates one-third of cases of bacteraemia in infants and is more likely when more than 1000 colony-forming units of infecting organisms per millilitre are recovered from blood cultures (Dietzman et al. 1974). Two-thirds of cases of meningitis are associated with bacteraemia (Klein and Marcy 1976). Babies with malformations such as meningomyelocoele or congenital dermal sinus are vulnerable. Goldacre (1976) found that bacterial meningitis was more common in the first week and month of life than at any other time. The incidence of neonatal meningitis was 0.2 per 1000 livebirths, 43% were fatal.

In a review of meningitis in infants under 1 year in England and Wales, De Louvois et al. (1991) found infection in 423 neonates, an incidence of 0.32 per 1000; 19.8% were fatal. Post-neonatal fatality was 5.4%. Mortality was higher in neonates with positive CSF cultures than in those with CSF pleocytosis only. Ventriculitis, hydrocephalus or convulsions were complications of 33% of infected newborns, and 5% relapsed after treatment. Causative organisms are shown in Table 13.12. Group B streptococci were found in 28% of

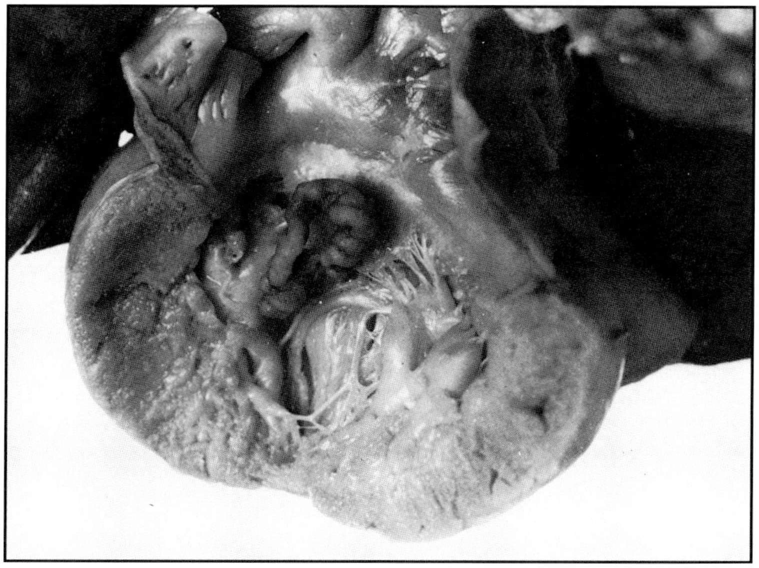

Fig. 13.3. Endocarditis with vegetations composed of *Candida albicans* mycelium in a pretern baby following chronic vascular cannulation. (Courtesy of Dr. S.A.S. Knowles, Adelaide)

cases, *E. coli* were documented in 18% and *L. monocytogenes* and *Strep. pneumoniae* in 5% each. Viruses were isolated in 4% of cases. A wide range of organisms was associated with neonatal disease. *Neisseria meningitidis*, *H. influenzae* and *Strep. pneumoniae* together account for only 10% of neonatal sepsis, whereas in post-neonatal infants these bacteria were associated with 70% of infections.

Table 13.12. Meningitis in neonates in England and Wales 1985–1987

Causative organism	Number of reports
Group B β haemolytic streptococci	118 (28)
Escherichia coli	78 (18)
Listeria monocytogenes	23 (5)
Haemophilus influenzae	9 (2)
Neisseria meningitidis	11 (3)
Streptococcus pneumoniae	19 (5)
Other Gram-positive bacteria	15 (4)
Other Gram-negative bacteria	28 (7)
Viruses	16 (4)
Mycoplasma hominis	3 (<1)
Candida albicans	4 (1)
Other microorganisms	5 (1)
Cerebrospinal fluid sterile or not collected	92 (22)
Unknown	2 (<1)
Total	423

Adapted from de Louvois et al. 1991.
Figures in parenthesis are % of total number of reports.

Respiratory Tract Infection

Klein (1990) found the incidence of pneumonia at perinatal necropsies was 15%–38% in stillbirths and 20%–32% in liveborn infants. Incidence was similar in preterm and mature babies. Bacterial species responsible were vaginal flora.

Early-onset group B streptococcal disease is often clinically indistinguishable from hyaline

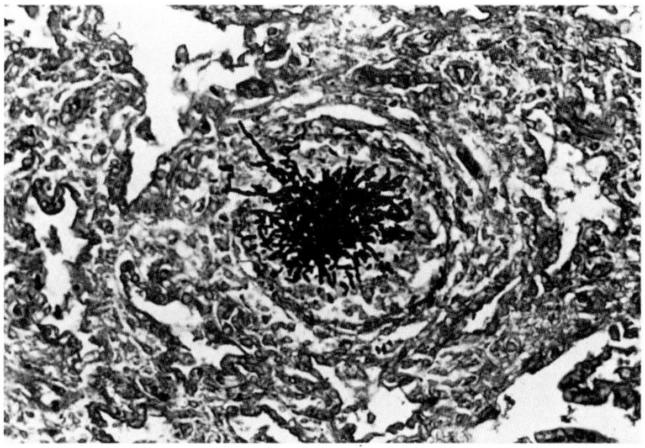

Fig. 13.4. Same case as Fig. 13.3. Mycotic emboli are present in many pulmonary arteries and mural invasion is widespread.

membrane disease. Infection must be distinguished from colonisation of the nose and throat. Detection of group B streptococcal antigen in blood or urine helps make this distinction.

Enteric Gram-negative bacilli such as *E. coli* and Klebsiella are acquired from the maternal birth canal and cause invasive infection particularly in neonates requiring intensive care. Colonisation leading to infection by *Pseudomonas* species and a range of Gram-negative bacteria including Acinetobacter, Citrobacter and Serratia may be the result of antibiotic selection or contamination of ventilators (Stone and Das 1986; Nicolle 1988).

Staph. aureus infection is usually postnatally acquired and far less common now than 20 years ago. It is an occasional cause of neonatal pneumonia with lung abscess and pneumatocoele formation, particularly in babies with severe congenital defects (George 1982).

Gastrointestinal Infection

During the 1970s, epidemics of diarrhoeal disease in newborn nurseries caused by specific serotypes of enteropathogenic *E. coli* (EPEC) were documented. Mortality was high, between 24% and 50% (Jacobs et al. 1970). This disorder is now uncommon in the UK but is still a problem in South Africa and southern Brazil (Gurwith et al. 1978; Edelman and Levine 1983). Most of these organisms were neither invasive nor toxin-producing, although outbreaks of diarrhoea in special care nurseries caused by toxin-producing strains have occurred (Gross et al. 1976; Ryder et al. 1976). EPEC which adhere to villous epithelium and produce brush border damage have been isolated from infants. Adherence is associated with a specific plasmid critical to the production of diarrhoea (Baldini and Kaper 1983).

Neonatal infection with *Salmonella* species occurs in those countries where carriage is common in the population. Transmission occurs perinatally or during epidemics (Schroder et al. 1968). Neonatal salmonella infection in the UK is rare.

Campylobacter infection in pregnancy has resulted in fetal death despite antibiotic therapy (Eden 1966) and neonatal infection with meningitis has followed maternal disease. The prognosis is poor in babies born prematurely (Carpenter 1985).

Clostridium difficile Carriage

Up to 71% of neonates carry *C. difficile* and its cytotoxin in their stools and are usually asymptomatic. Infants in intensive care have high rates of colonisation reflecting frequent antibiotic use. Clustering of neonatal infection suggests that colonisation represents nosocomial spread rather than acquisition of maternal flora. A high frequency of colonisation in the very young has lead to scepticism about the pathogenicity of this organism (Welch and Marks 1982).

Necrotising Enterocolitis

Necrotising enterocolitis is a major cause of morbidity and mortality in low birthweight infants after the first week of life (Wilson et al. 1981). Mucosal injury often follows hypoxia or hypotension in preterm neonates. The pathogenesis of this disorder is complex (see Chapters 8, 14, 15). It is usually sporadic but outbreaks in neonatal intensive care units have led to a search for infective causes (Frantz et al. 1975). A wide variety of bacteria has been isolated, commonly bowel flora. Occasional viral isolates have been recorded (British Association for Perinatal Paediatrics and Communicable Disease Surveillance Centre 1983). Despite enormous efforts to identify specific infectious agents or toxins, no two reports have convincingly implicated the same pathogen (Robarts and Levin 1983).

Acute Neonatal Viral Infection

Enteroviral Infection

Serious infection of the neonate caused by Coxsackie and echovirus groups may be indistinguishable from acute bacterial sepsis. Viruses most frequently encountered are Coxsackie B serotypes 1–5 and echovirus 11, although a range of echoviruses have been responsible for occasional fatal infection. Coxsackie A is rarely a problem. The majority of neonatal enteroviruses are of maternal origin and the incidence reflects patterns of infection within the community (Table 13.13), although clusters of neonatal infection caused by a single

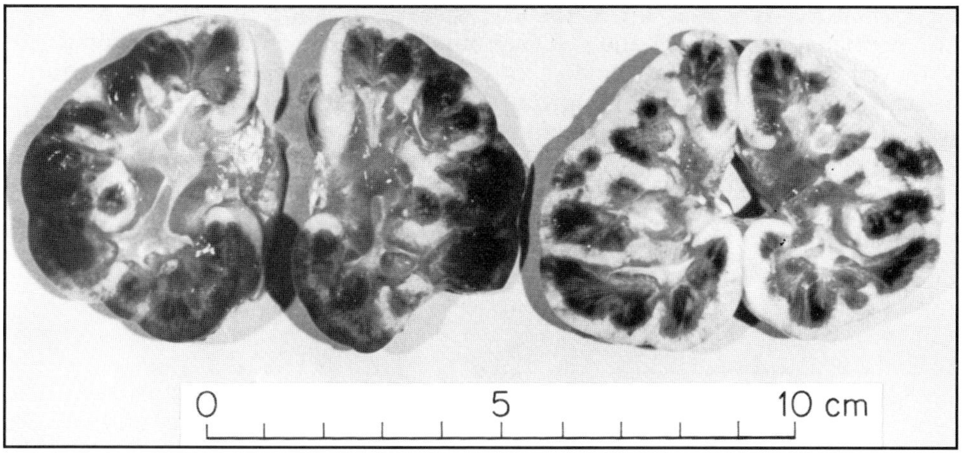

Fig. 13.5. Echovirus 11 infection: haemorrhagic infarction of the kidneys in a term baby who died at 5 days of age.

serotype have been recorded during community outbreaks (Modlin 1980). Severe neonatal disease usually occurs in the first week of life. Two clinical syndromes are described. The first, usually caused by Coxsackie B_{1-5} (Gear and Measroch 1973) but occasionally by echovirus 11 (Drew 1973), presents with encephalitis and myocarditis. The second is characterised by hypotension, haemorrhagic infarction of many organs (Fig. 13.5) and acute hepatic necrosis (Nagington et al. 1978). More than half of the cases are due to echovirus 11 (Berry and Nagington 1982); other serotypes have been isolated (Krous et al. 1973; Philip and Larson 1973).

Table 13.13. Enterovirus isolation in the neonate. Reports to the CDSC 1988–1990

	1988	1989	1990
Coxsackie A	3	1	8
Coxsackie B	8	7	22
Echo	29	42	18
Polio	1	—	1
Total	41	50	49

The encephalitis/myocarditis syndrome presents with tachycardia, heart failure, respiratory distress and CNS signs. Mortality is less than 50% (Modlin 1980). Presentation of the haemorrhage/hepatitis syndrome is nonspecific and often indistinguishable from acute bacterial sepsis. Illness progresses to bleeding diathesis and metabolic acidosis. Mortality is between 80% and 90%. Death follows uncontrollable haemorrhage, and hepatic or renal failure. Organ involvement is summarised in Table 13.14.

Table 13.14. Sites of haemorrhage found at necropsy in 12 neonates with fatal echovirus 11 infection (Berry and Nagington 1982)

Site	Neonates (n = 12)
Renal medulla	11
Adrenal	11
Gastrointestinal tract	8
Central nervous system	8
Pericardium	6
Bladder mucosa	4
Intrapulmonary	2
Subpleural	1
Capsule of thymus	1
Capsule of liver	1

In neonatal Coxsackie B myocarditis, early deaths (2–5 days) have left ventricular dilatation; endocardium and valves appear normal with myocardial pallor. In late infection (9–11 days) heart size is much increased by massive dilatation of the left and, occasionally, right ventricle. Myocardial necrosis is apparent. Initially, the inflammatory infiltrate is polymononuclear but by day 5–6 mononuclear cells predominate (Minor et al. 1990).

Respiratory Viral Infection

Respiratory tract viral infection is more common at this age than current reports suggest, probably reflecting incomplete investigation.

Reports of respiratory syncytial virus (RSV) isolation in neonates made to the CDSC outnumber the combined total for isolates of all other respiratory viruses in this age group (Table 13.15). Both parainfluenza and adenovirus infection may result in bronchiolitic symptoms in neonates.

Table 13.15. Viral and mycoplasma respiratory tract infection in infants less than 1 month of age. Reports to the CDSC 1988–1990

	1988	1989	1990
RSV	269	219	355
Adenovirus	30	26	11
Influenza A	1	9	13
Influenza B	3	—	1
Parainfluenza 1	1	2	1
Parainfluenza 2	2	1	—
Parainfluenza 3	4	2	7
Mycoplasma	2	—	4
Total	312	259	392

Rapid diagnosis of respiratory tract viral infection is possible using direct immunofluorescent antibody techniques on nasopharyngeal aspirates, or bronchoalveolar lavage. Routine investigations include tests for RSV, influenza A and B, parainfluenza 1 and 3 and adenovirus. Virus isolation takes 2–3 weeks. Retrospective diagnosis is made on a fourfold rise in antibody in paired sera or a single high specific antibody level.

Gastrointestinal Viral Infection

Ready availability of commercial kits (ELISA and latex agglutination systems) allows the diagnosis of diarrhoea caused by rotavirus to be undertaken by many laboratories (Madeley 1990). Rotavirus has been identified in up to 80% of hospitalised neonates (Walker-Smith 1978) and has caused outbreaks of diarrhoeal disease (Bishop et al. 1976). A personally investigated outbreak resulted in serious morbidity in neonates in an intensive care nursery. Adenovirus and small round viruses including astrovirus and calici virus have also been demonstrated in neonates with diarrhoea (Table 13.16).

Table 13.16. Viruses identified in neonatal diarrhoea in infants aged less than 1 month. Reports to the CDSC 1988–1990

	1988	1989	1990
Rotavirus	70	208	215
Adenovirus	16	28	33
SRSV	—	1	3
Calicivirus	—	2	1

SRSV = Small round structured viruses.

Other Infections

Chlamydial Pneumonia

Chlamydial pneumonia is seen in 3–10 per 1000 livebirths (Schachter and Grossman 1981). It usually has a benign course so few lung samples have been examined. There are a few reports of interstitial pneumonia both when *C. trachomatis* was isolated alone and with other pathogens such as CMV (Schachter and Grossman 1990). Neonatal infection is infrequent, and diagnosis is made by culture of *C. trachomatis* from nasopharyngeal aspirate or lung.

An occasional case of congenital infection with *Pneumocystis carinii* has been reported (Arvin et al. 1990).

Investigation of Infection

It is probable that the role of infection is underestimated both as an attendant cause and as a direct cause of perinatal death. Before necropsy begins information about clinical suspicion of infection, microbiological investigations undertaken, and results should be made available. Examination of clinical notes may alert the pathologist to the possibility of infection and indicate the type of investigations required. As certain microbiological investigations are not undertaken routinely, it is essential that appropriate information accompanies all samples. It is important that microbiology specimens should be taken early in the necropsy using full aseptic precautions. The extent to which routine microbiological investigations can be undertaken as part of a perinatal necropsy will depend on local resources. In most centres examination of bacteriology samples causes no problem as they comprise a small proportion of the diagnostic work load. Review of bacterial isolations suggests that samples for culture may not be appropriate for

Table 13.17. Samples for microbiological investigation

Likely diagnosis				
Rubella	CMV	Herpes simplex	Entero/Parvo/ Bacteria	Toxoplasma
Eye				
Lung	Lung	Lung	Lung	
Spleen } [a]	Spleen } [a]	Spleen } [a]	Spleen } [a]	
Liver	Liver	Liver	Liver	Liver
Kidney	Kidney		Kidney	
	Pancreas			
	Adrenal	Adrenal	Adrenal	
	Testis			
		Skin lesion if present		
Brain	Brain	Brain	Brain + meninges	Brain
			Myocardium	Myocardium + heart blood
			Intestinal contents	
				Skeletal muscle
Blood[b]	Blood[b]	Blood[b]	Blood[b]	Blood

A placental sample should be sent if available.
[a] Spleen and liver samples may be pooled.
[b] Blood samples should be collected in two ways: 2–3 ml clotted
1–2 ml in preservative-free heparin

every perinatal necropsy (Billson et al. 1993). Some selection of cases for virological investigation is appropriate. When determining the nature of microbiological investigations required, there is no substitute for good communication between the clinician and all pathologists involved. Only close collaboration between histopathologists and microbiologists can resolve the problems inherent in the postmortem diagnosis of infection.

Spontaneous Abortion

When spontaneous abortion is thought to result from systemic maternal infection, the products of conception should be examined microbiologically. The nature of maternal illness and appearance of the placenta help to determine the most useful investigations. Specimens for microbiological examination should include placental tissue and the samples of fetal organs in column four of Table 13.17.

Fetal samples should be divided and one snap frozen for future possible investigation. Virus isolation should be performed on the other sample. A maternal blood sample is extremely helpful.

When maternal rubella cannot be excluded, a rubella isolation must be specifically requested. Maternal and fetal sera can be tested for parvovirus IgG, IgM, and DNA can be extracted from fresh tissue (Clewley et al. 1987) and in formalin fixed paraffin-embedded material (Anderson et al. 1988). Maternal serology for rubella, toxoplasma and cytomegalovirus is useful.

When ascending infection seems likely following leakage of liquor amnii or offensive vaginal discharge, microbiological investigations should include examination for typical organisms (see Table 13.5)—usually genital and gastrointestinal tract flora.

Investigation of Congenital Infection

When clinical findings or previous investigations point to infection by a particular organism, appropriate samples for the diagnosis of specific viral infections are shown in the first three columns of Tables 13.17 and 13.18. When there are no specific pointers, samples in Table 13.17 column 4 should be investigated first.

Interpretation of Results

Interpretation of the results of microbiological investigations may be simple or cause much difficulty. It is useful to compare any antemortem microbiological results with necropsy

Table 13.18. Samples for demonstration of *Toxoplasma gondii* and *Treponema pallidum*

T. gondii		*T. pallidum*	
Brain	(20)	Liver	
Heart	(9)		bullous
Eye	(8)	Skin lesion	
Adrenal	(6)		vesicular
Striated muscle	(5)	Many other tissues show	
Lung	(4)	characteristic histological change	
Kidney	(4)	CNS	
Skin	(3)	Skeletal system	
Pancreas	(1)	Pancreas	
Spleen	(1)	Lung	
Liver	(0)		

Numbers in parentheses indicate the frequency of demonstration of the parasite, as seen in 21 cases of congenital toxoplasmosis.

samples to determine if these are consistent. Isolation of one or more organism from the placenta and membranes following abortion must be interpreted together with histopathological appearance of both fetus and placenta. A single bacterial species isolated from lung and heart blood of a neonate with histological evidence of pneumonia is usually relevant. Problems arise when several bacterial species are isolated from a variety of sites. Postmortem microbiological investigations carried out over a period of 4 years in the author's department found splenic culture extremely useful in ascertaining the significance of a specific organism. Bacteria isolated from the spleen plus one or more sites are likely to be significant. Review of cultures from all postmortem samples enables the significance of organisms present at a number of sites, in different combinations, to be determined. Where several organisms are found in three or more sites, particularly where this involves the spleen, they are likely to be significant.

When a virus is isolated from several sites it is likely to be significant. Distinction between organ infection and contamination can be a problem. Infection by culturally exacting viruses can give rise to diagnostic difficulties. Molecular biological techniques such as in vitro hybridisation, immunoblotting and polymerase chain reaction are more readily available so many of these problems will be resolved. Now that highly specific techniques are available close collaboration between histopathologists and microbiologists is even more important to enable appropriate investigations to be undertaken and to facilitate appropriate and accurate interpretation of results.

References

Ahlfors K, Harris S, Ivarsson S, Svanberg L (1981) Secondary maternal cytomegalovirus infection causing symptomatic congenital infection. N Engl J Med 305: 284

Alford CA, Neva FA, Weller TH (1964) Virologic and serologic studies on human products of conception after maternal rubella. N Engl J Med 271: 1275–1281

Alford CA, Stagno S, Reynolds DW (1974) Congenital toxoplasmosis: clinical, laboratory and therapeutic considerations with special reference to subclinical disease. Bull NY Acad Med 50: 160–181

Alford CA, Stagno S, Pass RF, Britt WJ (1990) Congenital and perinatal cytomegalovirus infections. Rev Infect Dis 12: S742–S753

Ancona RJ, Ferrieri P, Williams PP (1980) Maternal factors that enhance the acquisition of group B streptococci by newborn infants. J Med Microbiol 13: 273–280

Anderson LJ (1990) Human parvoviruses. J Infect Dis 161: 603–608

Anderson MJ, Khousani MN, Maxwell DJ, Gould SJ, Happerfield CC, Smith WJ (1988) Human parvovirus B_{19} and hydrops fetalis. Lancet i: 535

Arvin A, Ruskin J, Yeager A (1990) Protozoon and helminth infections (including *Pneumocystis carinii*). In: Remington JS, Klein JO (eds) Infectious diseases of the fetus and newborn infant, 3rd edn. Saunders, Philadelphia, pp 528–573

Baker CJ, Edwards M (1990) Group B streptococcal infection. In: Remington JS, Klein JO (eds) Infectious diseases of the fetus and newborn infant, 3rd edn. Saunders, Philadelphia, pp 742–811

Baker CJ, Edwards MS, Kasper DL (1981) Role of antibody to maternal type II polysaccharide of Group B strep in infant infection. Pediatrics 68: 544–549

Baldini MM, Kapper JB (1983) Plasmid mediated adhesion in enteropathogenic *Escherichia coli*. J Pediatr Gastroenterol 2: 534–538

Bates T (1955) Poliomyelitis in pregnancy, fetus and newborn. Am J Dis Child 90: 189–195

Berkovich S, Smithwick EM (1968) Transplacental infection due to ECHO virus type 22. J Pediatr 72: 94–96

Berry PJ, Nagington J (1982) Fatal infection with echovirus 11. Arch Dis Child 57: 22–29

Best JM, Banatvala JE, Morgan-Capner P, Miller E (1989) Fetal infection after maternal reinfection with rubella: criteria for defining reinfection. Br Med J 299: 773–775

Billson V, Masterton RG, Keeling JW (1993) How useful is postmortem bacteriological investigation? J Pathol 169 suppl 120A

Bishop RF, Hewstone AS, Davidson GP et al. (1976) An epidemic of serotypes of *E. coli* diarrhoea in human neonates involving a reovirus-like agent and enteropathogenic serotypes of *E. coli*. J Clin Pathol 29: 46–49

Blanc WA (1981) Pathology of the placenta, membranes and umbilical cord in bacterial, fungal and viral infections in man. In: Naeye RL, Kissane JM, Kaufman N (eds) Perinatal disease. Williams and Wilkins, Baltimore, pp 67–132

Blattner RJ (1963) Intra-uterine infection with poliovirus type 1. J Pediatr 62: 625–627

Boué A, Loffredo V (1970) Avortment causé par le virus de l'herpes type II. Isolement du virus à partir de cultures de tissues zygotiques. Presse Med 78: 103–106

Boué A, Nicolas A, Montagnin B (1971) Reinfection with rubella in pregnant women. Lancet i: 1251–1253

Boyer KM, Papiernak CK, Gazala CA et al. (1984) Trans-

placental passage of IgG antibodies to Group B Streptococcus serotype 1a. J Pediatr 104(4): 618–620
Brightman VJ, Scott TFM, Westphal M, Boggs TR (1966) An outbreak of Coxsackie B5 virus infection in a newborn nursery. J Pediatr 69: 179–192
British Association for Perinatal Paediatrics and Communicable Disease Surveillance Centre (1983) Surveillance of necrotising enterocolitis 1981–2. Br Med J 287: 824–826
Brown GC, Karunas RS (1972) Relationship of congenital anomalies and maternal infection with selected enteroviruses. Am J Epidemiol 95: 207–217
Brown T, Anand A, Ritchie DL, Clewley JP, Reid TMS (1984) Intrauterine parvovirus infection associated with hydrops fetalis. Lancet ii: 1033–1034
Brunell PA (1967) Varicella-zoster infections in pregnancy. JAMA 199: 315–317
Buitrago B, Hadler SC, Popper H et al. (1986) Epidemiologic aspects of Santa Marta hepatitis over a 40-year period. Hepatology 6: 1292–1296
Burch GE, Sun SC, Chu KC, Sohal RS, Colcolough HL (1968) Interstitial and Coxsackie B myocarditis in infants and children. JAMA 203: 1–8
Carpenter C (1985) Other pathogenic viruses. In: Mandell G. Douglas JE, Bennett RG (eds) Principles and practice of infectious diseases, 2nd edn. Wiley, Chichester, pp 1218–1226
Catalano LW, Sever JL (1971) The role of viruses as causes of congenital diseases. Annu Rev Microbiol 25: 255–282
Caul EO, Usher MJ, Burton PA (1988) Intra-uterine infection with a human parvovirus; a light and electron microscopy study. J Med Virol 24: 55–66
Centre for Disease Control (1988) Guidelines for the prevention and control of congenital syphilis. MMWR 37: 1–13
Centre for Disease Control (1989) Risks associated with human parvovirus B_{19} infection. MMWR 38: 81–87
Cherry JD (1990) Enteroviruses. In: Remington JS, Klein JO (eds) Infectious diseases of the fetus and newborn infant, 3rd edn. Saunders, Philadelphia, pp 325–366
Cherry JD, Soriano F, Jahn CL (1968) Search for perinatal viral infection. A prospective virologic and serologic study. Am J Dis Child 116: 245–250
Clewley JP, Cohen B, Field A (1987) Detection of parvovirus B_{19} DNA, antigen and particles in the human fetus. J Med Virol 23: 367–376
Coffey VF, Jessop WJE (1959) Maternal influenza and congenital deformities. A prospective study. Lancet ii: 935–938
Corey L (1982) The diagnosis and treatment of genital herpes. JAMA 248: 1041–1049
Corey L, Adams HG, Brown ZA, Holmes KK (1983) Genital herpes simplex virus infection, clinical manifestation, course and complication. Ann Int Med 98: 958–972
Cossart YE (1974) Acquisition of hepatitis B antigen in the newborn period. Postgrad Med 50: 334–337
Covell G (1950) Congenital malaria. Trop Dis Bull 47: 1147–1167
Cowan MJ, Hellman D, Chudwin D, Wara DW, Chang RS, Ammann AJ (1984) Maternal transmission of acquired immune deficiency syndrome. Pediatrics 73: 382–386
Das BC, Lakhani P, Kurts JB et al. (1989) Congenital rubella after previous maternal immunity. Arch Dis Child 65: 545–546
Davies PA, Gothefors L (1984) "Bacteraemia". Infections of central nervous and respiratory systems. In: Bacterial infections in the fetus and newborn infant. Saunders, Philadelphia, pp 122–142
De Louvois J, Blackbourn J, Hurley R, Harvey D (1991) Infantile meningitis in England and Wales: a two year study. Arch Dis Child 66: 603–607
Derso A, Boxall EH, Tarlow MJ, Flewett TH (1978) Transmission of HBsAg from mother to infant in four ethnic groups. Br Med J i: 949–952
Desmonts G, Couvreur J (1974) Toxoplasmosis in pregnancy and its transmission to the fetus. Bull NY Acad Med 50: 146–159
Desmonts G, Couvreur J (1979) Congenital toxoplasmosis: a prospective study of the offspring of 542 women who acquired toxoplasmosis during pregnancy. Pathophysiology of congenital disease. In: Thalhammer O, Baumgarten K, Pollak A (eds) Proceedings of the sixth European congress on perinatal medicine, Vienna, 1978. Thieme, Stuttgart, pp 51–60
Desmonts G, Naot Y, Remington JS (1981) Immunoglobulin M-immunosorbent agglutination assay for diagnosis of acute congenital diseases: diagnosis of acute congenital and acquired toxoplasmosis infections. J Clin Microbiol 14: 486–491
Dietzman DE, Matthew EB, Madden DL et al. (1972) The occurrence of epidemic hepatitis in chronic carriers of Australia antigen. J Pediatr 80: 577–582
Dietzman DE, Fischer GW, Schoenknecht FD (1974) Neonatal *E. coli* septicaemic-bacterial counts in blood. J Pediatr 85: 128–130
Dimusto JC, Bohjalian D, Millar M (1973) *Mycoplasma hominis* type 1 infection and pregnancy. Obstet Gynecol 41: 33–37
Doll R, Hill AB, Sakula J (1960) Asian influenza in pregnancy and congenital defects. Br J Prev Soc Med 14: 167–172
Drew JH (1973) Echo 11 virus outbreak in a nursery associated with myocarditis. Aust J Paediatr 9: 90–95
Dupuy JM, Frommel D, Alagille D (1975) Severe viral hepatitis type B in infancy. Lancet i: 191–194
Easmon CSF, Hastings MJG (1985) Group B streptococcal colonisation in mothers and babies. Antibiot Chemother 35: 28–39
Edelman R, Levine MM (1983) Summary of a workshop on enteropathogenic *E. coli*. J Infect Dis 147: 1108–1118
Eden AN (1966) Perinatal mortality caused by *Vibrio fetus*. Review and analysis. J Pediatr 68: 297–304
Embree JE, Krause VW, Embil JA, MacDonald S (1980) Placental infection with *Mycoplasma hominis* and *Ureaplasma urealyticum*: clinical correlation. Obstet Gynecol 56: 475–481
Epstein H, King CR (1985) Diagnosis of congenital syphilis by immunofluorescence following fetal death in utero. Am J Obstet Gynecol 152: 689–690
Eschenbach D (1977) Significance for the fetus of sexually acquired maternal infection with Mycoplasma, Chlamydia and *N. gonorrhoeae*. Semin Perinatol 1(1): 11–23
European Collaborative Study (1991) Children born to women with HIV_1 infection: natural history and risk of transmission. Lancet 337: 253–260
Falloon J, Pizzo P (1990) Acquired immunodeficiency syndrome in the infant. In: Remington JS, Klein JO (eds) Infectious diseases of the fetus and newborn infant, 3rd edn. Saunders, Philadelphia, pp 306–324
Fawaz KA, Grady GF, Kaplan MM, Gellis SS (1975) Repetitive maternal–fetal transmission of fatal hepatitis B. N Engl J Med 293: 1357–1359
Finland M (1973) Mumps. In: Charles D, Finland M (eds) Obstetric and perinatal infections. Lea and Febiger, Philadelphia, pp 333–353
Fiumara NJ, Lessell S (1970) Manifestations of late con-

genital syphilis. An analysis of 271 patients. Arch Dermatol 102: 78–83
Fleck DG (1979) Perinatal and neonatal infections: toxoplasmosis. J Antimicrob Chemother 5 (Suppl A): 87–89
Florman AL, Gerson AA, Blackett PR, Nahmias AJ (1973) Intrauterine infection with herpes simplex virus: resultant congenital malformations. JAMA 225: 129–132
Foy HM, Kenny GE, Wentworth BB (1970) Isolation of *Mycoplasma hominis*, T. strains and cytomegalovirus from the cervix of pregnant women. Am J Obstet Gynecol 106: 635–643
Frantz ID, L'heureux P, Engel RR et al. (1975) Necrotising enterocolitis. J Pediatr 86: 259–263
Freedman PS (1979) Echovirus 11 infection and intrauterine death. Lancet i: 96–97
Gauntt CJ, Gudvangen RJ, Brans YW, Marlin AE (1985) Coxsackievirus group B antibodies in the ventricular fluid of infants with severe anatomic defects in the central nervous system. Pediatrics 76: 64–68
Gazala E, Karplus M, Liberman JR, Sarov I (1985) The effect of maternal measles on the fetus. Pediatr Infect Dis 4: 203–204
Gear JH, Measroch V (1973) Coxsackie virus infections of the newborn. Prog Med Virol 15: 42–63
George R (1982) Infections in the neonate. In: Barson AJ (ed) Fetal and neonatal pathology. Praeger, Eastbourne, pp 247–255
Gershon AA (1975) Varicella in mother and infant: problems old and new. In: Krugman S, Gershon AA (eds) Infections of the fetus and the newborn infant. Progress in clinical and biological research, vol 3. Alan R Liss, New York, pp 79–95
Gershon A (1990) Chickenpox, measles and mumps. In: Remington JS, Klein JO (eds) Infectious diseases of the fetus and newborn infant, 3rd edn. Saunders, Philadelphia, pp 395–445
Gill P (1988) Is listeriosis often a foodborne illness? J Infect Dis 17: 1–5
Goldacre MJ (1976) Acute bacterial meningitis in childhood. Incidence and mortality in a defined population. Lancet i: 28–31
Gregg NM (1941) Congenital cataract following German measles in the mother. Trans Ophthalmol Soc Aust 3: 35–46
Griffiths PD, Baboonian C (1984) A prospective study of primary cytomegalovirus infection during pregnancy, final report. Br J Obstet Gynaecol 91: 307–315
Griffiths PD, Ronalds CJ, Heath RB (1980) A prospective study of influenza infection during pregnancy. J Epidemiol Community Health 34: 124–128
Griffiths PD, Baboonian C, Rutter D, Peckham C (1991) Congenital and maternal CMV infections in a London population. Br J Obstet Gynaecol 98: 135–140
Gross RJ, Rowe B, Henderson A et al. (1976) A new *Escherichia coli* O-group 0159 associated with outbreaks of enteritis in infants. Scand J Infect Dis 137: 292–297
Gurwith M, Hinde D, Gross R, Rowe B (1978) A prospective study of enteropathogenic *Escherichia coli* in endemic diarrhoeal disease. J Infect Dis 137: 292–297
Gutman LT, Holmes K (1990) Gonococcal infection. In: Remington JS, Klein JO (eds) Infectious diseases of the fetus and newborn infant, 3rd edn. Saunders, Philadelphia, pp 848–865
Hall S (1983) Congenital toxoplasmosis in England and Wales, and N. Ireland. Some epidemiological problems. Br Med J 287: 453–455
Hanshaw JB, Dudgeon JA, Marshall WC (1985) Rubella. In: Viral diseases of the fetus and newborn, 2nd edn. Saunders, Philadelphia, 13–91
Harger JH, Paz GF, Armstrong JA, Breinig MC, Ho M (1983) Characteristics and management of pregnancy in women with genital herpes simplex virus infection. Am J Obstet Gynecol 145: 784–791
Harris JW (1919) Influenza in pregnant women. JAMA 72: 978–981
Harrison HR, Alexander ER, Weinstein L, Lewis M, Nash M, Sim DA (1983) Cervical *Chlamydia trachomatis* and mycoplasma infections in pregnancy. Epidemiology and outcome. JAMA 250: 1721–1727
Heiber JP, Dalton D, Shorey J, Combs B (1977) Hepatitis and pregnancy. J Pediatr 91: 545–549
Hindi RD, Azimi PH (1980) Congenital malaria due to *Plasmodium falciparum*. Pediatrics 66: 977–979
Hira SK, Kamanga J, Bhat GJ et al. (1989) Perinatal transmission of HIV_1 in Zambia. Br Med J 299: 1250–1252
Holliman RC (1990) The diagnosis of toxoplamosis: serodiagnosis and immunotherapy. J Infect Dis 4: 83–93
Horn P (1955) Poliomyelitis in pregnancy, a 20 year report from Los Angeles County, California. Obstet Gynecol 6: 121–137
Hutto C, Arvin A, Jacobs R et al. (1987) Intra-uterine herpes simplex virus infection. J Pediatr 110: 97–101
Ingall D, Dobson S, Musher D (1990) Syphilis. In: Remington JS, Klein JO (eds) Infectious diseases of the fetus and newborn infant, 3rd edn. Saunders, Philadelphia, pp 367–394
Jacobs SI, Holzel A, Wolman B et al. (1970) Outbreak of infantile gestroenteritis caused by *Escherichia coli* 0114. Arch Dis Child 45: 656–663
Jespersen CS, Littauer J, Sagild U (1977) Measles as a cause of fetal defects. Acta Paediatr Scand 66: 367–372
Johnstone FD, MacCallum L, Brettle R, Inglis JM, Peutherer JF (1988) Does infection with HIV affect the outcome of pregnancy? Br Med J 296: 467
Jones MJ, Kolb M, Votava HJ, Johnson RL, Smith TF (1980) Intra-uterine echovirus type 11 infection. Mayo Clin Proc 55: 509–512
Jovaisas E, Koch MA, Schäffer A, Stauber M, Löwenthal D (1985) LAV HTLV III in 20 week fetus. Lancet 2: 1129
Joynson DHM, Payne R (1988) Screening for toxoplasmosis in pregnancy. Lancet ii: 795–796
Kampelmacher EH, Van Noorle-Jansen L (1972) Further studies on the isolation of *L. monocytogenes* in clinically healthy individuals. Zentralbl Bakteriol Mikrobiol Hyg [A] 221: 70–77
Kass EH (1960) Bacteriuria and pyelonephritis of pregnancy. Arch Intern Med 105: 194–198
Kass EH (1982) Infectious disease and perinatal morbidity. Yale J Biol Med 55: 231–237
Kattamis CA, Demetrios D, Matsaniotis NS (1974) Australia antigen and neonatal hepatitis syndrome. Pediatrics 54: 157–164
Kaye BM, Rosner DC, Stein I (1953) Viral diseases in pregnancy and their effect upon the embryo and fetus. Am J Obstet Gynecol 65: 109–119
Kibrick S, Benirschke K (1956) Acute septic myocarditis and meningoencephalitis in the newborn child infected with Coxsackie virus group B, type 3. N Engl J Med 255: 883–889
Klein JO (1990) Bacterial infection of the respiratory tract. In: Remington JS, Klein JO (eds) Infectious diseases of the fetus and newborn infant, 3rd edn. Saunders, Philadelphia, pp 658–673
Klein JO, Marcy SM (1976) Bacterial infection. In: Remington JS, Klein JO (eds) Infectious diseases of the fetus and newborn infant. Saunders, Philadelphia, pp 747–802

Klein JO, Marcy M (1990) Bacterial sepsis and meningitis. In: Remington JS, Klein JO (eds) Infectious diseases of the fetus and newborn infant, 3rd edn. Saunders, Philadelphia, pp 602–656

Klein JO, Buckland D, Finland M (1969) Colonisation of newborn infants by mycoplasma. N Engl J Med 280: 1025–1030

Knott PD, Welply GA, Anderson MJ (1984) Serologically proved intrauterine infection with parvovirus. Br Med J 284: 1660

Krous HF, Dietzman D, Ray CG (1973) Fatal infections with Echovirus types 6 and 11 in early infancy. Am J Dis Child 126: 842–846

Kucera J (1970) Down's syndrome and infectious hepatitis. Lancet i: 569–570

Kundsin RB, Driscoll SG (1970) Mycoplasmas and human reproductive failure. Surg Gynecol Obstet 131: 89–92

Kurtz B, Tomlinson AH, Pearson J (1982) Mumps virus isolated from a fetus. Br Med J 284: 471

Kurtzman GJ, Gascon P, Caras M, Cohen B, Young NS (1988) B_{19} parvovirus replicates in circulatory cells of acutely infected patients. Blood 71: 1448–1454

Lamont RJ, Postlethwaite R (1986) Carriage of *Listeria monocytogenes* and related species in pregnant and non pregnant women in Aberdeen, Scotland. J Infect Dis 13: 187–193

Lamprecht C, Schauf V, Warren D, Nelson K, Northrop R, Christiansen M (1982) An outbreak of congenital rubella in Chicago. JAMA 247: 1129–1133

Landsman JB, Grist NR, Ross CA (1964) Echo 9 virus infection and congenital malformations. Br J Prev Soc Med 18: 152–156

Lapointe N, Michaud J, Pekovic D, Chausseau JP, Dupuy JM (1985) Transplacental transmission of HTLV III virus. N Engl J Med 312: 1325–1326

Leck I (1963) Incidence of malformations following influenza epidemics. Br J Prev Soc Med 17: 70–80

Lee AKY, Ip HMH, Wong VCW (1978) Mechanisms of maternal–fetal transmission of hepatitis B virus. J Infect Dis 138: 668–671

Lundstrom R (1962) Rubella during pregnancy. A follow-up study of children born after an epidemic of rubella in Sweden 1951. Acta Pediatr Scand [Suppl] 133: 1–110

MacGregor JD, Avery JG (1974) Malaria transmission and fetal growth. Br Med J 3: 433–436

Madeley CR (1990) Viruses associated with acute diarrhoeal disease. In: Zuckerman AJ, Banatvala JE, Pattison JR (eds) Principles and practice of clinical virology, 2nd edn. Wiley, Chichester, pp 173–209

Manson MM, Logan WPD, Loy RM (1960) Rubella and other virus infections during pregnancy. Reports on Public Health and Medical Subjects 110. HMSO, London

Marion RW, Wiznia AA, Hutcheon RG, Rubinstein A (1986) Human T-cell lymphotropic virus type III (HTLV III) embryopathy. A new dysmorphic syndrome associated with intrauterine HTLV III infection. Am J Dis Child 140: 633–640

Marion RW, Wiznia AA, Hutcheon RG, Rubinstein A (1987) Correlation between severity of dysmorphism and age at diagnosis of immunodeficiency. Am J Dis Child 141: 429–431

Martin DH, Koutsky L, Eschenbach DA et al. (1982) Prematurity and perinatal mortality in pregnancies complicated by maternal *Chlamydia trachomatis* infection. JAMA 250: 1585–1588

Maupas P, Barin F, Chiron JP et al. (1981) Efficacy of hepatitis B vaccine in prevention of early HBsAg carrier state in children. Lancet 1: 289–292

McCracken GH, Sarff LD, Glode MP, Mize SG (1974) Relation between *Escherichia coli* K, capsular polysaccharide antigen and clinical outcome in neonatal meningitis. Lancet ii: 246–250

McLaughlin J, Audurier A, Taylor AG (1986) Aspects of the epidemiology of human *Listeria monocytogenes* infection in Britain 1967–84; use of serotyping and phage typing. J Med Microbiol 22: 367–377

Menser MA, Forrest JM (1974) High incidence of defects in children considered normal at birth. Med J Aust 1: 123–126

Merrill DA, Dubois RS, Kohler PF (1972) Neonatal onset of the hepatitis associated antigen carrier state. N Engl J Med 287: 1280–1282

Miller E (1990) Rubella reinfection. Arch Dis Child 65: 820–821

Miller E, Cradock-Watson JE, Pollock TM (1982) Consequences of confirmed maternal rubella at successive stages of pregnancy. Lancet ii: 781–784

Miller E, Waight PA, Vurdien JE et al. (1991) Rubella surveillance to December 1990: a joint report from the PHLS and National Congenital Rubella Surveillance Programme. Communicable Disease Report 1: R33–R37

Minor PD, Morgan-Capner P, Schild GC (1990) The enteroviruses. In: Zuckerman AJ, Banatvala JE and Pattison JR (eds) Principles and practice of clinical virology, 2nd edn. Wiley, Chichester, pp 389–409

Modlin JF (1980) Fatal echovirus 11 disease in premature neonates. Pediatrics 66: 775–780

Monif GRG, Sowards DL, Eitzman DL (1972) Serologic and immunologic evaluation of neonates following maternal influenza infection during the second and third trimesters of gestation. Am J Obstet Gynecol 114: 239–249

Morbidity and Mortality Weekly Report (1991) Increase in rubella and congenital rubella syndrome—United States 1988–1990 MMWR 40: 3–99

Morey AL, Keeling JW, Porter HJ, Fleming KA (1992) Clinical and histopathological features of parvovirus B_{19} infection in the human fetus. Br J Obstet Gynaecol 99: 566–574

Morgan-Capner P (1986) Does rubella reinfection matter? In: Mortimer, PP (ed) Public Health Virology 12 reports. Public Health Laboratory Service, London, pp 50–62

Mortimer PP (1980) Hepatitis A and its virus. In: Waterson AP (ed) Recent advances in clinical virology 3. Churchill Livingstone, Edinburgh, pp 1–15

Mulder CJ, Van Alphen L, Zanen H (1984) Neonatal meningitis caused by *Escherichia coli* in the Netherlands. J Infect Dis 150: 935–940

Munday PE, Porter R, Folder PF et al. (1984) Spontaneous abortion, an infectious aetiology. Br J Obstet Gynaecol 91(12): 1177–1180

Naessens A, Foulon W, Volckaert M, Amy JJ, Lauwers S (1983) Cervical and placental colonisation by *Ureaplasma urealyticum* in pregnant women and fetal outcome. J Infect Dis 148: 333

Naeye RL (1979) Coitus and associated amniotic-fluid infections. N Engl J Med 301: 1198–1199

Nagington J, Wreghitt TG, Gandy G, Roberton NRC, Berry PJ (1978) Fatal echovirus 11 infections in outbreak in special care baby unit. Lancet ii: 725–728

Nahmias AJ, Josey WE, Naib ZM, Freeman MG, Fernandex RJ, Wheeler JH (1971) Perinatal risk associated with maternal genital herpes simplex virus infection. Am J Obstet Gynecol 110: 825–837

Nahmias AJ, Keyserling HL, Kerrick GM (1983) Herpes simplex. In: Remington JS, Klein JO (eds) Infectious diseases of the fetus and newborn infant, 2nd edn. Saunders, Philadelphia, pp 636–678

Newton L, Hall MS, Pelerin M, McLauchlin J (1990) Listeriosis surveillance. Communicable Disease Report, 1: R110–R113

Nicolle LE (1988) Prior antimicrobial therapy and resistance of Enterobacter, Citrobacter and Serratia to third generation cephalosporins. J Hosp Infect 11: 321–327

Norden CW, Kass CH (1968) Bacteriuria of pregnancy—a critical appraisal. Am Rev Med 19: 431–470

Okada K, Kamiyama I, Inomata M, Imai M, Miyakawa Y, Mayumi M (1976) e Antigen and anti-e in the serum of asymptomatic carrier mothers as indicators of positive and negative transmission of hepatitis B virus to their infants. N Engl J Med 294: 746–749

Pantelakis SN, Chryssostomidou O-M, Alexiou D, Valaes T, Doxiadis SA (1970) Sex chromatin and chromosome abnormalities among 10 412 liveborn babies. Arch Dis Child 45: 87–92

Parjani SG, Arvin A (1986) Intra-uterine infection with varicella zoster virus after maternal varicella. N Engl J Med 314: 1542–1546

Pass RF, Stagno S, Myers GJ, Alford CA (1980) Outcome of symptomatic congenital CMV infection; results of long term longitudinal follow up. Pediatrics 66: 758–762

Peckham CS, Chin KS, Coleman JC, Henderson K, Hurley R, Preece PM (1983) Cytomegalovirus infection in pregnancy. Preliminary findings from a prospective study. Lancet i: 1352–1355

Philip AGS, Larson EJ (1973) Overwhelming neonatal infection with ECHO 19 virus. J Pediatr 82: 391–397

Plager H, Beebe R, Miller JK (1962) Coxsackie B5 pericarditis in pregnancy. Arch Intern Med 110: 735–738

Pleydell MJ (1960) Anencephaly and other congenital abnormalities. Br Med J i: 309–315

Porter HJ, Quantrill AM, Fleming KA (1988) B_{19} parvovirus infection of myocardial cells. Lancet i: 535–536

Preblud S, Cochi S, Orenstein W (1986) Varicella-zoster infection in pregnancy. N Engl J Med 315: 1415–1417

Prober CY, Sullender WM, Yasukawa LL, Au DS, Arvin AM (1987) Low risk of herpes simplex virus infection in neonates exposed to the virus at the time of vaginal delivery to mothers with recurrent genital herpes simplex infection. N Engl J Med 316: 240–244

Public Health Laboratory Service Working Party on Fifth Disease (1990) Br Med J 300: 1166–1170

Public Health Laboratory Service (1991) The unlinked anonymous HIV prevalence monitoring programme in England and Wales: preliminary results. Communicable Disease Report 1: R69–R75

Puck J, Glezen WP, Frank AI (1980) Protection of infants from infection with influenza A virus by transplacentally acquired antibody. J Infect Dis 142: 844–849

Quinn TC, Jacobs RF, Mertz GJ et al. (1982) Congenital malaria: A report of 4 cases and a review. J Paediatr 101: 229–232

Quinn PA, Shewchuk AB, Shuber J et al. (1983) Serologic evidence of *Ureaplasma urealyticum* infection in women with spontaneous pregnancy loss. Am J Obstet Gynecol 145: 245–250

Ransome-Kuti O (1972) Malaria in childhood. Paediatrics 19: 319–340

Rantasalo I, Penttinen K, Saxen L, Ojala A (1960) ECHO 9 virus antibody status after an epidemic period and the possible teratogenic effect of the infection. Ann Pediatr Fenn 6: 175–184

Reinhardt MC (1980) Effects of parasitic infections in pregnant women. In: Ciba Foundation Symposium 77. Perinatal infections. ASP Elsevier Excerpta Medica, Amsterdam, pp 149–161

Remington JS (1973) Toxoplasmosis. In: Charles D, Finland M (eds) Obstetric and perinatal infections. Lea and Febiger, Philadelphia, p 27

Remington J, Desmonts G (1990) Toxoplasmosis. In: Remington JS, Klein JO (eds) Infectious diseases of the fetus and newborn infant, 3rd edn. Saunders, Philadelphia, pp 89–195

Rettig PJ (1988) Perinatal infections with *Chlamydia trachomatis*. Clin Perinatol 15: 321–350

Reuman PD, Ayoub EM, Small PA (1987) Effect of passive maternal antibody in influenza illness in children: a prospective study of influenza A in mother—infant pairs Pediatr Infect Dis 6: 398–403

Ricci JM, Fojaco RM, O'Sullivan MJ (1989) Congenital syphilis. The University of Miami Jackson Memorial Medical Centre experience 1986–1988. Obstet Gynaecol 74: 687–693

Robarts HA, Levin MJ (1983) How contagious is necrotising enterocolitis? Pediatr Infect Dis 2: 406–408

Robbins JB, McCracken GH, Gorschlick EC et al. (1984) *Escherichia coli* K, capsular polysaccharide antigen associated with neonatal meningitis. N Engl J Med 290: 1216–1220

Ross JM, Furr PM, Taylor-Robinson D, Altman DG, Coid CR (1981) The effect of genital mycoplasma on human foetal growth. Br J Obstet Gynaecol 88: 749–755

Rotimi VO, Duerden BI (1981) The development of the bacterial flora in normal neonates. J Med Microbiol 14: 51–62

Rudd P, Peckham C (1988) Infection of the fetus and the newborn: prevention, treatment and related handicap. Baillière's Clin Obstet Gynaecol 2: 55–71

Rutter D, Griffiths PD, Trompeter RS (1985) Cytomegalic inclusion disease after recurrent maternal infection. Lancet ii: 1182

Ryder RW, Wachsmuth IK, Buxton AE et al. (1976) Infantile diarrhoea produced by heat stable enterotoxigenic *E. coli*. N Engl J Med 295: 849–853

Ryder RW, Nsa W, Hassig SE et al. (1989) Perinatal transmission of the human immunodeficiency virus type 1 to infants of seropositive women in Zaire. N Engl J Med 320: 1637–1642

Sarff LD, McCracken GH, Schiffer MS et al. (1975) Epidemiology of *Escherichia coli* K, in healthy and diseased newborns. Lancet i: 1099–2004

Saulsbury FT, Raldolph F, Wykoff MPH, Boyle RJ (1987) Transfusion acquired human immunodeficency virus infection in twelve neonates, epidemiologic clinical and immunological features. Pediatr Infect Dis 6: 544–548

Savage WF, Hajj SN, Kass EH (1967) Demographic and prognostic characteristics of bacteriuria in pregnancy. Medicine 46: 385–407

Schachter J, Grossman M (1981) Chlamydial infection. Annu Rev Med 32: 41–61

Schachter J, Grossman M (1990) Chlamydia. In: Remington JS, Klein JO (eds) Infectious diseases of the fetus and newborn infant, 3rd edn. Saunders, Philadelphia, pp 465–473

Schachter J, Grossman M, Sweet RL, Holt J, Jordan C, Bishop E (1986) Prospective study of perinatal transmission of *Chlamydia trachomatis*. JAMA 255: 3374–3377

Schaeffer M, Fox MJ, Li CP (1954) Intra-uterine poliomyelitis infection. JAMA 155: 248–250

Schroder SA, Aseroff B, Brackman PS (1968) Epidemic salmonellosis in hospitals and institutions. N Engl J Med 279: 674–678

Schuchat A, Swaminathan B, Broume CV (1991) Epidemiology of human listeriosis. Clin Microbiol Rev 4: 169–183

Schweitzer IL, Dunn AE, Peters RL, Spears RL (1973) Viral hepatitis in neonates and infants. Am J Med 55: 762–771

Schwer M, Moosa A (1978) Effects of hepatitis A and B in pregnancy on the mother and fetus. S Afr Med J 54: 1092–1095

Scott GB, Fischl N, Klimas M et al. (1985) Mothers of infants with acquired immunodeficiency syndrome. Outcome of subsequent pregnancies. Abstracts of 1st international conference on acquired immunodeficiency syndrome, Atlanta, Georgia, April 1985. Report ISSN0025729X

Seeliger HPR, Finger H (1983) Listeriosis. In: Remington JS, Klein JO (eds) Infectious diseases of the fetus and newborn infant, 2nd edn. Saunders, Philadelphia, pp 333–365

Selwyn PA, Schoenbaum EE, Davenny K et al. (1989) Prospective study of human immunodeficiency virus infection and pregnancy outcome in intravenous drug users. JAMA 261: 1289–1294

Sever J, White LR (1968) Intrauterine viral infections. Annu Rev Med 19: 471–486

Sever JL, Ellenberg JH, Evans D (1978) Urinary infections during pregnancy: maternal and paediatric findings. In: Kass EH, Brumfitt HW (eds) Infections of the urinary tract. University of Chicago Press, Chicago, pp 19–21

Shelokov A, Weinstein L (1951) Poliomyelitis in the early neonatal period, report of a case of possible intra-uterine infection. J Pediatr 38: 80–84

Siegal M (1973) Congenital malformation following chickenpox, measles, mumps and hepatitis. Results of a cohort study. JAMA 226: 1513–1524

Siegal M, Fuerst HT (1966) Low birth weight and maternal virus diseases. A prospective study of rubella, measles, mumps, chickenpox and hepatitis. JAMA 197: 680–684

Siegal M, Greenberg M (1956) Poliomyelitis in pregnancy: effect on fetus and newborn infant. J Pediatr 49: 280–288

Siegal M, Fuerst HT, Peress NS (1966) Comparative fetal mortality in maternal virus disease. A prospective study on rubella, measles, chickenpox and hepatitis. N Engl J Med 274: 768–771

South MA, Tompkins WAF, Morris R, Rawls WE (1969) Congenital malformations of the central nervous system associated with genital type (type 2) herpes infection. J Pediatr 75: 13–18

Spencer JAD (1987) Perinatal listeriosis. Br Med J 295: 349

Stagno S (1980) Congenital toxoplasmosis. Am J Dis Child 134: 635–637

Stagno S (1990) Cytomegalovirus. In: Remington JS, Klein JO (eds) Infectious diseases of the fetus and newborn infant, 3rd edn. Saunders, Philadelphia, pp 241–281

Stagno S, Whitley RJ (1985a) Current concepts, herpesvirus infection of pregnancy. Cytomegalovirus and Epstein–Barr virus infections. N Engl J Med 313: 1270–1274

Stagno S, Whitley RJ (1985b) Herpesvirus infection of pregnancy. Herpes simplex virus and varicella zoster virus infections. N Engl J Med 313: 1372–1330

Stagno S, Reynolds DW, Amos CS et al. (1977) Auditory and visual defects resulting from symptomatic and subclinical congenital cytomegaloviral and Toxoplasma infections. Pediatrics 59: 669–678

Stagno S, Pass RF, Cloud G et al. (1986) Primary CMV infection in pregnancy. Incidence, transmission to fetus and clinical outcome. JAMA 256: 1904–1908

Stoller A, Collmann RD (1965) Evidence of infective hepatitis followed by Down's syndrome nine months later. Lancet ii: 1221–1223

Stone JH, Das BC (1986) Investigation of an outbreak with *Acinetobacter calcoaceticus* in a special care baby unit. J Hosp Infect 7: 42–47

Stringer J, Crees-Morris A, Young S et al. (1981) Group B streptococcal systemic disease in Great Britain. J Infect 3: 385–391

Thaler M, Park CK, Landers DV et al. (1991) Vertical transmission of hepatitis C virus. Lancet 338: 17–18

Tong MJ, Thursby M, Rakela J, McPeak C, Edwards VM, Mosley JW (1981) Studies on the maternal–infant transmission of the viruses which cause acute hepatitis. Gastroenterology 80: 999–1004

Walker-Smith J (1978) Rotavirus gastroenteritis. Arch Dis Child 53: 355–362

Weiland HT, Vermey-Keers CHR, Salimans MM, Fleuren GJ, Verwey RA (1987) Parvovirus B_{19} associated with fetal abnormality. Lancet i: 682–683

Welch DF, Marks MT (1982) Is *C. difficile* pathogenic in infants? J Pediatr 100: 393–396

Whitley R (1990) Herpes simplex virus infections. In: Remington JS, Klein JO (eds) Infectious diseases of the fetus and newborn infant, 3rd edn. Saunders, Philadelphia, pp 282–305

Whitley R, Arvin A, Prober C et al. (1991) Predictions of morbidity and mortality in neonates with herpes simplex virus infections. N Engl J Med 324: 450–454

Williams JD, Reeves DS, Condie AP et al. (1978) Significance of bacteriuria in pregnancy. In: Kass EH, Brumfitt HW (eds) Infections of the urinary tract. University of Chicago Press, Chicago, pp 8–18

Wilson CB, Remington JS, Stagno S, Reynolds DW (1980) Development of adverse sequelae in children born with subclinical congenital Toxoplasma infection. Pediatrics 66: 767–774

Wilson R, Kauto WP, McCarthy VSJ et al. (1981) Epidemiologic characteristics of necrotising enterocolitis: a population based study. Am J Epidemiol 114: 880–887

Wood PL, Hobson D, Rees E (1984) Genital infection with *Chlamydia trachomatis* in women attending an antenatal clinic. Br J Obstet Gynaecol 91: 1171–1176

Wright DJ, Berry CL (1974) Liver involvement in congenital symphilis. Br J Vener Dis 50: 241 (letter)

Wyler DJ (1983) Malaria—resurgence, resistance and research. N Engl J Med 308: 875–878, 934–940

Zeldis JB, Crumpacker C (1990) Hepatitis. In: Remington JS, Klein JO (eds) Infectious diseases of the fetus and newborn infant, 3rd edn. Saunders, Philadelphia, pp 574–600

Zuckerman A (1990) Hepatitis E virus. Br Med J 300: 1475–1476

Chapter 14

Iatrogenic Disease

Jean W. Keeling

Introduction

The realisation that medical treatment can be harmful to the patient is not new. Injury to the fetus during instrumental delivery is well recognised (Fedrick and Butler 1971), but still occurs. A review of obstetric cases coming to litigation found that failure to observe or act on signs of fetal distress, mismanagement of the use of forceps and inadequate supervision of junior medical staff were common factors (Ennis and Vincent 1990). The authors thought these cases should not be dismissed as isolated incidents but reflect a more general problem. The increasing use of invasive antenatal investigations and the availability of sophisticated neonatal intensive care has resulted in an increased in both the incidence and range of iatrogenic disease in the fetus and neonate. It is important that the pathologist recognises the manifestations of iatrogenic disease when he undertakes the necropsy examination of babies. By so doing he contributes to safer, more effective management of both pregnancy and the neonatal period. If he is to do this, he must be aware of investigations and procedures which have been undertaken and of medication prescribed during both the pregnancy and in postnatal life before he begins his examination. To this end, it is important that the clinical notes are available and all drain tubes and catheters are left in situ after death.

Maternal Medication During Pregnancy

The concept of the placenta as a barrier between mother and fetus is inappropriate as far as drugs are concerned. The concentration of the drug in the maternal plasma is an important factor, and diffusion across the placenta will take place if this is sufficiently high. Only a small number of drugs are destroyed or altered by passage through the placenta. It follows, therefore, that medication in pregnant women should be kept to a necessary minimum and self-medication discouraged.

Only those drugs which result in recognisable morphological or histological abnormality are briefly described here. A more detailed account of the effect of drugs on both fetus and infant is given by Ashton (1981).

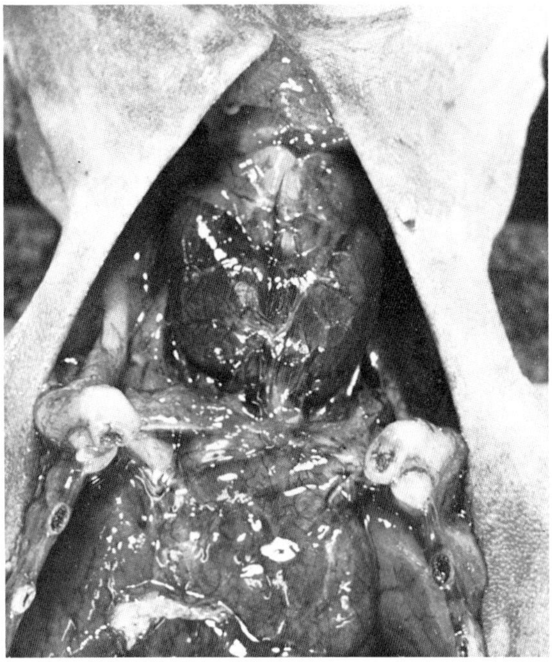

Fig. 14.1. Thyroid enlargement in fetus at 20 weeks' gestation related to maternal carbimazole medication.

Teratogenic Effects

Drugs can only produce teratogenic effects when administered during the period of embryogenesis, i.e. the 3rd to the 8th weeks of intrauterine life. It is likely that the embryo is most sensitive to environmental effects during the first half of this period.

Teratogenicity in man is difficult to prove, and convincing evidence of teratogenic effect exists for only a very small number of drugs. Few would dispute the effects of folate antagonists (Thiersch 1952) or thalidomide (Leck and Millar 1962; Lenz 1962) on the fetus. It is now thought likely that anticonvulsant drugs (congenital heart disease, cleft lip and palate), warfarin (nasal hypoplasia, stippled epiphyses, microcephaly, mental retardation), inhalation anaesthetics (CNS and musculoskeletal abnormalities) and psychotropic drugs (cardiovascular anomalies) are causally related to malformation in the fetus. Administration of steroid hormones undoubtedly produces virilisation of the fetus and diethylstilboestrol has a transplacental carcinogenic effect in females. Steroid hormones may also result in increase in non-random associations of malformations of the VACTERL type (vertebral, anal, cardiac, tracheo-oesophageal, renal, limb deformities) in the exposed fetus (Nora and Nora 1973; Harlap et al. 1975).

Second and Third Trimester Medication

Antithyroid Drugs

Antithyroid drugs readily cross the placenta and many produce thyroid enlargement in the fetus (Fig. 14.1). This is thought to result from an increase in TSH secretion by the fetus in response to inhibition of thyroxine production by the drug.

Sulphonamides

Sulphonamides and other drugs which compete with bilirubin for protein binding sites will produce jaundice and kernicterus in the neonate if given to the mother late in pregnancy (see Chap. 17; Chap. 24).

Salicylates

Salicylate administration late in pregnancy has been related to neonatal haemorrhage (Stirrat and Beard 1973).

Local Anaesthetics

Inadvertent fetal injection with prilocaine hydrochloride (Citanest) during vulval infiltration prior to episiotomy can cause methaemoglobinaemia (Menahem 1988).

Prenatal Diagnosis

Several invasive techniques are currently practised to facilitate prenatal diagnosis. Amniocentesis is most frequently used. Sampling of the amniotic fluid is usually undertaken transabdominally using a long, narrow-gauge needle, and is undertaken during the second trimester of pregnancy to facilitate the diagnosis of many different inherited disorders and malformations. It has been performed during the third trimester in management of rhesus incompatibility and to assess fetal lung maturity when early delivery is indicated for any reason. Amniocentesis has an established rôle in antenatal management, but the potential hazard of any invasive investigation should not be forgotten. Maternal complications of amniocentesis are infrequent (see Keeling 1987 for review).

Chorion villus biopsy, undertaken between the 7th and 12th weeks of pregnancy, involves the aspiration of villi either vaginally with catheter or transabdominally with a long needle, both done with ultrasound guidance. It is used to obtain tissue for antenatal diagnosis, chromosome analysis, investigation of genetic metabolic disease or to provide material for DNA restriction analysis for the diagnosis of disorders such as thalassaemia or sickle cell disease. The advantages of this technique are the relatively early stage of gestation at which the test can be undertaken and the more rapid tissue culture because of the much greater volume of cells obtained compared with amniocentesis.

Fetoscopy has a limited rôle in antenatal diagnosis. It requires the passage of a wider bore instrument than does amniocentesis and is more prone to complications. Its use is restricted to the few situations which need specific fetal tissue for prenatal diagnosis.

Percutaneous fetal blood sampling from an umbilical cord vessel under ultrasound control is undertaken in the second or third trimester of pregnancy for a variety of investigations. A pure sample of fetal blood is obtained. It appears to carry low risk to the fetus (Daffos et al. 1983) but acute, sometimes fatal, fetal distress can occur (Benacerraf 1987).

Complications of Amniocentesis

The experience of collaborative studies in Canada (Simpson et al. 1976), Europe (Galjaard 1976) and the USA (NICHD 1976) found no increase in fetal wastage over the natural level expected at that stage of gestation, and the American study found no increase in problems during delivery or the neonatal period. In the UK, the Medical Research Council Collaborative Study (MRC 1978) found an increase in fetal loss of 1%–1.5% over controls and a similar increase in infant morbidity. The high quality of ultrasound imaging available during sampling and accumulated experience with amniocentesis have combined to reduce the miscarriage rate to about 1% (Tabor et al. 1986). The serious nature of the complications reported indicates the need for continued scrupulous attention to detail by clinical and laboratory personnel.

Midtrimester Amniocentesis

Abortion following amniocentesis seems likely to be related to mechanical damage to the gestation sac during the procedure. The recent MRC trial (MRC 1991) found that most post amniocentesis spontaneous abortions occurred in the week following the procedure. The MRC (1978) study found premonitory signs of such damage in the form of heavy blood staining of the fluid sample or loss of fetal movements or heart beats in 10 of 15 women who aborted in the 4-week period following amniocentesis. Half of these women had vaginal bleeding or leakage of amniotic fluid preceding abortion. The NICHD (1976) study found that post-amniocentesis abortion was significantly associated with use of a needle larger than 18 gauge, and that procedures requiring more than one needle insertion were also associated with abortion, whilst there was no relationship with the volume of fluid removed.

The MRC (1978) study identified an increase in late complications of amniocentesis in the form of antepartum haemorrhage from either placenta praevia or abruption, an increase in respiratory problems in the neonatal period and in the number of deaths from hyaline membrane disease. This study also found an increase in postural deformities (congenital dislocation of the hip and severe talipes) amongst the amniocentesis group. It was suggested that all the fetal problems encountered resulted from removal of amniotic fluid, perhaps compounded by subsequent leakage of liquor amnii.

Fetal injury following mid-trimester amniocentesis is not common. Skin puncture with healing to form small scars or dimples is the most frequently recorded injury (Karp and Hayden 1977; see Chap. 4, p. 120). Internal injury has been reported, in the form of fatal haemothorax (Rushton 1981), ileal atresia and peritoneal adhesions (Therkensen and Rehder 1981) and intestinal cutaneous fistula and ileal atresia (Rickwood 1977). Youroukos et al. (1980) reported temporal and occipital skin lesion and porencephalic cysts following amniocentesis. Limb abnormalities have been observed, in the form of gangrene in the arm secondary to supraclavicular puncture (Lamb 1975) and distal limb constrictions and amputations secondary to amniotic bands (Rehder 1978).

Third Trimester Amniocentesis

The most frequently encountered complication of third trimester amniocentesis, after failure to obtain a fluid sample, is premature rupture of membranes. Brinsmead (1976) reported this in 8% of reviewed cases in which amniocentesis had been undertaken as part of the management of pregnancies complicated by rhesus disease. In more than half of the cases where membrane rupture occurred it was followed by premature delivery of the fetus; neonatal deaths from problems of prematurity were observed. Amnionitis leading to perinatal death is reported following third trimester amniocentesis by both Liley (1960) and Brinsmead (1976).

Haemorrhage from puncture of umbilical cord during amniocentesis is recorded by Ryan et al. (1972), Grove et al. (1973) and Gassner and Paul (1976). This is more likely during the third trimester as the relatively small amount of liquor at this stage makes it more difficult for the cord to float away from the needle point. Puncture of a large subchorionic vessel was observed by Kalbac and Newman (1974), and massive fetomaternal haemorrhage following placental puncture has been reported by Misenhimer (1966).

Fetal injury during third trimester amniocentesis is related to the large size and relative immobility of the fetus. Fatal intracranial haemorrhage is reported by Creasman et al. (1968) and Portman and Brouillette (1982) and occular trauma necessitating enucleation by Cross and Maumenee (1972). Fatal haemothorax and haemopericardium is recorded at 31 weeks' gestation by Berner et al. (1972) and pneumothorax following amniocentesis at term by Creasman et al. (1968), Grove et al. (1973), Hyman et al. (1973) and Hamid (1975).

The high quality of ultrasound imaging currently available to monitor sampling procedures has made this type of injury uncommon.

Chorion Villus Sampling

In the MRC trial of chorion villus sampling (CVS) (MRC 1991) more spontaneous fetal losses before 28 weeks' gestation and more neonatal death followed first trimester CVS when compared with second trimester amniocentesis. More women needed a second diagnostic test following CVS (100) than was the case following amniocentesis (35). This was largely due to failure to obtain an adequate sample. CVS was less accurate than amniocentesis because of identification of chromosomal mosaicism which was subsequently shown to be confined to the placenta.

Intra-amniotic Injection

Intra-amniotic injection of methylene blue dye as an aid to detection of premature rupture of membranes has resulted in haemolytic jaundice in the neonate (Crooks 1982). Its use for this purpose or even in some circumstances for reversal of methaemoglobinaemia in the newborn is questioned in view of the seriousness of hyperbilirubinaemia in the neonate (Menahem 1988).

Intrapartum Monitoring

The use of scalp electrodes for continuous intrapartum fetal heart rate monitoring may often result in abrasions or puncture of the scalp (Fig. 14.2) and may sometimes be complicated by more extensive scalp laceration, abscess or osteomyelitis (Chan et al. 1973; Overturf and Balfour 1975). Ashkenazi et al. (1985) reported serious complications in only 1.5% of more than 500 babies. D'Souza et al. (1982) recognised an increase in neonatal jaundice following extensive scalp bruising related to use of a spiral monitoring scalp electrode. Fatal herpes simplex infection was related to intrapartum monitoring at 34 weeks' gestation by Goldkrand (1982).

Breech Delivery

Breech presentation has long been associated with increased mortality and morbidity amongst babies delivered vaginally (Butler and Bonham

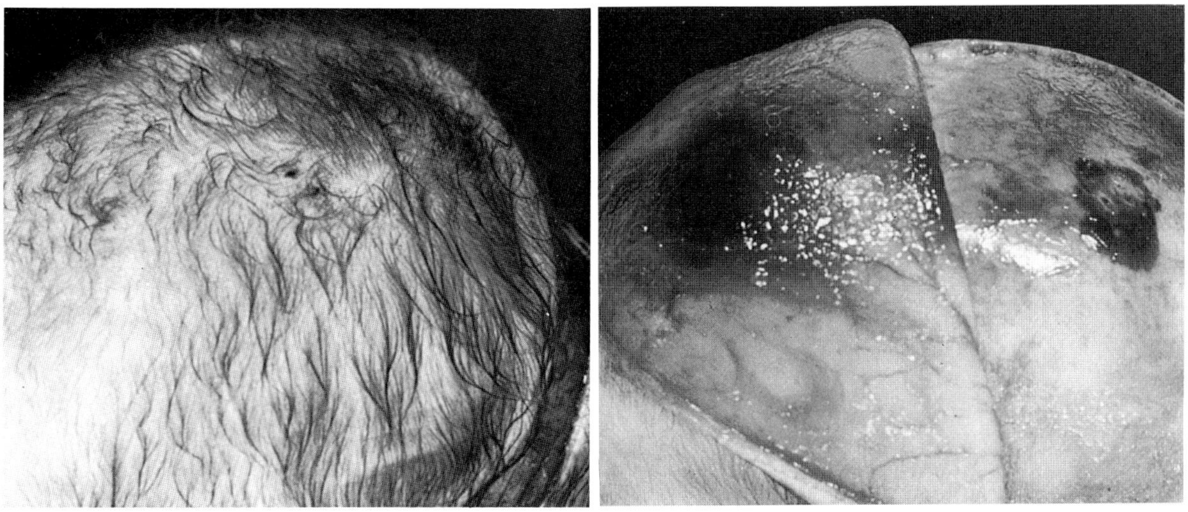

a b

Fig. 14.2. **a** Two puncture marks in scalp of term neonate following use of scalp clip for intrapartum monitoring. **b** Reflection of scalp reveals scalp and subperiosteal haemorrhage.

1963). Whilst cerebral hypoxic injury is a well-recognised hazard, other types of injury may go undetected without modification of necropsy techniques. Occipital osteodiastases, described by Wigglesworth and Husemeyer (1977), results from pressure on the lower half of the squamous portion of the occipital bone and its inwards dislocation in respect of the lateral portions. The baby's occiput appears flatter than normal. Displacement tears underlying venous sinuses and catastrophic haemorrhage ensues. Unless the scalp is reflected downwards as far as the foramen magnum and the occipital bone fully exposed, then this injury and its relationship to cranial haemorrhage is likely to be missed.

Injury to the cervical region of the spinal cord may also occur if the neck is overextended during delivery. There may be direct injury to the cord or hypoxic damage following injury to the cervical portion of the vertebral arteries (Yates 1959). It is necessary to excise the cervical portion of the vertebral column with the spinal cord in situ and examine the whole for evidence of injury by slicing the specimen transversely after fixation and possibly following a short period of decalcification (see Chap. 1, p. 27).

Haemorrhage into muscles of the buttocks and legs readily occurs during breech delivery as a result of hypoxic injury to small blood vessels; this may result in significant hypovolaemia and, later, as haemoglobin is broken down, in hyperbilirubinaemia serious enough to warrant treatment. Whilst bruising of the overlying skin is usual, the extent of haemorrhage will not be appreciated at necropsy unless muscles are deliberately incised.

Testicular interstitial haemorrhage may occur during breech delivery if the testes have descended (Dunn 1975). Tubular loss and interstitial fibrosis follow (Fig. 14.3). Tiwary (1989) found genital injuries in 19 of 34 male infants who presented by the breech and were delivered vaginally. Ten babies (6.5%) had testicular injury; only three were normal to palpation later. It seems likely that this may lead to infertility. Tiwary suggests that careful attention be paid to perinatal events in the husband before expensive investigations are contemplated when couples present with infertility.

Rona and Tanner (1977) noted a higher incidence of both breech presentation and forceps delivery amongst children with growth hormone deficiency than was found amongst babies in the British Perinatal Mortality Study of 1958, although they did not consider the two to be causally related. However, Piccolo et al. (1979) reviewed the obstetric histories of their patients with growth hormone deficiency and found that 19.6% had presented by the breech, compared with only 1.6% of a control group of children. These authors postulated that intrapartum hypoxic damage to the pituitary resulted in growth hormone deficiency.

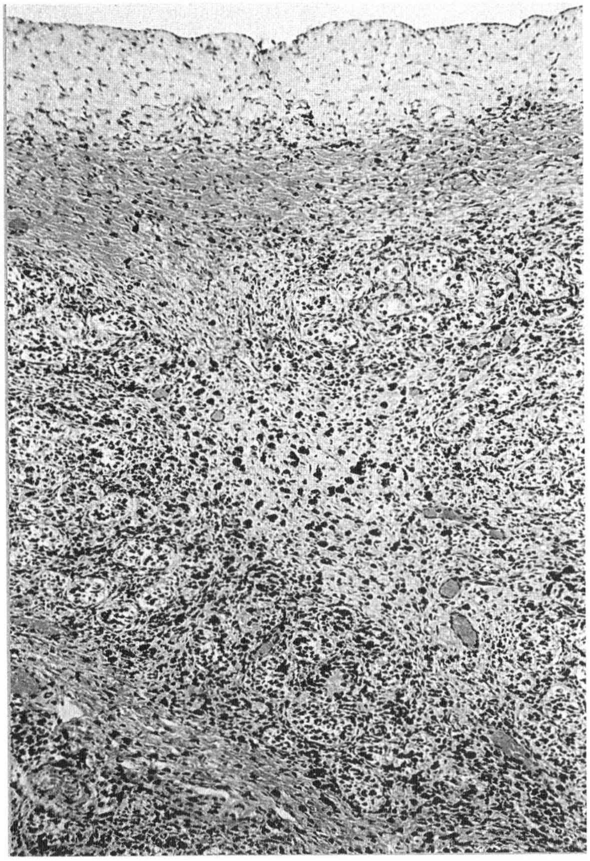

Fig. 14.3. Breech delivery at term; baby died at age 3 weeks. Testis with loss of tubules and fibrosis. Iron pigment is present within macrophages.

Neonatal Intensive Care

Many iatrogenic lesions in the neonate are related to the need to maintain adequate tissue oxygenation in the face of respiratory distress and apnoea of prematurity. Others result from manoeuvres to monitor Po_2 as clinicians strive to maintain oxygen levels within the narrow confines of adequacy and safety, bearing in mind the damaging effects of both hypoxia and the prolonged use of high concentrations of oxygen to many fetal organs.

Ventilation

At the present time, ventilation is the basis of treatment of severe respiratory distress of prematurity and may be required for several days and even weeks. It is sometimes required in other clinical situations in the neonatal period. The problems arising as a result of ventilation may be conveniently considered in three groups: those related to contact with the apparatus used, those attributable to the pressure of the ventilating gases and those related to the gas mixture itself.

Apparatus

The poorly keratinised skin of the premature infant withstands friction poorly. Ulceration around the nose or mouth can easily occur if the endotracheal tube or face mask is not securely fixed (Fig. 14.4). Irregular primary dentition, common in children who were of low birthweight is thought to be the result of pressure of the endotracheal tube on the gingeval margin (Fearne et al. 1985). Midline palatal grooving (Erenberg and Nowak 1984) and clefting (Duke et al. 1976) is described in preterm babies following long-term orotracheal intubation. These authors propose that pressure from long-term contact with the tube was responsible for the palatal abnormality; how-

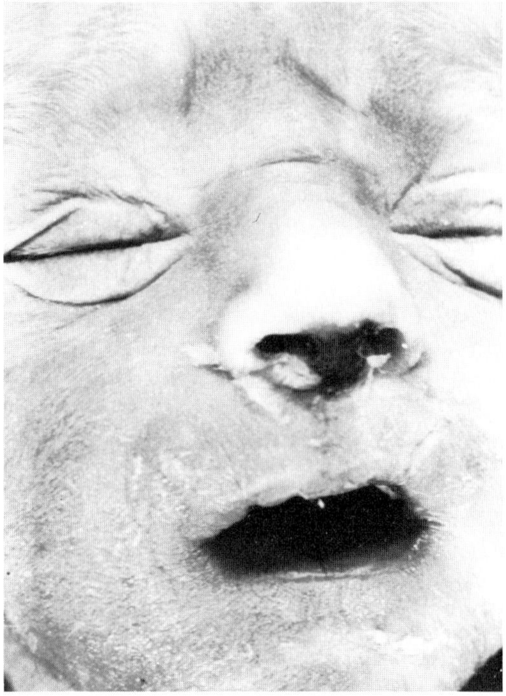

Fig. 14.4. Ulceration of nasal septum after endotracheal intubation.

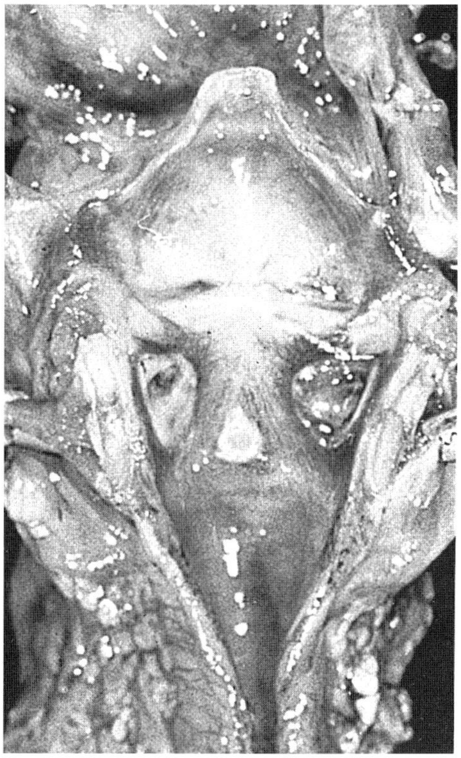

Fig. 14.5. Larynx opened posteriorly. Ulceration is apparent in the midline anteriorly and bilaterally below the vocal cords following endotracheal intubation.

ever, Carrillo (1985) suggested that the mechanism may be interference with normal tongue pressure on the palate by the tube resulting in unopposed growth of the lateral palate and ridges, as described by Hanson et al. (1976) in babies with poor neuromuscular coordination. It is difficult to envisage how this process alone could produce clefting, although it may accentuate any groove produced by pressure. Even the use of adhesive tape may produce erythema or ulceration in the very premature infant. These may lead to permanent changes in pigmentation. Secure fastening of face masks by means of a 2.5 cm (1 in) Velcro band may lead to deformity of the skull and cerebellar haemorrhage (Pape et al. 1976). Histologically, the cerebellar lesions appear to be venous infarcts.

Whilst skin ulceration is unsightly and may induce parental anxiety, the damage to the upper respiratory tract resulting from pressure and friction against an endotracheal tube is of a potentially more serious nature. Ulceration of the vocal chords or subglottic region (Fig. 14.5) is frequently seen. Whilst many lesions are superficial and apparently heal without sequel once the tube is removed, deep ulceration provokes fibrosis, and shrinkage during maturation of the fibrous scar may result in narrowing of the airway necessitating tracheostomy or operative repair. Perichondritis and chrondromalacia affecting the arytenoid and cricoid cartilages are described as a sequel to prolonged intubation (Gould and Howard 1985). O'Neill (1984) estimated that laryngeal or tracheal stenosis occurred in 1.5% of the population at risk and that intubation for longer than 4 weeks' duration was a predisposing factor.

In the trachea, a vertical row of shallow ulcers may be found in the midline anteriorly over tracheal rings following endotracheal intubation. Squamous metaplasia of the anterior half of the tracheal epithelium may develop in the length of trachea in contact with the tube (Fig. 14.6). Theoretically this might interfere with bronchial toilet and so predispose to infection.

Perforation of the trachea (Reynolds and Taghizadeh 1974), bronchus (Holcomb and Templeton 1989) or oesophagus (Clarke et al. 1980) is an infrequent complication of endotracheal intubation.

Necrotising Tracheobronchitis

This lesion has been recognised following the introduction of high-frequency jet ventilation (see Chap. 17, p. 420).

Pressure of Ventilating Gases

The gas pressures used for ventilation are the minimum necessary to achieve alveolar expansion and permit adequate gas exchange. If pulmonary compliance falls, then an increase in ventilating pressure becomes necessary. Immature or hypoplastic lungs are fragile and passage of gas into the interstitial tissue occurs readily. It accumulates along interlobular septa and beneath the pleura. It is readily seen as small bubbles beneath the pleural surfaces (Fig. 14.7). Larger volumes of gas accumulate in interlobular fissures and track into the mediastinum and occasionally into retroperitoneal tissues, where they must be distinguished in radiographs from the sequelae of necrotising enterocolitis. Gas may extend via the mediastinum into subcutaneous

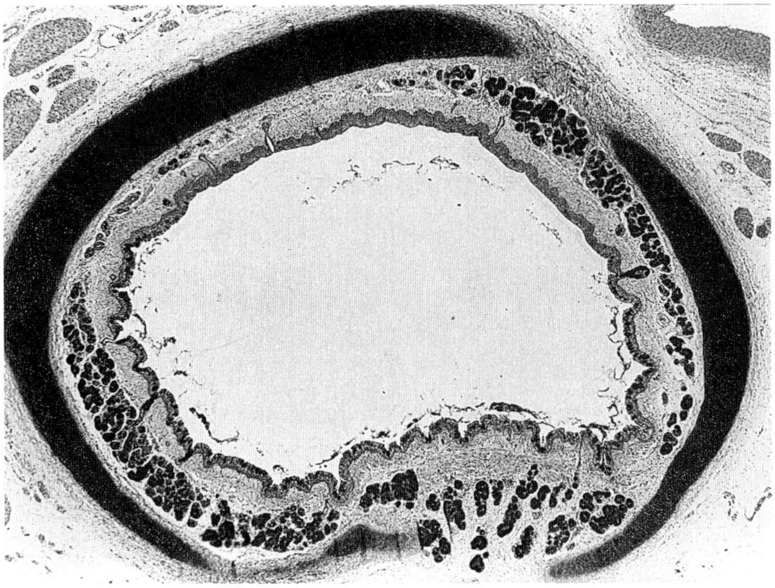

Fig. 14.6. Cross-section of trachea. Anteriorly, there is squamous metaplasia of the epithelium and loss of goblet cells. (Keeling 1981)

tissues over the head and neck, when the crepitant texture of subcutaneous tissues is readily apparent.

Large amounts of gas may accumulate in the interstitium of one lobe of lung (Fig. 14.8) and result in respiratory embarrassment and mediastinal shift. Lobectomy may occasionally be necessary (Drew et al. 1978).

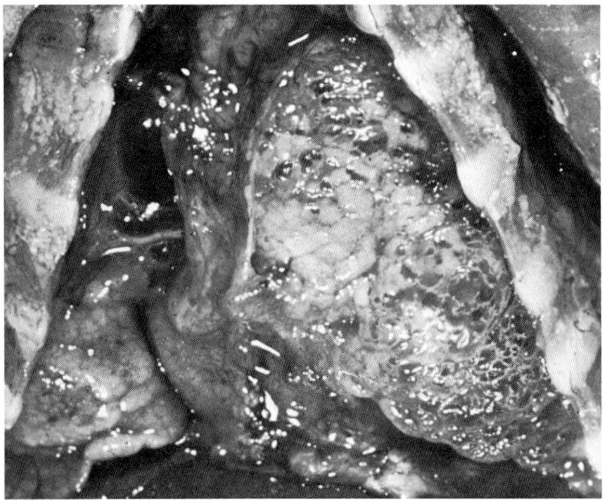

Fig. 14.7. Interstitial emphysema involving both lobes of left lung. Many gas bubbles are seen through the pleura. There is a larger accumulation of gas at the hilus on the *right*. (Keeling 1981)

Pneumothorax is a common and life-threatening sequel of interstitial emphysema (Fig. 14.9). Its frequency in a particular unit is not just related to the skill of the neonatologist and type of apparatus available but also to the admissions policy of the unit. Moessinger et al. (1978) recognised pneumothorax in 13.4% of 209 consecutive admissions in their unit, and Lindroth et al. (1980) observed pneumothorax in 20% of babies receiving intermittent positive pressure ventilation for hyaline membrane disease. Rates are higher when babies less than 1500 g birthweight are ventilated, Whitelaw et al. (1983) found pneumothorax in 52% of their patients.

The use of chest drains in the management of pneumothorax is not without hazard; perforation of the lung may complicate the procedure (Fig. 14.10). The frequency of this complication is related to the type of drain used, the use of a metal trocar to introduce the drain and the inexperience of the operator. Moessinger et al. (1978) found lung perforation in 25% of their patients whose pneumothorax was treated. Serious scarring with muscle and breast involvement can follow the anterior insertion of chest drains (Cartlidge et al. 1990). Diaphragmatic paralysis, thought to be the result of injury to both phrenic nerves by chest drains, is described by Arya et al. (1991).

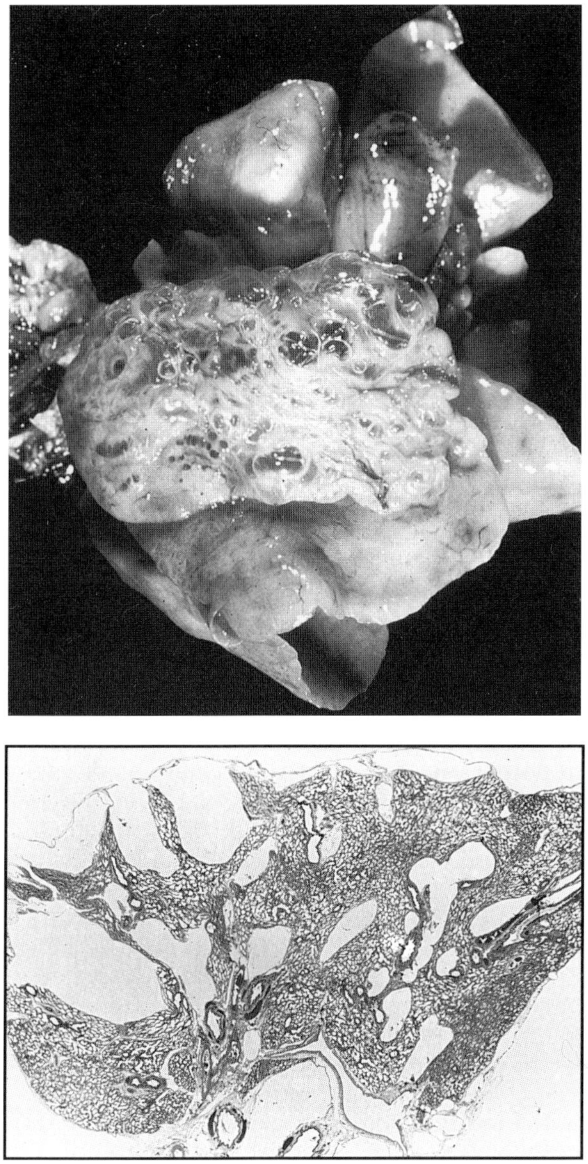

a

b

Fig. 14.8. **a** Large accumulations of gas are present beneath the upper lobe pleura. **b** Histological section shows distortion of lung architecture and compression of parenchyma by gas bubbles. (Keeling 1981)

Oxygen Toxicity

The organs of the preterm neonate which are vulnerable to oxygen toxicity are the eye and the lung. In the immature baby an elevated Po_2 for any period of time stimulates vasobliteration and subsequent neovascularisation of the retina (Ashton 1954). If the stimulus persists, these vessels extend into the vitreous. Retinal

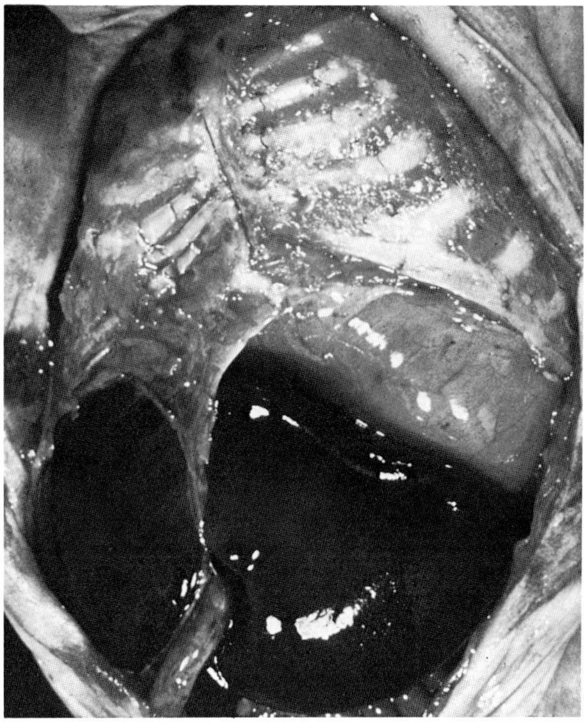

Fig. 14.9. A large left-sided pneumothorax has depressed the left hemidiaphragm and elevated and separated the ribs on that side. (Keeling 1981)

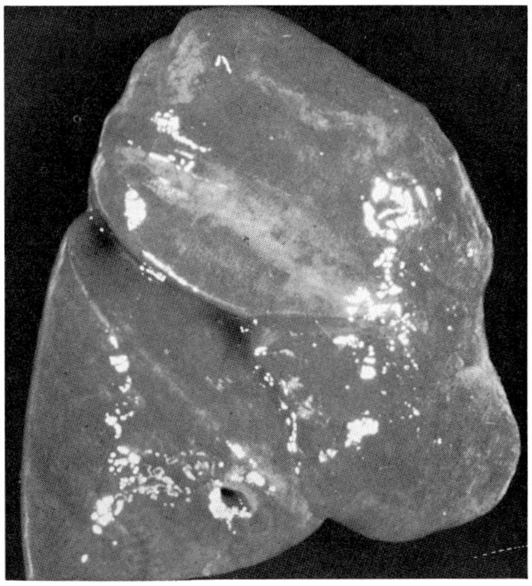

Fig. 14.10. Collapsed lung of hyaline membrane disease. Perforation of the lower lobe complicated the use of a chest drain for pneumothorax. (Keeling 1981)

detachment and fibroblast proliferation in the vitreous ensue (see Chap. 28, p. 679).

Chronic lung damage following hyaline membrane disease was first described by Northway et al. in 1967 (Fig. 14.11). The effect of high oxygen concentration on the premature lung is initially to damage the lining cells of alveoli and intrapulmonary airways of all sizes. Following this initial damage, thickening of alveolar walls occurs, first as a result of interstitial oedema and then by fibroblast infiltration. Hyperplastic regeneration of airways epithelium occurs. These are the histological appearances of bronchopulmonary dysplasia. Some regard this as a manifestation of oxygen damage alone (Bonikos et al. 1976; Edwards et al. 1977), whereas Taghizadeh and Reynolds (1976) related its development to a mode of ventilation using high peak airways pressure and high ventilation rates. Animal studies (deLemos et al. 1969; Bonikos et al. 1975) have shown that all the histological features of human bronchopulmonary dysplasia can be produced in animals who are exposed to high levels of oxygen, without the need for ventilation. Brown et al. (1978) have suggested that pulmonary interstitial oedema plays an important role in the development of this condition (see also Chaps. 8 and 17).

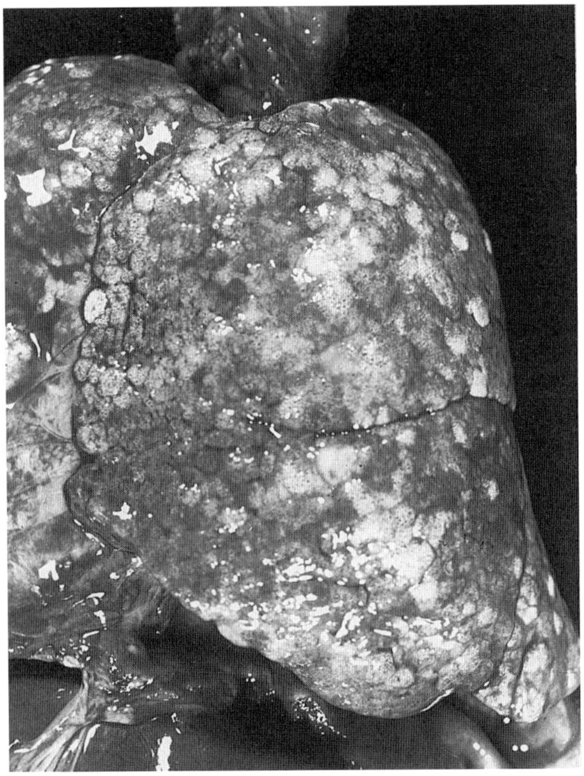

Fig. 14.11. Bronchopulmonary dysplasia. Preterm baby died at age 3 months. The lungs are bulky and fill the chest. Overdistended terminal air spaces are seen as small bubbles through the pleura; some lobules are collapsed. (Keeling 1981)

Extracorporeal Membrane Oxygenation

Extracorporeal membrane oxygenation (ECMO) was introduced into neonatal intensive care about 12 years ago for the short-term support of babies with respiratory failure. It is still only undertaken in a few centres. The procedure involves cannulation of a carotid artery and jugular vein to channel a large proportion of the infant's blood volume to a membrane oxygenator. Blood is rewarmed and returned to the baby. The most common complication of ECMO is intracranial haemorrhage which occurs in about one-third of patients (Cilley et al. 1986; Taylor et al. 1987a). Intracranial haemorrhage is a predictable problem if one considers the likely effect of intracranial pressure changes consequent on jugular vein ligation and anoxia/hypotension which would follow changes in circulating blood volume or equipment failure, in an infant who is heparinised and whose platelets are at risk of damage by the oxygenator. Infants who are preterm or of low birthweight are at particular risk of intracranial haemorrhage during this procedure.

A variety of intracranial lesions is described in babies following the use of ECMO. Parenchymal haemorrhage alone or in combination is the commonest, most often in the occipital region. Some babies have only subarachnoid or germinal matrix haemorrhage (Taylor et al. 1987a). A thalamostriatal haemorrhage was found in a mature baby (Cilley et al. 1986). The distribution of lesions suggests prior cerebral ischaemic insult.

Several ischaemic cerebral lesions are described both in babies who die and survivors (Taylor et al. 1987a,b). They include porencephaly, cerebral atrophy, sagittal sinus thrombosis, infarction, periventricular leukomalacia and cerebellar haemorrhage. Chronic problems include cerebral palsy, low intelligence and microcephaly (Andrews et al. 1986).

Fibrin thrombi or thromboemboli were found in 16 of 19 babies at necropsy following ECMO treatment shortly before death (Vogler et al. 1988). They were commonest in brain and lung but were found in kidney, heart, liver and spleen as well. All organs contained basophilic emboli. Some were shown to contain aluminium thought to originate from the blood warmer. Aluminium-containing material appeared to be the origin of some emboli. These authors noted infarction in the right middle cerebral artery territory in three babies whose right carotid artery had been cannulated.

Oxygen Monitoring

The observation of a high frequency of blindness in infants who had been born prematurely prompted investigations which linked it with oxygen therapy for respiratory distress syndrome. Subsequent investigation of the pathogenesis of retinopathy of prematurity (ROP) (Ashton et al. 1954) confirmed an association with tissue hyperoxia. It is apparent now that the aetiology of ROP is more complex than originally thought (Lancet 1992). This does not eliminate the need to measure arterial Po_2 when oxygen-enriched gas mixtures are used. Initially this was done intermittently, either by repeated sampling from peripheral arteries or using samples withdrawn from an indwelling catheter inserted into the aorta via an umbilical artery. Intermittent sampling is unsatisfactory by its very nature. When peripheral arteries are sampled the number of tests is limited by the availability of sampling sites. The sampling procedure may result in an incorrect reading because of the trauma involved.

Continuous Po_2 monitoring using a continuous recording electrode in the tip of a catheter which could also be used for infusion or blood sampling was clearly an improvement from the point of view of the data obtained. A disadvantage of this method is the large external diameter of the catheter, particularly when the patient is of low birthweight, when it fills the common iliac artery.

The problems encountered with methods of Po_2 monitoring which required arterial blood samples stimulated the development of a transcutaneous oxygen electrode which heats the skin to stimulate capillary dilatation and measures oxygen diffusion across the capillary/cutaneous barrier (Huch et al. 1974).

Whilst iatrogenic lesions may complicate the use of all of these methods of Po_2 monitoring, those associated with the use of transcutaneous oxygen electrodes are much less serious than those associated with other monitoring methods.

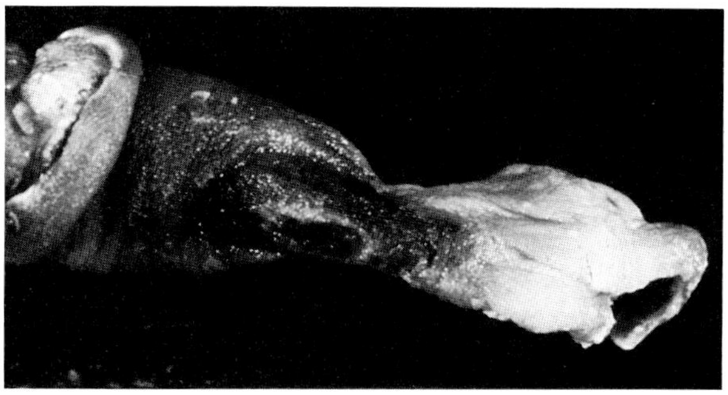

Fig. 14.12. Gangrene of the forearm following brachial and radial artery puncture led to amputation. (Keeling 1981)

Peripheral Artery Sampling

Undesirable sequelae of peripheral artery sampling have been recorded for most sampling sites used. The slow development of contralateral hemiplegia over several months following temporal artery puncture (Simmons et al. 1978) led these authors to recommend discontinuation of the practice.

Radial artery sampling may be complicated by carpal tunnel syndrome caused by local haematomas (Koenigsberger and Moessinger 1977), whilst others have reported only minor complications in the form of bruising (Adams and Rudolph 1975), even following loss of radial pulse after the procedure. Rarely, more serious sequelae are seen, in the form of ulceration of the forearm and even gangrene, necessitating amputation (Fig. 14.12).

Catheterisation of the posterior tibial artery as a multi-use sampling site was suggested by Spahr et al. (1979), in view of the problems associated with temporal or radial artery sampling. In their hands complications were limited to transient cyanosis of the toes, which was alleviated in all cases by removal of the cannula.

Monitoring with an Indwelling Aortic Catheter

The complications encountered when indwelling aortic catheters are used are similar to those encountered when the aorta is catheterised for any reason (p. 334).

Transcutaneous Electrode

Local cutaneous erythema is common when transcutaneous oxygen electrodes are used (see

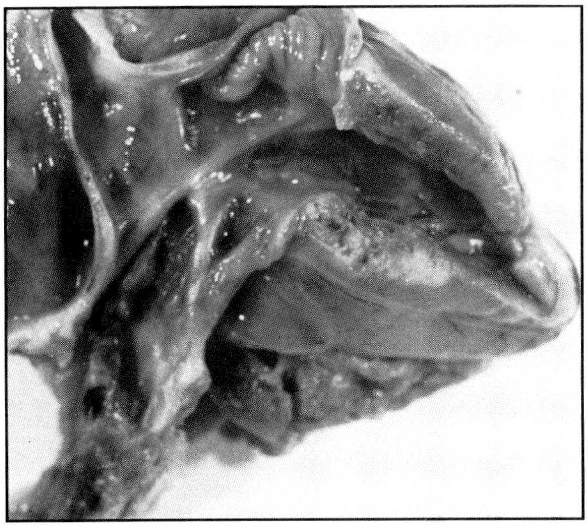

Fig. 14.13. Thrombus in the inferior vena cava and right atrium following umbilical venous catheterisation.

Fig. 1.6, p. 9). Ulceration does not usually occur, but minor scarring may be apparent more than a year later (Cartlidge et al. 1990). Local injury is readily apparent and the electrode can be moved to a fresh area of skin; any breech of epidermal continuity should be taken seriously as infection may occur and be the instigator of systemic infection. Particularly vulnerable are preterm babies whose handling of many organisms is defective.

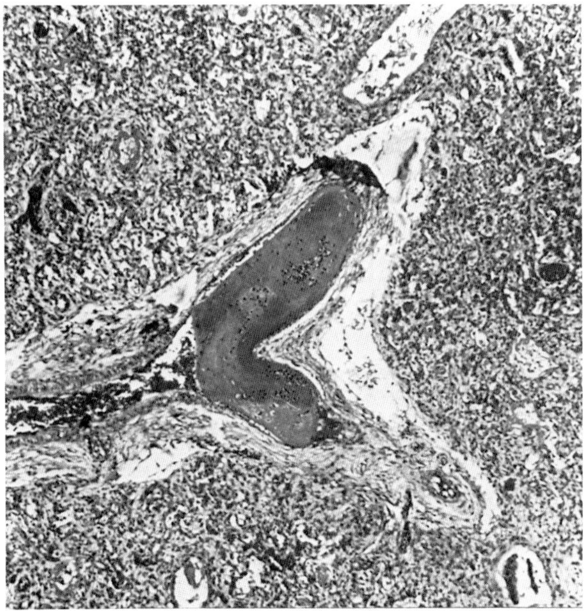

Fig. 14.14. Thromboembolus straddles a pulmonary artery bifurcation following umbilical venous catheterisation. (Keeling 1981)

Catheterisation of Umbilical Vessels

Because of their large size and easy accessibility, catheterisation of umbilical vessels, both arteries and vein, has been undertaken for a variety of reasons in the neonatal period. They have been used to permit blood transfusion, exchange transfusion, infusion of drugs, electrolyte solutions and nutrients and for angiographic studies. Systemic infection is a potential hazard when cannulation of vessels is undertaken for any length of time. Fungal infection may be a problem in the preterm neonate who has also received antibiotics (Smith and Congdon 1985).

Venous Catheterisation

Catheterisation of the umbilical vein was formerly undertaken more frequently than at present because of the relative ease of the procedure compared with the difficulties encountered during cannulation of the umbilical arteries. The procedure is now rarely performed because of the high frequency of complications.

Umbilical vein thrombosis was extremely common and particularly likely to follow the infusion of hypertonic solutions (Kitterman et al. 1970), presence of the catheter for longer than 2 days and failure to ensure that the tip of the catheter was in the inferior vena cava (Larroche 1970). As a result of extension (Fig. 14.13) or detachment of the thrombus, patchy hepatic necrosis and pulmonary thromboembolism (Fig. 14.14) were frequently early complications of umbilical venous catheterisation (Scott 1965). Massive hepatic necrosis accompanying portal vein thrombosis was observed in some cases (Larroche 1970; see Fig. 16.26, p. 395). Traumatic injury to the liver is occasionally encountered (see Fig. 16.22, p. 392). An infrequent late complication of umbilical venous catheterisation is portal hypertension presenting with splenomegaly or haematemesis (Junker et al. 1976; Lauridsen et al. 1978). Necrotising enterocolitis was reported by Corkery et al. (1968) and Orme and Eades (1968) following umbilical venous catheterisation for exchange transfusion in the management of rhesus disease.

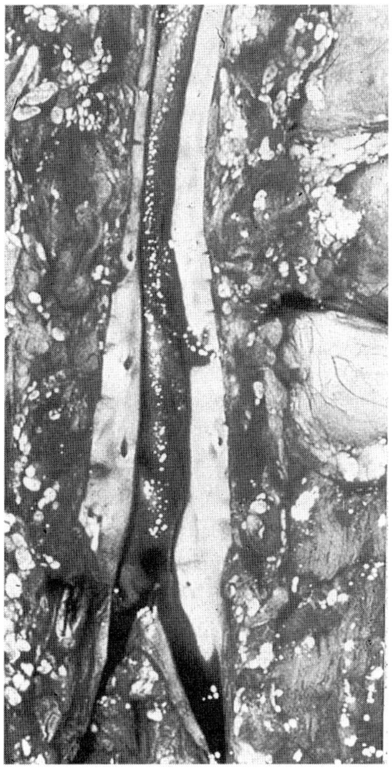
a

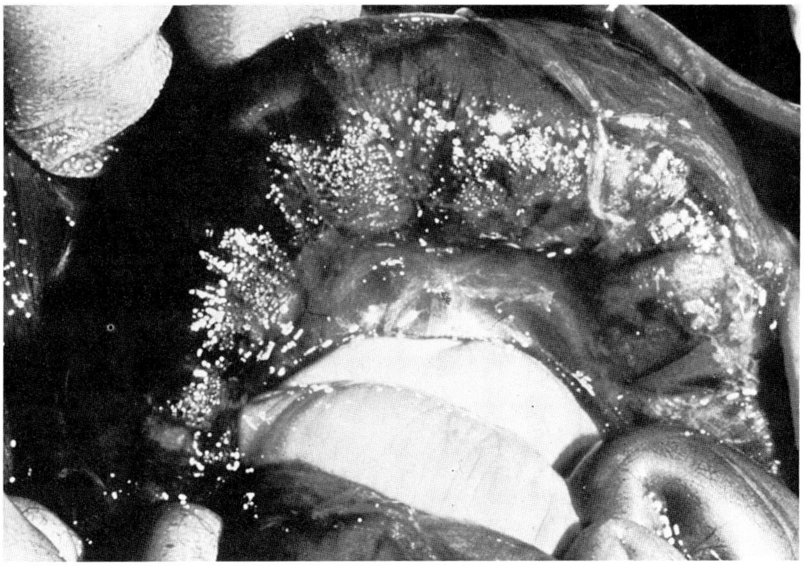
b

Fig. 14.15. **a** Massive aortic thrombosis following umbilical arterial catheterisation, which resulted in infarction of the colon (**b**). (Keeling 1981)

Arterial Catheterisation

Whilst complications of umbilical arterial catheterisation are recognised and some are of a particularly serious nature, the incidence of serious lesions is not as common as has been observed following umbilical venous catheterisation. The most commonly reported complications of umbilical arterial catheterisation are aortic or iliac artery thrombosis. The frequency varies between 24% and 95% amongst infants investigated by angiography and is reported in from 3.5% to 48% of cases coming to necropsy (see Wesstrom et al. 1979). My own experience is similar. In most cases the thrombus does not occlude the aortic lumen. A cylindrical thrombus may form around the catheter, indicating the original level of the catheter tip. When the catheter remains in situ, a shred of clot connects the tip of the catheter and the aortic wall. Massive aortic thrombosis is infrequent (Fig. 14.15a) and may be fatal, as infarction of viscera (Fig. 14.15b) or gangrene of the lower limbs (Fig. 14.16) are likely to accompany thrombosis of this magnitude; Wesstrom (1980) found only 2% of serious sequelae amongst his cases.

It is important to remember that not all aortic thrombosis or thromboembolism in

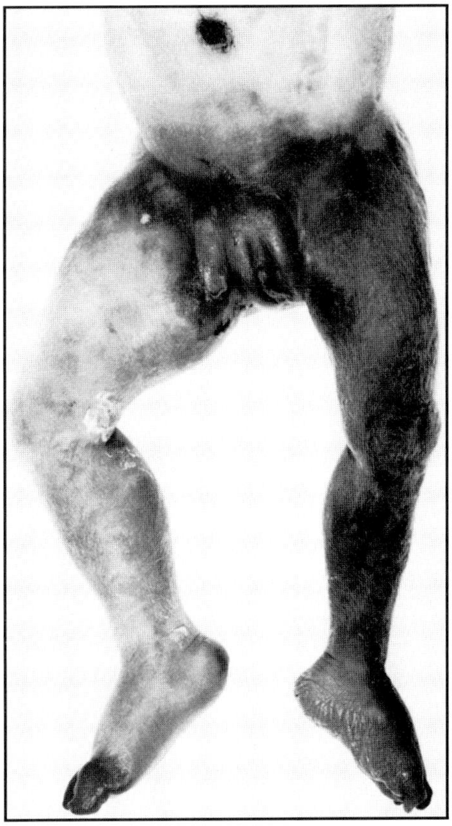

Fig. 14.16. Gangrene of perineum and lower limbs caused by massive aortic thrombosis.

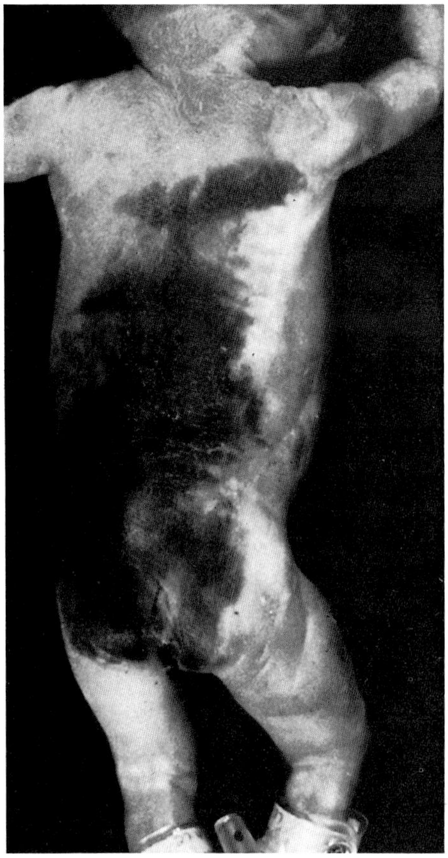

Fig. 14.17. Dorsal cutaneous necrosis following prolonged contact with an alcoholic solution of a skin-cleansing agent.

the neonate is iatrogenic. Knowlson and Marsden (1978) drew attention to massive aortic thrombosis as a result of propogation of thrombus in the ductus arteriosus. The aortic end of the ductus should be examined with care in any baby with thromboembolism of vessels arising beyond the ductus or with massive aortic thrombosis.

Wesstrom et al. (1979) found a correlation between the use of side-hole catheters and thrombosis, implicating the dead space at the catheter tip as site of origin of the thrombus. These workers also found that low siting of the catheter and its use for parenteral nutrition predisposed to thrombosis; long duration of catheterisation was also related to the development of thrombosis.

Aortic aneurysm is an infrequent complication of aortic catheterisation; damage to the aortic wall by the catheter tip in the presence of septicaemia is postulated as its cause. False aneurysms of the aorta have been described by Rajs et al. (1976), Malloy and Nichols (1977) and Spangler et al. (1977). All were in preterm neonates who had concurrent staphylococcal septicaemia. Rupture of the aortic wall permitted communication between the aortic lumen and a cavity within surrounding organising haematoma. In the case described by Rajs et al. (1976), the aneurysm ruptured into the oesophagus with massive, fatal haematemesis. Colclough and Barson (1981) describe a true aneurysm of the aorta following umbilical arterial catheterisation in a preterm infant whose course was complicated by pseudomonas septicaemia, the organism being isolated from the catheter tip as well as from blood cultures.

A late, infrequent, but serious complication of umbilical arterial catheterisation is systemic hypertension. Eight of ten infants with hypertension seen by Plumer et al. (1976) had undergone umbilical arterial catheterisation in the neonatal period; five subsequently died after failure to respond to medical management.

Other complications of umbilical arterial catheterisation include interstitial haemorrhage around the umbilical arteries or aorta following technically difficult insertion of the catheter and damage to vasa vasorum of the cannulated vessel. Although usually inconsequential, blood staining of ascitic fluid may give rise to diagnostic difficulties, and resorption of larger haematomas may result in jaundice. Displacement of the catheter may lead to serious haemorrhage at the umbilicus.

Inadvertent urachal catheterisation is reported (Egan and Eitzman 1971). Vordermark et al. (1980) report avulsion of the urachus giving rise to urinary ascites following umbilical arterial catheterisation.

Gluteal skin necrosis as a complication of umbilical arterial catheterisation was described by Mann (1980), but others (Wilkinson et al. 1981; Harpin and Rutter 1982) have implicated alcohol-based skin-cleansing agents as its cause (Fig. 14.17).

Venepuncture

Asnes and Arendar (1966) reported septic arthritis complicating femoral venepuncture in the perinatal period and emphasised the need for scrupulous aseptic technique when undertaking any invasive procedure. Rey et al. (1987) described a false aneurysm of the brachial artery which they attributed to inadvertent arterial puncture in an infant requiring multiple venepuncture in the neonatal period.

Injection into Umbilical Arteries

Gangrene of the perineum or buttocks has been described following a single injection into the umbilical artery at birth, by Bonifazi and Meneghini (1980). Both infants survived and angiography was not undertaken, but the authors postulated that spasm of a branch of the internal iliac artery followed the injection.

Medication

The side effects of some drugs might be predicted from their structure and should be sought when a particular drug has been used. However, the pathologist should very carefully record all pathological findings and try to explain them. This is particularly important when new treatment regimens are introduced, in order that unwanted side effects may be recognised at the earliest opportunity.

Topical Preparations

Neonates, particularly those who are born prematurely or small for gestational age, have a higher surface to volume ratio than mature infants. This, together with the incomplete state of keratinisation of the epidermis, contributes to undesirable absorption of some topical preparations.

Hexachlorophene

Hexachlorophene was at one time used widely as a bacteriostatic agent, usually applied to the umbilical cord area. Later it was used as a whole-body application for cleansing purposes. Neuropathological abnormalities were first identified in rats (Kimbrough and Gaines 1971), when spongy degeneration of both brain and spinal cord was described following the observation of spasticity in the hind limbs after repeated topical applications of hexachlorophene. Hart (cited by Lockhart 1972) applied 3% hexachlorophene emulsion to the skin of infant monkeys and they all developed widespread spongy degeneration of the central nervous system. Spongiform encephalopathy in humans was first described by Powell et al. (1973) in the brains of six preterm infants who had received at least four whole-body exposures to hexachlorophene. These authors described symmetrical bubbly change in myelinated fibres in the medial longitudinal fasciculus, medial lemniscus and cerebellar peduncles; they considered excessive absorption of hexachlorophene to be related to prematurity, low birthweight and the presence of pathological abnormalities of the skin. Shuman et al. (1974) found similar abnormalities in the brains of 17 of 248 babies who were all of low birthweight and had been subjected to repeated whole-body applications of 3% hexachlorophene. They speculated that the poor cutaneous keratinisation and relatively large surface area of these babies would more readily permit transcutaneous absorption of drugs than might occur in the mature infant.

Alcohol-based Cleansing Solutions

Dorsal superficial skin necrosis has been observed in babies who have undergone umbilical arterial catheterisation and was initially ascribed to the procedure (Mann 1981). We observed similar skin damage following umbilical arterial catheterisation and initially considered spasm of dorsal arteries as a response to trauma during the procedure to be the cause; however, we were puzzled by the distribution of the damage (Fig. 14.17), which did not conform to known cutaneous arterial distribution (cf. Fig. 14.16), and by its superficial nature, being confined to the skin and sparing underlying connective tissue and muscle. Subsequent investigation (Wilkinson et al. 1981) incriminated the generous use of an alcoholic solution of 0.5% chlorhexidine, which had resulted in babies lying in a pool of the solution whilst umbilical arterial catheterisation was carried out. Subsequently, Harpin and Rutter (1982) described similar skin damage following the use of industrial methylated spirit and found dangerously high blood levels of both ethanol and methanol in some of their babies.

Systemic Medication

Koren et al. (1986) described drug overdose resulting from computation errors and stressed

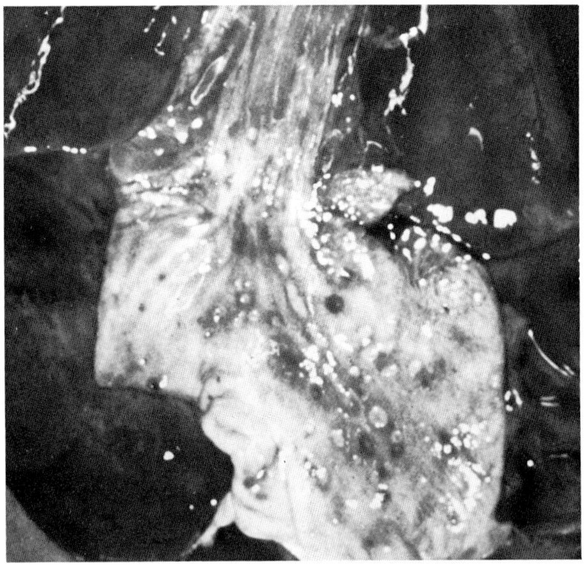

Fig. 14.18. Multiple, discrete ulcers in the gastric mucosa. At necropsy, the stomach and duodenum were filled with blood. (Keeling 1981)

the need for awareness of dosage ranges when prescribing for infants.

Tolazoline

Tolazoline is an alpha-adrenergic blocking agent used in the management of pulmonary hypertension in the neonate. Its chemical structure is related to both histamine and sympathomimetic amines. Gastrointestinal ulceration and haemorrhage is a predictable side effect. It was observed by Goetzman et al. (1978) in 6 of 21 of their patients. Multiple discrete ulcers measuring up to 3 mm in diameter were present in the gastric mucosa (Fig. 14.18). Concomitant haemorrhage may be life-threatening.

Prostaglandin E_1

This drug is widely used to maintain short-term patency of the ductus arteriosus in neonates. Pulmonary arteritis was observed in three infants after its use and a causal relationship proposed (Heffelfinger et al. 1987). Similar vascular changes have been produced in beagle pups using prostaglandin E_1 in physiological doses (Goddard-Finegold et al. 1989).

Blood Transfusion

The risk of transmission of infection by transfusion of blood or blood products is well recognised. The particular susceptibility of the neonate to transfusion-associated problems has become apparent since the introduction of active management of major malformations and the problems of prematurity in the neonatal period. Sometimes blood transfusion is required simply to replace blood taken during the course of investigations. Balin et al. (1989) suggest that this might be avoided to some extent by centrifugation of the blood sample whilst still in the syringe and replacement of red cells when only plasma is required for investigations.

Cytomegalovirus Infection

Transmission of cytomegalovirus (CMV) may complicate the transfusion of even very small amounts of blood. Although in most cases infection is asymptomatic, disseminated serious infection may occur in immunologically incompetent individuals. The preterm infant belongs to this group. Fatal neonatal infection may follow transfusion with CMV-positive blood in the neonatal period (Benson et al. 1979). Yeager (1974) followed up 77 infants treated with blood products in the neonatal period and found that 25% were excreting virus at 7 months of age compared with 11% of 74 infants from the same nursery who had not been transfused. Benson et al. (1979) found that 4 of 11 infants became infected following transfusion of a small amount of CMV-positive blood and that transmission of CMV infection was prevented by the use of CMV-negative blood in the transfusion of neonates. Yeager et al. (1981) found that 13.5% of infants of CMV-negative mothers who were transfused with CMV-positive blood developed CMV infection, and this proportion was increased to 24% when more than 50 ml of packed red cells were transfused. Serious or fatal illness was observed in half of the infected babies.

Hepatitis A Infection

Hepatitis A infection may be transmitted by transfused blood from donors incubating the disease. This has been clearly documented in a baby who underwent exchange transfusion for rhesus incompatibility (Seeberg et al. 1981). The baby was asymptomatic but transmitted the disease to her mother and nurses on a subsequent hospital admission.

Acquired Immune Deficiency Syndrome

The neonate may become infected with acquired immune deficiency syndrome (AIDS)-associated retrovirus either directly as a result of blood transfusion (Ammann et al. 1983) or indirectly following maternal transfusion for intrapartum haemorrhage (Ziegler et al. 1985). Virus transmission to the infant was presumed to have occurred through breast milk, although passage as a result of other forms of intimate contact could not be ruled out.

Intravenous Alimentation

Intravenous alimentation was first introduced into paediatric practice in the management of infants who had undergone surgery, particularly following major intestinal resection (Wilmore and Dudrick 1968). It then began to be used in the intensive care nursery to supplement oral feeding in very small infants with inappropriate weight gain and in the conservative management of necrotising enterocolitis.

The mixture infused consists of amino acids, sugars, vitamins and minerals, with or without the addition of lipid emulsion to increase calorific value without introducing an unacceptable fluid load. Problems have been encountered which have been related to both amino acid mixtures and lipid emulsions.

Amino Acid Mixtures

Amino acid mixtures produce serious tissue necrosis if there is any leakage from infusion into a peripheral vessel. The injuries produced are serious, slow to heal and may necessitate skin grafting. For this reason, amino acids are usually given by infusion into the vena cava or aorta.

Cholestasis in infants given amino acids by infusion was first reported by Peden et al. (1971), and a number of other reports followed. In 1977, Bernstein et al. described the histological appearance of the liver in five infants who became jaundiced during the administration of amino acid and hyperosmolar sugar solution intravenously. They found cholestasis, hepatocellular damage and giant cell transformation of hepatocytes, and prominence of Kupffer cells, which contained PAS-positive material and pigment (Fig. 14.19). No hepatocytic fatty change was observed in any of the biopsies.

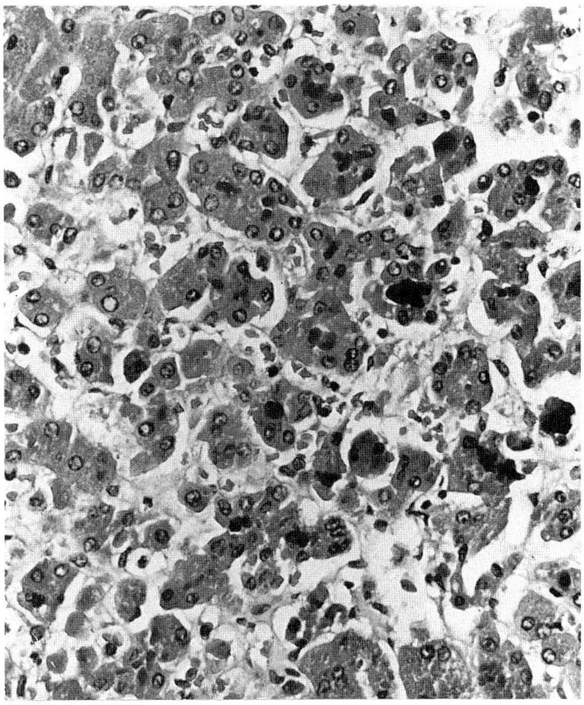

Fig. 14.19. Liver following parenteral amino acid infusion. Bile plugging, sinusoidal dilatation and prominence of Kupffer cells are apparent. (Keeling 1981)

Fat Emulsions

Koga et al. (1975) demonstrated fat and pigment in Kupffer cells and hepatocytes in infants given intravenous alimentation which involved the use of lipid emulsions (see Fig. 16.23, p. 392). Whitington and Black (1980) described cholelithiasis in preterm infants given a mixture of amino acids and lipids who were treated with frusemide. They speculated that parenteral nutrition was the initiating factor, producing cholestasis, and that frusemide may have contributed to the formation of gallstones by reducing bile salts, independent of bile flow, and/or by enhancing the secretion of calcium into the bile.

Whilst in most infants the liver returns to normal both functionally and histologically

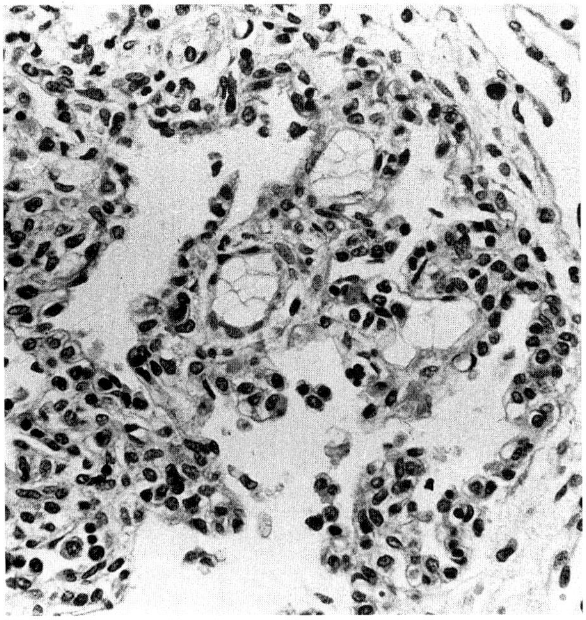

Fig. 14.20. Lipid globules fill pulmonary capillaries following lipid emulsion infusion. (Courtesy of Dr. A.J. Barson, Manchester; Keeling 1981)

when intravenous alimentation is discontinued, in some babies liver abnormalities persist; there is expansion of portal areas, which show fibrosis and cellular infiltration that, in a few cases, may go on to cirrhosis.

Pulmonary lipid embolism (Fig. 14.20) was first described by Barson et al. (1978) in both preterm and mature infants. They thought that provoking factors were the rate of administration, which was periodically in excess of that recommended, and severe acidosis from either respiratory distress or septicaemia. Levene et al. (1980) described fat emboli in pulmonary capillaries in preterm neonates when the rate of administration of lipid emulsions had always been below the maximum recommended; plasma lipaemia was not observed. In some of their cases, lipid embolism was sufficiently widespread to produce pulmonary infarction.

Dahms and Halpin (1980) describe lipid accumulation in the intima of pulmonary arteries with involvement of the media and adventitia in a few babies. The vessels also showed changes of pulmonary hypertension and these were compatible with the clinical course of the patient. They speculated that lipid accumulates only in the walls of previously damaged arteries and in a retrospective study were unable to demonstrate arterial lipid accumulation unless both pulmonary hypertension and lipid emulsion administration had occurred.

Lipid droplets in macrophages can be demonstrated throughout the baby's reticuloendothelial system following lipid emulsion administration. In animals, lipid accumulation results in defective neutrophil and macrophage function (Fischer et al. 1980). These authors postulate that the administration of such emulsions to neonates may overload the reticuloendothelial system and compromise handling of bacteria, which could contribute to the development or worsening of infection in these infants.

Nutritional Rickets

Nutritional rickets occurs in premature infants with respiratory problems and is probably the result of a low intake of both calcium and vitamin D compounded by the administration of sodium bicarbonate and use of frusemide (Chudley et al. 1980; Oppenheimer and Snodgrass 1980). These infants develop expansion of epiphyses and costochondral junctions; rib fractures and bizarre angulation also occur (Fig. 14.21). This problem is easily prevented by dietary supplementation.

Necrotising Enterocolitis

Necrotising enterocolitis is an ischaemic necrosis commencing in the mucosa and extending through the intestinal wall towards the serosa. It usually affects the small intestine, but colon and stomach may also be involved. There appears to have been a real increase in the incidence of this condition in the past two decades (Goldman 1980), and it is an important cause of mortality and morbidity in the neonatal period. A variety of iatrogenic factors have been implicated in the development of this condition since it was first described. The first reported cases of necrotising enterocolitis as a complication of treatment were those following exchange transfusion via umbilical vessels for the management of rhesus disease in the neonatal period (Waldausen et al. 1963; Corkery et al. 1968; Orme and Eades 1968). Ischaemia

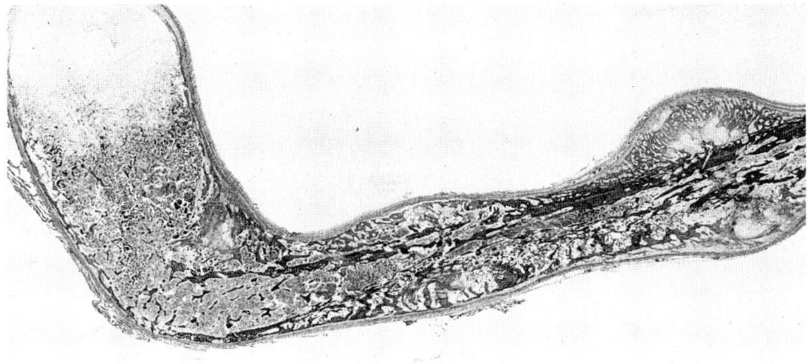

Fig. 14.21. Rib with irregularity and expansion of the costochondral junction. Angulation of the rib is the result of fracture; periosteal elevation by callus at the site of a healing fracture is present on the *right*. (Keeling 1981)

was thought to be the result of rapid changes in pressure in the splanchnic circulation during exchange transfusion.

As the number of exchange transfusions performed for rhesus disease in the neonatal period has declined following the introduction of anti-D antibody administration to susceptible mothers postpartum, the commonest victim of necrotising enterocolitis is now the preterm neonate (see Chap. 8, p. 213). It is likely that intestinal ischaemia is the result of splanchnic shutdown in response to periodic systemic hypotension (Lloyd 1969). Many of the infants had undergone umbilical arterial catheterisation; Bunton et al. (1977) found longer duration of catheterisation and more frequent changes of catheter in infants who develop NEC compared with a control group.

Cooke et al. (1980) have described necrotising enterocolitis in term neonates following aortic catheterisation and angiography in the investigation of congenital heart disease. Whilst catheterisation and the injection of contrast media may induce vascular spasm, it is postulated that reduced splanchnic blood flow may accompany hyperviscosity of the blood following the use of hyperosmolar contrast medium, which also has a diuretic effect. An association between hyperviscosity of blood and necrotising enterocolitis in neonates of low birthweight was described by Hakanson and Oh (1977).

Intestinal obstruction, perhaps provoking localised intestinal mucosal ischaemia may be a factor in some cases of necrotising enterocolitis (Dunn 1963; Cook and Rickam 1969). Goldman (1980) found a relationship between the introduction of a regimen of rapidly increasing volume of feed and development of necrotising enterocolitis and suggested that postprandial bradycardia led to hypotension and splanchnic shutdown.

Some studies have implicated particular organisms in "outbreaks" of necrotising enterocolitis in some units, for example salmonellae (Stein et al. 1972) and *Clostridium butyricum* (Howard et al. 1977). Generally, however, a variety of organisms, usually normal intestinal flora, have been isolated. The clinical presentation and pathological appearance are described in Chapter 16 (see p. 357).

References

Adams JM, Rudolph AJ (1975) The use of indwelling radial artery catheters in neonates. Pediatrics 55: 261–265

Ammann AJ, Cowan MJ, Wara DW, et al. (1983) Acquired immunodeficiency in an infant: possible transmission by means of blood products. Lancet I: 956–958

Andrews AF, Nixon CA, Cilley RE, Roloff DW, Bartlett RH (1986) One- to three-year outcome for 14 neonatal survivors of extracorporeal membrane oxygenation. Pediatrics 78: 692–698

Arya H, Williams J, Ponsford SN, Bissenden JG (1991) Neonatal diaphragmatic paralysis caused by chest drains. Arch Dis Child 66: 441–442

Ashkenazi S, Metzker A, Merlob P, Ovadia J, Reisner SH (1985) Scalp changes after fetal monitoring. Arch Dis Child 60: 267–269

Ashton HE (1981) Disorders of the foetus and infant. In: Davies DM (ed) Textbook of adverse drug reactions, 2nd edn. Oxford University Press, Oxford, pp 64–80

Ashton N (1954) Pathological basis of retrolental fibroplasia. Br J Ophthalmol 38: 385–396

Ashton N, Ward B, Serpell G (1954) Effect of oxygen on developing retinal vessels with particular reference to the problem of retrolental fibroplasia. Br J Ophthalmol 38: 397–432

Asnes RS, Arendar GM (1966) Septic arthritis of the hip: a complication of femoral venepuncture. Pediatrics 38: 837

Balin A, Koren G, Hasu M, Zipursky A (1989) Evaluation of a new method for the prevention of neonatal anemia. Pediatr Res 25: 274–275
Barson AJ, Chiswick ML, Doig CM (1978) Fat embolism in infancy after intravenous fat infusions. Arch Dis Child 53: 218–223
Benacerraf BR, Barss VA, Saltzman DH, Greene MF, Penso CA, Frigoletto FD Jr (1987) Acute fetal distress associated with percutaneous umbilical blood sampling. Am J Obstet Gynecol 156: 1218–1220
Benson JWT, Bodden SJ, Tobin JO'H (1979) Cytomegalovirus and blood transfusion in neonates. Arch Dis Child 54: 538–541
Berner HW, Seisler EP, Barlow J (1972) Fetal cardiac tamponade. A complication of amniocentesis. Obstet Gynecol 40: 599–604
Bernstein J, Chang CH, Brough AJ, Heidelberger KP (1977) Conjugated hyperbilirubinaemia in infancy associated with parenteral alimentation. J Pediatr 90: 361–367
Bonifazi E, Meneghini C (1980) Perinatal gangrene of the buttock; an iatrogenic or spontaneous condition? J Am Acad Dermatol 3: 596–598
Bonikos DS, Bensch KG, Ludwin SK, Northway WH (1975) Oxygen toxicity in the newborn. The effect of prolonged 100 per cent O_2 exposure on the lungs of newborn mice. Lab Invest 32: 619–635
Bonikos DS, Bensch KG, Northway WH, Edwards DK (1976) Bronchopulmonary dysplasia: the pulmonary pathologic sequel of necrotising bronchiolitis and pulmonary fibrosis. Hum Pathol 7: 643–666
Brinsmead MW (1976) Complications of amniocentesis. Med J Aust 1: 379–385
Brown ER, Stark A, Sosenko I, Lawson EE, Avery ME (1978) Bronchopulmonary dysplasia: possible relationship to pulmonary edema. J Pediatr 92: 982–984
Bunton GL, Durbin GM, McIntosh N, et al. (1977) Necrotising enterocolitis. Controlled study of 3 years' experience in a neonatal intensive care unit. Arch Dis Child 52: 772–777
Butler NR, Bonham DG (1963) Perinatal mortality. The first report of the 1958 British Perinatal Mortality Study. Livingstone, Edinburgh, p 148
Carrillo P (1985) Palatal groove formation and oral endotracheal intubation. Am J Dis Child 139: 859–880
Cartlidge PH, Fox PE, Rutter N (1990) The scars of newborn intensive care. Early Hum Dev 21: 1–10
Chan WH, Paul RH, Toews J (1973) Intrapartum fetal monitoring: maternal and fetal morbidity, and perinatal mortality. Obstet Gynecol 41: 7–13
Chudley AE, Brown DR, Holzman IR, Oh KS (1980) Nutritional rickets in 2 very low birthweight infants with chronic lung disease. Arch Dis Child 55: 687–690
Cilley RE, Zwischenberger JB, Andrews AF, Bowerman RA, Roloff DW, Bartlett RH (1986) Intracranial hemorrhage during extracorporeal membrane oxygenation in neonates. Pediatrics 78: 699–704
Clarke TA, Coen RW, Feldman B, Papile L (1980) Esophageal perforations in premature infants and comments on the diagnosis. Am J Dis Child 134: 367–368
Colclough AB, Barson AJ (1981) Infantile aortic aneurysm complicating umbilical arterial catheterisation. Arch Dis Child 56: 795–797
Cook RCM, Rickham PP (1969) Neonatal intestinal obstruction due to milk curds. J Pediatr Surg 4: 599–605
Cooke RWI, Meradji M, de Villenueve VH (1980) Necrotising enterocolitis after cardiac catheterisation in infants. Arch Dis Child 55: 66–68
Corkery JJ, Dubowitz V, Lister J, Moosa A (1968) Colonic perforation after exchange transfusion. Br Med J II: 345–349
Creasman WT, Lawrence RA, Thiede HA (1968) Fetal complications of amniocentesis. JAMA 204: 91–94
Crooks J (1982) Haemolytic jaundice in a neonate after intraamniotic injection of methylene blue. Arch Dis Child 57: 872–873
Cross HE, Maumenee AE (1972) Ocular trauma during amniocentesis. N Engl J Med 287: 993–994
Daffos F, Capella-Pavlovsky M, Forestier F (1983) Fetal blood sampling via the umbillical cord using a needle guided by ultrasound. Prenat Diagn 3: 271–277
Dahms BB, Halpin TC (1980) Pulmonary arterial lipid deposit in newborn infants receiving intravenous lipid infusion. J Pediatr 97: 800–805
deLemos R, Wolfsdorf J, Nachman R, et al. (1969) Lung injury from oxygen in lambs: the role of artifical ventilation. Anesthesiology 30: 609–618
Drew JH, Landau LI, Acton CM, Kent M, Campbell PE (1978) Pulmonary interstitial emphysema requiring lobectomy. Complication of assisted ventilation. Arch Dis Child 53: 424–426
D'Souza SW, Black P, MacFarlane T (1982) Fetal scalp damage and neonatal jaundice: a risk of routine fetal scalp electrode monitoring. J Obstet Gynaecol 2: 161–164
Dunn PM (1963) Intestinal obstruction in the newborn with special reference to transient functional ileus associated with respiratory distress syndrome. Arch Dis Child 38: 459–467
Dunn PM (1975) Testicular birth trauma. Arch Dis Child 50: 744–745 (abstract)
Edwards DK, Dyer WM, Northway WH (1977) Twelve years' experience with bronchopulmonary dysplasia. Pediatrics 59: 839–845
Egan EA, Eitzman DV (1971) Umbilical vessel catheterisation. Am J Dis Child 121: 213–218
Ennis M, Vincent CA (1990) Obstetric accidents: a review of 64 cases. Br Med J 300: 1365–1367
Erenberg A, Nowak AJ (1984) Palatal groove formation in neonates and infants with orotracheal tubes. Am J Dis Child 138: 974–975
Fearne J, Bryan E, Elliman A, Elliman A (1985) Enamel defects in deciduous dentition of low birthweight infants. Presented to the Paediatric Research Societies in Europe, Munich, 1985
Fedrick J, Butler NR (1971) Certain causes of neonatal death V. cerebral birth trauma. Biol Neonate 18: 321–329
Fischer GW, Hunter KW, Wilson SR, Mease AD (1980) Diminished bacterial defences with intralipid. Lancet II: 819–820
Galjaard H (1976) European experience with prenatal diagnosis of congenital disease: a survey of 6121 cases. Cytogenet Cell Genet 16: 453–467
Gassner CB, Paul RH (1976) Laceration of umbilical cord vessels secondary to amniocentesis. Obstet Gynecol 48: 627–630
Goddard-Finegold J, Langston C, Hawkins EP, Michael LH, Ou CN (1989) Prostaglandin E_1—associated pathology of pulmonary microvasculature in newborn pups: similarity to findings in prostaglandin E_1-treated human newborns. Pediatr Pathol 9: 251–260
Goetzman BW, Sunshine P, Johnson JD, et al. (1976) Neonatal hypoxia and pulmonary vasospasm: response to tolazoline. J Pediatr 89: 617–621
Goldkrand JW (1982) Intrapartum innoculation of herpes simplex virus by fetal scalp electrode. Obstet Gynecol 59: 263–265

Goldman HI (1980) Feeding and necrotising enterocolitis. Am J Dis Child 134: 553–555
Gould SJ, Howard S (1985) The histopathology of the larynx in the neonate following endotracheal intubation. J Pathol 146: 301–311
Grove CS, Trimbetta GC, Amstey MS (1973) Fetal complications of amniocentesis. Am J Obstet Gynecol 115: 1154
Hakanson DO, Oh W (1977) Necrotising enterocolitis and hyperviscosity in the newborn infant. J Pediatr 90: 458–461
Hamid TK (1975) Pneumothorax and surgical emphysema in a newborn baby caused by amniocentesis. Br J Obstet Gynecol 82: 170–171
Hanson JW, Smith DW, Cohen MM (1976) Prominent lateral palatine ridges: developmental and clinical relevance. J Pediatr 89: 54–58
Harlap S, Prywes R, Davies AM (1975) Birth defects with oestrogens and progesterones in pregnancy. Lancet I: 682–683
Harpin V, Rutter N (1982) Percutaneous alcohol absorption and skin necrosis in a preterm infant. Arch Dis Child 57: 477–479
Heffelfinger S, Hawkins EP, Nihill M, Langston C (1987) Pulmonary vascular changes associated with prolonged prostaglandin E_1 treatment. Pediatr Pathol 7: 165–173
Hobbins JC, Grannum PA, Romero R, Reece EA, Mahoney MJ (1985) Percutaneous umbilical blood sampling. Am J Obstet Gynecol 152: 1–6
Holcomb GW, Templeton JM Jr (1989) Iatrogenic perforation of the bronchus intermedius in a 1100 g neonate. J Pediatr Surg 24: 1132–1134
Howard FM, Flynn DM, Bradley JM, Noone P, Szawatkowski M (1977) Outbreaks of necrotising enterocolitis caused by *Clostridium butyricum*. Lancet II: 1099–1102
Huch R, Lubbers DW, Huch A (1974) Reliability of transcutaneous monitoring of arterial Po_2 in newborn infants. Arch Dis Child 49: 213–218
Hyman CJ, Depp R, Pakravan P, Stinson DA, Allen AC (1973) Pneumothorax complicating amniocentesis. Obstet Gynecol 41: 43–46
Junker P, Egeblad M, Nielson O, Kamper J (1976) Case report. Umbilical vein catheterisation and portal hypertension. Acta Paediatr Scand 65: 499–504
Kalbac RW, Newman RL (1974) Amniotic fluid analysis in complicated pregnancies. Obstet Gynecol 44: 814–818
Karp LE, Hayden PW (1977) Fetal puncture during midtrimester amniocentesis. Obstet Gynecol 49: 115–117
Keeling JW (1981) Iatrogenic disease in the newborn. Virchows Arch [A] 394: 1–29
Keeling JW (1987) Pathological aspects of sampling the amniotic fluid. In: Fox H (ed) Haines and Taylor's obstetrical and gynaecological pathology. Churchill Livingstone, Edinburgh pp 1088–1120
Kimbrough RD, Gaines TB (1971) Hexachlorophene effects on the rat brain. Arch Environ Health 23: 114
Kitterman JA, Phibbs RH, Tooley WH (1970) Catheterisation of umbilical vessels in newborn infants. Pediatr Clin North Am 17: 895–912
Knowlson GT, Marsden HB (1978) Aortic thrombosis in the newborn period. Arch Dis Child 53: 164–166
Koenigsberger MR, Moessinger AC (1977) Iatrogenic carpal tunnel syndrome in the newborn infant. J Pediatr 91: 443–445
Koga Y, Swanson VL, Hayes DM (1975) Hepatic "intravenous fat pigment" in infants and children receiving lipid emulsions. J Pediatr Surg 10: 641–648
Koren G, Barzilay Z, Greenwald M (1986) Tenfold errors in administration of drug doses: a neglected iatrogenic disease in pediatrics. Pediatrics 77: 848–849
Lamb MP (1975) Gangrene of a fetal limb due to amniocentesis. Br J Obstet Gynecol 82: 829–830
Lancet (1992) Editorial. Oxygen restriction and retinopathy of prematurity 339: 961–963
Larroche JC (1970) Umbilical catheterisation: its complications. Biol Neonate 16: 101–116
Lauridsen UB, Enk B, Gammeltoft A (1978) Oesophageal varices as a late complication to neonatal umbilical vein catheterisation. Acta Paediatr Scand 67: 633–636
Leck IM, Millar ELM (1962) Incidence of malformations since the introduction of thalidomide. Lancet II: 16–20
Lenz W (1962) Thalidomide and congenital abnormalities. Lancet I: 45
Levene MI, Wigglesworth JS, Desai R (1980) Pulmonary fat accumulation after intralipid infusion in the preterm infant. Lancet II: 815–818
Liley AW (1960) The technique and complications of amniocentesis. NZ Med J 59: 581–586
Lindroth M, Svenningsen NW, Ahlstrom H, Jonson B (1980) Evaluation of mechanical ventilation in newborn infants. Acta Paediatr Scand 69: 143–149
Lloyd JR (1969) Etiology of gastrointestinal perforations in the newborn. J Pediatr Surg 4: 77–84
Lockhart JD (1972) How toxic is hexachlorophene? Pediatrics 50: 229–235
Malloy MH, Nichols MM (1977) False abdominal aortic aneurysm: an unusual complication of umbilical arterial catheterisation. J Pediatr 90: 285–286
Mann NP (1980) Gluteal skin necrosis after umbilical artery catheterisation. Arch Dis Child 55: 815–817
Menahem S (1988) Neonatal cyanosis, methaemoglobinaemia and haemolytic anaemia. Acta Paediatr Scand 77: 755–756
MRC (1978) An assessment of the hazards of amniocentesis. Br J Obstet Gynaecol 85: 1–41 (suppl 2)
MRC Working Party on the Evaluation of Chorion Villus Sampling (1991) Medical Research Council European trial of chorion villus sampling. Lancet 337: 1491–1499
Misenhimer HR (1966) Fetal haemorrhage associated with amniocentesis. Am J Obstet Gynecol 94: 1133–1135
Moessinger AC, Driscoll JM Jr, Wigger H (1978) High incidence of lung perforation by chest tube in neonatal pneumothorax. J Pediatr 92: 635–637
NICHD (1976) National Registry for Amniocentesis Study Group. Midtrimester amniocentesis for prenatal diagnosis: safety and accuracy. JAMA 236: 1471–1476
Nora JJ, Nora AH (1973) Birth defects and oral contraceptives. Lancet I: 941–942
Northway WH, Rosan RC, Porter DY (1967) Pulmonary disease following respirator therapy of hyaline-membrane disease. N Engl J Med 276: 357–368
O'Neill JA Jr (1984) Experience with iatrogenic laryngeal and tracheal stenoses. J Pediatr Surg 19: 235–238
Oppenheimer SJ, Snodgrass GJAI (1980) Neonatal rickets. Histopathology and quantitative bone changes. Arch Dis Child 55: 945–949
Orme RL'E, Eades SM (1968) Perforation of the bowel in the newborn as a complication of exchange transfusion. Br Med J 4: 349–351
Overturf GD, Balfour G (1975) Osteomyelitis and sepsis: severe complications of fetal monitoring. Pediatrics 55: 244–247
Pape KE, Armstrong DL, Fitzhardinge PM (1976) Central nervous system pathology associated with mask ventilation in the very low birthweight infant: a new aetiology

for intracerebellar haemorrhages. Pediatrics 58: 473–483
Peden VH, Witzleben CL, Skelton MA (1971) Total parenteral nutrition. J Pediatr 78: 180
Piccolo F, Pasquino AM, Boscherini B, Taggi F, Pasquino P (1979) Hypopituitary dwarfism and breech delivery. Arch Dis Child 54: 485–486
Plumer LB, Kaplan GW, Mendoza SA (1976) Hypertension in infants—a complication of umbilical arterial catheterisation. J Pediatr 89: 802–805
Portman MA, Brouillette RT (1982) Fatal intracranial haemorrhage complicating amniocentesis. Am J Obstet Gynecol 144: 731–733
Powell H, Swarner O, Gluck L, Lampert P (1973) Hexachlorophene myelinopathy in premature infants. J Pediatr 82: 976–981
Rajs J, Finnstrom O, Wesstrom G (1976) Case report. Aortic aneurysm developing after umbilical artery catheterisation. Acta Paediatr Scand 65: 495–498
Rehder H (1978) Fetal limb deformities due to amniotic constrictions (a possible consequence of preceding amniocentesis). Pathol Res Pract 162: 316–326
Rey C, Marache P, Watel A, Francart C (1987) Iatrogenic false aneurysm of the brachial artery in an infant. Eur J Pediatr 146: 438–439
Reynolds EOR, Taghizadeh A (1974) Improved prognosis of infants mechanically ventilated for hyaline membrane disease. Arch Dis Child 49: 505–515
Rickwood AMK (1977) A case of ileal atresia and ileocutaneous fistula caused by amniocentesis. J Pediatr 91: 312
Robinson A, Bowes W, Drogemueller W, et al. (1973) Intrauterine diagnosis: potential complications. Am J Obstet Gynecol 116: 937–941
Rona RJ, Tanner JM (1977) Aetiology of idiopathic growth hormone deficiency in England and Wales. Arch Dis Child 52: 197–208
Rushton DI (1981) Examination of products of conception from previable human pregnancies. J Clin Pathol 34: 819–835
Ryan GT, Ivy FCR, Pearson JW (1972) Fetal bleeding as a major hazard of amniocentesis. Obstet Gynecol 40: 702–707
Scott JM (1965) Iatrogenic lesions in babies following umbilical vein catheterisation. Arch Dis Child 40: 426–429
Seeberg S, Brandberg A, Hermodsson S, Larsson P, Lundgren S (1981) Hospital outbreak of hepatitis A secondary to blood exchange in a baby. Lancet I: 1155–1156
Shuman RM, Leech RW, Alvord EC (1974) Neurotoxicity of hexachlorophene in the human: I. A clinicopathologic study of 248 children. Pediatrics 54: 689–695
Simmons MA, Levine RV, Lubchenco LO, Guggenheim MA (1978) Warning: serious sequelae of temporal arterial catheterisation. J Pediatr 92: 284
Simpson NE, Dallaire L, Miller JR, et al. (1976) Prenatal diagnosis of genetic disease in Canada: report of a collaborative study. Can Med Assoc J 115: 739–746
Smith H, Congdon P (1985) Neonatal systemic candidiasis. Arch Dis Child 60: 365–369
Spahr RC, MacDonald HM, Holzman IR (1979) Catheterisation of the posterior tibial artery in the neonate. Am J Dis Child 133: 945–946
Spangler JG, Kleinberg F, Fulton RE, Barnhorst DA, Ritter DG (1977) False aneurysm of the descending aorta. A complication of umbilical arterial catheterisation. Am J Dis Child 131: 1258–1259
Stein H, Beck J, Solomon A, Schmaman A (1972) Gastroenteritis with necrotising enterocolitis in premature babies. Br Med J I: 616–619
Stirrat GM, Beard RW (1973) Drugs to be avoided or given with caution in the second and third trimester of pregnancy. Prescrib J 13: 135
Tabor A, Philip J, Madsen M, Bang J, Obel EB, Nørgaard-Pedersen B (1986) Randomised controlled trial of genetic amniocentesis in 4606 low-risk women. Lancet 1: 1287–1293
Taghizadeh A, Reynolds EOR (1976) Pathogenesis of bronchopulmonary dysplasia following hyaline membrane disease. Am J Pathol 82: 241–258
Taylor GA, Fitz CR, Miller MK, Garin DB, Catena LM, Short BL (1987a) Intracranial abnormalities in infants treated with extracorporeal membrane oxygenation: imaging with US and CT. Radiology 165: 675–678
Taylor GA, Glass P, Fitz CR, Miller MK (1987b) Neurologic status in infants treated with extracorporeal membrane oxygenation: correlation of imaging findings with developmental outcome. Radiology 165: 679–682
Therkensen AJ, Rehder H (1981) Intestinal atresia caused by second trimester amniocentesis. Br J Obstet Gynaecol 88: 559–562
Thiersh JB (1952) Therapeutic abortions with folic acid antagonist, 4-aminopteroglutamic acid (4-amino PGA) administered by the oral route. Am J Obstet Gynecol 63: 1298–1304
Tiwary CM (1989) Testicular injury in breech delivery: possible implications. Urology 34: 210–212
Vogler C, Sotelo-Avila C, Lagunoff D, Braun P, Schreifels JA, Weber T (1988) Aluminium-containing emboli in infants treated with extracorporeal membrane oxygenation. N Engl J Med 319: 75–79
Vordermark JS, Buck AS, Dresner ML (1980) Urinary ascites resulting from umbilical artery catheterisation. J Urol 124: 751
Waldhausen JA, Herenden T, King H (1963) Necrotising colitis of the newborn: common cause of perforation of the colon. Surgery 54: 365–372
Wesstrom G (1980) Umbilical artery catheterisation in newborns. V. A clinical follow-up study. Acta Paediatr Scand 69: 371–376
Wesstrom G, Finnstrom O, Stenport G (1979) Umbilical artery catheterisation in newborns. I. Thrombosis in relation to catheter type and position. Acta Paediatr Scand 68: 575–581
Whitelaw A, Placzek M, Dubowitz L et al. (1983) Phenobarbitone for prevention of periventricular haemorrhage in very low birthweight infants. Lancet 98: 1168–1170
Whitington PF, Black DD (1980) Cholelithiasis in premature infants treated with parenteral nutrition and furosemide. J Pediatr 97: 647–649
Wigglesworth JS, Husemeyer RP (1977) Intracranial birth trauma in vaginal breech delivery: the continued importance of injury to the occipital bone. Br J Obstet Gynaecol 84: 684–691
Wilkinson A, Baum JD, Keeling JW (1981) Gluteal skin necrosis after umbilical arterial catheterisation. Arch Dis Child 56: 237–238 (letter)
Wilmore DW, Dudrick SJ (1968) Growth and development of an infant receiving all nutrients exclusively by vein. J Am Med Assoc 203: 860
Yates PO (1959) Birth trauma to the vertebral arteries. Arch Dis Child 34: 436–441
Yeager AS (1974) Transfusion-acquired cytomegalovirus infection in newborn infants. Am J Dis Child 128: 478–483

Yeager AS, Grumet FC, Hafleigh EB, Arvin AM, Bradley JS, Prober CG (1981) Prevention of tranfusion-acquired cytomegalovirus infections in newborn infants. J Pediatr 98: 281–287

Youroukos S, Papadelis F, Matsaniotis N (1980) Porencephalic cysts after amniocentesis. Arch Dis Child 55: 814–815

Ziegler JB, Cooper DA, Johnson RO, Gold J (1985) Postnatal transmission of AIDS-associated retrovirus from mother to infant. Lancet I: 896–897

Chapter 15

The Gastrointestinal Tract and Exocrine Pancreas

Dick Variend

Development

The gut derives from that part of the secondary yolk sac which becomes enclosed by the head, tail and lateral folds of the embryonic plate at around the 20th day of development. The head and tail folds enclose the fore- and hindgut respectively. The intermediate portion of the intraembryonic yolk sac forms the midgut which connects through a wide communication with the extraembryonic part of the secondary yolk sac (the definitive yolk sac). This communication becomes progressively reduced by better definition of the head, tail and lateral folds of the embryo (Fig. 15.1); by 28 days the communication is via a narrow vitelline duct and the umbilical cord is clearly visible. At about this time the primitive foregut and hindgut come into contact with rostral and caudal invaginations, the stomodeum and proctodeum. Most of the epithelium and glands of the digestive tract originate from embryonic endoderm, while the epithelium of the cranial and caudal ends is derived from the stomodeum and proctodeum respectively. In the foregut, two lateral ridges appear and grow towards each other in the midline, separating an anterior diverticulum which becomes the larynx and trachea, from the oesophagus. The stomach appears as a fusiform expansion towards the caudal end of the foregut in the cervical region of the embryo. The oesophagus elongates rapidly during the 6th to 7th weeks, reaching its final relative length by the end of this time. The original lining of the oesophagus is simple ciliated pseudostratified columnar epithelium, which is replaced progressively by squamous epithelium from the 5th intrauterine month.

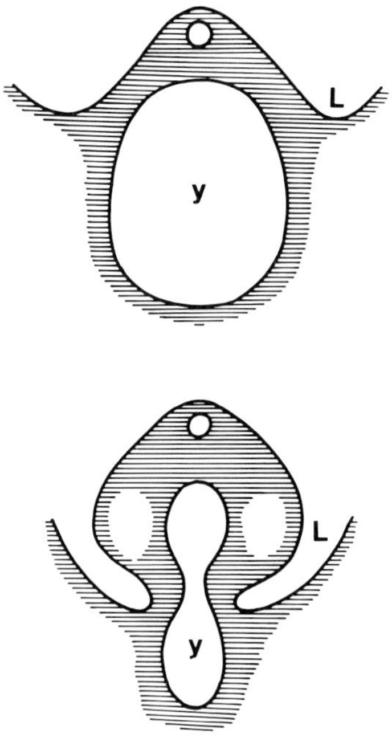

Fig. 15.1. Transverse slice through embryo illustrates diagrammatically the vitelline duct. (*Y*, yolk sac; *L*, lateral fold).

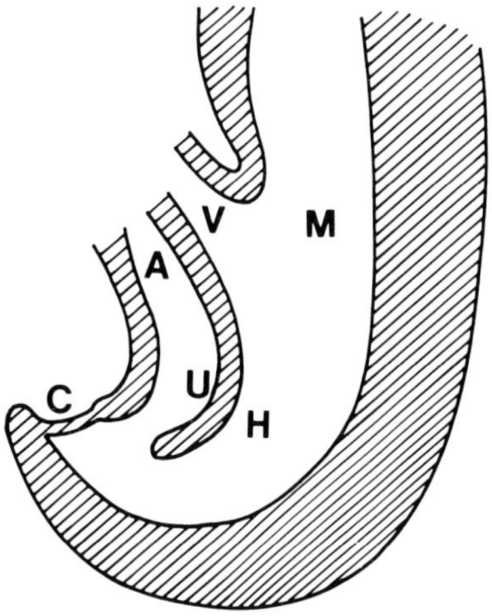

Fig. 15.2. Division of the cloaca into urogenital sinus and rectum. (*U*, urorectal septum; *A*, allantois; *H*, hindgut; *C*, cloacal membrane; *V*, vitelline duct; *M*, midgut).

At about the 4th week the intestine is almost a straight tube suspended by a mesentery from the dorsal body wall. Because the abdominal cavity is too small to accommodate the enlarging liver and growing intestine the midgut herniates into the extraembryonic coelom in the base of the umbilical cord. Between 10 and 11 weeks, the midgut withdraws from the umbilical cord and returns to the abdominal cavity. A 180° counterclockwise rotation occurs late in this stage and, as a result of a further 90° counterclockwise rotation, the caecum lies in the right upper quadrant. From the 12th week to birth, the caecum descends to its final location in the right lower quadrant.

At the 5th week of gestation a group of neuroblasts appears bilaterally along the vagal trunks at the level of the pharynx (Okamoto and Ueda 1967). They appear around the oesophagus at 6 weeks and reach the cephalic limb of the midgut by 7 weeks. By 12 weeks they are present throughout the alimentary tract down to the rectum. The early neurons appear first in the myenteric plexus, and then migrate across the circular muscle to populate the submucosa. A more caudal neural crest origin for the distal enteric neurons has also been suggested (Andrew 1971).

The cloaca, the dilated terminal part of the primitive hindgut, receives the allantois ventrally and the mesonephric ducts laterally. The urorectal septum develops in the angle between the allantois and the midgut and divides the cloaca into urogenital sinus and rectum (Fig. 15.2). Recent work (van der Putte 1986) suggests that the urorectal septum is not important in the subdivision of the cloaca and that fusion between the urorectal septum and the cloacal membrane does not normally occur. The dorsal cloacal membrane and its mesenchymal component descend towards the tail groove, and subsequently its attenuation and disintegration causes the formation of separate anorectal and urogenital orifices.

Oral Cavity

Cleft lip and cleft palate are among the most common developmental abnormalities of the oral cavity.

Microstomia comprises severe hypoplasia of the mandible accompanied by hypoplasia of the mouth. A broad oral cavity is known as macrostomia. Both of these anomalies are frequent components of malformation syndromes (Smith 1982).

The tongue may be abnormally large (macroglossia); causes include Beckwith–Wiedemann syndrome, trisomy 21, glycogenosis type 2 and lymphangioma.

A lingual thyroid is a localised midline mass in the posterior third of the tongue that results from maldescent of the thyroid primordium. Thyroglossal duct remnants, commonly manifesting as cysts, may also occur at this site. Dermoid cysts rarely present in the floor of the mouth (Howell et al. 1972). Congenital epulis (Fuhr and Krogh 1972) is a benign soft tissue tumour that, on microscopy, shows a striking resemblance to granular cell myoblastoma. It usually arises from the alveolar mucosa of the premaxilla, and females are predominantly affected. A teratoma arising from the basicranium, tonsillar area or soft palate may protrude through the mouth (Gonzalez-Crussi 1980); they are usually benign but may obstruct the airway (see Fig. 12.4, p. 280).

The most common infection of the mouth in the newborn is moniliasis; there may be an associated maternal vulvovaginitis. It is also a frequent complication of antibiotic therapy in the neonate.

Malformations of the salivary glands are very uncommon. Absence of the parotid is rarely reported. A ranula is a retention cyst of the sublingual or submaxillary gland ducts elevat-

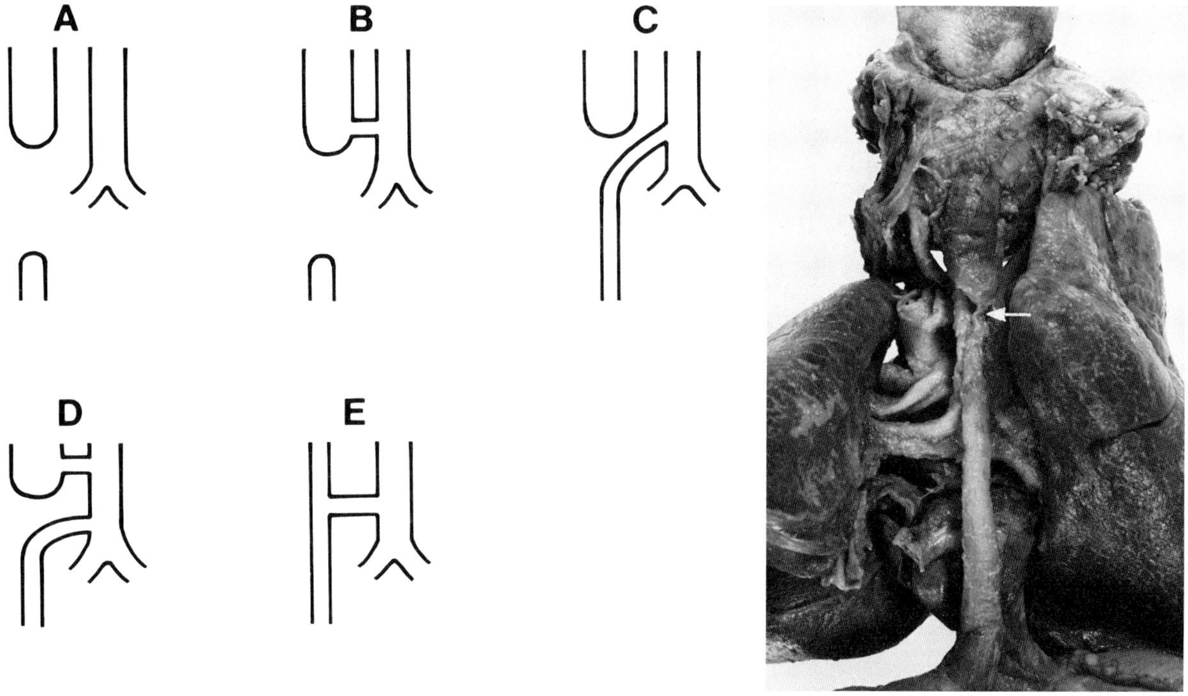

a b

Fig. 15.3. **a** Anatomical types of oesophageal atresia and tracheo-oesophageal fistula. **b** Commonest type of defect (*C* in **a**): dissection of thoracic viscera from back. The atretic segment (*arrow*) is short.

ing the buccal epithelium. The cyst is usually unilocular and lined by mucus-secreting epithelium. Cytomegalovirus (CMV) infection often involves the salivary glands but is trivial compared with its effects on other organs. The most common tumour of the parotid in the neonate is a capillary haemangioma (Martinez-Mora et al. 1971). Rare neoplasms, designated choristoma (Tang et al. 1979) and embryoma (Vawter and Tefft 1966) have been described in the neonatal period.

Oesophagus

Foci of ciliated pseudostratified columnar epithelium may persist within the oesophagus and be identified in the neonatal period; it is more likely to be encountered in preterm babies. Gastric heterotopia may occur in the anterior subcricoid area of the oesophagus (Rector and Connerley 1941).

Mucosal erosions of the upper oesophagus are a common histological finding among babies dying in the neonatal period (Merriam and Benirschke 1959). Only a proportion of cases can be explained on the basis of intubation.

Oesophageal Atresia

Oesophageal atresia may take one of several forms (Fig. 15.3a); the commonest is that where the upper oesophagus ends as a blind pouch and the lower oesophagus joins the respiratory tract through a fistula near the tracheal bifurcation (Fig. 15.3b); Waterston et al. 1962). This variety accounts for over 80% of cases. Atresia of the oesophagus without tracheo-oesophageal fistula is the next most common variety. Less common variants are shown in Fig. 15.3a. Associated anomalies are found in 48% of cases and commonly involve the cardiovascular system (Weaver et al. 1986) and gastrointestinal tract, including anal atresia (Holder et al. 1964). Mortality is adversely affected by low birthweight and associated malformations.

Other anomalies that may rarely affect the oesophagus are mucosal webs and diaphragms. Absence of the oesophagus and double oesophagus are rarely reported.

The VATER association (Quan and Smith 1973; Temtamy and Miller 1974) is the acronym applied to a non-random combination of vertebral anomalies (V), anal atresia (A), tracheo-oesophageal fistula (T–E) with atresia, renal defects (R) and radial limb dysplasia (R). A mesodermal defect operating in early development has been suggested as the basis for this association.

Stomach

Microgastria

Microgastria is a rare condition in which the stomach is considerably reduced in size and may retain a mid-sagittal position normally observed in the early embryo (Blank and Chisolm 1973). Asplenia may be associated. Clinical presentation is usually related to feeding problems.

Infantile Hypertrophic Pyloric Stenosis

The incidence of pyloric stenosis in the UK is approximately 3 in 1000 live births, but present evidence suggests that it is becoming more common. It is up to four times more common in boys than girls and familial cases are reported. Vomiting is the commonest presenting symptom and usually starts after the first week of life. Because of the excellent prognosis that follows current management, the pathologist is unlikely to encounter this abnormality as a cause of upper intestinal obstruction. The pathogenesis is unknown, but current theories implicate work hypertrophy and abnormalities of the myenteric plexus, muscle enzymes and excessive gastrin production (Spicer 1982).

The pylorus is increased in length and external diameter, the stomach is dilated and the antrum is hypertrophic. The circular muscle layer is up to four times normal thickness and the longitudinal muscle is attenuated. Evidence of previous pyloromyotomy is sometimes seen in infants dying from other causes. A longitudinal brown line about 1.5 cm in length is visible in the anterior wall of the pylorus. Residual myohypertrophy may be present.

Spontaneous Gastric Perforation

The predominant symptom of spontaneous gastric perforation is the sudden onset of abdominal distension during the first week; there is a high incidence of prematurity. The majority of perforations occur high on the greater curvature (Parrish et al. 1964). Theories of pathogenesis include tissue ischaemia secondary to hypoxia (Touloukian 1973), congenital absence of musculature, mechanical disruption, stress ulcers and perforations from feeding catheters (Holgersen 1981). Gastric perforation related to distal obstruction should not be included in this category.

Peptic Ulceration

Gastric and duodenal ulcers are both unusual in the neonatal period; duodenal ulcers are slightly more common (Nacheff et al. 1964; Bell et al. 1981). No single aetiological factor seems to be responsible. Perforation or haemorrhage, or both, are the usual clinical presentations. Of all cases reported in children, peptic ulcer in the neonate accounts for approximately 10%. Peptic ulcers in the newborn are always acute and microscopy shows little evidence of inflammatory reaction. Neonatal gastric ulceration may be iatrogenic; it is a reported complication of tolazoline administration (see Chap. 14, p. 338). Mucosal erosions of the neonatal stomach are far more common and are usually seen in association with severe asphyxia or overwhelming sepsis.

Small Intestine

Intestinal Duplication

Intestinal duplication or enterogenous cysts are spherical or tubular structures possessing the basic pattern of the enteric wall. Any part of the alimentary tract may be affected but duplications are usually intra-abdominal. The small intestine is most commonly involved, particularly the distal ileum (Dohn and Povlsen 1951; Grosfeld et al. 1970). Of the foregut duplications, those associated with the oesophagus are most common (Bissler and Klein 1988); gastric duplications are usually located

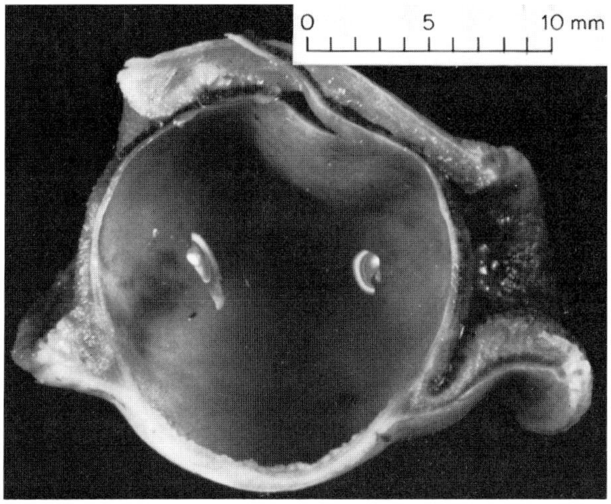

Fig. 15.4. Ileal duplication impinging on bowel lumen. Infant presented with intestinal obstruction in the neonatal period.

on the greater curvature and are twice as common in females.

A variety of mechanisms have been invoked to explain the origin of duplication cysts. These include failure of recanalisation of the bowel lumen following the so-called solid epithelial phase of intestinal development (Bremer 1944), persistence of epithelial outpouchings described in embryonic intestine (Bremer 1944) and intestinal ischaemia in early intrauterine life (Favara et al. 1971). A mechanism currently popular, especially when vertebral defects coexist, implicates persistent connections between the notochord and intestinal endoderm (Veeneklaas 1952; Fallon et al. 1954).

Foregut duplications often cause respiratory distress while those of the mid- and hindgut are associated with a palpable mass, or intestinal obstruction caused by direct mechanical pressure (Fig. 15.4) (Grosfeld et al. 1970). Rectal duplications are rare and may present as a sacrococcygeal mass (Lemire et al. 1971). Those containing gastric mucosa are vulnerable to ulceration, accompanied by perforation and haemorrhage. Intussusception occasionally occurs (Cunningham et al. 1980).

Most duplication cysts are located close to the mesenteric border of the intestine, often lying within the mesentery and sharing a common blood supply, or are situated within the muscularis propria (Fig. 15.4). Occasionally, they are more widely separated from the intestine and lie in the retroperitoneum. Cysts are usually single and exceptionally communicate with the bowel lumen. A smooth muscle coat, which sometimes contains a neural plexus, is always present. The mucosal lining may be that of the contiguous alimentary organ or resemble that of a more distant site. Many duplication cysts, irrespective of location, contain gastric mucosa.

Sometimes, duplications or their fibrous connections pass through the diaphragm producing bizarre symptoms (McLetchie et al. 1954; Goldberg and Johnson 1962). Some duplication cysts, particularly those in the mediastinum, may be attached directly or via a fibrous cord to a spinal defect of some sort; vertical clefts, hemivertebrae and anterior spina bifida are all described. The lower cervical and upper thoracic vertebrae are usually involved. Mediastinal and abdominal cysts may coexist (Fallon et al. 1954).

Split Notochord Syndrome

A spectrum of rare anomalies, ranging from dorsal cysts to bowel herniating between incomplete vertebral arches, has been reported. Clefts of vertebral bodies and vertebral arch defects are invariably present (Bentley and Smith 1960; Smith 1960). Related malformations have been described by Esterley and Baghdassarian (1963) and Denes et al. (1967). It has been suggested that a common pathogenetic mechanism involves localised division of the notochord and persistence of connections between notochord and endoderm. These abnormalities may be part of a spectrum which embraces duplication cysts, intestinal diverticulae and neuroenteric fistulae.

Vitellointestinal Duct Remnants

A spectrum of anomalies can be related to persistence of part or all of the vitellointestinal duct (Smith 1960). The commonest anomaly is Meckel's diverticulum. It is the commonest congenital anomaly of the gastrointestinal tract and is present in 2% of the population; boys are more commonly affected. It is the result of failure of obliteration of the intestinal end of the duct.

The diverticulum is sited on the antimesenteric border of the terminal ileum and is usually of the same diameter as the intestine from which it arises. It is usually lined by small intestinal mucosa, but pancreatic and gastric

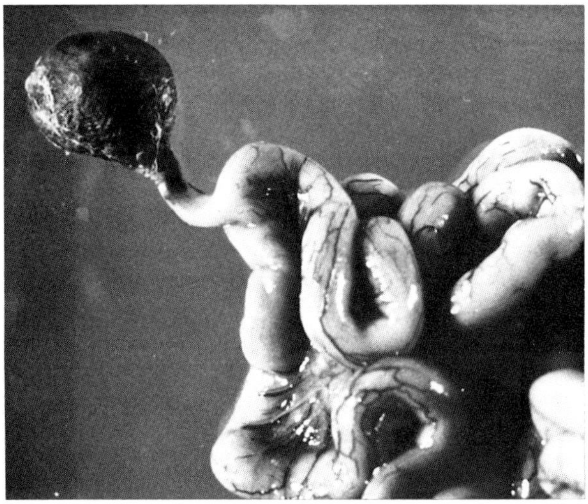
a

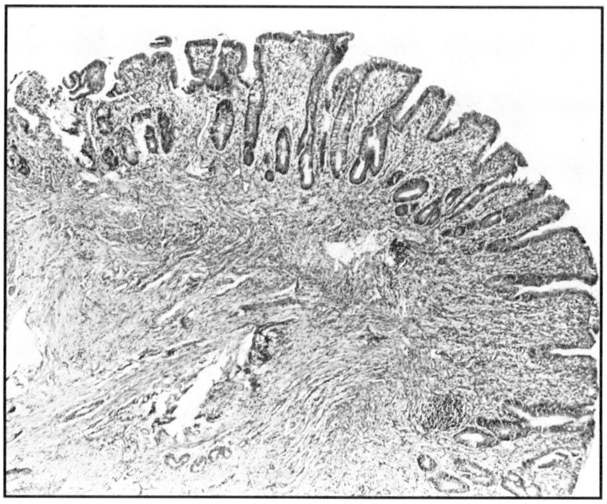
b

Fig. 15.5. Vitellointestinal remnant in a neonate. **a** Nodule attached to a diverticulum protruded at the umbilicus. **b** It comprises small intestinal mucosa with fibromuscular stroma.

heterotopic foci may be present. Peforation, haemorrhage, volvulus and intussusception are recognised complications but they are rarely symptomatic in the neonatal period.

A fibrous cord may connect the ileum or a Meckel's diverticulum to the abdominal wall at the umbilicus. It may cause volvulus and intestinal obstruction. A cyst may occur at any point along the course of the original vitelline duct. Persistence of intestinal mucosa at the umbilicus (vitelline sinus, enterocystoma) may require excision because of mucus secretion or haemorrhage (Fig. 15.5).

Exceptionally, the entire vitellointestinal duct remains patent, and meconium leaks from the umbilicus shortly after birth (Jackson and Bird 1961). Ileal intussusception through a patent vitellointestinal duct is rare; everted small bowel may mimic a ruptured exomphalos or gastroschisis (Moore and Schumacker 1952).

Abnormalities of Intestinal Rotation

Failure of the intestine to undergo rotation during and after its return to the abdominal cavity may be complete. More commonly, however, the initial anticlockwise 180° rotation takes place, but the final stage of rotation may arrest at that time or any stage before the caecum has descended to the right iliac fossa (Fig. 15.6).

When intestinal rotation does not occur (non-rotation), the entire colon is on the left side of the abdomen with the small bowel lying on the right. This is the pattern usually associated with diaphragmatic hernia and exomphalos but may be an incidental finding at necropsy.

When intestinal rotation is incomplete (malrotation), the caecum may lie in the upper central abdomen anterior to the duodeno-jejunal junction (Snyder and Chaffin 1954). The mesenteric attachment of the midgut is short, rendering the intestine unduly mobile, and midgut volvulus is a frequent complication. This may present in the neonatal period as intestinal obstruction and gangrene (Fig. 15.7), or may result in small intestinal atresia or meconium peritonitis if volvulus occurs in utero.

When caecal descent is incomplete, the peritoneal bands that normally run between

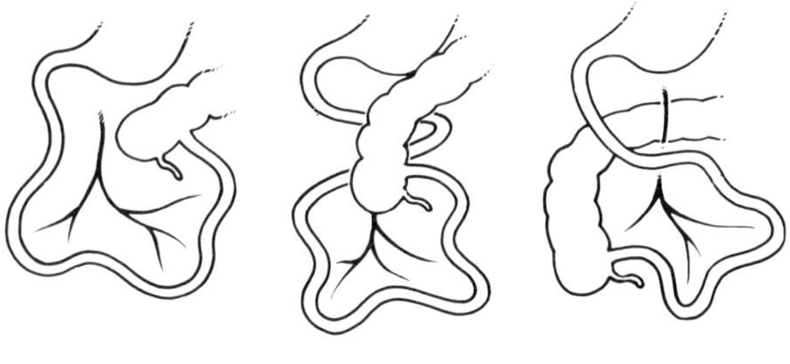

Fig. 15.6. Different patterns of rotational abnormality of the bowel (*A*, non-rotation; *B*, malrotation; *C*, reversed rotation).

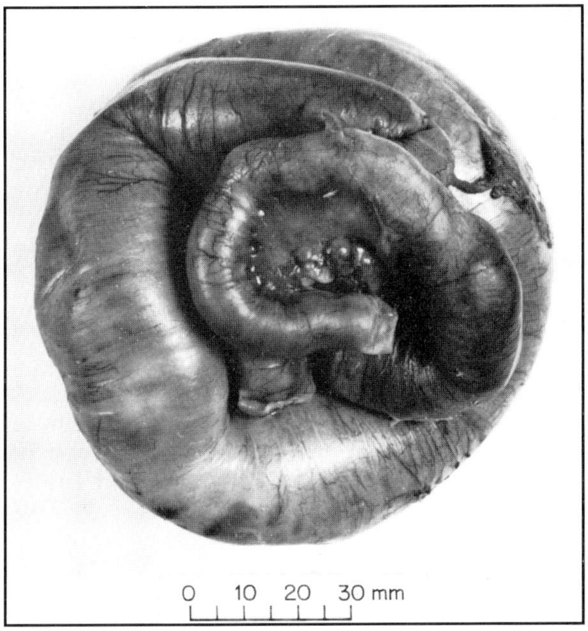

Fig. 15.7. Gangrenous bowel secondary to volvulus complicating malrotation of the intestine.

the right peritoneal gutter and right colon after resorption of the right mesocolon and effect colonic fixation, are abnormal in length and situation. They persist as Ladd's bands, which cross anterior to the duodenum and may cause extrinsic obstruction (Stewart et al. 1976).

Reversed rotation occurs when the intestine rotates in a clockwise direction rather than counter-clockwise. The superior mesenteric artery passes anterior to, and may obstruct, the transverse colon, with the duodenum lying anterior to the artery (Kiesewetter and Smith 1958).

Congenital Short Intestine

Short small bowel has been described in association with omphalocele (Reiquam et al. 1965) and gastroschisis, conditions known to be associated with prenatal volvulus. Bowel infarction with resorption of the infarcted length of bowel and anastomosis of the lumen has been suggested as the underlying cause. A similar mechanism has been proposed for reduced intestinal length in babies with jejunal or ileal atresia (Benson et al. 1960). Congenital short intestine is occasionally reported as an isolated defect (Yutani et al. 1973).

Intestinal Atresia and Stenosis

Atresia is a loss of continuity of the bowel lumen and is accompanied by intestinal obstruction, whilst stenosis is a localised luminal narrowing which may produce a partial obstruction to passage of intestinal contents. The duodenum is most commonly affected, its incidence being about 1 in 5000 live births. Involvement of the jejunum and ileum are less common, whilst atresias of the colon are rare. Antral mucosal web is a rare cause of gastric outlet obstruction (Bell et al. 1978); there is a high incidence of associated congenital anomalies. Its relationship to atresia occurring at other levels of the intestine is unclear.

Presenting symptoms are vomiting, abdominal distension and failure to pass meconium. There is a recognised association between atresia and maternal polyhydramnios, especially with proximal bowel atresias.

Duodenal Atresia

Extraintestinal anomalies and prematurity are more commonly associated with duodenal atresia than with distal intestinal atresias, and there is a recognised association between duodenal atresia and Down's syndrome (Young and Wilkinson 1968; Fonkalsrud et al. 1969). The associated defects are usually cardiac malformations; anorectal anomalies are also described.

Duodenal atresia, unlike more distal intestinal atresias, appears to be the result of defective embryogenesis. The suggestion that it is the result of failure of recanalisation of the intestinal lumen following florid epithelial proliferation about the 8th week of gestation is probably correct (Tandler 1900, cited by Santulli and Blanc 1961). The duodenum is the only point in the intestine where epithelial proliferation completely occludes the lumen. Duodenal atresia is often accompanied by annular pancreas, which adds further support to the concept of locally defective embryogenesis.

Jejunal and Ileal Atresia

Three forms of atresia are described (Santulli and Blanc 1961; Fig. 15.8):

1. The muscularis propria is uninterrupted and a diaphragm composed of connective tissue

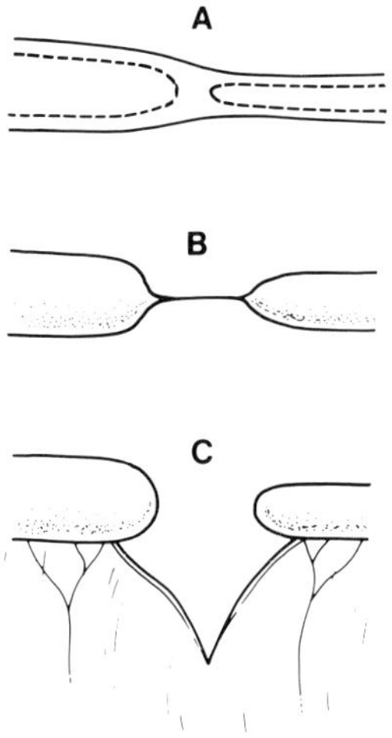

Fig. 15.8. Different types of intestinal atresia.

covered on both sides by mucosa separates the dilated proximal bowel from the distal collapsed segment (Fig. 15.9). Sometimes the occluding diaphragm may have a central perforation.

2. There is loss of continuity of intestine, and the proximal dilated segment is separated from the distal intestine by a fibrous cord.
3. There is a gap between the proximal and distal segments and a wedge-shaped defect in the mesentery is frequently present.

Atresias are multiple in 15% of cases and two or more of the three types described may coexist in the same patient. Type 3 is the most common.

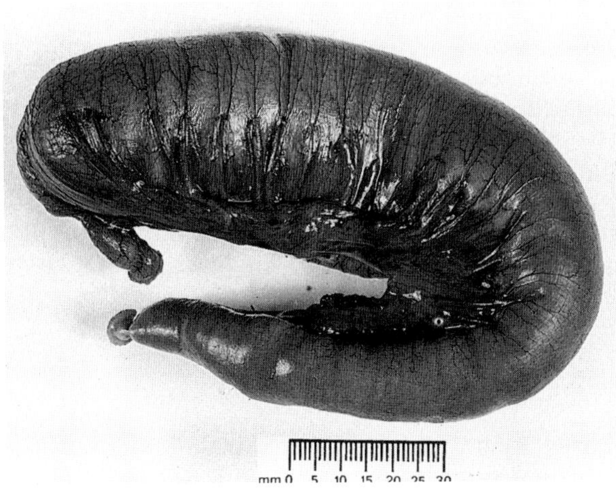

Fig. 15.9. Type 1 atresia of ileum with considerable dilatation of proximal loop.

Previous theories of pathogenesis have implicated failure of recanalisation of the solid stage at the end of the second embryonic month. However, all three forms of atresia and stenosis have been produced experimentally in dogs by occlusion of branches of the superior mesenteric artery, so rendering the intestine ischaemic in utero (Louw 1966). The presence of fetal squamae and lanugo hairs in the lumen distal to the atresia provides evidence that the atresia develops after patency of the bowel lumen and peristalsis have become established (Santulli and Blanc 1961). Evidence of fetal bowel infarction at operation was found in 42% of cases of jejunoileal atresia by deLorimier et al. (1969), and peritonitis was observed in 48% of jejunoileal atresias by Nixon and Tawes (1971). Malrotation of the intestine, volvulus, gastroschisis, intussusception and umbilical attachment are associations also described by these authors. Jejunoileal atresias or stenosis accompany meconium ileus.

The bowel proximal to the atresia is always bulbous and its vascularity may be seriously impaired; perforation is a recognised complication. The distal bowel is contracted and has a narrow lumen.

A rare variant of intestinal atresia is the "Christmas tree", "maypole" or "apple peel" deformity (Weitzmann and Vanderhoof 1966; Dickson 1970). The lesion comprises a duodenal or high jejunal atresia and absence of the dorsal mesentery. The distal small bowel is considerably reduced in length and it is twisted round a marginal artery. This variety of intestinal atresia has been reported in families (Blyth and Dickson 1969).

Meconium Ileus

Meconium ileus is the earliest manifestation of cystic fibrosis (mucoviscidosis). Its incidence is reported in between 7% and 25% of affected individuals. The majority of affected babies are born at term. Intestinal obstruction associated with failure to pass meconium is apparent in the first few hours or days after birth and is always present from birth. Babies who survive the neonatal period eventually develop other signs and symptoms of mucoviscidosis which are largely related to malabsorption and recurrent respiratory infection. Maternal polyhydramnios has been reported in 20% of cases (Holsclaw et al. 1965). Radiological examination of the abdomen shows a mottled granular or ground-

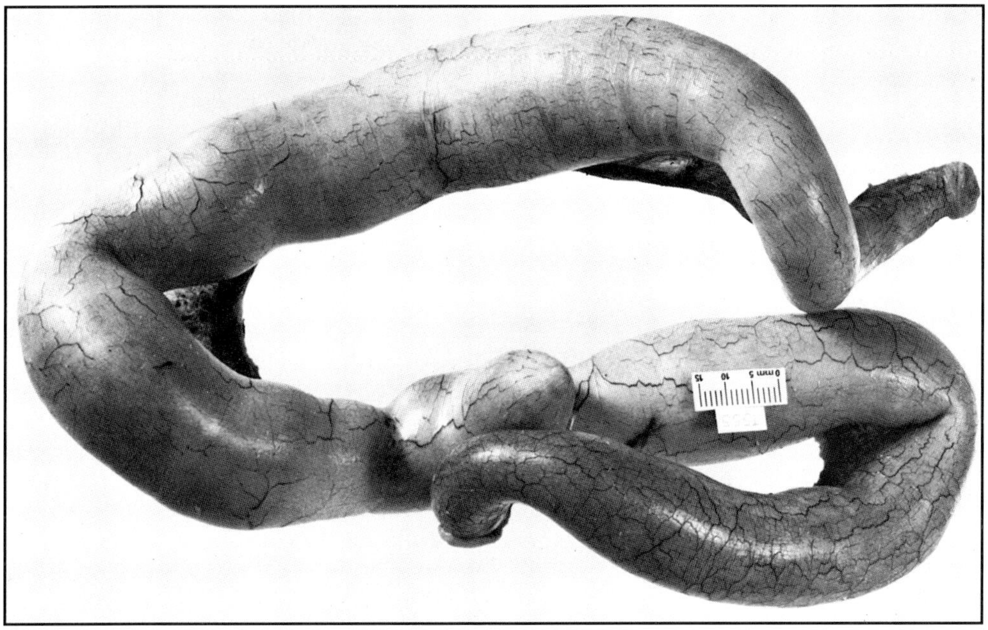

Fig. 15.10. Surgically resected ileum impacted with meconium from infant with neonatal intestinal obstruction and meconium ileus.

glass appearance and a characteristic paucity of fluid levels (Kopel 1972). Intestinal obstruction is due to an intraluminal bolus of abnormally viscid meconium. There is a dilated loop of bowel, often rigid because of impacted meconium (Fig. 15.10), which, when removed, forms a cast of the bowel lumen (Fig. 15.11). The more proximal bowel is dilated and its wall may be hypertrophied. The colon is very small, and, because of failure of significant passage of meconium beyond the level of obstruction, there may be tiny concretions of grey inspissated meconium with a consistency of dried putty scattered along the colon.

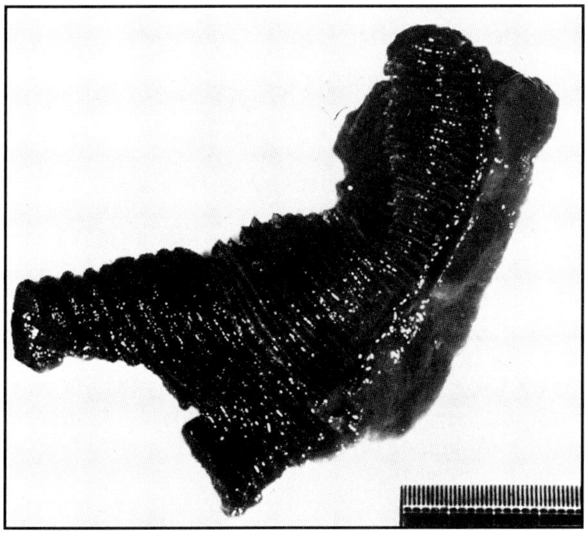

Fig. 15.11. Meconium cast removed from surgically resected ileum in infant with meconium ileus.

Two factors may explain the altered consistency of the meconium: pancreatic insufficiency resulting in deficient protein digestion, and abnormally viscid tenacious mucus produced by intestinal goblet cells which is not released into the lumen in normal amounts. As the pancreas in the neonate may be normal or show only minimal abnormality in individuals with meconium ileus, it is thought that abnormality of the intestinal mucous glands is more important (Thomaidis and Arey 1963).

Mucosal glands of the small intestine contain masses of acidophil secretion (Fig. 15.12) and may be cystically dilated. Brunner's glands may be similarly dilated by "stringy" mucus.

The incidence of associated congenital abnormalities is no different from that in the general population (Holsclaw et al. 1965; Donnison et al. 1966). On the other hand, atresia, stenosis, volvulus, peritoneal bands, gangrene and perforation, which are fairly frequent, are considered secondary mechanical complications (Oppenheimer and Esterly 1962).

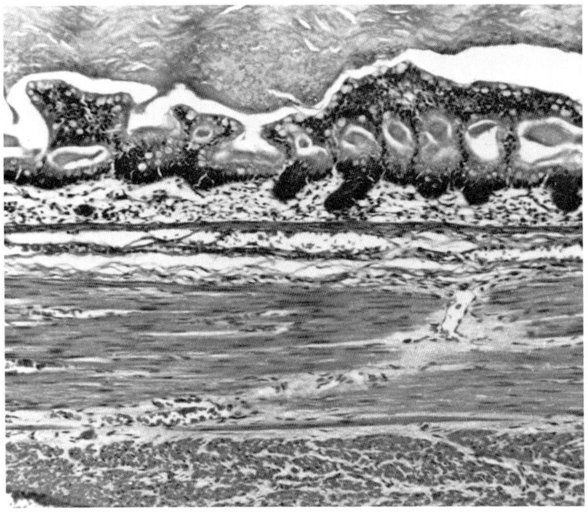

Fig. 15.12. Post-mortem specimen of small intestine to show retention of acidophilic secretion within crypt lumina. (H&E, ×90)

Intestinal atresia and stenosis in meconium ileus may be the result of localised pressure on the intestinal wall from inspissated meconium producing ulceration, granuloma formation and scarring, or prenatal volvulus of meconium-loaded loops of small bowel may occur (Bernstein et al. 1960).

The incidence of cystic fibrosis amongst patients with intestinal atresia is about 10% (Nixon and Tawes 1971), but cystic fibrosis should be excluded in all cases of atresia of the distal bowel as the prognosis is much worse and the implications for future pregnancies very serious.

Meconium Plug Syndrome

Intestinal obstruction caused by plugs of sticky meconium blocking the distal small bowel and proximal colon in the neonate was reported in the absence of cystic fibrosis by Rickham and Boeckman (1965). Sporadic reports followed, and Vinograd et al. (1981) reported seven cases in infants of very low birthweight whose sweat tests were subsequently shown to be normal. These cases differed from the typical infant with meconium ileus both radiologically and because intestinal obstruction was not present from birth. A similar clinical presentation in six fatal cases was reported by King et al. (1986) in preterm babies with respiratory problems and sepsis who passed meconium in the first 3 days of life but subsequently exhibited intestinal obstruction. At necropsy the small intestine was distended by abnormal meconium. The colon was small. Inspissated secretions were present in gland crypts. Within the pancreas, acinar and ductular dilatation, focal acinar atrophy and patchy fibrosis were apparent. Similar changes were present in salivary glands of some babies. Immunoreactive trypsin levels were normal in six babies. These authors suggested that fluid restriction, uraemia and sepsis may be important in the development of this condition. They questioned the specificity of the necropsy findings in meconium ileus.

Obstruction caused by sticky meconium involving more distal colon and rectum has been designated "meconium plug syndrome" (Clatworthy et al. 1956). Clinically and radiologically this condition may mimic Hirschsprung's disease, but ganglion cells are normal. A transient disturbance of colonic mobility, designated "small left colon syndrome", has been reported in infants of diabetic mothers and seems to be a related condition (Philippart et al. 1975).

Blockage of the distal small bowel caused by impacted milk curd is occasionally reported (Cook and Rickham 1969). Clinical obstruction is usually manifest during the second week after birth. The condition appears to be associated with early high-calorie formula feeds. It is not associated with cystic fibrosis and ganglion cells appear normal.

Meconium Peritonitis

Meconium peritonitis is a sterile chemical peritonitis following prenatal or perinatal perforation of the bowel, usually associated with intestinal obstruction (Rickham 1955; White 1956). The perforation may occur at any time from the 5th month of fetal life until bacterial colonisation of the intestine takes place after birth. Abdominal distension may be present at birth or develop during the first 24 h.

The most useful investigation is a plain abdominal radiograph, which reveals an opaque ground-glass appearance speckled with calcification. Calcification within the bowel lumen or wall and involvement of peritoneal surfaces is seen in a high proportion of cases. Radiological demonstration of calcification in the scrotum is considered pathognomonic and is due to the passage of

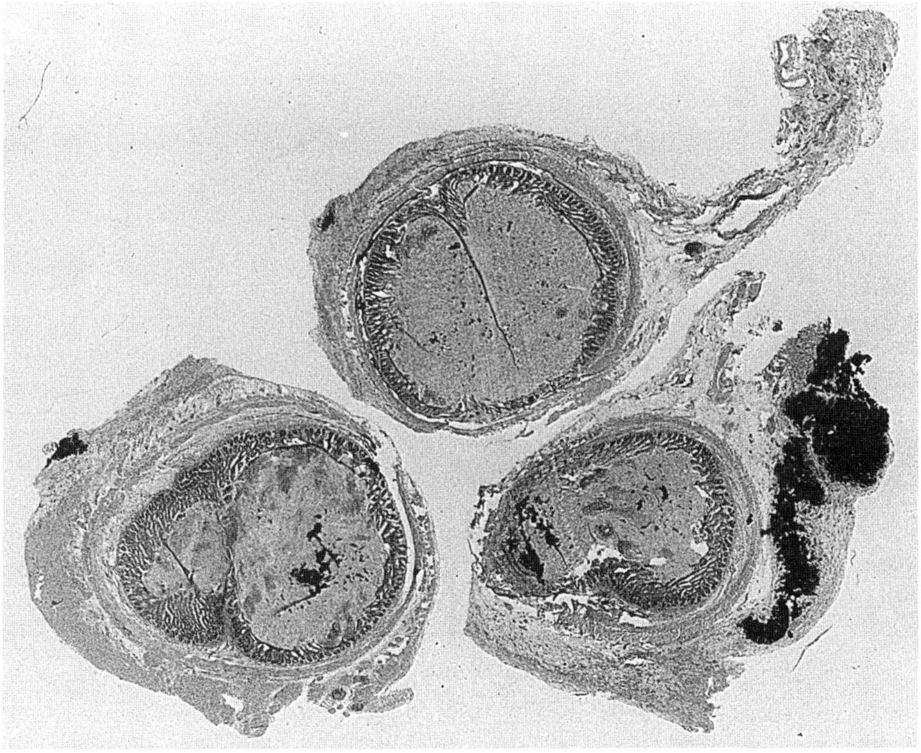

Fig. 15.13. Section of small intestine from an infant with meconium peritonitis and meconium ileus. The subserosa is irregularly thickened and calcified. Intraluminal calcification is also seen. (H&E, ×11)

meconium and exudate down a patent processus vaginalis; hard calcified nodules may develop in the scrotum or inguinal region subsequently (Forouhar 1982).

The pathology of this condition depends largely on the time at which the perforation occurs and may be classified as fibroadhesive, cystic or generalised (Lorimer and Ellis 1966). In the fibroadhesive form, which is probably related to early prenatal perforation, a fibroplastic reaction seals off the intestine at the site of the perforation. Calcification is common (Fig. 15.13) and perforation may not be detected at operation or post mortem. In the cystic type, a thick-walled cyst which is isolated from the remainder of the abdominal viscera forms around the perforation. The cyst is filled with exudate and its lining is calcified.

When perforation occurs in the perinatal period prior to or during birth, a generalised form of peritonitis develops, with meconium-stained viscid exudate distributed widely throughout the peritoneal cavity.

Jejunoileal atresia and meconium ileus, singly or combined, account for the majority of cases (Smith and Clatworthy 1961). Meconium peritonitis complicating cystic fibrosis carries a poor prognosis, while the prognosis of meconium peritonitis from other causes is similar to that of the underlying anomaly.

Necrotising Enterocolitis

Necrotising enterocolitis has become increasingly common and usually affects small premature infants, in particular those weighing less than 2000 g (Dudgeon et al. 1973), but mature babies are also affected (Rodin et al. 1973). It is usually apparent during the first 2 weeks of life, but may be seen later in small preterm babies. The increasing incidence is partly explained by survival of very small, preterm babies. Pallor, lethargy, vomiting, abdominal distension, diarrhoea and blood-stained stools are the usual clinical features.

Pneumatosis intestinalis is the radiological hallmark of the condition (Mizrahi et al. 1965), but intestinal dilatation may be the only abnormality. Pneumoperitoneum on the radiograph almost always indicates intestinal perforation, a frequent complication. Gas is

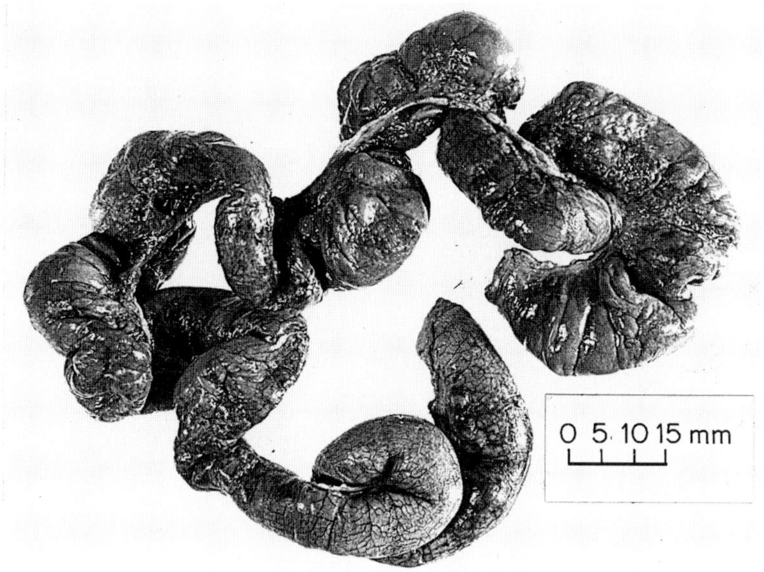

Fig. 15.14. Segment of small bowel removed at surgery for neonatal necrotising enterocolitis. Gas blebs are visible beneath the serosa.

seen occasionally in the portal vein or liver (Dudgeon et al. 1973). "Appendicitis" in the neonate is almost always due to necrotising enterocolitis (Santulli et al. 1975; Bax et al. 1980).

Pneumatosis may result from intraluminal gas diffusing through ischaemic mucosa or may be liberated by organisms colonising devitalised tissue (Stevenson et al. 1969). Both intramural and intraluminal gas from affected neonates comprise more than 30% hydrogen (Engel et al. 1973).

Necrotising enterocolitis is still incompletely understood (Kliegman 1990). Factors in the pathogenesis of this condition include mucosal ischaemia, oral feeding and bacterial colonisation of the bowel lumen. A wide variety of bacteria has been isolated from affected infants and there is some evidence that severity is related to the type of organism (Howard et al. 1977). Ischaemia may be related to an "overshooting" of the normal physiological response to hypoxia in the perinatal period resulting in splanchnic shutdown. A high incidence of perinatal asphyxia has been reported in one series (Lloyd 1969). Necrotising enterocolitis has been reported to occur prior to oral feeding (Marchildon et al. 1982). These infants were generally of lower birthweight and maturity and had a higher incidence of perinatal asphyxia and respiratory distress syndrome than those who developed necrotising enterocolitis after feeding. A proportion of these infants also had pneumatosis. The development of necrotising enterocolitis in the absence of feeding suggests that ischaemia has a more significant role.

Aminophylline, a xanthine derivative, is often employed as a stimulant in the management of neonates with episodes of apnoea. Aminophylline decreases gastrointestinal motility and promotes intraluminal bacterial overgrowth. Its role as a factor in some cases of necrotising enterocolitis has been questioned (Grosfeld et al. 1983).

Necrotising enterocolitis has been described following exchange transfusion (Corkery et al. 1968), umbilical arterial catheterisation (Franz et al. 1975), cardiac catheterisation (Bunton et al. 1977) and hyperviscosity (Hakanson and Oh 1977).

The terminal ileum and proximal colon are affected most commonly, but more proximal or distal gut may be involved. Rarely, the entire intestinal tract below the duodenum is affected. The bowel wall may be thickened and congested and later becomes thin and friable. Perforation, which may be single or multiple, often occurs along the antimesenteric border. Gas blebs may be visible beneath the serosa (Fig. 15.14). Histological appearances are related to the stage and severity of the disease. Initially, oedema, haemorrhage, coagulation necrosis, inflammation and pneumatosis predominate (Fig. 15.15). These changes may be

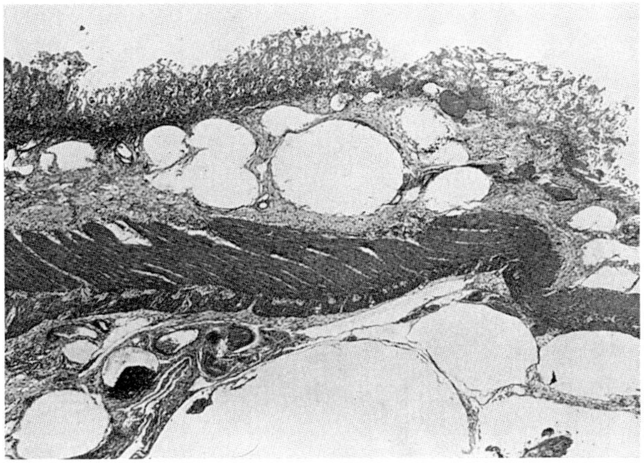

Fig. 15.15. Section of ileum showing extensive necrosis and pneumatosis in necrotising enterocolitis. (H&E, ×50)

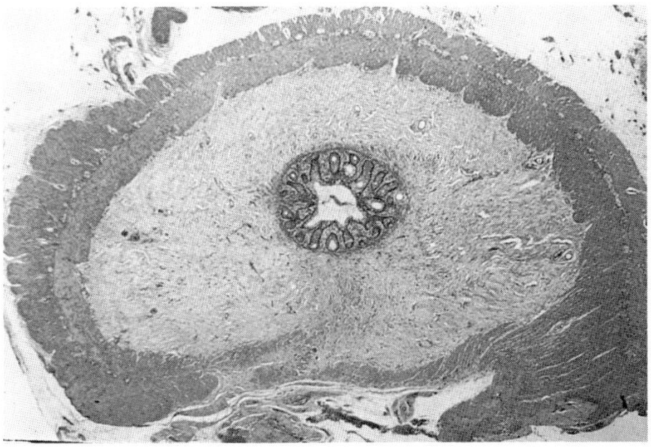

Fig. 15.16. Marked luminal stenosis of the colon following earlier episode of necrotising enterocolitis. (H&E, ×15)

limited to the mucosa or extend deeper to involve submucosa and muscle. Pneumatosis may involve all layers of the intestinal wall but frequently accumulates in the loose connective tissue of the submucosa. Ganglion cells are generally spared. Localised perforation of the bowel wall with little or no reaction in the adjacent tissue has been described (Lloyd 1969; Marchildon et al. 1982).

Epithelial regeneration and granulation characterise the repair phase, and residual damage in the form of fibrosis and mural thickening frequently results in luminal obstruction (Fig. 15.16).

Bowel Ischaemia Associated with Thromboembolic Disease

Extensive infarction of the small bowel and colon may occur as a result of thrombosis of the superior mesenteric artery (Rothschild et al. 1953) or aorta. The origin of the thrombus may not be apparent or may follow umbilical arterial catheterisation (Cochran et al. 1968; Neal et al. 1972; Fig. 14.16).

Colon and Rectum

Hirschsprung's Disease

Hirschsprung's disease is a disorder characterised by aganglionosis of the distal rectum with involvement of the bowel in continuity with it proximally for a variable extent. Aganglionosis interrupts peristalsis and so produces intestinal obstruction.

Its exact incidence is not known. Figures ranging from 1 in 1000 to 1 in 30 000 live births have been quoted (Lister and Rickham 1980). Males are more commonly affected than females in proportions varying from 3:1 to 5:1. The condition accounts for approximately 15% of all cases of neonatal intestinal obstruction (Santulli and Amoury 1967). In one large American series (Kleinhaus et al. 1979), only 15% of all cases of Hirschsprung's disease were detected during the first month of life, but in the UK the figure is considerably higher (Lister and Rickham 1980). Around 7% of patients with Hirschsprung's disease have a positive family history; this is more common when a long segment of colon is involved. Prematurity among affected neonates is uncommon (Klein et al. 1984). There is a recognised association between Hirschsprung's disease and Down's syndrome. The incidence of other associated anomalies is low, but includes colonic and ileal atresia (Currie et al. 1983; Gauderer et al. 1984).

Failure of completion of migration of neuroblasts from the cephalic neural crest down the alimentary tract is probably the embryological basis of this disorder. The earlier neuronal migration ceases, the longer the aganglionic segment will be. Classification depends on the length of the aganglionic segment: short-segment disease involves rectum and sigmoid colon; in long-segment disease aganglionosis extends more proximally than the sigmoid colon. Rarely, the entire intestinal tract is

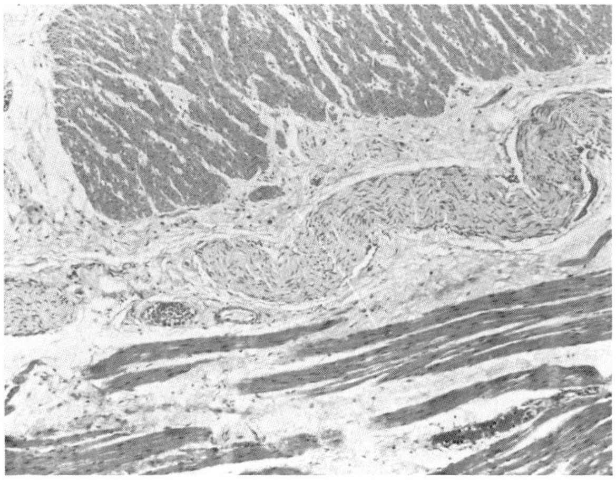

Fig. 15.17. Thickened nerve fascicles in myenteric plexus from a child with Hirschsprung's disease. (H&E, ×60)

aganglionic. The aganglionic segment is confined to the rectosigmoid region in about 70% of cases. There is poor correlation between the degree of obstruction and the length of the segment affected (Garrett et al. 1969).

The use of rectal suction submucosal biopsies to replace full-thickness biopsies marked an important advance in the management of Hirschsprung's disease. Suction biopsy does not require general anaesthesia, is associated with a lower incidence of complications, and, being superficial, does not interfere with subsequent pull-through procedures.

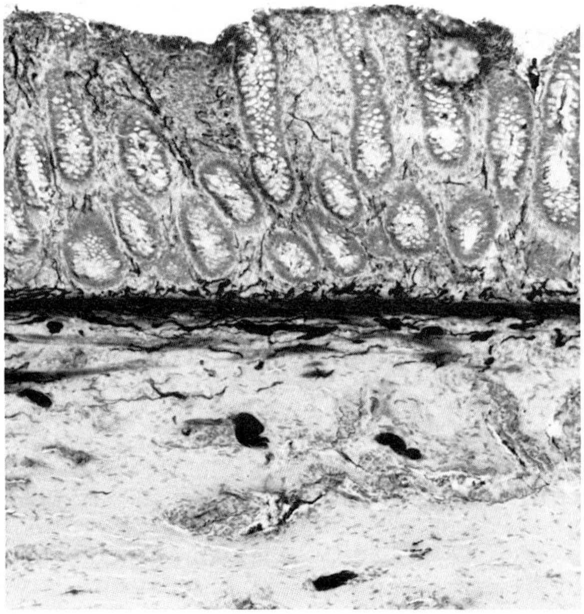

Fig. 15.18. Acetylcholinesterase staining to show intense fibre staining within the muscularis mucosae and submucosa in a case of Hirschsprung's disease. (AChE, ×75)

The diagnosis of Hirschsprung's disease presupposes a knowledge of normal innervation of the lower rectum and anal canal. Normally there is a 2–3 cm long aganglionic zone immediately above the mucocutaneous junction of the anus (Weinberg 1975). Biopsies taken from this area may be wrongly diagnosed as Hirschsprung's disease. Absence of ganglion cells above this level, often accompanied by thickened nerve fascicles, is required for diagnosis (Fig. 15.17), so that the adequacy of the biopsy is important. The thickened nerve fascicles represent sacral parasympathetic outflow and are consequently observed only up to the level of the splenic flexure, even when aganglionosis is present more proximally when the plane of the plexus is empty. A transitional zone of variable length comprising hypoganglionosis and thickened nerve fascicles often intervenes between distal aganglionic segment and normally innervated bowel.

The acetylcholinesterase reaction has substantially facilitated evaluation of suction biopsies. The technique is carried out fairly rapidly and the results are usually easy to interpret. Cholinergic fibres, particularly in the muscularis mucosae and the submucosa, are increased in number, thickness and intensity of staining (Fig. 15.18). This appearance extends into the physiological aganglionic zone. In addition, ganglion cells which are normally easily demonstrated by this method are absent. Many acetylcholinesterase-positive fibres are present in the lamina propria, although they may be absent in the early neonatal period (Huntley et al. 1982; Goto et al. 1984). Although this is an effective screening method for Hirschsprung's disease, false-negative and equivocal results were encountered in 6% of biopsies by Barr et al. (1985). False-negative results are more likely when the biopsy does not include muscularis mucosae or is taken too high in very short segment disease. One false-negative result has been encountered in 758 tests carried out in this Department since 1981, amongst which were 96 cases of Hirschsprung's disease. The false-negative case was subsequently found to have total intestinal aganglionosis.

Enterocolitis, the most serious complication of Hirschsprung's disease, carries significant

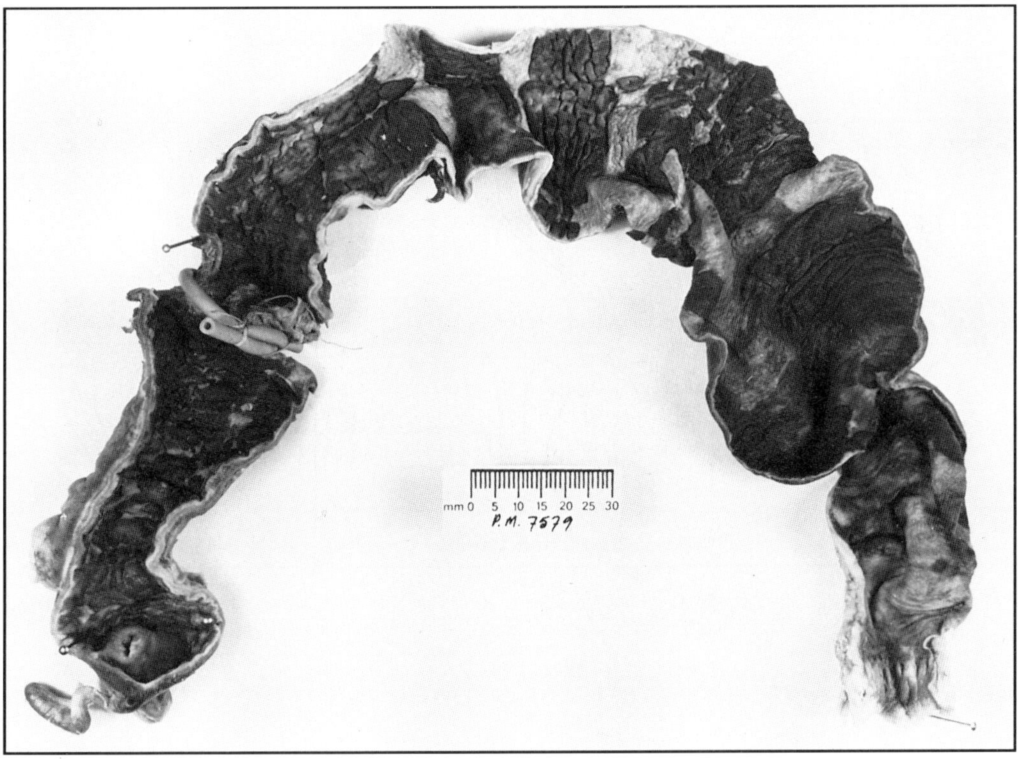

Fig. 15.19. Colon and rectum from an infant who died from enterocolitis complicating Hirschsprung's disease. There is extensive mucosal congestion and ulceration. The mucosa of the distal aganglionic segment is comparatively well preserved.

morbidity and mortality. The complication is likely to develop when surgical decompression of the colon is delayed and is more common with long-segment disease (Kleinhaus et al. 1979). Extensive necrosis and ulceration of the colonic mucosa (Fig. 15.19) of normally innervated bowel with marked dilatation and variable involvement of the terminal small bowel is the usual finding. Toxic shock, septicaemia, perforation and peritonitis are common. The mucosa of the aganglionic segment is surprisingly well preserved.

Ischaemia following mechanical obstruction (Bill and Chapman 1962), a Schwartzmann reaction involving bacterial antigens and the toxin of *Clostridium difficile* (Thomas et al. 1986) have been suggested as pathogenetic mechanisms (Berry and Fraser 1968).

Necrotising (ischaemic) enterocolitis has been reported as a complication of neonatal Hirschsprung's disease (Teich et al. 1986). It is indistinguishable from the usual form of necrotising enterocolitis apart from the low incidence of pneumatosis intestinalis. It is a more serious complication than the enterocolitis usually associated with Hirschsprung's disease. The appendix rarely perforates in the neonatal period secondary to distal colonic obstruction due to Hirschsprung's disease (Martin and Perrin 1967).

So-called ultra-short-segment Hirschsprung's disease is probably a functional defect of the internal anal sphincter; diagnosis is not made on rectal biopsy as there is no aganglionic segment (Neilson and Yazbeck 1990).

Colonic Neuronal Dysplasia

Colonic neuronal dysplasia is a rare condition characterised by aberrant innervation and clinically may simulate Hirschsprung's disease (Meier-Ruge 1974). The usual microscopic features are hyperplasia of the intramural plexuses and giant ganglia. Isolated ganglion cells may be seen in the lamina propria and within the muscularis mucosae. Rarely, the whole colon is involved (Dickson and Variend 1983). Colonic neuronal dysplasia occasionally coexists with Hirschsprung's disease (Scharli

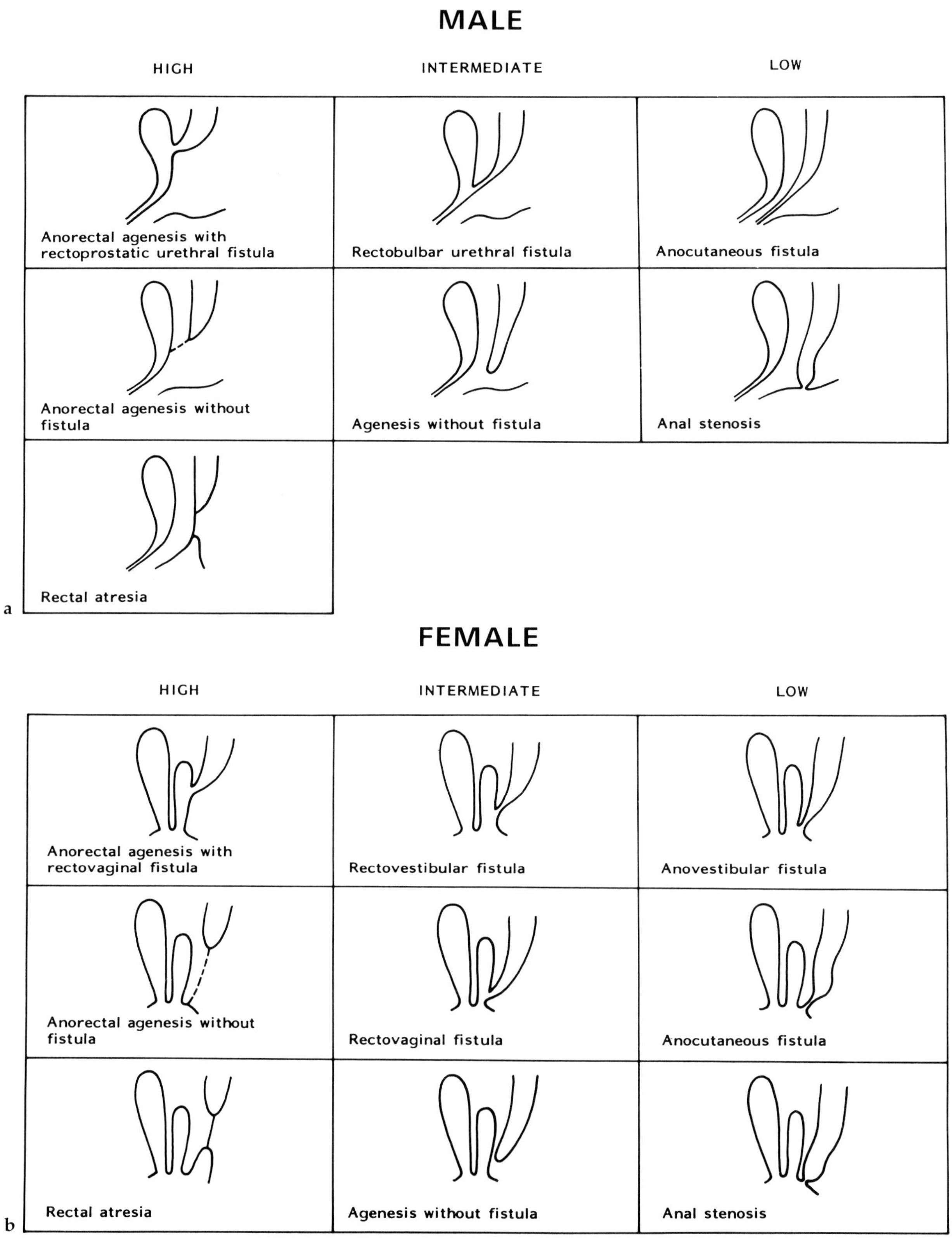

Fig. 15.20. Classification of anal atresia in males (**a**) and females (**b**). (After Stephens and Durham Smith 1986)

and Meier-Ruge 1981) and may explain some cases of residual intestinal obstruction found after the definitive pull-through procedure.

Megacystis-Microcolon-Intestinal Hypoperistalsis Syndrome (MMIHS)

MMIHS is a rare cause of intestinal obstruction in the newborn (Wiswell et al. 1979). The outcome is almost always fatal. The abdominal distension is caused by a non-obstructed distended bladder. A malrotated microcolon is associated with normal or increased numbers of ganglion cells. The condition is probably a manifestation of visceral myopathy (Puri et al. 1983).

Anorectal Malformations

Anorectal malformations are amongst the most common congenital abnormalities of the gut, the incidence being approximately 1 in 5000 live births (Partridge and Gough 1961). Males are more frequently affected. No general agreement exists as to the most satisfactory classification. A core classification agreed at an international workshop meeting in Wisconsin in 1984 is presented in Fig. 15.20.

Abnormalities may be categorised generally as high, intermediate or low, relative to the level of the puborectalis sling of the levator ani. All types may be associated with fistulae, which may open into the bowel, the perineum, vagina, urethra or, rarely, the bladder, depending on sex and the level of the lesion.

Other congenital abnormalities are more common with high malformations, frequently involving the genitourinary system, heart and skeleton (Gough 1961; Partridge and Gough 1961). Approximately one-third of rectal cases have a serious urological problem (Durham Smith 1968). Abnormalities of the lumbosacral spine are found in over 50% of the "high anomaly" group and include sacral agenesis or hemisacral anomalies. The inclusion of anorectal malformation in the VATER association has been alluded to earlier (see p. 350).

Recent investigation (van der Putte 1986) suggests that a defect in the dorsal cloacal membrane interferes with its migration towards the tail groove and that different types of anomalies are produced, depending on the form and size of the defect. Thus, superficial defects cause low malformations such as stenotic anus and ectopic anus, while deeper defects cause anal and anorectal agenesis, with and without fistulae. Agenesis of the whole cloacal membrane rarely results in absence of anorectal and urethral orifices. Other anomalies such as high anorectal and rectal atresias cannot be readily explained on this basis and may be the result of ischaemic insult in utero.

Abdominal Wall Defects and Hernias

Exomphalos

An exomphalos is a hernia at the base of the umbilical cord. Its sac is formed from amniotic membrane and peritoneum. About 1 in 3500 live births are affected. A small exomphalos is also called "hernia of the umbilical cord". Small defects contain only loops of small intestine, whilst other viscera, particularly the liver, are frequently present within the sac of a large defect (Fig. 15.21).

The defect results from failure of the midgut to return from the extraembryonic coelom (physiological hernia) to the abdomen, and rectus abdominus muscles are displaced laterally when the defect is large. The diameter of the sac is often larger than the abdominal wall defect as it contains no muscle and is easily stretched.

The sac may rupture before, during or after birth (Aitken 1963). When antenatal rupture occurs, loops of bowel are often oedematous, friable and matted together. It is important to distinguish between antenatal rupture of an exomphalos and gastroschisis, as malformations in other systems, particularly cardiac defects (Greenwood et al. 1974) and chromosome anomalies (Mann et al. 1984; Nicolaides et al. 1986), frequently accompany exomphalos, whereas they are rarely seen with gastroschisis, and will influence choice of treatment and survival. Exomphalos is frequently seen in trisomies 13, 18 and 21 and Beckwith–Wiedemann syndrome.

Gastroschisis

Gastroschisis is much less common than exomphalos. Preterm delivery is common and

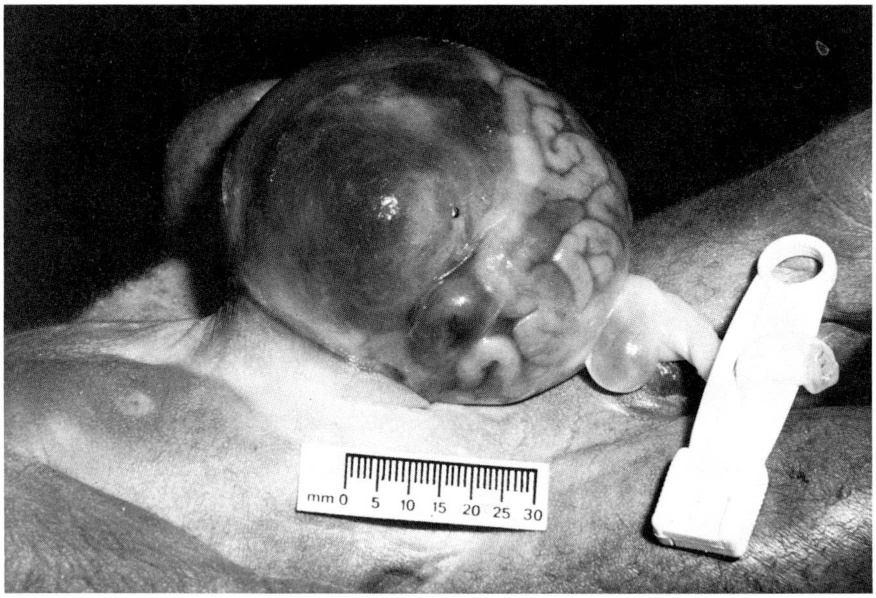

Fig. 15.21. A large defect of the ventral abdominal wall in newborn with exomphalos.

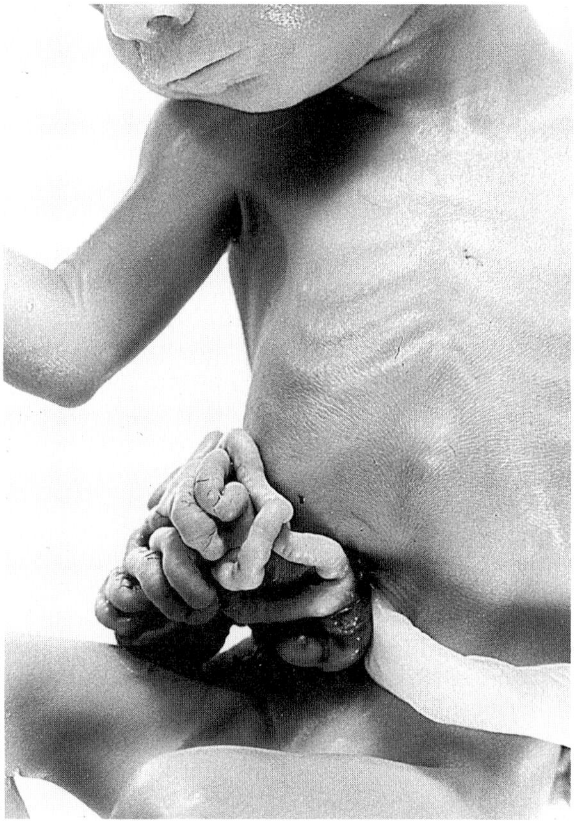

Fig. 15.22. Evisceration of a large segment of intestine through a small paraumbilical abdominal wall defect in a fetus with gastroschisis.

chromosomal analysis is usually normal. Antenatal ultrasound examination now provides an effective method of prenatal diagnosis (Nakayama et al. 1984). Theories of pathogenesis include rupture of a small exomphalos (Nakayama et al. 1984), premature involution of the right umbilical vein (deVries 1980) and interruption of the omphalomesenteric artery during early embryonic development (Hoyme et al. 1981).

There is a full-thickness defect of the anterior abdominal wall usually just to the right of the midline (Shaw 1975; King et al. 1980; Fig. 15.22), generally measuring less than 5 cm in diameter. No sac or sac remnant is present at its margin. A narrow strip of skin often separates the defect from the umbilical cord. Intestinal loops prolapse through the defect and float freely in the amniotic cavity. At birth, eviscerated bowel is encased in a peel of fibrin. The liver is usually intra-abdominal.

Associated defects are confined to the intestine and include jejunal or ileal atresia and stenosis (Amoury et al. 1977). These abnormalities are probably ischaemic in origin and are directly related to the abdominal wall defect. Bowel length is often reduced and intestinal rotation is incomplete. These abnormalities are all secondary to the abdominal wall defect; anomalies of other organs are uncommon and usually of a minor nature.

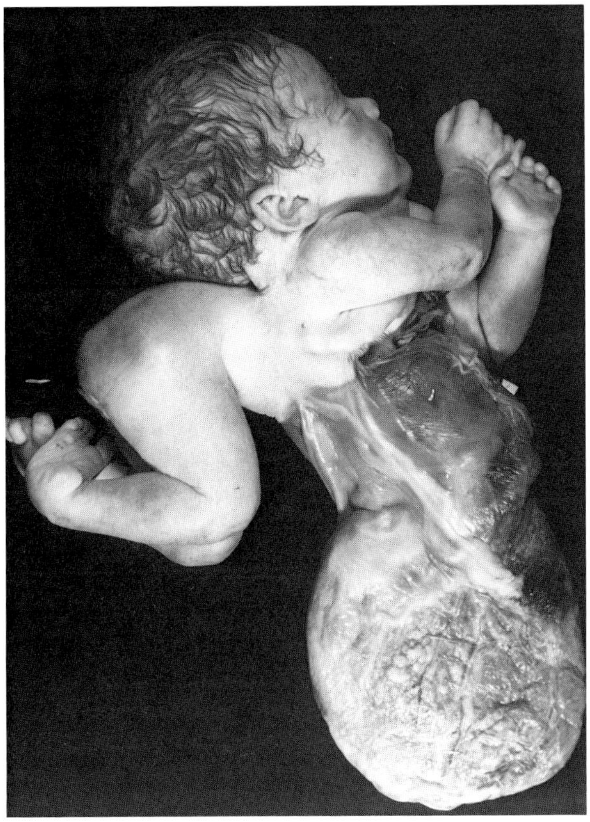

Fig. 15.23. Body-stalk abnormality in which the fetus is closely applied to the chorionic plate. Umbilical cord is absent.

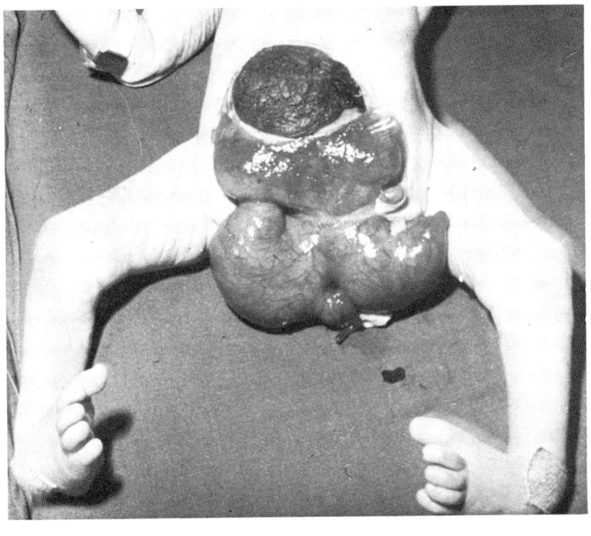

Fig. 15.24. Vesicointestinal fissure with exomphalos, exstrophy of the bladder, and everted caecum and appendix.

Other Abdominal Wall Defects

Large abdominal wall defects may occur either above or below the umbilicus as manifestations of early amnion rupture (Higginbottom et al. 1979; see Chap. 4, p. 134). In the so-called body-stalk anomaly, the fetus is closely applied to the chorionic plate (Fig. 15.23). Umbilical vessels are short and abdominal viscera are exteriorised. The pelvis and lower limbs are usually hypoplastic, and major spinal deformity is usual. The condition is incompatible with postnatal life. Abnormalities referred to as "limb/body wall deficiency" (Miller et al. 1981) and "limb body wall malformation complex" (Hartwig et al. 1989) are probably related disorders.

In vesicointestinal fissure (lower midline defect) exstrophic hemibladders, each with a ureteric orifice, lie on either side of a central zone of intestinal mucosa with upper and lower orifices (Fig. 15.24) communicating with proximal and distal intestine (Jones 1963; Johnston and Penn 1966). Length of the small intestine is usually reduced and an exomphalos is usually present above the defect. The anus is imperforate and abnormalities of the urogenital system are common. The condition has been referred to erroneously as cloacal extrophy.

An upper midline defect is frequently accompanied by defects in the lower sternum, pericardium and anterocentral part of the diaphragm together with cardiac displacement (Cantrell et al. 1958; Toyama 1972). A large exomphalos may be present.

It is important to recognise this group of disruption deformities which may be accompanied by exomphalos as, despite their major proportion, familial recurrence is unlikely.

Diaphragmatic Hernia

A defect in the posterolateral part of the diaphragm (foramen of Bochdalek) is due to failure of the pleuroperitoneal canal to close, resulting in persistent communication between the pleural and peritoneal cavities (Fig. 15.25a; Avery et al. 1981). The majority of diaphragmatic hernias are left sided (about 80%), perhaps related to earlier closure of the right pleuroperitoneal canal. Occasionally, the defect is bilateral. Abdominal viscera become displaced upwards into the pleural cavity when the physiological hernia reduces. The pleural cavity on the affected side contains small

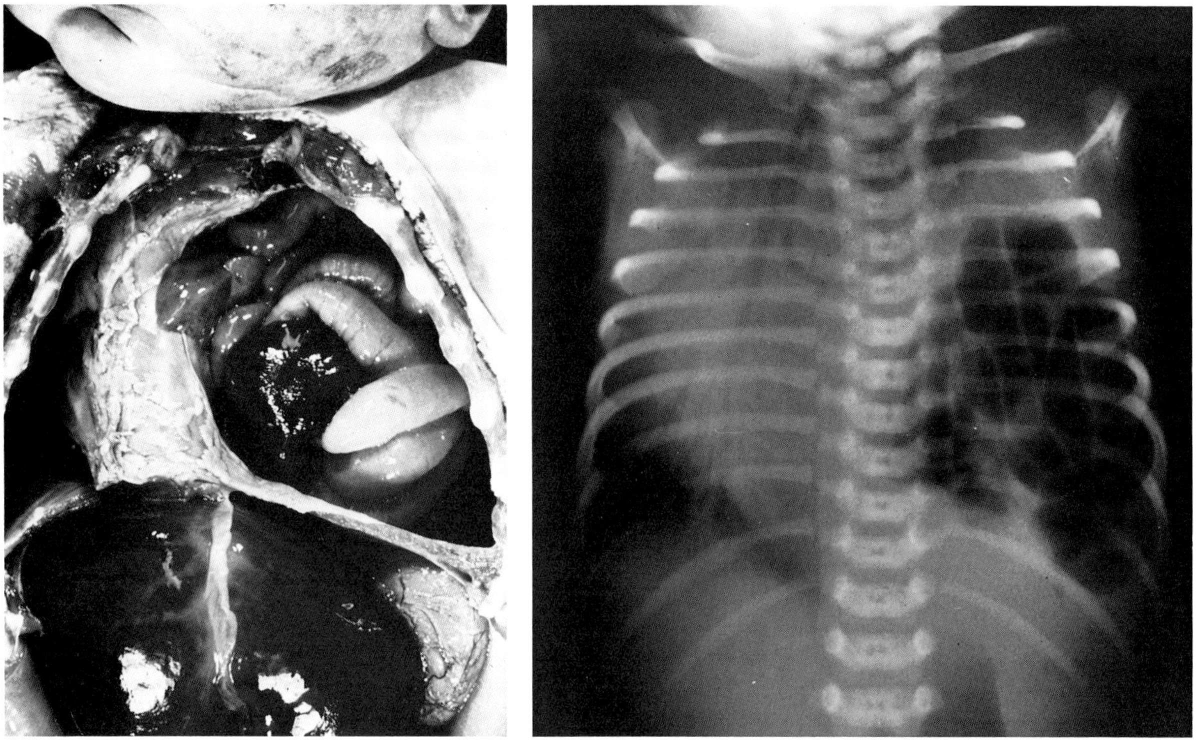

Fig. 15.25. **a** Mature neonate with large, left-sided diaphragmatic hernia. There is mediastinal shift, and the spleen and small intestine lie in the left pleural cavity. **b** Radiograph shows displacement of gas-filled loops of intestine into left pleural space in newborn with diaphragmatic hernia. The trachea is deviated to the right.

intestine, proximal colon, stomach, spleen and, when the defect is large, the left lobe of the liver. The heart is displaced to the opposite side. Pulmonary hypoplasia is usual and, although it is more severe on the side of the defect, the contralateral lung is frequently affected; survival is dependent on the degree of pulmonary hypoplasia. Underdevelopment of the left side of the heart due to intrauterine compression may also be an important factor in mortality (Siebert et al. 1984). With appreciable displacement of viscera into the chest the abdomen is scaphoid.

Presentation is related to the size of the defect and degree of pulmonary hypoplasia. Large left-sided defects are often recognised at birth because of difficulty in establishing respiration, and others become apparent during the first 24 h of life as air swallowing increases the volume of the displaced viscera and produces respiratory embarrassment (Fig. 15.25b). Right-sided defects are often small and, partly protected by the liver, may be asymptomatic; however, when the liver is displaced upwards through a large defect, obstruction to the fetoplacental circulation may result in hydrops (see Chap. 11, p. 262).

Those infants who require emergency surgery before 24 h of age have a mortality rate approaching 50%.

Parasternal diaphragmatic hernias (Morgagni hernias) are far less common and are rarely symptomatic in the newborn (Pokorny et al. 1984).

Eventration of the diaphragm, when the upwardly displaced abdominal viscera are covered by a sac consisting of abnormally thinned central part of the diaphragm, is occasionally seen.

Exocrine Pancreas

Development

The pancreas develops from the dorsal and ventral outpouchings of the most caudal part of the embryological foregut. Unequal growth of the circumference of the duodenum and rotation carry the dorsal primordium to the left. The ventral primordium initially comes to lie on the right and, with further differential growth of the duodenal wall, joins the dorsal pancreas. Fusion of the two segments occurs in the second intrauterine month. The bulk of the pancreas is formed by the dorsal segment, while the ventral segment forms the uncinate process and the inferior part of the pancreatic head.

Developmental Anomalies

Pancreas Divisum

Pancreas divisum results from failure of fusion of the ventral and dorsal primordia, so that the bulk of the gland (dorsal segment) drains separately through the duct of Santorini, while the isolated ventral pancreas drains through the ampulla of Vater. An association between this malformation and pancreatitis in later life has been reported (Cotton 1980). Rarely, the dorsal or the ventral primordium fails to develop.

Annular Pancreas

Annular pancreas is an uncommon abnormality; a ring of pancreatic tissue partially or completely encircles the second part of the duodenum. The lesion is encountered at all ages and may be found incidentally at necropsy (Morrell and Keynes 1981). It frequently accompanies duodenal stenosis or atresia and may rarely cause extrinsic duodenal obstruction. Associated defects are those encountered in duodenal atresia (Jackson 1963).

Ectopic Pancreatic Tissue

Ectopic pancreatic tissue consists of nodules of pancreatic acini within the wall of stomach or small intestine and are a common histological finding in the wall of a Meckel's diverticulum. They are often submucosal in site, but subserosal nodules may be encountered in pylorus and duodenum in trisomies 13 and 18. Focal dysplasia comprising ill-defined areas of immature stroma containing sparse acini and distorted ducts are described in trisomy 18 (Rohde et al. 1964). Inclusions of splenic tissue in the tail of the pancreas are not uncommon. However, they are unduly frequent, in association with microcysts and ducts lined by goblet cells, in trisomy 13 (Hashida et al. 1983).

Other Anomalies

Isolated congenital cysts of the pancreas have been described, and microcysts of the pancreas may be seen in association with infantile polycystic disease of the kidneys (Cruickshank 1986).

Vestigial pancreas (Elliott and Knight 1974) and congenital absence of the pancreas (Lemons et al. 1979) have also been reported. In the latter condition, intrauterine growth retardation is usually due to the absence or deficiency of insulin, which is an important fetal growth factor.

Mucoviscidosis (Fibrocystic Disease of Pancreas)

The most important disease of the neonatal pancreas is found in cystic fibrosis. The disease affects exocrine glands throughout the body. Its incidence is around 1 in 2000 births in the UK and its inheritance is autosomal recessive. The gross appearance of the pancreas in the neonatal period is usually unremarkable and histologically the parenchyma is often normal (Oppenheimer and Esterly 1975). These authors reported normal histology in 25% of cases aged up to 6 weeks. The remainder of cases show mostly early changes that comprise inspissated eosinophilic material within acini and ducts associated with epithelial flattening (Fig. 15.26). Fibrosis is not usually a prominent feature at this age. This appearance may not be specific for mucoviscidosis, particularly in preterm neonates (King et al. 1986).

The pancreas is commonly involved in generalised CMV infection, and the typical inclusion-bearing cells may be seen in the acinar and islet cells. In erythroblastosis the pancreas is often the seat of marked erythropoiesis. The organ is usually affected in congenital leukaemia. There is heavy iron deposition in the exocrine glands in neonatal haemochromatosis, an idiopathic neonatal iron-storage disorder (Blisard and Barton 1986).

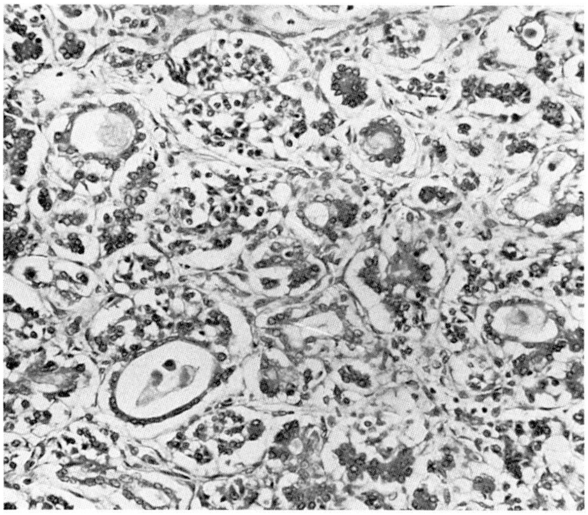

Fig. 15.26. Pancreas showing a mild degree of acinar and ductular dilatation with inspissated intraluminal material from infant with cystic fibrosis who died 2 weeks after birth. (H&E, ×160)

References

Aitken J (1963) Exomphalos. Analysis of a 10 year series of 32 cases. Arch Dis Child 38: 126–129

Amoury RA, Ashcraft KW, Holder TM (1977) Gastroschisis complicated by intestinal atresia. Surgery 82(3): 373–381

Andrew A (1971) The origin of intramural ganglia. IV The origin of enteric ganglia: a critical review and discussion of the present state of the problem. J Anat 108(1): 169–184

Avery ME, Fletcher BD, Williams RG (1981) The lung and its disorders in the newborn infant, 4th edn. Saunders, Philadelphia

Barr LC, Booth J, Filipe MI, Lawson JON (1985) Clinical evaluation of the histochemical diagnosis of Hirschsprung's disease. Gut 26:393–399

Bax NMA, Pearse RG, Dommering N, Molenaar JC (1980) Perforation of the appendix in the neonatal period. J Pediatr Surg 15(2): 200–202

Bell MJ, Ternberg JL, Keating JP, Moedjona S, McAlister W, Shackelford GD (1978) Prepyloric gastric antral web: a puzzling epidemic. J Pediatr Surg 13(3): 307–313

Bell MJ, Keating JP, Ternberg JL, Bower RJ (1981) Perforated stress ulcers in infants. J Pediatr Surg 16(6): 998–1002

Benson CD, Lloyd JR, Smith JD (1960) Resection and primary anastomosis in the management of stenosis and atresia of the jejunum and ileum. Pediatrics 26:265–272

Bentley JFR, Smith JR (1960) Developmental posterior enteric remnants and spinal malformations. The split notochord syndrome. Arch Dis Child 35: 76–86

Bernstein J, Vawter G, Harris GBC, Young V, Hillman LS (1960) The occurrence of intestinal atresia in newborns with meconium ileus. AMA J Dis Child 99: 804–818

Berry CL, Fraser GC (1968) The experimental production of colitis in the rabbit with particular reference to Hirschsprung's disease. J Pediatr Surg 3: 36–42

Bill AH, Chapman ND (1962) The enterocolitis of Hirschsprung's disease. Am J Surg 103: 70–74

Bissler JJ, Klein RL (1988) Alimentary tract duplications in children: case and literature review. Clin Pediatr 27: 152–157

Blank E, Chisolm AJ (1973) Congenital microgastria, a case report with a 26 year follow-up. Pediatrics 51(6): 1037–1041

Blisard KS, Barton SA (1986) Neonatal haemochromatosis. Hum Pathol 17: 376–383

Blyth H, Dickson JAS (1969) Apple peel syndrome (congenital intestinal atresia). A family study of seven index patients. J Med Genet 6(3): 275–277

Bremer JL (1944) Diverticula and duplications of the intestinal tract. Arch Pathol 38: 132–140

Bunton GL, Durbin GM, McIntosh N et al. (1977) Necrotising enterocolitis. Arch Dis Child 52: 772–777

Cantrell J R, Haller JA, Ravitch MM (1958) A syndrome of congenital defects involving the abdominal wall, sternum, diaphragm, pericardium and heart. Surg Gynecol Obstet 107: 602

Clatworthy HW, Howard WHR, Lloyd J (1956) The meconium plug syndrome. Surgery 39: 131–142

Cochran WD, Davis HT, Smith CS (1968) Advantages and complications of umbilical artery catheterisation in the newborn. Pediatrics 42: 769–777

Cook RCM, Rickham PP (1969) Neonatal intestinal obstruction due to milk curds. J Pediatr Surg 4(6): 599–605

Corkery JJ, Dubowitz V, Lister J, Moosa A (1968) Colonic perforation after exchange transfusion. Br Med J II: 345–349

Cotton PB (1980) Congenital anomaly of pancreas divisum as cause of obstructive pain and pancreatitis. Gut 21: 105–114

Cruickshank AH (1986) Pathology of the pancreas. Springer, Berlin Heidelberg New York

Cunningham P, Rose JS, Sokol A, Bleicher MA (1980) A case of neonatal intussusception. J Pediatr Surg 15(2): 203–204

Currie ABM, Hemalatha AH, Doraiswamy NV, Cos SA (1983) Colonic atresia associated with Hirschsprung's disease. J R Coll Surg Edinb 28: 31–34

deLorimier AA, Fonkalsrud EW, Hays DM (1969) Congenital atresia and stenosis of the jejunum and ileum. Surgery 65(5): 819–827

Denes J, Honti J, Leb J (1967) Dorsal herniation of the gut: a rare manifestation of the split notochord syndrome. J Pediatr Surg 2(4): 359–363

deVries P (1980) The pathogenesis of gastroschisis and omphalocele. J Pediatr Surg 15(3): 245–251

Dickson JAS (1970) Apple peel small bowel: an uncommon variant of duodenal and jejunal atresia. J Pediatr Surg 5(6): 595–600

Dickson JAB, Variend S (1983): Colonic neuronal dysplasia. Acta Paediatr Scand 72: 635–637

Dohn K, Povlsen O (1951) Enterocystomas. Report of six cases. Acta Chir Scand 102: 21–35

Donnison AB, Shwachman H, Gross RE (1966) A review of 164 children with meconium ileus seen at the Children's Hospital Medical Center, Boston. Pediatrics 37(5): 833–850

Dudgeon DL, Coran AG, Lauppe FA, Hodgman Joan E, Rosenkrantz JG (1973) Surgical management of acute necrotising enterocolitis in infancy. J Pediatr Surg 8: 607–614

Durham Smith E (1968) Urinary anomalies and complications in imperforate anus and rectum. J Pediatr Surg 3(3):

337–349
Elliott K, Knight J (1974) Size at birth. Ciba Found Symp 27: 202–203
Engel RR, Virnig NL, Hunt CE, Levitt MD (1973) Origin of mural gas in necrotising enterocolitis. Pediatr Res 7: 292
Esterly JR, Baghdassarian OM (1963) Presacral neuroenteric cyst: an unusual malformation resulting from persistence of the neuroenteric canal. Bull Johns Hopkins Hosp 113: 202–210
Fallon M, Gordon ARG, Lendrum AC (1954) Mediastinal cysts of foregut origin associated with vertebral abnormalities. Br J Surg 41: 520–533
Favara BE, Franciosi RA, Akers DR (1971) Enteric duplications. Thirty seven cases: a vascular theory of pathogenesis. Am J Arch Dis Child 122: 501–506
Fonkalsrud EW, deLorimier AA, Hays DM (1969) Congenital atresia and stenosis of the duodenum. Pediatrics 43(1): 79–83
Forouhar F (1982) Meconium peritonitis. Am J Clin Pathol 78: 208–213
Franz ID, L'Heureux P, Engel RR, Hunt CE (1975) Necrotising enterocolitis. J Pediatr 86: 259–263
Fuhr AH, Krogh PHJ (1972) Congenital epulis of the newborn. J Oral Surg 30: 30–35
Garrett JR, Howard ER, Nixon HH (1969) Autonomic nerves in rectum and colon in Hirschsprung's disease. A cholinesterase and catecholamine histochemical study. Arch Dis Child 44: 406–417
Gauderer MWL, Rothstein FC, Izant RJ (1984) Ileal atresia with long-segment Hirschsprung's disease in a neonate. J Pediatr Surg 19(1): 15–17
Goldberg HM, Johnson TP (1962) Posterior abdominothoracic enteric duplications. Br J Surg 50: 445–449
Gonzalez-Crussi F (1980) Extragonadal teratomas. Armed Forces Institute of Pathology, Washington DC
Goto S, Ikeda K, Toyohara T (1984) Histochemical confirmation of the acetylcholinesterase-activity in rectal suction biosy from neonates with Hirschsprung's disease. Z Kinderchir 39: 246–249
Gough MH (1961) Congenital abnormalities of the anus and rectum. Arch Dis Child 36: 146–151
Greenwood RD, Rosenthal A, Nadas AS (1974) Cardiovascular malformations associated with omphalocele. J Pediatr 85(6): 818–821
Grosfeld JL, O'Neill JA, Clatworthy HW (1970) Enteric duplications in infancy and childhood: an 18 year review. Ann Surg 172(1): 83–90
Grosfeld JL, Dalsing MC, Hull M, Weber TR (1983) Neonatal apnea, xanthines, and necrotising enterocolitis. J Pediatr Surg 18(1): 80–84
Hakanson DO, Oh W (1977) Necrotising enterocolitis and hyperviscosity in the newborn infant. J Pediatr 90: 458–461
Hartwig NG, Vermeij-Keers CHR, deVries HE, Kagie M, Kragt H (1989) Limb body wall malformation complex: an embryologic etiology? Hum Pathol 20(11): 1071–1077
Hashida Y, Jaffe R, Yunis EJ (1983) Pancreatic pathology in trisomy 13: specificity of the morphologic lesion. Pediatr Pathol 1: 169–178
Higginbottom MC, Jones KL, Hall BD, Smith DW (1979) The amniotic band disruption complex: timing of amniotic rupture and variable spectra of consequent defects. J Pediatr 95(4): 544–549
Holder TM, Cloud DT, Lewis JE, Pilling GP IV (1964) Esophageal atresia and tracheoesophageal fistula. Pediatrics 34: 542–549
Holgersen LO (1981) The etiology of spontaneous gastric perforation of the newborn: a reevaluation. J Pediatr Surg 16(4, 1): 608–613
Holsclaw DS, Eckstein HB, Nixon HH (1965) Meconium ileus. A 20 year review of 109 cases. Am J Dis Child 109: 101–113
Howard FM, Flynn DM, Bradley JM, Noone P, Swawatkowski M (1977) Outbreak of necrotising enterocolitis caused by *Clostridium butyricum*. Lancet II: 1099–1102
Howell WE, Stein H, Romaro AJ (1972) Sublingual dermoid cyst in infant: report of case. J Oral Surg 30: 437–441
Hoyme HE, Higginbottom MC, Jones KL (1981) The vascular pathogenesis of gastroschisis: intrauterine interruption of the omphalomesenteric artery. J Pediatr 98(2): 228–231
Huntley CC, Shaffner L, Challa VR, Lyerly AD (1982) Histochemical diagnosis of Hirschsprung disease. Pediatrics 69(6): 775–761
Jackson JM (1963) Annular pancreas and duodenal obstruction in the neonate. A review. Arch Surg 87: 379–383
Jackson RH, Bird AR (1961) Meckel's diverticulum in childhood. Br Med J II: 1399–1402
Johnston JH, Penn IA (1966) Exstrophy of the cloaca. Br J Urol 38: 302–307
Jones PG (1963) Exomphalos (syn. omphalocele). A review of 45 cases. Arch Dis Child 38: 180–187
Kiesewetter WB, Smith JE (1958) Malrotation of the midgut in infancy and childhood. AMA Arch Surg 77: 483–491
King A, Mueller RF, Heeley AR, Roberton NRC (1986) Diagnosis of cystic fibrosis in premature infants. Pediatr Res 20: 536–541
King DR, Savrin R, Boles ET (1980) Gastroschisis update. J Pediatr Surg 15(4): 553–557
Klein MD, Coran JAG, Wesley JR, Drongowski RA (1984) Hirschsprung's disease in the newborn. J Pediatr Surg 9(4): 370–374
Kleinhaus S, Boley SJ, Sheran M, Sieber WK (1979) Hirschsprung's disease. A survey of the members of the surgical section of the American Academy of Pediatrics. J Pediatr Surg 14(5): 588–597
Kliegman RM (1990) Neonatal necrotising enterocolitis: bridging the basic science with the clinical disease. J Pediatr 117: 833–835
Kopel FB (1972) Gastrointestinal manifestations of cystic fibrosis. Curr Clin Concepts 62(3): 483–491
Lemire RJ, Graham CB, Beckwith JB (1971) Skin-covered sacrococcygeal masses in infants and children. J Pediatr 79(6): 948–954
Lemons JA, Ridenour R, Orsini EN (1979) Congenital absence of the pancreas and intrauterine growth retardation. Pediatrics 64(2): 255–257
Lister J, Rickham PP (1980) Hirschsprung's disease. In: Rickham PP, Lister J, Irving IM (eds) Neonatal surgery, 2nd edn. Butterworths, London, pp 441–455
Lloyd JR (1969) The etiology of gastrointestinal perforations in the newborn. J Pediatr Surg 4: 77–84
Lorimer WS, Ellis DG (1966) Meconium peritonitis. Surgery 60(2): 470–475
Louw JH (1966) Jejunoileal atresia and stenosis. J Pediatr Surg 1(1): 8–23
McLetchie NGB, Purves JK, Saunders RLdeCH (1954) The genesis of gastric and certain intestinal diverticula and enterogenous cysts. Surg Gynecol Obstet 99: 135–141
Mann L, Feguson-Smith MA, Desai M, Gibson AAM, Raine PAM (1984) Prenatal assessment of anterior abdominal wall defects and their prognosis. Prenat Diagn 4: 427–435
Marchildon MB, Buck BE, Abdenour G (1982) Necrotising

enterocolitis in the unfed infant. J Pediatr Surg 17: 620–623
Martin LW, Perrin EV (1967) Neonatal perforation of the appendix in association with Hirschsprung's disease. Ann Surg 166(5): 799–802
Martinez-Mora J, Boix-Ochoa J, Tresserra L (1971) Vascular tumours of the parotid region in children. Surg Gynecol Obstet 133: 973–977
Meier-Ruge W (1974) Hirschsprung's disease: its aetiology, pathogenesis and differential diagnosis. Curr Top Pathol 59: 131–179
Merriam JC, Benirschke K (1959) Esophageal erosions in the newborn. Lab Invest 8: 39–47
Miller ME, Graham JM, Higginbottom MC, Smith DW (1981) Compression-related defects from early amnion rupture: evidence for mechanical teratogenesis. J Pediatr 98(2): 292–297
Mizrahi A, Barlow O, Berdon W, Blanc WA, Silverman WA (1965) Necrotising enterocolitis in premature infants. J Pediatr 66: 697–706
Moore TC, Schumacker HB (1952) Intussusception of ileum through persistent omphalomesenteric duct. Surgery 31: 278–284
Morrell MT, Keynes M (1981) Annular pancreas. In: Keynes WM, Keith RG (eds) The pancreas. Heinemann, London, pp 159–168
Macheff M, Morgan R, Einsenstein EM (1964) The surgical treatment of perforated duodenal ulcer in the newborn. Am J Surg 108: 717–723
Nakayama DK, Harrison MR, Gross BH et al. (1984) Management of the fetus with an abdominal wall defect. J Pediatr Surg 19: 408–413
Neal WA, Reynolds JW, Jarvis CW, Williams HJ (1972) Umbilical artery catheterisation: demonstration of arterial thrombosis by aortography. Pediatrics 50: 6–13
Neilson IR, Yazbeck S (1990) Ultrashort Hirschsprung's disease: myth or reality. J Pediatr Surg 25(11): 1135–1138
Nicolaides KH, Rodeck CH, Fosden CM (1986) Rapid karyotyping in non-lethal fetal malformations. Lancet I: 283–287
Nixon HH, Tawes R (1971) Etiology and treatment of small intestinal atresia: analysis of a series of 127 jejunoileal atresias and comparison with 62 duodenal atresias. Surgery 69: 41–51
Okamoto E, Ueda T (1967) Embryogenesis of intramural ganglia of the gut and its relation to Hirschsprung's disease. J Pediatr Surg 2(5): 437–443
Oppenheimer EH, Esterly JR (1963) Observations in cystic fibrosis of the pancreas. II Neonatal intestinal obstruction. Bull Johns Hopkins Hosp 111: 1
Oppenheimer EH, Esterly JR (1975) Pathology of cystic fibrosis. Review of literature and comparison with 146 autopsied cases. In: Rosenberg HS, Bolande RP (eds) Perspectives in pediatric pathology, vol 2. Year Book Medical Publishers, Chicago, pp 241–278
Parrish RA, Sherman RT, Wilson H (1964) Spontaneous rupture of the gastro-enteric tract in the newborn: a report of 13 cases and description of a characteristic x-ray finding. Ann Surg 159: 244–251
Partidge JP, Gough MH (1961) Congenital abnormalities of the anus and rectum. Br J Surg 49: 37–49
Philippart AI, Reed JO, Geargeson KE (1975) Neonatal small left colon syndrome: intramural not intraluminal obstruction. J Pediatr Surg 10: 733–739
Pokorny WJ, McGill CW, Harberg FJ (1984) Morgagni hernias during infancy: presentation and associated anomalies. J Pediatr Surg 19(4): 394–397
Puri P, Lake BD, Gorman F, O'Donnell B, Nixon HH (1983) Megacystis-microcolon-intestinal hypoperistalsis syndrome: a visceral myopathy. J Pediatr Surg 18(1): 64–69
Quan L, Smith DW (1973) The VATER association. J Pediatr 82(1): 104–107
Rector LE, Connerley ML (1941) Aberrant mucosa in the esophagus in infants and in children. Arch Pathol 31(3): 285–294
Reiquam CW, Allen RP, Akers DR (1965) Normal and abnormal small bowel lengths. An analysis of 389 autopsy cases in infants and children. Am J Dis Child 109: 447–451
Rickham PP (1955) Peritonitis in the neonatal period. Arch Dis Child 30: 23–31
Rickham PP, Boeckman CR (1965) Neonatal meconium obstruction in the absence of mucovisicidosis. Am J Surg 109: 173–177
Rodin AE, Nichols MM, Hsu FL (1973) Necrotising enterocolitis occurring in full-term neonates at birth. Arch Pathol 96: 335–338
Rohde RA, Hodgman JE, Cleland RS (1964) Multiple congenital anomalies in the E1-trisomy (Group 16–18) syndrome. Pediatrics 33: 258–270
Rothschild HB, Storck A, Myers B (1953) Mesenteric occlusion in a newborn infant. J Pediatr 43: 569–572
Santulli TV, Amoury RA (1967) Congenital anomalies of the gastrointestinal tract. Pediatr Clin North Am 14: 21–45
Santulli TV, Blanc WA (1961) Congenital atresia of the intestine: pathogenesis and treatment. Am Surg 151: 939–948
Santulli TV, Schullinger JN, Heird WC et al. (1975) Acute necrotising enterocolitis in infancy: a review of 64 cases. Pediatrics 55: 376–387
Scharli AF, Meier-Ruge W (1981) Localized and disseminated forms of neuronal intestinal dysplasia mimicking Hirschsprung's disease. J Pediatr Surg 16(2): 164–170
Shaw A (1975) The myth of gastroschisis. J Pediatr Surg 10(2): 235–241
Siebert JR, Beckwith JB (1984) Left ventricular hypoplasia in congenital diaphragmatic hernia. J Pediatr Surg 19(5): 567–571
Smith B, Clatworthy HW (1961) Meconium peritonitis: prognostic significance. Pediatrics 27: 967–970
Smith DW (1982) Recognizable patterns of human malformation. Saunders, Philadelphia
Smith JR (1960) Accessory enteric formations. Arch Dis Child 35: 87–89
Snyder WH, Chaffin L (1954) Embryology and pathology of the intestinal tract: presentation of 40 cases of malrotation. Ann Surg 140: 368–379
Spicer RD (1982) Infantile hypertrophic pyloric stenosis: a review. Br J Surg 69: 128–135
Stephens FD, Durham Smith E (1986) Classification, identification and assessment of surgical treatment of anorectal anomalies. Pediatr Surg Int 1: 200–205
Stevenson JK, Graham CB, Oliver TK, Goldenberg VE (1969) Neonatal necrotising enterocolitis—a report of twenty-one cases with fourteen survivors. Am J Surg 118: 260–272
Stewart DR, Colodny AL, Dagget WC (1976) Malrotation of the bowel in infants and children: a 15 year review. Surgery 79(6): 716–720
Tang TT, Glicklich M, Siegesmund KA, Oechler HW, McCreadie SR (1979) Neonatal cystic choristoma in submandibular salivary gland simulating cystic hygroma. Arch Pathol Lab Med 103: 537–539
Teich S, Schisgall RM, Anderson KD (1986) Ischemic enterocolitis as a complication of Hirschsprung's disease.

J Pediatr Surg 21(2): 143–145
Temtamy SA, Miller JD (1974) Extending the scope of the VATER association: definition of the VATER syndrome. J Pediatr 85(3): 345–349
Thomaidis TS, Arey JB (1963) The intestinal lesions in cystic fibrosis of the pancreas. J Pediatr 63: 444–453
Thomas DFM, Fernie DS, Bayston R, Spitz L, Nixon HH (1986) Enterocolitis in Hirschsprung's disease: a controlled study of the etiologic role of *Clostridium difficile*. J Pediatr Surg 21(1): 22–25
Touloukian RJ (1973) Gastric ischaemia: the primary factor in neonatal perforation. Clin Paediatr 12: 219–225
Toyama WM (1972) Combined congenital defects of the anterior abdominal wall, sternum, diaphragm, pericardium, and heart: a case report and review of the syndrome. Pediatrics 50(5): 778–792
van der Putte SCJ (1986) Normal and abnormal development of the anorectum. J Pediatr Surg 21(5): 434–440
Vawter GF, Tefft M (1966) Congenital tumours of the parotid gland. Arch Pathol 82: 242–245
Veeneklaas GMH (1952) Pathogenesis of intrathoracic gastrogenic cysts. Am J Dis Child 83: 500–507
Vinograd I, Mogle P, Peleg O, Alpan G, Lernau OZ (1981) Meconium disease in premature infants with very low birth weight. J Pediatr 103: 963–966
Waterston DJ, Bonham Carter RE, Aberdeen E (1962) Oesophageal atresia: tracheo-oesophageal fistula. A study of survival in 218 infants. Lancet I: 819–822
Weaver DD, Mapstone CL, Yu P (1986) The Vater association. Analysis of 46 patients. Am J Dis Child 140: 225–229
Weinberg AG (1975) Hirschsprung's disease—a pathologist's view. In: Rosenberg HS, Bolande RP (eds) Perspectives in pediatric pathology, vol 2. Year Book Medical Publishers, Chicago, pp 207–239
Weitzman JJ, Vanderhoof RS (1966) Jejunal atresia with agenesis of the dorsal mesentery. Am J Surg 111: 443–449
White RB (1956) Meconium peritonitis: a surgical emergency. J Pediatr 48: 793–796
Wiswell TE, Rawlings JS, Wilson JL, Pettett G (1979) Megacystis-microcolon-intestinal hypoperistalsis syndrome. Pediatrics 63(5): 805–808
Young DG, Wilkinson AW (1968) Abnormalities associated with neonatal duodenal obstruction. Surgery 63(5): 832–836
Yutani C, Sakurai M, Miyaji T, Okuno M (1973) Congenital short intestine. Arch Pathol 96: 81–82

Chapter 16

Liver and Gall Bladder

D. Ian Rushton

Embryology

The embryology of the liver has been described in detail by Elias (1955) and Du Bois (1963). The hepatic anlage first appears about the 18th day of embryonic life as an endodermal diverticulum, arising from the duodenum. By the 25th day it forms a T-shaped outgrowth which is invaded by vessels derived from the vitelline and umbilical veins. The larger cephalad portion of the diverticulum, the pars hepatica, gives rise to the parenchymal cells and hepatic ducts, while the smaller caudal portion, the pars cystica, forms the gall bladder. The pars intermedia, linking the two portions, forms the cystic duct. It is now believed that the rudimentary bile ducts of the liver are derived from the parenchymal cells (Koga 1971; Ruebner et al. 1990) and are not, as was previously held, invaded by the developing duct system. The latter authors using immunohistological techniques to demonstrate cytokeratins, carcinoembryonic antigen (CEA) and epithelial membrane antigen (EMA) have suggested there may be stages in the development of the interlobar bile ducts from the hepatocytes. Initially the ductal plate hepatocytes become flattened and show increased staining for cytokeratins. In the second phase these cells become cuboidal CEA negative and strongly EMA positive.

The cells in the pars hepatica grow into the septum transversum, isolating groups of mesenchymal cells which form endothelialised spaces containing erythropoietic foci. These fuse, forming a vascular plexus which joins that derived from the vitelline and umbilical veins. The left umbilical vein is linked to the right hepatocardinal vein by the ductus venosus, and the right umbilical vein atrophies. The parenchymal cells in the septum transversum form branching cords which acquire a central lumen; this tubular pattern is characteristic of the fetal and neonatal liver. Normally this matures to the platelike arrangement of the adult postnatally, but under certain pathological conditions the tubular pattern may persist or even reappear.

Between the 6th and 7th weeks mesoderm surrounding the extrahepatic bile ducts migrates into the liver to invest branches of the portal vein and hepatic ducts to form the portal tracts. The portal vein forms as the result of remodelling of anastomotic channels between the vitelline veins (Hamilton et al. 1972). Initially it was believed the liver was symmetrical, and that disparity in the growth rates of the two halves of the organ, possibly as a result of the asymmetrical blood supply, leads to dominance of the right lobe. However more recent data suggest the right lobe is dominant from its first appearance (Hutchins and Moore 1988). While the fetus remains in utero, the liver receives blood from the umbilical vein, the portal vein and the hepatic artery. As a result of atrophy of the right umbilical vein the right lobe of the liver receives a direct blood supply from the portal vein and the left lobe from the left umbilical vein. These two veins are linked by the sinus intermedius (Barclay et al. 1944), which permits flow in either direction. As a result the left lobe is better oxygenated and therefore contains less erythropoietic tissue than the right lobe, since during fetal life flow in the sinus intermedius is from left to right. Postnatally the cessation of the umbilical venous circulation and closure of the ductus venosus reverses the flow in the sinus intermedius, which then forms the left branch of the portal vein. This redistribution of the blood supply may further accentuate the disparity in the size of the lobes of the liver.

Physiology

While the fetus is in utero many of the normal metabolic functions of the liver are performed by the placenta and thus the need to develop the metabolic capability for a postnatal existence may be obtunded. Haemoglobin broken down in the reticuloendothelial system is transported to the liver in the unconjugated lipid soluble form. In utero the placenta actively transports unconjugated bilirubin from the fetus to the mother, only a small proportion being conjugated in the liver and secreted in the bile, whereas after delivery secretion is confined to the latter route. The fetal and neonatal liver differs in several important respects from the adult organ in the way it handles bile salts and in its capability to conjugate bilirubin. The latter is limited by relative deficiencies of certain enzymes responsible for conjugation and detoxification, e.g. glucuronyl transferase, tyrosine transaminase and tryptophan pyrolase. The loss of the placental route of transfer to the neonate, particularly the premature neonate, may, in the face of these deficiencies, lead to a transient unconjugated hyperbilirubinaemia, the so-called physiological jaundice of the newborn. Since in these circumstances the liver has little or no functional reserve, any further noxious influences may result in severe jaundice (Table 16.1).

Table 16.1. Neonatal Jaundice

Unconjugated hyperbilirubinaemia	Conjugated hyperbilirubinaemia
Increased bilirubin production	*Acquired*
Physiological jaundice/ prematurity	Sepsis
Blood group incompatibility	Infection
Internal haemorrhage	Drugs
Polycythaemia	Parenteral feeding
Sepsis	Severe haemolytic disease (including rhesus disease)
Haemoglobinopathies	*Idiopathic*
Abnormalities of erythrocytes	Neonatal hepatitis syndrome
Drugs	Extrahepatic biliary atresia
Late clamping of umbilical cord	Paucity of intrahepatic bile ducts
Impaired transport and uptake	Choledochal cyst
Decreased hepatic perfusion	*Metabolic*
Hypoalbuminaemia	Galactosaemia
Hypoxia	Fructose intolerance
Acidosis	Tyrosinaemia
Parenteral feeding	α_1 Antitrypsin deficiency
Physiological jaundice	Cystic fibrosis
Inadequate conjugation	Neimann–Pick disease
Transient familial hyperbilirubinaemia	Wolman's disease
Physiological jaundice	Gaucher's disease
High intestinal obstruction	Zellweger's syndrome
Hypothyroidism (cretinism)	Abnormalities of cholic acid synthesis
Drugs	*Familial*
Crigler–Najjar syndrome	Cholestatic jaundice and lymphoedema
Breast milk jaundice	Cholestatic jaundice with hepatosteatosis with hypercholesterolaemia (Byler's disease)
Abnormal enterohepatic circulation	Arteriohepatic dysplasia
Low intestinal obstruction (anatomical or mechanical)	*Other*
Cystic fibrosis	Chromosomal abnormalities (trisomies 13, 18, 21, 45XO)
Altered bacterial flora in gut	Hepatic tumours

The secretion of bilirubin in bile is dependent on the metabolism of bile salts (bile acids) which are derived from cholesterol. Bile has three major constituents, bile salts, bilirubin and organic cations, all of which are actively transferred across the cell membrane of the hepatocyte into the canaliculi by different mechanisms. The flow of bile is dependent on the osmotic drive of the bile salts (bile salt dependent) and the osmotic drive of other solutes (bile salt independent), the former being the more important mechanism in man. Bile salt independent flow is believed to be related to the active transport of sodium ions since it may be largely eliminated by ethacrynic acid and ouabain. Following secretion into the canaliculi the bile is modified by the addition of solutes, particulary chloride and bicarbonate. This process of modification is secretin dependent (Jorpes 1965). Between a third and a half of canalicular and intrahepatic bile consists of bile salts. The major bile acids are cholic and chenodeoxycholic acids, which are conjugated with taurine in the fetus, rather than with glycine, as occurs in the adult liver. These bile salts form a metabolic pool of which about 10% is lost and resynthesised daily, the remainder constituting the enterohepatic circulation that provides the major osmotic drive to bile flow. In the full-term neonate this pool is approximately half that of the adult, while in the premature infant it may only be equivalent to one-quarter of that in the adult (Watkins et al. 1973). As a result, the concentration of bile salts in the duodenum of premature neonates may be only one-fifth of that in term babies, explaining in part the limited ability of such infants to absorb fats (Katz and Hamilton 1974). The pattern of bile salt secretion in the bile is influenced by the bacterial flora of the bowel which metabolise the major bile acids so that in adults up to one-third may be deoxycholate. Deoxycholate is found in both the bile (Poley et al. 1964) and the cord blood (Sandberg 1970) of the newborn and is believed to originate from the maternal circulation via the placenta. Bacterial degradation of chenodeoxycholate in the adult leads to the formation of lithocholic acid, which has also been found in meconium (Sharp et al. 1971), where it is believed to be the end product of an alternative mitochondrial metabolic pathway in the fetal liver (Back 1973). Also present in meconium is beta hydroxy-5-cholenic acid (Back and Ross 1973). Both these metabolites are toxic to the liver in experimental animals, in which they may induce cholestasis, ductular proliferation, hepatocellular necrosis and irreversible liver damage (Silverberg et al. 1971; Palmer 1972; Palmer and Heywood 1974). It is possible that they may play a role in the aetiology of cholestasis and hepatocellular damage in the neonate.

In addition to these embryological and biochemical parameters of liver development and function there are two further gestation-related variants of liver morphology which may be of value to the pathologist. Haemopoiesis commences in the fetal liver at about the 6th week of pregnancy, peaks during the 12th and 16th weeks and continues until about the 36th week, though on a progressively declining scale, as judged from the proportion of haemopoietic tissue in the liver. It is, however, not uncommon to find small collections of erythroid and or myeloid cells in early infancy. Myelopoiesis predominates in the portal tracts, while erythropoiesis is largely intrasinusoidal. There may be significant variations in the content of the two lobes of the liver (see p. 393). The pathological assessment of variations in haemopoietic activity is crude but it may be aided by the demonstration of extrahepatic erythropoiesis in other organs such as the spleen, kidneys, pancreas etc. or by other abnormalities such as excess iron storage. Generally only relatively gross abnormalities can be reliably detected by routine histological techniques. Rhesus incompatibility is discussed further in Chapter 22 (see p. 537).

Glycogen is stored within the liver in small quantities from the first trimester, but major synthesis and storage does not occur until late pregnancy (Devos and Hers 1974). From about the 36th week of pregnancy glycogen storage within hepatocytes is progressive and by term the normal fetal liver contains abundant deposits. During the transition phase between minimal and maximal storage two populations of hepatocytes may be apparent within lobules—smaller intensely eosinophilic cells with minimal glycogen content and large clear cells with granular cytoplasm containing abundant glycogen (Fig. 16.1). Such variations in the morphology of hepatocytes should not be misinterpreted as evidence of liver disease.

Classification of Fetal and Neonatal Liver Disease

Transient disturbances of liver function are the rule rather than the exception in the newborn, and the vast majority are of no clinical consequence. In the premature infant such disturbances may be of greater importance and necessitate specific clinical treatment either to protect distant organs (e.g. brain) from kernicterus, or to correct deficiencies which might be life threatening (e.g. liver-dependent coagulopathies). Since the metabolic capabilities of the liver are so closely related to fetal maturity, the parameters of liver function of value in later life are usually inappropriate. Normal ranges related to gestation are as yet not fully defined and the distinction between

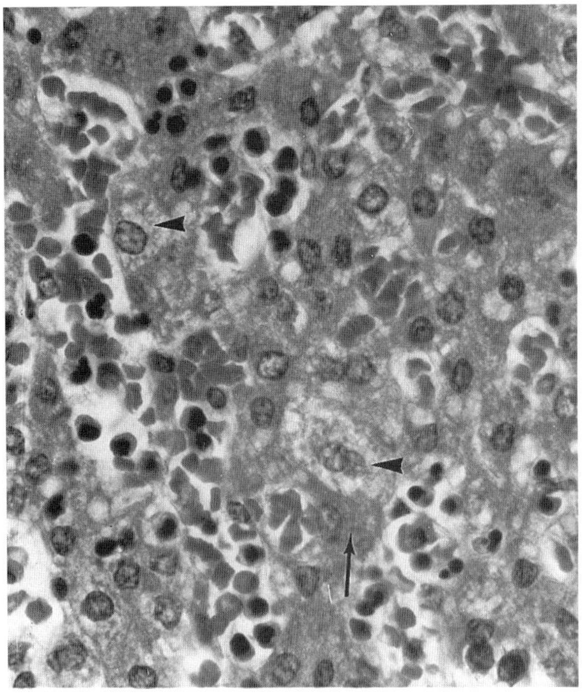

Fig. 16.1. Partial glycogenation of hepatocytes in 28-week fetus. The glycogen-containing hepatocytes are larger (*arrowheads*), while the non-glycogenated ones stain intensely with eosin (*small arrow*). (H&E, ×390)

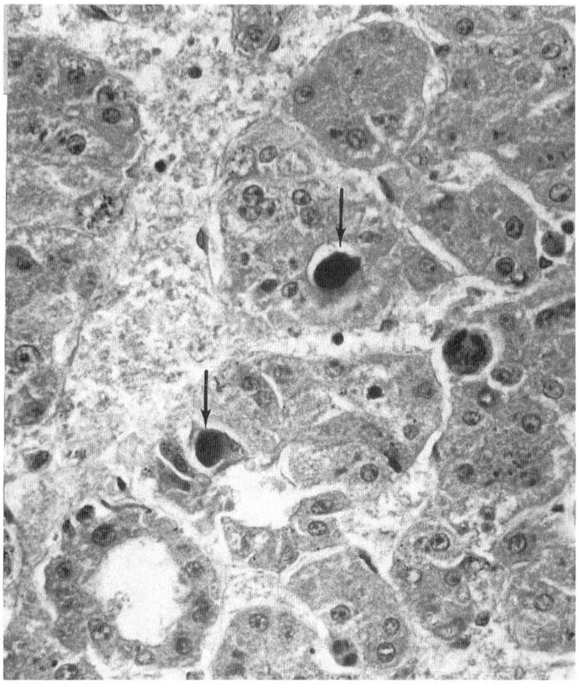

Fig. 16.2. Canalicular cholestasis around hepatic vein. The hepatocytes have a tubular pattern and surround bile plugs in dilated canaliculi (*arrows*). (H&E, ×365)

physiological variation and pathological disturbance is blurred. The most important indicator of liver disease in this age group is jaundice. This may be subdivided biochemically into unconjugated and conjugated forms. The former is more important in the short term, largely because of the toxic effects of unconjugated bilirubin on other organs, particularly the brain, whilst the latter is frequently an indicator of serious liver disease. Inevitably there is an overlap between the two types of jaundice and they may coexist in the same patient (Table 16.1). The majority of disorders which result in unconjugated hyperbilirubinaemia do not result in specific pathognomonic lesions in the liver. Liver biopsy is rarely indicated, and the pathological effects on the liver are usually only seen at autopsy. These frequently reflect circulatory or metabolic disorders and include glycogen depletion, fatty metamorphosis, sinusoidal dilatation, hypoxic damage and necrosis which is characteristically centrilobular in distribution. If severe, unconjugated jaundice may overload the secretory ability of the liver and result in canalicular cholestasis with biochemical evidence of obstructive jaundice. This may occur in up to 10% of cases of rhesus haemolytic disease as the inspissated bile syndrome (Hsai et al. 1972), when it may persist for several months after birth.

Conjugated hyperbilirubinaemia has a graver implication and, if persistent, requires detailed clinical investigation. In spite of the diverse aetiology of conjugated jaundice there are two major pathological manifestations, cholestasis and neonatal giant cell hepatitis. To these may be added more specific features which allow a definitive diagnosis to be obtained.

Cholestasis

The accumulation of bile pigments in hepatocytes and plugging of the canaliculi are the hallmarks of cholestasis. The latter typically affects the centrilobular zones (Fig. 16.2). It is a very common lesion in the liver of premature neonates dying after receiving modern neonatal intensive care. Associated pathological changes include pigmentation of the Kupffer cells, tubular transformation of the periportal hepatocytes and inflammation of the portal tracts. The inflammation occurs as the result of leakage of bile from ductules and may lead to fibrosis which extends into adjacent lobules (Fig. 16.3). If there is extrahepatic obstruction of the biliary tract, bile lake formation associated with liver cell necrosis, and bile duct proliferation may ensue, with half of the cases also showing giant cell change (Fig. 16.4). Isolated cholestasis occurs most frequently in association with physiological jaundice in extremely premature infants but is also found in association with some forms of intestinal obstruction, prolonged parenteral feeding, drug-induced jaundice and in the Crigler–Najjar syndrome. Other causes are listed in Table 16.2.

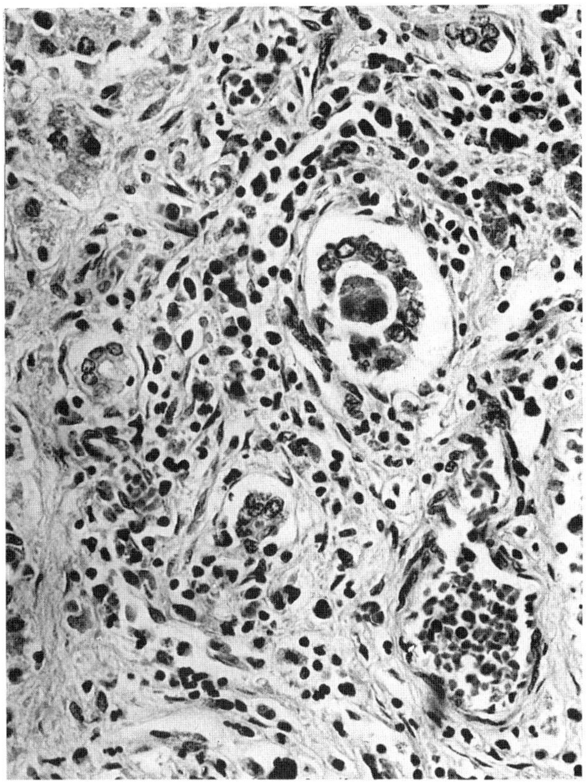

Fig. 16.3. Portal tract. There is severe cholestasis with plugging of bile ducts, portal fibrosis and a predominantly lymphocytic infiltrate within the tract. (Rushton 1981.) (H&E, ×262)

Table 16.2. Cholestasis in the fetus and neonate (after Finegold 1976)

Primary liver disease
Extrahepatic biliary atresia
Paucity of intrahepatic bile ducts
Extrahepatic obstruction of biliary tract
Familial and recurrent forms of cholestasis
Systemic disease of genetic origin
Galactosaemia
α_1 Antitrypsin deficiency
Tyrosinaemia
Fructose intolerance
Chromosomal anomalies (i.e. trisomy 18)
Cystic fibrosis
Cerebrohepatorenal syndrome (Zellweger)
Lipidoses
Systemic disease with secondary liver involvement
Haemolytic disease
Infection
Parenteral nutrition
Haemolytic anaemia
Drugs
Histiocytosis X

The aetiology of cholestasis is not yet fully understood, but a combination of the effects of the loss of the placenta, changes in the hepatic circulation, inadequate alimentation leading to a reduction in the secretin-dependent component of bile flow, the presence of potentially hepatotoxic metabolites in the meconium and the low concentration of bile salts in the small bile salt pool of the premature neonate are all believed to contribute to a reduction in the

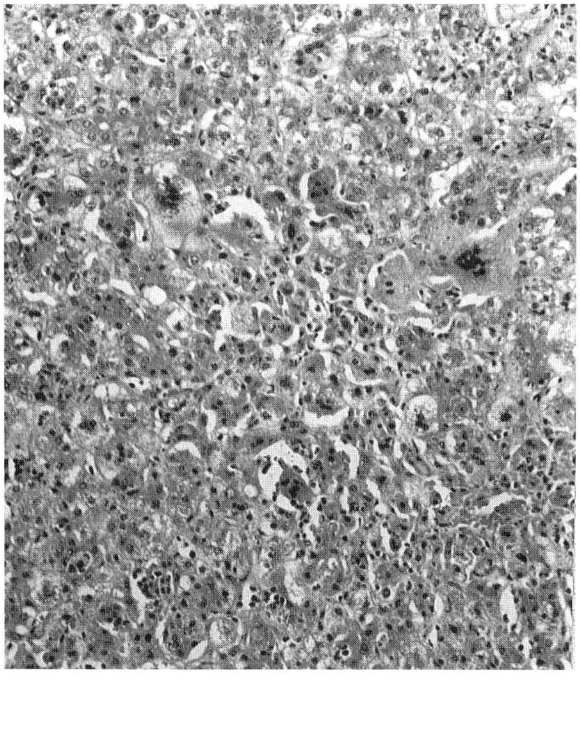

Fig. 16.4. Neonatal giant cell hepatitis. The hepatocytes are very variable in size, but several giant cells are evident. The lobular architecture is not clearly identifiable. (H&E, ×106)

flow of bile within the liver, resulting in the accumulation of the constituents of bile in the blood, hepatic parenchyma and biliary tract. At necropsy cholestasis may be evident to the naked eye, the cut surface of the liver having a greenish tinge. This becomes very much more prominent after fixation in formalin.

Neonatal Giant Cell Transformation

First described by Craig and Landing (1952) as giant cell hepatitis, it is now accepted that it is not primarily an inflammatory disorder but is an nonspecific response to liver damage associated with conjugated hyperbilirubinaemia, hence the preferred term "neonatal hepatocellular giant cell transformation" (GCT). However, the role of viruses in some cases must not be totally dismissed (Aterman 1989). The histological diagnosis depends on the demonstration of multiple hepatocytes containing three or more nuclei. The multinucleate cells frequently contain haemosiderin, lipofuschin and bilirubin as well as abundant glycogen and elevated levels of acid phosphatase and glucose-6-phosphatase.

GCT rarely occurs in isolation, and associated lesions include tubular transformation of the liver plates (Fig. 16.5), canalicular cholestasis and a scanty chronic inflammatory cellular infiltrate of lymphocytes and macrophages.

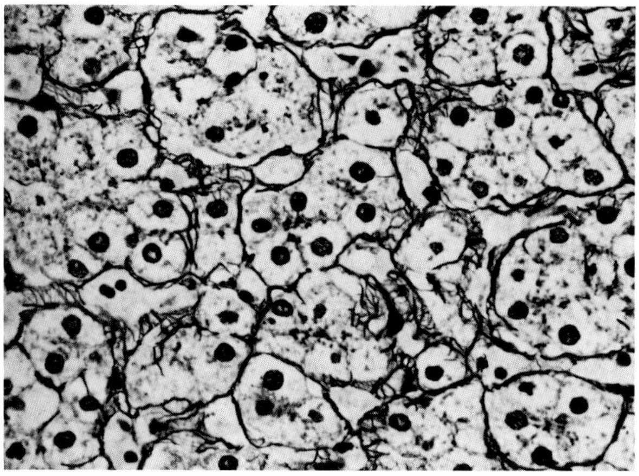

Fig. 16.5. Tubular pattern of hepatocytes in 26-weeks fetus. The reticulin outlines each group of liver cells. (Reticulin ×270)

Conjugated Hyperbilirubinaemia

Conjugated hyperbilirubinaemia occurs in between 1 in 2000 and 1 in 5000 neonates (Danks 1965; Cottral et al. 1974), about half the cases having obstructive lesions in the biliary tract, most commonly extrahepatic biliary atresia (EHBA). The combination of GCT, cholestasis and the other abnormalities of the liver described above is often described clinically as the neonatal hepatitis syndrome, a misnomer in that there is no convincing evidence that it is an inflammatory process in the majority of cases. Table 16.3 shows the breakdown of cases of neonatal and infantile liver disease by aetiology in several series from various parts of the world. Because EHBA and neonatal hepatitis are not entirely distinct in their aetiology and pathogenesis, Landing (1974) introduced the term "infantile obstructive cholangiopathy", which, though more informative and scientifically accurate, has not been widely accepted. GCT is found in about half the cases of EHBA and in the majority of cases without evidence of obstructive lesions. The aetiology of neonatal hepatitis with GCT is unknown in the vast majority of cases (70%)

Table 16.3. Liver disease in various parts of the world in neonates and infants

	Greece[a]	UK[b]	Australia[c]
Total number of cases	27	137	171
Extrahepatic biliary atresia	4	32	55
Intrahepatic biliary atresia	0	0	11
Neonatal hepatitis	23	103	105
Unknown aetiology	0	71	69
Presumed infection:	22	5	22
Hepatitis A	5	0	0
Hepatitis B	13	2	0
Rubella	0	2	3
Toxoplasmosis	0	1	0
CMV	1	1	15
Syphilis	0	0	1
Other viruses	0	0	3
Sepsis	3	0	0
Metabolic:			
α_1 Antitrypsin deficiency	0	24	8
Galactosaemia	0	1	6
Tyrosinaemia	0	1	0
Fructose intolerance	1	0	0

[a] Kattamis et al. (1974)
[b] Mowat et al. (1976)
[c] Danks et al. (1977a)

whilst the remainder have a multiplicity of underlying causes (Montgomery and Ruebner 1976). The clinically unexplained cases are classified as idiopathic neonatal hepatitis syndrome (INHS). This occurs both sporadically and in families, where the risk of recurrence may be about one in seven (Danks et al. 1977a,b). It is more common in males and carries a mortality of about 40%.

Extrahepatic Biliary Atresia

EHBA is rarely familial and there is a female predominance. Up to 25% of cases have associated anatomical abnormalities (Dimmick et al. 1975) though the only consistent anatomical abnormality appears to be polysplenia (Witzleben 1979; Maksem 1980).

As has been indicated, there is a considerable overlap in the pathology of EHBA and neonatal hepatitis, although the differential diagnosis can usually be made on histological grounds alone. There is almost invariably additional biochemical evidence available which may aid the diagnosis. In a review of 158 biopsies from babies between 6 days and 40 weeks of age with conjugated hyperbilirubinaemia, Brough and Bernstein (1974) found that GCT and inflammatory lesions in the portal tracts were of little value in differentiating EHBA and hepatitis. However, uniform proliferation of the interlobular ducts was a consistent and reliable indicator of EHBA (Fig. 16.6). The most common error in this series was overdiagnosis of EHBA as a result of overreading of mild degrees of duct hyperplasia, often of uneven distribution, which occurs in both neonatal hepatitis and neonatal α_1 antitrypsin deficiency. The major pathological differences between EHBA and hepatitis are listed in Table 16.4. It should be emphasised that the pathological response of the liver to extrahepatic obstruction is the same, whatever the cause; therefore the features described in EHBA are not pathognomonic.

The cause of EHBA is unknown, although it is widely held to be a destructive process which affects the developed biliary tract rather than a primary failure in the development of the duct system. Since hepatocytes are thought to be derived from the rudimentary duct system and, in the early stages of the disease, they show little abnormality other than the effects of obstruction, it can be argued that the duct system must have developed normally. There is no evidence of a systemic upset in utero in babies that develop EHBA, in that intrauterine growth is normal, whereas babies with idiopathic neonatal hepatitis are frequently growth retarded. Among associated or implicated causes are viruses (Witzleben 1979), bacteria (Becroft 1972) and abnormal cilia (Teichberg et al. 1982) in cases with polysplenia. Histological examination of tissues

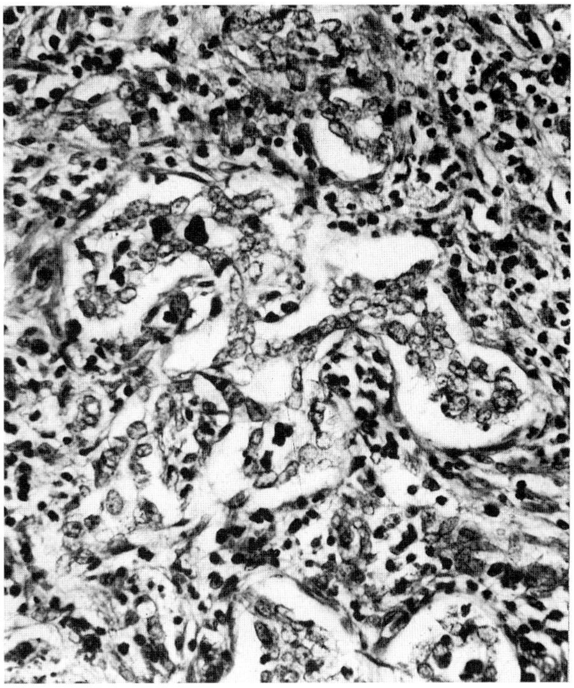

Fig. 16.6. Portal tract. There is bile duct proliferation of a mild degree which was associated with prolonged cholestasis. (Rushton 1981.) (H&E, ×230)

Table 16.4. Pathological features of extrahepatic biliary atresia and neonatal hepatitis

Extrahepatic biliary atresia	Neonatal hepatitis
Widened portal tracts	Hepatocellular necrosis
Distorted angular elongated bile ducts	Inflammation of parenchyma
Normal lobular architecture	Disturbed hepatic architecture
Cholestasis (canalicular and ductular)	Cholestasis (particularly intracellular)
Giant cell transformation (50%)	Giant cell transformation
Inflammation of portal tracts	Inflammation of portal tracts
Fibrosis of portal tracts	
Bile lakes	

obtained from the biliary tract at laparotomy in EHBA show intense inflammation, epithelial necrosis and fibrosis, the inflammatory exudate consisting initially of a few polymorphs, numerous lymphocytes, plasma cells and frequently eosinophils. Later, mononuclear cells and eosinophils may predominate (Witzleben et al. 1978). These features suggest that EHBA is an acquired disorder. This is further confirmed by the occasional examples with late onset of the jaundice. The timing of the evolution of the lesions in EHBA has been determined (Landing et al. 1985). Rapid bile duct proliferation occurs for about 200 days and then regression follows with a rapid phase for a further 200 days. Fibrosis follows a similar but slower pattern and appears to be independent of the ductular proliferation.

It is of paramount importance to elucidate the causes of conjugated hyperbilirubinaemia, since persistence of jaundice is associated with progressive and eventually irreversible liver damage. If surgical intervention to correct EHBA is to be performed, then operation should be carried out before the infant is 60 days of age (Howard and Mowat 1977). The most important role of liver biopsy in this age group is to confirm or exclude the diagnosis of EHBA. Biopsy is usually carried out at about 4–6 weeks of age (Witzleben 1981). If biopsy is combined with biochemical assessment of liver function, then the correct diagnosis is possible in virtually all cases (Mowat et al. 1976; Manolaki et al. 1983). Thus unnecessary laparotomies may be prevented in babies with neonatal hepatitis, since laparotomy is a procedure which may increase mortality in this group (Lawson and Boggs 1974).

Paucity of the Intrahepatic Bile Ducts

The term "paucity of the intrahepatic bile ducts" (PIBD) has come to replace the older "intrahepatic biliary atresia" and "hypoplasia of the intrahepatic bile ducts" as the preferred term to describe infants with a patent extrahepatic biliary tract, obstructive jaundice, absence of neonatal GCT and either a reduction or absence of bile ducts in the portal tracts. The aetiology is obscure, though it is possible bile salts may contribute to the disorder. The jaundice in patients with PIBD may be reduced or resolved if the enterohepatic circulation of bile salts is reduced either by treatment with cholestyramine, which binds bile salts in the gut, or by draining the bile from the common bile duct to the exterior (Finegold 1976). Alagille and Odievre (1978) divided PIBD into syndromatic and non-syndromatic types, the former being associated with a constellation of other abnormalities and the latter being found in association with a variety of diseases (see below).

The major problems confronting the pathologist are (1) that reduction in the number of bile ducts within the liver is not uniform and (2) that there are no universally acceptable criteria to assess the adequacy of the bile ducts within portal tracts. Diagnosis on the basis of a single needle biopsy is not reliable and open biopsy is recommended (Witzleben 1981). The number of portal tracts which must be examined is disputed, ranging from 6 (Henricksen et al. 1977) to 20 (Alagille et al. 1975). Alagille et al. (1975) found the normal ratio of bile ducts to portal tracts to be 0.9–1.8. Clearly the more portal tracts that can be evaluated the more accurate the diagnosis. However, the diagnosis is often reached by consensus after interpretation of the histological findings in the light of biochemical and clinical data.

The outcome of PIBD is variable, and both benign and progressive forms are described. At least two forms of benign PIBD have been delineated that commence in the first 3 months of life (Alagille et al. 1975). Only one of these syndromes is well described; it is remarkable, in that, despite a gross deficiency in the number of bile ducts within portal tracts, i.e. less than half the lower limit of normal, there is no evidence of progressive liver disease. The syndrome has been described as intrahepatic biliary dysgenesis with cardiac malformations (Greenwood et al. 1976) and arterohepatic dysplasia (Watson and Miller 1973). The deficiency in ducts is present from birth and is associated with peripheral stenoses in the pulmonary arteries. Other abnormalities involving the skeletal, nervous and genital systems are less consistent, though the facies are said to be characteristic. Eye abnormalities are common. It is said to be the commonest syndrome associated with PIBD, though Mueller et al. (1981) were only able to find 62 cases reported in the literature. The evolution of syndromatic PIBD has been described by

Hashida and Yunis (1988). These authors found that both reduced numbers of portal tracts and an increased number of portal tracts devoid of bile ducts were more characteristic than a paucity of interlobular bile ducts in infancy. Later portal fibrosis is uneven in distribution, being more extensive near the hilum of the liver.

Non-syndromatic PIBD may occur either sporadically or in families and may be found in association with other hepatic disorders such as α_1 antitrypsin deficiency and cholestasis associated with defective formation of cholic acid (Isenberg et al. 1976). The latter has certain similarities with Zellweger's syndrome. Many cases occur in the absence of known metabolic disorders (Alagille et al. 1975), but examples have been reported with cytomegalovirus (CMV), rubella and hepatitis B infections, EHBA, cystic fibrosis, graft verus host disease and chromosomal abnormalities, e.g. trisomies 18 and 21 and 45XO (Witzleben 1982).

Infectious Causes of Conjugated Hyperbilirubinaemia

The liver is the first major organ in the fetus to receive blood returning from the placenta and is therefore commonly involved in transplacental infections. After birth, umbilical infection may ascend the remnant of the vein to the liver or be introduced by a catheter, hence the need to examine the remnants of the umbilical vessels at necropsy, particularly where death is due to infection. Many organisms are either known to cross the placenta or suspected of doing so, though not all cause liver disease (Klein et al. 1976). In any case where infection is suspected as a cause of liver disease it is essential that both the baby and mother are investigated, and, where appropriate, tissues obtained at necropsy should be submitted for microbiological investigation.

Overwhelming infections involving the liver of the neonate may present atypical clinical pictures; thus massive hepatic necrosis may result in the acute onset of a bleeding diathesis with fatal haemorrhage. As with other forms of neonatal hepatitis, both cholestasis and GCT may be present and have been described in association with rubella, CMV, herpes simplex, hepatitis B and Coxsackie virus infections.

The advent of the polymerase chain reaction and of DNA probes combined with immunoperoxidase techniques should allow retrospective diagnosis of specific infections as well as aiding the diagnosis of new cases of hepatitis.

Infectious and Serum Hepatitis

Acute infectious hepatitis (hepatitis A) and serum hepatitis (hepatitis B) are rare in this age group, only being found in association with active maternal disease. If the mother acquires hepatitis B in the third trimester the risk of neonatal hepatitis is approximately 50% (Cossart 1974), with a similar risk if the mother is infected in the first 2 months after delivery (Schweitzer et al. 1972). Australia antigen (Hb_sAg) may be transmitted from the carrier mother to the baby, probably at the time of delivery, when it comes into contact with maternal blood (Lancet 1980). While affected babies are not clinically ill, they may show biochemical evidence of disturbed liver function (Derso et al. 1978). Liver biopsies from Hb_sAg-positive infants aged 3–27 months show a remarkably consistent pattern. The lobular architecture is preserved, but the hepatocytes are enlarged with a polyhedral shape and hydropic cytoplasm. Small groups undergo lysis in the presence of aggregates of macrophages (Schweitzer et al. 1972). These authors also noted that about a third of babies born to mothers acquiring hepatitis B during pregnancy were small for dates. Rarely, hepatitis B may cause fulminating hepatitis in the neonate (Ewing and Davidson 1985). Of ten infants under 4 months of age with severe Hb_sAg-positive hepatitis, four developed cirrhosis while two died in hepatic coma (Kattamis et al. 1974). Histological changes in the livers included GCT, cholestasis, collapse of the lobular reticulin framework, bile duct proliferation and periportal fibrosis.

There is a striking ethnic variation in the transmission of Hb_sAg from carrier mothers to their offspring. Thus 64% of infants of Chinese extraction were infected, while only 31% of Negroes and none of the Europeans were affected; this pattern of infection reflects the frequency of the e antigen in the respective ethnic groups (Derso et al. 1978). The same variation in the transmission of Hb_sAg also occurs in those ethnic groups where the mother acquires hepatitis B in the first and second trimesters of pregnancy. As has been indicated, vertical transmission of Hb_SAg is usually of little consequence to the infant; however, the long-term consequences are uncertain, and it has been suggested that there may be a relationship with the later development of hepatocellular carcinoma (Lancet 1980).

Cytomegalovirus Hepatitis

Congenital CMV infection is associated with multiple stigmata (see Chapter 13, p. 296), the majority of which are usually present if the liver is involved. The only specific lesion in the liver is the presence of the characteristic inclusions most typically seen in the bile duct epithelium (Fig. 16.7). Other lesions include fatty metamorphosis, cholestasis, occasionally GCT and interstitial and periportal fibrosis (Medearis 1964). Calcification may be evident in the liver either radiologically or to the naked eye as fine white lines beneath the capsule. The liver is usually enlarged and contains excess erythropoietic tissue. Hepatic fibrosis has been reported with fetal ascites and pulmonary hypoplasia in association with congenital CMV infection (Chen-Chih et al. 1990).

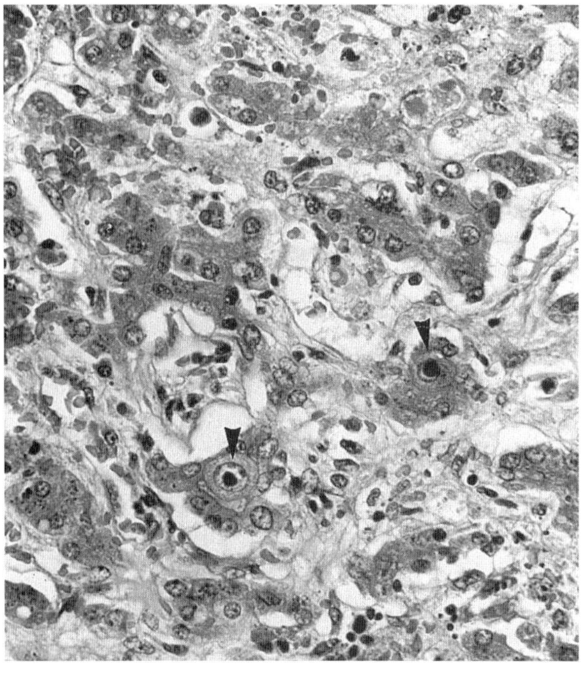

Fig. 16.7. CMV infection. Two cells with intranuclear inclusions are *arrowed*. There is focal hepatocellular necrosis and an increase in fibrous tissue at the margin of the lobules. (H&E, ×250)

Herpes Simplex Hepatitis

Liver involvement is a consistent finding in disseminated neonatal infection with herpes simplex virus (HSV; Nahamias et al. 1970). Most infections are believed to be acquired either as a result of ascending infection via ruptured membranes or as a result of contamination during passage through the mother's genital tract. Indeed, the growth of special clinics to treat HSV infections has led to a policy of operative delivery of such pregnancies if the mother is excreting HSV from her lower genital tract when delivery is due. The typical herpetic lesion is 1–2 mm in diameter with a pale centre and prominent surrounding haemorrhagic rim (Fig. 16.8). The pale central zone consists of necrotic hepatocytes with numerous hyperchromatic fragments of nuclear debris but with a minimal inflammatory cellular response. The peripheral zone consists of distorted hepatocytes with irregular nuclei, some of which contain the characteristic inclusion bodies (Fig. 16.9). The sinusoids are dilated and distended with red cells. Cholestasis and GCT may be present. The serious nature of the disseminated disease in the neonatal period usually allows the diagnosis to be established clinically. Liver biopsy is considered inappropriate because of the risk of haemorrhage in the neonate, but in older infants and children biopsy may be helpful (Raga et al. 1984).

Varicella-Zoster Viruses

Approximately 1 in 2000 mothers acquires chicken pox while pregnant (Young 1976). Transplacental infection associated with a villitis may lead to intrauterine death or neonatal chicken pox. In either case liver involvement is common. The lesions closely resemble those of HSV; indeed, their distinction may only be possible by virological isolation. Calcification of the liver may be prominent and visible on the post-mortem radiograph.

Enteroviruses

Enteroviruses comprise three major groups: the polio viruses, which affect the central nervous

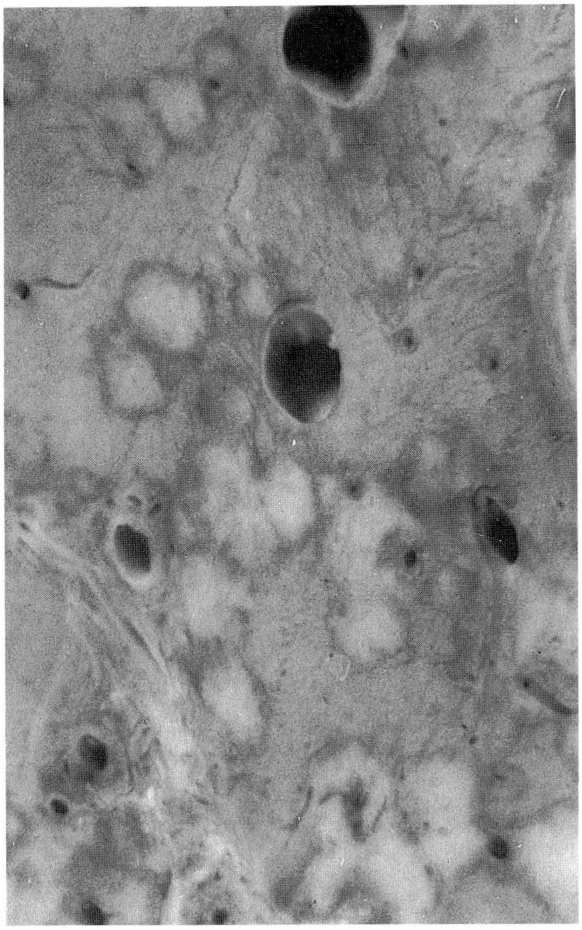

Fig. 16.8. Herpes simplex infection. The cut surface of the liver reveals multiple pale foci, some of which are coalescing, surrounded by a distinct hyperaemic zone. (Approx. ×3)

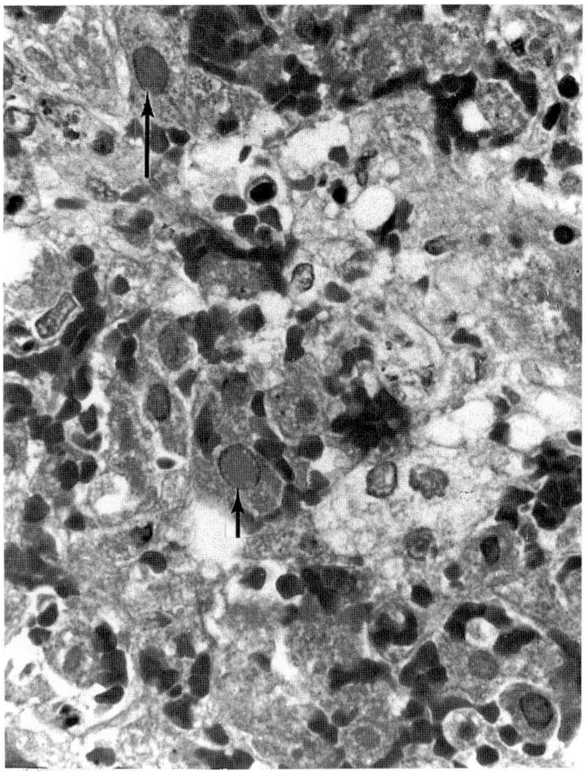

Fig. 16.9. Herpes simplex infection. Hepatocytes at the margin of an area of necrosis contain typical intranuclear inclusions (*arrows*). (H&E, ×405)

system (CNS); the Coxsackie viruses, which characteristically affect the heart and CNS but may involve other organs such as the liver (Hosier and Newton 1958; Kilbrick and Benirschke 1958; Wright et al. 1963; Montgomery and Ruebner 1976); and the echoviruses. These are of particular concern in the neonatal period since they may result in fulminant necrotising hepatitis, which commonly manifests itself as a haemorrhagic diathesis involving the CNS, kidneys, lungs or gut. Though sporadic cases may be acquired transplacentally or during delivery, the virus can spread rapidly within neonatal intensive care units with disastrous results. Types 11 (Krous et al. 1973; Nagington et al. 1978; Berry and Nagington 1982) and 19 (Philip and Larson 1973; Bacon and Sims 1976; Purdham et al. 1976) appear to be particularly dangerous in this respect, though severe liver disease has been reported with type 9 (Rawls et al. 1964) and type 14 (Hughes et al. 1972). However, these are not the only types that may affect the liver (Cherry 1976).

Gross examination of the liver shows a mottled or variegated subcapsular and cut surface (Fig. 16.10), while on microscopy there is massive central and mid-zonal necrosis with little or no inflammatory response (Fig. 16.11). Since similar lesions may occur in association with shock, it is important to perform virological studies on suspect livers. If echoviruses are responsible they are generally readily isolated from necropsy tissues.

Non-viral Infections

Liver function may be disturbed in the neonate by any serious infection, including septicaemia, without direct involvement of the hepatic

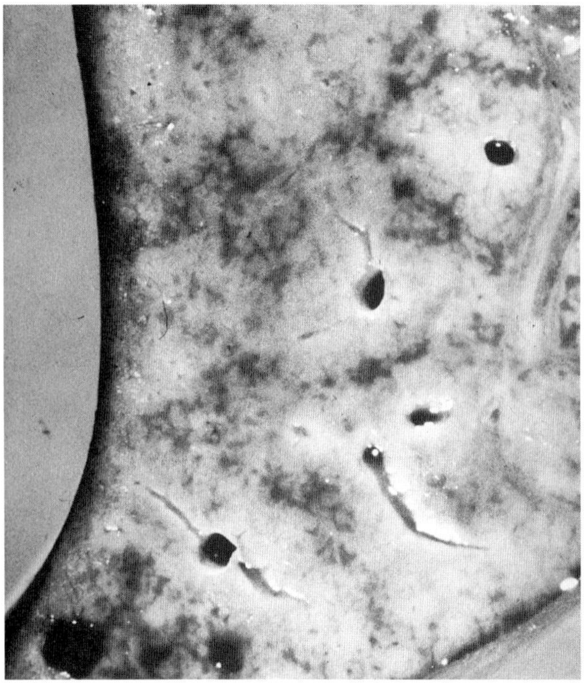

Fig. 16.10. Massive hepatic necrosis associated with echovirus infection. (×3.4)

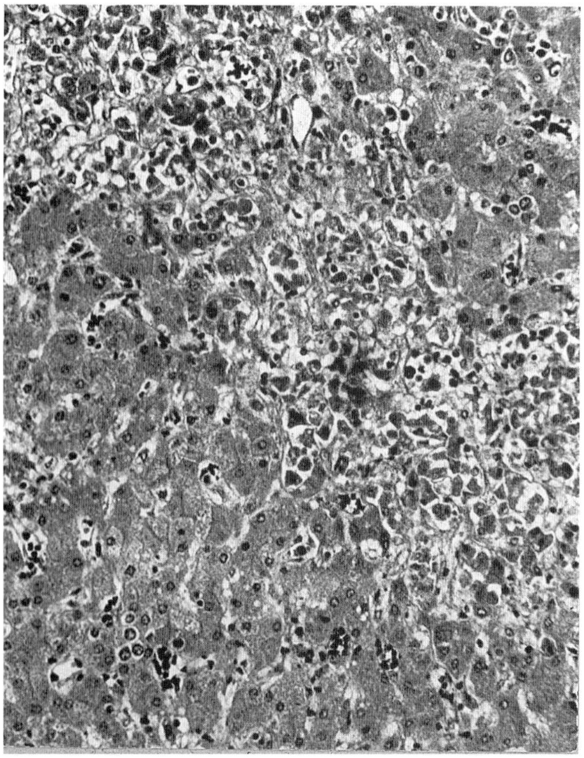

Fig. 16.11. Mix-zonal and centrilobular necrosis associated with echovirus infection. There is a minimal inflammatory response. (H&E, ×106)

parenchyma (Hamilton and Sass-Korstak 1963). Ascending infection, via the umbilical vein, is associated with focal necrosis and abscess formation, though in the early stages the only abnormality may be distention of the sinusoids with polymorphonuclear leucocytes. Focal necrosis and abscess formation may also complicate septicaemia.

There are a small number of non-viral infections that may directly affect the liver, of which the most important are listeriosis, syphilis, tuberculosis, toxoplasmosis and candidiasis. Rarely, anthrax, brucellosis, histoplasmosis, leptospirosis, tularaemia or typhoid may be encountered, although it is likely the diagnosis will be made in the mother before the fetal liver is available for examination.

Listeriosis

Listeria monocytogenes is a short, motile, predominantly Gram-positive rod which in histological material is best stained by the Levaditi technique. The characteristic lesions are miliary granulomas usually a few millimetres in diameter which lack the characteristic peripheral flare seen in herpes virus infections (Fig. 16.12). Macroscopically they appear sharply defined, although histologically there is a gradual transition from the central necrotic zone to the surrounding unaffected liver. Initially there is a minimal cellular reaction, the lesion consisting of ghost-like hepatocytes with variable quantities of fibrin in the sinusoids. Eventually a polymorph response occurs, this being most striking at the periphery of the lesions (Fig. 16.13). There are also variable numbers of histiocytes and lymphocytes. Levaditi staining usually reveals numerous organisms. Liver involvement is invariably a component of a disseminated infection with multiorgan disease and placentitis. Prenatal listeriosis has also been reported in association with biliary atresia (Becroft 1972).

Syphilis

Congenital syphilis is less common than in the past but it has by no means been eradicated; sporadic cases are encountered in most large maternity units. Liver involvement is common and is reflected clinically in jaundice and hepatomegaly. The essential lesion is an increase in hepatic connective tissue which

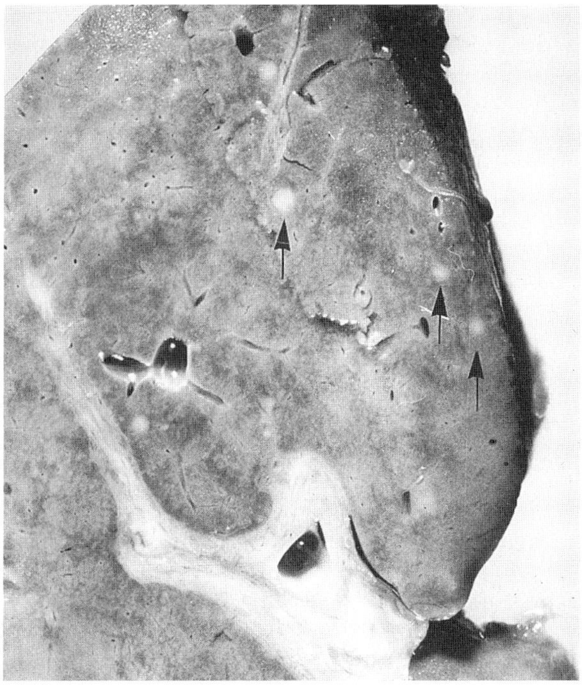

Fig. 16.12. Congenital listeriosis. The slice of liver contains multiple discrete white foci of necrosis (*arrows*) which do not have a peripheral hyperaemic zone. (Rushton 1981.) (Approx. ×2)

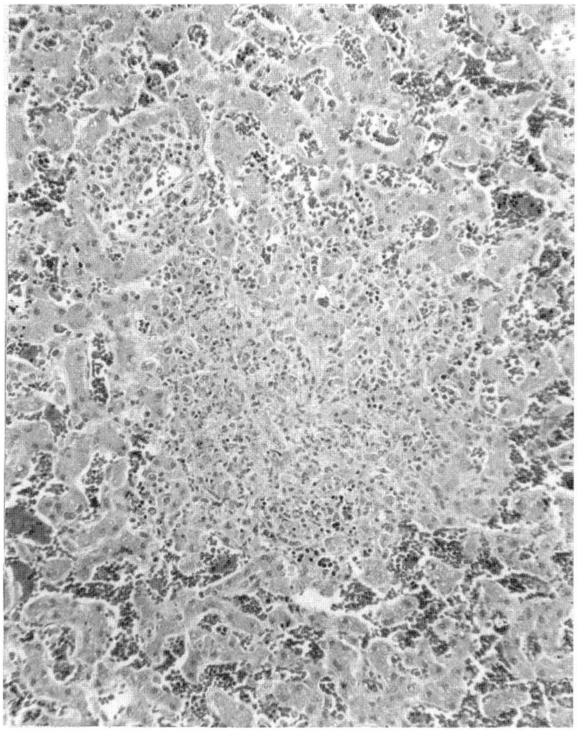

Fig. 16.13. Congenital listeriosis. An early lesion with a focus of necrosis of the hepatic parenchyma. The ghost-like hepatocytes are still evident and there is a scanty polymorphonuclear infiltrate. (H&E, ×92)

involves both the portal tracts and the lobules of the liver. This fibrous scarring is most common in the right lobe adjacent to the ductus venosus (Potter and Craig 1976). Destruction of the liver parenchyma and shrinkage of the scar tissue eventually results in the deeply fissured hepar lobatum. The relation of treponemal infiltration to the inflammation and fibrosis is not clear since heavy infiltration may be found in livers that appear normal on routine haematoxylin and eosin staining (Wright and Berry 1974). The inflammatory response involves all parts of the liver but is particularly prominent around vessels, which may show endarteritic changes. Lymphocytes and plasma cells predominate (Fig. 16.14). Erythropoiesis is frequently increased. The fibrosis very rarely progresses to a cirrhotic pattern (Oppenheimer and Hardy 1971).

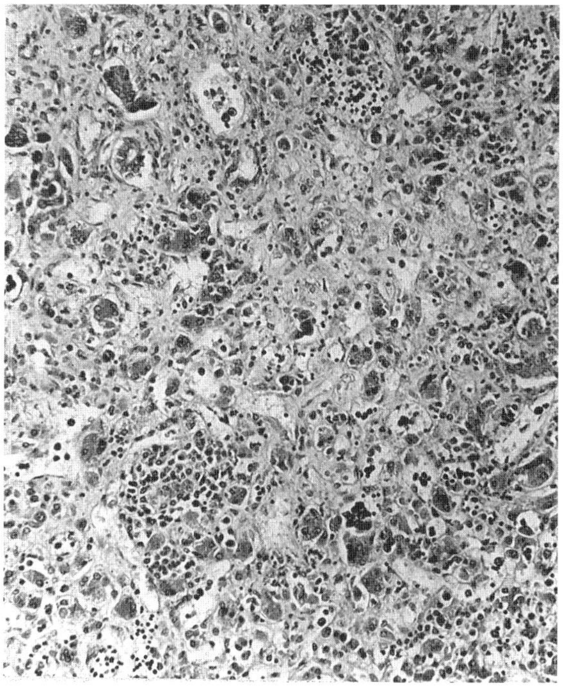

Fig. 16.14. Congenital syphilis. There is diffuse destruction of hepatocytes, interstitial fibrosis and focal erythropoiesis. (H&E, ×316)

Tuberculosis

Congenital tuberculosis is rare; however; if it is transplacental it invariably involves the liver, particularly the left lobe, which prior to delivery has a higher oxygen tension preferred by the tubercle bacillus. Organisms are usually demonstrable with appropriate staining, though fully developed caseating granulomas are uncommon.

Toxoplasmosis

Liver involvement is usually only a minor manifestation of congenital infection but may be associated with hepatomegaly, excessive erythropoiesis and iron deposition, an increase in lipofuscin in the hepatocytes and canalicular cholestasis. Periportal fibrosis may be prominent.

Metabolic Disorders

Metabolic disorders account for only a small proportion of cases of hyperbilirubinaemia. The majority are unlikely to be diagnosed in the neonatal period. Many will, as the result of persistent unexplained jaundice be referred to specialist centres for diagnosis. Although few of the disorders are amenable to treatment, many are genetically determined and therefore require diagnosis to enable appropriate counselling to be given to the parents.

Although rare, these disorders may be overlooked at necropsy, particularly in stillbirths, if routine histological examination of the internal organs, including the liver, is omitted. If they are suspected, special arrangements may be required to obtain tissue for histochemical, immunohistochemical, electron microscopical or biochemical investigation. During life, liver biopsy is rarely essential since diagnosis can be made by biochemical or histological methods using more accessible tissues or cells such as skin, rectal or gingival tissue, or blood (Tarlow 1979). A few of the disorders may respond to dietary measures (e.g. galactosaemia, tyrosinaemia and fructose intolerance); therefore, early diagnosis is essential, although none requires liver biopsy to confirm the diagnosis. Of the inherited disorders of bilirubin reviewed by Finegold (1976) and Berthelot and Dhumeaux (1978), only Crigler–Najjar disease may present with evidence of disturbed liver function in the neonatal period. This disorder is associated with a deficiency of uridine diphosphoglucuronyl transferase. Liver histology is usually normal and the hyperbilirubinaemia is of the unconjugated type. Certain drugs may mimic this disorder by depressing the level of the enzyme.

The liver may be involved in Niemann–Pick disease, Letterer–Siwe disease, gargoylism, cystinosis and disorders of the urea cycle, but the hepatic manifestations are of little clinical importance in the perinatal period (Potter and Craig 1976; Zimmermann et al. 1987; Rutledge 1988).

α_1 Antitrypsin Deficiency

α_1 Antitrypsin is a protease inhibitor active against several proteolytic enzymes and constitutes approximately 90% of serum α_1 globulin. It is synthesised in the liver and in α_1 antitrypsin deficiency accumulates in the cisternae of the rough endoplasmic reticulum of the hepatocytes (Aagenaes et al. 1974), particularly in the periportal zones. Starch gel electrophoresis has shown it to be polymorphic, and although coded by a single locus at least 24 different alleles have been identified, the most common being M, S and Z (Tarlow 1979), with frequencies of 0.86–0.99, 0.03 and 0.01–0.03 respectively. The biochemistry and clinical manifestations of the disease have been extensively reviewed by Morse (1978a,b).

The majority of affected individuals have a PiZZ phenotype, though only 10%–20% of the 1 in 2000 infants with this phenotype are clinically affected. It has been estimated that between 200 and 250 affected infants are delivered in England and Wales annually (Cook 1974). Jaundice may begin in the second week of life, the hepatic conjugated hyperbilirubinaemia being associated with evidence of hepatocellular damage including both cholestasis and GCT. At this stage it may be mistaken for EHBA or idiopathic neonatal hepatitis. The classic pathological features, diastase-resistant PAS-positive globules 2–20 μm in diameter in the peripheral and paraseptal hepatocytes (Fig. 16.15), are not apparent in the neonatal period but are usually demonstrated over the age of 3 months (Talbot and Mowat 1975; McPhie et al. 1976). They may be demonstrated by immunofluorescence or immunoperoxidase

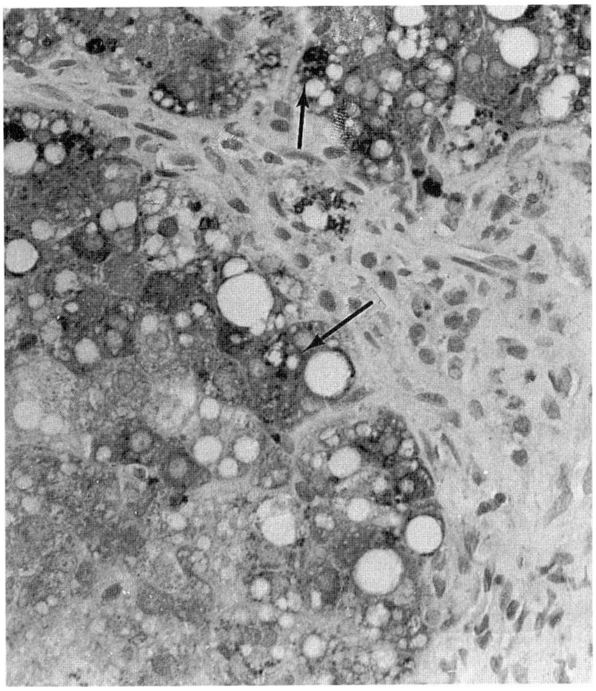

Fig. 16.15. α_1 Antitrypsin deficiency. Hepatocytes surrounding a portal tract show fatty vacuolation and contain darkly staining material (*arrows*) staining positively for α_1 antitrypsin. (Courtesy of Dr. W.R. Shortland-Webb, Birmingham.) (Immunoperoxidase ×416)

techniques and electron microscopy and are present in PiZZ individuals whether or not they show evidence of liver disease clinically. In the fetus the liver architecture is normal but granular deposits may be demonstrated in hepatocytes (Malone et al. 1989). It is important not to mistake material with similar staining properties within macrophages or Kupffer cells as α_1 antitrypsin, since such accumulations are not uncommon in the neonatal liver, particularly if parenteral feeding has occurred.

The ultimate prognosis of neonates and infants presenting with liver disease associated with the PiZZ phenotype is very variable, as might be anticipated, since the majority of them appear to be entirely unaffected. It has been suggested that liver biopsy in the early cholestatic phase may provide clues to the eventual outcome (Hadchouel and Gautier 1976). Thus cholestasis, hepatocellular damage and mild portal fibrosis in the absence of bile duct proliferation were associated with a good prognosis, whereas when bile duct proliferation was present in association with marked portal fibrosis the prognosis was poor, the patients going on to develop cirrhosis. In a proportion of cases cholestasis was associated with ductular hypoplasia. These children suffered prolonged jaundice, pruritis and hypercholesterolaemia. It is of interest in this respect that Odievre et al. (1976) and Heathcote et al. (1976) have described paucity of the intrahepatic bile ducts in association with α_1 antitrypsin deficiency. Liver abnormalities have also been described in association with the PiMM and PiSZ phenotypes (Wilkinson et al. 1974; Talbot and Mowat 1975). In the former, GCT may be present, while in the latter congenital cirrhosis has been described. Since congenital cirrhosis is extremely rare, every fetus or infant with cirrhosis should be investigated as a possible case of α_1 antitrypsin deficiency and Pi phenotype determined.

Galactosaemia

Galactosaemia is due to a deficiency of galactose-1-phosphate uridyl transferase and was first identified by Reuss in 1908. The disease only becomes manifest when either galactose or lactose are introduced into the diet, and clinically it affects many organs. Hepatomegaly, persistent jaundice and biochemical evidence of hepatocellular damage are associated with failure to thrive and a bleeding diathesis or mental retardation and blindness caused by cataract formation. When challenged with galactose such infants may become hypoglycaemic. The diagnosis is made by assay of the enzyme in red cells. It is estimated that 1 in 110000 births in the UK may be affected (Levy 1973); inheritance is autosomal recessive.

Histologically diffuse fatty metamorphosis is associated with cholestasis and ductular proliferation within portal tracts. There may be GCT in the early stages (Hardwick and Dimmick 1976). Tubular transformation of the hepatocytes is progressive (Fig. 16.16) and is followed by degeneration of the hepatocytes, collapse of the reticulin network, regeneration, fibrosis and finally an irregular macronodular cirrhosis. An appropriate dietary regimen introduced early in life can prevent the development of these complications.

Hereditary Tyrosinaemia

Hereditary tyrosinaemia is a rare autosomal-recessive disorder associated with failure to thrive, cyclical vomiting, diarrhoea and ab-

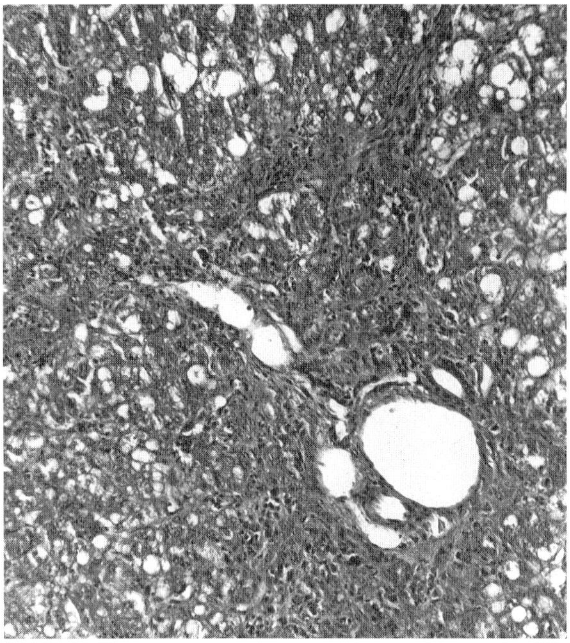

Fig. 16.16. Galactosaemia. The liver architecture is disturbed and there is very extensive fatty change. The portal tract appears enlarged because of loss of hepatocytes and fibrosis. At a higher magnification the hepatocytes showed a tubular arrangement. (H&E, ×99)

dominal distension with hypertyrosinaemia and tyrosyluria (la Du and Gyessing 1972). The genetic disease may be closely mimicked by neonatal hepatitis in the premature infant (Yu et al. 1971), which is a transient disorder. The pathological changes in the liver are very similar to those described in galactosaemia.

Hereditary Fructose Intolerance

Deficiency of fructose-1-phosphate aldolase occurs in about 1 in 30 000 births and becomes manifest on the introduction of fructose into the diet. A fructose challenge results in a consistent and often profound hypoglycaemia. The liver lesions are similar to those described in galactosaemia.

Cystic Fibrosis

The liver is rarely involved to any significant degree in the fetus or neonate in cystic fibrosis, though occasionally persistent jaundice may develop in the neonatal period. Liver biopsy findings are non-specific, with cholestasis and fatty metamorphosis (Valman et al. 1971). Three types of liver lesion have been reported (Oppenheimer and Esterley 1975) in infants under 1 year of age:

1. Focal biliary cirrhosis with inspissation of bile and mucus within the portal bile ducts, fibrosis and ductular proliferation
2. Periportal fibrosis, oedema and inflammation, with excess mucus in the bile ducts, most commonly in the larger ducts at the porta hepatis
3. As in 2, without mucus accumulation

Only the last is likely to be encountered in the neonatal period and is not, in isolation, diagnostic of cystic fibrosis.

Glycogen Storage Disease

Multiple enzyme deficiencies have been described that involve the metabolism of glycogen. The clinical management of these disorders is dependent on elucidating the specific enzyme deficiency, and therefore diagnosis is biochemical rather than histological. Indeed the information obtained by routine histological examination is minimal (Lake 1981); thus liver biopsy must be undertaken in conjunction with units capable of performing appropriate enzyme assays. Both alcohol and non-alcoholic fixatives are required, but stains performed on fixed tissues are unreliable since the various forms of glycogen have differing solubilities; thus frozen sections from fresh tissue are considered essential. Types I, III and VI are the most common forms affecting the liver, though the rarer Type IV is associated with cirrhosis and bile stasis. Only Type I is likely to be encountered in the neonatal period. Liver function tests are usually normal or only mildly disturbed. Hypoglycaemia and acidosis may be associated with hyperlipaemia and hyperuricaemia. The liver is enlarged and fatty and the hepatocytes contain both fat and glycogen, the former often predominating (Fig. 16.17).

Gaucher's Disease

Liver involvement is usually mild in Gaucher's disease and is due to collections of Gaucher cells distorting the hepatic architecture as they accumulate in sinusoids and around central veins. The cells are polyhedral, varying from 40–80 μm in diameter, with an eccentric

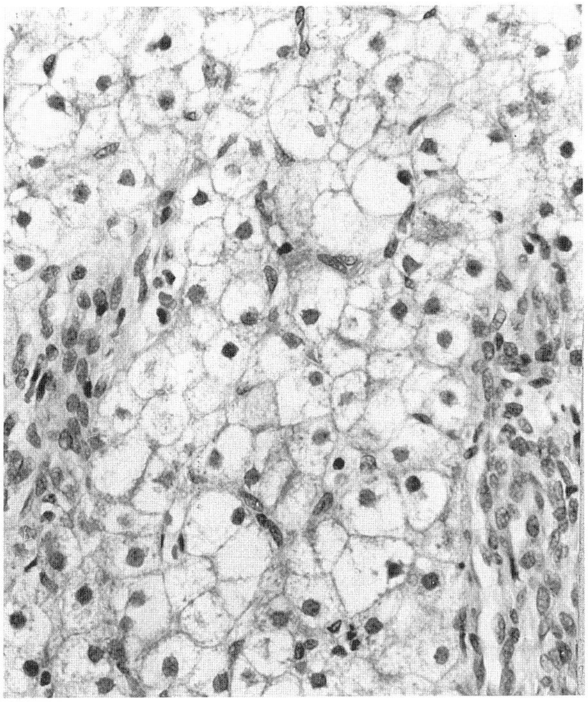

Fig. 16.17. Glycogen storage disease, Type I. The hepatocytes appear empty and contain small featureless nuclei. (Formalin fixed; H&E, ×262)

nucleus and reticulated cytoplasm. They are both PAS and Sudan positive.

Perinatal Haemochromatosis

Though uncommon, perinatal haemochromatosis is said to be the commonest form of end-stage liver disease in the uninfected neonate (Silver et al. 1989). It is presumed to be a metabolic disorder but as yet no specific biochemical defect has been identified and thus it is possible that the pathological changes are the final outcome of more than one disease process. It has been described in both the fetus and the newborn where it is rapidly fatal. (Goldfischer et al. 1981; Blisard and Bartow 1986; Silver et al. 1987; Knisely et al. 1987).

Iron storage is characteristically within hepatocytes with sparing of the reticuloendothelial system, though other organs such as the heart, pancreas, kidneys, stomach and thyroid may be involved.

The liver is of firm consistency and may be enlarged and bile stained. Microscopy reveals focal necrosis and shrinkage of hepatocytes which retain a fetal acinar pattern. Fibrosis is diffuse and cholestasis often pronounced. Regeneration nodules, giant cell transformation and haemopoietic tissue may be identified.

Clinically, neonates are growth retarded and may show muscle weakness resulting in respiratory and swallowing problems. (The latter may result in polyhydramnios.) Liver failure may be manifest as a coagulopathy, hypoalbuminaemic oedema or ascites as well as jaundice.

Cirrhosis, Fibrosis and Cystic Disease

Cirrhosis is extremely rare in the fetus and neonate. With the exception of isolated cases suspected of being due to α_1 antitrypsin deficiency (Wilkinson et al. 1974), erythroblastosis (Craig 1950) and cardiac disease (Craig et al. 1952) the aetiology is obscure, though viral and metabolic disorders come under suspicion. The largest congenital neonatal and early infantile series was reported by Thaler (1964), who stressed that GCT was not a feature of cirrhosis, although other authors question this (Witzleben 1981). Occasional examples are encountered in the fetus (Rushton 1981).

The reasons for the rarity of cirrhosis in this age group are obscure, although the short duration of underlying disease processes and the powers of regeneration of the hepatic parenchyma may be important. The increasing use of ultrasound in the diagnosis of fetal disorders will undoubtedly provide new data, since fetuses with gross ascites and small livers are being diagnosed and terminated before they die in utero and undergo maceration.

Hepatic fibrosis is uncommon in isolation and is usually associated with infantile polycystic disease of the kidneys (Blyth and Ockenden 1971), where it is of minor importance. It may also be found in association with adult polycystic disease of the kidneys in the fetus or neonate together with a neural tube defect (NTD) and limb abnormalities—the Meckel–Gruber syndrome, which is an autosomal-recessive disorder (Opitz and Howe 1969; Crawfurd et al. 1978). The NTD is usually an occipital encephalocele, but examples of anencephaly have been recorded (Fried et al. 1971). It is therefore important to examine both the kidneys and liver in all fetuses with NTDs (Seller 1978). In the fetal and neonatal period

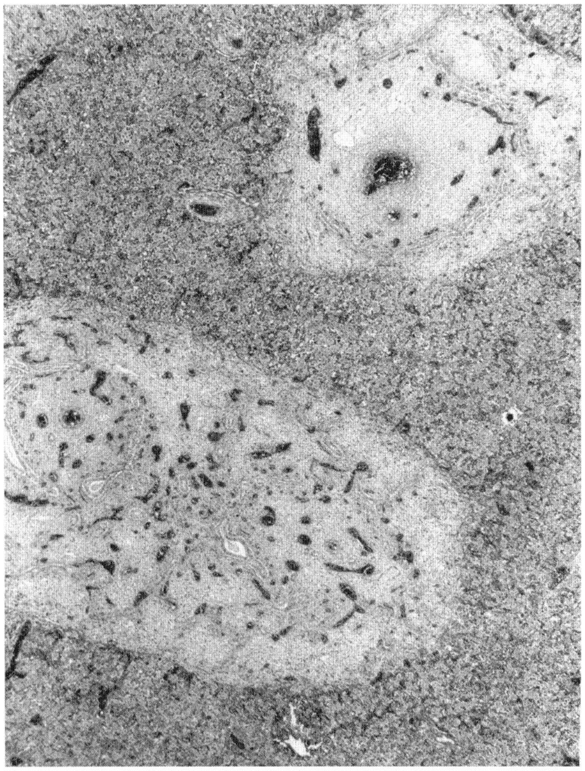

Fig. 16.18. Congenital hepatic fibrosis. Two enlarged portal tracts containing dilated bile ducts which are arranged in a concentric manner. The lobular architecture is normal. (H&E, ×24)

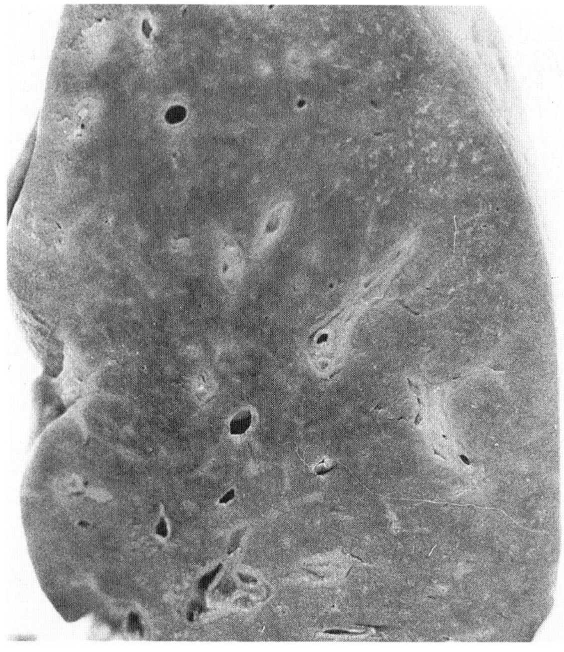

Fig. 16.19. Congenital hepatic fibrosis. Cut surface of the liver. There are fine fibrous bands dividing the parenchyma, but a lobular architecture is still apparent. (Approx. ×2.9)

the fibrosis is rarely associated with cystic dilatation of the biliary tract visible to the naked eye, though it is readily apparent on microscopy (Fig. 16.18). The liver is usually abnormally firm in consistency and an interlacing network of white fibrous strands may be visible through the capsule. The cut surface reveals the expanded portal tracts, which may link up to form more extensive masses of fibrous tissue (Fig. 16.19). The lobular architecture of the liver is well preserved. Hepatic fibrosis has also been reported in association with renal dysplasia (Ivemark et al. 1959), trisomy 18 (Alpert et al. 1969) and 3–14 translocation (Hardwick and Dimmick 1976).

It is as yet uncertain whether these disorders of liver, which are characterised by proliferation and cystic dilatation of the bile ducts and fibrosis of the portal tracts in association with a normal lobular architecture, are separate entities or parts of a spectrum of abnormalities with a common underlying aetiology. Jorgensen (1977), in a review of the embryology and pathology of these disorders, emphasises the importance of the differentiation of the cells closest to the future portal vein branches, the so-called ductal plate which forms the ducts that connect the centrifugally expanding hilar ducts to the bile capillaries, and suggests that disturbances in its development may be responsible for these lesions. Peters (1981) has suggested that these disturbances may be vascular in origin. Jorgensen (1977) concluded that there were differences in the morphology of the ductal plate derivatives in infantile polycystic disease and isolated congenital hepatic fibrosis. Landing et al. (1980) found that the varying forms of hepatic polycystic disease were indistinguishable when quantitative morphometric techniques were used. They noted that isolated congenital hepatic fibrosis did not differ from infantile polycystic disease—a conclusion contrary to that of Adams et al. (1974). It would therefore seem that, while a unified embryological approach is not yet fully acceptable, it has not been totally excluded; further studies are necessary to elucidate this problem.

Trauma and Iatrogenic Disease

The liver is rarely traumatised as the result of accidental or deliberate injury in the neonatal

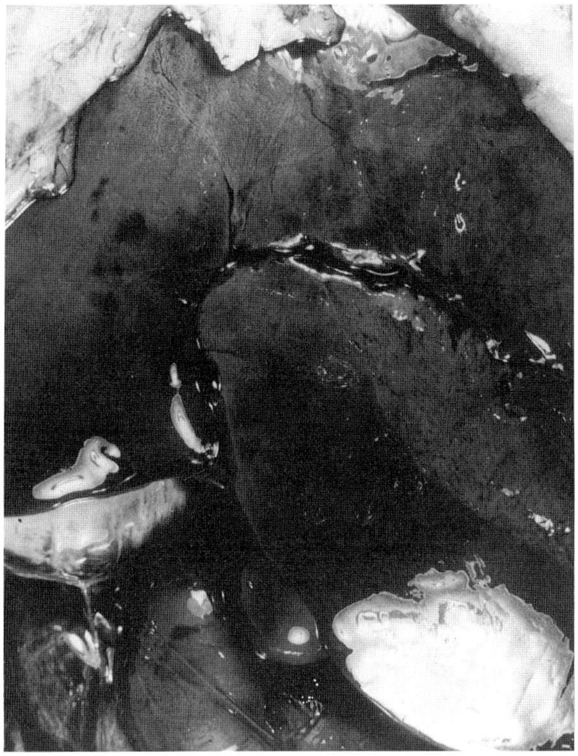

Fig. 16.20. Ruptured liver. There is a transverse tear in the liver at the site of disruption by the lower border of the ribs in an infant that became impacted in the pelvis in a folded transverse position. (Approx. ×1.8)

period, but injuries sustained during delivery are not uncommon. Fatal intraperitoneal haemorrhage may follow rupture of the liver during delivery. This, in the present author's experience, is most common in premature infants with abnormal intrauterine positions, in particular a transverse lie. As the fetus is folded in utero the lower border of the rib cage may be driven into the substance of the liver (Fig. 16.20). Commoner than physical disruption of the liver as a cause of intra-abdominal bleeding is the subcapsular haematoma (Fig. 16.21). This may arise as the result of the combination of the effects of trauma, hypoxia and vascular congestion. It is most common in the premature breech delivery. The haematoma may rupture in utero or it may enlarge after delivery and rupture spontaneously or following abdominal palpation. Haematomas may form in any part of the liver but are most common on the anterior surface of the right lobe. Other causes of bleeding from the liver are inappropriately sited umbilical vein catheters (Fig. 16.22), paracentesis and intrauterine transfusion. In intrauterine transfusion it is necessary to determine the relative proportions of fetal and adult blood in the haemorrhage and in the fetal blood to confirm that haemorrhage has occurred. Umbilical vein

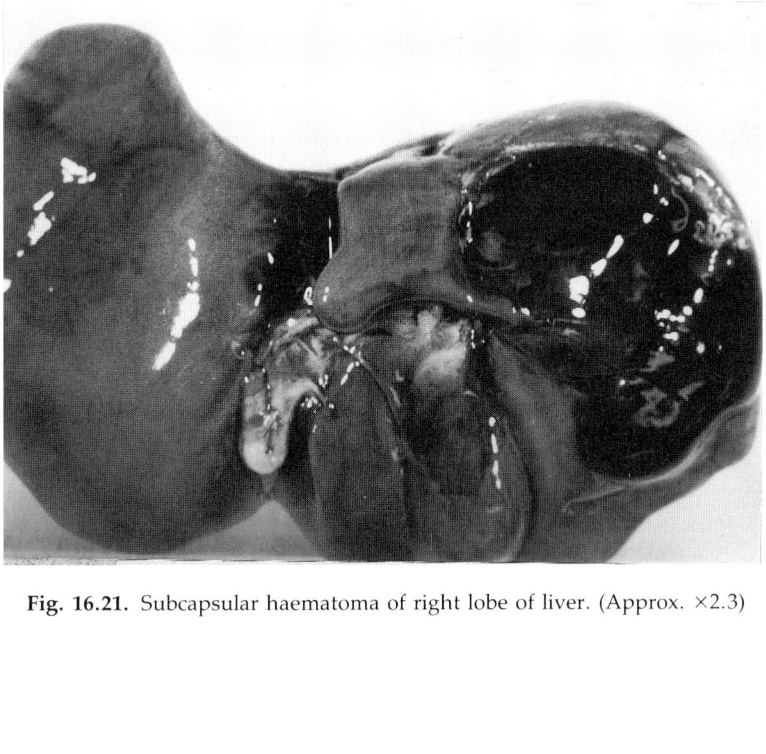

Fig. 16.21. Subcapsular haematoma of right lobe of liver. (Approx. ×2.3)

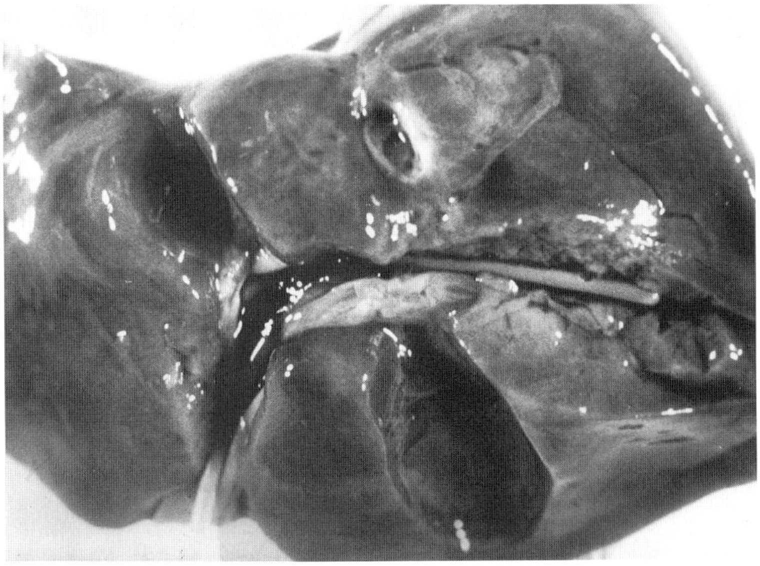

Fig. 16.22. Disruption of the liver by an umbilical vein catheter thought to be in the ductus venosus. (Rushton 1981.) (Approx. ×2.3)

catheterisation may result in portal vein thrombosis, hepatic infarction and necrosis as well as the occasional introduction of infection (Larroche 1977).

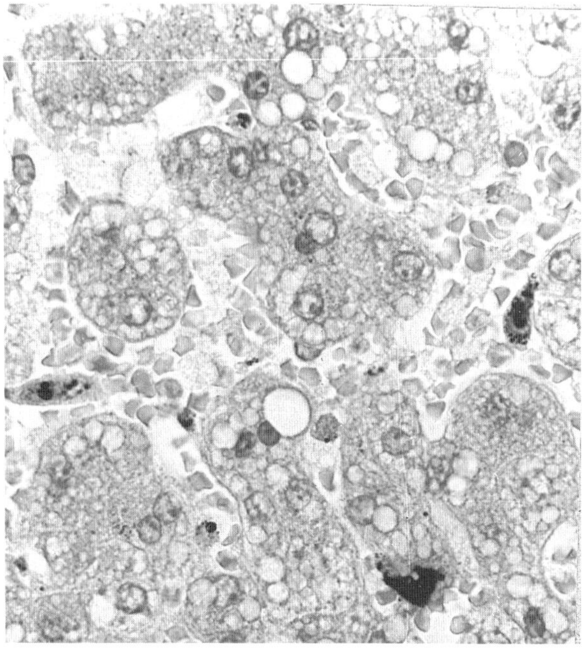

Fig. 16.23. Prolonged parenteral feeding (6 weeks). The hepatocytes show a tubular configuration with very extensive fatty vacuolation. The Kupffer cells contain black pigment derived from Intralipid. (Sudan black, ×254)

Parenteral Feeding

Total parenteral nutrition (TPN) is commonly used in the treatment of sick, predominantly premature neonates, and it is probable that its usage will increase as smaller and smaller babies are kept alive. A proportion of these, almost a quarter in one series (Beale et al. 1979), develop evidence of liver dysfunction (Peden et al. 1971; Touloukian and Downing 1973; Postuma and Trevenen 1979). Although liver function may be disturbed within a few days or starting TPN, a longer history of exposure is more characteristic. Liver function usually returns to normal after cessation of therapy, although this may take several months. Rarely, liver damage may be irreversible and progress to cirrhosis (Finegold 1976). However, there is considerable individual variation in the response to TPN because of factors that are ill understood; thus liver function requires careful monitoring in these patients.

The histological changes in the liver (Fig. 16.23) include fatty metamorphosis; centrilobular, canalicular and hepatocellular cholestasis; tubular transformation of the liver plates; scattered GCT; bile duct proliferation; and portal fibrosis. The Kupffer cells frequently contain PAS-positive, diastase-resistant material which stains positively with Sudan black in

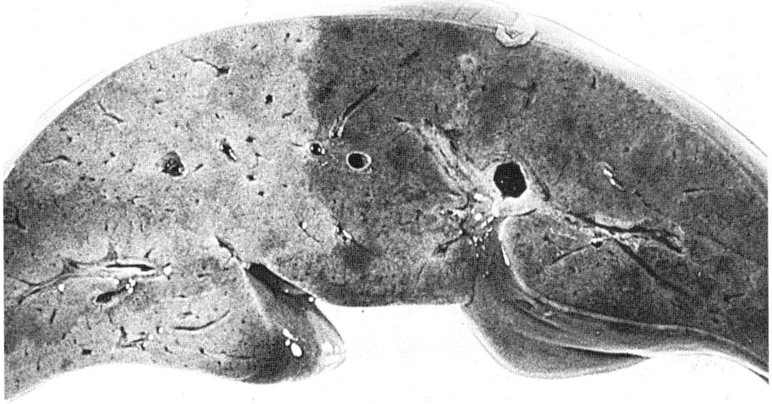

Fig. 16.24. Two-tone liver. The right lobe is pale. The line of demarcation, though sharp, is not straight. (Rushton 1981.) (Approx. actual size)

paraffin-embedded tissues. Similar deposits may be found in macrophages in the portal tracts, lymph nodes and spleen.

The pathogenesis of TPN-induced liver damage is disputed, but suppression of the secretin-dependent component of bile may be a critical factor. The absence of the luminal stimulation of secretin by bowel contents (Rager and Finegold 1975) and high blood sugar levels will both depress secretin production. The constituents of the bile salt pool and thus the enterohepatic circulation may also be modified by use of antibiotics which alter the bacterial flora of the gut. There might also be a direct toxic effect on the liver, though how this is mediated is unknown.

Circulatory Disorders

The anatomy of the fetal hepatic blood supply inevitably results in unequal oxygenation of the left and right lobes of the liver. In utero the right lobe is less well oxygenated, and as a result there is frequently more erythropoietic tissue when compared with the left lobe (Emery 1956). The lower oxygen tension may also be associated with reduced glycogen storage in later pregnancy. However, this may be a simplistic explanation, since experimental evidence suggests that stable perfusion of the liver is more important than a steady oxygen tension in the blood (Edelstone et al. 1984). It would appear that, if the liver is well perfused, oxygen uptake by the hepatocytes can be adjusted, within certain limits, to allow for variations in the oxygen tension. Whatever the pathophysiological mechanisms involved, hepatic anoxia will result in glycogen depletion, fatty metamorphosis and eventually necrosis, the severity and distribution of these lesions being determined, at least in part, by the anatomy of the hepatic circulation and the physiological adaptation that occurs after birth. The high content of glycogen in the full-term infant's liver—two to three times that found in the adult liver weight for weight—are almost certainly a provision to compensate for the stresses of labour and delivery. The much lower levels in the premature infant are a further hazard to this high-risk group. It is believed that glycogen depletion and fatty metamorphosis may develop very rapidly, particularly in the centrilobular zones (i.e. within hours), and they are therefore frequently interpreted as indicating fetal distress.

Hemilateral degeneration of the liver or two-tone liver (Emery 1955) is said to occur in about 5% of perinatal necropsies (Daamen and Schaberg 1969); however, in the present author's experience the incidence has declined in recent years, possibly as the result of more intensive monitoring of the fetus in utero and the greater willingness of the obstetrician to perform caesarean sections for early fetal distress. On macroscopic examination (Fig. 16.24) the right lobe of the liver is paler and softer than the left lobe, the yellowish colour of the former contrasting with the dark red of the latter. The line of demarcation between the two lobes is irregular, though sharp, and lies within

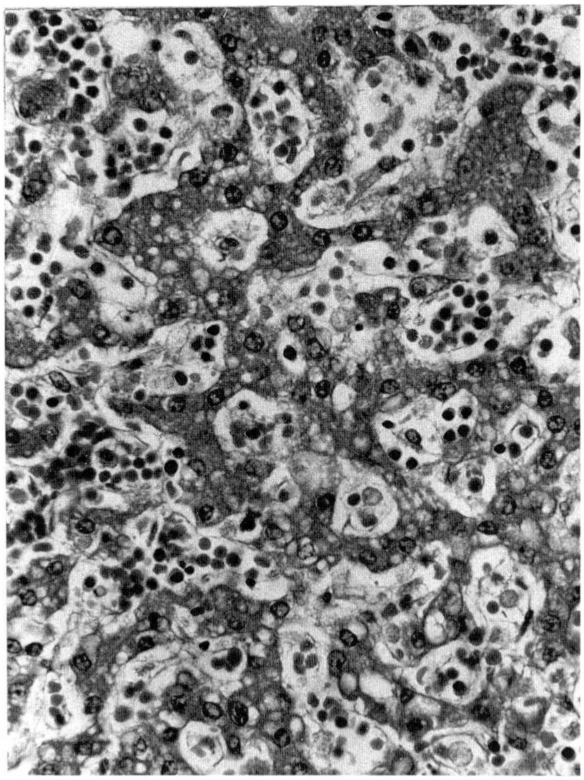

Fig. 16.25. Hypoxic liver. The hepatocytes are shrunken, forming narrow trabeculae around the dilated sinusoids. They show pronounced fatty vacuolation. (H&E, ×219)

1–2 cm of the midline on the right of the falciform ligament. Microscopic examination shows greater glycogen depletion and more extensive fatty change in the right lobe, though the left lobe is rarely entirely devoid of these changes. Daamen and Schaberg (1969) noted that differential deposition of iron also occurred in about one-third of cases and that iron deposition only occurred in the right lobe in rhesus isoimmunisation. In those infants who survive to develop cholestasis, canalicular cholestasis is more marked in the right lobe. It is therefore important that histological material be obtained from both lobes of the liver at necropsy (Ghosh and Emery 1970).

Necrosis, usually focal or centrilobular, is common among perinatal deaths; thus Emery (1952) demonstrated that as many as 50% of livers may show necrosis. It must be emphasised that necrosis of the liver is not always the result of hypoxia or ischaemia. Thus some of the infections discussed earlier may produce massive hepatic necrosis. Initially the hepatocytes form shrunken strands surrounding dilated sinusoids (Fig. 16.25), which may coalesce to form blood lakes (peliosis hepatis). Fibrin deposition may occur either as the result of local thrombosis, as occurs in association with hyaline membrane disease (Wade-Evans 1961) or following embolisation after insertion of an umbilical vein catheter. The latter may lead to massive hepatic necrosis (Fig. 16.26). Emboli may also arise in the placenta during intrauterine life.

Cardiac failure, particularly when associated with cyanotic heart disease or abnormalities of the left heart (e.g. hypoplasia, coarctation of the aorta), may result in hepatic necrosis (Shiraki 1970), when the mid-zone of the lobule may be most affected. Periportal and portal haemorrhage with focal necrosis of hepatocytes may be found in livers of infants dying after intraventricular haemorrhage (Shiraki 1970; Rushton 1981), although the mechanisms by which these lesions arise are obscure.

Hepatomegaly, particularly if massive, as is found in severe rhesus isoimmunisation or some storage diseases, may be associated with irregular areas of necrosis.

Lesions of the hepatic veins are extremely rare in the neonate, as is emphasised by the first report of thrombosis manifest as ascites at birth, which led to the development of the Budd–Chiari syndrome at 4 months of age (Jaffe and Yunis 1983).

Liver Disease in Babies of Diabetic Mothers

The effects of maternal diabetes on the fetal liver are very variable and have been reviewed by Haust (1981). The differences are at least partly explained by the severity of the diabetes and the quality of management during pregnancy. While small-for-dates babies may occur in association with diabetes, presumably as a result of both uteroplacental ischaemia and impaired placental function, the more typical offspring of a diabetic mother is large and cherubic.

Naeye (1965), in a quantitative morphological study of infants of diabetic mothers, found striking differences between these two groups of diabetic infants. The weight of the livers of growth-retarded infants was, on average, about 20% below that of normal controls,

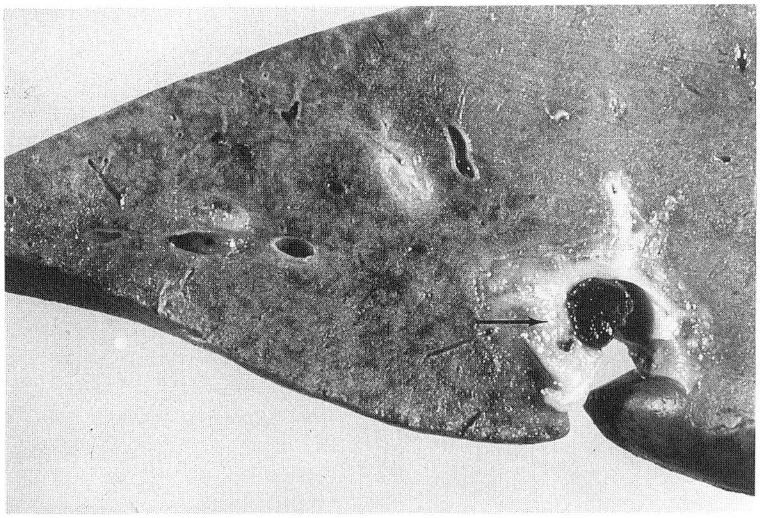

Fig. 16.26. Infarction of the left lobe of the liver caused by an umbilical vein catheter; this resulted in thrombosis of the umbilical and portal veins (*arrows*). (Approx. actual size)

almost entirely because of a reduction in the number of hepatocytes; the individual cells were hypertrophied and contained 60% more cytoplasm than normal. There was also a striking excess erythropoietic tissue. The livers of the large babies were about 50% above the weight of normal controls because of an increase in both cell numbers and cell size. Erythropoiesis was also increased, though to a lesser degree than in the growth-retarded fetuses. Singer (1986) found that erythropoietic activity in normally grown babies of diabetic mothers was normal, only the large babies showing an increased activity. The excess erythropoietic activity is believed to be due to chronic hypoxia subsequent to the placental lesions. The increased erythropoietic tissue appears to be associated with reduced hepatic iron storage.

In addition to the effect on the size of the liver and on the content of erythropoietic tissue within the liver there may also be increased glycogen and fat within hepatocytes, often concurrently, and in the enlarged livers there may be areas of focal necrosis (Fig. 16.27), presumably of ischaemic origin.

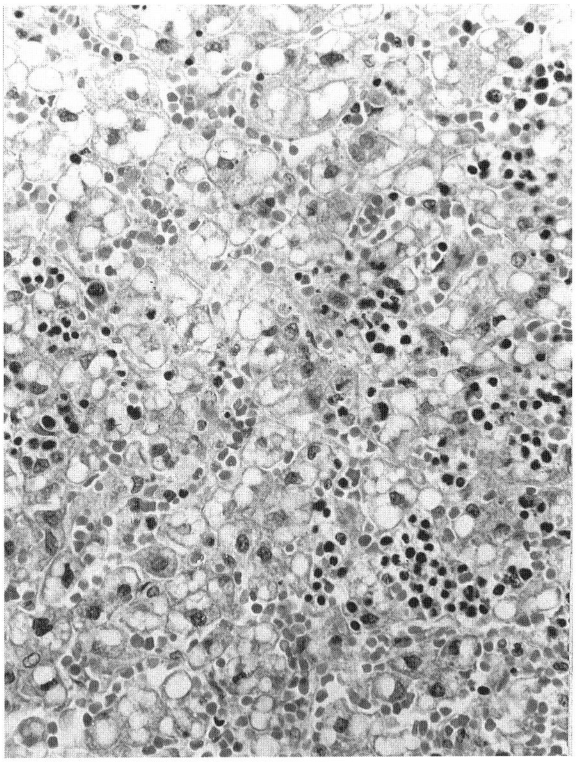

Fig. 16.27. Liver from a diabetic cherub of 38 weeks' gestation. The liver was twice the expected weight and shows excessive erythropoietic activity and fatty vacuolation. On frozen section it also contained abundant glycogen. (H&E, ×200)

Malformations of the Liver

The most common malformations of the liver are abnormalities of shape and lobation and are

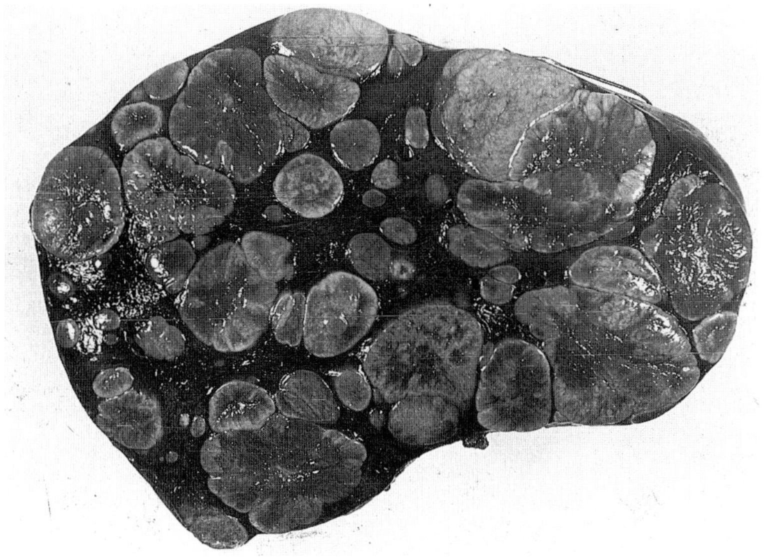

Fig. 16.28. Hepatoblastoma. Slice of liver of an infant with a multinodular tumour, the nodules having a variegated appearance. (Courtesy of Dr. A.H. Cameron, Birmingham; Rushton 1981)

found in diaphragmatic hernias and defects of the ventral body wall. The liver may be reversed in situs inversus.

Abnormalities of the liver are described in several chromosomal anomalies (Witzleben 1982), including trisomies 18, 21 and 45XO. These include paucity of the intrahepatic bile ducts and proliferative lesions with periportal fibrosis. They are not consistent associations, and the isolated reports suggest they may be fortuitous.

Tumours

Tumours of the livers are rare in the perinatal period and usually present as silent abdominal masses, though they may occasionally lead to intrauterine complications (Benjamin et al. 1981). They have been comprehensively reviewed by Dehner (1978).

Hepatoblastoma

Hepatoblastoma may occur in isolation or in association with other abnormalities, e.g. hemihypertrophy and sexual precocity. An elevated serum alphafetoprotein level is common in affected infants. There is a pronounced male predominance (6M:1F).

The extent of liver involvement is variable, from a local lesion in one lobe to massive involvement in about one-third of patients. The tumours are frequently nodular, the nodules having a fleshy cut surface (Fig. 16.28). Growth results in compression of the surrounding liver distoring the biliary tree and producing local obstruction and cholestasis or necrosis by interrupting the blood supply. There is no true capsule around the nodules.

Although the tumours have been divided into epithelial and mesenchymal subgroups the majority contain both elements (Keeling 1971). Embryonic and fetal subtypes of the epithelial groups are described (Ishak and Glunz 1967).

The embryonic pattern is characterised by rosette-like collections of cells (Fig. 16.29), often with numerous mitoses and scattered tumour giant cells. The fetal pattern shows plates of primitive hepatocytes around sinusoids, which frequently contain abundant erythropoietic tissue. The mesenchymal component consists of loose spindle cells, often with numerous mitoses. Metaplasia is common and may affect both the epithelial and mesenchymal elements, though metastases are usually of epithelial origin.

Hamartoma

About 20% of tumours in this age group are hamartomas, the most common being the

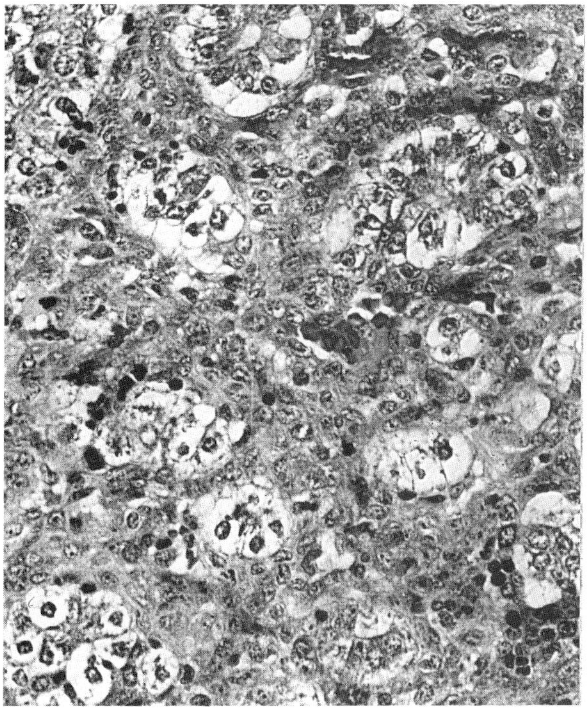

Fig. 16.29. Hepatoblastoma. Embryonic pattern with tubular and rosette-like arrangement of cells. (Courtesy of Dr. A.H. Cameron, Birmingham; Rushton 1981.) (H&E, ×190)

cavernous haemangioma; this is usually an incidental discovery at necropsy. Hamartomas form a spectrum of lesions varying from predominantly vascular (Fig. 16.30) to mixed fibrovascular through to a predominantly fibrotic form.

Haemangioendothelioma may present clinically as a haemorrhagic diathesis caused by sequestration of platelets within the lesion, as cardiac failure caused by arteriovenous shunting or as haemoperitoneum caused by rupture. It frequently presents within the first 6 months of life (Dehner and Ishak 1971), although rarely in the neonatal period. Many affected infants also have cutaneous haemangiomas. Calcification may be apparent on the radiograph. Single or multiple lesions may occur and they vary in consistency from soft and spongy to firm and fibrous. They typically consist of empty vascular channels lined by plump sometimes pleomorphic endothelial cells. The stromal component is frequently myxomatous and may contain bile ducts.

Fibrotic hamartomas may be cystic. They occur most commonly in the right lobe of the liver and may contain numerous endothelial lined channels resembling those seen in lymphangiomas.

Gall Bladder and Extrahepatic Bile Ducts (Excluding EHBA)

Malformations

Malformations of the gall bladder are rare, the most common being agenesis. Absent gall bladder occurs in isolation in about 25% of cases, the vast majority being associated with multiple malformations, cardiovascular malformations or malformations of the anterior abdominal wall (Turkel et al. 1983). Rudimentary or hypoplastic gall bladders may

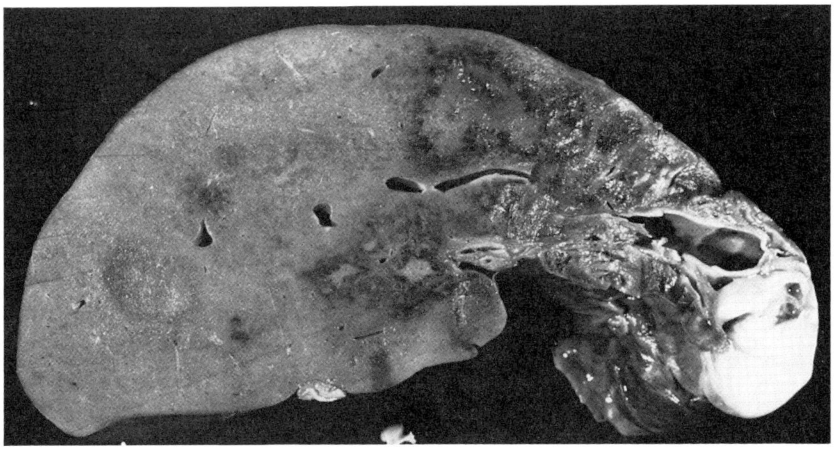

Fig. 16.30. Vascular hamartoma replacing the left lobe of the liver from a 3-day-old neonate. (Courtesy of Dr. J.W. Keeling)

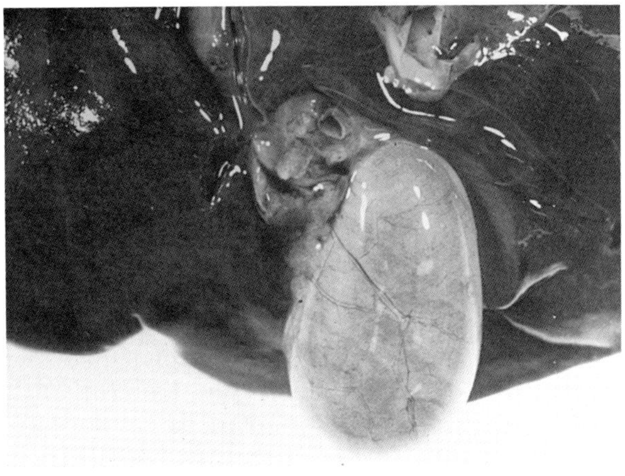

Fig. 16.31. Distended gall bladder containing "white bile" in a neonate with septicaemia, pneumonia and meningitis. (Approx. ×1.7)

be totally buried within the substance of the liver; thus complete absence requires histological confirmation.

Choledochal cyst, a developmental abnormality of the common bile duct, rarely presents in the neonatal period, usually with jaundice, acholic stools and an abdominal mass (Kobayashi and Ohbe 1977). It is predominantly a disorder of females and is very much more common in Japanese than in Caucasians (Lee et al. 1969). Three types are described (Alonso-Lej et al. 1959):

1. Segmental enlargement of the common bile duct, the dilated portion being in continuity with the normal duct
2. A cystic diverticulum arising from a normal or dilated duct
3. Choledochocele lying within the intraduodenal portion of the duct

The vast majority are of the first type. The aetiology and pathogenesis are obscure though both developmental (Mlyano et al. 1984) and acquired mechanisms (Dimmick 1990) are proposed.

Acquired Lesions

Few acquired lesions of the gall bladder are described in the literature. Marked distension of the gall bladder has been noted in septic neonates (Peevy and Wiseman 1982), and the present author has observed several examples, the bile usually being almost colourless (Fig. 16.31).

Other lesions described in the neonatal and infantile age group include cholelithiasis (Jeffrey et al. 1984), empyema of the gall bladder (Jamieson and Shaw 1975) and spontaneous perforation of the common bile duct (Howard et al. 1976).

References

Aagenaes Ø, Fagerhol M, Elgjo K, Monthe E, Hovig T (1974) Pathology and pathogenesis of liver disease in α_1 antitrypsin deficient individuals. Postgrad Med J 50: 365–375

Adams M, Danks DM, Campbell PE (1974) Comments upon the classification of infantile polycystic diseases of the liver and kidney, based upon three dimensional reconstruction of the liver. J Med Genet 11: 234–243

Alagille D, Odievre M. (1978) Liver and biliary tract disease in children. Wiley Flammarion, New York, pp 1–16

Alagille D, Odievre M, Gautier M, Dommergues JP (1975) Hepatic ductular hypoplasia associated with characteristic facies, vertebral malformations, retarded physical, mental and skeletal development, and cardiac murmur. J Pediatr 86: 63–71

Alonso-Lej F, Rever WB, Pessagno DJ (1959) Congenital choledochal cyst with a report of two and analysis of 94 cases. Surg Gynecol Obstet 108: 1–30

Alpert LI, Strauss L, Hirschorn K (1969) Neonatal hepatitis and biliary atresia in association with trisomy 17–18 syndrome. N Engl J Med 280: 16–20

Aterman K (1989) Neonatal hepatitis–a viral disease. Pediatr Pathol 9: 243–250

Back P (1973) Synthesis and excretion of bile acids in a case of extrahepatic biliary atresia. Helv Med Acta 37: 193–200

Back P, Ross K (1973) Identification of 3 beta OH 5 cholenoic acid in human meconium. Hoppe Seylers Z Physiol Chem 354: 83–89

Bacon CJ, Sims DG (1976) Echovirus 19 infection in infants under six months. Arch Dis Child 51: 631–633

Barclay AE, Franklin KJ, Prichard MML (1944) The foetal circulation. Blackwell, Oxford

Beale E, Nelson R, Bucciarelli R, Donnelly W, Eitzman D (1979) Intrahepatic cholestasis associated with parenteral nutrition in premature infants. Pediatrics 64: 342–347

Becroft DMO (1972) Biliary atresia associated with prenatal infection by *Listeria monocytogenes*. Arch Dis Child 47: 656–660

Benjamin E, Lendon M, Marsden HB (1981) Hepatoblastoma as a cause of intrauterine fetal death. Br J Obstet Gynaecol 88: 329–332

Berry PJ, Nagington J (1982) Fatal infection with Echovirus 11. Arch Dis Child 57: 22–29

Berthelot P, Dhumeaux D (1978) New insights in the classification and mechanisms of hereditary chronic non haemolytic hyperbilirubinaemias. Gut 19: 474–480

Blisard KS, Bastow SA. (1986) Neonatal haemochromatosis. Hum Pathol 17: 376–383

Blyth H, Ockenden BG (1971) Polycystic disease of kidneys and liver presenting in childhood. J Med Genet 8: 257–284

Brough AJ, Bernstein J (1974) Conjugated hyperbilirubinaemia in early infancy. A reassessment of liver biopsy. Hum Pathol 5: 507–518

Chen-Chih J, Sun G, Keene L, Nagey D A (1990) Hepatic fibrosis in congenital cytomegalovirus infection with fetal ascites and pulmonary hypoplasia. Pediatr Pathol. 10. 641–646

Cherry JD (1976) Enteroviruses. In: Remington JS, Klein BO (eds) Infectious diseases of the fetus and newborn infant. Saunders, Philadelphia, pp 366–413

Cook PJL (1974) Genetic aspects of the Pi system. Postgrad Med J 50: 362–364

Cossart YE (1974) Acquisition of hepatitis B antigen in the newborn period. Postgrad Med J 50: 334–337

Cottrall K, Cook PJL, Mowat AP (1974) Neonatal hepatitis syndrome and α_1 antitrypsin deficiency: an epidemiological study in South-east England. Postgrad Med J 50: 376–379

Craig JM (1950) Sequences in the development of cirrhosis of the liver in cases of erythroblastosis fetalis. Arch Pathol Lab Med 49: 665–686

Craig JM, Landing BH (1952) A form of hepatitis in the neonatal period simulating biliary atresia. Arch Pathol 54: 321–333

Crawfurd Md'A, Jackson P, Kohler HG (1978) Case report. Meckel's syndrome (dysencephalia splanchnocystica) in two Pakistani sibs. J Med Genet 15: 242–245

Daamen CBF, Schaberg A (1969) Hemilateral liver degeneration in perinatal death. J Pathol 97: 29–34

Danks DM (1965) Prolonged obstructive neonatal hepatitis. A survey of modern concepts. Clin Pediatr 4: 499–510

Danks DM, Campbell PE, Jack I, Rogers J, Smith AL (1977a) Studies of the aetiology of neonatal hepatitis and biliary atresia. Arch Dis Child 52: 360–367

Danks DM, Campbell PE, Smith AL, Rogers L (1977b) Prognosis of babies with neonatal hepatitis. Arch Dis Child 52: 368–372

Dehner LP (1978) Hepatic tumours in the pediatric age group. A distinctive pathological spectrum. In: Rosenberg HS, Bolande RP (eds) Perspectives in pediatric pathology, vol 4. Year Book Medical Publishers, Chicago, pp 217–268

Dehner LP, Ishak KG (1971) Vascular tumours of the liver in infants and children. A study of 30 cases and review of the literature. Arch Pathol 92: 101–111

Derso A, Boxall EH, Tarlow MJ, Flewet TH (1978) Transmission of Hb_sAg from mother to infant in four ethnic groups. Br Med JI: 949–952

Devos P, Hers HG (1974) Glycogen metabolism in the liver of the fetal rat. Biochem J 140: 331–340

Dimmick JE (1990) Liver disease in the perinatal infant. In: Wigglesworth JS, Singer DB (eds) Textbook of fetal and perinatal pathology, vol 2. Blackwell Scientific Publications, Oxford, pp 992–993

Dimmick JE, Bove KE, McAdams AJ (1975) Extrahepatic biliary atresia and the polysplenia syndrome. J Pediatr 86: 644–645

Du Bois AM (1963) The embryonic liver. In: Roullier C (ed) The liver, vol 1. Academic, New York, pp 1–40

Edelstone DI, Pavlone ME, Holzman IR (1984) Hepatic oxygenation during arterial hypoxemia in neonatal lambs. Am J Obstet Gynecol 150: 513–518

Elias H (1955) Origin and early development of the liver in various vertebrates. Acta Hepatol 3: 1–56

Emery JL (1952) Degenerative changes in the left lobe of the liver in the newborn. Arch Dis Child 27: 558–561

Emery JL (1955) Asymmetrical liver disease in infancy. J Pathol Bacteriol 69: 219–224

Emery JL (1956) The distribution of haemopoietic foci in the infantile human liver. J Anat 90: 293–297

Ewing CI, Davidson DC (1985) Fatal hepatitis B in infant born to a HB_cAg carrier with HB_eAb. Arch Dis Child 60: 265–267

Finegold MJ (1976) Cholestatic syndromes in infancy. In: Rosenberg HS, Bolande RP (eds) Perspectives in pediatric pathology, vol 3. Year Book Medical Publishers, Chicago, pp 41–84

Fried K, Liban E, Lurie M, Friedman S, Reisner SH (1971) Polycystic kidneys associated with malformations of the brain, polydactyly and other birth defects in newborn sibs. A lethal syndrome showing autosomal recessive inheritance. J Med Genet 8: 285–290

Ghosh ML, Emery JL (1970) The connective tissue in livers of children. J Clin Pathol 23: 599–603

Goldfischer S, Grotsky HW, Chang CH et al. (1981) Idiopathic neonatal iron storage involving the liver, pancreas, heart, endocrine and exocrine glands. Hepatology 1: 58–64

Greenwood DR, Rosenthal A, Crocker AC, Nadas AS (1976) Syndrome of intrahepatic biliary dysgenesis and cardiovascular malformations. Pediatrics 58: 243–247

Hadchouel M, Gautier M (1976) Histopathologic study of liver in the early cholestatic phase of α_1 antitrypsin deficiency. J Pediatr 89: 211–215

Hamilton JR, Sass-Korstak A (1963) Jaundice associated with severe bacterial infection in young infants. J Pediatr 63: 121–132

Hamilton WJ, Boyd JD, Mossman HW (1972) Human embryology. Heffer, Cambridge, p 342

Hardwick DF, Dimmick JE (1976) Metabolic cirrhoses of infancy and early childhood. In: Rosenberg HS, Bolande RP (eds) Perspectives in pediatric pathology, vol 3. Year Book Medical Publishers, Chicago, pp 103–144

Hashida Y, Yunis EJ (1988) Syndromatic paucity of interlobular bile ducts. Hepatic histopathology of the early and endstage liver. Pediatr Pathol 8: 1–15

Haust DM (1981) Maternal diabetes—Effects on the fetus and placenta. In: Naeye RL, Kissane JH, Kaufman N (eds) Perinatal diseases. Williams and Wilkins, Baltimore, p 223

Heathcote J, Deodhar KP, Scheuer PJ, Sherlock S (1976) Intrahepatic cholestasis in childhood. N Engl J Med 295: 801–805

Henricksen NT, Langmark F, Sørland SJ, Fausa O, Landaas S, Aagenaes Ø (1977) Hereditary cholestasis combined with peripheral pulmonary stenosis and other anomalies. Acta Paediatr Scand 66: 7–15

Hosier DM, Newton WA (1985) Serious Coxsackie infection in infants and children. Am J Dis Child 96: 251–259

Howard ER, Mowat AP (1977) Extrahepatic biliary atresia. Recent developments in management. Arch Dis Child 52: 825–827

Howard ER, Johnson DI, Mowat AP (1976) Spontaneous perforation of the common bile duct in infants. Arch Dis Child 51: 883–886

Hsai DY-Y, Patteson P, Allen FH, Diamond LK, Gellis SS (1952) Prolonged obstrutive jaundice in infancy. 1. General survey of 156 cases. Pediatrics 10: 245–252

Hughes JR, Wilfert CM, Moore M, Benirschke K, Hoyosguevara E (1972) Echo virus 14 infection associated with fatal neonatal hepatic necrosis. Am J Dis Child 123: 61–67

Hutchins GM, Moore GW (1988) Growth and asymmetry of the human liver during the embryonic period. Pediatr Pathol 8: 17–24

Isenberg JN, Hanson RF, Williams G, Szczepanik E, Klein

PD, Sharp HL (1976) A clinical experience with familial paucity of intrahepatic bile ducts associated with defective metabolism of trihydroxycoprostanic acid to cholic acid. In: Alagille D (ed) Liver Diseases in children. Institut National de la Santé et de la Recherche Medical, Paris, pp 43–56

Ishak KG, Glunz PR (1967) Hepatoblastoma and hepatocarcinoma in infancy and childhood. Report of 47 cases. Cancer 20: 396–422

Ivemark BI, Oldfelt V, Zetterstrom RI (1959) Familial dysplasia of kidneys, liver and pancreas: a probably genetically determined syndrome. Acta Paediatr Scand 48: 1–11

Jaffe R, Yunis EJ (1983) Congenital Budd–Chiari syndrome. Pediatr Pathol 1: 187–192

Jamieson PN, Shaw DG (1975) Empyema of gall bladder in an infant. Arch Dis Child 50: 482–484

Jeffrey I, Lund RJ, Whitelaw A (1984) Cholelithiasis in a preterm infant. Pediatr Pathol 2: 207–214

Jorgensen MJ (1977) The ductal plate malformation. Acta Pathol Microbiol Scand [A] 257: 1–87

Jorpes JE (1965) The influence of secretin and cholecystokinin on bile flow. In: Taylor W (ed) The biliary system. Blackwell, Oxford, pp 293–301

Kattamis CA, Demetrios D, Matsaurotis NS (1974) Australia antigen and neonatal hepatitis syndrome. Pediatrics 54: 157–164

Katz L, Hamilton JR (1974) Fat absorption in infants of birth weight less than 1300 grams. J Pediatr 85: 608–614

Keeling JW (1971) Liver tumours in infancy and childhood. J Pathol 103: 69–86

Kilbrick S, Benirschke K (1958) Severe generalised disease (encephalo-hepato-myocarditis) occurring in the newborn period and due to infection with Coxsackie virus group B. Pediatrics 22:857–875

Klein JO, Remington JS, Marcy SM (1976) An introduction to infection of the fetus and newborn infant, In: Remington JS, Klein JO (eds) Infectious disease of fetus and newborn infants. Saunders, Philadelphia, pp 1–32

Knisely AS, Magid MS, Dische MR, Cutz E (1987) Neonatal haemochromatosis. Birth Defects 23: 75–102

Kobayashi A, Ohbe Y (1977) Choledochal cyst in infancy and childhood. Arch Dis Child 52: 121–128

Koga A (1971) Morphogenesis of intrahepatic bile ducts of the human fetus. Z Anat Entwicklungs 135: 156–184

Krous HF, Dietzman D, Ray CG (1973) Fatal infection with echovirus types 6 and 11 in early intancy. Am J Dis Child 126: 842–846

la Du BM, Gjessing LY (1972) Tyrosinosis and tyrosinaemia. In: Stanbury JB, Wyngaarden JB, Fredickson DS (eds) The metabolic basis of inherited disease. McGraw Hill, New York, 256–267

Lake BD (1981) Metabolic disorders. General considerations. In: Berry CL (ed) Paediatric pathology. Springer, Berlin Heidelberg New York, pp 632–635

Lancet (1980) Leading article. Hepatitis B in mothers and babies. Lancet I: 237–238

Landing B (1974) Considerations on the pathogenesis of neonatal hepatitis, biliary atresia and choledochal cysts—the concept of infantile obstructive cholangiopathy. In: Bill AH, Kasai M (eds) Progress in paediatric surgery, vol 6. University Park Press, Baltimore, pp 113–139

Landing BH, Wells TR, Claireaux AE (1980) Morphometric analysis of liver lesions in cystic disease of childhood. Hum Pathol 11: 549–560

Landing BH, Wells TR, Ramicone E (1985) Time course of the intrahepatic lesion of extrahepatic biliary atresia. A morphometric study. Pediatr Pathol 4: 309–319

Larroche JC (1977) Umbilical catheterisation. In: Developmental pathology of the neonate. Excerpta Medica, Amsterdam, pp 233–241

Lawson E, Boggs J (1974) Long term follow up of neonatal hepatitis: safety and value of surgical exploration. Pediatrics 53: 650–655

Lee SS, Min PC, Kim GS, Hong PW (1969) Choledochal cyst. A report of nine cases and review of the literature. Arch Surg 99:19–28

Levy HL (1973) Massachusetts department of public health: new born screening for metabolic disorders. N Engl J Med 288: 1299–1300

McPhie JL, Birnie S, Brunt PW (1976) α_1 Antitrypsin deficiency and infantile liver disease. Arch Dis Child 51: 584–588

Maksem JA (1980) Polysplenia syndrome and splenic hypoplasia associated with extrahepatic biliary atresia. Arch Pathol Lab Med 104: 212–214

Malone M, Mieli-Vergani G, Mowat AP, Portmann B (1989) The fetal liver in PIZZ, antitrypsin deficiency. A report of five cases. Pediat Pathol 9: 623–631

Manolaki AG, Larcher VF, Mowat, AP, Barrett JJ, Portmann B, Howard ER (1983) The prelaparotomy diagnosis of extrahepatic biliary atresia. Arch Dis Child 58: 591–594

Medearis DN (1964) Observations concerning human cytomegalovirus infection and disease. Bull Johns Hopkins Hosp 114: 181–211

Miyano T, Suruga, K, Shimomura H, Nittono H, Matsumoto M. (1984) Choledochopopancreatic elongated common channel disorders. J. Pediat Surgery 19: 165–170.

Montgomery CK, Ruebner BH (1976) Neonatal hepatocellular giant cell transformation. A review. In: Rosenberg HS, Bolande RP (eds) Perspectives in pediatric pathology, vol 3. Year Book Medical Publishers, Chicago, pp 85–101

Morse JO (1978a) Alpha $_1$ antitrypsin deficiency I. N Engl J Med 299: 1045–1048

Morse JO (1978b) Alpha $_1$ antitrypsin deficiency II. N Engl J Med 299: 1099–1105

Mowat AP, Psacharopoulos HT, Williams R (1976) Extrahepatic biliary atresia versus neonatal hepatitis. Review of 137 prospectively investigated patients. Arch Dis Child 51: 763–770

Mueller RF, Pagon RA, Hass JE, Stephan MJ (1981) Arteriohepatic dysplasia: potentially lethal disorder of intrahepatic cholestasis and/or congenital heart disease. Am J Hum Genet 33: 87A (abstract)

Naeye RL (1965) Infants of diabetic mothers: a quantitative morphologic study. Pediatrics 35: 980–988

Nagington J, Wreghitt TG, Gandy G, Roberton NRC, Berry PJ (1978) Fatal Echo 11 infections in outbreak in special care baby unit. Lancet II: 725–728

Nahamias A, Alford CA, Korones SB (1970) Infection of the newborn with herpesvirus hominis. Adv Pediatr 17: 185–226

Odievre M, Martin JP, Hadchouel M, Alagille D (1976) a_1 Antitrypsin deficiency and liver disease in children: phenotypes, manifestations and prognosis. Pediatrics 57: 226–231

Opitz JM, Howe JJ (1969) The Meckel syndrome (dysencephalia splanchnocystica, the Gruber syndrome). Birth Defects 5: 167–179

Oppenheimer EH, Esterly JR (1975) Hepatic changes in young infants with cystic fibrosis: possible relation to focal biliary cirrhosis. J Pediatr 86: 683–689

Oppenheimer EH, Hardy JB (1971) Congenital syphilis in the newborn infant: clinical and pathological obser-

vations in recent cases. Johns Hopkins Med J 129: 63–82
Palmer AK, Heywood R (1974) Pathological changes in the rhesus fetus associated with the oral administration of chenodeoxycholic acid. Toxicology 2: 239–242
Palmer RH (1972) Bile acids, liver injury and liver disease. Arch Intern Med 130: 606–617
Peden VH, Witzleben CL, Skelton MA (1971) Total parenteral nutrition. J Pediatr 78: 180–181
Peevy KJ, Wiseman HJ (1982) Gall bladder distension in septic neonates. Arch Dis Child 57: 75–76
Peters R L (1981) Early development of the liver: a review. In: Fisher MM, Roy CC (eds) Pediatric liver disease. Plenum Press, New York, pp 1–16
Philip AGS, Larson EJ (1973) Overwhelming neonatal infection with ECHO 19 virus. J Pediatr 82: 391–397
Poley JR, Dower JC, Owen CA, Stickler GB (1964) Bile acids in infants and children. J Lab Clin Med 63: 838–846
Postuma R, Trevenen C (1979) Liver disease in infants receiving total parenteral nutrition. Pediatrics 63: 110–115
Potter EL, Craig JM (1976) Pathology of the fetus and the infant, 3rd edn. Year Book Publishers, New York, pp 393–425
Purdham DR, Purdham PA, Wood BSB, George, RH, Martin AJ (1976) Severe Echo 19 virus infection in a neonatal unit. Arch Dis Child 51: 634–636
Raga J, Chrystal V, Coovadia HM (1984) Usefulness of clinical features and liver biopsy in diagnosis of disseminated herpes simplex infection. Arch Dis Child 59: 820–824
Rager R, Finegold H (1975) Choiestasis in immature newborn infants. Is parenteral alimentation responsible? J Pediatr 86: 264–269
Rawls, WE, Shorter RG, Hermann EC (1964) Fatal neonatal illness associated with ECHO 9 (Coxsackie A-23) virus. Pediatrics 33: 278–280
Reuss A von (1908) Zuckerauscheidung im Sauglingsalter. Wien Med Wochenschr 58: 799–803
Ruebner BH, Blankenberg TA, Burrows DA, Soohoo W, Lund JK (1990) Development and transformation of the ductal plate in the developing human liver. Pediatr Pathol 10: 55–68
Rushton DI (1981) Fetal and neonatal liver disease. Diagn Histopathol 4: 17–48
Rutledge JC (1989) Progressive neonatal liver failure due to type C Niemann Pick disease. Pediatr Pathol 9: 779–784
Sandberg DH (1970) Bile acid concentrations in serum during infancy and childhood. Pediatr Res 4: 262–267
Schweitzer IL, Wing A, McPeak C, Spears, RL (1972) Hepatitis and hepatitis associated antigen in 56 mother infant pairs. JAMA 220: 1092–1095
Seller MJ (1978) Meckel syndrome and prenatal diagnosis of neural tube defects. J Med Genet 15: 462–465
Sharp HL, Peller J, Carey JB, Krivit W (1971) Primary and secondary bile acids in meconium. Pediatr Res 5: 274–279
Shirake K (1970) Hepatic cell necrosis in the newborn. Am J Dis Child 119: 395–400
Silver MM, Beverly DW, Valberg LS, Cutz E, Phillips MJ, Shahed WA (1987) Perinatal hemochromatosis. Clinical morphologic and quantitative iron studies. Am J Pathol 128: 538–554
Silver MM, Cave CT, Kirpalani H (1989) Perinatal hemochromatosis. Pediatr Pathol 9: 203–210
Silverberg J, Solomon L, Erlich JC (1971) The hepatotoxic effects of lithocholic acid in the newborn hamster. Gastroenterology 60: 753(A)
Talbot IC, Mowat AP (1975) Liver disease in infancy. Histological features and relationship to a_1 antitrypsin phenotype. J Clin Pathol 28: 529–536
Tarlow MJ (1979) Metabolic liver disease. In: Chandra RK (ed) The liver and biliary system in infants and children. Churchill-Livingstone, Edinburgh, pp 196–218
Teichberg S, Markowitz J, Silverberg M et al. (1982) Abnormal cilia in a child with the polysplenia syndrome and extrahepatic biliary atresia. J Pediatr 100: 399–401
Thaler M (1964) Fatal neonatal cirrhosis. Entity or end result? A comparative study of 24 cases. Pediatrics 33: 721–734
Touloukian R, Downing S (1973) Cholestasis associated with long term parenteral hyperalimentation. Arch Surg 106: 58–63
Turkel SB, Swanson V, Chandrasoma P (1983) Malformations associated with congenital absence of the gall bladder. J Med Genet 20: 445–449
Valman HB, France NE, Wallis PG (1971) Prolonged neonatal jaundice in cystic fibrosis. Arch Dis Child 46: 805–809
Wade-Evans T (1961) Thrombi in the hepatic sinusoids of the newborn and their relation to pulmonary hyaline membrane formation. Arch Dis Child 36: 282–292
Watkins JB, Ingall D, Szczepanik P, Klein PD, Lester R (1973) Bile salt metabolism in the newborn. N Engl J Med 298: 431–434
Watson GH, Miller V (1973) Arteriohepatic dysplasia: familial pulmonary arterial stenosis with liver disease. Arch Dis Child 48: 459–466
Wilkinson EJ, Raab K, Browning CA, Hosty TA (1974) Familial hepatic cirrhosis in infants associated with a_1 antitrypsin ZS phenotype. J Pediatr 85: 159–164
Witzleben C (1979) Extrahepatic biliary atresia: concepts of cause, diagnosis and management. In: Rosenberg HS, Bolande RP (eds) Perspectives in pediatric pathology, vol 5. Masson, New York, pp 41–62
Witzleben CL (1981) Neonatal liver disease. In: Naeye RL, Kissane JM, Kaufman N (eds) Perinatal diseases. Williams and Wilkins, Baltimore, pp 346–368
Witzleben CL (1982) Bile duct paucity ("intrahepatic atresia"). In: Rosenberg HS, Bernstein J (eds) Perspectives in pediatric pathology, vol 7. Masson, New York, pp 185–201
Witzleben C, Buck B, Schnaufer L, Broszko L (1978) Studies in the pathogenesis of biliary atresia. Lab Invest 38: 525–532
Wright DJM, Berry CL (1974) Liver involvement in congenital syphilis. Br J Vener Dis 50: 241
Wright HT Jr, Okuyama K, McAllister RM (1963) An infant fatality associated with Coxsackie B1 virus. J Pediatr 63: 428–431
Young NA (1976) Chickenpox, measles and mumps. In: Remington JS, Klein JO (eds) Infectious diseases of the fetus and newborn infant. Saunders, Philadelphia, pp 521–586
Yu SS, Walker-Smith JA, Burnard ED (1971) Neonatal hepatitis in premature infants simulating hereditary tyrosinosis. Arch Dis Child 46: 306–309
Zimmermann A, Bachman C, Colombo JP (1981) Ultrastructural pathology in congenital defects of the urea cycle: ornithine transcarbamylase and carbamyl phosphate synthetase deficiency. Virchows Arch [Pathol Anat] 393: 321–331

Chapter 17

The Respiratory System

Steve J. Gould

Introduction

One of the most critical events of birth is the conversion of the fluid-filled lung, unimportant to fetal intrauterine existence, into a hollow organ distended with air and capable of gaseous exchange sufficient to support life. Indeed, it has been argued that the major determinant of perinatal survival is respiratory function (Wigglesworth and Desai 1982).

The failure to make this conversion adequately may lead, directly or indirectly, to infant death and the pathologist will often need to assess the contribution made by respiratory inadequacy to the sequence of events leading to death. In the preterm infant, problems are mainly related to pulmonary immaturity and associated therapy. In the mature infant, birth asphyxia primarily results in cerebral damage but can engender significant respiratory complication when associated with aspiration of meconium. Even in stillbirths, where primary pulmonary pathology is rarely a cause of death, poor lung growth and maturation may point to the presence of pathology elsewhere. Consequently, adequate pathological investigation of the fetal or infant respiratory system is critical in any perinatal autopsy.

Examination of the Respiratory System

Pneumothoraces can be identified by radiology, although some caution is needed in interpretation of other pulmonary changes because of post-mortem absorption of air. Where this is not available, the more conventional approach to diagnosing pneumothorax can be used by releasing pleural air under water. This can often be achieved easily by immersing the whole infant thorax under water.

Choanal patency can be tested by passing a probe through each of the nares in turn and ensuring it reaches the nasopharynx. Inspection of the mouth may reveal palatal clefts and whether they involve the hard or soft portions. The larynx and major airways can be opened conventionally by a posterior longitudinal incision, but where histology will be important, it is frequently of value to fix the larynx whole, and cut it transversely into three or four blocks for processing and step or serial histological sectioning (Gould and Howard 1985).

Lungs should be removed with the heart to allow inspection of the pulmonary arterial and venous system. The lower borders of the lungs and heart should be approximately at the same level; if they are not, it is often an indication of lung hypoplasia. Lung weights followed by calculation of lung to body weight ratios are the simplest and most useful guide to the normality of lung growth or otherwise (see below). Inflating the lung with formalin instilled through the airways can be valuable, particularly in assessing maturity. The precise diagnosis of lung pathology macroscopically is difficult and histology is mandatory, with at least one block from each main lobe.

Normal Development

The respiratory system can be divided developmentally into upper and lower tracts. Whilst histoanatomic discussion inevitably dominates the approach to respiratory development, it is important to consider the maturation of vital biochemical pathways, the immaturity of which contribute significantly to the postnatal morbidity and mortality of preterm infants.

Upper Respiratory Tract

The nose and mouth commence development at 5 weeks post-conceptional age and are derived from five main facial processes; a fused pair of frontonasal prominences, paired maxillary processes and paired mandibular processes. The maxillary processes fuse with the frontonasal processes and their medial point of fusion becomes the philtrum of the upper lip. Caudally, the mandibular processes fuse and the intervening space between mandibular and maxillary processes becomes the primitive mouth, or stomatodeum. On either side of the midline of the frontonasal process, thickening of the epithelium forms circular nasal discs or placodes, each of which recedes from the surface due to a combination of active invagination and proliferation of surrounding mesenchyme. Ultimately this burrowing activity forms the anterior nares (Ferguson 1991). The newly developed nasobuccal membrane separating the nose from the mouth breaks down posteriorly at 7 weeks to form the communicating posterior choanal space. Anteriorly, the bucconasal membrane ultimately remains as the primary palate, the remainder being replaced by the secondary or definitive palate derived from horizontal palatine processes. Fusion commences at the primary palate and extends rostrally.

The larynx develops separately but at the same time from the endodermal lining of the laryngotracheal tube and the mesenchyme of the 4th to 6th branchial arches. A diverticulum forms in the ventromedial aspect of the foregut at day 20, and gives rise to the larynx, trachea and lungs. Separation of the larynx and trachea from the oesophagus occurs by ingrowth of tissue to form the tracheo-oesphageal septum. During development, proliferation of mesenchyme in the lateral wall of the larynx partially obliterates the lumen for a time. Final recanalisation occurs between the 8th and 10th weeks of gestation (Hamilton et al. 1972; Zaw-Tun 1988).

Lower Respiratory Tract

As described above, the trachea becomes separated from the oesophagus by the tracheo-oesophageal septum. After initial branching, the bronchial tree forms by dichotomous division, which is completed by 17 weeks of gestation.

Conventionally, fetal lung development is divided into three main phases (Hislop and Reid 1974) although more recent data would argue for a fourth.

Pseudoglandular phase (7–17 weeks). Major lung components develop including bronchial glands, cartilage and, towards the end of this period, ciliated epithelium. The preacinar branching is completed by 17 weeks, faster in the right than the left lung, but airways terminate in blind-ending tubes, and are lined by low columnar or cuboidal epithelium containing glycogen (Fig. 17.1). Mesenchyme is abundant but capillaries are sparse and not closely apposed to epithelium. Respiration is not possible at this stage.

Canalicular phase (17–24 weeks). Tubules begin to dilate and the mesenchymal tissues become more vascularised. The epithelial cells are characterised by abundant glycogen initially but from about 20 weeks, and associated with differentiation, glycogen diminishes. Type 1 pneumocytes, stretched over capillaries, are identifiable by 22 weeks and type 2 cells shortly afterwards (McDougal and Smith 1975) (Fig. 17.2). By the end of this period, capillaries are pushing into the airways, the first blood–air barriers are forming and respiration just becomes possible (Fig. 17.3).

Terminal sac phase (24 weeks–term). This designation was based on the concept that true alveoli did not develop until after birth. However, it is now recognised that alveoli are present from about 32 weeks' gestation and up to 20%–30% of the adult number have developed by term (Langston et al. 1984; Hislop et al. 1986). Arguably, therefore, an alveolar or fourth

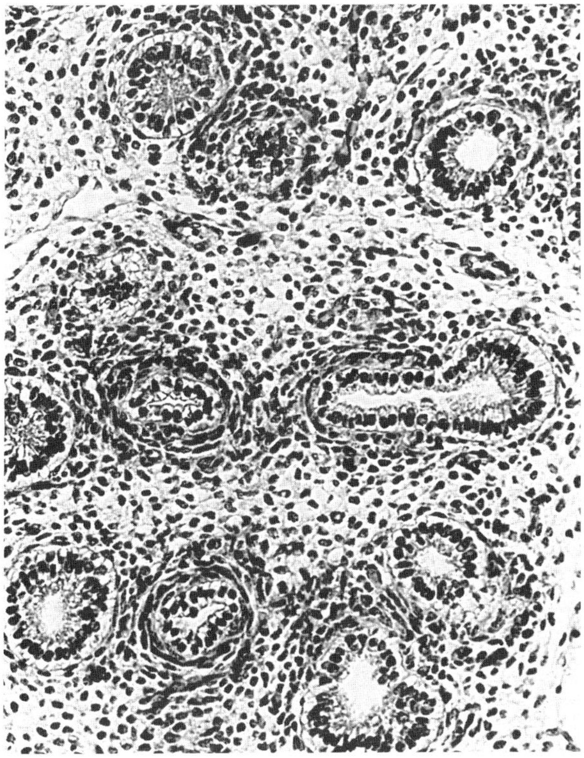

Fig. 17.1. Lung from a 13-week spontaneous abortion showing pseudoglandular development.

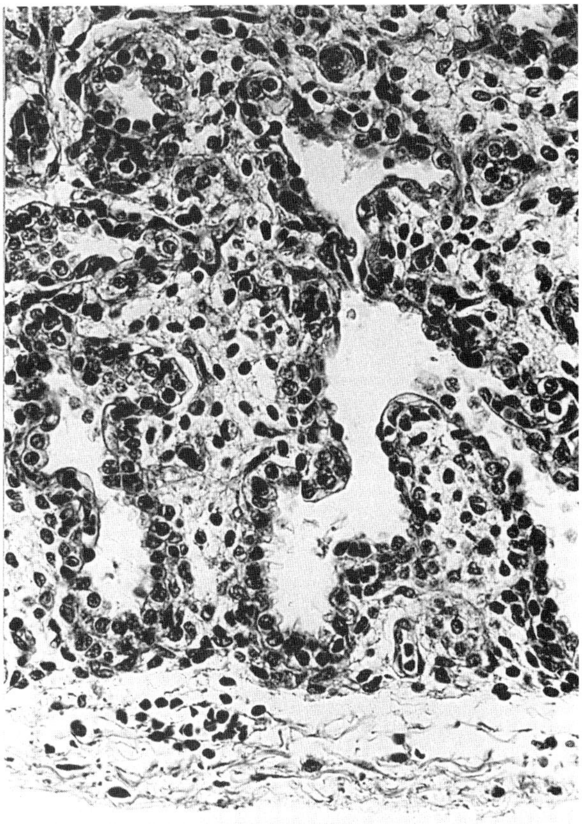

Fig. 17.3. Late canalicular stage lung at 23 weeks' gestation. Capillaries are starting to push into the airways, pulmonary epithelium is becoming attenuated and blood–air barriers are recognisable. Epithelium at distal sites, adjacent to the pleura remain cuboidal.

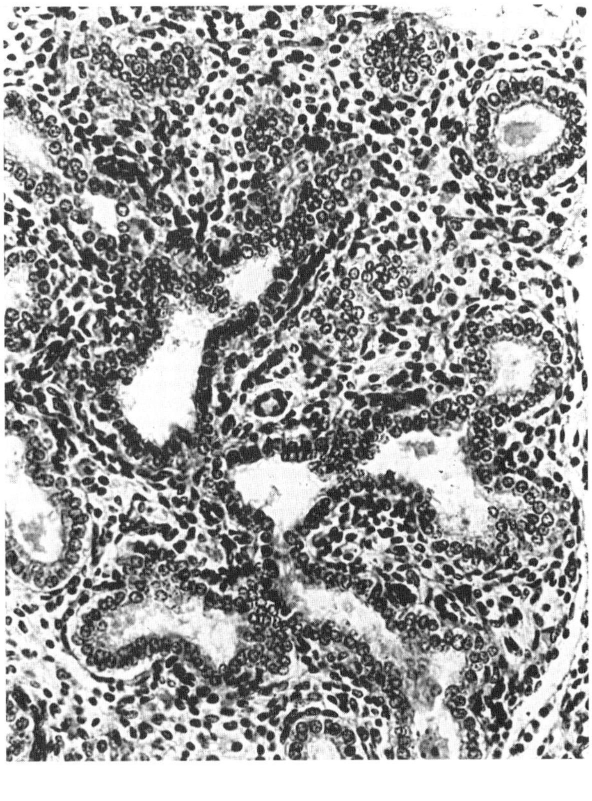

Fig. 17.2. Early canalicular stage of development at 17 weeks' gestation. Vascularity is still poor and there is no blood–air barrier formation.

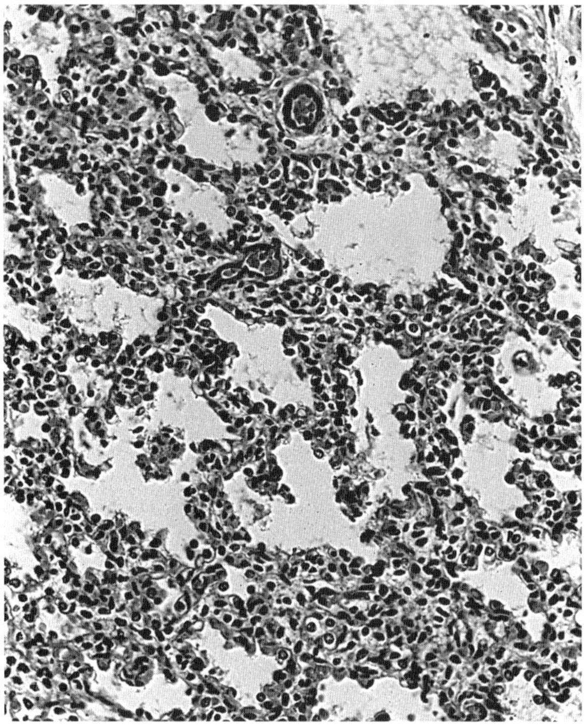

Fig. 17.4. Terminal sac development at 28 weeks' gestation. Mesenchyme is less prominent and vascularisation more marked.

phase of lung development could be considered to start at 32 weeks of gestation. It continues to about 8 years of age.

A characteristic of the terminal sac phase is the rapid differentiation of type 1 and type 2 pneumocytes (Fig. 17.4). The development of the former is reflected in the increasing numbers of blood–air barriers and surface area available for gaseous exchange, the latter in production of surfactant, a complex surface active secretion formed of phospholipid and protein. The lung interstitium diminishes and by term, there is little residual mesenchyme between respiratory units.

Biochemical and Physiological Maturation

It is clear that the simple physical process of blood–air barrier formation permitting rapid diffusion of gases to and from the pulmonary vasculature, and recognisable microscopically, is an important prerequisite for the transition to extrauterine life. However, successful transition is also dependent on the concurrent maturation of specific biochemical enzyme systems. Whilst not readily assessable by the pathologist, an awareness of them can assist in the understanding of the problems of early neonatal life which produce respiratory difficulties, particularly in the preterm infant. Three main systems have been studied, although only a brief outline will be presented.

Surfactant. Synthesised by type 2 pneumocytes, surfactant is a compound formed mainly of phospholipid (80%; 50% of which is dipalmitoylphosphatidylcholine), cholesterol (10%), and protein (10%). Glucocorticoids, possibly acting synergistically with thyroid hormones, stimulate pulmonary fibroblasts to produce fibroblast pneumocyte factor (FPF). FPF causes pulmonary epithelia to differentiate into type 2 pneumocytes, indicated by an increased capacity to produce surfactant (Smith and Post 1989). In vitro this occurs rapidly (<60 min), suggesting a post-translational effect. Glucocorticoids may also stimulate the de novo synthesis of fatty acids, used by type 2 pneumocytes to produce surfactant (Rooney 1989). Of interest, androgens appear to block FPF production and this might partly account for the increased risk of respiratory distress in male infants.

Type 2 pneumocytes store surfactant in lamellar bodies which are secreted onto the alveolar surface by exocytosis to form a monolayer of surface active material. Production and secretion appears to be further stimulated after birth by mechanical factors such as lung expansion (Wright and Clements 1987). Once secreted, turnover is rapid and approximately 10%–30% is replaced per hour. The means by which surfactant is removed is not clear but there is evidence that alveolar macrophages are involved and recycling occurs (Mendelson and Boggaram 1989).

Lung liquid secretion. The fetal lung is filled by a liquid, the production of which starts early in gestation and normally terminates only in the early stages of labour. Pulmonary epithelium actively secretes chloride ions into the duct lumen and this passage of negative ions is accompanied by sodium and water (Olver and Strang 1974). At birth, lung liquid secretion needs to cease and that already present to be absorbed. Adrenaline, to which pulmonary epithelium becomes increasingly sensitive as term approaches, appears to control this latter aspect (Brown et al. 1983). Its action on chloride transport is unclear, but adrenaline may open sodium channels and stimulate active sodium transport from the alveolar lumen (Walters and Ramsden 1987). Where there is a failure of this process, persistence of lung liquid may cause transient neonatal respiratory distress. Of greater importance to the pathologist, is the evidence which indicates that the secretion of lung liquid and its *gradual* loss into the amniotic fluid is vital to normal lung growth (Nicolini et al. 1989).

Anti-oxidant enzymes. Oxygen, even at normal inspired concentrations, is damaging to lung epithelium and endothelium because of the production of toxic radicals. Evolution has provided a number of defence mechanisms including some vitamins (A, C and E), and enzymes such as superoxide dismutase, catalase and glutathione peroxidase. Under normal circumstances, fetal lung is only exposed to low oxygen tensions, and consequently antioxidant enzyme levels are relatively low. In parallel with those of surfactant, antioxidant enzyme systems mature with gestation and reach a peak at term (Frank and Sosenko 1987). Recent evidence suggests that resistance/susceptibility to oxygen is determined less by baseline levels of anti-oxidant enzymes than the response of those enzymes to hyperoxia. A deficient response has been detected in the prematurely born (Frank and Sosenko 1991).

Pulmonary Vascular Changes at Birth

Only some 10%–12% of cardiac output passes through the pulmonary vasculature in utero, most bypassing it via the ductus arteriosus and foramen ovale. Intrapulmonary arteries are thick-walled and endothelial cells are plump and overlap. At birth, the closure of the ductus and foramen ovale is associated with a rapid increase in pulmonary blood flow. To cope with this, and partly under the influence of increased oxygen tensions, pulmonary arteries dilate, vessel walls become thinner and endothelial cells are stretched and appear flatter. More muscular arteries are "recruited" to the pulmonary circulation so that the cross-sectional area of the precapillary bed rises. This allows an increase in cardiac output through the pulmonary vasculature, but without a parallel rise in pulmonary vascular resistance. Over a period of weeks, these changes are "fixed" structurally, by smooth muscle hyperplasia, increases in the connective tissue of the media and an increase in the internal elastic lamina (Haworth 1988).

Developmental Anomalies

Upper Respiratory Tract

Anterior and Posterior Nares

Total absence of the nose may result from failure of development of the nasal placodes or occur as part of a wider range of cerebrocranial abnormalities (Gifford et al. 1972). More often the nose is replaced by a blind-ending proboscis or lies superior to a single fused orbit. Many of these midline defects are associated with trisomy 13 (p. 561).

Attempts at passing a probe through the nares into the nasopharynx may reveal the presence of choanal atresia which may be unilateral. It can be an isolated finding or be part of a wide range of anomalies including those of the ear, eye, cardiac defects such as Fallot's tetralogy and cerebral abnormalities (CHARGE association) (Pagon and Graham 1981).

Lips and Palate

Clefts of the lip and palate are frequently seen together although they may occur in isolation. Failure of the maxillary process to fuse with the nasal prominence gives rise to a lateral cleft and involvement of the alveolar margin can also be found. As with many midline facial lesions, trisomy 13 is a frequent underlying cause although there is a considerable list of potential associations and syndromes (Winter et al. 1988) (p. 564).

Larynx

Laryngeal atresia. This may occur at any level within the larynx (Smith and Bain 1965), although there always appears to be some involvement of the supraglottic region. Atresias have been classified in different ways (Smith and Bain 1965; Zaw-Tun, 1988) but the classifications are based on the varying

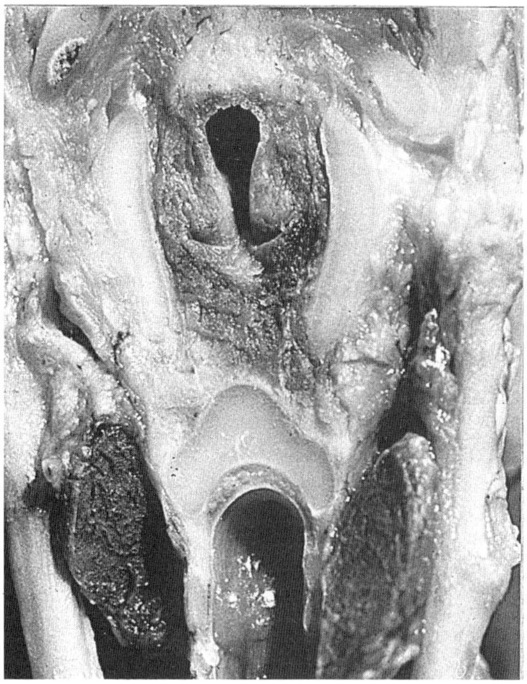

Fig. 17.5. Laryngeal stenosis. Coronal slice through the larynx shows an abnormal bar of cartilage obstructing the lumen. (Courtesy of Dr S. Knowles.)

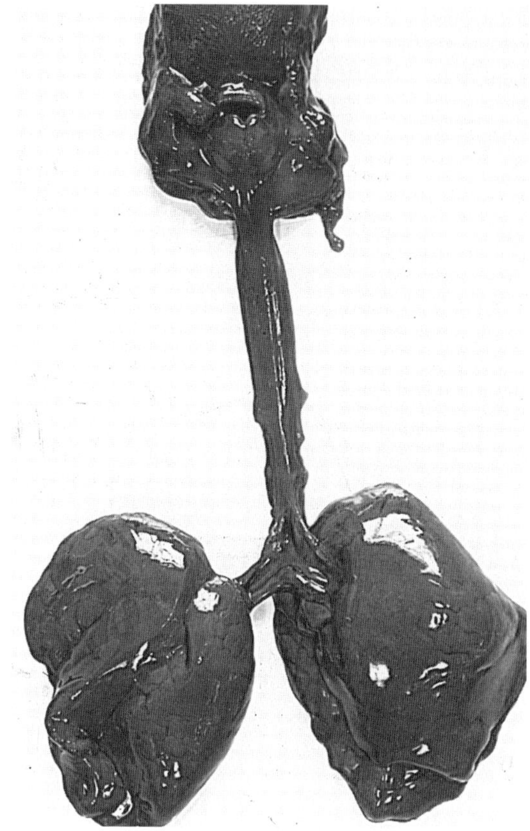

Fig. 17.6. Tracheal agenesis in a 34-week gestation stillbirth. Laryngeal inlet appears relatively normal despite the absence of airway below the cricoid and the bronchi are arising directly from the oesophagus. Both lungs are of normal size.

presence of recognisable laryngeal structures and the extent of any lumen. Laryngeal atresia represents an arrest of normal development when there is failure of recanalisation of the lumen during the 8th to 10th weeks of gestation, after it has been obliterated by proliferation of pharyngeal mesoderm (Zaw-Tun 1988). The most common type (type 3), representing a late failure of recanalisation, is a "web" at the level of the vocal cords but which sometimes includes the false cords. Of interest, the lungs in the severe forms of atresia may be hyperplastic due to failure of lung liquid to eflux normally from the developing alveoli (p. 415).

Laryngeal stenosis. Excluding laryngeal webs, which for pathogenetic reasons are discussed under atresia, most laryngeal stenoses are below the true vocal cords in the subglottis. Stenosis may be soft, due to fibrous tissue and mucous gland overgrowth, or hard (Fig. 17.5), due to cricoid cartilage overgrowth (McMillan and Duvall 1968), an abnormally shaped cricoid or even a displaced first tracheal ring (Tucker et al. 1979). The laryngeal inlet may appear normal (Fig. 17.6).

Laryngeal clefts. Occasionally, clefts are anterior but most laryngeal clefts are in the midline posteriorly and represent a failure of fusion of the tracheo-oesophageal septum. They have been classified into: type 1, involving larynx only; type 2, partial cleft involving larynx and upper trachea; type 3, complete cleft involving trachea as far down as the carina (Lim et al. 1979). Neonates often suffer from stridor and/or respiratory distress. Mortality is high and surgery is required for type 2 and 3 clefts for survival. Up to 40% of type 1 clefts are associated with a tracheo-oesophageal fistula.

Laryngeal cysts. Laryngeal cysts may present with neonatal stridor (90%) or respiratory distress (55%) usually on the first day of life (Mitchell et al. 1987). They have been classified as either saccular when they are present in the laryngeal saccule or ductal, when they result from distention of obstructed ducts (De Santo et al. 1970).

Laryngomalacia. A frequent clinical though rare pathological diagnosis, laryngomalacia is one of the commonest causes of congenital laryngeal stridor (Friedman et al. 1990). Sometimes stated to be due to a soft cartilaginous framework of the larynx (Cotton and Richardson 1981), the pathology is very poorly defined and the histology may be normal. It has been suggested that stridor may result from a mild localised form of hypotonia due to neuromuscular dysfunction (Belmont and Grundfast 1984). Laryngomalacia usually resolves spontaneously during the second year.

Trachea

There are about 22 cartilaginous rings between the lower border of the larynx and the carina. Most are simple "C-shaped" transverse rings, open posteriorly, but a significant number of half-rings or Y-shaped structures are present even in normal infants (Landing and Wells 1973).

Tracheal agenesis. Tracheal agenesis may be total or segmental, usually of the lower part, and is rare, with fewer than 50 cases reported. Displacement of the tracheo-oesophageal septum either ventrally or dorsally appears to result in failure of the trachea to form and bronchi to arise from the oesophagus (Fig. 17.6) (Diaz et al. 1989). It is commonly associated with tracheo-oesophageal fistulae (Floyd et al. 1962; Bray and Lamb 1988) and other congenital abnormalities, particularly in the cardiac or genitourinary systems (McNie and Pryse-Davies 1970; Diaz et al. 1989).

Tracheal stenosis. Tracheal stenosis may present as stridor or respiratory distress in the neonate or recurrent peumonia in the older infant (Loeff et al. 1990). It can result from an intrinsic abnormality of the trachea such as a complete cartilaginous tracheal ring or a solid, funnel-shaped cartilaginous "tube". Associated anomalies are common. More frequent than intrinsic tracheal stenosis is extrinsic compression from a vascular ring encircling the trachea, such as a double aortic arch, or an abnormal vessel such as an aberrant left pulmonary artery (Fig. 17.7).

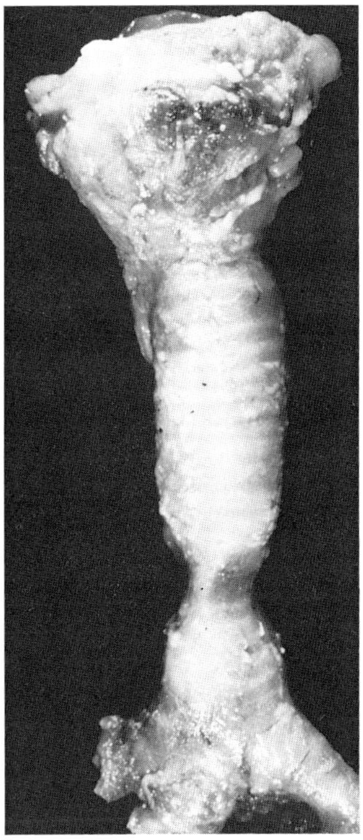

Fig. 17.7. Localised tracheal stenosis in a baby with aortic arch anomalies and congenital heart disease.

Tracheo-oesophageal fistula. A tracheo-oesophageal fistula is the most common congenital abnormality to affect the trachea, which almost invariably demonstrates abnormalities of the tracheal cartilages similar to those found in tracheomalacia. The usual variant of tracheo-oesophageal fistula is a blind-ending, upper oesophageal pouch associated with a fistulous connection between the lower oesophagus and the trachea (Holder and Wooler 1970). Tracheo-oesophageal fistula is discussed more fully in Chap. 15 (p. 349).

Tracheo- and bronchomalacia. This is due to an inadequacy of the respective cartilaginous frameworks and causes a loss of airway patency at some point in the respiratory cycle. It may present clinically as stridor and/or respiratory distress and diagnosis is made bronchoscopically by visualising airway collapse, usually during expiration. As the problem can resolve spontaneously, and is more frequent in preterm infants, it has been attributed to "immaturity" of tracheal or bronchial cartilages (Cogbill et al. 1983), implying abnormally thin or floppy cartilage. A deficit in the cartilaginous rings may be present (Gupta et al. 1968; Landing and Wells 1973). Benjamin (1984), describing the normal cartilage to soft tissue ratio as 4.5:1, states that the C-shaped cartilages in tracheomalacia are smaller and the ratio may fall to 2:1. The increase in the soft tissue posteriorly, allows anteroposterior collapse of the airway. Familial malacia is recorded (Agosti et al. 1974) and an association with other congenital abnormalities, particularly congenital heart disease, is common.

Secondary tracheomalacia, in this context implying acquired damage to the trachea, is a rare complication of chronically ventilated preterm infants. Damage to the cartilaginous framework is presumed to occur from recurrent tracheal infection or possibly trauma from the endotracheal tube (Sotomayer et al. 1986).

Lower Respiratory Tract

Bronchial Abnormalities

Abnormalities of bronchial segmentation may be extra- or intrapulmonary. Invariably associated with congenital heart disease and/or other malformations (Landing 1984; Stewart et al. 1984; Devine et al. 1991), the commonest extrapulmonary anomaly is that of isomerism in which bronchial development is similar on both sides (either left or right). Bronchial stenosis is usually caused by pressure from or enlargement of another viscus. Atresia is rare but apical if it occurs. The lung distal to an atresia may show changes akin to type 3 adenomatoid malformation.

Pulmonary Agenesis

Total pulmonary agenesis is extremely rare (Ostor et al. 1978) but unilateral agenesis is encountered occasionally (Booth and Berry 1967; Engellener et al. 1989). Congenital anomalies of the VACTERL type are common associations and, it has been suggested, unilateral pulmonary agenesis may "replace" tracheo-oesophageal fistula as a component of the syndrome (Knowles et al. 1988). The solitary lung may show the normal bronchial divisions but a compensatory increase in alveolar number may produce mediastinal shift.

Pulmonary Cystic Disease

A wide variety of pulmonary abnormalities can lead to a clinical diagnosis of a congenital pulmonary cyst or cysts. The timing and nature of their clinical presentation are extremely variable, and some may be an incidental discovery at autopsy. Rarely, congenital pulmonary cystic lesions have been associated with the late development of malignant neoplasia (Ueda et al. 1977; Domitzio et al. 1990).

Bronchogenic Cysts

These are usually an incidental finding in the perinate. Considered to result from an abnormal "late" budding of the primitive tracheobronchial tree, they may be intrapulmonary, anterior mediastinal or occasionally apposed to the trachea in the neck (Ramenofsky et al. 1979). The epithelium is ciliated columnar, but squamous metaplasia can be present. Although some searching may be necessary, bronchial glands or cartilage in the cyst wall is the most reliable histological means of distinguishing bronchogenic from oesophageal cysts (Salyer et al. 1977).

Congenital Lobar Emphysema

This presents postnatally with respiratory distress due to lobar overexpansion and compression of adjacent tissues. It is usually attributed to a defect in the cartilaginous framework of the local bronchial tree. Intracardiac defects are a common association (Buntain et al. 1974).

Cystic Adenomatoid Malformation

Congenital cystic adenomatoid malformation (CCAM) may present postnatally with respiratory distress or as an incidental radiographic finding. It may sometimes be visualised in utero during routine second trimester fetal ultrasonography or as part of the investigation of fetal hydrops.

Stocker et al. (1978) have provided the classification by which most adenomatoid malformations are typed. In some cases, classification is difficult, with histology inconsistent with any of the main subtypes (Fisher et al. 1982) or

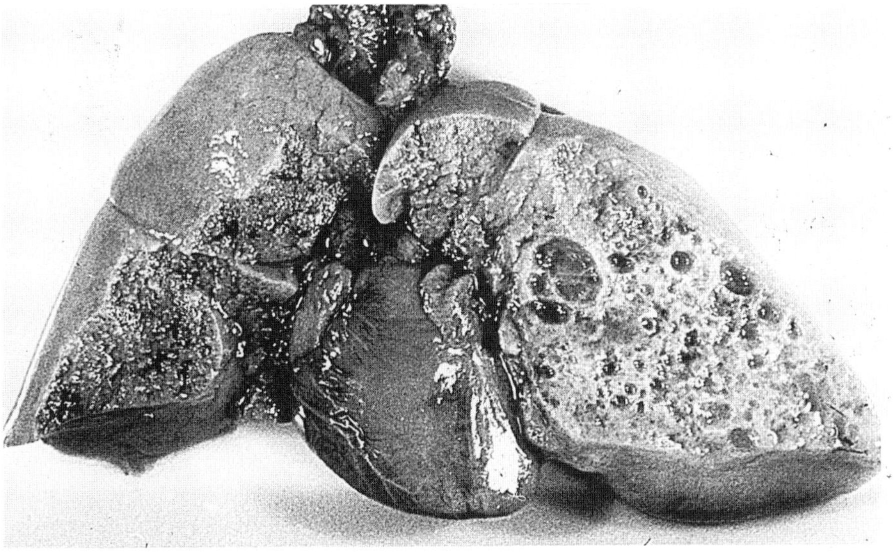

Fig. 17.8. Cystic adenomatoid malformation type 1 (CCAM, type 1) affecting most of the left lower lobe in an 18-week gestation fetus. Cysts are of variable size.

showing resemblances to other pulmonary anomalies (Bale 1979). The cyst sizes quoted below may not be appropriate to preterm infants or fetuses.

Type 1. Multiple large cysts, or single predominant cyst, usually 3–7 cm in diameter but occasionally up to 10 cm diameter, and affecting one or more lobes of one lung (Fig. 17.8). Smaller cysts may blend with adjacent normal lung and cysts communicate with the bronchial tree but distention and compression of adjacent tissue may cause mediastinal shift. Microscopically, cysts are lined by respiratory type ciliated columnar epithelium (Fig. 17.9), which may be flattened, or a mucigenic epithelium. The wall comprises a thin fibromuscular layer and small islands of cartilage may be present (Fig. 17.10). Cysts with the appearance of enlarged alveoli are interspersed between the larger cysts.

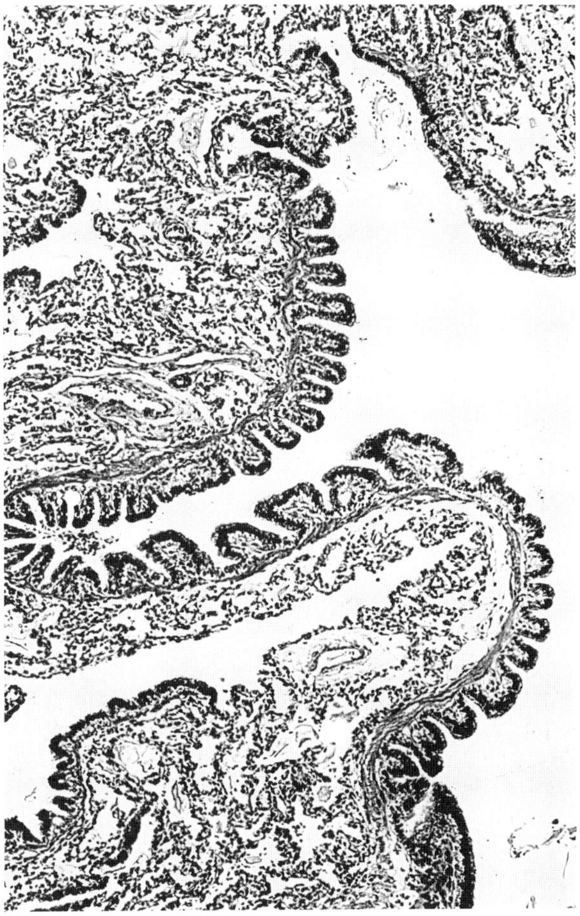

Fig. 17.9. Part of a large cyst from stillborn infant with type 1 CCAM.

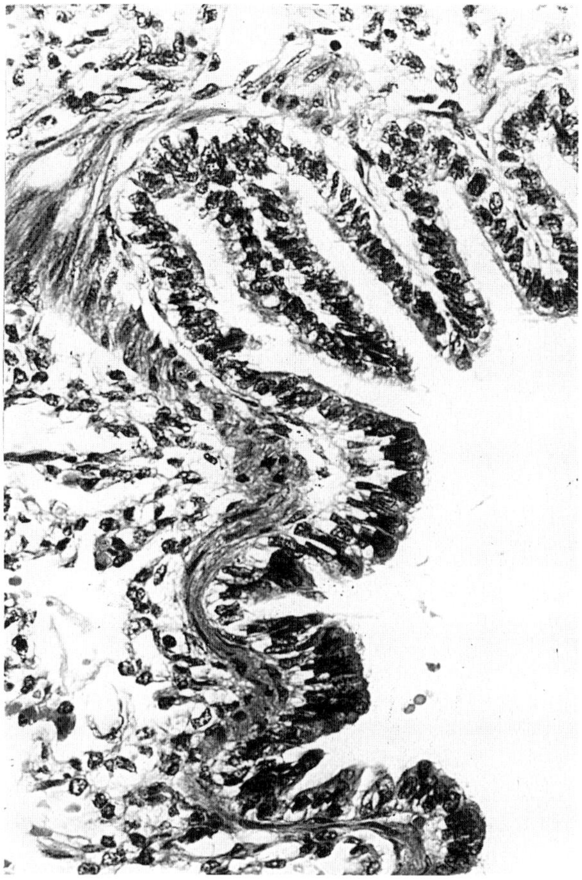

Fig. 17.10. Type 1 CCAM cyst wall. The epithelium is respiratory and a thin layer of fibrous tissue is present within the wall.

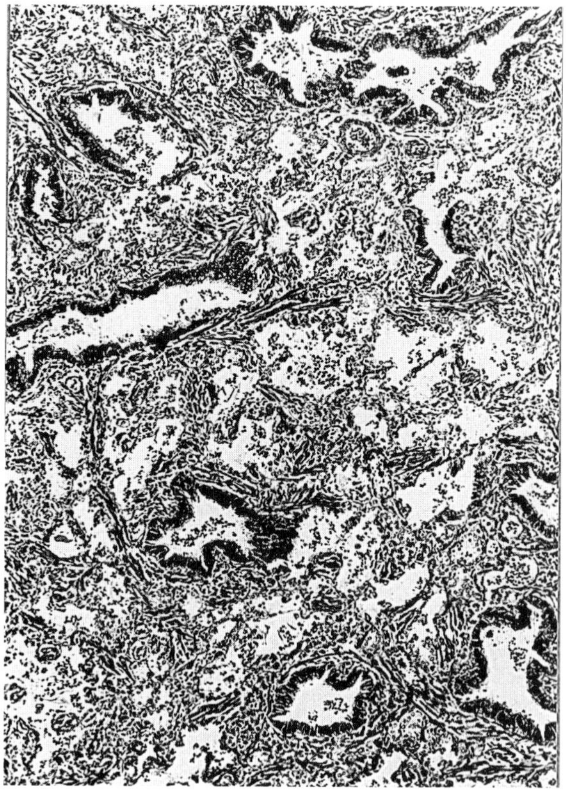

Fig. 17.11. Type 2 CCAM. Under the low power, the cysts might be mistaken for a slightly excessive number of bronchioles.

Type 2. Multiple, evenly spaced cysts, usually less than 1.2 cm, which communicate with the bronchial tree and occupy an entire lobe or, rarely, a whole lung. The cyst lining is very similar to bronchiolar epithelium and may be difficult to distinguish from normal structures except that they are present to excess (Fig. 17.11). The cyst wall is formed of a thin fibromuscular layer, but cartilage is not seen. Very occasionally striated muscle may be found, randomly distributed throughout the malformation (Fig. 17.12). Of the three main subtypes, type 2 is most commonly associated with malformation elsewhere, especially of the renal tract.

Type 3. This subtype is formed of small cysts less than 0.5 cm in diameter, involving an entire lobe. Cyst lining is ciliated cuboidal epithelium on a very thin fibromuscular layer with no cartilage or mucigenic cells. Due to the overall size of the affected lung, type 3 CCAM invariably produces mediastinal shift and carries a poor prognosis.

Lymphangiectasia

Lymphagiectasia, or cystic dilatation of pulmonary lymphatics, may be primary or secondary. The former is rare and probably results from failure of pulmonary lymphatics to establish connections with the thoracic duct (Laurence 1959; France and Brown 1971). Secondary lymphangiectasia is usually associated with cardiac malformations, particularly anomalous pulmonary venous drainage (Esterly and Oppenheimer 1970). In contrast to interstitial emphysema, which it grossly resembles and in which air is trapped in the interstitial tissues, the lungs are firm, inelastic and heavy. Bilateral pleural effusions are usual and these may

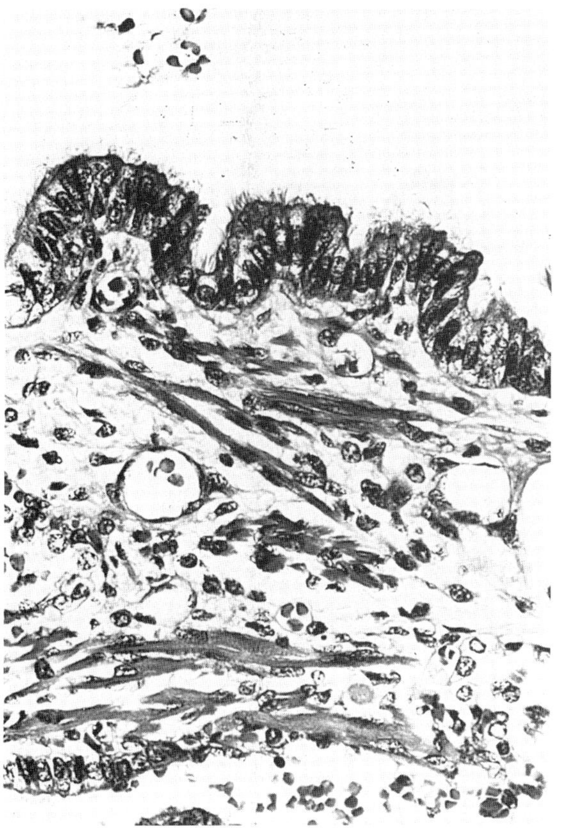

Fig. 17.12. Type 2 CCAM. The wall of this cyst contains a number of large muscle cells, the striations of which are visible.

be chylous. Histologically, dilated lymphatic spaces are present within interlobular septa, beneath the pleura and between large vessels at the hilus of the lung.

Pulmonary Sequestration

In its classic forms, sequestered lobes are abnormal masses of pulmonary tissue which do not communicate with the main pulmonary bronchial tree and are supplied by an anomalous artery arising from the descending aorta. Sequestration may be intrapulmonary, when the abnormal mass is within normal lung parenchyma, usually the left lower lobe, or extrapulmonary, when the sequestered lobe is invested by its own pleura; this can be subdiaphragmatic. Presentation of intrapulmonary sequestration is unusual in the neonatal period but extrapulmonary lobes may come to attention when associated with abnormalities such as diaphragmatic hernia. A wide range of bronchial connection, arterial supply and venous drainage is described and should be allowed for in the dissection of sequestrations (Clements and Warner 1987). The embryological origin of pulmonary sequestration is a matter of debate although there does appear to be a consensus that other bronchopulmonary abnormalities may be related (Heithoff et al. 1976; Landing and Dixon 1979; Clements and Warner 1987).

Pulmonary Heterotopias/Hamartomas

Solid hamartomas are rare anomalies and may contain cartilage and adrenal tissue (Bozic 1974). Glial and skeletal muscle masses are sometimes seen in anencephaly. Rhabdomyomatosis or diffuse heteroplasia of skeletal muscle is described and is usually associated with a cardiovascular malformation (Chi and Shong 1982; Chellam 1988; Chen et al. 1991).

Lung Hypoplasia

Although lung hypoplasia is a congenital condition, it is not a malformation, and is almost invariably secondary to pathology outside the respiratory tract. It is considered at some length, first because it is one of the most common abnormalities encountered in perinatal pathology, secondly, because of its varied pathogenesis, and thirdly, because of the impact the study of lung hypoplasia has had on the study of normal lung growth.

Lung hypoplasia is common and occurs in up to 14% of perinatal autopsies (Wigglesworth and Desai 1982). In stillbirths, it may be an incidental finding but is an important cause of death in a neonate, often within minutes or hours of birth. Occasionally, a clinical diagnosis of lung hypoplasia is not associated with immediate death and postnatal changes in the lung may make pathological confirmation of the diagnosis difficult or impossible.

In most instances, however, diagnosis is straightforward, with macroscopically small lungs in a small thoracic cage (Fig. 17.13). After removal as a block, the inferior surface of the lungs is not in line with the apex of the heart (Fig. 17.14). Another readily available

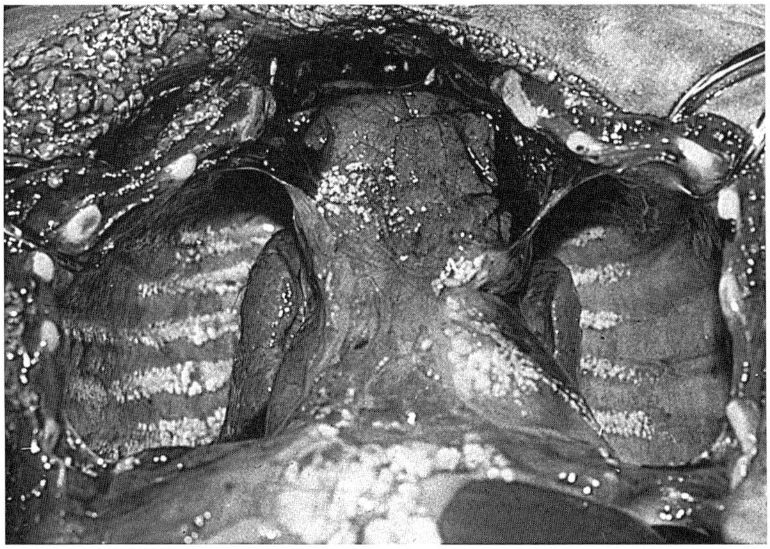

Fig. 17.13. Thoracic contents of a 33-week early neonatal death with idiopathic fetal hydrops. The pleural effusions have been removed to show marked bilateral pulmonary hypoplasia.

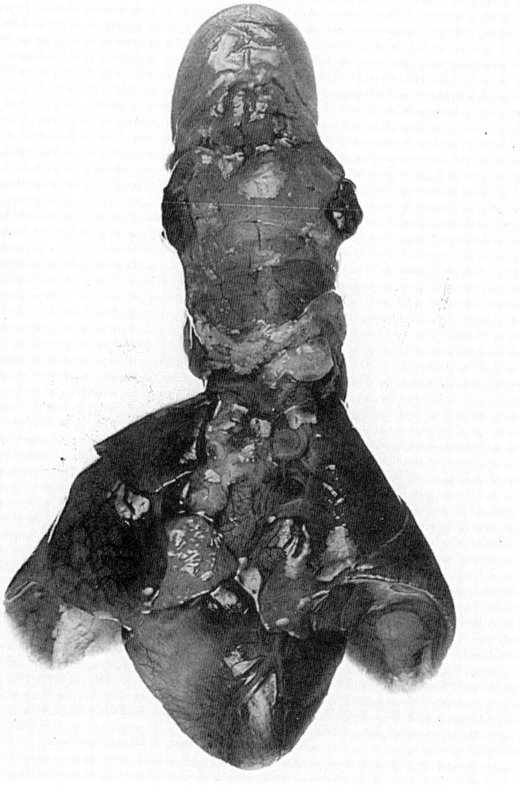

Fig. 17.14. Hypoplastic lungs in relation to the size of the heart. Normally, the inferior surfaces of the lungs and apex of the heart should all be at approximately the same level. From an early neonatal death at 26 weeks of gestation with renal agenesis.

measure is lung to bodyweight ratio. Below 28 weeks' gestation, a lung to bodyweight ratio of <0.015 and one of <0.012 at 28 weeks of gestation or more, is indicative of hypoplasia. The lungs should always be greater than 1.2% of bodyweight (Askenazi and Perlman 1979; Wigglesworth and Desai 1981). However, ratios need to be interpreted cautiously in the presence of pathology such as infection or significant postnatal survival.

Histomorphometrically, hypoplastic lungs demonstrate reduced radial alveolar counts (Emery and Mithal 1960) although this may be a difficult assessment as a "one-off" procedure and normal standards may vary (Cooney and Thurlbeck 1982).

Broadly, two patterns of histology in lung hypoplasia have been described (Wigglesworth et al. 1981). In oligohydramnios, the lungs appear immature as well as poorly grown. This manifests itself as narrow airways, retardation of epithelial differentiation and delay in development of blood–air barriers. Evidence suggests that this is due to failure of differentiation of undifferentiated cells into type 1 pneumocytes. The percentage of type 2 pneumocytes is similar in oligohydramnios-associated hypoplastic lungs compared with normal controls, although evidence of deficient surfactant production in the former suggests there may be functional impairment of this cell type (Haidar et al. 1991). In lung hypoplasia *not* associated with

Table 17.1. Mechanisms and causes of lung hypoplasia

Reduction in thoracic volume	Skeletal dysplasias	Thanatophoric dysplasia Achondrogenesis Asphyxiating thoracic dysplasia
	Pleural space lesions	Diaphragmatic hernia Pleural effusions e.g. in hydrops
Impairment of fetal breathing	CNS damage	Anencephaly involving brain stem Hypoxic-ischaemic injury
	Congenital muscular disease	Congenital muscular dystrophy
Oligohydramnios	Reduced production	Renal agenesis Renal cystic dysplasia Urinary tract obstruction
	Increased loss	Prolonged rupture of membranes

oligohydramnios, maturation is appropriate for the gestation of the infant.

Mechanisms and Causes of Lung Hypoplasia

At first glance, the long list of associations and causes of lung hypoplasia show little in common, but study of these seemingly disparate pathologies has contributed significantly to our understanding of normal lung growth (Wigglesworth, 1987a,b) such that they can be classified in a more logical manner (Table 17.1).

Adequacy of thoracic volume. Not surprisingly, for lung to grow normally it must have sufficient space in which to do so. Reduction in thoracic volume can be caused by poor rib growth, e.g. skeletal dysplasias; any space-occupying lesion e.g. an abnormal viscus associated with diaphragmatic hernia (Areechon and Reid 1963) or pleural effusion associated with hydrops.

Fetal breathing. In utero, the fetus normally makes bursts of rapid but low amplitude breathing movements, primarily diaphragmatic in origin. It is not entirely clear how or why such movements should be important to lung growth, but that they are is strongly suggested by lung hypoplasia in conditions associated with their absence, or by experimental work in which the effects of fetal breathing are negated (Liggins et al. 1981). It has been suggested they allow influx of amniotic fluid or generate important pressure changes within the thorax (Kitterman 1984; Wigglesworth 1987a).

Oligohydramnios. Oligohydramnios due either to insufficient production or excessive loss of fluid (Hislop et al. 1979; Nimrod et al. 1984), is probably the commonest recognised cause of lung hypoplasia although the mechanism is unclear. Previously thought to result from compression of the fetal thorax by the uterus, recent evidence suggests that in oligohydramnios a larger than normal pressure gradient between fetal lung and amniotic sac occurs and the efflux of fetal lung liquid is too rapid (Nicolini et al. 1989; Harding et al. 1990). Lung liquid, retained within fetal airways and developing respiratory units, might act as a "stent" around which alveoli form. The importance of intra-alveolar pressure can be seen in a rare combination of abnormalities sometimes found in Fraser's syndrome—laryngeal atresia or stenosis with renal agenesis. Despite the oligohydramnios due to renal agenesis which would be expected to cause lung hypoplasia, the lungs are not hypoplastic but are either of normal size or even hyperplastic. The laryngeal anomaly prevents the rapid loss of fetal lung liquid (Wigglesworth et al. 1987; Silver et al. 1988).

Idiopathic or primary. It is rare for a specific cause of lung hypoplasia not to emerge from careful study although instances of "primary" pulmonary hypoplasia are recorded (Swischuk et al. 1979). Before a diagnosis of idiopathic or primary lung hypoplasia is entertained, some aspects of a case may be worth reassessing. In particular, the face (Potter's facies) or placenta (amnion nodosum) for evidence of oligohydramnios and radiographs for possible skeletal dysplasia. Pathology or malformation involving the brain stem should also be specifically sought.

In some instances there is evidence that there is a genetic basis for the poor lung growth; hypoplasia has been associated with chromosomal abnormality (Page and Stocker 1982), recorded in families and sets of twins.

Acquired Pathology

Broadly, the acquired pathology of the respiratory tract can be related either to pulmonary immaturity with its associated therapy, or the consequences of birth asphyxia or infection.

Pathology of Immaturity

As discussed above, there are two aspects of pulmonary immaturity which together lead to respiratory problems: physical immaturity with inadequate surface area for efficient gaseous exchange and, as importantly, biochemical immaturity. Surfactant production may be inadequate and a lack of anti-oxidant defences may increase susceptibility to injury.

The lungs of most immature infants will demonstrate pathological changes but occasionally will be histologically normal. This is usually confined to the extremely preterm infant of around 23–25 weeks of gestation, in whom death has occurred within minutes or hours of birth. Death may be attributable to pulmonary immaturity alone.

Respiratory Distress Syndrome

The terms respiratory distress syndrome (RDS) and hyaline membrane disease are frequently used interchangeably. However, RDS should be used strictly as a clinical term describing a constellation of symptoms: increased respiratory rate, sternal and subcostal recession, cyanosis and grunting which does not resolve within 24 hours. Radiographically there may be pulmonary collapse and an air bronchogram.

The majority of cases (75%–80%) are associated with hyaline membrane disease, but, among others, it can be caused by infection, birth asphyxia, massive pulmonary haemorrhage and cerebral intraventricular haemorrhage (Wigglesworth 1977). It is possible that some babies die from other major problems before hyaline membranes develop.

Hyaline Membrane Disease

Hyaline membrane disease (HMD) is a pathological term describing the presence of eosinophilic amorphous material lining the terminal airways of the neonate. It is usually seen in the lungs of very preterm infants (Farrell and Avery 1975) and is most commonly associated with surfactant deficiency. However, it can also be associated with severe acute asphyxia, some forms of pulmonary infection and pulmonary haemorrhage. It is almost invariably accompanied by respiratory distress although the clinical syndrome may be obscured if the infant is ventilated.

HMD associated with surfactant deficiency usually presents an hour or so after birth with respiratory distress. Except the most immature, the majority of infants will survive with appropriate ventilatory therapy, unless additional pathology such as intraventricular haemorrhage supervenes. Ventilation is often required for a few days but towards the end of the first week, and presumably reflecting a resurgence in surfactant levels, ventilatory requirements decrease.

Should infants die within a few hours of onset of the disease, the lungs are collapsed, heavy and red/purple in colour, their texture resembling that of liver. Microscopically, the lungs are collapsed, but with many dilated terminal airways. Necrotic bronchial or bronchiolar epithelium is the earliest feature and may be seen before hyaline membranes develop (de la Monte et al. 1986). They may become dislodged and plug more distal airways. The eosinophilic hyaline membranes lining the terminal airways are present within an hour or so of birth and often contain nuclear debris of necrotic epithelium (Fig. 17.15). Membranes are not usually seen in the terminal sacs, which are collapsed. After a few hours the presence of a few polymorphs and macrophages is typical.

In infants dying at a day or two of age, the lungs show evidence of repair and regeneration. Macrophages ingest membrane (membranophages) but also accompany the fibroblasts proliferating beneath the hyaline membranes. Subsequently, regenerating cuboidal epithelium (type 2 pneumocytes) is apparent, often growing over residual hyaline membranes which are incorporated into the bronchiolar walls.

In some cases, the hyaline membranes may be bright yellow, particularly on the luminal surface. This is due to the incorporation of albumin-bound bilirubin into the hyaline membranes; jaundice is not always present (Blanc 1976).

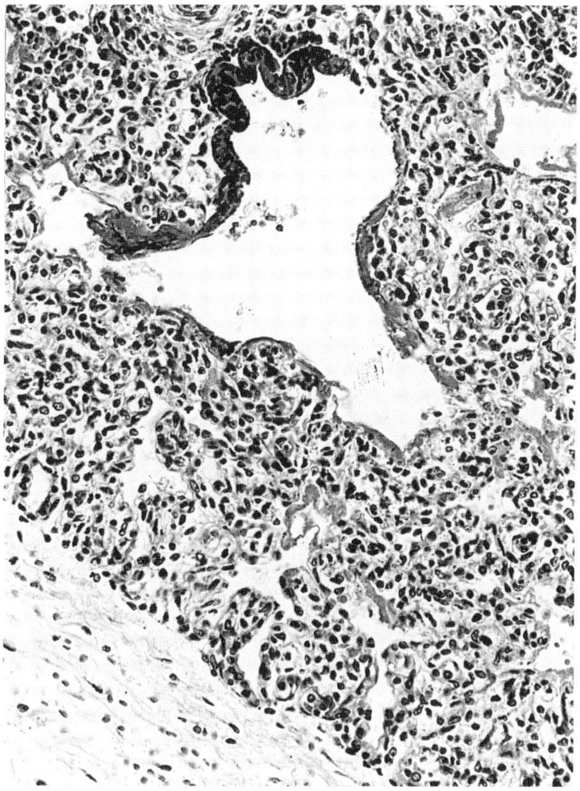

Fig. 17.15. Hyaline membrane disease in a 26-week gestation neonate dying at 12 hours of age. Necrotic respiratory bronchiolar epithelium lines part of a dilated airway. Hyaline membrane is also present at this level and more distally. In the most distal part of the lung, the air sacs adjacent to the pleura are collapsed but do not contain membrane.

Pathogenesis of Hyaline Membrane

Hyaline membranes are composed of necrotic debris and a proteinaceous precipitate of plasma, including some fibrin. The acute transudation from capillaries adjacent to the terminal airways reflects damage to epithelium and endothelium at this point, whose integrity is necessary to form an impermeable barrier between the vasculature and the airways. What produces the damage is not entirely clear. It is presumed that either in the infant's attempts to breathe or because of the positive pressure from the ventilator, the terminal airways expand and shear forces damage the lining epithelium (Robertson 1991). The toxic effect of oxygen might also contribute or the epithelial damage may reflect a "reflow" injury following a period of local ischaemia (de la Monte et al. 1986). That ischaemia may be contributory in some instances is suggested by evidence of increased pulmonary intravascular coagulation (Schmidt et al. 1992). The very terminal parts of the respiratory units, i.e. the air sacs, fail to expand because surface tension, which acts to collapse these small "spheres", is too great to overcome in the absence of surfactant.

Bronchopulmonary Dysplasia: Chronic Lung Disease

Perhaps the most intractable problem which the immature neonate may develop, usually as a consequence of HMD, is chronic ventilatory dependence. The infant may eventually die after many months either because support is withdrawn or because of the development of pulmonary hypertension and cor pulmonale. Although still in widespread use, the term bronchopulmonary dysplasia (BPD), as described by Northway et al. (1967), is not always entirely appropriate to lungs of infants with long-term ventilatory dependence. In recent years the "bronchial" component of the pathology is often minimal or even absent, and the pathology is dominated by the interstitial or vascular changes.

A more severe acute episode of respiratory disease is often the prelude to developing BPD. Although the early ventilatory requirements may fall, pulmonary permeability fails to return to normal and the infant continues to require ventilatory support. Clinically, the age at which an infant is labelled as having BPD is ill defined, as the transition from acute to chronic lung disease is gradual, but one set of criteria has been provided by O'Brodovich and Mellins (1985). An infant with BPD is one requiring some form of assisted ventilation and/or supplementary oxygen to maintain life at greater than 28 days of life, which began with an acute lung injury in the first 2 weeks of life, and in whom there are significant clinical (tachypnoea, retractions, etc.), radiological (hyperinflation or pulmonary cystic change) and blood gas abnormalities.

Pathology

Bronchiolar injury. Bronchiolar damage is characterised by an obliterative bronchiolitis often associated with squamous metaplasia and collapse of lung tissue distal to the obstructed

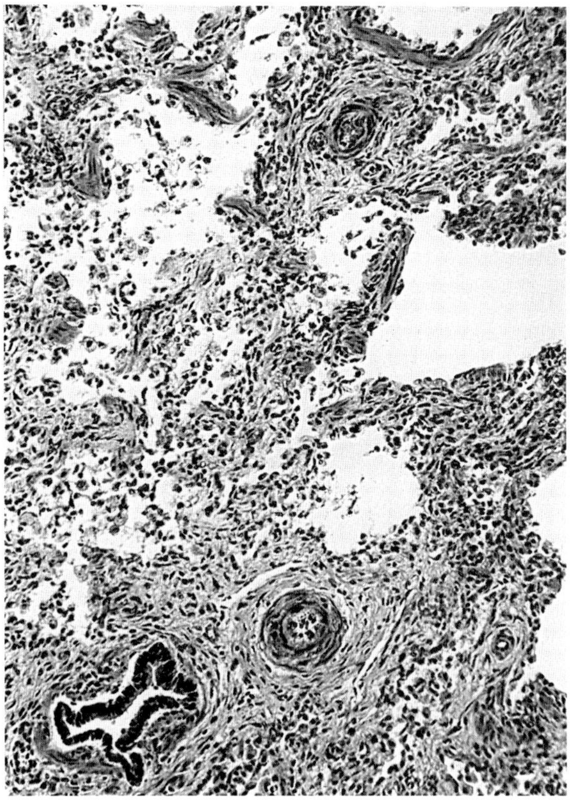

Fig. 17.16. Bronchopulmonary dysplasia in an infant dying at 3 months of age. Interstitium shows striking fibrous thickening and the small pulmonary artery is thick-walled. The adjacent terminal bronchiole is normal.

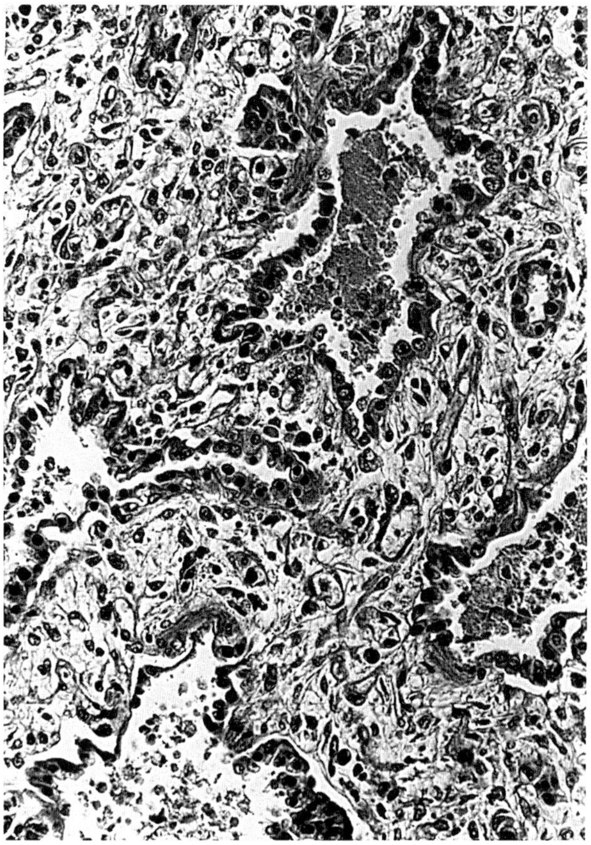

Fig. 17.17. Striking cuboidal metaplasia associated with bronchopulmonary dysplasia.

airway (Bonikos et al. 1976; Taghizadeh and Reynolds 1976). Its frequency in earlier descriptions of BPD probably reflects ventilatory management then current and the relatively high inflationary pressures. In infants who now die with chronic lung disease and demonstrate an obliterative bronchiolitis a history of severe difficulty in maintaining ventilation can usually be obtained. Morphometric study suggests that the major persistent airway lesions identifiable are bronchial gland hyperplasia and peribronchiolar smooth muscle hyperplasia (Hislop and Haworth 1989; Margraf et al. 1991).

Interstitium. The most prominent component of the lung injury is a widespread but occasionally patchy interstitial fibrosis (Fig. 17.16) associated with cuboidal metaplasia (Fig. 17.17). Fibrosis is accompanied by emphysema (Fig. 17.18) and alveoli will frequently contain macrophages. Special stains will show increase in the elastic tissue, usually in the form of thick plaques at points of bronchiolar or alveolar duct division. The interstitial damage forms a continuum with the repair processes associated with the acute lung injury.

Vasculature. Arterial muscular hypertrophy and adventitial thickening of small pulmonary arteries may be the most significant component of lung damage in ventilator-dependent infants (Fig. 17.16) (Hislop and Haworth 1990). In some cases, there is evidence of a reduction in peripheral arterial density, possibly due to failure of normal postnatal recruitment (Gorenflo et al. 1991). Eventually, pulmonary hypertension and cor pulmonale develop, although there may not always be good correlation between the occurrence of cardiac complications and the pulmonary histology.

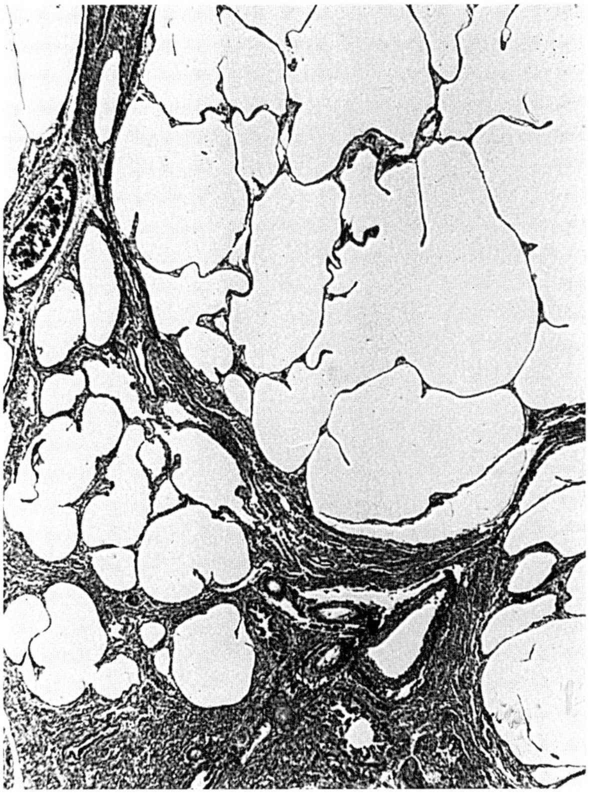

Fig. 17.18. Bronchopulmonary dysplasia. An area of emphysema.

Pathogenesis

BPD as a distinct entity emerged primarily following the introduction of ventilatory support. Two main pathogenetic factors are recognised—barotrauma and oxygen toxicity.

Barotrauma. As indicated above, high inflationary pressure may well be the most significant factor in the bronchiolar lesions although it is probably impossible to dissociate entirely the action of high pressures and oxygen toxicity (Taghizadeh and Reynolds 1976; Saugstad 1990).

Oxygen toxicity. Cellular metabolism produces oxygen-related toxic radicals such as OH^- and O_2^- and singlet oxygen. In the lung, there are probably two main sources of toxic radicals: from neutrophils or macrophages as a product of inflammation, and as a by-product of normal pulmonary epithelial or endothelial metabolism. Tissue production of free radicals will be enhanced in the presence of high oxygen concentrations and damage accentuated in the absence of normal cellular antioxidant defences. The precise mechanism by which tissue damage leads to interstitial fibrosis is unclear, but it may cause an increase in capillary permeability, and fluid leakage with subsequent organisation. Platelet-derived growth factor may be produced by the interstitium in response to hyperoxia and stimulate early fibroblast hyperplasia (Han et al. 1992). Inactivation of surfactant may also be important (Merritt 1982; Saugstad 1990).

Pulmonary Haemorrhage

In preterm infants dying during the acute phase of lung injury, some pulmonary haemorrhage is a common finding in the terminal sacs and pulmonary interstitium. Haemorrhage may also occur into the dilated pulmonary lymphatics. In some cases massive haemorrhage is a terminal event. Although the pathogenesis is not certain, pulmonary haemorrhage may represent a haemorrhagic pulmonary oedema (Cole et al. 1973) and reflect terminal heart failure.

Pathology of Therapy

Intubation

Significant acquired pathology presenting in nose, palate, larynx and trachea, other than infection, is almost confined to the trauma of endotracheal intubation.

Nasotracheal intubation can cause nasal septal deviation, ulceration or even perforation (Abbott 1968). With orotracheal intubation the palate may show grooving and clefting (Duke et al. 1976; Erenberg and Nowak 1984). Pressure from long-term contact with the tube could be responsible, although a contributing mechanism might be interference with tongue pressure on the palate by the tube, resulting in unopposed growth of the lateral palate and ridges (Hanson et al. 1976; Carillo 1985).

The larynx generally bears the brunt of the damage from the endotracheal tube, primarily because it is the narrowest part of the intubated airway. The tube lies posteriorly, directed by the triangular shape of the lumen at the vocal cords. Pressure results in ischaemic necrosis of epithelium over the arytenoid cartilages within hours of starting intubation (Bozic 1969; Rasche and Kuhns 1972; Gould and Howard 1985). Similar changes are seen in the subglottis at the level of the cricoid cartilage, because here there is a complete cartilaginous ring. Associated with the ulceration, an acute perichondritis, whose aetiology is unknown, may develop on the outer surface of the cartilages (Bozic 1969; Gould and Howard 1985).

Ulcer healing usually occurs even with the tube still in situ and thick metaplastic squamous epithelium replaces the normal respiratory epithelium (Fig. 17.19). Healing may be delayed by further trauma during tube replacement or from infection. Very preterm infants with small airways are particularly susceptible.

The most significant long-term complication of endotracheal intubation is subglottic stenosis. The pathology is poorly described but is comprised primarily of circumferential occlusion of the airway by fibrous scar tissue (Gould and Howard 1988). A possible contributing factor is severe damage to the cricoid ring leading to collapse of the cartilaginous framework (Harley 1971; Boriewiecki and Croft 1977; Gould 1988).

The trachea may also show similar lesions with ulceration followed by healing and squamous metaplasia. It is possible that some squamous metaplasia may be generated by the high inspired oxygen concentrations used in therapy. A more serious complication, though fortunately very rare, is tracheal perforation by the endotracheal tube (Serlin and Daily 1975; Schild et al. 1976).

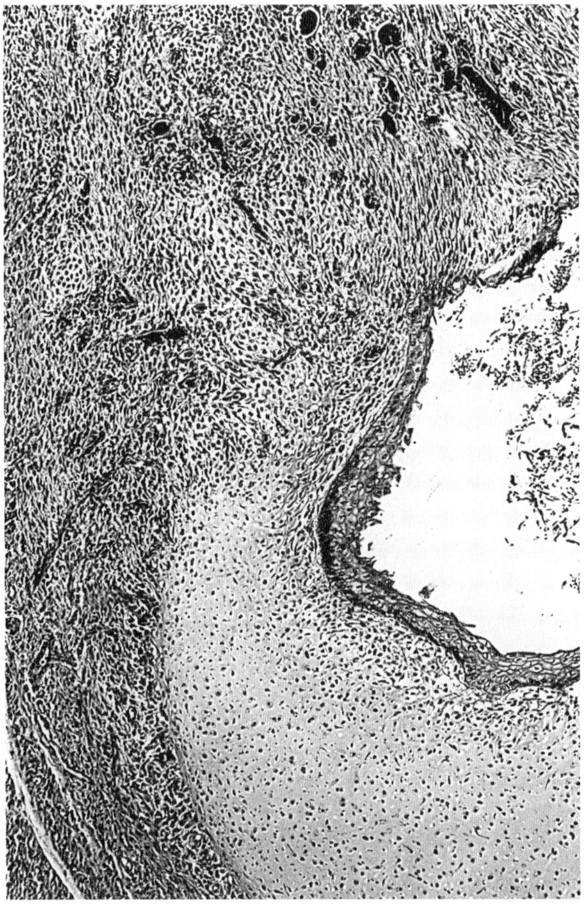

Fig. 17.19. Subglottis in an infant dying at 44 days of age having been intubated since birth. Metaplastic squamous epithelium grows almost directly onto the cricoid cartilage which has been partly destroyed.

Necrotising Tracheobronchitis

Necrotising tracheobronchitis is a relatively recently described lesion, mainly in North America, associated with the use of high-frequency jet ventilation, a technique not established in the United Kingdom for treating neonates. The lower trachea and main bronchi show superficial necrosis and inflammation distal to the tip of the endotracheal tube. The pathogenesis is not clear but may be related to excessive drying of these tissues (Boros et al. 1986; Metlay et al. 1987).

Air Leaks

The use of positive pressure to maintain lung inflation during hyaline membrane disease, may lead to tearing of delicate respiratory tissues. Air leakage into the pleural cavities can be a cause of sudden collapse (Fig. 17.20). Particularly if under tension, a pneumothorax can interfere with venous return and seriously impair cardiac output, causing intracerebral complications. Rapid drainage of air is important, but occasionally drains may damage pulmonary parenchyma.

Pulmonary interstitial emphysema (PIE), when air passes into pulmonary tissues, may track in pulmonary lymphatics and, by compression of adjacent lung, seriously impair ventilation (Fig. 17.21). Clinically, it may produce a dilemma as excessive ventilatory pressure may exacerbate PIE, whereas the same pressure may be necessary to maintain

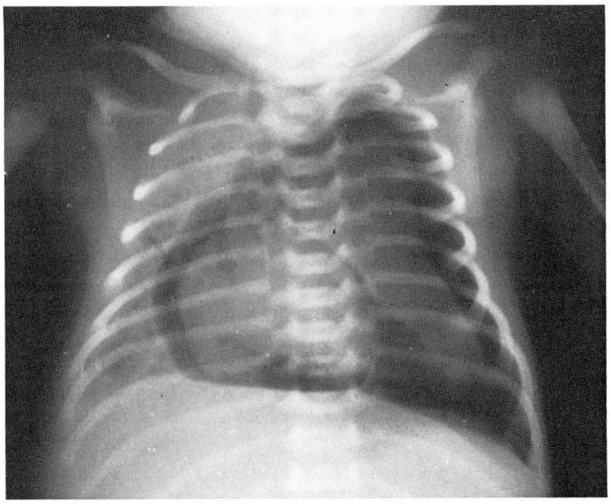

Fig. 17.20. Chest radiograph from a baby at 28 weeks' gestation; there is air within the left pleural and pericardial cavities.

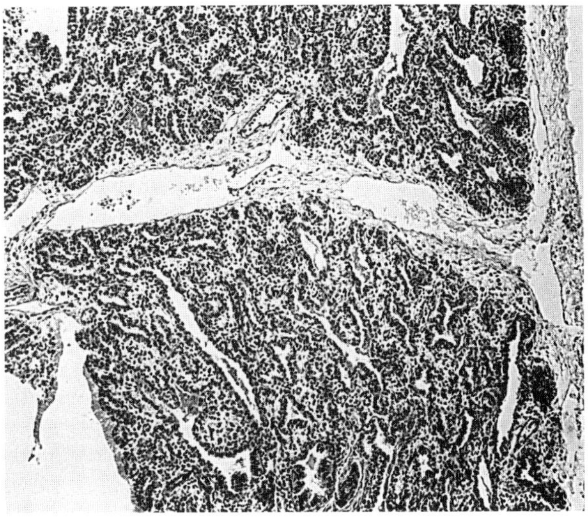

Fig. 17.21. Lung from a 25-week early neonatal death showing emphysema and air within septal lymphatics tracking to the subpleural region.

lung expansion elsewhere. Persistent PIE may loculate and stimulate a giant cell reaction and fibrosis (Fig. 17.22). Often at post-mortem, due to resorption, PIE is less impressive than the ante-mortem radiographs might lead one to expect.

Intra-Lipid Embolism

Neonates who receive intralipid as a component of parenteral nutrition may show lipid within pulmonary capillaries. Although best demonstrated by fat stains on frozen material, its presence can often be detected without special techniques. Capillaries are round and distended but are empty of red cells. On close inspection, slightly refractile material can be seen. It is probable that it has little deleterious effect in most circumstances, although there is some evidence it can interfere with oxygenation (Stahl et al. 1992) or increase the risk of BPD (Cooke 1991).

Pathology of Birth Asphyxia

Birth asphyxia typically presents in the term neonate, but may occur in the premature infant and compound the effects of organ immaturity. In stillborns, evidence of acute asphyxia may also be observed in the lungs.

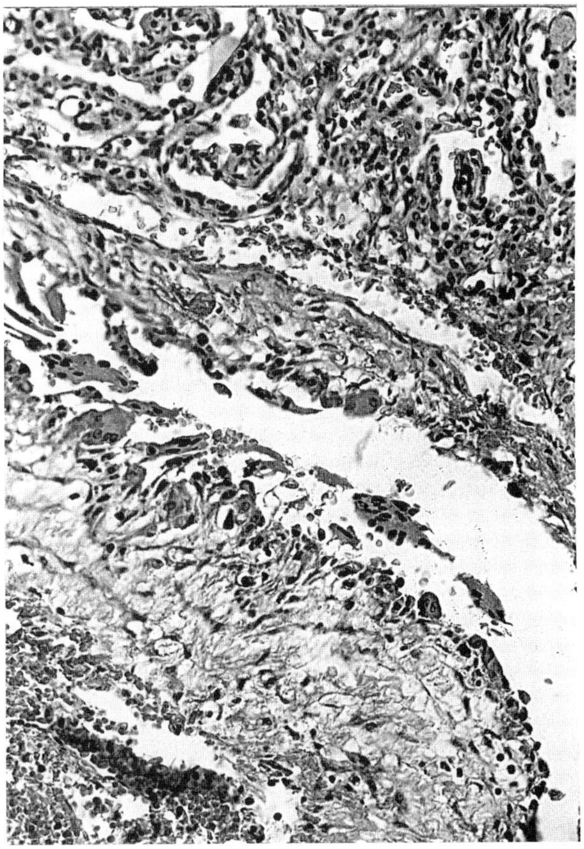

Fig. 17.22. Partially collapsed old cyst resulting from interstitial emphysema. Cyst wall is formed of thick fibrous tissue and lined by macrophages including giant cells.

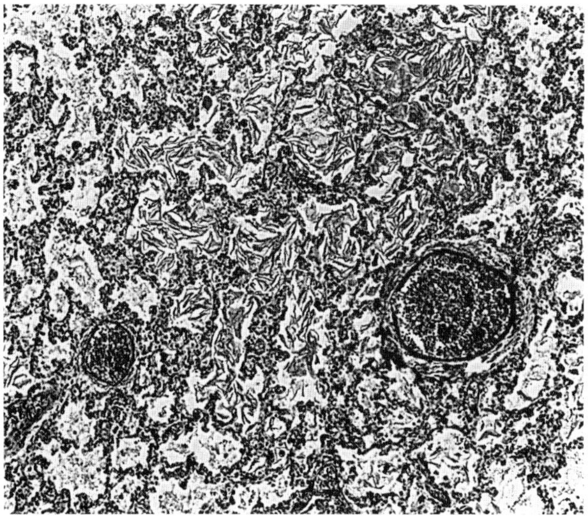

Fig. 17.23. Lung from a fresh stillbirth at 37 weeks' gestation. Airways are unexpanded and aspirated squames are present in air spaces.

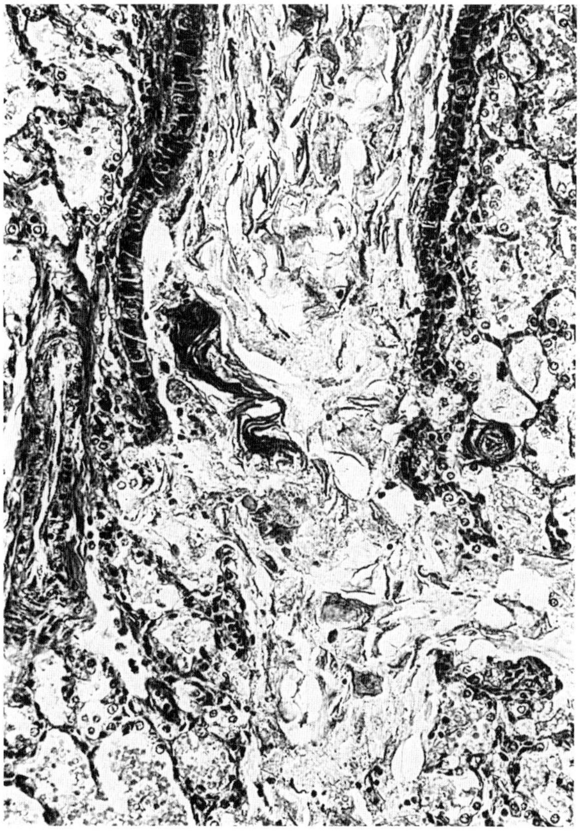

Fig. 17.24. Terminal bronchiole from term infant containing squames and mucin, typical of meconium aspiration. Other amorphous granular material is also present.

Acute hypoxia causes two reflex responses in the mature infant. First, anal relaxation allows meconium to pass into the amniotic liquor. Second, deep gasping movements result in amniotic fluid aspiration. At necropsy, asphyxia is suggested by petechial haemorrhages, sometimes confluent, on the pleura but the cut surfaces may be normal. Where substantial meconium aspiration has occurred, however, the lungs are heavy and mottled, and careful inspection may reveal areas of overdistension with yellow-green meconium expressible from airways.

Microscopically, amniotic fluid inhalation is indicated by squames plugging the main airways, and sometimes extending into more distal sites (Fig. 17.23). This is commonly the only indication of acute asphyxia in the stillborn. Deep aspiration of meconium is more a feature of the neonate, as intrauterine gasping does not allow large volume shifts of such viscid material. The initial gasps are critical in the extent to which meconium penetrates into the lung. Histologically, the plugs of meconium comprise squames, mucus and eosinophilic, granular material sometimes containing small yellow "meconium bodies" (Fig. 17.24). Hyaline membranes, which may be patchy, can occur rapidly associated with the acute hypoxia. If the infant survives a few days, acute inflammation may develop in association with the meconium plugs, but this is an indication of subsequent infection. Meconium does not generate a chemical pneumonitis.

Persistent Pulmonary Hypertension

Persistent pulmonary hypertension of the newborn reflects a failure to reduce or maintain a reduction in the normal postnatal fall in pulmonary vascular resistance. Cyanosis and respiratory distress may develop after birth, although there may be an initial period of apparent normality. There is right-to-left intrapulmonary shunting but also across the foramen ovale and the ductus arteriosus (if it remains patent). Because of this latter feature, the condition is often referred to as persistent fetal circulation (Gersony 1973).

It can be associated with other abnormalities such as congenital heart disease or congenital alveolar capillary dysplasia (Janney et al. 1981). This latter condition may be more common than previously realised but appears to be due to a malposition of the intrapulmonary veins associated with reduced capillary numbers and blood–air barriers (Wagenvoort 1986; Cater et al. 1989; Langston 1991).

A more common association is lung hypoplasia where, it is assumed, there is a failure of the normal development of the pulmonary circulation and a reduced vascular cross-sectional area. It may also occur in association with sepsis, pneumonia, hyperviscosity, acute hypoxia with meconium aspiration and hypoglycaemia. Rarely, it may be idiopathic.

This latter form is characterised microscopically by extension of medial smooth muscle distally, such that most precapillary arteries have muscular walls (Haworth and Reid 1976). In a recent study, nerve fibres were also found at a more distal location than normal (Raine et al. 1991). It has been suggested that in the idiopathic form there may be an antenatal increase in peripheral pulmonary artery muscularity.

Infection

The newborn infant is susceptible to infection, particularly if very preterm or suffering from growth retardation. Infection may be acquired in utero, intrapartum or in the neonatal period and, whilst the lung may not always demonstrate the most significant pathology, pulmonary involvement is frequent. In utero, transmission to the fetus is by two main routes—ascending through the maternal uterine os and transplacentally from the maternal circulation (Zaaijman et al. 1986).

Ascending Infection

Evidence of an ascending infection is a common feature of spontaneous abortions, particularly before 24 weeks of gestation, and chorioamnionitis may be found in up to 20%–30% of cases. A few aspirated maternal polymorphs within airways and terminal sacs may be present, or, at a later stage, an interstitial response with polymorphs and bronchocentric aggregates of lymphocytes.

The infecting organism may be a common gastrointestinal commensal such as *E. coli* and *Clostridium* species, or a vaginal commensal such as Group B streptococcus. Frequently, especially in abortuses, no organism is cultured despite florid histological evidence of infection. Mycoplasmas, ureaplasmas or even chlamydias (Gravett et al. 1986; Lamont et al. 1987) may be involved in a proportion of cases.

Bacterial Infection

Most bacterial infection produces a typical non-specific bronchopneumonia although some organisms produce characteristic features.

Group B streptococcus (*GBS*), normally an innocuous vaginal commensal, is a particularly virulent organism in the neonate and can be acquired antepartum, intrapartum or neonatally. Death may be very rapid following acute collapse but developing pulmonary infection may cause respiratory distress, indistinguishable clinically and radiographically from surfactant-deficient hyaline membrane disease (Ablow et al. 1976). Subsequent problems include pulmonary hypertension, reduced cardiac output and systemic hypotension. Many of the cardiovascular effects of GBS may be mediated by tumour necrosis factor (Gibson et al. 1991). Although usually sensitive to antibiotics, deterioration and death from GBS may supervene before effective control has been achieved.

If onset of infection and death are very rapid, the lungs may show surprisingly little pathology other than congestion and oedema. Small patches of inflammation within major airways may be suggestive and careful examination with a Gram stain, may reveal a few organisms. Longer survival is associated with the more typical picture of bronchopneumonia although hyaline membranes, often containing abundant stainable organisms giving a blue tinge to the membranes, may dominate some areas.

Pseudomonas is a frequent coloniser of neonates but can cause a severe pneumonia. Histologically, areas of more typical pneumonia contain foci of necrosis and haemorrhage due to infarction. In disseminated *Listeria monocytogenes* infection the lung may show the typical granulomatous abscesses involving parenchyma and vessels as seen in other tissues (Vawter 1981; Khong et al. 1986).

Congenital syphilis is not common in most developed countries, but should be considered as a cause of a congenital pneumonia where

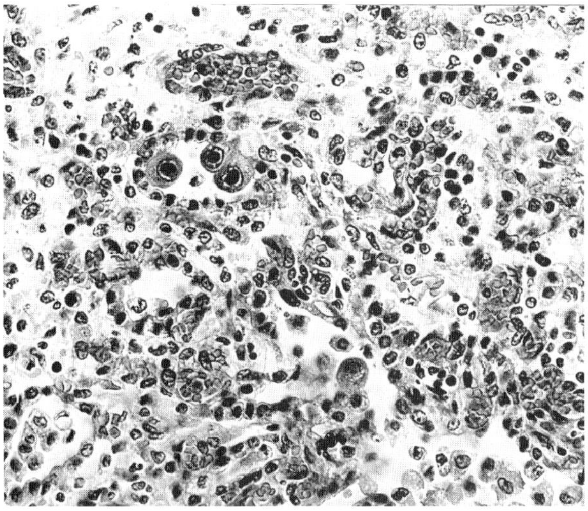

Fig. 17.25. Cytomegalovirus inclusions in the lung of an infant dying from chronic lung disease. The infection was not congenital and was acquired whilst on the infant was on the neonatal unit.

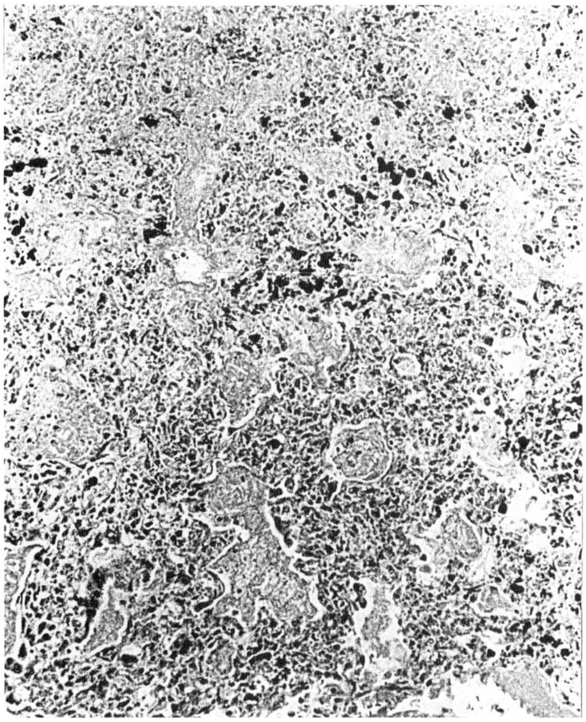

Fig. 17.26. Lung, immunostained for herpes simplex virus, from a term infant dying at 10 days of age from disseminated infection. On the *right*, considerable interstitial thickening is apparent together with HMD (*top right*), primarily the consequence of ventilator therapy rather than the virus. To the *left*, the lack of nuclear staining reflects an area of bland necrosis at the margins of which are virally affected cells stained intensely positive by specific antibody. Of note, there is no inflammatory infiltrate and, even under high power, viral inclusions are not apparent.

there are interstitial infiltrates of lymphocytes, plasma cells and "onion-skinning" of pulmonary arteries (Oppenheimer and Dahms 1981). This "pneumonia alba" will usually only be one manifestation of the disease and histological evidence of syphilis is likely to be present elsewhere, such as in the liver or pancreas.

Fungal Infection

Pulmonary Candida occurs either as a manifestation of an ascending infection and amniotic fluid infection, or as a component of systemic candidiasis (Keller et al. 1977; Kassner et al. 1981; Whyte et al. 1982). In the former case, the infection is a typical bronchopneumonia in which fungal hyphae can be identified. In the latter situation, the vasculature will usually be the prime site of infection from septic emboli.

Viral Infection

Most viral infections can affect the lungs, but other tissues or organs will often demonstrate more characteristic or extensive damage. Particularly in abortuses or stillbirths, however, pulmonary histology may be better preserved than elsewhere.

Congenital Cytomegalovirus (*CMV*) may produce a pulmonary interstitial infiltrate of mononuclear cells associated with the typical inclusions in macrophages and epithelial cells. More commonly, CMV is encountered in infants who have been long-term residents of the neonatal unit, having required ventilation for chronic lung disease. The inclusions may be sparse, and while the infection may have contributed to the pulmonary damage, in most situations it is probable that the infection is incidental (Fig. 17.25).

Herpes simplex may be acquired antenatally or during passage through the birth canal. The organs most typically affected and showing virally induced necrosis are the liver and adrenals, but the lungs also may be involved. Necrosis is often bland and the extent of the viral infection not readily apparent unless specific immunohistology is performed (Fig. 17.26).

References

Abbott TR (1968) Complications of prolonged nasotracheal intubation in children. Br J Anaesth 40: 347–353

Ablow RC, Driscoll SG, Effman EL et al. (1976) A comparison of early onset Group B streptococcal neonatal infection and the respiratory distress syndrome of the newborn. N Engl J Med 294: 65–70

Agosti E, Filippi G, Chiussi F (1974) Generalized familial bronchomalacia. Acta Pediatr Scand 63: 616–618

Areechon W, Reid L (1963) Hypoplasia of lung with congenital diaphragmatic hernia. Br Med J 1: 230–233

Askenazi SS, Perlman M (1979) Pulmonary hypoplasia: lung weight and radial alveolar count as criteria of diagnosis. Arch Dis Child 54: 614–618

Bale PM (1979) Congenital cystic malformation of the lung. Am J Clin Pathol 71: 411–442

Belmont JR, Grundfast K (1984) Congenital laryngeal stridor (laryngomalacia). Etiologic factors and associated disorders. Ann Otol Rhinol Laryngol 93: 430–437

Benjamin B (1984) Tracheomalacia in infants and children. Ann Otol Rhinol Laryngol 93: 438–442

Blanc WA (1976) Commentary: yellow lung in premature infants. J Pediatr 89: 131–132

Bonikos DS, Beusch KG, Northway WH Jr, Edwards DKE (1976) Bronchopulmonary dysplasia: the pulmonary pathologic sequel of necrotizing bronchiolitis and pulmonary fibrosis. Hum Pathol 7: 643–666

Booth JB, Berry CL (1967) Unilateral pulmonary agenesis. Arch Dis Child 42: 361–374

Boriewiecke B, Croft CB (1977) Experimental animal model of subglottic stenosis. Ann Otol Rhinol Laryngol 86: 835–840

Boros SJ, Mammel MC, Lewallen PK, Coleman JM, Gordon MJ, Ophoven J (1986) Necrotizing tracheobronchitis: a complication of high-frequency ventilation. J Pediatr 109: 95–100

Bozic C (1969) Lésions dues a l'intubation endotrachéale des nouveau-nés. Helv Paediatr Acta 24: 458–462

Bozic C (1974) Ectopic fetal adrenal cortex in the lung of the newborn. Virchows Arch (Pathol Anat) 363: 371–374

Bray RJ, Lamb WH (1988) Tracheal stenosis or agenesis in association with tracheo-oesophageal fistula and oesophageal atresia. Anaesthesia 43: 654–658

Brown MJ, Olver RE, Ramsden CA, Strang LB, Walters DV (1983) Effects of adrenaline and of spontaneous labour on the secretion and absorption of lung liquid in the fetal lamb. J Physiol 344: 137–152

Buntain WL, Isaacs H Jr, Payne VC, Lindesmith GG (1974) Lobar emphysema, cystic adenomatoid malformation, pulmonary sequestration, and bronchogenic cyst in infancy and childhood: a clinical group. J Pediatr Surg 9: 85–93

Carrillo P (1985) Palatal groove formation and oral endotracheal intubation. Am J Dis Child 139: 859–880

Cater G, Thibeault DW, Beatty EC Jr, Kilbride HW, Huntrakoon M (1989) Misalignment of lung vessels and alveolar capillary dysplasia: a cause of persistent pulmonary hypertension. J Pediatr 114: 293–300

Chellam VG (1988) Rhabdomyomatous dysplasia of the lung: a case report with review of the literature. Pediatr Pathol 8: 391–394

Chen MF, Onerheim R, Wang NS, Huttner I (1991) Rhabdomyomatosis of the newborn lung. Pediatr Pathol 11: 123–129

Chi JG, Shong Y-K (1982) Diffuse striated muscle heteroplasia of the lung. An autopsy case. Arch Pathol Lab Med 106: 641–644

Clements BS, Warner JO (1987) Pulmonary sequestration and related congenital bronchopulmonary-vascular malformations: nomenclature and classification based on anatomical and embryological considerations. Thorax 42: 401–408

Cogbill TH, Moore FA, Accurso FJ, Lilly JR (1983) Primary tracheomalacia. Ann Thorac Surg 35: 538–541

Cole VA, Normand ICS, Reynolds EOR, Rivers RPA (1973) Pathogenesis of haemorrhagic pulmonary edema and massive pulmonary haemorrhage in the newborn. Pediatrics 51: 175–186

Cooke RWI (1991) Factors associated with chronic lung disease in preterm infants. Arch Dis Child 66: 776–779

Cooney TP, Thurlbeck WM (1982) The radial alveolar count method of Emery and Mithal: a reappraisal. Thorax 37: 580–583

Cotton RT, Richardson MA (1981) Congenital laryngeal anomalies. Otolaryngol Clin North Am 14: 203–218

de la Monte SM, Hutchins GM, Moore GW (1986) Respiratory epithelial cell necrosis is the earliest lesion of hyaline membrane disease of the newborn. Am J Pathol 123: 155–160

DeVine WA, Debich DE, Anderson RH (1991) Dissection of congenitally malformed hearts, with comments on the value of sequential segmental analysis. Pediatr Pathol 11: 235–260

De Santo LW, De Vine KD, Weiland LH (1970) Cysts of the larynx. Classification. Laryngoscope 80: 145–176

Diaz EM, Adams JM, Hawkins HK, Smith RJH (1989) Tracheal agenesis. A case report and literature review. Arch Otolaryngol Head Neck Surg 115: 741–745

Domitzio P, Liesner RJ, Dicks-Mireaux C, Risdon RA (1990) Malignant mesenchymoma associated with a congenital lung cyst in a child. Case report and review of the literature. Pediatr Pathol 10: 785–797

Duke PM, Coulson JD, Santos JI, Johnson JD (1976) Cleft palate associated with prolonged orotracheal intubation in infancy. J Pediatr 89: 990–991

Emery JL, Mithal A (1960) The number of alveoli in the terminal respiratory unit of man during late intrauterine life and childhood. Arch Dis Child 35: 544–547

Engellener W, Kaplan C, Van de Vegte GL (1989) Pulmonary agenesis association with non-immune hydrops. Pediatr Pathol 9: 725–730

Erenberg A, Nowak AJ (1984) Palatal groove formation in neonates and infants with orotracheal tubes. Am J Dis Child 138: 974–975

Esterly JR, Oppenheimer EH (1970) Lymphangiectasis and other pulmonary lesions in the asplenia syndrome. Arch Pathol 90: 553–560

Farrell PM, Avery ME (1975) Hyaline membrane disease. Am Rev Resp Dis 3: 657–688

Ferguson MWJ (1991) The orofacial region. In: Wigglesworth JS, Singer DB (eds) Textbook of fetal and perinatal pathology. Blackwell Scientific Publications, Oxford, pp 843–880

Fisher JE, Nelson SJ, Allen JE, Holzman RS (1982) Congenital cystic adenomatoid malformation of the lung. A unique variant. Am J Dis Child 136: 1071–1074

Floyd J, Campbell DC, Dominey DE (1962) Agenesis of the trachea. Am Rev Resp Dis 86: 557–560

France NE, Brown RJK (1971) Congenital pulmonary lymphangiectasis. Arch Dis Child 46: 528–532

Frank L, Sosenko IRS (1987) Development of lung antioxidant enzyme system in late gestation: possible implications for the prematurely born infant. J Pediatr

110: 9–14
Frank L, Sosenko IRS (1991) Failure of premature rabbits to increase antioxidant enzymes during hyperoxic exposure: increased susceptibility to pulmonary oxygen toxicity compared with term rabbits. Pediatr Res 29: 292–296
Friedman EM, Vastola P, McGill TJI, Healy GB (1990) Chronic pediatric stridor: etiology and outcome. Laryngoscope 100: 277–280
Gersony WM (1973) Persistence of the fetal circulation. A commentary. J Pediatr 82: 1103–1106
Gibson RL, Redding GJ, Henderson WR, Truog WE (1991) Group B Streptococcus induces tumor necrosis factor in neonatal piglets. Am Rev Resp Dis 143: 598–604
Gifford GH Jr, Swanson L, MacCollum DW (1972) Congenital absence of the nose and anterior nasopharynx. Plast Reconstr Surg 50: 5–12
Gorenflo M, Vogel M, Obladen M (1991) Pulmonary vascular changes in bronchopulmonary dysplasia: a clinical pathologic correlation in short and long term survivors. Pediatr Pathol 11: 851–866
Gould SJ (1988) The pathology of neonatal endotracheal intubation and its relationship to subglottic stenosis. J Laryngol Otol [Suppl] 17: 3–6
Gould SJ, Howard S (1985) The histopathology of the larynx in the neonate following endotracheal intubation. J Pathol 146: 301–311
Gould SJ, Howard S (1988) Long term pathological sequelae of neonatal endotracheal intubation. J Laryngol Otol 103: 622–625
Gravett MG, Nelson P, DeRouen T, Critchlow C, Eschenbach DA, Holmes KK (1986) Independent associations of bacterial vaginosis and *Chlamydia trachomatis* infection with adverse pregnancy outcome. JAMA 256: 1899–1903
Gupta CM TG, Goldberg SJ, Lewis E, Fonkalsrud EW (1968) Congenital bronchomalacia. Am J Dis Child 115: 88–90
Haidar A, Ryder TA, Wigglesworth JS (1991) Epithelial cell morphology and airspace size in hypoplastic human fetal lungs associated with oligohydramnios. Pediatr Pathol 11: 839–850
Hamilton WJ, Boyd JD, Mossman HW (1972) Human embryology. Williams and Wilkins, Baltimore, pp 291–377
Han RNN, Buch S, Freeman BA, Post M, Tanswell AK (1992) Platelet-derived growth factor and growth-related genes in rat lung. II. Effect of exposure to 85% O_2 Am J Physiol 262:L140–146
Hanson JW, Smith DW, Cohen MM (1976) Prominent lateral palatine ridges: developmental and clinical relevance. J Pediatr 89: 54–58
Harding R, Hooper SB, Dickson KA (1990) A mechanism leading to reduced lung expansion and lung hypoplasia in fetal sheep during oligohydramnios. Am J Obstet Gynecol 163: 1904–1913
Harley HRS (1971) Laryngotracheal obstruction complicating tracheostomy or endotracheal intubation with assisted respiration. A critical review. Thorax 26: 493–533
Haworth SG (1988) Pulmonary vascular remodeling in neonatal pulmonary hypertension. State of the art. Chest 93: 133S–138S
Haworth SG, Reid L (1976) Persistent fetal circulation: newly recognized structural features. J Pediatr 88: 614–620
Heithoff KB, Sane SM, Williams HJ (1976) Bronchopulmonary foregut malformations. A unifying etiological concept. Am J Roentgenol 126: 46–55
Hislop AA, Howarth SG (1989) Airway size and structure in the normal fetal and infant lung and the effect of premature delivery and artificial ventilation. Am Rev Resp Dis 140: 1717–1726
Hislop AA, Howarth SG (1990) Pulmonary vascular damage and the development of cor pulmonale following hyaline membrane disease. Pediatr Pulmonol 9: 152–156
Hislop A, Reid L (1974) Growth and development of the respiratory system—anatomical development. In: Davis JA, Dobbing J (eds) Scientific foundations of paediatrics. Heinemann Medical, London, pp 214–254
Hislop A, Hey E, Reid L (1979) The lungs in congenital bilateral renal agenesis and dysplasia. Arch Dis Child 54: 32–38
Hislop AA, Wigglesworth JS, Desai R (1986) Alveolar development in the human fetus and infant. Early Hum Dev 1: 1–12
Holder MP, Wooler GH (1970) Tracheo-oesophageal fistula and oesophageal atresia: results of 30 years' experience. Thorax 25: 406–412
Janney CG, Askin FB, Kuhn C 3rd. (1981) Congenital alveolar capillary dysplasia: an unusual cause of respiratory distress in the newborn. Am J Clin Pathol 76: 722–727
Kassner EG, Kauffman SL, Yoon JJ, Semiglia M, Kozinn PJ, Goldberg PL (1981) Pulmonary candidiasis in infants: clinical, radiologic, and pathologic features. Am J Roentgenol 137: 707–716
Keller MA, Sellers BB, Melish ME, Kaplan GW, Miller KE, Mendoza SA (1977) Systemic candidiasis in infants. Am J Dis Child 131: 1260–1263
Khong TY, Frappell J, Steel HM, Stewart CM, Burke M (1986) Perinatal listeriosis. A report of six cases. Brit J Obstet Gynecol 93: 1083–1087
Kitterman JA (1984) Fetal lung development. J Dev Physiol 6: 67–82
Knowles S, Thomas RM, Lindenbaum RH, Keeling JW, Winter RM (1988) Pulmonary agenesis as part of the VACTERL sequence. Arch Dis Child 63: 723–726
Lamont RF, Taylor-Robinson D, Wigglesworth JS, Furr PM, Evans RT, Elder MG (1987) The role of mycoplasmas, ureaplasmas and chlamydiae in the genital tract of women presenting in spontaneous early preterm labour. J Med Microbiol 24: 253–257
Landing BH (1984) Five syndromes (malformation complexes) of pulmonary symmetry, congenital heart disease, and multiple spleens. Pediatr Pathol 2: 125–151
Landing BH, Dixon LG (1979) Congenital malformations and genetic disorders of the respiratory tract. Am Rev Resp Dis 120: 151–185
Landing BH, Wells TR (1973) Tracheobronchial anomalies in children. In: Rosenberg HS, Bolande RP (eds) Perspectives in pediatric pathology, vol 1. Year Book Medical Publishers, Chicago, pp 1–32
Langston C, Kida K, Reed M, Thurlbeck WM (1984) Human lung growth in late gestation and in the neonate. Am Rev Respir Dis 129: 607–613
Langston C. (1991) Misalignment of pulmonary veins and alveolar capillary dysplasia. Pediatr Pathol 11: 163–170
Laurence KM (1959) Congenital pulmonary lymphangiectasis. J Clin Pathol 12: 62–69
Liggins GC, Vilos GA, Campos GA, Kitterman JA, Lee CH (1981) The effect of bilateral thoracoplasty in lung development in fetal sheep. J Dev Physiol 3: 275–282
Lim TA, Spanier SS, Kohut RI (1979) Laryngeal clefts: a histopathologic study and review. Ann Otol Rhinol Laryngol 88: 837–845
Loeff DS, Filler RM, Vinograd I et al. (1990) Congenital tracheal stenosis: a review of 22 patients from 1965–1987.

J Pediatr Surg 25: 492–495
McDougall J, Smith JF (1975) The development of the human type 2 pneumocyte. J Path 115: 245–251
McMillan WG, Duvall AJ (1968) Congenital subglottic stenosis. Arch Otolaryngol 87: 272–278
McNie DJM, Pryse-Davies J (1970) Tracheal agenesis. Arch Dis Child 45: 143–144
Margraf LR, Tomashefski JF Jr, Bruce MC, Dahms BB (1991) Morphometric analysis of the lung in bronchopulmonary dysplasia. Am Rev Resp Dis 143: 391–400
Mendelson CR, Boggaram V (1989) Regulation of pulmonary surfactant protein synthesis in fetal lung: a major role of glucocorticoids and cyclic AMP. Trends in Endocrinol Metabol 1: 20–25
Merritt TA (1982) Oxygen exposure in the newborn guinea pig lung lavage cell populations, chemotactic and elastase response: a possible relationship to neonatal bronchopulmonary dysplasia. Pediatr Res 16: 798–805
Metlay LA, Macpherson TA, Doshi N, Milley JR (1987) Necrotizing tracheobronchitis in intubated newborns: a complication of assisted ventilation. Pediatr Pathol 7: 575–584
Mitchell DB, Irwin C, Bailey CM, Evans NG (1987) Cysts of the infants larynx. J Laryngol Otol 101: 833–837
Nicolini U, Fisk NM, Rodeck CH, Talbert DG, Wigglesworth JS (1989) Low amniotic pressure in oligohydramnios. Is this the cause of pulmonary hypoplasia? Am J Obstet Gynecol 161: 1098–1101
Nimrod C, Varela-Gittings F, Machin G, Campbell D, Wesenberg R (1984) The effect of prolonged membrane rupture on fetal development. Am J Obstet Gynecol 148: 540–543
Northway WH, Rosan RC, Porter DY (1967) Pulmonary disease following respirator therapy of hyaline membrane disease. Bronchopulmonary dysplasia. N Engl J Med 276: 357–368
O'Brodovich HM, Mellins RB (1985) Bronchopulmonary dysplasia. Am Rev Resp Dis 132: 694–709
Olver RE, Strang LB (1974) Ion fluxes across the pulmonary epithelium and the secretion of lung liquid in the foetal lamb. J Physiol 241: 327–357
Oppenheimer EH, Dahms BB (1981) Congenital syphilis in the fetus and neonate. In: Rosenberg HS, Bernstein J (eds) Perspectives in pediatric pathology, vol 6. Year Book Medical Publishers, Chicago, pp 112–138
Ostor AG, Stillwell R, Fortune DW (1978) Bilateral pulmonary agenesis. Pathology 10: 243–248
Page DV, Stocker JT (1982) Anomalies associated with pulmonary hypoplasia. Am Rev Resp Dis 125: 216–221
Pagon RA, Graham JM (1981) Coloboma, congenital heart disease and choanal atresia with multiple anomalies: CHARGE association. J Pediatr 99: 223–227
Raine J, Hislop AA, Redington AN, Haworth SG, Shinebourne EA (1991) Fatal persistent pulmonary hypertension presenting late in the neonatal period. Arch Dis Child 66: 398–402
Ramenofsky ML, Leape LL, McCauley RGK (1979) Bronchogenic cyst. J Ped Surg 14: 219–224
Rasche RFH, Kuhns LR (1972) Histopathologic changes in airway mucosa of infants after endotracheal intubation. Pediatrics 50: 632–637
Robertson B (1991) The origin of neonatal lung injury. Pediatr Pathol 11: iii–vi (editorial)
Rooney SA (1989) Fatty acid synthesis in developing fetal lung. Am J Physiol 257: L195–L207
Salyer DC, Salyer WR, Eggleston JC (1977) Benign developmental cysts of the mediastinum. Arch Pathol Lab Med 101: 136–139
Saugstad OD (1990) Oxygen toxicity in the neonatal period. Acta Paediatr Scand 79: 881–892
Schild JP, Wuilloud A, Kollberg H, Bossi E (1976) Tracheal perforation as a complication of nasotracheal intubation in the neonate. J Pediatr 4: 631–632
Schmidt B, Vegh P, Weitz J, Johnson M, Caco C, Roberts R (1992) Thrombin/antithrombin III complex formation in the neonatal respiratory distress syndrome. Am Rev Resp Dis 145: 767–770
Serlin SP, Daily WJR (1975) Tracheal perforation in the neonate: complication of endotracheal intubation. J Pediatr 86: 596–597
Silver MM, Thurston WA, Patrick JE (1988) Perinatal pulmonary hyperplasia due to laryngeal atresia. Hum Pathol 19: 110–113
Smith II, Bain AD (1965) Congenital atresia of the larynx. A report of nine cases. Ann Otol Rhinol Laryngol 74: 338–349
Smith BT, Post M (1989) Fibroblast pneumocyte factor. Am J Physiol 257: L174–L178
Sotomayor JJ, Godinez RI, Borden S, Wilmott RW (1986) Large airway collapse due to acquired tracheobronchomalacia in infancy. Am J Dis Child 140: 367–371
Stahl GE, Spear ML, Hamosh M (1992) Lipid Infusions and pulmonary function abnormalities. In: Polin RA, Fox WW (eds) Fetal and neonatal physiology. Saunders, London, 346–352
Stewart PA, Becker AE, Wladimiroff JW, Essed CE (1984) Left atrial isomerism associated with asplenia: prenatal echocardiographic detection of complex congenital cardiac malformations. J Am Coll Cardiol 4: 1015–1020
Stocker JT, Drake RM, Madewell JE (1978) Cystic and congenital lung disease in the newborn. In: Rosenberg HS, Bolande RP (eds) Perspectives in pediatric pathology, vol 4. Year Book Medical Publishers, Chicago, pp 93–148
Swischuk LE, Richardson CJ, Nichols MM, Ingman MJ (1979) Primary pulmonary hypoplasia in the neonate. J Pediatr 95: 573–577
Taghizadeh A, Reynolds EOR (1976) Pathogenesis of bronchopulmonary dysplasia following hyaline membrane disease. Am J Pathol 82: 241–264
Tucker GF, Ossoff RH, Newman AN, Holinger LD (1979) Histopathology of congenital subglottic stenosis. Laryngoscope 89: 866–876
Ueda K, Gruppo R, Unger F, Martin L, Bove K (1977) Rhabdomyosarcoma of the lung arising in a congenital adenomatoid malformation. Cancer 40: 383–388
Vawter GF (1981) Perinatal listeriosis. In: Rosenberg HS, Bernstein J (eds) Perspectives in pediatric pathology, vol 6. Year Book Medical Publishers, Chicago, 153–156
Wagenvoort CA (1986) Misalignment of lung vessels: a syndrome causing persistent neonatal pulmonary hypertension. Hum Pathol 17: 727–730
Walters DV, Ramsden CA (1987) The secretion and absorption of fetal lung liquid. In: Walters DV, Strang LB, Geubelle F (eds) Physiology of the fetal and neonatal lung. MTP Press Ltd, England, pp 61–75
Whyte RK, Hussain Z, De Sa DJ (1982) Antenatal infections with candida. Arch Dis Child 57: 528–535
Wigglesworth JS (1977) Pathology of neonatal respiratory distress. Proc R Soc Med 70: 861–863
Wigglesworth JS (1987a) Factors affecting fetal lung growth. In: Walters DV, Strang LB, Geubelle F (eds) Physiology of the fetal and neonatal lung. MTP Press Ltd, England, pp 25–36
Wigglesworth JS (1987b) Pathology of the lung in the fetus and neonate, with particular reference to problems of

growth and maturation. Histopathology 11: 671–689
Wigglesworth JS, Desai R (1981) Use of DNA estimation for growth assessment in normal and hypoplastic fetal lungs. Arch Dis Child 56: 601–605
Wigglesworth JS, Desai R (1982) Is fetal respiratory function a major determinant of perinatal survival? Lancet i: 264–267
Wigglesworth JS, Desai R, Guerrini P (1981) Fetal lung hypoplasia: biochemical and structural variations and their possible significance. Arch Dis Child 56: 606–615
Wigglesworth JS, Desai R, Hislop AA (1987) Fetal lung growth in congenital laryngeal atresia. Pediatr Pathol 7: 515–525
Winter RM, Knowles SAS, Bieber FR, Baraitser M (1988) The malformed fetus and stillbirth. Wiley, New York
Wright JR, Clements JA (1987) Metabolism and turnover of pulmonary surfactant. Am Rev Resp Dis 136: 426–444
Zaaijman J du T, Wilkinson AR, Keeling JW, Mitchell RG, Turnbull AC (1986) Spontaneous premature rupture of the membranes: bacteriology, histology and neonatal outcome J Obstet Gynecol 2: 155–160
Zaw-Tun HIA (1988) Development of congenital laryngeal atresias and clefts. Ann Otol Rhinol Laryngol 97: 353–358

Chapter 18

The Cardiovascular System

Jerry N. Cox and Jakob Briner

Introduction

The embryonal and structural development of the cardiovascular system is gradually unwoven as emphasis has shifted from the study of structures and their relation as they develop to the study of the molecular mechanisms governing the changes during the process. The role that genes or gene families play in controlling cell differentiation (activation/regression), behaviour and interaction to influence morphological events and finally give rise to definite structures is becoming more apparent (Icardo 1988; Potts and Runyan 1989; Gammage and Franklyn 1991). Expansion in the use of the many new and perfected radiological techniques for examining intrauterine growth patterns and perinatal morphology, especially of the cardiovascular system, continues to give new insights into the normal constituents of mature structures as well as the possible variations of cardiac abnormalities, some of which may be associated with chromosome anomalies, teratogens or environmental factors.

These advances have led to the earlier diagnosis and better understanding of cardiac malformation leading to a more precise nomenclature, often before serious functional disturbances appear, thus enabling early surgical repair with favourable outcome (Pexieder 1982; Allan et al. 1985; Gerlis 1985; Gembruch et al. 1990; Rao 1990). In this chapter, we will endeavour to outline briefly some of the major pathological conditions most frequently encountered in the perinatal period and a simple approach to their study.

Development of the Heart

There are few organs in the body whose development has aroused so much controversy as the heart. New techniques employed in the study of its organogenesis are shedding light on important aspects of development and our understanding of how some major malformations occur. A brief review of our current understanding of the heart is given below, but there are major problems still to be solved. (Pexieder et al. 1989; Bartelings 1990; Moscoso and Pexieder 1990).

In the second week of gestation, there is coalescence of endothelial blood islands, forming channels between the embryo and extraembryonic membranes. These channels make contact with the cardiogenic mesoderm and join the angioblastic cells, which have now formed two parallel tubes, the primary heart tubes. These invaginate the pericardial coelom carrying with them a myocardial mantle.

Gradually there is fusion of the tubes, beginning in the future ventricular outlet region and progressively extending throughout the cardiac primordium within the newly formed pericardial cavity.

By the third week, the heart is a straight unitubular structure with four dilated segments: sinus venosus, most distal; primitive atrium; primitive ventricle; and arterial segment, separated by three well-defined constrictions. Shortly thereafter, looping begins and is accompanied by cell shape changes and modulation of cell contact. The primitive atrium moves posteriorly and upwards to be located finally superior to the ventricular mass. The latter is now anterior and separated into an inlet portion to the left, and an outlet portion on the right. During this process, the conotruncus remains in the midline and superior to all other segments (Fig. 18.1a).

The ventricles are derived from the primitive ventricle. It divides into two parts, an *outlet*, forming the right ascending limb and supporting the conotruncus, and an *inlet*, forming the left descending limb facing the atrioventricular canal. From the greater curvature, two trabeculated expansions appear and progress rapidly downwards to form well-defined trabecular pouches. One pouch, taking its origin from the inlet portion, gives rise to the trabecular zone of the left ventricle, while the other pouch, arising from the outlet portion, develops into the trabecular zone of the right ventricle. Soon a trabecular septum forms between the two ventricular pouches by apposition of medial walls of both.

The attachment of the inferior atrioventricular endocardial cushion to the posterior extent of the trabecular septum prepares the formation of the inlet septum and the alignment of the atrioventricular orifices to their respective

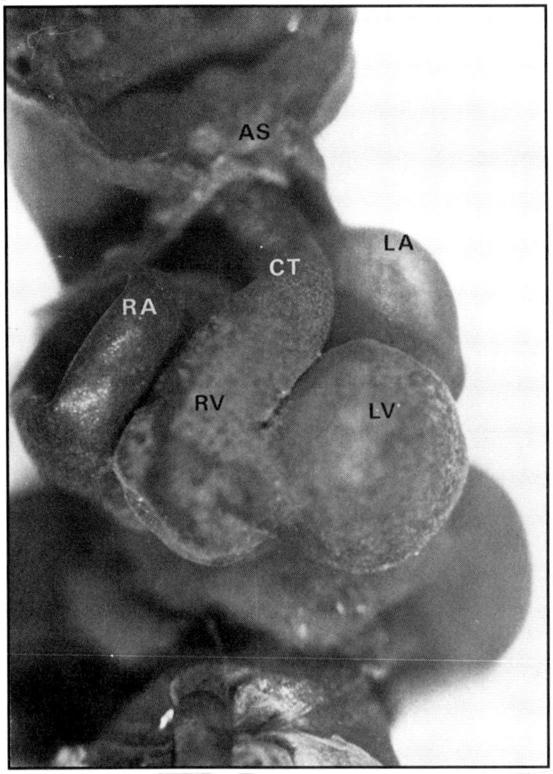

a

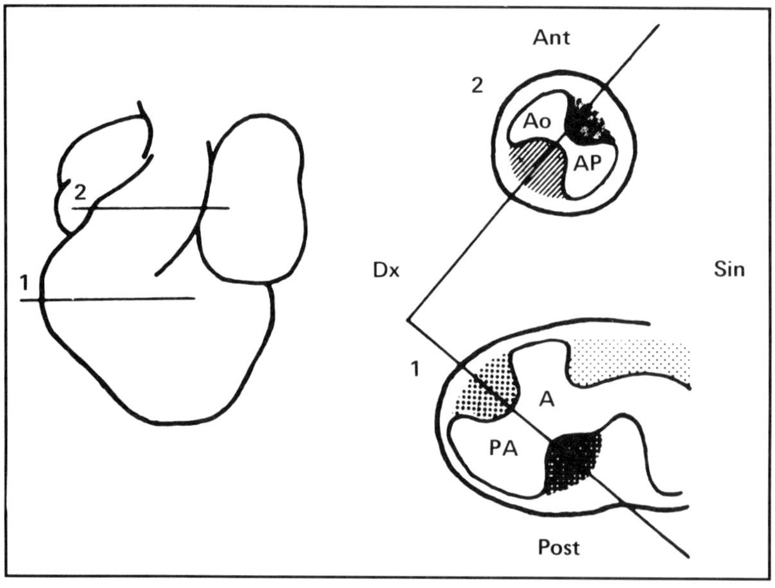

b

Fig. 18.1. **a** Human embryonic heart; day 28. *AS*, aortic sac; *CT*, conotruncus; *LA*, left atrium; *LV*, left ventricle; *RA*, right atrium; *RV*, right ventricle. (Courtesy of Prof. T. Pexieder, Lausanne.) **b** Orientation of the conotruncus cushions. *Dx*, right; *Sin*, left; *Ant*, anterior; *Post*, posterior; *A*, aorta; *PA*, pulmonary trunk. (Courtesy of Prof. T. Pexieder, Lausanne).

ventricles. In the meantime, fusion of the superior and inferior endocardial cushions in the region of the atrioventricular canal separates the future mitral and tricuspid orifices, although atrioventricular valves are not formed until after septation of the ventricles. Fusion of the right bulbar ridge with the superior endocardial cushion aligns the outlet septum to the inlet septum.

The ventricular septum develops from three distinct components: a muscular septum between the trabecular pouches, an outlet septum from fusion of bulbar ridges and an inlet septum derived from the posterior part of the muscular septum. An outgrowth of cushion tissue and sulcus tissue will form the membranous septum and close the temporary communications between the ventricles.

Endocardial thickening forming the right and left conotruncus ridges continues distally into the outlet component of the primary heart tube, where they join with the aortopulmonary septum originating in the peribranchial mesenchyme, separating the pulmonary artery anteriorly from the aorta posteriorly (Fig. 18.1b).

The normal development of two atria from the primitive atrium depends largely on extensive remodelling and reorganisation of the fetal venous system. The sinuatrial orifice, a midline structure at this stage of development, enters the posterior wall of the primitive atrium, whilst its anteroinferior aspect gives rise to the atrioventricular canal. The sinus venosus, guarded by flap valves, gradually shifts to the right as it is progressively separated from the septum transversum. These changes take place at the same time as the right cardinal vein (future superior vena cava) and right vitelline vein (inferior vena cava) open into the enlarged right sinus horn; the left sinus horn remains relatively small. Finally the sinus venosus becomes incorporated into the right side of the right atrium. As the primitive atrium expands, it is restricted in the midline anteriorly and superiorly; its anterior protrusions give rise to the right and left atrial appendages.

With the shift of the sinus venosus to the right, the septum primum appears as an indentation of the primitive atrial wall and grows downwards to fuse with the atrioventricular endocardial cushions, whilst the ostium secundum forms in its superior portion. The ostium secundum is eventually covered by the septum secundum, which takes origin from the roof of the atrium to the right of the plane of the septum primum. The left atrial roof forming the definitive left atrium arises from the union of the proximal pulmonary vein, outgrowth of the left atrium, and the intrapulmonary veins draining the splanchnic plexus around the lung buds. These structures are absorbed into the wall of the left atrium, which then receives four separate pulmonary veins.

The ventricular outlet is made up of three parts: conus (proximal bulbus); truncus (distal bulbus), situated between the aortic sac and the conus; and the integrated portion of the aortic sac (ventral aorta). The union of these three zones and of their respective septal anlage provides for separation of the pulmonary trunk from the aorta (Fig. 18.1b), the septum between the two being a combination of different processes. In the region of the ventricular outlet corresponding to the bulbus (conotruncus), the septum is formed by fusion of a pair of conotruncus cushions and a pair of truncus ridges, whilst in the aortic sac region the septum is derived from masses of mesenchyma migrating from either side of the branchial region towards the cardiac tube. The three pairs of anlage which form the septum are arranged in different geometric planes, frontal and sagittal, and their gradual progress towards each other in a spiral fashion and their fusion effects separation of the great vessels (Fig. 18.2). Failure of this intricate process better explains the pathogenesis of malformations such as aortopulmonary window, persistent truncus anteriosus communis and perhaps, transposition of great arteries. The aortic and pulmonary semilunar valves are formed from the distal portion of the truncal ridges.

The relationship of the aorta and the ventricles is a much disputed topic. It would appear from recent studies that the extracardiac aorta is always to the right and behind the pulmonary artery. With rapid growth of the lateral border of the right ventricle to the right and distal progression of trabecular transformation of the bulbar wall, the greater portion of the atrioventricular canal remains associated with the left ventricle and thus initially there is no aortomitral continuity. The aorta is not transferred into the left ventricle but is in continuity , connected by its infundibulum (Fig. 18.3).

From these observations it is clear that, from the outset, the anterior wall of the pulmonary artery is complete, whilst its posterior wall is

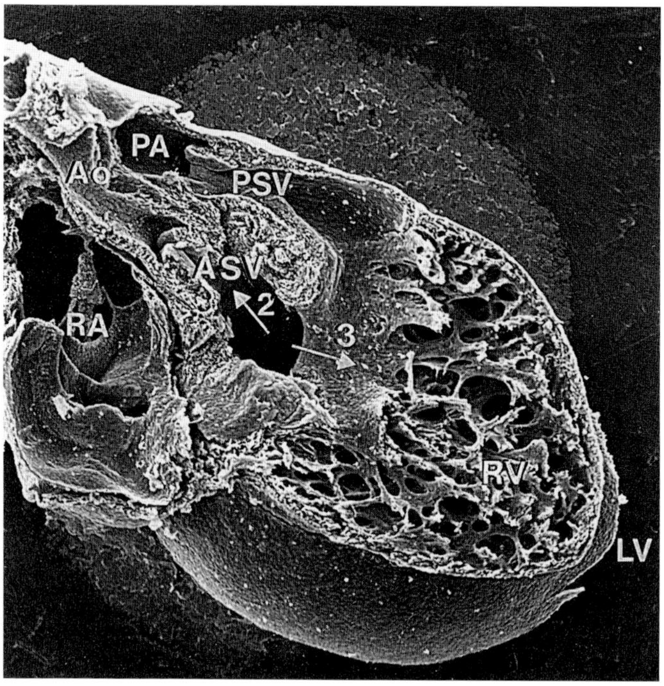

Fig. 18.2. Human embryonic heart; day 45. *Ao*, aorta; *ASV*, aortic semilunar valves; *LV*, left ventricle; *PA*, pulmonary artery; *PSV*, pulmonary semilunar valves; *RA*, right atrium; *RV*, right ventricle; 2, foramen interventriculare secundum (aortic infundibulum); 3, foramen interventriculare tertium. (Courtesy of Prof. T. Pexieder, Lausanne).

made from the bulbus ridge by fusion of the anterior surfaces of conotruncus cushions. Meanwhile, the aorta is incomplete between the distal part of the truncus and the left ventricle. This is the future infundibular region. Its posterior wall is formed by fusion of the superior and inferior atrioventricular cushions and its anterior part by fusion of the conotruncus cushions (Fig. 18.3). At this stage the aortic infundibulum is in communication with the left ventricle by way of the foramen interventriculum secundum, whose closure between the 35th and 67th days of gestation completes cardiac development.

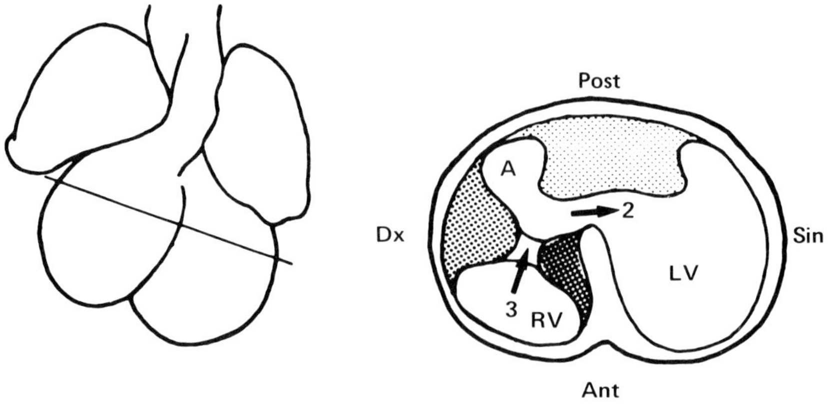

Fig. 18.3. Continuation of the aorta into the left ventricle. *Ant*, anterior; *Post*, posterior; *Dx*, right; *Sin*, left; *RV*, right ventricle; *LV*, left ventricle; *A*, aorta; 2, foramen interventriculare secundum; 3, foramen interventriculare tertium. The *dotted shaded* areas represent the conotruncus and atrioventricular cushions. (Courtesy of Prof. T. Pexieder, Lausanne).

Changes in the Circulation at Birth

Modifications to the fetal circulation occur at birth, when there is transfer of gas exchange from placenta to lungs. Systemic vascular resistance increases as that in the pulmonary system falls; there is closure of the ductus arteriosus, foramen ovale and ductus venosus.

During intrauterine life, oxygenated blood leaving the placenta by way of the umbilical vein passes through the inferior vena cava into the right atrium, where most of it is directed into the left atrium and ventricle through the foramen ovale. Left ventricular blood is directed to the aorta to perfuse the head and neck and coronary arteries. Blood drains from the head and neck into the right atrium through the superior vena cava and most is directed to the right ventricle and pulmonary artery. Vascular resistance in the pulmonary circulation is high, and only a small part of right ventricular flow goes to the lungs; most passes through the ductus arteriosus into the aorta and thence to the placenta, where vascular resistance is low (Rigby and Shinebourne 1981).

By extrapolating results from animal studies, it is estimated that 60% of blood volume arriving at the heart through the inferior vena cava goes through the foramen ovale into the left atrium; the remaining 40% mixes with unsaturated blood from the head and neck. Very little (3%) mixed blood passes through the foramen ovale; most goes via the right ventricle to the pulmonary artery. About 8% goes through the lungs; the remainder (52%) is shunted across the ductus arteriosus into the aorta to return to the placenta.

Of the 40% of total cardiac output leaving the left ventricle, 20% goes to the head and neck, 4% to the coronary arteries and the remaining 16% through the aortic isthmus (Fig. 18.4).

At birth, gaseous exchange is taken over by the lungs as placental circulation is eliminated. This results in a rise in systemic peripheral resistance and contraction of the umbilical arteries. A concomitant rise in oxygen tension within the main pulmonary artery is accompanied by progressive lowering of pulmonary resistance and increased pulmonary blood flow. Right atrial pressure falls as a result of this, and cessation of umbilical venous return

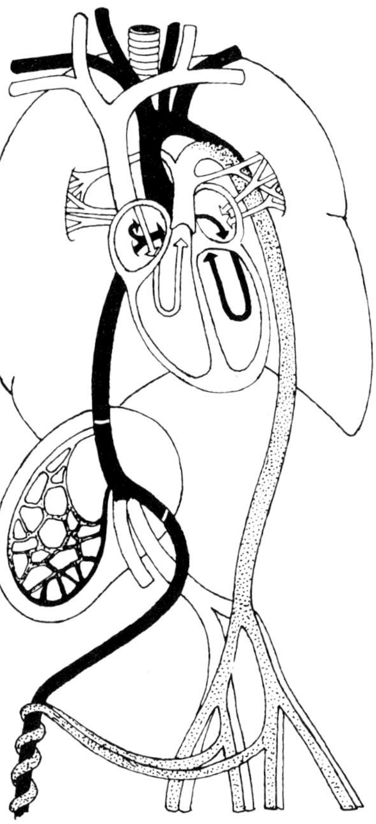

Fig. 18.4. The fetal circulation. *Black shading*, oxygenated blood at high Po_2; *stippled shading*, desaturated blood at relatively low Po_2. (After Rigby and Shinebourne 1981).

and the rise in left atrial pressure closes the foramen ovale. Rising pulmonary artery oxygen tension and circulatory pressure changes result in closure of the ductus arteriosus and ductus venosus.

Persistent Fetal Circulation

PFC, also referred to as persistent pulmonary arterial hypertension in the newborn, presents clinically as congestive heart failure with cyanosis in the neonate with left to right shunting and an increased pulmonary blood flow. Morphologically, the foramen ovale remains open, the ductus arteriosus largely patent and the right ventricle is hypertrophied and dilated. The main histological changes are found in the lung where the peripheral nonmuscular arteries and their branches become muscularised (peripheral muscularisation).

This can be demonstrated immunohistochemically by specific staining with α-smooth muscle actin antibody. The activated pericytes of the arteries and capillaries appear to proliferate, under as yet unidentified stimuli, and undergo transformation towards smooth muscle cells. The capillaries of the placenta villi are also thickened, suggesting intrauterine hypoxia.

Examination of the Heart

The need for careful and systematic dissection of the cardiovascular system in all perinatal and neonatal necropsies cannot be overemphasised (see Chap. 1, p. 19). Within the last decade, much has been done to simplify and standardise the nomenclature of congenital cardiac malformation, culminating in the sequential segmental approach detailed by Anderson and his collaborators, as well as others (Becker and Anderson 1981; Anderson et al. 1984; Devine et al. 1991; Jouk 1991), which is universally applicable.

The heart is considered in terms of three segments—atrial chambers, ventricular mass and great arteries. Identification of the morphology and position of the atrial chambers is followed by examination of their relationships and connections with the atrioventricular junctions and ventricular mass. The relationships and connections of the ventricles and ventriculoarterial junctions are then established.

Atrial morphology is determined almost exclusively by the shape of the atrial appendage. A morphologically right atrium has a blunt, cone-shaped appendage; its broad junction with the venous atrial component is identified by the crista terminalis. A morphologically left atrium has an appendage which is smaller, narrower, hook-shaped and somewhat scalloped; its junction with the venous part of the atrium is narrow; there is no crista terminalis.

Atrial morphology determines atrial situs as follows:

Situs solitus: The morphological right atrium is on the anatomical right and the morphological left atrium is on the left. This is the usual arrangement. The liver is on the right side, with stomach and spleen on the left. The right main stem bronchus, eparterial, is short, almost vertical, and superior to the right pulmonary artery. The other bronchus, hyparterial, is long, oblique and inferior to the left pulmonary artery. The right lung has three lobes and the left two.

Situs inversus: The morphological right atrium is on the anatomical left and the morphological left atrium is on the right. The hyparterial bronchus is on the right and the eparterial on the left. There is reversal of thoracoabdominal viscera.

Right atrial isomerism: Both atria are of morphological right type. Both main bronchi are eparterial. This situation is associated with asplenia and a midline liver.

Left atrial isomerism: Both atria are of morphological left type. There is associated polysplenia and a midline liver. Atrial isomerism is accompanied by abnormal morphology or situation of the thoracoabdominal organs (situs ambiguous). The bronchial tree is symmetrical and pulmonary veins are abnormally connected.

Juxtaposition: The atria are morphologically different but are situated on the same side, either right or left, of the arterial trunks. This uncommon situation is always associated with major cardiac malformations.

Once atrial situs is established, it is necessary to determine atrioventricular connections; this requires a knowledge of ventricular morphology. Each ventricle is made up of three component parts: an inlet portion guarded by the atrioventricular valve, a trabecular component which forms the major part of the ventricular mass and an outlet portion supporting the arterial valves. The morphological right ventricle has coarse trabeculations, while trabeculation of a morphological left ventricle is fine.

The possible connection of atria and ventricles are as follows:

Atrioventricular concordance: Right atrium to right ventricle, left atrium to left ventricle (normal heart).

Atrioventricular discordance: Right atrium to left ventricle, left atrium to right ventricle.

Ambiguous atrioventricular connection: Right or left atrial isomerism in continuity with ventricle of right or left morphology.

Double-inlet ventricle: Both atria in connection with one ventricle (right, left or indeterminate), univentricular heart.

Absent connection: One atrium has no connection with the corresponding ventricle.

The next step is to establish ventriculoarterial connections. The possible connections are as follows:

Ventriculoarterial concordance: The pulmonary trunk arises from a morphological right ventricle and the aorta from a morphological left ventricle, behind and to the left.

Ventriculoarterial discordance: The pulmonary trunk arises from a morphological left ventricle and the aorta from a morphological right ventricle: transposition of great arteries. An aortic valve to the right of the pulmonary valve is *d*-transposition, to the left of the pulmonary valve *l*-transposition.

Double-outlet connection: More than half of both great arteries arise from one ventricle, which may be right, left, rudimentary or indeterminate.

Truncus arteriosus: A single arterial trunk may arise from both ventricular chambers (overriding) or from a morphological right or left ventricle.

Single aortic trunk: The aorta arises from the ventricle with an atretic pulmonary trunk.

Single pulmonary trunk: The pulmonary trunk arises from ventricles with an atretic aorta. In either situation (single aortic trunk, single pulmonary trunk) the single trunk over-rides a septal defect.

Once this sequential segmental examination is accomplished, anomalies of any part of the heart and vascular connections can be described in an accurate and concise manner.

Congenital Heart Disease

Anomalies of Systemic Veins

Amongst the anomalies of the systemic veins, persistent left superior vena cava is the most common, comprising 2%–5% of congenital heart disease (Bankl 1977; Buirsky et al. 1986). It is often associated with other cardiac defects (tetralogy of Fallot 20%, Eisenmenger syndrome 8%). It is due to failure of obliteration of the left anterior cardinal vein. When connected to the right atrium, a left superior vena cava has no functional significance; the vessel runs obliquely, posterior to the left atrium and drains to the coronary sinus, which dilates. When it empties into the left atrium (8% of cases), it effects a right to left shunt. Sometimes, the innominate or left brachiocephalic vein may follow an anomalous course passing below the aortic arch to enter the superior vena cava below the orifice of the azygos vein (Gerlis and Ho 1989).

Rare anomalies of the inferior vena cava are described, including interruption below the hepatic vein and diversion via a dilated azygos vein into the superior vena cava.

Anomalies of Pulmonary Veins

Anomalous pulmonary venous connection occurs when the common pulmonary vein, an outgrowth of the left atrium, fails to establish connection with the intrapulmonary venous plexus or the connection becomes atretic at a very early stage of development. The anomalous pulmonary venous return may be total or partial, unilateral or bilateral.

In total anomalous pulmonary venous connection, all pulmonary veins drain into the systemic circulation above or below the diaphragm either by way of the left innominate vein, the coronary sinus, right atrium, right superior vena cava, portal system or by multiple sites (Sapire et al. 1986; Lucas et al. 1988; Rammos et al. 1990). The pulmonary veins thus continue to drain in the primitive foregut plexus (umbilicovitelline venous system).

Drainage of the aberrant supracardinal pulmonary venous connections to the innominate (left brachiocephalic) vein occurs in over 35% of cases and to the superior vena cava in about 13%. The cardiac type drains to the right atrium (15%) or coronary sinus (16%). In the infracardiac type, drainage is to the portal vein (6%) or the ductus venosus (3%) by a long trunk running in front of the oesophagus (Fig. 18.5). In 5%–9% of cases multiple connections may be present. Obstruction and stenosis of aberrant pulmonary veins is common at their junction with the systemic circulation and may result in pulmonary congestion and hypertension. In one-third of cases, major structural cardiac anomalies are present, and in 25%–30% extracardiac malformations are seen.

Since in total anomalous pulmonary venous connection, all pulmonary veins drain into the systemic circulation (Lucas et al. 1988), there is massive left to right shunting with hypertrophy

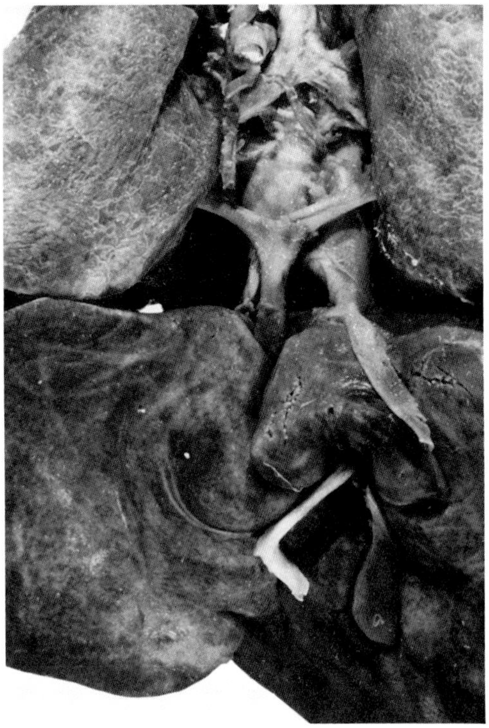

Fig. 18.5. Total anomalous pulmonary venous return to the portal vein; confluence of pulmonary veins viewed from the back.

and dilatation of the right atrium and ventricle, dilatation of the pulmonary artery and hyperperfusion of the lungs. The left side of the heart is hypoplastic. In this condition, circulation is maintained only by a large posterior atrial septal defect, which is always present. Prognosis is poor, with 50% of those affected dying by the age of 3 months, 70% by 6 months and 80% by 1 year if left untreated. Early diagnosis is important, as in many cases the common pulmonary trunk lies immediately behind the left atrium and surgical correction is simple.

Partial anomalous pulmonary venous return is twice as common as total anomalous connection and is usually right sided. It is compatible with long life.

Anomalies of Atrial Chambers

At birth, the rise in pressure within the left atrium causes the flap of the foramen ovale to close. It remains probe patent in about 30% of individuals, and it is important to distinguish between a guarded patent foramen ovale and a true atrial septal defect (ASD). In the latter the flap is too small to cover the entire foramen ovale.

Atrial Septal Defect

ASD is one of the commonest types of congenital heart disease and observed in about 10% of perinatal necropsies. It is functionally important only when very large or associated with other cardiac defects, as it is in approximately 15% of cases. There may be extracardiac anomalies. Several types of ASD are described. Secundum defect (ASD II, fossa ovalis type) is due to failure of the septum secundum to occlude the foramen secundum within the septum primum; it comprises 66% of ASDs. Defects involving the atrioventricular region (septum primum defects) comprise 26% of ASDs and are described on p. 437. Sinus venosus defects (vena cava superior defect) comprise 5% and inferior vena cava defects 1% of defective interatrial septa. The different types of defect may be present in combination.

ASD II is the most common type and is due to defective development of the flap of the foramen ovale (Fig. 18.6). It varies in size from a few millimetres to occupy most of the septum, so that only a small ring of septal tissue remains (cor triloculare, biventriculare).

The sinus venosus type of ASD is located in the inlet portion of the atrium, just beneath the superior vena cava. It is associated with anomalous connection of the right pulmonary veins.

Inferior caval defects are usually large and located posteriorly.

Atrial Septal Aneurysm

Congenital atrial septal aneurysm occurs in the interatrial septum mainly at the level of the foramen ovale with bulging into the cavity of either the left or right atrium or both. It is associated mainly with atrial septal defects and may become clinically apparent only when there is shunting across the defect, evidence of atrial tachyarrhythmias, or in association with Marfan's syndrome. It is commonly encountered in association with complex congenital cardiac abnormalities such as hypoplastic right ventricle, double-outlet right ventricle, Ebstein's anomaly and ventricular septal defects (Belkin and Kisslo 1990).

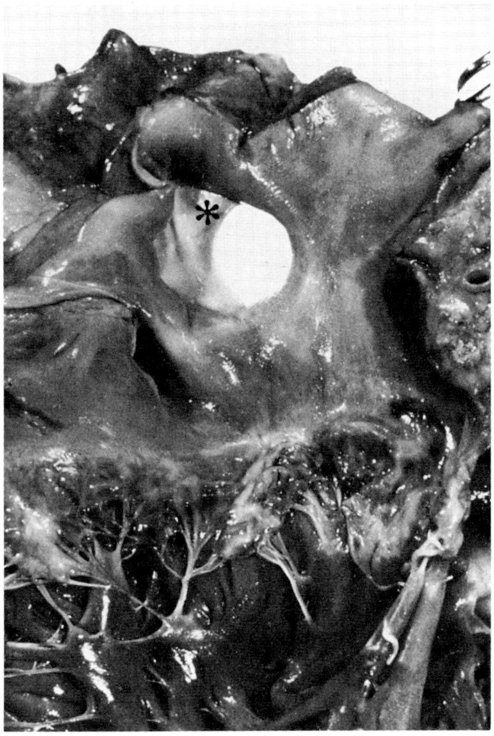

Fig. 18.6. ASD, secundum type, viewed from the right side. *Asterisk*, flap valve.

Premature Closure of the Foramen Ovale

Adhesion of the flap of the foramen ovale to the atrial septum during intrauterine life interrupts fetal circulation. This results in hypoplasia of the left heart and hypertrophy and dilatation of the right ventricle. Right ventricular failure can lead to hydrops in the fetus or neonate.

Cor Triatriatum Sinister

Defective incorporation of the common pulmonary vein into the left atrium results in the formation of a dorsocranial accessory atrial chamber which receives pulmonary venous return. This chamber is often dilated and exhibits endocardial thickening (fibroelastosis). It is separated from the caudal chamber, which gives rise to the atrial appendage and communicates with the mitral orifice by a thick fibromuscular membrane which is in continuity with the atrial septum. An ASD of secundum type is often present between the caudal atrial chamber and the right atrium. In over 90% of cases there is a communication between the two left-sided atrial chambers through a diaphragm, a tunnel-shaped orifice or a tubular structure. If the orifice is less than 3 mm in diameter, obstruction to venous return gives rise to pulmonary hypertension, and cardiac failure follows within the first year of life.

Anomalies of Atrioventricular Junctions

Atrioventricular (AV) septal defects and double-inlet ventricle are the most important malformations. Since endocardial cushions form the AV valves as well as the lower part of the atrial septum and the upper part of the ventricular septum (muscular and membranous components), any developmental anomaly of this region can produce a range of defects which are related to the timing of the insult (Silverman et al. 1986).

Atrioventricular Septal Defects (Endocardial Cushion Defects)

Three types are usually distinguished, depending on the extent of the lesion: ostium primum defect (ASD I, partial AV canal); incomplete persistent, common AV canal; and complete persistent, common AV canal.

Ostium primum defect. This is the least severe form of endocardial cushion defect and is situated in the lower portion of the atrial septum. The tricuspid and mitral valves are separate but sometimes have a cleft septal leaflet. The lesion is rare and comprises about 1% of congenital heart disease. It is often associated with a secundum ASD (17%), left superior vena cava (15%) and pulmonary stenosis (5%).

Incomplete persistent, common AV canal. This defect is similar to the preceding one, but additionally there is bridging of valve tissue from the anterior to the posterior portion of the valves. Two AV orifices are clearly defined. There is female predominance (3:1); trisomy 21 is present in 15%–20% and asplenia or polysplenia in 15%–25% of cases.

Complete persistent, common AV canal. This is the most severe variety of endocardial cushion defect. There is a single large AV orifice common to both ventricles. The anterior and

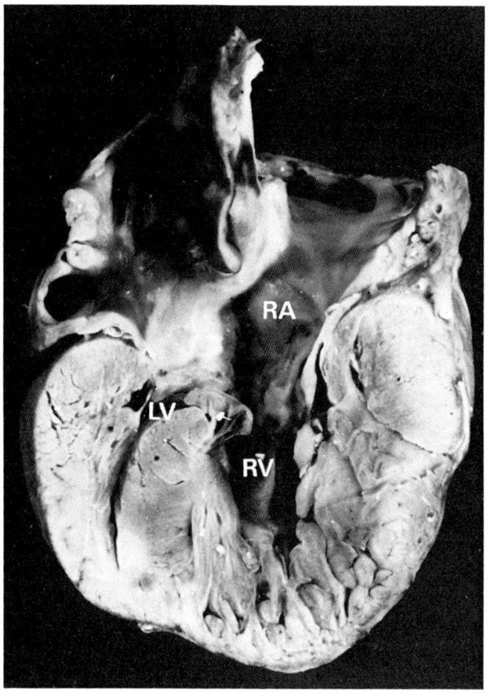

Fig. 18.7. Complete persistent common AV canal with hypertrophy of the right atrium and ventricle. Hypoplasia of the left atrium and ventricle with coarctation of the aorta and patent ductus arteriosus in Di George syndrome. *LV*, left ventricle; *RA*, right atrium; *RV*, right ventricle.

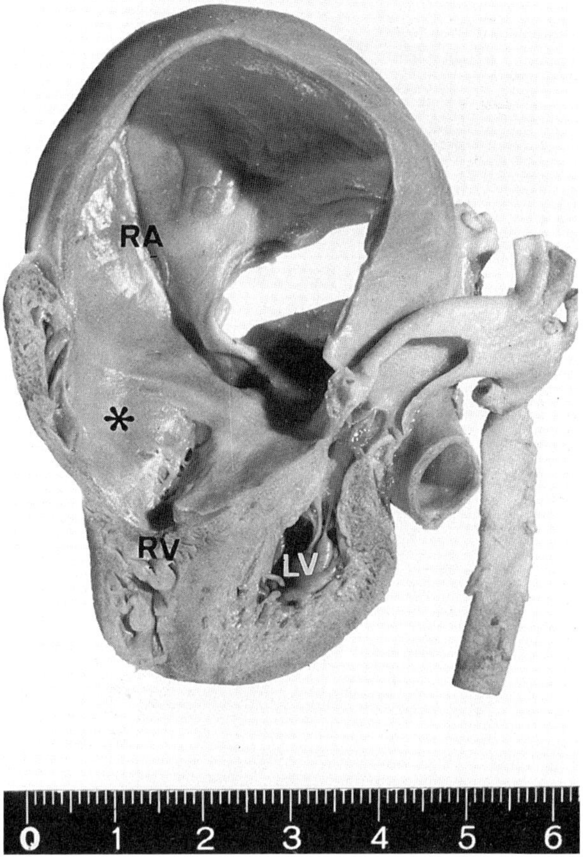

Fig. 18.8. Ebstein's anomaly. The tricuspid valve leaflets (*) are displaced downwards into the right ventricle (RV). The latter is reduced in volume and the right atrium (RA) is markedly dilated. LV, left ventricle.

posterior parts of the septal valve leaflets are fused over a large perimembranous ventricular septal defect (VSD; Fig. 18.7). This lesion comprises 5%–6.5% of congenital heart disease and is a common finding in trisomy 21 (40%–60%).

The large communication between all four chambers results in a left to right shunt with volume overload and elevated pressure in the right side of the heart. Pulmonary hypertension is an early consequence with death in infancy or childhood.

Double-inlet Ventricle

In the condition of double-inlet ventricle both AV valves open into a single ventricular chamber which may display right or left morphological features or may be of indeterminate type. When the main ventricle has determinate morphology a second small rudimentary chamber lacking an inlet portion is connected to the main chamber. The presence of this rudimentary chamber is often apparent on external inspection of the heart, as the descending branches of the coronary artery are a useful surface marker of the position of the interventricular septum. There is a high incidence of associated lesions.

Ebstein's Anomaly

In Ebstein's anomaly there is displacement of the attachment of the tricuspid valve leaflets from the AV junction into the inlet and trabecular portions of the right ventricle. The attachment of the valve leaflet is variable, and in its severest form the inlet portion of the ventricle is incorporated into the right atrium (Fig. 18.8). Involvement of both tricuspid and mitral valves may simultaneously occur (Dusmet et al. 1987). VSDs and occasionally AVSDs and other complex cardiac malforma-

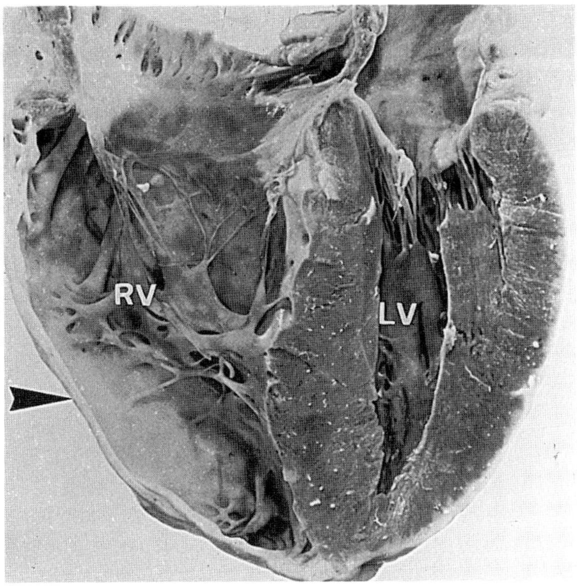

Fig. 18.9. Uhl's anomaly. The right ventricular wall is thin, fibrous (parchment) and dilated. RV, right ventricle; LV, left ventricle.

tions may be associated with this anomaly, but ASDs and pulmonary stenosis or atresia are the commonest additional malformations.

Uhl's Anomaly

In Uhl's anomaly (parchment right ventricle) there is marked dilatation of the thin-walled right ventricle whose wall is composed essentially of endocardium and epicardium, or separated by thin bands of connective tissue englobing islets or bands of myocardium, but the valve leaflets are normal (Fig. 18.9). The right atrium or both may be involved. The left ventricle is usually hypertrophied and there are often associated cardiovascular malformations.

Atrioventricular Valve Atresia

Atresia of tricuspid or mitral valves is always associated with reduced size of the corresponding ventricle. In a minority of cases, configuration of the small ventricle is normal (true hypoplasia) lying below an imperforate atrioventricular membrane. In most cases, however, there is only a rudimentary chamber which lacks an inlet portion (univentricular heart). There is absence of the atrioventricular connection. The floor of the blind-ending atrium is usually muscular and separated from the ventricle by the AV sulcus. In either case, interruption of circulation results in reduction of size of both the corresponding ventricle and the corresponding arterial trunk. These combinations are often called hypoplastic left or right heart syndrome (see p. 443). The noncommunicating atrium is poorly developed as blood is shunted to the opposite atrium through a widely patent foramen ovale or ASD. Due to the complex nature of the associated anomalies (atrial, ventricular and atrioventricular valves) in this condition, it is always important to establish the morphological details of the systemic and pulmonary venous connections, the atrioventricular junction, the infundibular morphology and the ventriculoarterial connection in order to arrive at an accurate nomenclature (Wenink and Ottenkamp 1987; Rigby et al. 1990; Anderson and Tynan 1991).

Absent Tricuspid Valve

Absent tricuspid valve (unguarded tricuspid orifice) is rare. The tricuspid leaflets are absent. In the case that we have seen there was marked dilatation of the right ventricle and anasarca.

Congenital Blood Cysts of AV Valves

Blood cysts of the free borders of tricuspid and mitral valves are an extremely common necropsy finding in the neonate Fig. 18.10. Cysts are variable in size and number and appear to be the result of ventricular endothelial infoldings in the base of the valve leaflet. They are of no clinical significance (Zimmerman et al. 1983).

Anomalies of Ventricular Chambers

Apart from VSD and Fallot's tetralogy, most ventricular lesions are associated with abnormal atrioventricular or ventriculoarterial connections.

Ventricular Septal Defect

VSD is one of the most common cardiac malformations, comprising about 20% of congenital

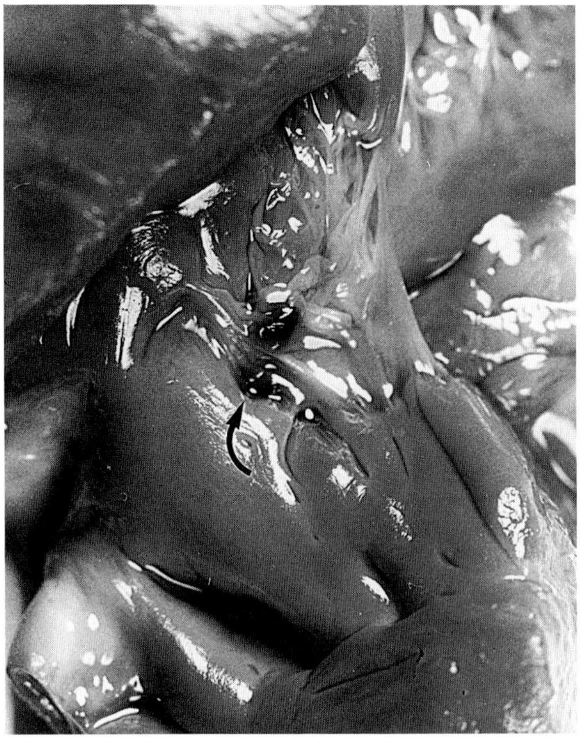

Fig. 18.10. Blood cysts on tricuspid valve in a 32 weeks premature baby.

heart disease, but has little significance in the perinatal period when present as an isolated lesion. It often accompanies other major cardiac malformations. A VSD may involve any part of the interventricular septum, either inlet, trabecular, outlet or membranous parts or a combination of these (Soto et al. 1989; Van Praagh et al. 1989). Most defects involving predominantly the membranous part extend to other portions and are classified as perimembranous; their border is formed in part by the central fibrous body (Fig. 18.11).

The second most common type is the muscular septal defect. Its border is formed by myocardial tissue only. It may be central in position but is often present in the anteroapical part of the septum.

Subarterial or infundibular defects lie directly under the pulmonary and aortic orifices which form part of the edge of the defect. The relationship of the defect to the cardiac conduction system depends on the type of VSD present. The bundle of His is posteroinferior to the perimembranous defect and its position is variable (Ueda and Becker 1985); it is anterosuperior to a muscular defect and unrelated to the infundibular septal defect.

Haemodynamic changes depend mainly on the size of the VSD. Small defects (5 mm or less) are of little significance and close spontaneously in up to 60% of cases. Large defects, on the other hand, are responsible for left to right shunts resulting in right ventricular hypertrophy and pulmonary hypertension, which are usually reversible before the age of 2 years.

Tetralogy of Fallot

Fallot's tetralogy, the most common cause of congenital heart disease, is in its classic form characterised by subvalvular pulmonary

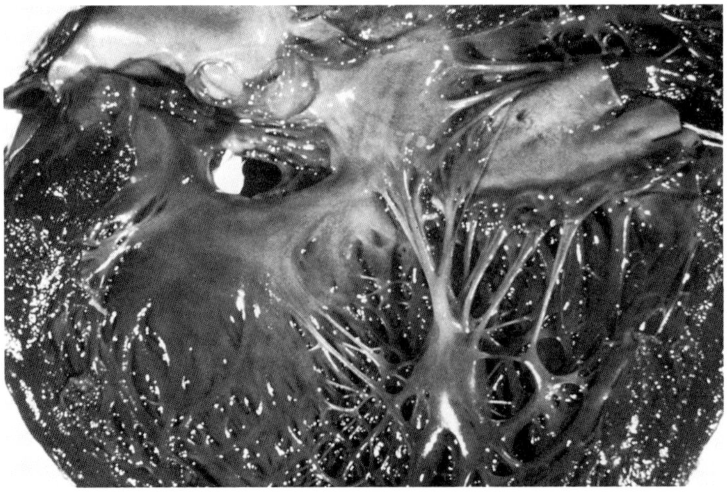

Fig. 18.11. Perimembranous VSD viewed from the left ventricle.

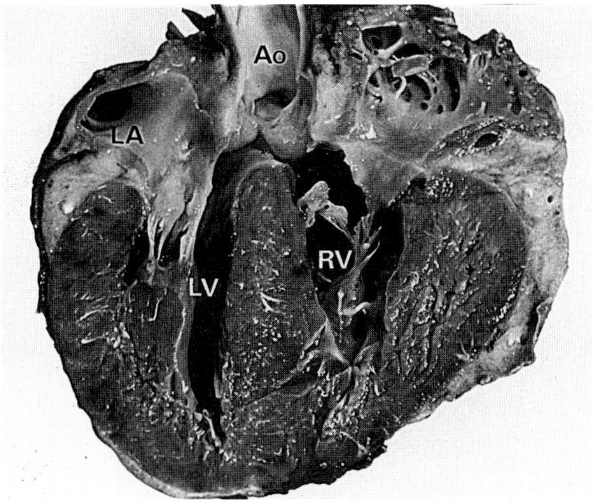

Fig. 18.12. Tetralogy of Fallot with over-riding aorta; there is marked right ventricular hypertrophy. *Ao*, aorta; *LA*, left atrium; *LV*, left ventricle; *RV*, right ventricle.

stenosis, VSD, overriding aorta and hypertrophy of the right ventricle (Fig. 18.12). It is rarely fatal in the perinatal period, but the more extreme maninfestations may be fatal in the neonatal period, when pulmonary outflow obstruction is compounded by valvular atresia or when associated with other serious malformations (Howell et al. 1990; Suzuki et al. 1990).

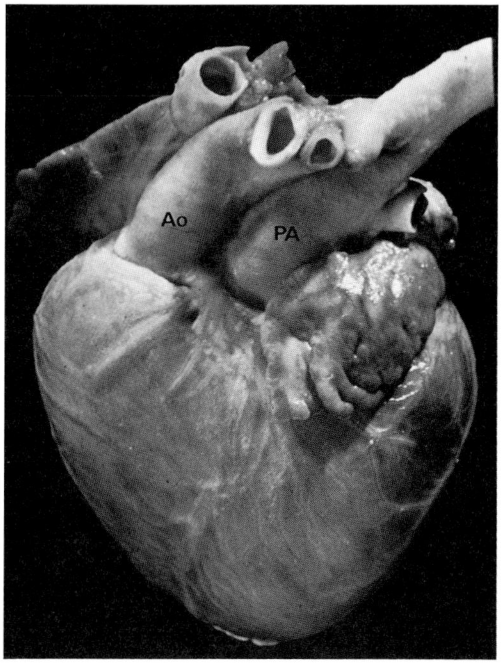

Fig. 18.13. TGA. *Ao*, aorta; *PA*, pulmonary artery.

Ventricular Aneurysm

Aneurysm of the left ventricle free wall or its apex in neonates is documented more freqently with the new radiological techniques. Histologically the wall is made up of fibrous tissue with little or no myocardium. The condition is sometimes associated with fetal and perinatal dysrhythmia.

Subaortic Muscular Stenosis (Hypertrophic Cardiomyopathy)

The abnormality known as subaortic muscular stenosis is only rarely described in newborns (Maron et al. 1982). In recent years this disorder has been diagnosed prenatally and confirmed on histological examination of the heart (Allan et al. 1985; Gerlis 1985). The histological diagnosis must not be confused with that of infants of diabetic mothers.

Aortic Valvular Stenosis

Aortic valvular stenosis is seldom seen as an isolated finding in the newborn; this anomaly and aortic valve atresia are most commonly seen as part of hypoplastic left heart syndrome.

Anomalies of Great Arteries and Conotruncus

Anomalies of the great arteries and conotruncus are an important group of cardiac malformations and comprise most of the defects which are present in the neonatal period. The main lesions are transposition of the great arteries (TGA), persistent truncus arteriosus, coarctation, interrupted aortic arch and aortic or pulmonary atresia.

Transposition of Great Arteries

TGA is characterised by a discordant ventriculo-arterial communication, with either a discordant atrioventricular (corrected transposition) or concordant atrioventricular (complete transposition) connection. In its most common form, the aorta arises anteriorly from the right ventricle (Fig. 18.13). It has a muscular conus, whilst fibrous continuity is present between the mitral valve and the abnormally positioned pulmonary trunk, which arises from the left ventricle.

In situs solitus with atrioventricular concordance, systemic venous blood returns to the right atrium and is conducted by the right ventricle to the aorta and systemic circulation. Oxygenated blood from the pulmonary veins recirculates to the lungs through the left atrium and ventricle and pulmonary trunk. Life is dependent on a communication between systemic and pulmonary circulation through the foramen ovale, ASD, VSD or patent ductus arteriosus. Creation of an artificial shunt by balloon septostomy (Rashkind procedure) serves as a palliative measure until surgical correction is possible.

Several variations of transposition depending on the relationship of aorta and pulmonary valve and cardiac situs have been described. TGA is relatively common, accounting for 16%–21% of congenital heart disease at necropsy (Bankl 1977).

Double-Outlet Right Ventricle

In this condition both the aorta and pulmonary trunk take their origin principally from the right ventricle with the aorta to the right of the pulmonary trunk and parallel to it. The position of the septal defect to both vessels is quite variable, thus giving rise to a heterogenous group of abnormalities. When the pulmonary trunk overrides or is in close relation to the septal defect the condition is referred to as the Taussig–Bing anomaly.

Truncus Arteriosus

In the anomaly of truncus arteriosus a single arterial trunk leaves the base of the heart via a single semilunar valve and gives rise to systemic and pulmonary arteries (Crupi et al. 1977). It is the result of failure of septation of the primitive truncus arteriosus. A VSD is always present; the single semilunar valve which comprises two to six cusps overrides the defect and the truncus receives blood from both ventricles.

A classification based on the origin of the pulmonary arteries was proposed by Collett and Edwards (1949). A single pulmonary trunk arises from the aorta in Type I. In Type II, both pulmonary arteries take their origin separately from the posterior wall of the trunk (Fig. 18.14) or from the lateral (Type III) aspect of the common trunk. In Type IV, the lungs are supplied by bronchial arteries arising from the descending aorta; this type is probably better considered as a variety of pulmonary atresia. Associated anomalies include absent ductus arteriosus (50%), abnormal coronary artery distribution and right-sided aortic arch.

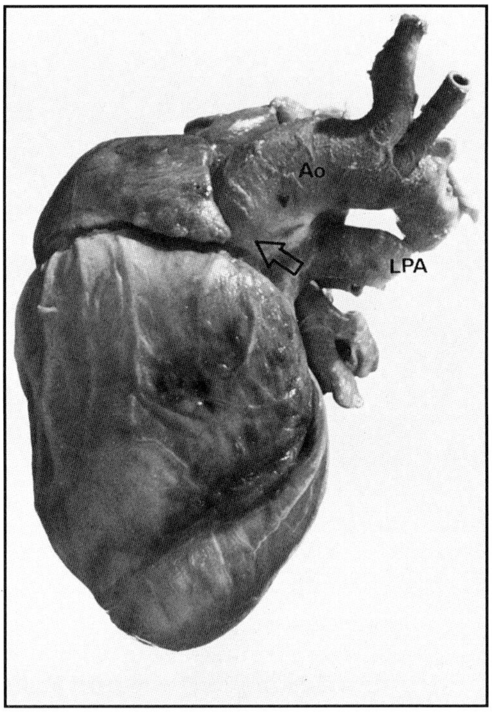

Fig. 18.14. Truncus arteriosus communis Type I with an associated membranous ventricular septal defect. *Open arrow*, truncus; *Ao*, aorta; *LPA*, left pulmonary artery.

Coarctation

The isthmus of the aorta in the normal neonate is always narrower than the ascending aorta, reaching only about two-thirds of the diameter of the ascending trunk. This physiological narrowing should be distinguished from coarctation.

The usual form of coarctation seen in the neonate is uniform tubular narrowing of the distal aortic arch (tubular hypoplasia) (Fig. 18.15). A localised constriction proximal to the entry of the ductus arteriosus (juxtaductal coarctation) is more commonly seen in infancy or childhood. Anatomical variations depend largely on the localisation and extent of involve-

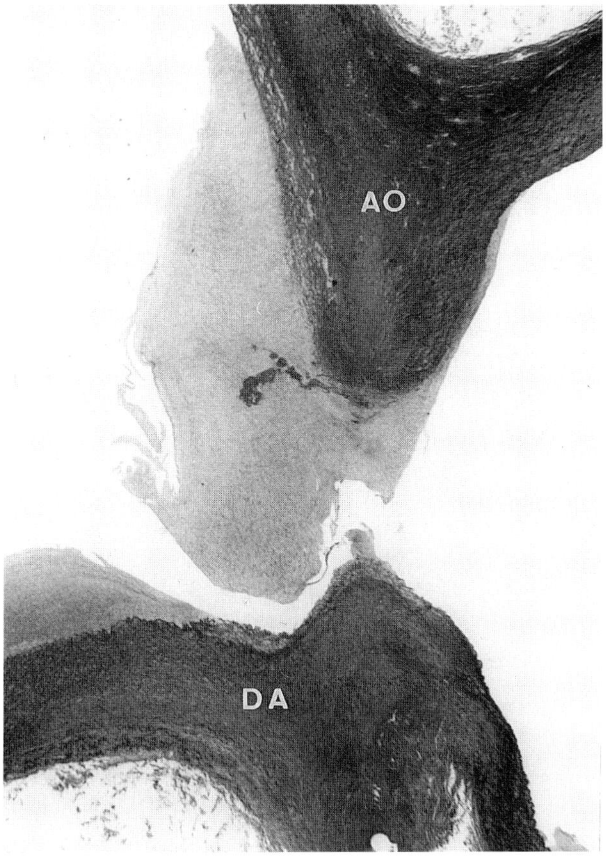

a

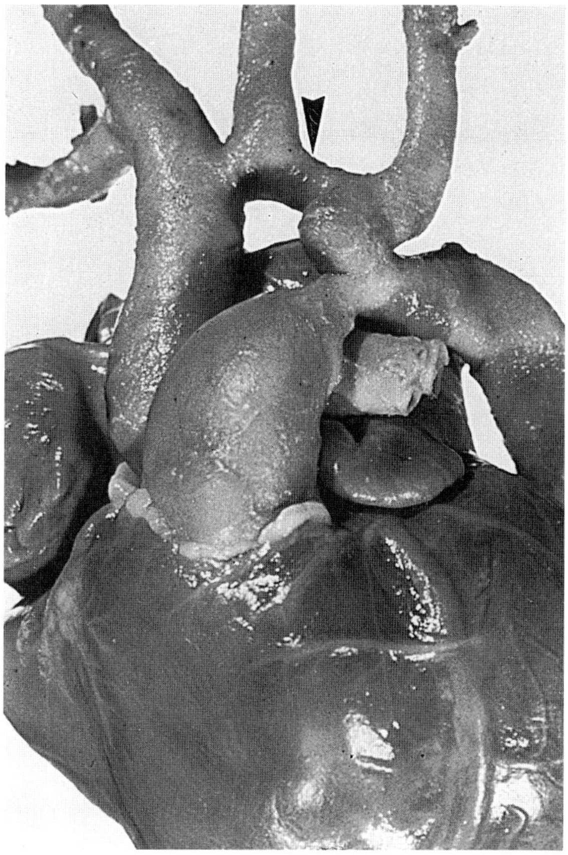

b

Fig. 18.15. **a** Aortic coarctation—histology: the upper portion of the aortic wall (AO) is folded, recovered by a dense layer of intimal thickening, obliterating almost completely the lumen and pointing towards the ductus arterious (DA). **b** Aortic coarctation with tubular narrowing (tubular hypoplasia) of the aortic arch.

ment of ductal tissue. This may determine both choice of treatment and outcome.

Coarctation may be associated with other cardiac anomalies including hypoplastic left heart syndrome (Ho and Anderson 1979; Elzenga and Gittenberger-de Groot 1985; Pellegrino et al. 1985). Perfusion of the trunk and legs occurs via a patent ductus arteriosus, and in most cases an intracardiac malformation which diverts blood flow to the right ventricle is also present; a bicuspid aortic valve of occurs in 46%–85% of cases or a variety of aortic outflow obstructions. The ascending aorta and aortic arch usually show some degree of hypoplasia.

Interrupted Aortic Arch

Regression or atrophy of the proximal left dorsal aorta or the fourth aortic arch leads to complete interruption of the aortic arch. Classification is related to the segment involved (Fig. 18.16). Most common are Type A (immediately distal to the left subclavian artery, 44%) and Type B (between left subclavian artery and left carotid artery, 52%). Type C, proximal to the left carotid artery, is rare (4%). Perfusion of the trunk and legs occurs via a patent ductus arteriosus. Surgical correction is difficult; 70% of affected infants die within the first month of life.

Aortic Atresia (Hypoplastic Left Heart Syndrome)

Aortic atresia is one of the commonest causes of cardiac failure in the neonate. In most cases there is absent left atrioventricular connection (mitral atresia or stenosis) and the ventricular septum is intact (Thiene et al. 1981). The left

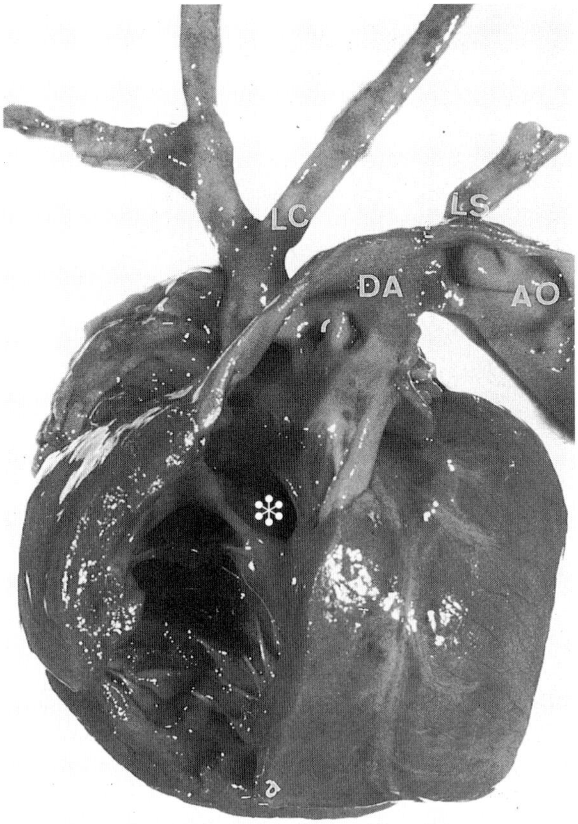

Fig. 18.16. There is interruption of the aortic arch between the left carotid (LC) and the left subclavian (LS) arteries. The aorta (AO) continues from the ductus arteriosus (DA). * = ventricular septal defect.

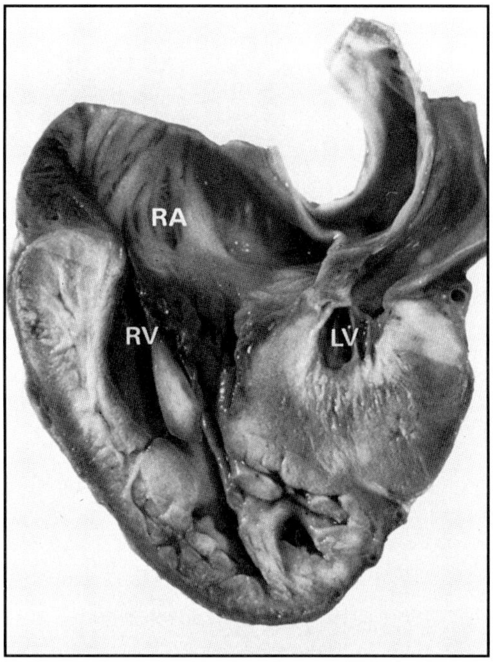

Fig. 18.17. Aortic valve atresia with hypoplasia and dysplasia of the mitral valve. The right ventricle is normally formed and dilated. The left ventricle is represented by a rudimentary inlet chamber with endocardial fibroelastosis. *RA*, right atrium; *RV*, right ventricle; *LV*, rudimentary left ventricle.

ventricle is rudimentary and the ascending aorta atretic or hypoplastic (Fig. 18.17). Systemic circulation depends on the hypertrophic right ventricle and a dilated ductus arteriosus or arterial canal. Cardiac perfusion is retrograde through the hypoplastic aortic arch and ascending aorta. Closure of the ductus arteriosus leads to irreversible, often fatal, cardiac failure within the first days of life. Coexistent cardiac abnormalities may be identified.

Pulmonary Atresia (Hypoplastic Right Heart Syndrome)

Pulmonary atresia with VSD constitutes the most severe form of Fallot's tetralogy. In cases where the ventricular septum is intact, there is a normally committed but small right ventricle (true hypoplastic right heart). In most cases, however, there is only a rudimentary right chamber present below the absent atrioventricular connection (tricuspid atresia) (Fig. 18.18). This is one type of univentricular heart. The pulmonary trunk is represented by a narrow fibrous remnant. The ascending aorta is very large and pulmonary perfusion is retrograde through a widely patent ductus arteriosus. Coronary arteries are often abnormal and communicate with the right ventricle through widely patent sinusoids.

Other Anomalies

Acardia

Acardia is an uncommon developmental anomaly and is found only in monozygotic twins where survival of the acardiac fetus is due to anastomoses with the circulation of the co-twin (see Chap. 9, p. 227).

Ectopia Cordis

Ectopia cordis may accompany defects of the sternum and thoracic wall (Cantrell et al. 1958; Poulias et al. 1982; Kaplan et al. 1985). Survival is dependent on both the extent of the abdominal wall defect and the nature of coexistent anomalies.

Metabolic Disorders

Among the many metabolic disorders affecting the heart in infancy and childhood, relatively few are seen in the neonate; however, as many of these conditions may be identified prenatally, early recognition of cardiovascular involvement in some of these disorders is likely.

Infants of Diabetic Mothers

Cardiomegaly with hypertrophy of the heart and visceromegaly in infants of diabetic mothers (IDMs) are well documented. The histological appearances often resemble those of hypertrophic cardiomyopathy (see p. 441). However, it is also important to note the increased risk and severity of congenital malformations in IDMs involving the cardiovascular, digestive, urinary and musculoskeletal systems, often associated with intrauterine death. Among the most common cardiovascular abnormalities are double-outlet right ventricle and truncus arteriosus (Ferencz et al. 1990; Johnson et al. 1991). A recent case we saw had, in addition to hypoplasia of the pulmonary trunk and its branches and the ductus arteriosus, also pulmonary stenosis with bicuspid valves, CIV and CIA, as well as severe caudal regression and imperforate anus (Fig. 18.19a,b).

Glycogen Storage Disease

Cardiac involvement is common in glycogen storage disease Type II (Pompe's disease, alpha-1, 4-glucosidase, acid maltase deficiency). In the infantile form there is generalised myocardial involvement, the myocardium being firm and pale with biventricular hypertrophy (Fig. 18.20a). Endocardial fibroelastosis is commonly present. Histological examination shows massive deposits of glycogen in the myocardium displacing myofibrils and nuclei towards the periphery of the cell (Fig. 18.20b). Liver, skeletal muscle, smooth muscle and the central nervous system are also involved.

A recently described disorder where excessive glycogen deposition is restricted to the heart has been identified (Eishi et al. 1985).

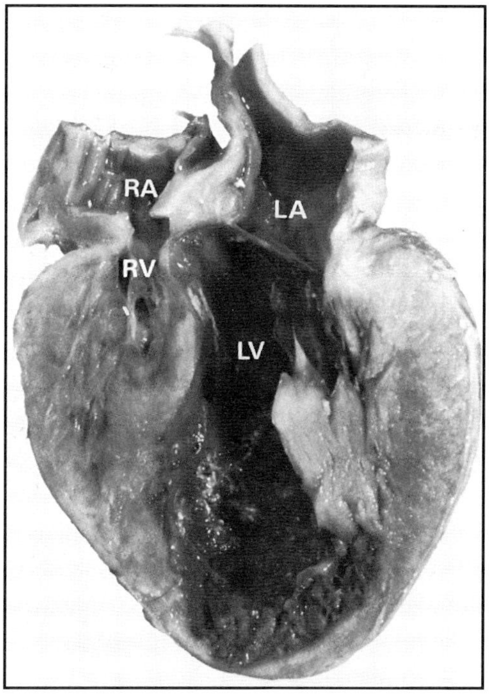

Fig. 18.18. Pulmonary valve atresia with tricuspid valve stenosis. There is a right-sided rudimentary ventricle. *RA*, right atrium; *RV*, right ventricle; *LA*, left atrium; *LV*, left ventricle.

Mucopolysaccharidoses

In lysosomal enzyme defects, the heart and vessels may be involved; however, relatively few cases are documented in the perinatal period, most frequently mucopolysaccharidoses (Hurler syndrome). There is marked accumulation of mucopolysaccharide within the myocardium, leading to cardiac failure. In Fabry's disease the abnormal deposits of glycosphingolipids can be demonstrated in myocardial cells by specific immunohistochemical techniques (Ogawa et al. 1989).

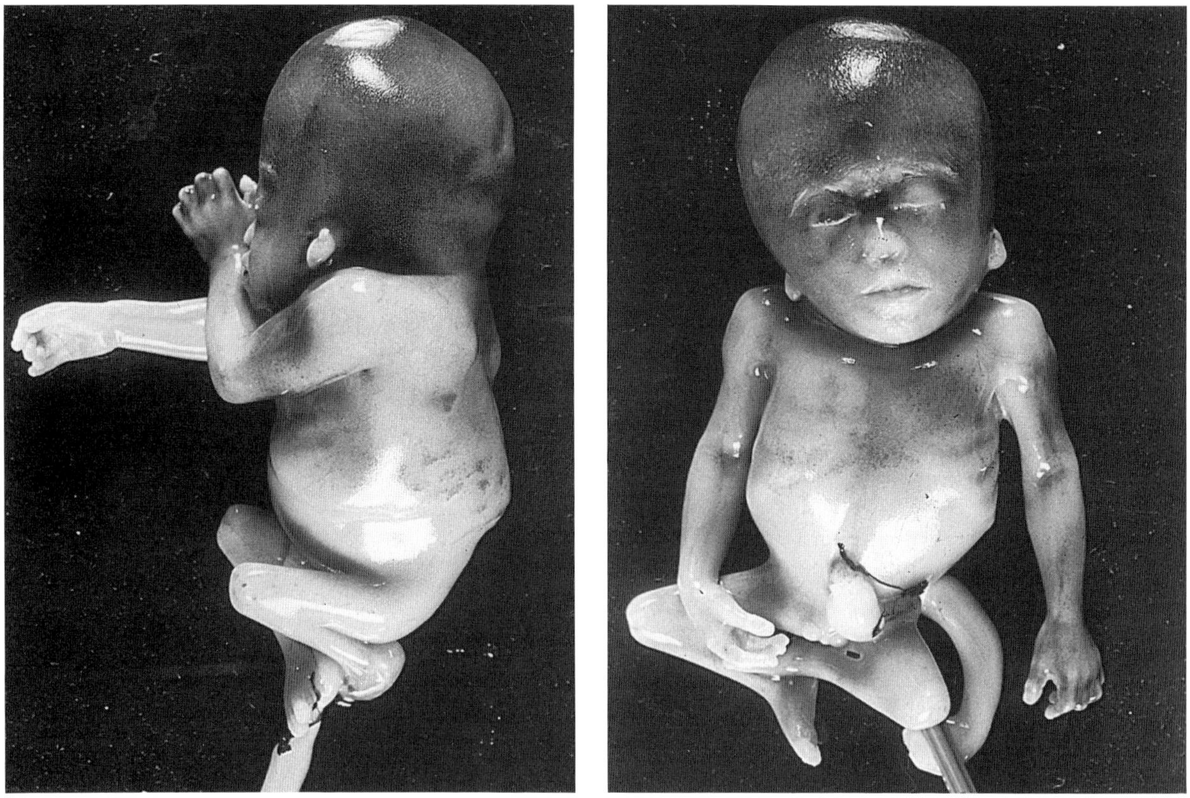

a b

Fig. 18.19. Fetus of diabetic mother with severe, complex cardiovascular malformation with **a** caudal regression and **b** characteristic "Buddha" presentation.

Other Cardiomyopathies

Many congenital myopathies may have associated cardiomyopathy (Stoeckel et al. 1981; Hübner and Grantzow 1983; Langes et al. 1985; Bertini et al. 1990). The heart is enlarged at birth and cardiac insufficiency may be the presenting symptom. The systemic form of carnitine deficiency may involve the neonatal myocardium often associated with anasarca (Steenhout et al. 1990; Rocchiccioli et al. 1990).

Histiocytoid or Lipid Cardiomyopathy

Histiocytoid or lipid cardiomyopathy is a rare condition which may present as neonatal heart failure (Zimmermann et al. 1982; Papadimitriou et al. 1984). The heart may be only slightly enlarged but contains bright yellow subendocardial nodules, mainly in the left ventricle, papillary muscles, chordae tendineae and valvular insertions. Histologically these foci are composed of large cells with well-defined borders and foamy lipid-rich cytoplasm (Fig. 18.21). This disorder is probably due to a defect of complex III (reduced coenzyme Q-cytochrome C reductase) in the respiratory chain in mitochondria of myocardial cells.

Infection

Endocarditis

Endocarditis, formerly considered rare in the neonate, has, in recent years, been observed with increasing frequency as the result of the more frequent use of indwelling catheters (umbilical and central venous) in the premature and severely asphyxiated newborn and of the frequent use of invasive cardiographic evaluation of potential cardiac malformations. The condition is known to complicate septicaemia, omphalitis, meningitis and severe hypoxia as well as congenital heart disease.

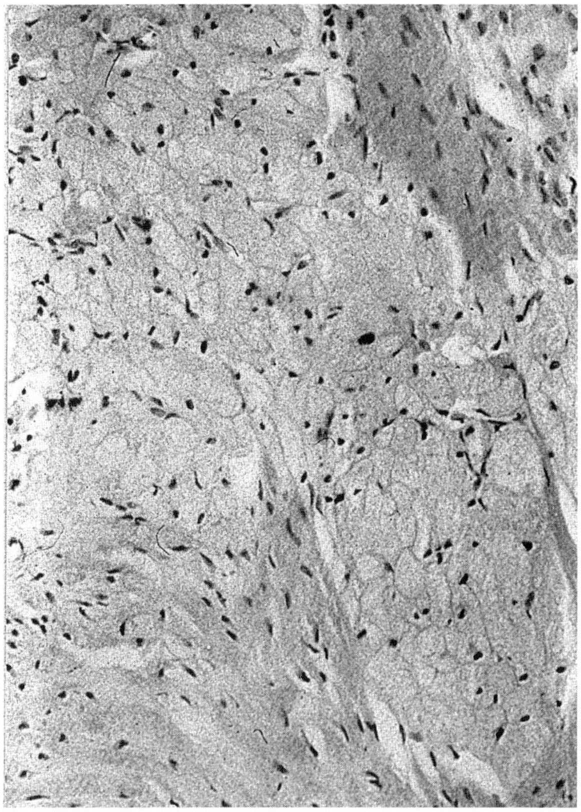

Fig. 18.21. Histiocytoid (oncocytic) cardiomyopathy. The myocardial cells are large, with a pale, foamy or granular cytoplasm due to a marked increased in number of mitochondria.

Bacterial endocarditis is uncommon; the main organisms implicated are *Staphylococcus aureus*, *Staph. epidermidis*, *Staph. viridans*, *Escherichia coli*, β-haemolytic streptococci and occasionally other organisms. Non-bacterial endocarditis is more prevalent and generally associated with the use of indwelling catheters, where endothelial trauma from the catheter evokes secondary infection.

In developing countries *Coxiella burnetii* and *Chlamydia trachomatis* (Laufer et al. 1986) are potential pathogens. The tricuspid valve is more frequently affected than is the mitral (Fig.

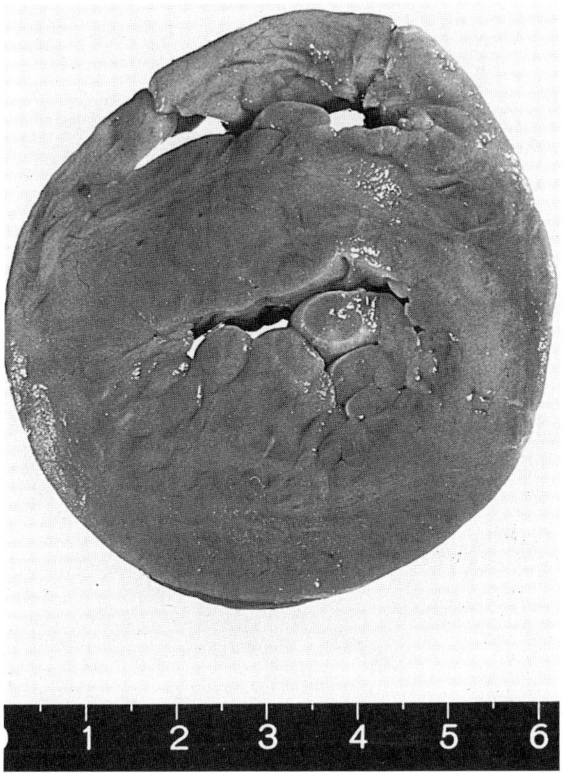

a

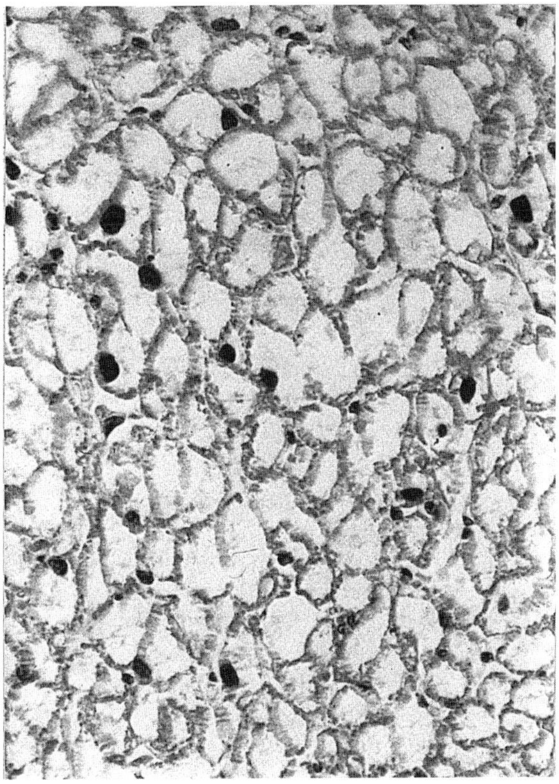

b

Fig. 18.20. Type II glycogenosis (Pompe's disease). **a** There is marked hypertrophy of both ventricles. **b** Histologically, there is vacuolisation of the myocytes with the myofibrils and nuclei pushed against the cell membrane.

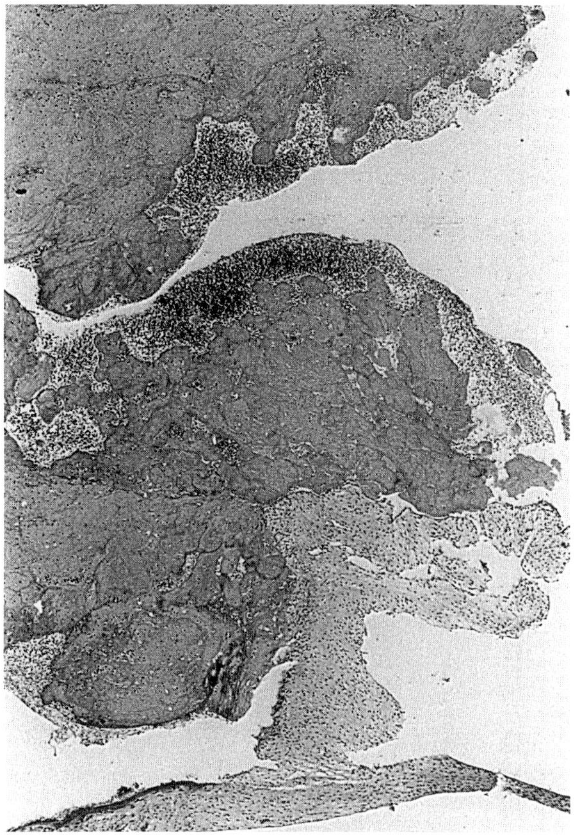

Fig. 18.22. Tricuspid valve endocarditis. Cauliflower-like fibrinous vegetation adhering to valve leaflet.

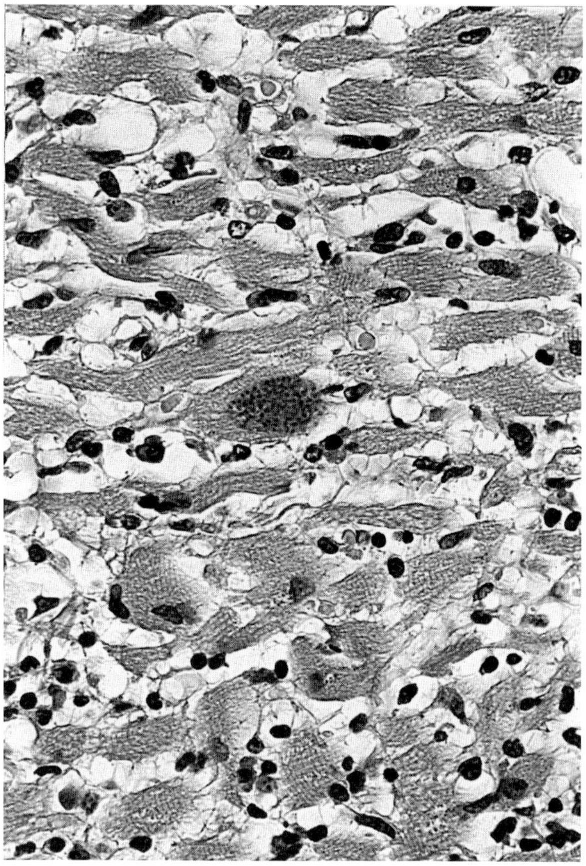

Fig. 18.23. Toxoplasma myocarditis. Toxoplasma pseudocyst in centre of field. Mild mononuclear cell infiltration.

18.22), and one or both atrial walls (McGinness et al. 1980; Oelberg et al. 1983; Vesikari et al. 1985) and the pulmonary valve may be involved (Ward et al. 1983).

Myocarditis

Myocarditis is rarely reported in the neonatal period and is often associated with endocarditis or is an incidental post-mortem finding. Whilst a variety of pathogens have been incriminated, the majority of recorded cases have been related to Coxsackie virus group B infection. In cases of congenital toxoplasmosis, cysts should be carefully sought in the myocardium (Fig. 18.23).

Cardiac chambers are usually dilated and flabby. Histologically there is isolated or focal eosinophilic degeneration of muscle fibres and round cell infiltration (DeSa 1985; Herreman et al. 1985). In one of our neonatal cases there was an accompanying psoas myositis.

Bacterial myocarditis has been reported complicating septicaemia (Fig. 18.24); multiple abscesses may be present (Oelberg et al. 1983). Mycotic infection may have a similar distribution.

Endocardial Fibroelastosis

Endocardial fibroelastosis—abnormal thickening of the endocardium, usually of one or both ventricles, by collagen and elastic tissue—may be primary or secondary.

Primary endocardial fibroelastosis occurs in an anatomically normal heart. The left ventricle is most severely affected. The endocardium is thick, whitish and opaque (Fig. 18.25). There

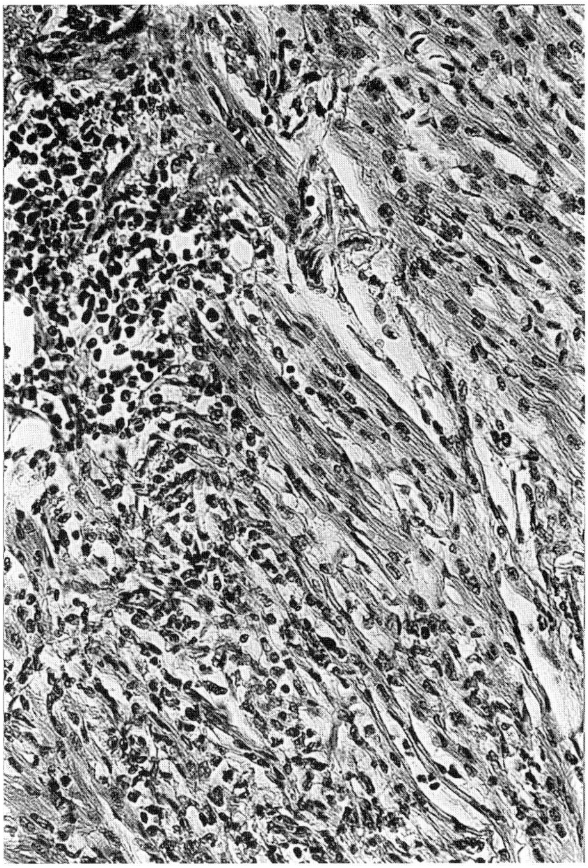

a

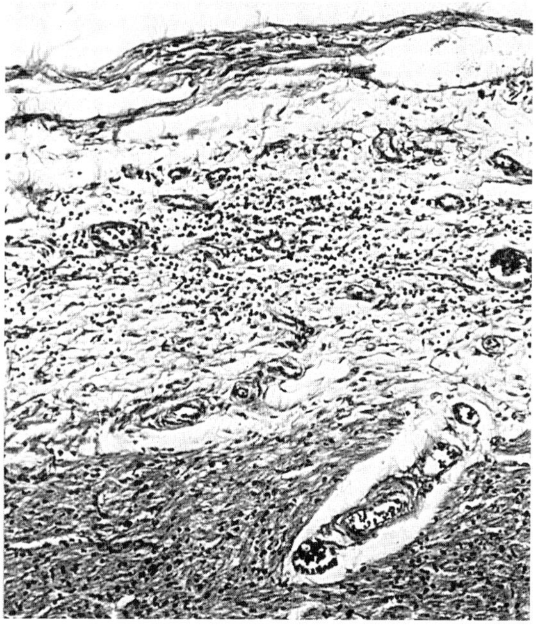

b

Fig. 18.24. **a** Septicaemia with diffuse mononuclear cell infiltration, microabscess and necrotic fibres of myocardium. **b** Inflammatory cell infiltration of the oedematous epicardium.

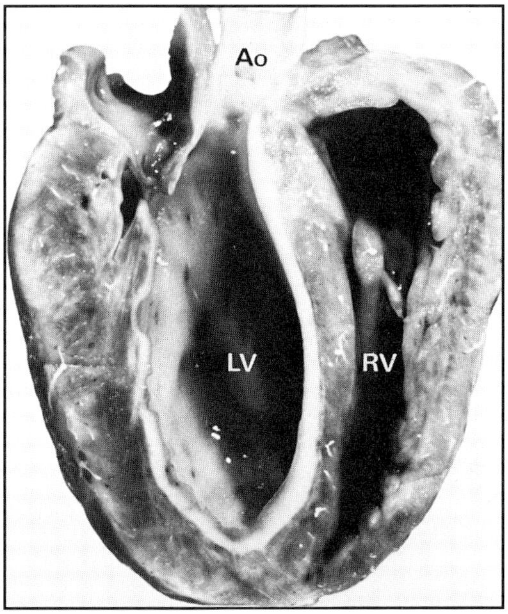

Fig. 18.25. Fibroelastosis of the left atrium and ventricle. There is stenosis of the aortic valve. *Ao*, aorta; *LV*, left ventricle; *RV*, right ventricle.

is marked hypertrophy of the myocardium, usually with dilatation of the ventricular cavity. A few cases with ventricular hypertrophy and contraction of the cavity have been described (Ursell et al. 1984). This condition has been described in the right ventricle in association with pulmonary hypertension (Larson et al. 1984). Both cavities may be involved simultaneously and present with congenital complete heart block (Rios et al. 1984; Huang et al. 1985). The aetiology and pathogenesis of this condition remain obscure, although intrauterine viral infection, metabolic and storage diseases, anomalous cardiac lymphatic drainage and maternal medication have all been incriminated (Ino et al. 1988; Stephan et al. 1989). Histologically the endocardium is markedly thickened and rich in connective tissue and elastic fibres (Fig. 18.26).

Secondary endocardial fibroelastosis is associated with cardiac malformation. It may be focal or confluent and is most commonly seen with aortic atresia or stenosis when the mitral valve is stenosed, in cases of anomalous

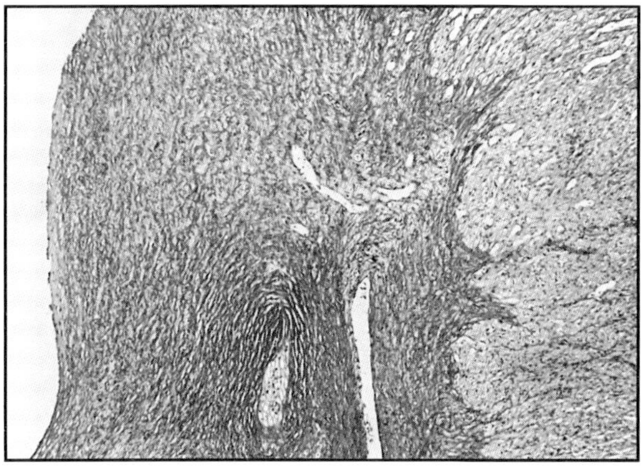

Fig. 18.26. Primary fibroelastosis. There is marked fibroelastic thickening of the endocardium. (Weigert's elastic Van Gieson).

origin of the left coronary artery from the pulmonary artery and aortic coarctation.

Myocardial Necrosis

Myocardial necrosis, once thought to be uncommon in the perinatal period, has recently been shown to be a relatively frequent event, especially amongst those coming to necropsy after severe perinatal asphyxia or prolonged mechanical ventilation (DeSa 1977; DeSa 1979; Kilbride et al. 1980; DeSa and Donnelly 1984). Previously described associations were cardiac malformations, especially those involving the coronary arteries (e.g. anomalous origin), and intrauterine viral infection.

Recent necrosis is seldom recognisable macroscopically, but focal whitish scar may identify older injury. When myocardial ischaemic damage is suspected, systematic sampling of all areas of the heart, as described by Donnelly et al. (1980), is essential. Special stains are often required to identify fresh necrosis; immunohistochemical methods may prove useful in this respect. The areas involved are principally the subendocardial region and papillary muscles (Fig. 18.27), but other areas may be involved. Focal calcification is common and may be widespread. Coronary arteries may be abnormal; subintimal haemorrhages, medial necrosis with or without aneurysm formation, disruption of the internal elastic lamina, thrombosis and intimal proliferation (Fig. 18.28) are described. Small necrotic foci in the atrioventricular node and bundle of His have also been identified (Sandhyamani and Chopra 1982; DeSa and Donnelly 1984).

Wolf et al. (1985) reported a case of acute prenatal myocardial infarction with cardiac tamponade caused by embolism from the

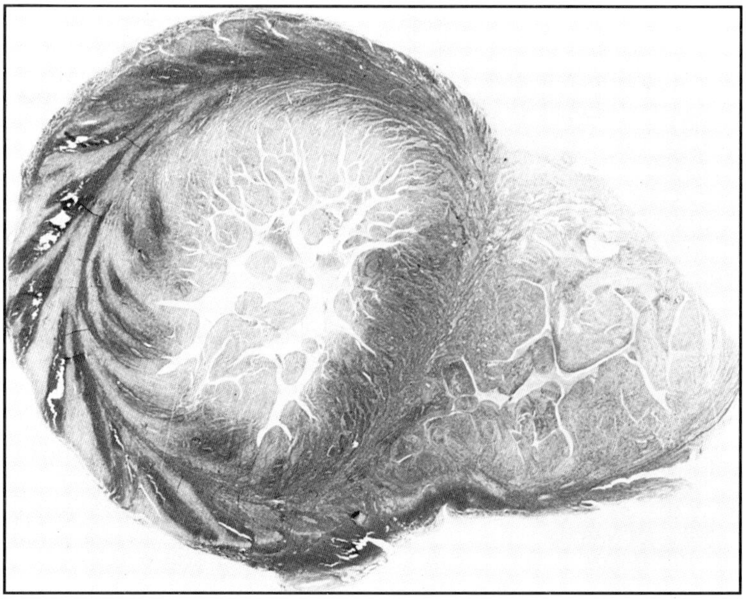

Fig. 18.27. Recent necrosis of the ventricular myocardium in a preterm infant ventilated after birth asphyxia. The damaged myocardium is darkly staining. (Courtesy of Dr. C. Bozic, Lausanne).

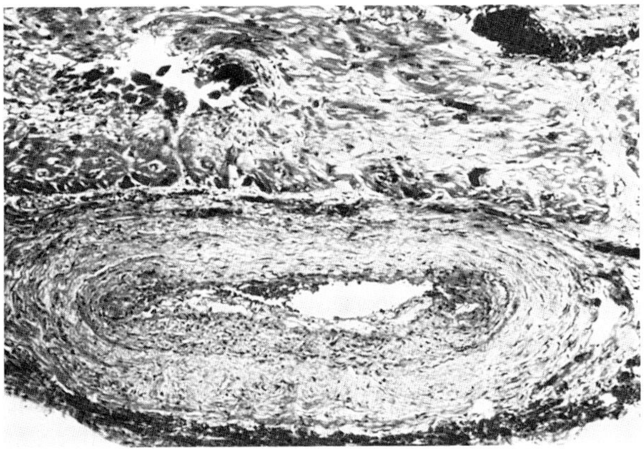

Fig. 18.28. Intrauterine hypoxia. Diffuse necrosis of the myocardium with calcification. Proliferative intimal thickening and thrombosis are present in an adjacent coronary artery.

placenta. Terhune et al. (1985) suggested that supraventricular aortic stenosis might be a predisposing factor for myocardial infarction in infancy.

Tumours

Primary tumours of the heart are uncommon in the neonatal period. However, use of new imaging techniques in this age group may result in more being diagnosed early in life. The majority of tumours are benign and of these rhabdomyoma is by far the most common, followed by fibroma, myxoma, haemangioma and intramural teratoma. Malignant tumours are extremely rare. Cyanosis, dyspnoea and tachyarrhythmia are the main presenting symptoms; haemodynamic disturbances are related to the size and location of the tumour (Arciniegas et al. 1980b; Schmaltz and Apitz 1981; Cox et al. 1983; Chan et al. 1985).

Rhabdomyoma

Rhabdomyomas are well-circumscribed, multiple, non-encapsulated nodules of variable size situated within the septum and ventricular wall and papillary muscles (Figs. 18.29, 18.30a). They may be the cause of non-immune hydrops and lead to intrauterine death (see Chap. 11). The atria may also be involved. About 50% of cases have other stigmata of tuberous sclerosis (Harding and Pagon 1990). The nodules are

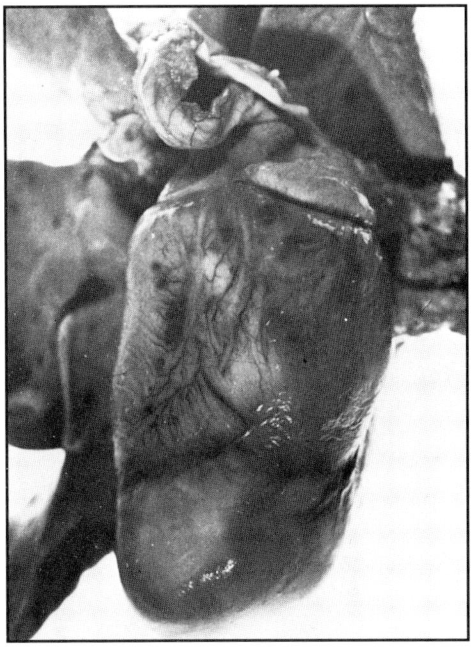

Fig. 18.29. Rhabdomyomas of the ventricular myocardium in a neonate.

composed of large round vacuolated cells with rays running from a central nucleus, giving them the classic spider-cell appearance (Fig. 18.30b). The cytoplasm is rich in glycogen. Calcium deposits are frequently observed.

Fibroma

Fibromas are usually single and located in either ventricle (intramural or intracavity) but most frequently located in the left ventricle or intraventricular septum. They are variable in size, rounded, whitish and firm. They are non-encapsulated and difficult to separate from the adjacent myocardium (Fig. 18.31a,b). Calcification is common.

Myxoma

Myxomas are rare in neonates (Dianzumba and Char 1982; Chan et al. 1985). They are located principally in the atria, but ventricles may be involved. About two-thirds of those reported at any age have been located in the left atrium attached to or in the vicinity of the foramen ovale. The tumours are often pedunculated, soft gelatinous yellowish or colourless masses

a
b
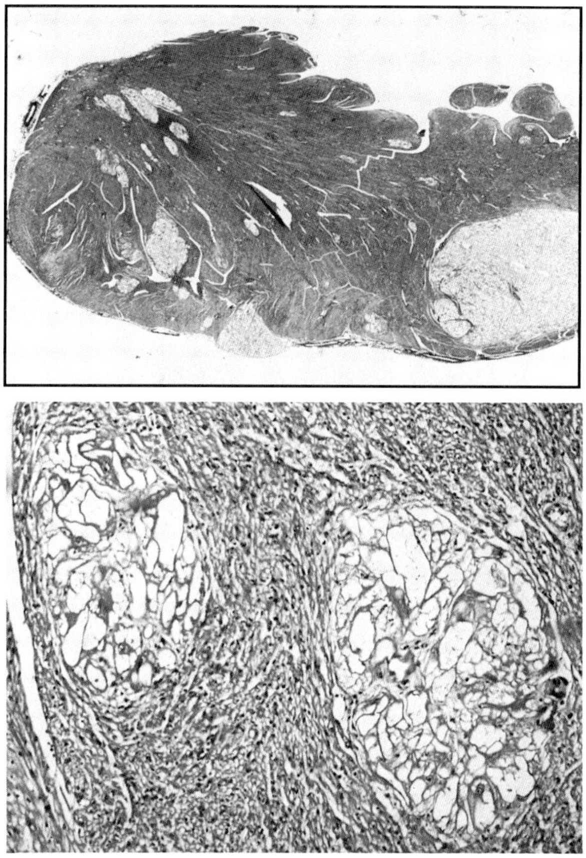

Fig. 18.30. **a** Rhadbomyomas of different size within the myocardium. **b** Glycogen-filled tumour cells vary in size but have a characteristic spider cell appearance. (Courtesy of Dr. C. Bozic, Lausanne).

and quite friable. Calcification is often extensive, and sometimes the entire tumour is calcified. Although the histological pattern is variable, the tumour consists of abundant pale eosinophilic matrix rich in proteoglycans containing scattered single or small groups of spindle or stellate cells (Fig. 18.32).

Haemangioma

Haemangioma is an uncommon myocardial tumour and only occasional cases are reported. Their vascular nature is indisputable (Ilbawi et al. 1982).

Ectopic Tissue

Thyroid tissue is encountered most frequently.

Teratoma

Teratomas involving the myocardium are rarely reported; they are histologically mature.

Malignant Tumours

Primary malignant tumours are rare at any age; rhabdomyosarcoma is the most common (Schmaltz and Apitz 1981; Small et al. 1985). We have observed a yolk sac tumour of the ventricular septum in a newborn (Fig. 18.33). Metastatic tumours to the heart and pericardium, although rare, have been observed in the perinatal period or infancy.

Tumours of the Atrioventricular Node

Tumours of the atrioventricular node are associated with conduction disturbances, usually partial or complete heart block, and may cause sudden death. Tumours described in this region are fibroma of the central fibrous body, rhabdomyoma (multifocal Purkinje cell tumour) and congenital polycystic tumour (mesothelioma, endothelioma; Travers 1982; James 1983; Nishida et al. 1985; Burke et al. 1990).

Conduction System

The time at which conducting tissue appears in the developing human heart and its derivation is controversial. It is assumed that some sort of conduction tissue exists when the heart tube begins to beat, but it is only around the 12th week of gestation that it has been identified with certainty. Immunohistochemical and other techniques may shed light on this important feature of cardiac development.

The sinus node is first located in junctional tissue between the sinus venosus and primitive atria within the sulcus terminalis. The atrioventricular node takes its origin from both the left sinus horn and the atrioventricular canal. These parts approximate and finally incorporate a block of specialised tissue from the atrial septum to form the node. Ventricular conduction tissues form in situ in the trabecular septum in the subendocardial region. Finally,

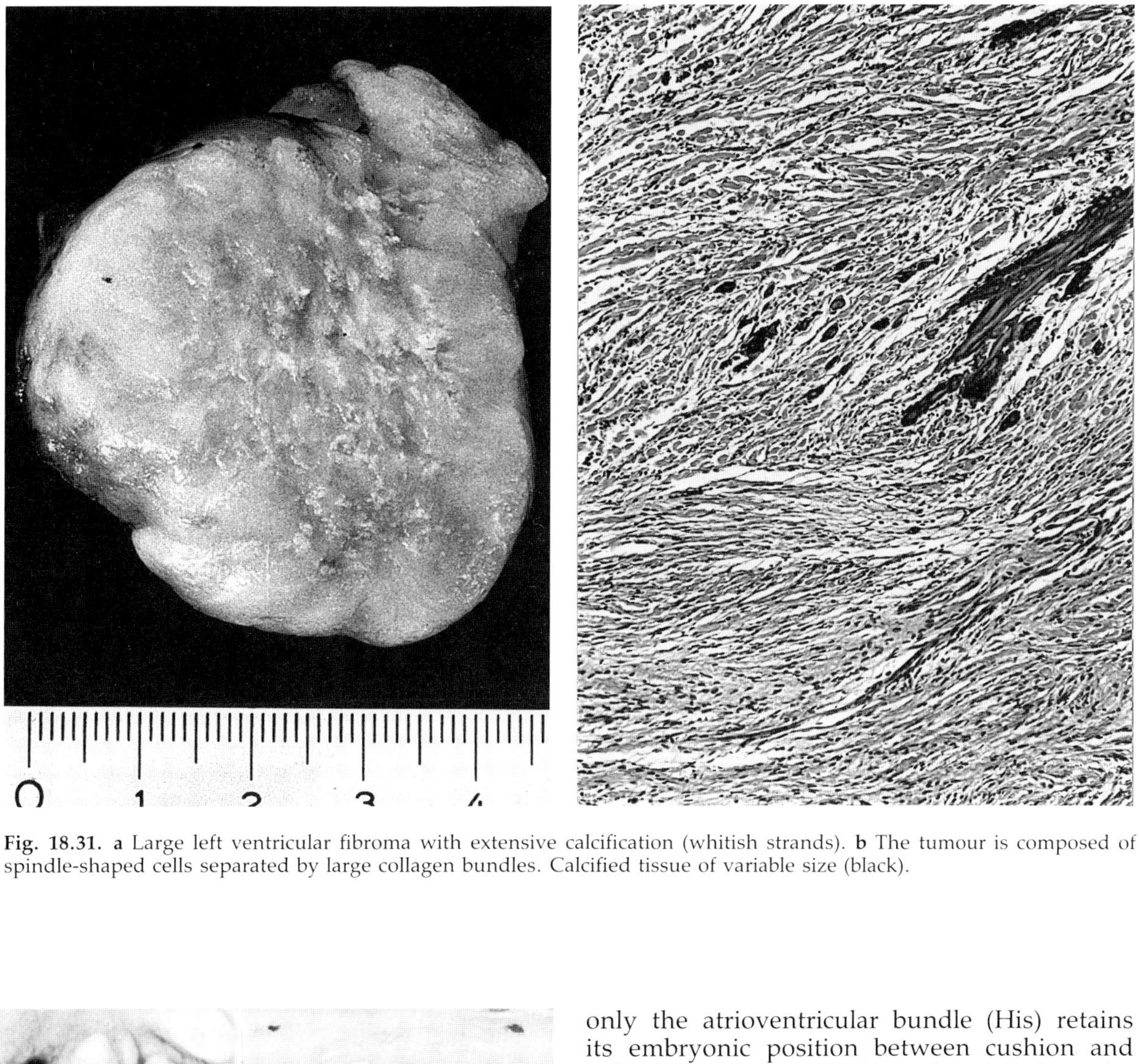

a b

Fig. 18.31. **a** Large left ventricular fibroma with extensive calcification (whitish strands). **b** The tumour is composed of spindle-shaped cells separated by large collagen bundles. Calcified tissue of variable size (black).

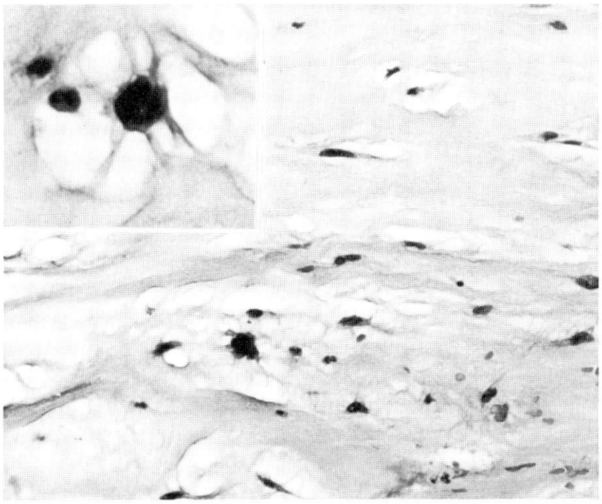

Fig. 18.32. Myxoma of the heart. Proteoglycan-rich stroma predominates the histological picture. Scattered cells, some stellate (*inset*), lie within it.

only the atrioventricular bundle (His) retains its embryonic position between cushion and sulcus tissue passing from the atria into the ventricular myocardium. There are accessory pathways and connections between the sinus node and the atrioventricular node. The position of these structures may vary, especially in the malformed heart, and may cause sudden death. Excessive fibrosis and the presence of cartilage (observed in one case) have also been described in association with this syndrome. They may also be damaged during cardiac surgery and provoke fatal outcome (Anderson and Taylor 1972; Forsgren et al. 1982; Anderson et al. 1983; Ho and Anderson 1988; Doménech-Mateu et al. 1991).

Besides this specialised tissue, the heart is innervated by both sympathetic and parasympathetic nerves. Immunohistochemical techniques have shown that nerves to the

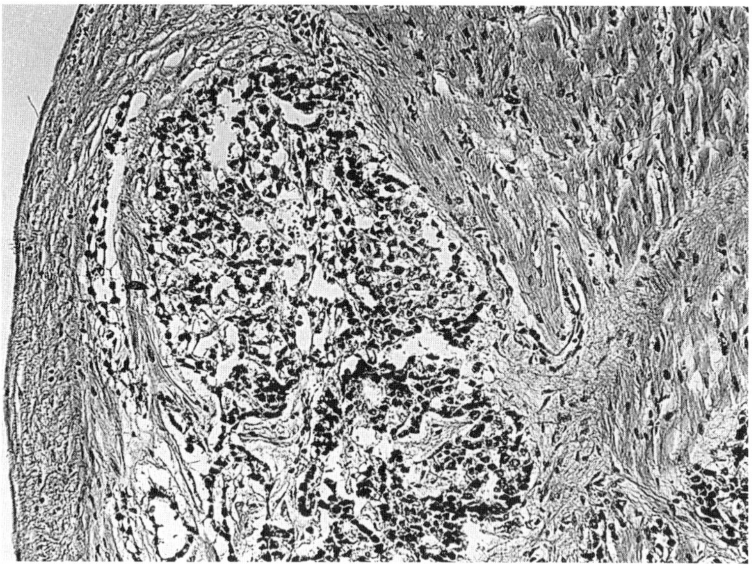

Fig. 18.33. Yolk sac tumour within the interventricular septum.

coronary arteries contain several different neuropeptides.

Recently it has been shown that atrial natriuretic peptide (ANP), a hormone first described in secretory granules of atrial myocytes (Fig. 18.34) is now known to be present in other tissues and has been identified in the conduction system, in atrial-like cardiocytes in the wall of the supradiaphragmatic portion of the vena cava, and in smaller quantities in the myocardium of the ventricles. There are presently three known subtypes (α-, β-, and γ-h ANP) which play an important role in the regulation of blood pressure, blood volume and excretion of water, sodium and potassium (Bierd et al. 1990; Sola et al. 1990; Mochizuki et al. 1991).

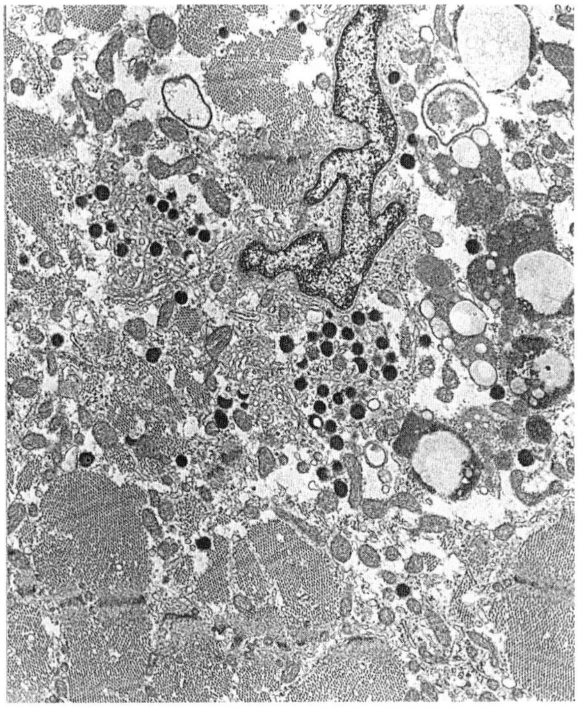

Fig. 18.34. Atrial natriuretic dense core granules in right atrium.

Complete Congenital Heart Block

The association of complete congenital heart block (CCHB) with the collagen diseases (particularly maternal systemic lupus erythematosus—SLE), as well as with abnormalities of the conducting system and other structural heart defects, is well documented. Focal myocarditis and fibrosis of the conducting system have been demonstrated in hearts from post-mortems on fetuses and neonates of mothers with SLE. The condition is due to an immune response and is associated with maternal antibodies (SSA/Ro-SSB/La) which can be demonstrated, not only in the myocardium, but in other organs (Buyon et al. 1988; Ross 1990; Schmidt et al. 1991; Silverman et al. 1991). In our material, IgG, fibrinogen and C_3 were demonstrated in the myocardium and vessel walls of both myocardium and liver. Fibrinogen was located in the vessel walls of the placenta.

Pericardium

Congenital defects of the pericardium are extremely rare and are occasional necropsy findings. Recently a number of cases have been detected by echocardiography (Kansal et al. 1985). They are usually associated with other anomalies of heart and lungs.

Pneumopericardium

Pneumopericardium is not uncommon amongst those neonates who have been subjected to over-zealous mechanical ventilation. There is usually pneumothorax and pneumomediastinum. The condition may occur spontaneously.

Pericardial Effusions

Pericardial effusions are generally a manifestation of congenital congestive cardiac failure. There may be anasarca, as in rhesus isoimmunisation, and severe vascular anomalies or perinatal infection. Some cases are idiopathic. The fluid may be chylous because of lymphatic abnormalities or obstruction. Occasionally, the fluid is blood stained, and in such cases infarction or/and trauma must be excluded.

Pericarditis

Pericarditis is rare in the neonatal period and generally observed in association with septicaemia (see Fig. 18.24b) or myocarditis.

Pericardial Cysts

Pericardial cysts are uncommon. They may be simple or multilocular, often pedunculated and contain clear fluid. The cavities are lined by flattened or cuboidal mesothelial cells. Large cysts may give rise to cardiorespiratory distress.

Pericardial Tumours

Pericardial tumours are rare abnormalities, the most common being teratoma (Arciniegas et al. 1980a; Agozzino et al. 1984).

Ductus Arteriosus

During intrauterine life, respiratory function is performed by the placenta, but at birth this is taken over by the lungs. Only a small amount of total blood volume from the right ventricle goes through the lungs during fetal life, the greater portion being shunted across the ductus arteriosus into the descending aorta. The ductus arteriosus thus maintains balance between ventricular loads during gestation; its patency during this period is under the constant influence of prostaglandins E_1 and E_2 as well as other vasoactive substances, which maintain its muscle tone.

The ductus is a muscular artery comprising intima, internal elastic lamina and muscle coat. Up to the 20th week of gestation, the intima is a monolayer overlying a thick continuous internal elastic lamina. Around this time focal endothelial proliferation is seen. These intimal cushions are composed of smooth muscle cell aggregates mixed with elastic fibres. The cushions are of variable size and dimension and become larger as gestation proceeds. Lacunae appear in the elastic lamina, which accumulate pools of acid mucopolysaccharides that are also observed in the intimal cushions. It has recently been suggested that the components of this accumulated extracellular material in the subendothelium play a role in directing the subsequent smooth muscle proliferation and migration, while other major extracellular matrix glycoproteins may influence the processes of proliferation, differentiation and migration of vascular cells (Boudreau and Rabinovitch, 1991). The media is made up of circularly arranged smooth muscle cells with occasional longitudinally arranged bundles in the inner part of the wall. Some elastic and reticulin fibres are present between muscle fibres. The ground substance

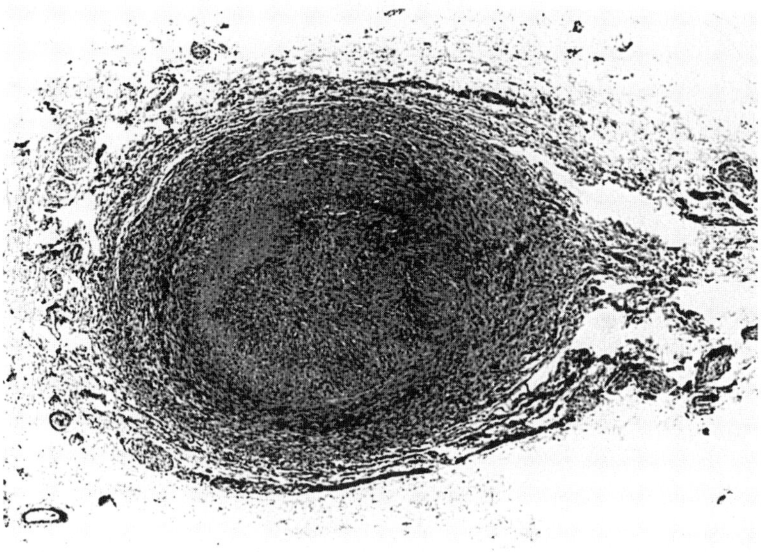

Fig. 18.35. Closure of the ductus arteriosus.

is rich in acid mucopolysaccharides. The outer half of the media contains capillary-like vasa vasorum. The entire vessel is surrounded by an adventitia composed of connective tissue containing elastic fibres, small blood vessels and nerves.

In longitudinal sections of the ductus, the elastic lamellae of adjacent aorta and pulmonary artery continue for a short distance into the media. At birth, there is physiological closure of the ductus as the lungs take over respiratory function and oxygen tension rises in the pulmonary artery and its branches. This rise in oxygen tension inhibits prostaglandin production, resulting in decreased muscle tone and closure. Anatomical closure is not complete for 2 or 3 weeks, after which the lumen becomes totally obliterated. Fibrin and thrombus in the lumen are invaded by and incorporated in proliferating cells from the intimal cushions and endothelium until the lumen is completely obliterated (Fig. 18.35). The process appears to be more active at the pulmonary side.

A persistent patent ductus arteriosus is usually encountered in preterm infants in intensive care units and in babies with cardiac anomalies. In the former, prostaglandin inhibitors (e.g. indomethacin) are administered to close the ductus, but their effectiveness is maturation dependent. Babies with respiratory distress syndrome with prolonged hypoxia and acidosis are frequent victims (Ho and Anderson 1979; Silver et al. 1981; Gittenberger-de Groot et al. 1985; Tada et al. 1985; Gersony 1986).

Dissecting Aneurysm

Aneurysms of the ductus are occasionally seen post mortem (Silver et al. 1981; Gillan et al. 1984; Fripp et al. 1985). Of the two cases seen by us, one was stillborn, the other lived for 18 h. The vessel was dilated, sacciform, firm and dark red. Histologically a tear in the elastic lamina and dissection of the media were identified. Rupture did not extend into adjacent tissue (Fig. 18.36).

Intrauterine Closure of the Ductus Arteriosus

Intrauterine closure of the ductus arteriosus is a rare finding and its cause is unknown. It has been described in maternal disorders (diabetes mellitus, chronic hypertension, pulmonary stenosis, chronic second trimester vaginal bleeding, disseminated intravascular coagulopathy) as well as with placental factors (placenta praevia, prolonged rupture of membranes, abruptio placentae) and with intrauterine exposure to prostaglandin synthetase

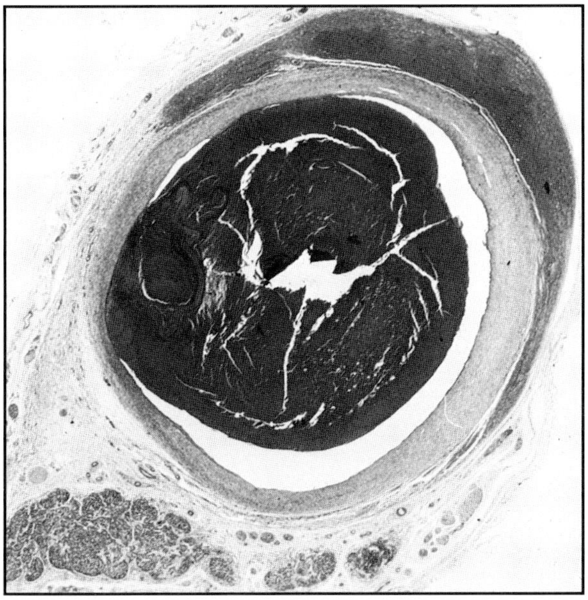

Fig. 18.36. Aneurysmal dilatation and thrombosis of the ductus arteriosus with mural haemorrhage suggestive of dissection.

inhibitors. The result is marked dilatation of the right side of the heart associated with anasarca (see Chap. 11).

Aorta and Peripheral Vessels

In the perinatal period the majority of lesions observed in the aorta and its branches and the venous system are iatrogenic and related to catheterisation of umbilical vessels (Keeling

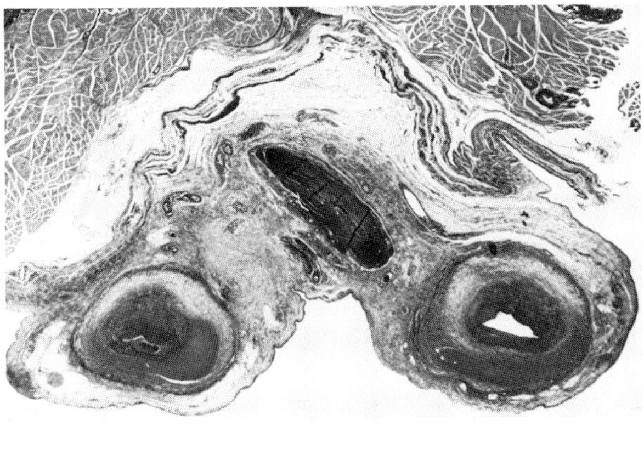

Fig. 18.37. Thrombosis of both umbilical arteries related to intimal traumatic injury following catheterisation.

1981). Catheterisation of the umbilical vein, a hitherto common procedure, is now generally replaced by catheterisation of the arteries because of the frequency of complications. Catheterisation of the umbilical vein may result in vascular trauma which causes perivascular oedema and haemorrhage. We have observed perforation of that vessel with haemorrhage into adjacent tissues. Hepatic necrosis of one or both lobes is described. Thrombosis is frequent and is related to the duration of catheterisation and infection; pulmonary thromboembolism may follow.

Catheterisation of the umbilical arteries is not without hazard. Damage to the endothelium and wall may result in thrombosis of these vessels (Fig. 18.37). Furthermore, neonates who present, in addition, inherited deficiencies of the coagulation system (deficits in protein C, protein S and antithrombin III) may quickly develop widespread thrombosis which could precipitate an unfavourable outcome. Iatrogenic aortic thrombosis and its sequelae are discussed in Chap. 14.

Single Umbilical Artery

In infants with a single umbilical artery the corresponding iliac artery is a large-diameter elastic artery, whilst the contralateral vessel is a small muscular artery.

Intimal Fibrous Plaques

Intimal fibrous plaques are encountered in the aorta and coronary or other systemic vessels in the neonate (Fig. 18.38a,b). They are physiological, overlying lacunae in the elastic lamina and frequently present at arterial bifurcations.

Idiopathic Infantile Arterial Calcification

Idiopathic infantile arterial calcification is a rare condition and its occurrence in siblings suggests heritable factors (Anderson et al. 1985; Van Reempts et al. 1991). There is focal or diffuse arterial calcification of the coronary arteries, the aorta and its branches and the pulmonary arteries (see Fig. 11.14, p. 264); cerebral arteries are often spared. Calcification is located principally in the elastic lamina, (Fig. 18.39) supporting the hypothesis of an inherent defect of elastic fibre as the primary abnor-

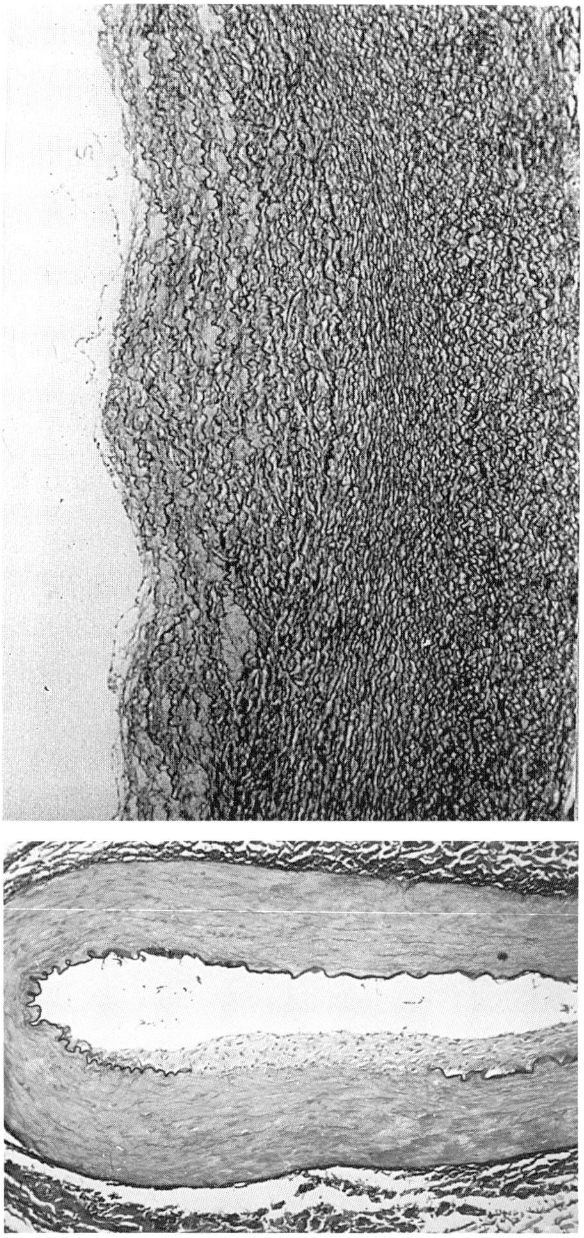

a

b

Fig. 18.38. **a** Intimal fibrous thickening of aorta in a 33-weeks premature baby (Van Gieson Elastine). **b** Intimal thickening overlying a gap in the internal elastic lamina of a muscular artery in a neonate (Weigert's elastic Van Gieson).

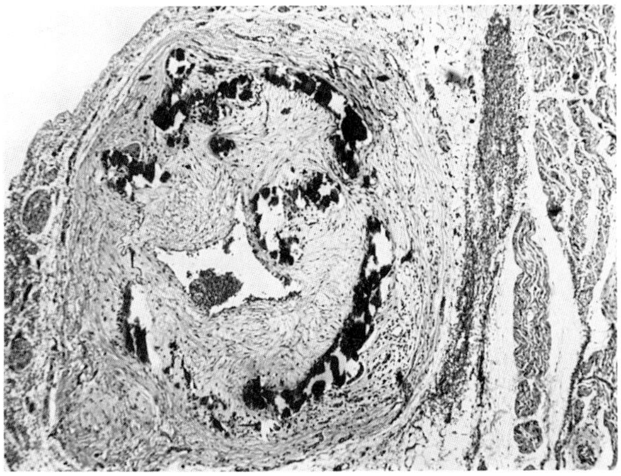

Fig. 18.39. Idiopathic infantile arterial calcification in the region of the internal elastic lamina with endothelial proliferation.

mality; however, deposits are also located in smooth muscle cells, fibroblasts and collagen fibres. Intimal proliferation is often present and may lead to arterial stenosis and thrombosis leading to secondary thromboembolus and infarction in various organs. Fetal hydrops may be the presenting feature (see p. 261). Cardiac ischaemia and hypertension in older infants are recorded complications. There has been clinical diminution of arterial calcification with appropriate treatment.

Marfan's Syndrome

Marfan's syndrome, an autosomal dominant inherited disorder with varying phenotypic manifestations and a high new mutation rate, is characterised by ocular, cardiovascular, musculoskeletal and pulmonary abnormalities. There is generally medial degeneration of the aorta and large arteries and accumulation of mucopolysaccharide substances within their walls. It has been documented in the perinatal period (Buchanan and Wyatt 1985; Schollin et al. 1988; Gross et al. 1989; Morse et al. 1990). A deficit in fibrillin, a constituent of microfibrillar fibres in connective tissue, appears to be associated to the condition, rather than an abnormality of the fibrillar and non-fibrillar collagens (Tsipouras 1990). It has now been clearly established that fibrillin is a major component of elastin-associated microfibrils in this syndrome and that the fibrillin gene is linked to chromosome 15q15-21. A second fibrillin gene has also been isolated on chromosome 5q23-21, suggesting that fibrillin mutations may be responsible for different forms and expressions of the Marfan syndrome (Lee et al. 1991; Maslen et al. 1991). Histological examination of the aorta and cardiac valves is necessary to make this diagnosis since skeletal and dysmorphic features are not always apparent.

It must be remembered however, that there is a spectrum of histochemical expression in tissues.

Ehlers–Danlos Syndrome

This is a genetically heterogeneous group of disorders affecting the connective tissue and is classified into at least 11 types. It has an autosomal dominant inheritance (phenotypically dominant or recessive pattern) or X-linked. Unlike Marfan's syndrome, the abnormality lies in the collagen fibres with systemic involvement of various organ systems (cardiovascular, gastrointestinal, respiratory, musculoskeletal and cutaneous). The morphological changes are therefore non-specific and, as a result, biochemical and molecular biological studies are mandatory to arrive at a correct diagnosis (Wenstrup et al. 1989; Utani et al. 1990, Kuivaniemi et al. 1991).

Coronary Arteries

Before the widespread use of coronary angiography and frequent surgery for congenital heart disease, congenital anomalies of the coronary arteries were considered mere curiosities. The origin and course of coronary arteries is important when cardiac surgery is mandatory for correction of anomalies.

Development of the Coronary Arteries

The first epicardial vessels appear about the time of trabecular septation of the heart as a series of plexuses communicating freely with the channels of the spongy myocardium. That in the anterior sulcus, about the first to appear, is destined to become the left anterior descending coronary artery. The right coronary and left circumflex coronary arteries appear much later. These epicardial vessels finally join up with the spongy anlagen surrounding the base of the conotruncus region before its division into aorta and pulmonary trunk. Buds later appear from the roots of the truncus arteriosus region from both aortic and pulmonary sinuses, but generally only those from the aortic portion will give rise to ostia of the coronary arteries and eventually link up with the remaining portions of the corresponding pedicular vessels.

Abnormalities at different stages of development could result in a number of abnormalities or combinations thereof. These are more prevalent in malformed hearts. Some have no clinical significance, whilst others can lead to congestive heart failure and even sudden death. The most commonly encountered anomalies are variations in number, location and level of the ostia; origin from the pulmonary trunk or a branch of the pulmonary artery; abnormal communications between the arteries; muscular ridges over a main branch, usually the left anterior descending; and abnormal course of one or both arteries.

Other Lesions

In myocarditis, inflammation of the arterial wall may occur. Aneurysmal dilatation, either saccular or fusiform, of the coronary arteries is rare and seen most often in Kawasaki disease (Fig. 18.40), when myocarditis, arteritis and pericarditis are prominent in the active phase. Stenosis and thrombosis are common complications with myocardial infarction. Arterial lesions may be observed in other sites or organs, suggesting a systemic arteritis. There is a strong belief that the condition is related to an infectious agent and recently both the Epstein–Barr virus and the adenovirus have been incriminated as possible pathogens (Okano et al. 1990, Naoe et al. 1991, Kikuta et al. 1992).

Lymphatics

The coronary lymphatics take their origin as an extensive subendocardial plexus, principally from the ventricles, and proceed through intramyocardial channels to form the subepicardial plexus from which the main surface collecting channels are derived. As the left coronary lymphatic leaves the base of the heart and travels upwards, it is usually joined by a right coronary channel to form the principal coronary lymphatic. Occasionally, the right-sided vessel does not join the left but goes directly to the thoracic duct. Generally, the principal coronary lymphatic passes under the pulmonary artery to the consistently placed pretracheal node immediately below the aortic arch, from where it continues upwards and to the right, dividing

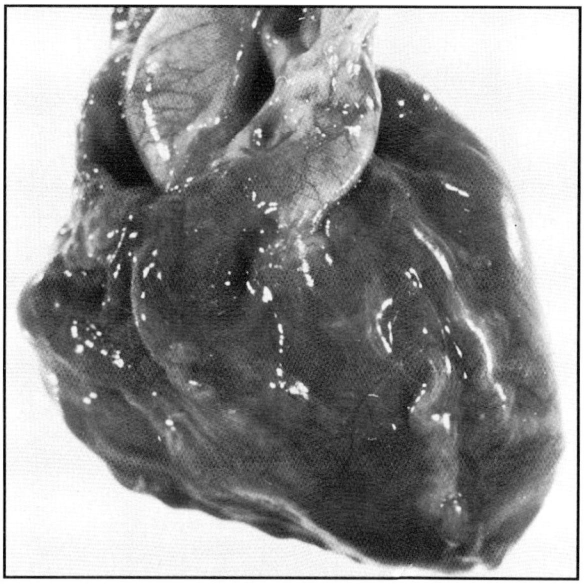

a

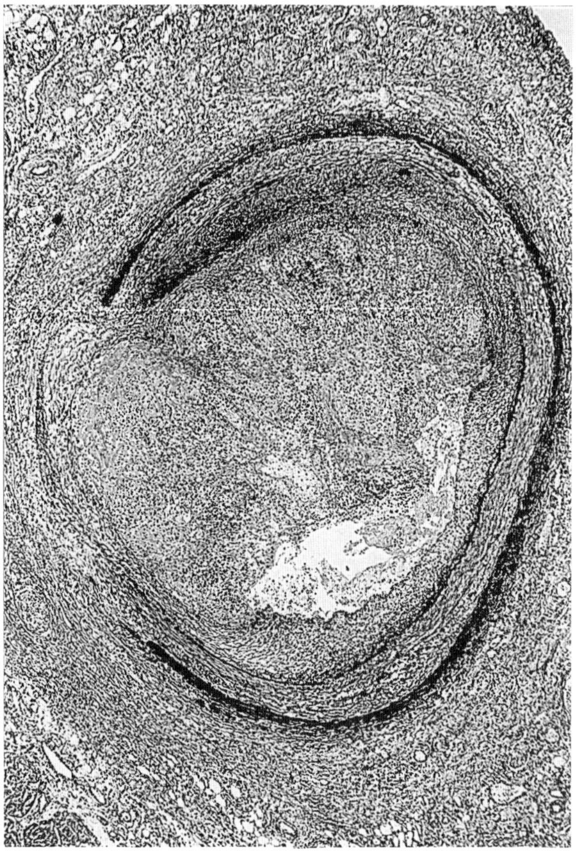

b

Fig. 18.40. **a** Kawasaki disease in a 3-month-old infant. Coronary arteries are tortuous, prominent and dilated (Courtesy of Prof. C. Nezelof, Paris). **b** Diffuse mononuclear cell infiltration of the vessel wall, the adventice and surrounding tissue; scarring of the media.

into two main branches as it proceeds to the cardiac lymph node. From that site one or more channels descend to the thoracic duct (Miller 1985).

Experimentally, acute and chronic obstruction to lymph flow results in ventricular endocardial changes. Chronic obstruction in Burmese and Siamese cats produces lesions similar to endocardial fibroelastosis (Zook and Paasch 1982).

References

Agozzino L, Vosa C, Arciprete P, De Leva F, Cotrufo M (1984) Intrapericardial teratoma in the newborn. Int J Cardiol 5: 21–28

Allan LD, Crawford DC, Anderson RH (1985) Spectrum of congenital heart disease detected echocardiographically in prenatal life. Br Heart J 54: 523–526

Anderson KA, Burbach JA, Fenton LJ, Jaqua RA, Barlow JF (1985) Idiopathic arterial calcification of infancy in newborn siblings with unusual light and electron microscopic manifestations. Arch Pathol Lab Med 109: 838–842

Anderson RH, Becker AE, Freedom RM et al. (1984) Sequential segmental analysis of congenital heart disease. Pediatr Cardiol 5: 281–288

Anderson RH, Taylor IM (1972) Development of atrioventricular specialized tissue in human heart. Br Heart J 34: 1205–1214

Anderson RH, Tynan M (1991) Description of complex forms of atrioventricular valvar atresia. Int J Cardiol 30: 243–247

Anderson RH, Ho SY, Becker AE (1983) The surgical anatomy of the conduction tissue. Thorax 38: 408–420

Arciniegas E, Hakimi M, Farooki ZQ, Green EW (1980a) Intrapericardial teratoma in infancy. J Thorac Cardiovasc Surg 79: 306–311

Arciniegas E, Hakimi M, Farooki ZQ, Truccone NJ, Green EW (1980b) Primary cardiac tumours in children. J Thorac Cardiovasc Surg 79: 582–591

Bankl H (1977) Congenital malformations of the heart and great vessels. Synopsis of pathology, embryology and natural history. Urban & Schwarzenberg, Baltimore

Bartelings MM (1990) The outflow tract of the heart—embryologic and morphologic correlations. Thesis, University of Leiden, Leiden

Bartelings MM, Gittenberger-de Groot AC (1989) The outflow tract of the heart—embryologic and morphologic correlations. Int J Cardiol 22: 289–300

Becker AE, Anderson RH (1981) Pathology of congenital heart disease. Butterworths, London, (Postgraduate pathology series)

Belkin RN, Kisslo J (1990) Atrial septal aneurysm: recognition and clinical relevance. Am Heart J 120: 948–957

Bertini E, Bosman C, Bevilacqua M et al. (1990) Cardiomyopathy and multicore myopathy with accumulation of intermediate filaments. Eur J Pediatr 149: 856–858

Bierd TM, Kattwinkel J, Chevalier RL et al. (1990) Interrelationship of atrial natriuretic peptide, atrial volume,

and renal function in premature infants. J Pediatr 116: 753–759
Boudreau N, Rabinovitch M (1991) Developmentally regulated changes in extracellular matrix in endothelial and smooth muscle cells in the ductus arteriosus may be related to intimal proliferation. Lab Inv 64: 187–199
Buchanan R, Wyatt GP (1985) Marfan's syndrome presenting as an intrapartum death. Arch Dis Child 60: 1074–1076
Buirsky G, Jordan SC, Joffe HS, Wilde P (1986) Superior vena caval abnormalities: their occurrence rate, associated cardiac abnormalities and angiographic classification in a paediatric population with congenital heart disease. Clin Radiol 37: 131–138
Burke AP, Anderson PG, Virmani R, James TN, Herrera GA, Ceballos R (1990) Tumor of the atrioventricular nodal region. Arch Pathol Lab Med 114: 1057–1062
Buyon JP, Ben-Chetrit E, Karp S et al. (1989) Acquired congenital heart block—pattern of maternal antibody response to biochemical defined antigens of the SSA/Ro-SSB/La system in neonatal lupus. J Clin Invest 84: 627–634
Cantrell JR, Haller JA, Ravitch MM (1958) A syndrome of congenital defects involving the abdominal wall, sternum, diaphragm, pericardium, and heart. Surg Gynecol Obstet 107: 602–614
Chan HSL, Sonley MJ, Moes CAF, Daneman A, Smith CR, Martin DJ (1985) Primary and secondary tumours of childhood involving the heart, pericardium, and great vessels. A report of 75 cases and review of the literature. Cancer 56: 825–836
Collett RW, Edwards JE (1949) Persistent truncus arteriosus: a classification according to anatomic types. Surg Clin N Am 29: 1245–1270
Cox JN, Friedli B, Mechmeche R, Ismail MB, Oberhaensli I, Faidutti B (1983) Teratoma of the heart: a case report and review of the literature. Virchows Arch [A] 402: 163–174
Crupi G, Macartney FJ, Anderson RH (1977) Persistent truncus arteriosus: a study of 66 autopsy cases with special reference to definition and morphogenesis. Am J Cardiol 40: 569–578
DeSa DJ (1977) Myocardial changes in immature infants requiring prolonged ventilation. Arch Dis Child 52: 138–145
DeSa DJ (1979) Coronary arterial lesions and myocardial necrosis in stillbirths and infants. Arch Dis Child 54: 918–930
DeSa DJ (1985) Isolated myocarditis in the first year. Arch Dis Child 60: 484–485
DeSa DJ, Donnelly WH (1984) Myocardial necrosis in the newborn. Perspect Pediatr Pathol 8: 295–311
Devine WA, Debich DE, Anderson RH (1991) Dissection of congenitally malformed hearts, with comments on the value of sequential segmental analysis. Pediatr Pathol 11: 235–259
Dianzumba SB, Char G (1982) Large calcified right atrial myxoma in a newborn. Rare cause of neonatal death. Br Heart J 48: 177–179
Doménech-Mateu JM, Arnó-Palau A, Martínez-Pozo A (1991) Study of the development of the atrioventricular conduction system as a consequence of observing an extra atrioventricular node in the normal heart of a human fetus. Anat Rec 230: 73–85
Donnelly WH, Bucciarelli RL, Nelson RM (1980) Ischemic papillary muscle necrosis in stressed newborn infants. J Pediatr 96: 295–300
Dusmet M, Oberhaensli I, Cox JN (1987) Ebstein's anomaly of the tricuspid and mitral valves in an otherwise normal heart. Br Heart J 58: 400–404
Eishi Y, Takemura T, Sone R et al. (1985) Glycogen storage disease confined to the heart with deficient activity of cardiac phosphorylase kinase: a new type of glycogen storage disease. Hum Pathol 16: 193–197
Elzenga NJ, Gittenberger-de Groot AC (1985) Coarctation and related aortic arch anomalies in hypoplastic left heart syndrome. Int J Cardiol 8: 379–389
Ferencz C, Rubin JD, McCarter RJ, Clark EB (1990) Maternal diabetes and cardiovascular malformations: predominance of double outlet right ventricle and truncus arteriosus. Teratol 41: 312–326
Forsgren S, Eriksson A, Kjörell U, Thornell LE (1982) The conduction system in the human heart at midgestation—immunohistochemical demonstration of the intermediate filament protein skeletin. Histochemistry 75: 43–52
Fripp RR, Whitman V, Waldhausen JA, Boal DK (1985) Ductus arteriosus aneurysm presenting as pulmonary artery obstruction: diagnosis and management. J Am Coll Cardiol 6: 234–236
Gammage MD, Franklyn JA (1991) Role of proto-oncogenes in the control of myocardial cell growth and function. Clin Science 80: 405–411
Gembruch U, Knöpfle G, Chatterjee M, Bald R, Hansmann M (1990) First-trimester diagnosis of fetal congenital heart disease by transvaginal two-dimensional and Doppler echocardiography. Obstet Gynecol 75: 496–498
Gerlis LM (1985) Cardiac malformations in spontaneous abortions. Int J Cardiol 7: 29–43
Gerlis LM, Ho SY (1989) Anomalous subaortic position of the brachiocephalic (innominate) vein: a review of published reports and report of three new cases. Br Heart J 61: 540–545
Gersony WM (1986) Patent ductus arteriosus in the neonate. Pediatr Clin N Am 33: 545–560
Geva T, Santini F, Pear W, Driscoll SG, Van Praagh R (1991) Cardiac rabdomyoma: rare cause of fetal death. Chest 99: 139–143
Gillan JE, Costigan DC, Keeley FW, Rose T, Cutz E, Rose V (1984) Spontaneous dissecting aneurysm of the ductus arteriosus in an infant with Marfan syndrome. J Pediatr 105: 952–955
Gittenberger-de Groot AC, Strengers JLM, Mentink M, Poelmann RE, Patterson DF (1985) Histologic studies on normal and persistent ductus arteriosus in the dog. J Am Coll Cardiol 6: 394–404
Gross DM, Robinson LK, Smith LT, Glass N, Rosenberg H, Duvic M (1989) Severe perinatal Marfan syndrome. Pediatrics 84: 83–89
Harding CO, Pagon RA (1990) Incidence of tuberous sclerosis in patients with cardiac rabdomyoma. Am J Med Genet 37: 443–446
Herreman G, Ferme I, Morel S, Batisse J, Phat VN, Meyer O (1985) Mort foetale par myocardité et bloc auriculo-ventriculaire congénital isolé. Presse Med 14: 1547–1550
Ho SY, Anderson RH (1979) Coarctation, tubular hypoplasia and the ductus arteriosus—histological study of 35 specimens. Br Heart J 41: 268–274
Ho SY, Anderson RH (1988) Conduction tissue and SIDS. In: Schwartz PJ, Southall DP, Valdes-Dapena M (eds) The sudden infant death syndrome—cardiac and respiratory mechanisms and interventions. Ann NY Acad Sci 533: 176–190
Howell CE, Ho SY, Anderson RH, Elliott MJ (1990) Variations within the fibrous skeleton and ventricular outflow tracts in tetralogy of Fallot. Ann Thorac Surg 50: 450–457
Huang TY, Hsueh Y, Tsung SH (1985) Endocardial fibroelastosis and myocardial calcification secondary to an anomalous right coronary artery arising from the

pulmonary trunk. Hum Pathol 16: 959–960
Hübner G, Grantzow R (1983) Mitochondrial cardiomyopathy with involvement of skeletal muscles. Virchows Arch [A] 399: 115–125
Icardo JM (1988) Heart anatomy and developmental biology. Experientia 44: 910–919
Ilbawi M, DeLeon S, Riggs T, Hernandez R (1982) Primary vascular tumors of the heart in infancy. Chest 81: 511–512
Ino T, Benson LN, Freedom RM, Rowe RD (1988) Natural history and prognostic risk factors in endocardial fibroelastosis. Am J Cardiol 62: 431–434
James TN (1983) The Mikano lecture: structure and function of the AV junction. Jpn Circ J 47: 1–47
Johnson P, Seller MJ, Morrish N, Neales K, Maxwell D (1991) Pancreatic and sacral agenesis in association with maternal diabetes mellitus: case report. Prenatal Diagn 11: 329–331
Jouk PS (1991) Analyse segmentaire et classification des malformations cardiaques. Méd Foetale et Echographie en Gynécologie 5: 4–21
Kansal S, Roitman D, Sheffield LT (1985) Two-dimensional echocardiography of congenital absence of pericardium. Am Heart J 109: 912–915
Kaplan LC, Matsuoka R, Gilbert EF, Opitz JM, Kurnit DM (1985) Ectopia cordis and cleft sternum: evidence for mechanical teratogenesis following rupture of the chorion or yolk sac. Am J Med Genet 21: 187–199
Keeling JW (1981) Iatrogenic disease in the newborn. Virchows Arch [A] 394: 1–29
Kikuta H, Nakanishi M, Ishikawa N, Konno M, Matsumoto S (1992) Detection of Epstein–Barr virus sequences in patients with Kawasaki disease by means of the polymerase chain reaction. Intervirology 33: 1–5
Kilbride H, Way GL, Merenstein GB, Winfield JM (1980) Myocardial infarction in the neonate with normal heart and coronary arteries. Am J Dis Child 134: 759–762
Kuivaniemi H, Tromp G, Prockop DJ (1991) Mutations in collagen genes: causes of rare and some common diseases in humans. FASEB J 5: 2052–2060
Langes K, Frenzel H, Seitz RJ, Kluitmann G (1985) Cardiomyopathy associated with Leigh's disease. Virchows Arch [A] 407: 97–105
Larson JE, McManus BM, Lofschire PJ, Colombo JL, Look CE (1984) Isolated endocardial fibroelastosis of the right ventricle associated with pulmonary hypertension. Am Heart J 107: 1286–1290
Laufer D, Lew PD, Oberhaensli I, Cox JN, Longson M (1986) Chronic Q fever endocarditis with massive splenomegaly in childhood: report of two cases. Pediatrics 108: 535–539
Lee B, Godfrey M, Vitale E et al. (1991) Linkage of Marfan syndrome and a phenotypically related disorder to two different fibrillin genes. Nature 352: 330–334
Lucas RV, Lock JE, Tandon R, Edwards JE (1988) Gross and histologic anatomy of total anomalous pulmonary venous connections. Am J Cardiol 62: 292–300
Maron BJ, Tajik AJ, Ruttenberg HD et al. (1982) Hypertrophic cardiomyopathy in infants: clinical features and natural history. Circulation 65 : 7–17
Maslen CL, Corson GM, Maddox K, Glanville RW, Sakai LY (1991) Partial sequence of a candidate gene for the Marfan syndrome. Nature 352: 334–337
McGuinness GA, Schieken RM, Maguire GF (1980) Endocarditis in the newbom. Am J Dis Child 134: 577–580
Miller AJ (1985) The study of the lymphatics of the heart: an overview. Microcirc Endothel Lymphat 2: 349–360
Mochizuki N, Sawa H, Yasuda H et al. (1991) Distribution of atrial natriuretic peptide in the conduction system and ventricular muscle of the human heart. Virchows Arch [A] 418: 9–16
Morse RP, Rockenmacher S, Pyeritz RE et al. (1990) Diagnosis and management of infantile Marfan syndrome. Pediatrics 86: 888–895
Moscoso G, Pexieder T (1990) Variations in microscopic anatomy and ultrastructure of human embryonic hearts subjected to three different modes of fixation. Pathol Res Pract 186: 768–774
Naoe S, Takahashi K, Masuda H, Tanaka N (1991) Kawasaki disease with particular emphasis on arterial lesions. Acta Pathol Jpn 41: 785–797
Nishida K, Kamijima G, Nagayama T (1985) Mesothelioma of the atrioventricular node. Br Heart J 53: 468–470
Oelberg DG, Fisher DJ, Gross DM, Denson SE, Adcock EW (1983) Endocarditis in high-risk neonates. Pediatrics 71: 392–397
Ogawa K, Sugamata K, Funamoto N et al. (1990) Restricted accumulation of globotriaosylceramide in the hearts of atypical cases of Fabry's disease. Hum Pathol 21: 1067–1073
Okano M, Thiele GM, Sakiyama Y, Matsumoto S, Purtilo DT (1990) Adenovirus infection in patients with Kawasaki disease. J Med Virol 32: 53–57
Papadimitriou A, Neustein HB, Dimauro S, Stanton R, Bresolin N (1984) Histiocytoid cardiomyopathy of infancy: deficiency of reducible cytochrome b in heart mitochondria. Pediatr Res 18: 1023–1028
Pellegrino A, Deverall PB, Anderson RH et al. (1985) Aortic coarctation in the first three months of life: an anatomopathological study with respect to treatment. J Thorac Cardiovasc Surg 89: 121–127
Pexieder T (1982) La solution de deux énigmes de l'organogenèse du coeur. Bull Fond Suisse Cardiol 13: 3–14
Pexieder T, Wenink ACG, Anderson RH (1989) A suggested nomenclature for the developing heart. Int J Cardiol 25: 255–264
Potts JD, Runyan RB (1989) Epithelial-mesenchymal cell transformation in the embryonic heart can be mediated, in part, by transforming growth factor β. Dev Biol 134: 392–401
Poulias GE, Raftopoulos J, Polemis L, Skoutas B, Katsouli R (1982) Total thoracic ectopia cordis with complete absence of sternum and pericardium and double diverticulum. Case report. J Cardiovasc Surg 23: 75–78
Rammos S, Gittenberger-de Groot AC, Oppenheimer-Dekker A (1990) The abnormal pulmonary venous connexion: a developmental approach. Int J Cardiol 29: 285–295
Rao PS (1990) Is the term "tricuspid atresia" appropriate? Am J Cardiol 66: 1251–1254
Rigby ML, Shinebourne EA (1981) Development of the cardiovascular system. Functional development. In: Davis JA, Dobbing J (eds) Scientific foundations of paediatrics. Heinemann Medical, London, pp 373–389
Rigby ML, Carvalho JS, Anderson RH, Redington A (1990) The investigation and diagnosis of tricuspid atresia. Int J Cardiol 27: 1–17
Rios B, Duff J, Simpson JW (1984) Endocardial fibroelastosis with congenital complete heart block in identical twins. Am Heart J 107: 1290–1293
Rocchiccioli F, Wanders RJA, Aubourg P et al. (1990) Deficiency of long-chain 3-hydroxyacyl-CoA dehydrogenase: a cause of lethal myopathy and cardiomyopathy in early childhood. Pediatr Res 28: 657–662

Ross BA (1990) Congenital complete atrioventricular block. Pediatr Clin North Am 37: 69–78

Sandhyamani S, Chopra P (1982) Acute myocardial infarction in the neonate. Indian J Med Res 75: 820–826

Sapire DW, Ho SY, Anderson RH, Rigby ML (1986) Diagnosis and significance of atrial isomerism. Am J Cardiol 58: 342–346

Schmaltz AA, Apitz J (1981) Primary heart tumors in infancy and childhood. Report of four cases and review of literature. Cardiology 67: 12–22

Schmidt KG, Ulmer HE, Silverman NH, Kleinman CS, Copel JA (1991) Perinatal outcome of fetal complete atrioventricular block: a multicenter experience. J Am Coll Cardiol 91: 1360–1366

Schollin J, Bjarke B, Gustavson KH (1988) Probable homozygotic form of the Marfan syndrome in a newborn child. Acta Paediatr Scand 77: 452–456

Shinebourne EA, Macartney FJ, Anderson RH (1976) Sequential chamber localisation—logical approach to diagnosis in congenital heart disease. Br Heart J 38: 327–340

Silver MM, Freedom RM, Silver MD, Olley PM (1981) The morphology of the human newborn ductus arteriosus. A reappraisal of its structures and closure with special reference to prostaglandin E_1 therapy. Hum Pathol 12: 1123–1136

Silverman NH, Zuberbuhler JR, Anderson RH (1986) Atrioventricular septal defects: cross-sectional echocardiographic and morphologic comparisons. Int J Cardiol 13: 309–331

Silverman E, Mamula M, Hardin JA, Laxer R (1991) Importance of the immune response of the Ro/La particle in the development of congenital heart block and neonatal lupus erythematosus. J Rheumatol 18: 120–124

Small EJ, Gordon GJ, Dahms BB (1985) Malignant rhabdoid tumor of the heart in an infant. Cancer 55: 2850–2853

Soberman MS, Plauth WH, Winn KJ, Forest GC, Hatcher CR, Sink JD (1988) Hemangioma of the right ventricle causing outflow tract obstruction. J Thor Cardiovasc Surg 96: 307–309

Sola C, Thibault G, Haile-Meskel H, Anand-Srivastava MB, Garcia R, Cantin M (1990) Atrial natriuretic factor in the vena cava and sinus node. J Histochem Cytochem 38: 1123–1135

Soto B, Ceballos R, Kirklin JW (1989) Ventricular septal defects: a surgical viewpoint. J Am Coll Cardiol 14: 1291–1297

Steenhout P, Elmer C, Clercx A et al. (1990) Carnitine deficiency with cardiomyopathy presenting as neonatal hydrops: successful response to carnitine therapy. J Inherited Metab Dis 13: 69–75

Stephan MJ, Stevens EL, Wenstrup RJ et al. (1989) Mucopolysaccharidosis I presenting with endocardial fibroelastosis of infancy. Am J Dis Child 143: 782–784

Stoeckel ME, Osborn M, Porte A, Sacrez A, Batzenschlager A, Weber K (1981) An unusual familial cardiomyopathy characterized by aberrant accumulations of desmin-type intermediate filaments. Virchows Arch [A] 393: 53–60

Suzuki A, Ho SY, Anderson RH, Deanfield JE (1990) Further morphologic studies on tetralogy of Fallot, with particular emphasis on the prevalence and structure of the membranous flap. J Thorac Cardiovasc Surg 99: 528–535

Tada T, Wakabayashi T, Nako Y et al. (1985) Human ductus arteriosus. A histological study of the relation between ductal maturation and gestational age. Acta Pathol Jpn 35: 23–34

Terhune PE, Buchino JJ, Rees A (1985) Myocardial infarction associated with supravalvular aortic stenosis. J Pediatr 106: 251–254

Thiene G, Daliento L, Frescura C, De Tommasi M, Macartney FJ, Anderson RH (1981) Atresia of left atrioventricular orifice. Anatomical investigation in 62 cases. Br Heart J 45: 393–401

Travers H (1982) Congenital polycystic tumor of the atrioventricular node. Possible familial occurrence and critical review of reported cases with special emphasis on histogenesis. Hum Pathol 13: 25–35

Tsipouras P (1990) Marfan syndrome: light at the end of the tunnel? Am J Hum Genet 46: 643–645

Ueda M, Becker AE (1985) Morphological characteristics of perimembranous ventricular septal defects and their surgical significance. Int J Cardiol 8: 149–157

Ursell PC, Neill CA, Anderson RH, Ho SY, Becker AE, Gerlis LM (1984) Endocardial fibroelastosis and hypoplasia of the left ventricle in neonates without significant aortic stenosis. Br Heart J 51: 492–497

Utani A, Tanaka T, Nishigori C et al. (1990) Another mechanism for the defect in type III collagen accumulation in Ehlers–Danlos syndrome type IV: increased intracellular degradation of the procollagen. Lab Invest 63: 181–188

Van Praagh R, Geva T, Kreutzer J (1989) Ventricular septal defects: how shall we describe, name and classify them? J Am Coll Cardiol 14: 1298–1299

Van Reempts PJ, Boven KJ, Spitaels SE, Roodhoft AM, Vercruyssen EL, Van Acker KJ (1991) Idiopathic arterial calcification of infancy. Calcif Tissue Int 48(1): 1–6

Vesikari R, Janas M, Gronroos P et al. (1985) Neonatal septicaemia. Arch Dis Child 60: 542–546

Ward KE, Matson JR, Chartrand SR, Wilson DA (1983) Successfully treated pulmonary valve endocarditis in a normal neonate. Am J Dis Child 137: 913–914

Wenink ACG (1981) Embryology of the ventricular septum. Separate origin of its components. Virchows Arch [A] 390: 71–79

Wenink ACG, Ottenkamp J (1987) Tricuspid atresia. Microscopic findings in relation to "absence" of the atrioventricular connexion. Int J Cardiol 16: 57–65

Wenstrup RJ, Murad SR (1989) Ehlers–Danlos syndrome type VI: clinical manifestations of collagen lysyl hydroxylase deficiency. J Pediatr 115: 405–409

Wolf PL, Jones KL, Longway SR, Benirschke K, Bloor C (1985) Prenatal death from acute myocardial infarction and cardiac tamponade due to embolus from the placenta. Am Heart J 109: 603–605

Zimmermann A, Diem P, Cottier H (1982) Congenital "histiocytoid" cardiomyopathy: evidence suggesting a development disorder of the Purkinje cell system of the heart. Virchows Arch [A] 396: 187–195

Zimmerman KG, Paplanus SH, Dong S, Nagle RB (1983) Congenital blood cysts of the heart valves. Hum Pathol 14: 699–703

Zook BC, Paasch LH (1982) Endocardial fibroelastosis: endocardial fibroelastosis in Burmese cats. Am J Pathol 106: 435–438

Chapter 19

The Urinary System

R. Anthony Risdon

Introduction

In the perinatal period congenital abnormalities of the kidneys and urinary tract are of major importance, while specific acquired lesions and tumours are comparatively rare.

Development

In vertebrates, including man, the development of the urinary (excretory) and genital (reproductive) systems are closely linked. Indeed, in the male embryo part of the system initially concerned with urinary excretion later becomes connected with the testis and forms part of the genital ducts: even in postnatal life the urethra forms a common channel for the urinary and genital systems. In the female embryo the primitive excretory ducts largely regress and the definitive reproductive tract develops from a pair of paramesonephric (Müllerian) ducts, wholly separate from the excretory system.

In the human embryo the kidney develops from an intermediate mass of mesoderm, the nephrogenic cord, between the lateral plate mesoderm and dorsal somites behind the intra-embryonic coelom. The appearance of the definitive kidney, the metanephros, is preceded by two transient excretory organs, the pronephros and mesonephros. The pronephros develops in the most cranial, cervicodorsal segments of the nephrogenic cord. In the human embryo only a few tubules differentiate and rapidly degenerate. The mesonephros develops in the intermediate, dorsolumbar segments of the nephrogenic cord, differentiating after the pronephros but before it completely disappears. A series of vesicles which form glomeruli and tubules develop and these join an excretory channel, the mesonephric or Wolffian duct, which gradually extends to join the cloaca at the 27–28 somite stage (4th post-conception week). Degeneration of the most cranial mesonephric nephrons commences before the caudal nephrons develop. The metanephros is derived in two parts: the renal parenchyma from the caudal, initially sacral, part of the nephrogenic cord and the excretory system (the collecting tubules, calyces, pelvis and ureter) from the ureteric bud. The latter forms as a posteromedial outgrowth from the Wolffian (mesonephric) duct near its junction with the cloaca at the 5 mm stage. Its proximal end extends dorsally to impinge on the metanephric blastema, whilst its distal end grows caudally with growth of the embryo.

The ureteric bud develops a dilated terminal portion, the ampulla, and on contact with the metanephric blastema this undergoes a series of dichotomous branchings, each branch developing a separate ampulla at its tip. The caudal

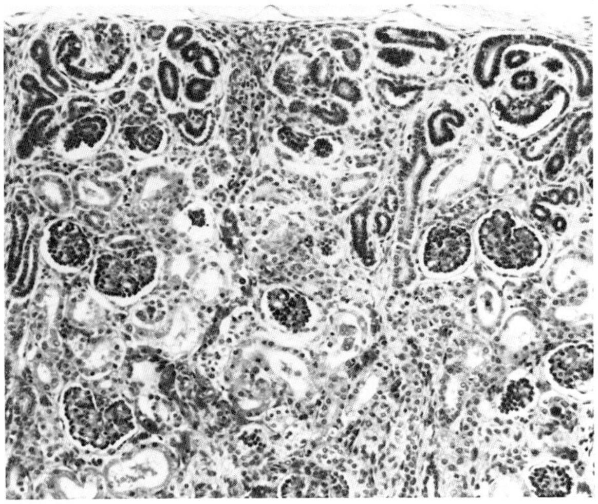

Fig. 19.1. The "nephrogenic zone" in the outer cortex of the kidney of a premature infant. (H&E, ×50)

unbranched portion of the ureteric bud forms the ureter. The first few generations of branches coalesce to form the renal pelvis and calyces, whilst subsequent divisions form the collecting ducts. From the end of the 7th week (18–20 mm stage) formation of the collecting system is accompanied by nephrogenesis. Oval condensations of metanephric blastemal cells become related to each ampulla. Some of these cells form a blastemal cap which accompanies the next subdivision of the ampulla, whilst others form a hollow vesicle. This elongates and becomes S-shaped. The lumen becomes continuous with that of the related ureteric bud branch, and at the other end capillary vessels develop in situ to form the glomerulus. The intervening portions develop into the proximal and distal convoluted tubules with the loop of Henle in the middle. Nephron attachment to the ampullae varies at different stages of organogenesis, as described by Osathanondh and Potter (1964) and summarised by Potter and Craig (1976). After the initial phase (7–14 weeks) branching of the ureteric bud ceases, and each ampulla becomes capable of inducing formation of a number of nephrons (14–22 weeks) which are joined together in a chain (nephron arcade). After the 22nd week in the outer cortex nephrons become attached singly behind the ampulla until new nephron formation stops at between the 32nd and 36th weeks. These last-forming nephrons can be recognised in the subcapsular cortex in sections of fetal kidneys of less than 36 weeks' gestation as a "nephrogenic zone", (Fig. 19.1), a reliable histological marker of prematurity. During its early development the metanephros is at the level of the upper sacral segments and it receives its blood supply from lateral sacral branches of the aorta. As the embryo increases in length the relative position of the developing kidney becomes progressively more cranial until by the 8th week it is in its definitive lumbar situation. This "ascent" is accompanied by medial rotation so that the renal pelvis, which is initially ventrally placed, comes to lie on the medial aspect of the kidney. During its ascent the kidney receives blood from stem arteries from the aorta at progressively higher levels until ultimately it is supplied by the definitive renal artery at the level of the 2nd lumbar vertebra.

The cloaca, marked externally by a shallow depression covered by the cloacal membrane, is continuous with three endodermal tubules: the hindgut, the allantois and the blind-ending diverticulum of the tail gut. At about the 5 mm stage a septum, the urogenital septum, extends down caudally from the angle between the allantois and the hindgut and ultimately fuses with the cloacal membrane at the 16 mm stage, thus dividing the cloaca into a smaller dorsal portion, the primitive rectum, and a larger ventral part, the primitive urogenital sinus. The terminal portions of the Wolffian (mesonephric) ducts beyond the origin of the metanephric ducts, now termed the common excretory ducts, join the urogenital sinus on the two sides dividing it into an upper portion above the ducts—the vesicourethral canal—and a lower portion below the ducts—the definitive urogenital sinus.

The vesicourethral canal, from which the bladder and upper urethra develop, is a slightly flattened cylinder, continuous cranially with the allantois. As the lower abdominal wall grows, the bladder segment of the vesicourethral canal enlarges and the urogenital sinus below it becomes flattened from side to side and elongates dorsiventrally. The common excretory ducts dilate and then become absorbed in the wall of the vesicourethral canal so that the metanephric and mesonephric ducts drain separately into the vesicourethral canal. As the bladder enlarges, the metanephric (now ureteric) orifices move gradually caudally and laterally in relation to the mesonephric ducts, which remain close together near the midline. In the male embryo the mesonephric ducts persist to form the epididymis, vas deferens, seminal vesicle and common ejaculatory duct. In the female the mesonephric duct degenerates from about the 30 mm stage and ultimately disappears, apart from the vestigial epoophoron, paroophoron and Gärtner's duct. The triangular zone and common ejaculatory duct between the ureteric orifices forms the trigone of the bladder, which is of mesodermal origin, unlike the rest of the bladder, which is derived from endoderm. The allantois regresses as the bladder enlarges and ultimately forms a solid fibrous cord, the urachus, extending from the bladder to the umbilicus.

In the female the primitive urethra, derived from the lower part of the vesicourethral canal, forms almost the whole of the definitive urethra. In the male this forms only the upper portion of the prostatic urethra and the membranous urethra is derived from the upper (pelvic) part of the definitive urogenital sinus, whilst the penile urethra is formed by the fusion of two urethral folds which form on each side of the ventral surface of the developing phallus. The urethral groove which lies between the two folds is formed by a plate of cells (the urethral plate) which extends forward from the lower (phallic) portion of the urogenital sinus. Fusion of the urethral folds starts posteriorly and extends forwards; it is marked posteriorly by the median raphe. Fusion extends forwards only as far as the circular coronary sulcus, which delineates the glans penis. A core of ectodermal cells grows backwards through the glans to join with the urethra. This later becomes canalised and is continuous with the urethral lumen, thus forming the terminal (glandular) part and the urethral meatus.

Malformations of the Kidney

Congenital renal abnormalities can be divided into (1) anomalies of position and form and (2) parenchymal maldevelopments.

Ectopia and Malrotation

Normal "ascent" and rotation of the kidney during development has been described above. Interference with, or arrest of, this process results in the permanent abnormal position of the kidney, which is often rounded or lobulated rather than reniform because of the different moulding effects of adjacent structures, and is normally malrotated with the renal pelvis pointing forwards instead of medially. Rarely, reversed rotation, or rotation through more than 90° results in a laterally or posteriorly directed renal pelvis. Most commonly, ectopic kidneys are located at the pelvic brim or in the pelvis. Often the ectopic kidney is supplied by a number of small arteries rather than a single vessel; these arise from the aorta near its bifurcation or from the iliac arteries. Not uncommonly, ectopic kidneys exhibit parenchymal maldifferentiation (renal dysplasia, see p. 470), and sometimes distortion or kinking of the renal pelvis or ureter may lead to hydronephrosis and predispose to renal infection and calculus formation. Occasionally, the ureter of an ectopic kidney is inserted ectopically in the bladder, vagina or seminal vesicle; sometimes it is subject to vesicoureteric reflux. Rarely, ectopic kidneys are located at a higher than normal level, even in the thorax in association with a diaphragmatic defect. High ectopia is almost always on the left side and is virtually confined to males.

Renal ectopia may be unilateral or bilateral and has an incidence of about 1 in 800. It is slightly commoner in females and on the left side. Rarely, unilateral renal ectopia is associated with absence (agenesis) of the contralateral kidney, and pelvic ectopia may accompany anorectal anomalies or absence of the vagina in females.

Crossed Ectopia

Crossed ectopia is a rare anomaly (with an incidence of about 1 in 8000) which is characterised by the presence of an ectopic kidney on the opposite side from the ureteric orifice, so that the ureter crosses the midline and both kidneys are situated on the same side of the body, the ectopic kidney lying below the orthotopic kidney. Almost always the two kidneys are fused. Dysplastic development of the crossed kidney is sometimes seen and the ureter may be dilated and subject to vesicouroteric reflux.

Fusion

The commonest variety of fusion is that of the lower poles of the two kidneys across the midline (the "horseshoe" kidney), which is seen in approximately 1 in 600 radiological examinations of the kidneys. The "ring" or "doughnut" kidney, where both poles are fused, is much rarer. Since fused kidneys are usually situated lower than normal they may also be regarded as ectopic. The renal pelves are usually anteriorly placed, and high insertion of the ureter into the pelvis at the pelviureteric junction may lead to hydronephrosis. Dysplastic development of part or all of the fused kidney may occur. Fusion is about twice as common in males, and there is an elevated incidence in Turner's syndrome and in association with other congenital urogenital anomalies.

Renal Agenesis

The condition of renal agenesis (Fig. 19.2a), in which the kidney and ureter are completely absent, is ascribed to a failure of development of the ureteric bud from the mesonephric duct (Burk and Beaudoin 1977), or to its early degeneration. The absence of the ureteric bud results in a failure of the metanephric blastema to develop; the corresponding trigonal area of

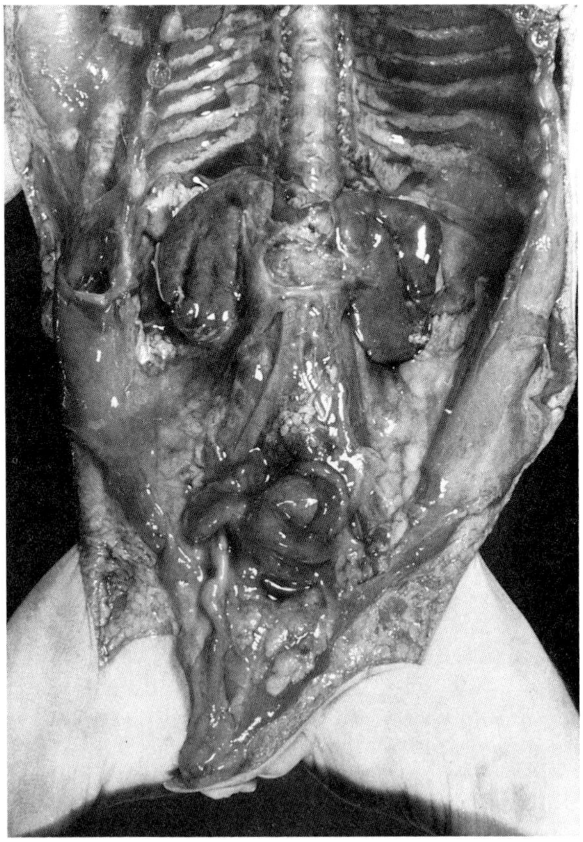
a

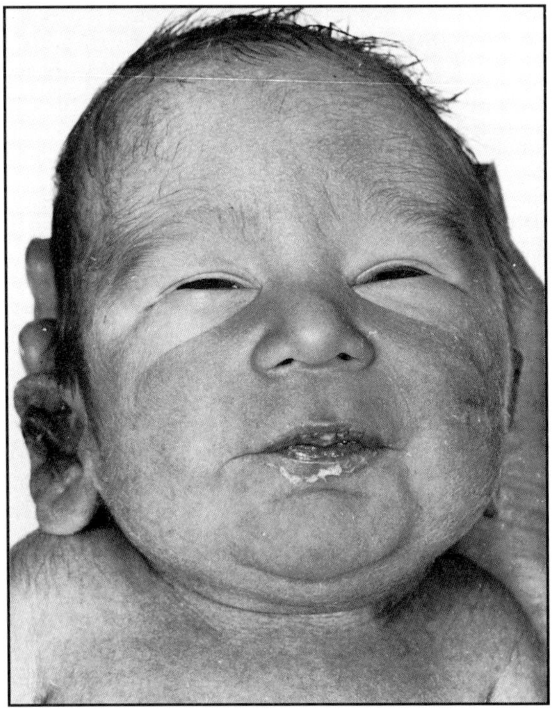
b

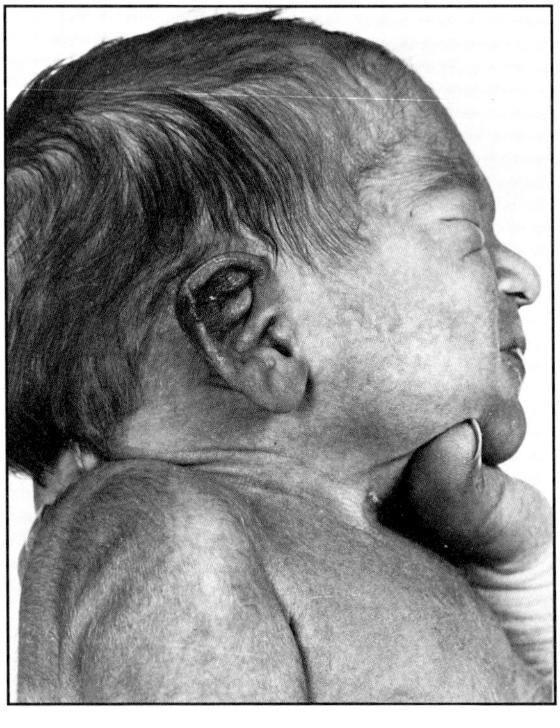
c

Fig. 19.2. Renal agenesis. **a** The kidneys are absent; the adrenals are disc-shaped and there is an associated bicornuate uterus (Risdon 1981a). **b,c** Potter's syndrome facies: **b** full face; **c** side view.

the bladder is also absent in the majority of cases.

Renal agenesis may be unilateral or bilateral. Unilateral agenesis has a frequency of about 1 in 1000 at necropsy and is slightly commoner in males. Other congenital urogenital tract anomalies are often associated. In the male, the testis often fails to descend and mesonephric duct derivatives such as the seminal vesicle and vas deferens are frequently absent. In the female paramesonephric (Müllerian) duct derivatives such as the fallopian tubes, uterine horn and upper vagina fail to develop or are abnormal. Outside the urogenital tract, anomalies such as an imperforate anus, oesophageal atresia and tracheo-oesophageal fistula, neural tube defects and congenital heart lesions are not infrequent.

Bilateral renal agenesis is comparatively rare (1 in 4000 births), and is twice as common in males as females. The condition is not compatible with life; death occurs in utero or in the neonatal period from respiratory insufficiency. Bilateral agenesis is associated with Potter's syndrome; pulmonary hypoplasia, low-set ears, beak-like nose, receding chin, large hands, bow legs and talipes (Potter 1946), which are attributed to oligohydramnios associated with this condition (Fantel and Shepard 1976). The typical Potter's syndrome facies is shown in Fig. 19.2b,c. The bladder and urethra are often absent, or the urethra is atretic and the bladder minute. Bilateral renal agenesis is also associated with lower limb deformities, particularly sirenomelia (posterior limb bud fusion with absence of the sacrum, hindgut, external genitalia, urethra and bladder).

Although usually sporadic, the occasional familial incidence of bilateral renal agenesis has been recognised for some time (Schmidt et al. 1952; Rizza and Dowling 1971). In recent years unilateral and bilateral agenesis, unilateral and bilateral renal dysplasia, or dysplasia of one kidney and agenesis of the other (renal adysplasia) have been recorded in various combinations in the same family (so-called familial renal adysplasia or the agenesis–dysplasia syndrome). The dysplastic kidneys in this syndrome are usually tiny and rudimentary (aplastic) or multicystic and the renal agenesis, though often accompanied by anomalies of mesonephric or paramesonephric duct derivatives, particularly ipsilateral ovarian or oviductal agenesis, is not associated with sirenomelia or caudal regression. Index cases usually present as perinatal deaths with bilateral renal agenesis. Family studies then reveal unilateral agenesis or dysplasia in parents or living siblings and perhaps other deaths from bilateral agenesis, dysplasia or adysplasia in other siblings; sometimes other generations of the family are found to have been affected. The studies of Buchta et al. (1973) indicate an autosomal dominant inheritance with variable expression, but the occasional instances of agenesis–dysplasia in siblings with normal parents indicate that other modes of inheritance may also operate.

Supernumerary Kidneys

"Extra" kidneys are very rare, and their definition requires complete separation of two kidneys on one side of the body with completely separate pelvicalyceal systems. The draining ureters may fuse or join the bladder separately.

Renal Hypoplasia

Normally there is close correlation between body size, age and renal weight throughout childhood (Coppoletta and Wolbach 1933; Landing and Hughes 1962; Table 19.1). Renal hypoplasia can thus be defined as the presence of a kidney that is congenitally small (i.e. less than 2 SD below the expected mean when correlated with age or the usual parameters of somatic growth). Clearly, reduction in renal size may be a result of contracture following acquired disease, but even in the neonatal period, when this is less of a problem, the definition may be hard to apply. This is because the great majority of congenitally small kidneys exhibit evidence of parenchymal maldifferentiation. Currently it is customary to label such kidneys as dysplastic and to retain the term "renal hypoplasia" for kidneys in which parenchymal differentiation is normal and which are abnormal only in terms of their small size, reduced nephron population and perhaps reduced number of lobules (reniculi). Defined strictly in this sense, pure renal hypoplasia without dysplasia is rare, although its exact incidence is difficult to judge since in the past many dysplastic kidneys have been called hypoplastic. In practice, the frequent coexistence of other urinary anomalies such as ureteral ectopia, ureterocele etc. is a useful pointer to a diagnosis of renal dysplasia.

Table 19.1. Mean normal kidney weights at various ages from birth to 12 years[a] (Risdon 1981a)

Age	Renal weight (g)		
	Right	Left	Combined
Birth to 3 days	13	14	27
3– 7 days	14	14	28
1– 3 weeks	15	15	30
3– 5 weeks	16	16	32
5– 7 weeks	19	18	37
7– 9 weeks	19	18	37
9–13 weeks	20	19	39
– 4 months	22	21	43
– 5 months	25	25	50
– 6 months	26	25	51
– 7 months	30	30	60
– 8 months	31	30	61
– 9 months	31	30	61
–10 months	32	31	63
–11 months	34	33	67
–12 months	36	35	71
–14 months	36	35	71
–16 months	39	39	78
–18 months	40	43	83
–20 months	43	44	87
–22 months	44	44	88
–24 months	47	46	93
– 3 years	48	49	97
– 4 years	58	56	114
– 5 years	65	64	129
– 6 years	68	67	135
– 7 years	69	70	139
– 8 years	74	75	149
– 9 years	82	83	165
–10 years	92	95	187
–11 years	95	96	189
–12 years	95	96	191

[a] Data of Coppoletta and Wolbach (1933).

Nevertheless, it is true that some ectopic or malrotated kidneys are smaller than expected, their reduced mass possibly being related to their anomalous blood supply, and in this sense may be regarded as hypoplastic. Such cases apart, unilateral simple hypoplasia is extremely infrequent, and one of the few acceptable cases described is that of Bernstein and Mayer (1964). So-called segmental hypoplasia (the Ask–Upmark kidney), often associated with hypertension in older children, is not now generally regarded as a developmental abnormality but rather a form of reflux nephropathy (Risdon 1981c).

Bilateral simple hypoplasia has been described in association with long-standing disease or congenital anomalies of the central nervous system (Roosen-Runge 1949). Since the numbers of renal lobules in these cases are usually not reduced, the possibility exists that their small size reflects a failure of postnatal growth rather than an intrinsic congenital insufficiency in renal mass. In addition there is a distinctive non-familial form of extreme bilateral hypoplasia termed "oligoméganéphronie" (oligonephronic hypoplasia) by Royer et al. (1962). In this condition the kidneys are tiny and often consist of only one or two lobules. Histologically, the nephron number is drastically reduced, but those present are markedly hypertrophied. On average, the cross-sectional areas of glomeruli are increased 12-fold, and microdissection studies show that proximal tubules are increased fourfold in length and 17-fold in volume (Fetterman and Habib 1969).

Congenital Nephromegaly

Compensatory growth and hypertrophy of one kidney may occur even in utero when the contralateral kidney is severely dysplastic or absent.

Bilateral nephromegaly is a feature of the Wiedemann–Beckwith syndrome (Wiedemann 1964; Beckwith 1969), an apparently autosomal-dominant trait (Engström et al. 1988) characterised by visceromegaly, hyperinsulinaemic hypoglycaemia due to islet cell hypertrophy, microcephaly, exomphalos, macroglossia and adrenal cytomegaly, as well as the similar, though genetically distinct, Perlman syndrome which appears to be autosomal-recessive (Perlman et al. 1975) and is characterised by an abnormal facies without macroglossia, visceromegaly and islet cell hyperplasia.

In both these conditions the kidneys are variably enlarged and show accentuated lobulation. The medullary pyramids are poorly defined and many exhibit ductal dysplasia. Superficial nodular nephroblastomatosis (see p. 477) is frequently present, and its malignant potential for the development of nephroblastoma is reflected in the increased incidence and common bilaterality of this tumour in patients with the Wiedemann–Beckwith and Perlman syndromes.

Renal Dysplasia

The term "renal dysplasia" defines a developmental abnormality of the kidney resulting from anomalous metanephric differentiation (Risdon 1971a). Almost invariably there are other associated congenital anomalies of the ureter or lower urinary tract. Histologically,

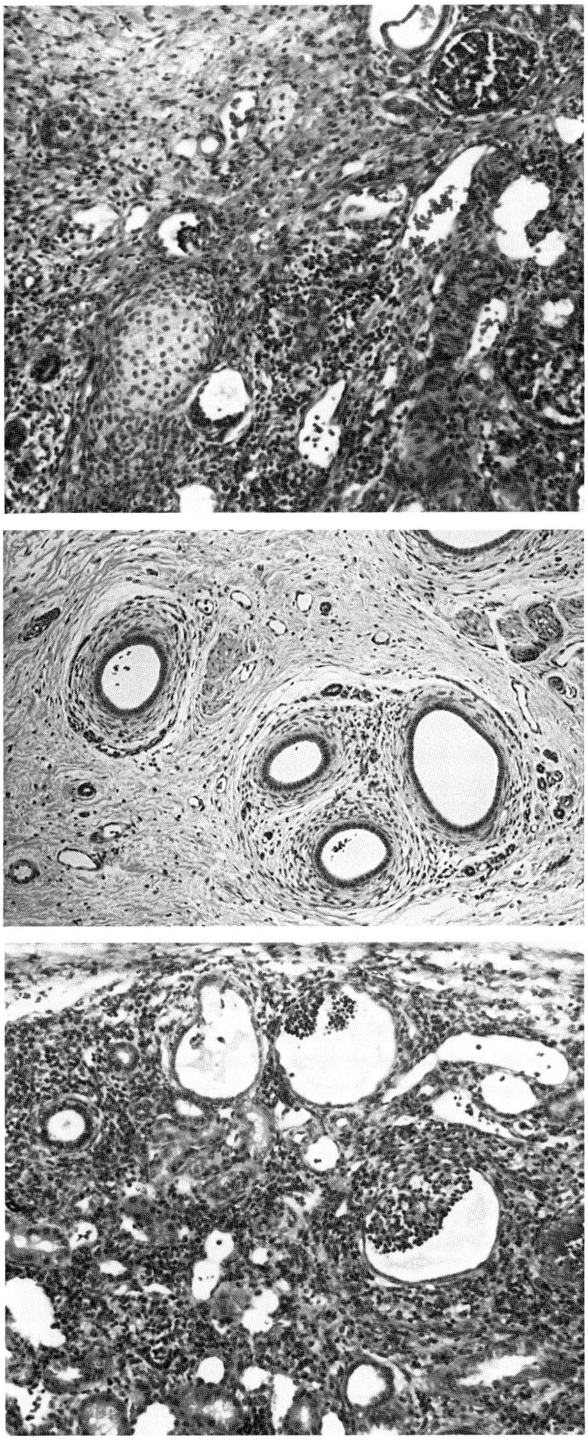

a

b

c

Fig. 19.3. Renal dysplasia. **a** Primitive glomeruli and bars of metaplastic cartilage. (H&E, ×80.) **b** Primitive ducts lined by columnar epithelium and surrounded by collars of mesenchymal cells (H&E, ×15.) **c** Primitive ducts and glomerular cysts (H&E, ×50)

dysplastic development is recognised by disorganisation of the renal parenchyma, often accompanied by cyst formation, and by the presence of immature nephronic and ductal structures resembling those seen in the fetal kidney (Fig. 19.3). The immature nephrons are often sparse in number and separated by loose mesenchyme. Occasionally, bars of metaplastic cartilage are present and there may be foci of extramedullary haemopoietic cells in the mesenchyme. Microdissection studies in severely dysplastic kidneys indicate that the anomaly results from diminished branching of the ureteric bud with partial failure of nephron induction. The larger cysts appear to represent ureteric bud branches which have failed to induce nephrons, whilst small cysts are derived from dilated tubular, ductal or glomerular structures.

Dysplastic renal development may affect the whole kidney or it may be focal or segmental in distribution, with part of the kidney developing normally. The pattern of dysplasia is related to the accompanying urinary tract anomalies, and this association is useful in classifying the condition (Risdon 1971a,b).

Renal dysplasia encountered in the neonatal period, and particularly in perinatal necropsies, is most commonly either of the multicystic or aplastic varieties; it may also occur in association with congenital lower urinary tract obstruction or rarely with syndromes of multiple malformations (see p. 476). Renal dysplasia associated with ureteric ectopia and sometimes with vesicoureteric reflux, which generally presents in older children, is described elsewhere (Risdon 1971a,b, 1981a, 1991; Risdon et al. 1975).

Multicystic and aplastic dysplasia are forms of severe generalised corticomedullary maldifferentiation affecting the whole of one or both kidneys. The multicystic dysplastic kidney is grossly cystic and as a result is enlarged to a variable extent. The largest cysts are distributed peripherally beneath the capsule of the kidney, where they distort its reniform shape (Fig. 19.4). The pelvicalyceal system is severely attenuated or absent, reflecting the diminution in branching of the ureteric bud during organogenesis. Examination of large, correctly orientated sections usually reveals some evidence of corticomedullary differentiation with scanty radially aligned primitive ducts, representing the diminished ureteric bud derivatives which extend from the hilus towards the capsule. These are lined by columnar epithelium and are sur-

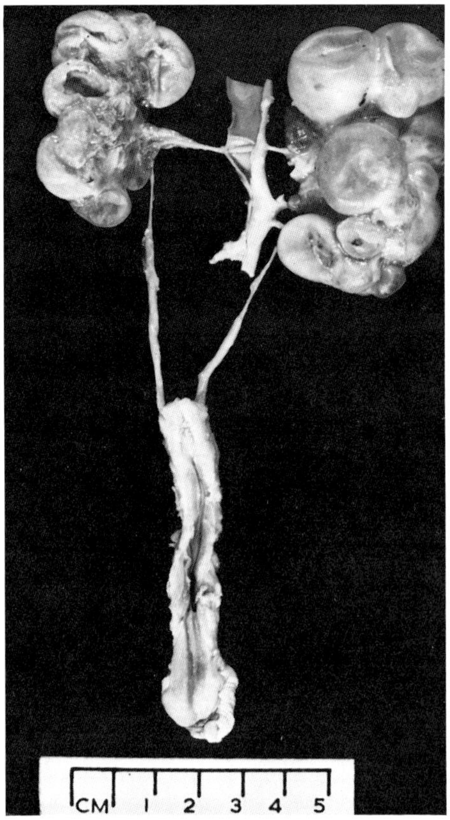

Fig. 19.4. Bilateral multicystic dysplasia. Note the atretic upper ureters.

rounded by mantles of mesenchymal spindle cells. Scanty immature ductal and nephronic elements are seen in the cortex, separated by loose mesenchyme. The nephron population is variably but usually severely diminished, and cyst formation is a prominent feature. The large subcapsular cysts have fibrous walls lined by flattened epithelium and are mostly derived from ureteric bud branches which have failed to induce nephron formation. Smaller cysts, representing dilated tubular, ductal and glomerular elements, are also seen. Occasionally, bars of metaplastic cartilage are present and are useful in diagnosis.

The aplastic kidney is an essentially similar malformation distinguished only by its much smaller size. It is extremely rudimentary consisting only of a nubbin of dysplastic renal tissue or a tiny collection of cysts.

With both multicystic and aplastic kidneys, the draining ureter is very thin or, rarely, it is completely absent. Usually the ureter is atretic for part (usually the upper third) or all of its length.

Bilateral multicystic or aplastic renal dysplasia are lethal malformations with clinical features like those of bilateral renal agenesis; Potter's syndrome is usually present. Clinically the only distinction is that with bilateral multicystic kidneys cystic loin masses may be palapable or may be demonstrated by ultrasonography.

Unilateral multicystic or aplastic dysplasia usually present in the perinatal period and may be associated with major congenital anomalies in other systems, most notably isolated ventricular septal defect, aortic coarctation, intestinal atresia and meningomyelocele. In addition, with unilateral disease there is an increased incidence of contralateral congenital ureteric stenosis and hydronephrosis (Pathak and Williams 1963).

Multicystic kidneys can be recognised in utero by fetal ultrasound and serial examinations have shown that the size and configuration of the cysts may alter with time (Avini et al. 1987) or even apparently disappear (Pedicelli et al. 1986). Since it is unlikely that a multicystic kidney will entirely regress, it is possible that the loss of the cystic ultrasound image denotes the progression of a multicystic to an aplastic kidney, and is further evidence that the two conditions are intimately related.

Renal Dysplasia with Congenital Lower Urinary Tract Obstruction

Anatomical or functional congenital lower urinary tract obstruction causes bilateral hydronephrosis and hydroureters and there may be additional dysplastic development of the kidneys (Fig. 19.5). The extent of both hydronephrosis and dysplasia is related to the degree of obstruction, and cases presenting in the perinatal period are usually the most severe. The commonest cause of obstruction in this age group is posterior urethral valves in infant boys (see p. 486), but occasionally there is urethral atresia, which is invariably accompanied by profound renal dysplasia. Functional obstruction, occurring in the megacystic-megaureter syndrome or as part of the "prune belly" syndrome (see p. 486), may also be associated with dysplastic renal development.

Whatever the cause of the obstruction, the changes in the kidney are similar and represent a combination of hydronephrosis and dysplastic differentiation. There is variable parenchymal

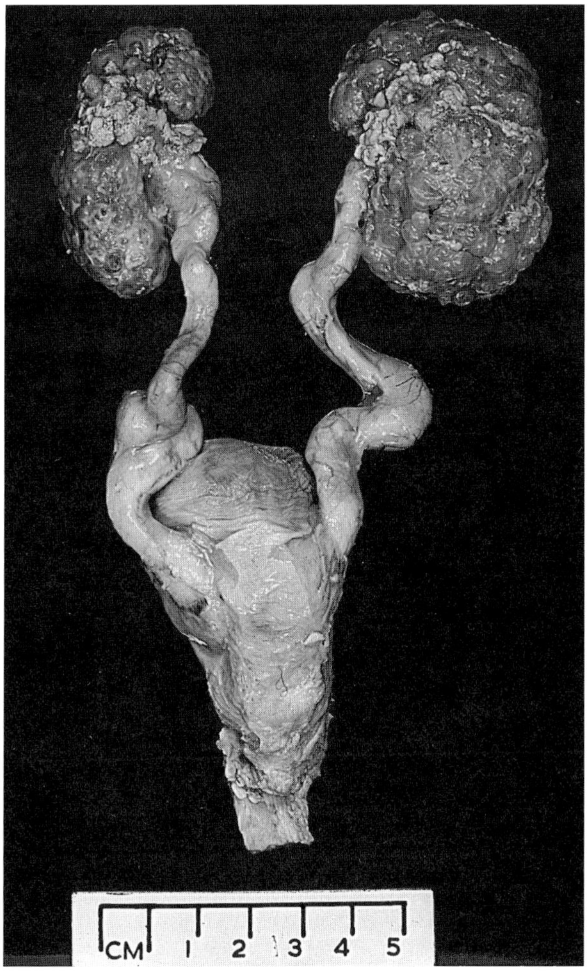

Fig. 19.5. Renal dysplasia associated with posterior urethral valves.

thinning with flattening of the medulla associated with calyceal dilatation. The flattened medulla contains a sparse system of ducts surrounded by mesenchymal connective tissue in a delta-like pattern. Cortical dysplasia is most marked peripherally beneath the capsule, affecting nephrons formed late in renal development. Glomerular and tubular elements of immature morphology are present, often separated by loose mesenchyme. Cyst formation may be prominent and occasional foci of metaplastic cartilage may also be present. Histological evidence of renal parenchymal infection may be superimposed.

The ureters are generally markedly dilated and tortuous, but occasionally ureteric atresia accompanied by profound multicystic dysplasia is seen in the perinatal period, mostly in association with urethral atresia.

Congenital Hydronephrosis

Hydronephrosis with varying degrees of pelvicalyceal dilatation, parenchymal atrophy and blunting of medullary pyramids may develop in utero, when it is usually associated with obstruction at the pelviureteric junction. This can be variously attributed, (1) to an intrinsic abnormality of the ureteric muscle bundles at this point, producing a narrow aperistaltic segment, possibly associated with aberrant segmental arteries crossing the pelviureteric junction; (2) to kinks, fibrous bands or adhesions producing abnormal angulation of the ureter against the renal pelvis; or rarely (3) to mucosal fold or polyps.

The condition may be unilateral or, in about 20% of cases, bilateral. The latter are more likely to present in infancy and in this age group boys are more frequently affected than girls. Occasionally extreme degrees of unilateral hydronephrosis (so-called giant hydronephrosis) present as large, easily palpable, cystic loin masses in the neonatal period. Parenchymal atrophy in such cases is extreme and may be associated with dysplastic changes.

Renal Cystic Disease

In this section the types of renal cystic disease encountered in the perinatal period are considered; for a full classification the reader is referred to Risdon (1981b; 1991).

Autosomal Recessive Polycystic Kidney Disease (ARPKD)

This rare, invariably bilateral and autosomal-recessive condition was previously termed infantile polycystic disease (Fig. 19.6). This is a less satisfactory description than ARPKD since it is now recognised to encompass a spectrum of renal and hepatic lesions, a minority of which may not become apparent until later childhood or even adult life. Classically, presentation is in infants who are stillborn or die in the neonatal period, often from respiratory insufficiency caused by pulmonary hypoplasia; Potter's syndrome is often present. Both

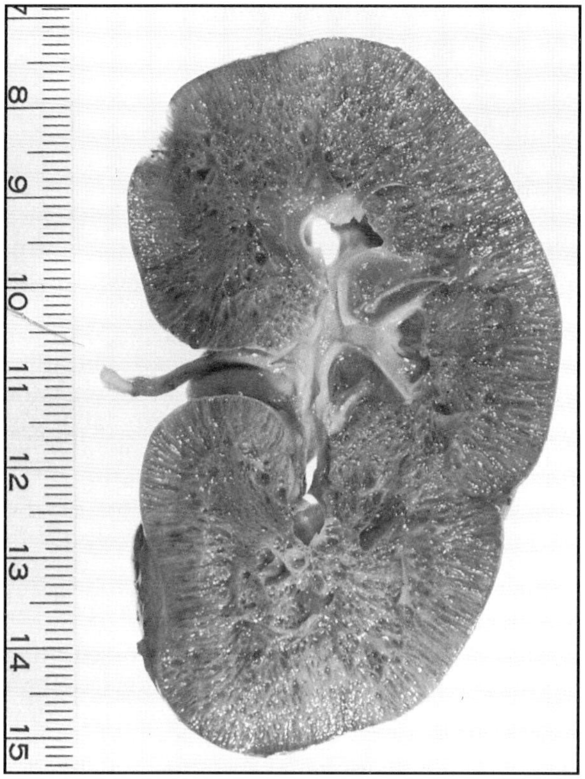
a

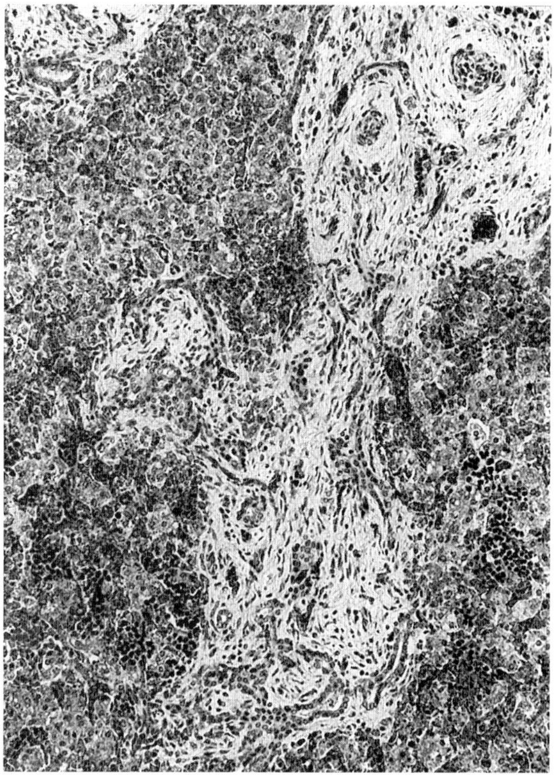
c

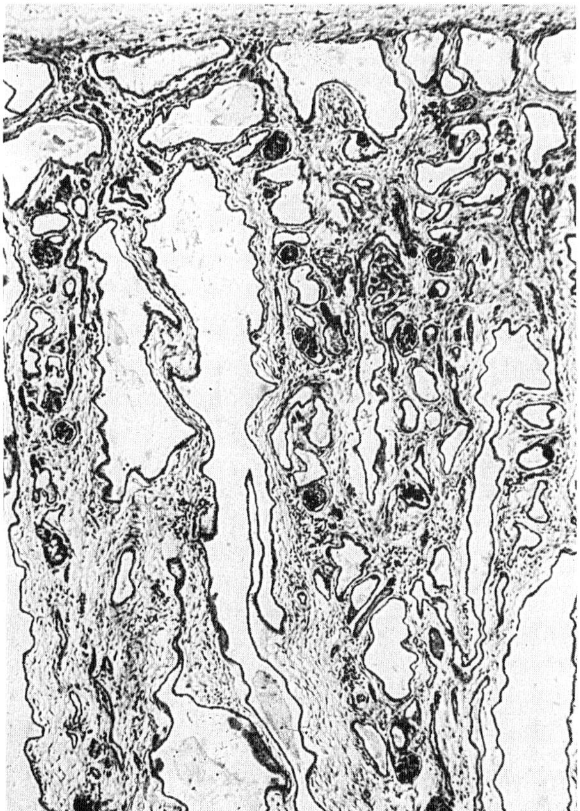
b

Fig. 19.6. Autosomal recessive polycystic disease. **a** The kidney showing radially aligned, fusiform cysts in the cortex and medulla. **b** Microscopic appearance of the kidney showing cystically dilated collecting ducts. (H&E, ×18.) **c** Microscopic appearance of the liver showing portal fibrosis and angulated branching bile ducts. (H&E, ×135)

kidneys are grossly enlarged, sometimes sufficiently to interfere with delivery. Despite their huge size, the reniform shape of the kidneys is preserved and fetal lobulation is often exaggerated. On slicing the kidney, the cortex and medulla resemble a sponge and contain innumerable radially arranged fusiform cysts. On histological examination these are seen to be cystically dilated collecting ducts, an impression that can be confirmed by the positive staining of their lining cells with peroxidase-labelled *Arachis hypogaea* (peanut) lectin (Faraggiana et al. 1985). Microdissection studies by Osathanondh and Potter (1964) in this type of renal cystic disease (Potter type 1) indicated the cysts to be due to dilatation and hyperplasia of the interstitial portions of ureteric bud branches. Ampullary function during organogenesis appears to be unimpaired in that branching is normal and nephron induction is unaffected.

In virtually every case of ARPKD the renal lesion is accompanied by congenital hepatic fibrosis. The latter is characterised by a varying degree of diffuse portal fibrosis and by intrahepatic bile ducts which appear to be increased in number, are often dilated and exhibit a characteristic angulated branching, the branches often surrounding portal veins. Reconstructions from serial sections indicate that the bile ducts in congenital hepatic fibrosis form interconnecting cisterns rather than tubules (Jørgensen 1972).

The above description encompasses cases of congenital hepatic fibrosis with classic infantile polycystic disease of the type encountered perinatally or in the preterm fetus. However, the complete spectrum of congenital hepatic fibrosis is more complex. Blyth and Ockenden (1971) have shown that some cases of ARPKD with congenital hepatic fibrosis present in later childhood and even in adult life. These variants exhibit less complete renal polycystic disease, affecting only a variable part of the two kidneys. Thus clinical presentation is more likely to be related to the hepatic lesions, the portal fibrosis leading eventually to portal hypertension and complications such as bleeding from oesophageal varices. Although in all such cases inheritance appears to be autosomal recessive in type, Blyth and Ockenden (1971) found that in an individual family the relative degrees of renal and hepatic involvement appeared to be constant. They suggested that a number of different mutant genes might operate and on this basis divided polycystic disease with hepatic fibrosis into four types (perinatal, neonatal, infantile and juvenile). Later studies, on the other hand, have shown that this distinction is not clear-cut and that siblings do not necessarily present at the same age, nor does the relative severity of the renal and hepatic lesions necessarily breed true (Six et al. 1975; Gang et al. 1986; Kaplan et al. 1988). In some cases renal cysts may be confined to the papillary collecting ducts; the radiographic appearances on intravenous urography are identical to the so-called medullary sponge kidney, the only distinction being the association with congenital hepatic fibrosis (Reilly and Newhauser 1960).

To add to the confusion, congenital hepatic fibrosis accompanies other forms of familial renal cystic disease, notably multicystic renal dysplasia in Meckel's syndrome and its variants (see p. 477) and also some cases of juvenile nephronophthisis (Delaney et al. 1978) and Jeune's thoracic dystrophy. In practical terms, whatever the associated lesions, the presence of congenital hepatic fibrosis suggests inherited disease with an autosomal-recessive transmission.

Increasingly, ARPKD is being diagnosed in utero by fetal ultrasonography which demonstrates enlarged, brightly echogenic kidneys in an affected fetus. Where termination of pregnancy is advised on the basis of fetal ultrasound it is essential that a proper examination of the fetus is made. Typical changes in the fetal kidneys and liver are recognisable by 18 weeks, gestation, but the author has insufficient experience to comment on changes at an early stage. It is worth noting that in some instances a diagnosis of ARPKD by fetal ultrasound has not been confirmed by pathological examination of the fetus and a genetic marker, like that being developed for ADPKD (see below) would be extremely helpful in making a more accurate diagnosis.

Autosomal Dominant Polycystic Kidney Disease (ADPKD) and Glomerulocystic Disease

ADPKD is much commoner than ARPKD. As with the term "infantile" polycystic kidney disease, the older description of ADPKD as "adult" polycystic disease is becoming outmoded following the recognition that a minority of patients with this condition may present clinically in childhood or even in infancy. In addition, improved diagnostic imaging techniques have allowed the recognition of affected members of an ADPKD kindred at an earlier, presymptomatic stage of their disease. The variability in expression of the disease has been further extended by the discovery that a significant proportion of affected individuals may have a normal lifespan with minimal renal impairment. The failure to recognise such cases in the past may be a significant factor in the apparent lack of a family history indicating an autosomal-dominant inheritance in some instances.

Recently the abnormal gene responsible for ADPKD has been found to be closely linked with the alpha-globin gene cluster and the phosphoglycolate gene on the short arm of chromosome 16 (Reeders et al. 1985, 1986; Breuning et al. 1987). This discovery has allowed prenatal diagnosis of ADPKD in a 9-week fetus by DNA analysis of a chorionic villus sample which demonstrated the same gene linkage as in other affected members of the same family (Reeders et al. 1986). However in some families with ADPKD, linkage of the mutant gene to chromosome 16 has not been identified (Kimberling et al. 1988; Romeo et al. 1988) indicating that at least two mutant genes exist for ADPKD, that on chromosome 16 being designated PCK-1 and the less frequent one unlinked to chromosome 16 as PCK-2.

In the context of this chapter, only those rare examples of ADPKD presenting problems in perinatal practice are considered. In these cases the kidneys vary in size from normal to considerably enlarged. Rounded cysts from a few mm up to about 3 cm in diameter may be seen in both cortex and medulla, with a variable distortion of the normal reniform shape. Unlike ARPKD, in ADPKD presenting in this age group there is always a considerable portion of normal renal parenchyma and the cysts may be derived from any part of the nephron as well as from the collecting ducts.

Often, dilatation of Bowman's spaces dominates the histological picture (Rapola and Kääriänen 1988) so that early-onset ADPKD represents one form of so-called glomerulocystic disease. This term, first used by Taxy and Filmer (1976), is now used loosely to describe a heterogeneous group of disorders which are linked only by the common feature of a variable cystic dilatation of Bowman's spaces, rather than a specific entity (Joshi and Kasznica 1984; Bernstein and Landing 1989).

Glomerular cysts occur in a wide variety of inherited and sporadic disorders including early-onset ADPKD (Fellows et al. 1976; Proesmans et al. 1982), Zellweger cerebro-renal–hepatic syndrome (Joshi and Kasznica 1984), tuberous sclerosis (Rolfes et al. 1985), trisomy 13 syndrome, Majewski-type short rib polydactyly syndrome (Joshi and Kasznica, 1984) oro-facio-digital syndrome (Stapleton et al. 1982), brachymesomelia–renal syndrome (Langer et al. 1983) and some examples of renal dysplasia. However, a significant proportion of cases of glomerulocystic disease occurring in infants have no abnormalities in other systems or syndromal associations and appear to be sporadic.

For the pathologist, a practical approach to this rather bewildering situation is as follows. An association of glomerular cysts with renal dysplasia is usually readily apparent from the histological appearances, except, perhaps, in very small and unrepresentative samples. Once renal dysplasia is excluded, the term glomerulocystic disease should only be applied when this is the predominant histopathological change. Evidence of syndromal associations should then be considered; most of these will be obvious, but special caution should be exercised in excluding tuberous sclerosis, since evidence of this in family members and the index case may be subtle. Bernstein et al. (1986) describe a patient with severe glomerulocystic disease at first thought to be sporadic but who was later found to have skin lesions of tuberous sclerosis.

About half the cases of glomerulocystic disease in infants are examples of early-onset ADPKD. In these the diagnosis can usually be confirmed by the recognition of other affected family members, which may require ultrasonic examination of the kidneys in asymptomatic subjects. Where the technique is available, the demonstration of the ADPKD-associated gene linkage on chromosome 16 by DNA analysis offers further confirmation of the diagnosis.

Renal Cystic Disease Associated with Syndromes of Multiple Malformations

Renal cysts are a component of a number of rare, often hereditary syndromes of multiple malformations, including the autosomal trisomy syndromes (Rohde et al. 1964; Mottet and Jensen 1965), the chromosomal translocation syndromes (Talvik et al. 1973), short rib polydactyly syndrome (Spranger et al. 1974), Ehlers–Danlos syndrome (Imahori et al. 1969), oro-facio-digital syndrome (Doege et al. 1964) and the lissencephaly syndrome (Dieker et al. 1969). The renal lesions are bilateral and range from minor focal microcystic changes to extensive diffuse cystic dysplasia. As stated above, in individual examples of some of these syndromes, the cysts may be predominantly glomerular.

Diffuse cystic dysplasia describes the occurrence of multiple, fairly regular and mainly cortical cysts ranging from a few mm up to several cm in diameter in both kidneys. The medullary pyramids are poorly formed and contain scanty primitive ducts. Ductal and nephronic structures are generally scanty and metaplastic cartilage very unusual. Whilst there is a superficial resemblance to multicystic dysplasia, diffuse cystic dysplasia can be distinguished by the invariably bilateral renal involvement and the presence of some degree of renal pelvic development with a patent ureter.

Whilst diffuse cystic dysplasia is sometimes an isolated anomaly of sporadic incidence, it is often part of an hereditary syndrome of multiple malformations of which the Meckel syndrome (Fig. 19.7) of microcephaly, posterior encephalocoele, polydactyly, hare lip and cleft palate and its variants is the most common (Opitz and Howe 1969; Bernstein 1976). Diffuse cystic dysplasia may also accompany the trisomy D (Mottet and Jensen 1965) and oro-facio-digital syndrome (Stapleton et al. 1982). The cystic changes in the kidney are variable in Zellweger's syndrome (Jan et al. 1970) of cerebral pachygyria and micropolygyria with ocular, genital and hepatic malformations, and in Jeune's syndrome (Cremin 1970) of osteochrondrodystrophic dwarfism and small thorax. The renal lesions range from minor focal microcystic changes to diffuse cystic renal dysplasia; involvement is bilateral. All three syndromes are inherited as autosomal-recessive traits and in all there are malformations of the intrahepatic bile ducts like those seen in infantile polycystic disease (see Figs. 16.18, 16.19, p. 390).

Tuberous sclerosis has been mentioned in the context of glomerulocystic disease (see page 476). In some cases of tuberous sclerosis, cysts of a more distinctive type may be seen. These are lined by large eosinophilic cells with granular cytoplasm resembling hyperplastic proximal tubular cells. In addition, curious, apparently microhamartomatous, glomerular lesions have recently been described (Nagashima et al. 1988). These are characterised by compact collections of large, clear polygonal cells containing lipid-filled vacuoles confined within the glomerular tufts and bordered by the glomerular basement membrane.

Tumours of the Kidney in the Neonate

Congenital Mesoblastic Nephroma

Congenital mesoblastic nephroma (Fig. 19.8) also referred to as mesenchymal hamartoma, fetal hamartoma and leiomyomatous hamartoma, is the tumour most frequently discovered in the neonatal period and clearly may arise in utero. Macroscopically the tumour is firm, rounded or spherical and usually about 5 cm in diameter. The cut surface is yellowish or white and shows a whorled appearance resembling a uterine fibroid. Microscopically it consists of interlacing bands of closely packed spindle cells with ultrastructural features resembling smooth muscle or mesenchymal cells. The tumour lacks a capsule, and structures in the adjacent normal renal parenchyma are trapped within its margin. Characteristically, foci of glomeruli and tubules, often immature in their morphological appearance, are scattered throughout. These probably represent structures entrapped within the developing tumour as it grows rather than intrinsic components of the tumour itself. Occasionally, foci of cartilage and small cysts may be seen, and mitoses in the in the tumour cells are not infrequent.

The particular features which separate this entity from nephroblastoma were first described by Bolande et al. (1967). The distinction is important since in the vast majority of cases mesoblastic nephroma is cured by surgery alone, local recurrence or metastatic spread being extremely rare. The previous inclusion of mesoblastic nephromas in series of nephroblastomas is probably reflected in the apparently very good prognosis ascribed to congenital nephroblastoma. Postoperative radiotherapy or chemotherapy appropriate to nephroblastoma is unnecessary with mesoblastic nephroma, and these forms of treatment themselves carry appreciable morbidity and mortality risks in very young children (Hilton and Keeling 1973).

Patients with mesoblastic nephroma may be hypertensive and immunoreactive renin can be demonstrated in glomerular arterioles entrapped within the tumour as well as in tumoral thin-walled vascular sinusoids (Cook et al. 1988).

Nephroblastomatosis

This may be defined as the persistence of metanephric blastema or its incompletely differentiated derivatives beyond 36 weeks' gestation.

Whilst nephroblastomatosis is seen in less than 1% of unselected infant kidneys at necropsy, it occurs in between 20% and 50% of kidneys harbouring nephroblastomas. When it occurs in association with nephroblastoma, the tumours are more likely to be multifocal or bilateral. In addition, nephroblastomatosis is seen in a number of genetic and teratological disorders strongly associated with the develop-

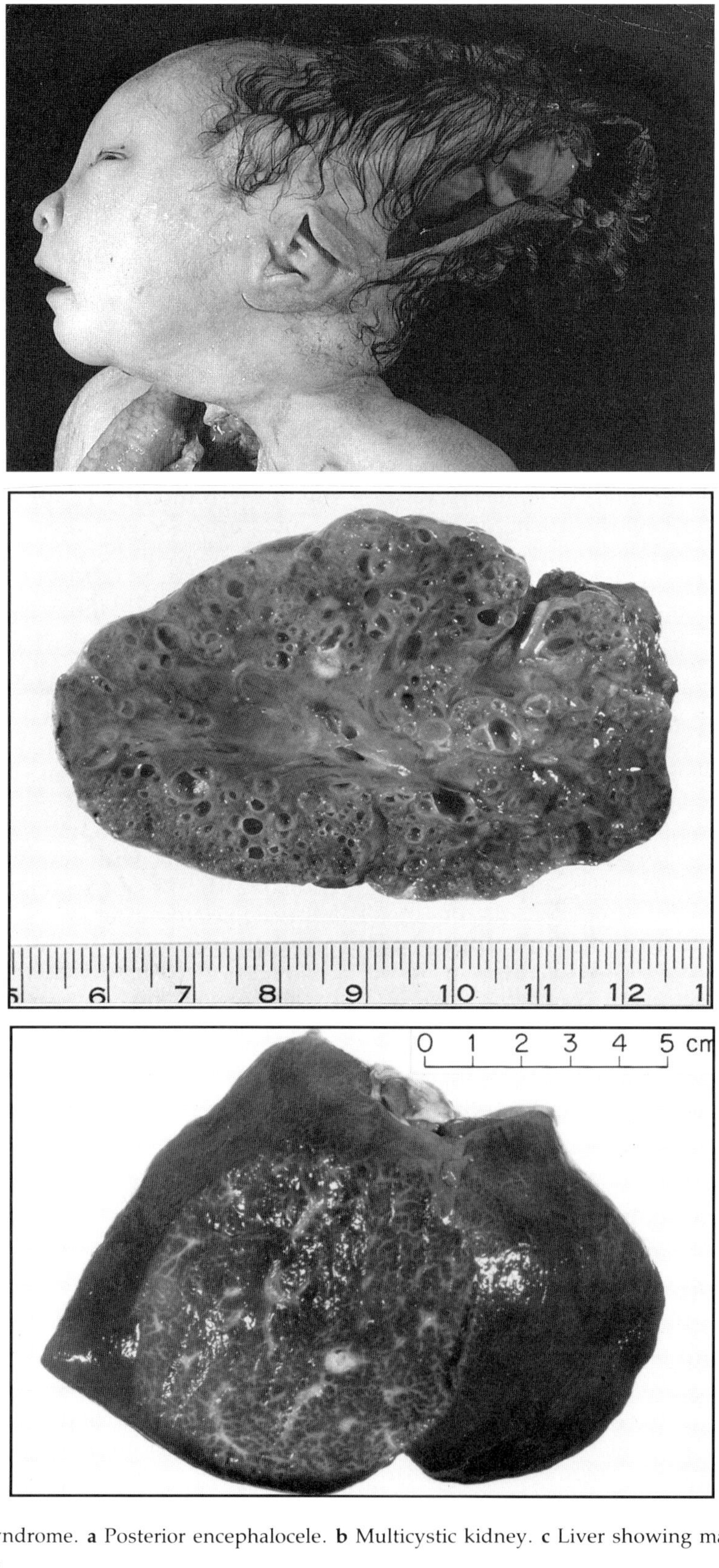

a b c

Fig. 19.7. Meckel's syndrome. **a** Posterior encephalocele. **b** Multicystic kidney. **c** Liver showing macroscopic evidence of diffuse portal fibrosis.

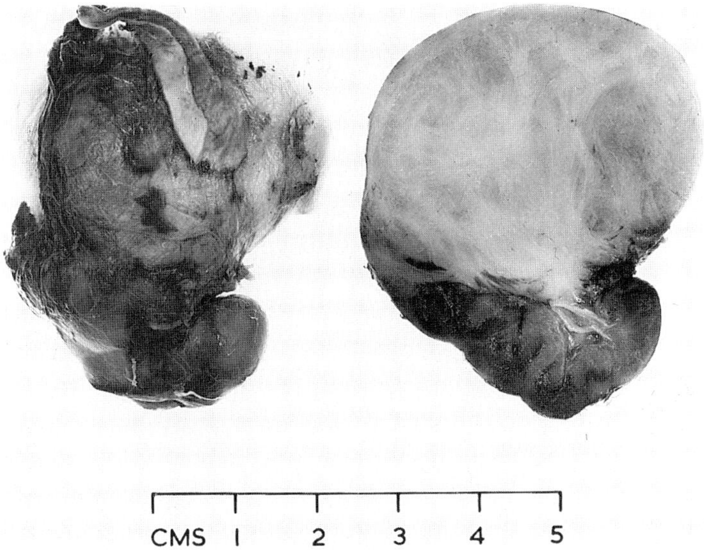

a

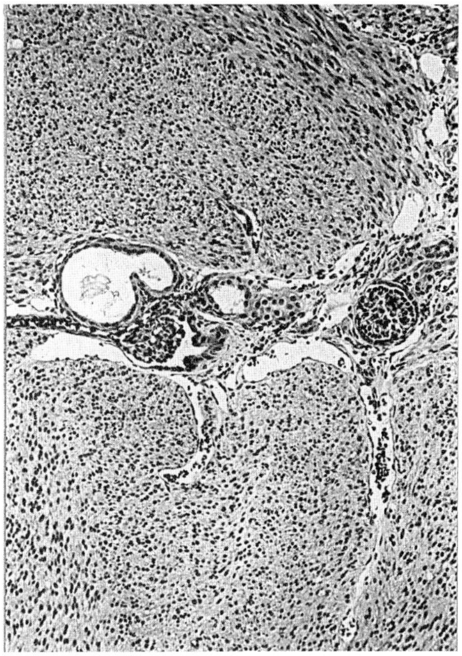

b

Fig. 19.8. Mesoblastic nephroma. **a** Macroscopic appearance showing a rounded tumour with a whorled cut surface. **b** Microscopic appearances showing interlacing sheets of spindle cells and entrapped tubular and glomerular elements. (H&E, ×58)

ment of nephroblastoma, such as Wiedemann–Beckwith, sporadic aniridia and the hemihypertrophy syndrome.

Nephroblastomatosis is classified in terms of its site and distribution within the kidney into (1) superficial (perilobular) nephroblastomatosis of multifocal or diffuse type and (2) deep (intralobular) nephroblastomatosis. Superficial nephroblastomatosis is the most common lesion in infancy and a third very rare, so-called panlobular variety also occurs in this age group.

Superficial nephroblastomatosis may occur as isolated, generally multiple, small nodules in the outer cortex beneath the renal capsule (multifocal type) or as a continuous subcapsular layer (diffuse type). In infants, the more common multifocal nodules (also termed "persistent nodular renal blastema" and "nephrogenic rests") occur as small, circumscribed unencapsulated or delicately encapsulated foci of metanephric blastema in which tubular formations can sometimes be seen. At this age the lesions are not usually visible macroscopically. In older children, the lesions tend to be larger and can be seen with the naked eye. They consist of well-formed tubules lined by small cells with darkly staining nuclei set in a collagenous stroma. These lesions have also been termed "sclerosing metanephric hamartomas" or "regressing nephrogenic rests".

As well as these regressive lesions, proliferative hyperplastic and potentially neoplastic components may be seen either separately or, more commonly, in association with regressive lesions. Putative neoplastic lesions consist of nodules (usually about 1.0–3.5 cm in diameter) and are of two types. The first, termed adenomatous neoplastic rests by Beckwith et al. (1990), consist of collections of embryonal tubular epithelial cells, usually distributed in a differentiated tubular or papillary pattern. Less commonly, nodular lesions are encountered which are composed of neoplastic epithelial elements indistinguishable from those in nephroblastoma, or even showing the full triphasic pattern of nephroblastoma. Mitotic activity may be prominent in these lesions, which are termed nephroblastomatous rests by Beckwith et al. (1990) or "Wilms' tumourlets" by other authors.

Panlobular nephroblastomasis is both extremely rare and incompatible with long survival and some familial cases are recorded. It describes bilateral involvement of virtually the whole renal parenchyma. The kidneys are enlarged and exhibit exaggerated lobulation. Histologically, coalescent nodules of blastemal tissue showing some tubular differentiation are apparent. Sometimes the tubular elements are cystic.

Nephroblastoma

True nephroblastoma is excessively rare in neonates, although fatal metastasising tumours have been described in this age group. With masses confined to the kidney, careful distinction from mesoblastic nephroma and nephroblastomatosis (see p. 477) is necessary (see also Chap. 12, p. 283).

Hereditary Abnormalities of Renal Tubular Transport

Although a number of hereditary disorders of renal tubular transport are recognised, the pathological changes seen in the kidney are seldom of help in diagnosis. A classification of these, based on that of Kissane (1973), is presented in Table 19.2.

Renal Hypoperfusion

Hypoperfusion of the kidneys in the perinatal period may result in renal tubular necrosis, renal cortical necrosis, renal medullary necrosis or renal vein thrombosis; combinations of these lesions frequently occur. Asphyxia and hypotension from any cause in the fetus and newborn may result in spasm of the splanchnic circulation and this appears to underlie the susceptibility to ischaemic lesions in the kidney as well as the intestine and adrenal in this age group. Intrapartum asphyxia, placenta praevia, severe haemolytic disease and some congenital heart lesions are potent causes in the perinatal period (Fig. 19.9).

In infancy, and particularly during the first 2 months of life, renal hypoperfusion is often complicated by renal vein thrombosis, and dehydration resulting from gastroenteritis is a common predisposing cause. Clinically, the condition is recognised by the presence of firm enlargement of the kidney in a sick, often dehydrated infant with oliguria and haematuria. Evidence of disseminated intravascular coagulation and thrombocytopenia may also be demonstrated.

Congenital Nephrotic Syndrome

Congenital nephrotic syndrome may be divided into the commoner, so-called "Finnish" type, and a less common lesion described as diffuse mesangial sclerosis or the "French" type. The "Finnish" type is inherited as an autosomal-recessive trait. Diffuse mesangial sclerosis has also been described in siblings, but its autosomal-recessive nature is less securely documented than "Finnish" congenital nephrotic syndrome. In the Finnish type, so-called because it was first described in families of Finnish origin, the nephrotic syndrome is recognised at or very soon after birth. The infant is generally premature and of low birthweight.

Table 19.2. Familial abnormalities of tubular transport (Risdon 1981a)

	Disorder	Inheritance	Functional abnormality	Morphological changes in kidneys	Clinical effects
1. Specific disorders of amino acid transport	a) Cystinuria	Autosomal recessive	Proximal tubular defect → increased urinary excretion of cystine, lysine, arginine and ornithine	—	Cystine calculi in the urinary tract
	b) Hartnup disease	Autosomal recessive	Proximal tubular defect → increased urinary excretion of alanine, glutamine, asparagine, histidine, serine, threonine, phenylalanine, tyrosine and tryptophan	—	Pellagra-like skin rash. Attacks of cerebellar ataxia
	c) Iminoglycinuria	Autosomal recessive	Proximal tubular defect → increased urinary excretion of glycine, proline and hydroxyproline	—	Urinary tract calculi

Table 19.2. *(continued)*

	Disorder	Inheritance	Functional abnormality	Morphological changes in kidneys	Clinical effects
2. Non-specific disorders of amino acid transport	a) Cystinosis (de Toni–Faconi–Lignac–Debré syndrome)				
	i) Childhood form	Autosomal recessive	Proximal tubular defect aminoaciduria, hyperphosphaturia, acidosis and hypokalaemia. May be proteinuria	Deposition of cystine crystals in tubules, glomerular epithelial cells and interstitium (as well as elsewhere in the body). Swan-neck deformity of nephrons on microdissection	Vomiting, fever, polyuria. Vitamin D-resistant rickets. Occasionally pitressin-resistant diabetes insipidus. Renal failure
	ii) Idiopathic form	Autosomal recessive and dominant described	Proximal tubular defect → glycosuria, aminoaciduria, hypophosphaturia	No cystine deposition	Milder disease than (i). Usually affects adults but may be present in childhood
	b) Lowe's syndrome	Sex-linked recessive	Proximal tubular defect → aminoaciduria hypophosphaturia. Acidosis, proteinuria and inability to concentrate the urine	Tubular atrophy and glomerulosclerosis	Congenital glaucoma, cataracts, mental retardation, rickets and renal failure
3. Tubular defects owing to endogenous poisons	a) Galactosaemia	Autosomal recessive	Galactose-l-phosphate uridyl transferase deficiency → galactose retention. Effect on proximal tubules → aminoaciduria and proteinuria	— —	Cataracts, mental deficiency, and hepatic cirrhosis
	b) Wilson's disease	Autosomal recessive	Defect of copper metabolism associated with reduced serum caeruloplasmin and deposition of copper. Effects on proximal tubules → aminoaciduria	— —	Extrapyramidal symptoms, Kayser–Fleischer rings, hepatic cirrhosis
4. Disorders of other transport mechanisms	a) Renal glycosuria	Autosomal dominant	Prominent tubular defect → glycosuria	—	—
	b) Vitamin D-resistant rickets	Sex-linked dominant	Increased clearance of phosphate owing to reduced reabsorption in the proximal tubules	— —	Rickets refractory to therapy with vitamin D
	c) Vasopressin-resistant diabetes insipidus	Probably sex-linked dominant with variable expressivity	Distal tubular defect resulting in unresponsiveness to vasopressin	Microdissection indicates diminution in proximal tubule convolutions	Vasopressin-resistant diabetes insipidus
	d) Primary renal acidosis i) Infantile form	Autosomal recessive	Distal tubular defect → inability to acidify urine	Reduction in renal size and nephrocalcinosis in some cases	Vomiting, failure to thrive, dehydration and hypotonia. Complete recovery following treatment usual. ? Failure in maturation of tubular function
	ii) Late form	Autosomal dominant with increased penetration in females	As in (i). Increased potassium loss in urine may occur	May be cortical scarring and urolithiasis	More serious disorder than (i). May develop periodic paralysis, rickets and renal stones

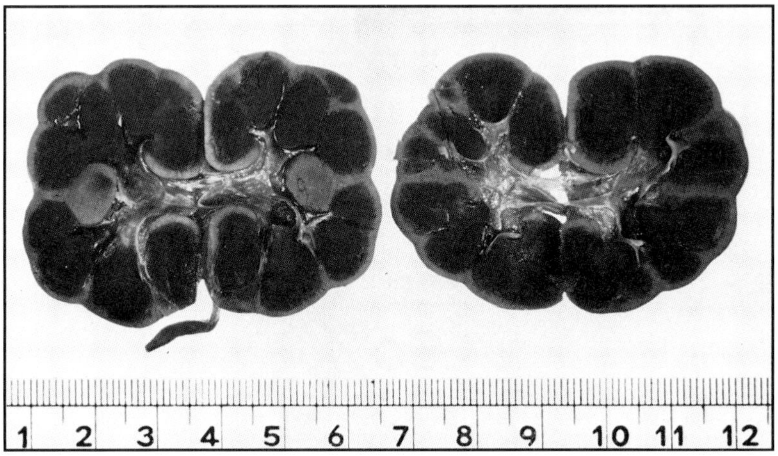

Fig. 19.9. Renal cortical and medullary necrosis in a child with cyanotic congenital heart disease.

Proteinuria can usually be recognised at birth and is associated with the development of oedema and hypoalbuminaemia in the first few days or weeks of life. Microscopic haematuria is often present and the placenta is large and oedematous, frequently constituting 25%–60% of the birthweight (Kouvalainen et al. 1962). The proteinuria fails to respond to corticosteroid or immunosuppressive therapy, which is contraindicated in any case because of the frequency of intercurrent infections and poor growth rate. Survival beyond the first year is uncommon, although the prognosis is improving as renal transplantation in the very young is becoming a therapeutic option. Histologically, the renal glomeruli appear immature and may exhibit mild to moderate mesangial hypercellularity early in the disease. Later, an increasing proportion of glomeruli show segmental or global sclerosis. Characteristically many tubules are cystically dilated ("microcystic" disease; Fig. 19.10). Immunofluorescence microscopy reveals no consistent glomerular deposition of immunoreactants and is generally completely negative. Electron microscopy fails to reveal evidence of immune complex deposition, but there is diffuse effacement of podocyte foot processes. This change is seen even in utero, indicating that proteinuria occurs at this stage. Levels of alpha-fetoprotein are raised in the amniotic fluid and maternal blood and this can be used for antenatal diagnosis where there is known to be a family history.

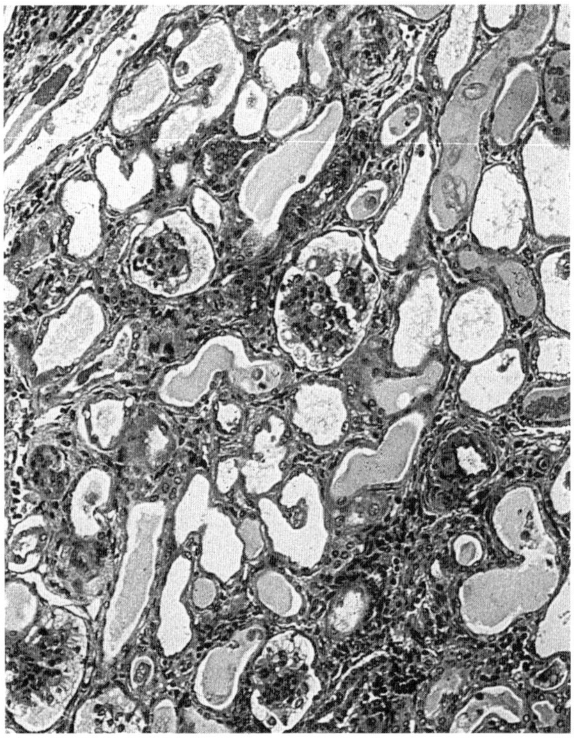

Fig. 19.10. Congenital nephrotic syndrome. Late stage "Finnish" type with microcystic tubular dilatation and glomerulosclerosis. (H&E, ×56)

Diffuse mesangial sclerosis, also referred to as "French" type congenital nephrotic syndrome, and so-called because it was first described in the French literature (Habib and Bois 1975), also presents in the first year of life, sometimes in the first weeks, but usually later than the Finnish type. The clinical course is characterised by progressive renal failure and death between the ages of 1 and 3 years.

Histologically, the fully developed glomerular lesion is characterised by diffuse mesangial sclerosis with a marked increase in mesangial matrix and obliteration of most tuft capillary lumina. The glomerular tuft is contracted to a rounded mass, often covered by hypertrophied and sometimes vacuolated podocytes. Tuft nuclei are surprisingly well preserved for the degree of sclerosis and because tufts are contracted they often appear superficially to be hypercellular. Capsular adhesions and crescents are uncommon, and silver staining may demonstrate focal double contouring of residual thickened peripheral tuft capillary walls. Examination of sections of the whole kidney show the most severely affected glomeruli to be in the mid to outer cortex; in the juxtamedullary cortex, glomeruli may show only increase in fibrillary mesangial matrix, or in early lesions may appear normal. In the extreme outer, subcapsular cortex, small immature and partly sclerosed glomeruli with a simplified lobular structure associated with small atrophic tubules often form a distinct layer.

Tubulointerstitial changes are generally marked, with tubular atrophy as well as dilated and often hypertrophied tubules containing eosinophilic proteinaceous casts associated with diffuse interstitial fibrosis. Immunofluorescence microscopy may reveal diffuse deposition of IgM and C_3 in the glomerular mesangium and along thickened tuft capillary walls.

In diffuse mesangial sclerosis, the increase in mesangial matrix is confirmed ultrastructurally and occasional mesangial interposition is seen corresponding to the double contours seen by light microscopy. Abnormalities of the glomerular basement membrane may be apparent focally. The membrane outside the normal lamina densa is thickened, with a wavy outer contour. Strands of lamina densa-like material delineate clear lacunae in the outer glomerular basement membrane to give an appearance superficially resembling that in Alport's syndrome. An intriguing feature of diffuse mesangial sclerosis is that exactly the same glomerular lesion is seen in the so-called Drash syndrome of male pseudohermaphroditism (MPH), nephropathy and nephroblastoma. In the Drash syndrome, nephrotic syndrome and renal failure often develop early, and incomplete forms without Wilms' tumour or occurring in genotypic females are described. This raises the possibility that the Drash syndrome in its various forms and congenital nephrosis with diffuse mesangial sclerosis are part of a continuum.

Renal Infection

Bacterial infection of the kidney is rarely demonstrated in perinatal necropsies. However, obstructive congenital anomalies of the urinary tract and vesicoureteric reflux are important predisposing factors in the development of the pyelonephritic scarring which may be seen in older children, and the mechanisms involved are discussed elsewhere (Risdon 1981c). It is important to recognise that in the presence of vesicoureteric reflux urinary infection may induce renal scarring very early in life, although this may not be recognised clinically until much later. In the perinatal period acute bacterial infection of the kidney sometimes complicates a generalised septicaemia and may also be seen with lower urinary tract obstruction, particularly with posterior urethral valves in infant boys, in whom the kidney often exhibits dysplastic changes in addition to those associated with infection (Risdon 1971b).

Viral and fungal infections of the kidney may also be recognised in the perinatal period. Haemorrhagic infarction of the renal medulla and inner adrenal cortex have been described in infants dying during an outbreak of echovirus 11 infection (Nagington et al. 1978). In congenital cytomegalovirus infections the typical nuclear inclusions can often be recognised in some proximal tubular cells in the kidneys if sought for carefully.

Intravenous feeding in neonates may be complicated by fungal infections, particularly with *Candida* species, and the organisms can often be recognised in sections of the kidney.

Renal Glomerular Lesions in Cyanotic Congenital Heart Disease

Glomerular enlargement, often associated with mesangial cell proliferation and occasionally with mesangial accumulation of PAS-positive fibrillary material, may be seen in infants dying of cyanotic congenital heart disease (Spear 1964). Clinical evidence of renal impairment or proteinuria are lacking and there is no increase in renal size. Hypoxia, polycythaemia and pulmonary hypertension are all factors which have been associated with the glomerular change. Similar changes may be encountered in patients with primary pulmonary hypertension and also in the twin–twin transfusion syndrome in the kidneys of the recipient twin, when there is significant polycythaemia.

Congenital Abnormalities of the Renal Pelvis and Ureter

Duplication

Duplication of the renal pelvis and ureter ranges from mere bifurcation of the extrarenal pelvis, through duplication of the pelvis and upper ureter joining to form a single ureter entering the trigone, to complete duplication of the whole system with two separate ureteric orifices. Minor duplications are common, but complete duplications are much rarer and very occasionally triplication or even quadruplication of the ureter is recognised. All these anomalies are due to premature division or duplication of the ureteric bud. Rarely, in partial ureteric duplication, one of the ureters ends blindly and does not communicate with the renal pelvis and kidney. This condition is also referred to as a diverticulum of the ureter.

Ureteric Ectopia

An ectopic ureter is inserted distally at a site other than the normal in the trigone of the bladder. The ectopic ureter may thus drain into the rectum, urethra, seminal vesicle or vagina. Minor degrees of lateral ectopia in the bladder may be associated with primary vesicoureteric reflux. Here the ureteric orifice is abnormal and the submuscosal tunnel, on which the efficacy of the valvular mechanism normally preventing vesicoureteric reflux depends, is deficient. In complete duplication of the ureter, with two ureteric oriflices, one or other (usually that draining the upper part of the kidney) may be ectopic. The part of the kidney drained by the ectopic ureter may be dysplastic, particularly if vesicoureteric reflux occurs.

Ureterocele

A ureterocele is a saccular expansion of the distal ureter about its orifice, involving the intramural segment in the bladder wall and the submucosal segment immediately above the orifice. Most commonly ureteroceles are associated with ectopic ureters and ureteral duplications. Ectopic ureterocele describes a complex anomaly where there is complete duplication of the ureter, the lower moiety being inserted normally in the trigone and the upper moiety, which is associated with the ureterocele, being inserted ectopically medially and below the lower moiety. The upper pole of the kidney drained by the ectopic ureterocele is frequently dysplastic. Obstruction by the ureterocele is usually accompanied by dilatation and tortuosity of the ureter and hydronephrosis of the kidney drained by it.

Retrocaval Ureter

In the rare anomaly of retrocaval ureter the upper part of the ureter passes behind the inferior vena cava and descends medially to it to the bladder.

Congenital Hydrocalycosis

Congenital obstruction of the infundibular portion of a renal calyx produces dilatation of the calyx and atrophy of the associated renal parenchyma (hydrocalycosis). One or several calyces may be affected and obstruction may be extrinsic, due, for example, to aberrant blood vessels, or intrinsic, due to congenital infundibular stenosis.

Congenital Hydronephrosis (see p. 473)

Ureteral Dilatation

Congenital ureteric dilatation is common and may be obstructed or non-obstructed. Obstruction due to congenital stenosis may occur at any point, but is usually seen in the lower, supravesical portion. Congenital obstruction of this type may occur in the contralateral ureter in unilateral multicystic dysplasia (see p. 472).

Non-obstructive ureteric dilatation is seen in association with vesicoureteric reflux and sometimes in the absence of a satisfactory anatomical explanation. It is important to recognise that the diameter of the ureter in the neonatal period is relatively greater than in older children and adults, a point to be remembered in assessing the normality or otherwise of the calibre of the ureter in this age group.

Congenital Abnormalities of the Bladder

Agenesis

Congenital absence of the bladder is an extremely rare anomaly. Affected infants are usually stillborn, and other congenital anomalies usually coexist. Ectopic insertion of the ureters into the vagina in females and into the rectum in males is described in the reported cases (Lepoutre 1939/40; Glen 1959).

Duplication

Bladder duplication may be complete or incomplete (Abrahamson 1961). In complete duplication two separate bladders with separate urethras lie side by side in a common adventitial sheath. Duplication of the hindgut is almost always present and a rectourethral fistula involving one bladder is present in over half the cases. Other rectal and genital anomalies commonly coexist. In partial duplication two bladders are joined at their base and have a single urethra.

Septation

Various types of septation of the bladder have been described. Sagittal septation may be complete or incomplete. When complete, one half of the bladder is separated from the urethra and hydronephrosis occurs on that side. Frontal septation divides the bladder into anterior and posterior compartments and is usually incomplete. The so-called hourglass bladder probably reflects a partial persistence of the urachus and may be considered as an exaggerated form of urachal diverticulum.

Urachal Anomalies

Persistence of the urachus results in a fistula from the bladder to the umbilicus. Partial persistence of the distal urachus forms a urachal diverticulum, and persistence of the mid-part of the urachus produces a urachal cyst.

Bladder Exstrophy

Bladder exstrophy is the commonest of a series of malformations which result from a failure in fusion of the mesodermal elements of the anterior abdominal wall below the umbilicus. These congenital anomalies range from minor degrees of epispadias (see p. 496) with exposure of the terminal penile urethra to gross ectopia vesicae with accompanying hindgut anomalies and often a vesicointestinal fistula.

In bladder exstrophy the abdominal wall below the umbilicus is shortened and there is a variably sized midline defect. This ranges from a small hole through which the bladder trigone protrudes on straining to a large defect through which the entire posterior wall of the bladder is exposed (ectopia vesicae). Some degree of pubic diastasis and epispadias, in which the urethra is open on the upper surface of the penis, invariably accompanies bladder exstrophy.

In surviving children secondary changes occur in the exposed bladder mucosa, such as squamous metaplasia, cystitis cystica and cystitis glandularis. Squamous or adenocarcinoma may develop in patients surviving childhood. In cases amenable to surgical correction, vesicoureteric reflux is usually demonstrable after surgery.

In cloacal exstrophy, an exstrophied bladder is in two separate halves, each with a ureteric orifice; these hemibladders are separated by exstrophied bowel. This has two openings; an upper orifice communicating with terminal ileum, which frequently prolapses as a tube covered by intestinal mucosa, and a lower orifice communicating with a blind-ending segment of colon. The anus is imperforate and there may be a separate appendicular orifice (or sometimes two, as the appendix is frequently duplicated). A large exomphalos above the exstrophy usually contains liver and intestine. An epispadiac penis is present in males and is frequently duplicated. The testes are undescended and the scrotum is absent. In females the vagina is septate, the uterus duplicated and the external genitalia are absent.

Covered exstrophy occurs with delayed closure of the abdominal wall defect following the formation of an exstrophy. The umbilicus is low and the abdomen below it consists of a paper-thin membrane formed from skin and anterior bladder wall. Epispadias is usual and the pubes are separated.

Congenital Abnormalities of the Urethra

Urethral Valves and Strictures

Posterior urethral valves in infant boys are the commonest cause of congenital urethral obstruction. The various types of posterior urethral valve have been described by Young and McKay (1929), the most frequent type appearing to be an accentuation of a pair of mucosal folds normally present in the male urethra, extending down laterally from the verumontanum to the urethral wall. Wigglesworth (1984) describes and illustrates a type of urethral obstruction in infant males in which there is a pinhole orifice at the verumontanum connecting the distended posterior urethra with the distal urethra. Wigglesworth regards this as the commonest variety he encounters in perinatal necropsies and suggests that this appearance might be transformed to the more classically described one by the passage of a catheter or by opening the urethra anteriorly at necropsy.

The consequences of posterior urethral valves depend largely on the degree of obstruction they cause. Most cases present in the first year of life, and those with the most severe obstruction in the neonatal period with urinary retention. Hydronephrosis is usual and renal dysplasia may be severe, particularly in the presence of vesicoureteric reflux (see p. 472).

Congenital urethral stenosis may result from strictures developing because of inadequate cooption of the genital tubercles (in males) or from mucosal diaphragms. The strictures may be single or multiple, and meatal strictures are the most common.

Prune Belly Syndrome

The combination of atrophy of the muscles of the anterior abdominal wall, undescended testes with bilateral hydronephrosis and hydroureter in infant male is termed the "prune belly" syndrome (Wigger and Blanc 1977) because of the prune-like wrinkling of the anterior abdominal skin consequent on the absent musculature.

Mechanical urethral obstruction is unusual, although occasionally there is atresia of the membranous urethra or urethral valves. More often there is tapering dilatation of the posterior urethra narrowing into the membranous urethra without obstruction, although clinical investigation indicates an abnormal functional resistance in the membranous urethra. The bladder is thick-walled, although usually not trabeculated. The trigone is abnormally wide and the ureteric orifices dilated and subject to vesicoureteric reflux. The ureters are dilated and tortuous; the kidneys are hydronephrotic and show varying degrees of dysplastic development (see p. 472).

Megacystis/Megaureter Syndrome

Megacystis/megaureter syndrome is characterised by the very large capacity, thin-walled bladder associated with gross bilateral vesicoureteric reflux, hydroureters and hydronephrosis. The kidneys are also often dysplastic (see p. 470). The bladder often appears persistently full, but this is because detrusor contraction at micturition tends to cause urine to flow retrogradely into the capacious ureters as well as through the urethra. When the bladder is emptied, it immediately refills when urine returns from the ureters by gravity.

Urethral Atresia

Urethral atresia is an uncommon condition characterised by a congenital absence of the urethral lumen, generally at the level of the membranous urethra. It may be accompanied by rectourethral or urachal fistula and is sometimes seen in the prune belly syndrome.

Urethral Duplication

Complete duplication of the urethra is seen in association with complete bladder duplication or diphallus. Rarely in males, the urethra divides along its course, with one normally placed meatus and a second meatus in the perineum.

Prostatic Utricle (Mullerian Duct) Cyst

This is a developmental cyst of Mullerian origin occurring in the midline of the urethra posteriorly, just above the prostate and below the bladder in males.

Polyp of the Verumontanum

This is a connective tissue polyp covered by urothelium arising from the floor of the prostatic urethra near the verumontanum.

Anterior Urethral Diverticulum

This occurs in males and describes a wide-mouthed (saccular) or narrow-mouthed (globular) diverticulum occurring anywhere from the membranous to the mid-penile urethra.

Hypospadias

This is a congenital abnormality of the male urethra in which the meatus is sited on the underside of the penis proximal to its normal site. The ventral foreskin is deficient and the penis is often short and curved downwards because of tethering bands of connective tissue (ventral chordee). The condition is classified according to the position of urethral meatus as glandular, coronal, distal, mid or proximal shaft, penoscrotal, scrotal and perineal.

References

Abrahamson J (1961) Double bladder and related anomalies, clinical and embryological aspects and a case report. Br J Urol 33: 195–214

Avini EF, Thoua Y, Lalmand B, Didier F, Droulle P, Schulman CC (1987) Multicystic dysplastic kidney: natural history from in utero diagnosis and postnatal follow-up. J Urol 138: 1420–1424

Beckwith JB (1969) Macroglossia, omphalocele, adrenal cytomegaly, giantism, and hyperplastic visceromegaly. Birth Defects 5: 188–196

Beckwith JB, Kiviat NB, Bonadio JF (1990) Nephrogenic rests, nephroblastomatosis, and the pathogenesis of Wilms' tumor. Pediatr Pathol 10: 1–36

Bernstein J (1976) A classification of renal cysts. In: Gardner KD Jr (ed) Cystic diseases of the kidney. Wiley, New York, p 7

Bernstein J, Landing BH (1989) Glomerulocystic kidney diseases. Prog Clin Biol Res 305: 27–43

Bernstein J, Meyer R (1964) Some speculations on the nature and significance of developmentally small kidneys (renal hypoplasia). Nephron 1: 137–143

Bernstein J, Robbins TO, Kissane JM (1986) The renal lesions of tuberous sclerosis. Semin Diagn Pathol 3: 97–105

Blyth H, Ockendon BG (1971) Polycystic disease of the kidneys and liver presenting in childhood. J Med Genet 8: 257–284

Bolande RP, Brough AJ, Izant RJ (1967) Congenital mesoblastic nephroma of infancy. A report of eight cases and the relationship to Wilms' tumor. Pediatrics 40: 272–278

Breuning MH, Reeders ST, Brunner H et al. (1987) Improved early diagnosis of adult polycystic disease with flanking DNA markers. Lancet 2: 1359–1361

Buchta RM, Viseskul C, Gilbert EF, Sarto GE, Opitz JM (1973) Familial bilateral renal agenesis and hereditary renal adysplasia. Z Kinderheilk 115: 111–129

Burk D, Beaudoin AR (1977) Arsenate induced renal agenesis in rats. Teratology 16: 247–259

Cook HT, Taylor GM, Malone R, Risdon RA (1988) Renin in mesoblastic nephroma: an immunohistochemical study. Hum Pathol 19: 1347–1351

Coppoletta JM, Wolbach SB (1933) Body length and organ weights of infants and children: study of body length and normal weights of more important organs of the body between birth and 12 years of age. Am J Pathol 9: 55–70

Cremin BJ (1970) Infantile thoracic dystrophy. Br J Radiol 43: 199–204

Delaney V, Mullaney J, Bourke E (1978) Juvenile nephronophthisis, congenital hepatic fibrosis and retinal hypoplasia in twins. Q J Med 186: 281–290

Dieker H, Edwards RH, ZuRhein G et al. (1969) The lissencephaly syndromes. In: Bergsma D (ed) Part II Malformation syndromes. Birth Defects 5(2): 93–101

Doege TC, Thuline HC, Priest JH, Norby DE, Bryant JS (1964) Studies of a family with the oro-facial-digital syndrome. N Engl J Med 271: 1073–1080

Engström W, Lindham S, Schofield P (1968) Wiedemann–Beckwith Syndrome. Eur J Pediatr 147: 450–457

Fantel AG, Shepard RH (1976) Potter syndrome: non renal features induced by oligoamnios. Am J Dis Child 129: 1346–1347

Faraggiana T, Bernstein J, Strauss L, Churg J (1985) Use of lectins in the study of histogenesis of renal cysts. Lab Invest 53: 575–579

Fellows RA, Leonidas JL, Beatty EC Jr (1976) Radiological features of "adult type" polycystic kidney disease in the neonate. Pediatr Radiol 4: 87–92

Fetterman GH, Habib R (1969) Congenital bilateral oligonephronic renal hypoplasia with hypertrophy of nephrons (oligoméganéphronie): studies by microdissection. Am J Clin Pathol 52: 199–207

Gang DL, Herrin JT (1986) Infantile polycystic disease of the liver and kidneys. Clin Nephrol 25: 28–36

Glen JF (1959) Agenesis of the bladder. JAMA 169: 2016–2018

Habib R, Bois E (1975) Congenital and infantile nephrotic syndrome. In: Strauss J (ed) Pediatric nephrology, vol 2. Stratton Intercontinental Medical Book Corp, New York, p 335

Hilton C, Keeling JW (1973) Neonatal renal tumours. Br J Urol 46: 157–161

Imahori S, Bannerman RM, Graf CJ, Brennan JC (1969) Ehlers–Danlos syndrome with multiple arterial lesions. Am J Med 47: 967–977

Jan JE, Hardwick DF, Lowry RB, McCormick AQ (1970) Cerebrohepato renal syndrome of Zellweger. Am J Dis Child 119: 274–277
Jørgensen M (1972) Three dimensional reconstruction of intrahepatic bile ducts in case of polycystic disease of the liver in an infant. Acta Pathol Microbiol Scand [A] 80: 201–206
Joshi VV, Kasznica J (1984) Clinicopathologic spectrum of glomerulocystic kidneys: report of two cases and a brief review of literature. Pediatr Pathol 2: 176–186
Kaplan BS, Kaplan P, de Chadarevian J-P, Jequier S, O'Regan S, Russo P (1988) Variable expression of autosomal recessive polycystic kidney disease and congenital hepatic fibrosis within a family. Am J Med Genet 29: 639–647
Kimberling WJ, Fain PR, Kenyon JB, Goldgar D, Sujansky E, Gabow PA (1988) Linkage heterogeneity of autosomal dominant polycystic kidney disease. N Engl J Med 319: 913–918
Kissane JM (1973) Hereditary disorders of the kidney. II. In: Rosenberg HS, Bolande RP (eds) Perspectives in pediatric pathology, vol 1. Year Book Medical Publishers, Chicago, pp 147–187
Kouvalainen K, Hjelt L, Hallman N (1962) Placenta in congenital nephrotic syndrome. Ann Paediatr Fenn 8: 181–188
Landing BH, Hughes ML (1962) Analysis of weights of kidneys in children. Lab Invest 11: 452–454
Langer LO Jr, Nishino R, Yamaguchi A et al. (1983) Brachymesomelia-renal syndrome. Am J Med Genet 15: 57–65
Lepoutre C (1939/40) Sur un cas d'absence congénital de la vessie (persistance du cloaque). Bull Soc Fr Urol 254–256
Mottet NK, Jensen H (1965) The anomalous embryonic development associated with trisomy 13–15. Am J Clin Pathol 43: 334–347
Nagashima Y, Yoshihara O, Tanaka Y, Misugi K, Horiuchi M (1988) A case of renal angiomyolipomas associated with multiple and various hamartomatous microlesions. Virchows Arch (Pathol Anat) 413: 177–182
Nagington J, Wreghitt TG, Gandy G, Robertson NRC, Berry PJ (1978) Fatal echovirus 11 infections in outbreak in special care baby unit. Lancet II: 725–728
Opitz JM, Howe JJ (1969) The Meckel syndrome (dysencephalia splanchnocystica, the Gruber syndrome). In: Proceedings of the first conference on the clinical delineation of birth defects. Birth Defects 5(2): 167–179
Osathanondh V, Potter EL (1964) Pathogenesis of polycystic kidneys: historical survey; type 1 due to hyperplasia of interstitial portions of collecting tubules; type 2 due to inhibition of ampullary activity; type 3 due to multiple abnormalities of development; type 4 due to urethral obstruction; survey of results of microdissection. Arch Pathol 77: 466–512
Pathak IG, Williams DI (1963) Multicystic and cystic dysplastic kidneys. Br J Urol 36: 318–331
Pedicelli G, Jequier S, Bowen A, Boisvert J (1986) Multicystic dysplastic kidneys. Spontaneous regression demonstrated with US. Radiology 160: 23–26
Perlman M, Levin M, Wittels B (1975) Syndrome of fetal giantism, renal hamartomas and nephroblastomatosis with Wilms' tumor. Cancer 35: 1212–1217
Potter EL (1946) Facial characteristics of infants with bilateral renal agenesis. Am J Obstet Gynecol 51: 885–888
Potter EL (1972) Normal and abnormal development of the kidneys. Year Book Medical Publishers, Chicago
Potter EL, Craig JM (1976) Pathology of the fetus and infant. 3rd edn. Year Book Publishers, Chicago, pp 434–475
Proesmans W, van Damme B, Caesar P, Marchal G (1982) Autosomal dominant polycystic kidney disease in the neonatal period. Association with cerebral arteriovenous malformation. Pediatrics 70: 971–975
Rapola J, Kääriäinen H (1988) Polycystic kidney disease. Morphologic diagnosis of recessive and dominant polycystic disease in infancy and childhood. Acta Pathol Microbiol Scand 96: 68–76
Reeders ST, Breuning MH, Davies KE et al. (1985) A highly polymorphic DNA marker linked to adult polycystic kidney disease on chromosome 16. Nature 317: 542–544
Reeders ST, Gal A, Propping P et al. (1986) Prenatal diagnosis of autosomal dominant polycystic kidney disease with a DNA probe. Lancet 2: 6–8
Reilly BJ, Neuhauser EBD (1960) Renal tubular ectasia in cystic disease of the kidney and liver. Am J Roentgenol 84: 546–554
Risdon RA (1971a) Renal dysplasia I. A clinicopathological study of 76 cases. J Clin Pathol 24: 57–65
Risdon RA (1971b) Renal dysplasia II. A necropsy study of 41 cases. J Clin Pathol 24: 65–71
Risdon (1981a) Diseases of the kidney and lower urinary tract. In: Berry CL (ed) Paediatric pathology. Springer, Berlin Heidelberg New York, pp 395–450
Risdon RA (1981b) Cystic diseases of the kidney and reflux nephropathy. In: Anthony PP, MacSween RNM (eds) Recent advances in histopathology (no 11). Churchill Livingstone, Edinburgh, pp 163–184
Risdon RA (1981c) Reflux nephropathy. Diagn Histopathol 1: 61–70
Risdon RA (1992) Development, Developmental defects and cystic diseases of the kidney. In: Heptinstall RH (ed) Pathology of the kidney, 4th edn. Little, Brown & Co, Boston, pp 93–167
Risdon RA, Young LW, Chrispin AR (1975) Renal hypoplasia and dysplasia. A radiological and pathological correlation. Pediatr Radiol 3: 213–225
Rizza JM, Dowling SE, (1971) Bilateral renal agenesis in two female siblings. Am J Dis Child 121: 60–63
Rohde RA, Hodgman JE, Cleland RS (1964) Multiple congenital anomalies in the E-trisomy (group 16–18) syndrome. Pediatrics 33: 258–270
Rolfes DB, Towbin R, Bove KE (1985) Vascular dysplasia in a child with tuberous sclerosis. Pediatr Pathol 3: 359–373
Romeo G, Costa G, Catizone L et al. (1988) A second genetic locus for autosomal dominant polycystic kidney disease. Lancet 2: 7–10
Roosen-Runge EC (1949) Retardation of post natal development of kidneys in persons with early cerebral lesions. Am J Dis Child 77: 185–200
Royer P, Habib R, Mathieu H, Cortecuisse V (1962) L'hypoplasie rénale bilatérale congénital avec réduction du nombre, et hypertrophie des néphrons chez l'enfant. Ann Pediatr 9: 133–146
Schmidt ECH, Hartley AA, Bower R (1952) Renal aplasia in sisters. Arch Pathol 54: 403–406
Scorer CG (1956) Incidence of incomplete descent of the testicle at birth. Arch Dis Child 31: 198–202
Six R, Oliphant M, Grossman H (1975) A spectrum of renal tubule ectasia and hepatic fibrosis. Radiology 117: 117–122
Spear GS (1964) The glomerulus in cyanotic congenital heart disease and primary pulmonary hypertension: a review. Nephron 1: 238–248
Spranger J, Grimm B, Weller M, Weissenbacher G, Hermann J, Gilbert E, Krepter R (1974) Short rib polydactyly (SRP) syndromes. Z Kinderheilkd 116: 73–94

Stapleton FB, Bernstein J, Koh G, Roy S III, Wilroy RS (1982) Cystic kidneys in a patient with oral-facial-digital syndrome type 1. Am J Kidney Dis 1: 288–293
Talvik T, Mikel'saar A-V, Mikel'saar R, Kaosaar M, Tuur S (1973) Inherited translocations in two families (t(14q+; 10q−) and t(13a−; 21a+)). Hum Genet 19: 215–226
Taxy JB, Filmer RB (1976) Glomerulocystic disease. Report of a case. Arch Pathol 100: 186–188
Wiedemann HR (1964) Complex malformatif familiale avec hernie ombilicale et macroglossie, un syndrome nouveau? J Genet Hum 13: 223–232
Wigger HJ, Blanc WA (1977) The prune belly syndrome. Pathol Annu 12(1): 17–39
Wigglesworth JS (1984) Perinatal pathology, Saunders, Philadelphia, pp 365–369
Young HH, McKay RW (1929) Congenital valvular obstruction of the prostatic urethra. Surg Gynecol Obstet 48: 509–535

Chapter 20

The Reproductive System

Jørn Müller and Niels Græm

Development

The gonads develop in two paired ridges of mesenchyme at the medial aspect of the mesonephros during the 5th–7th weeks of gestation (Byskov and Høyer 1988; Wartenberg 1989). The primordial germ cells originate from the yolk sac and migrate to the gonadal ridges. Regardless of the karyotype, all embryos have, after 6–7 weeks of gestation, indifferent gonads consisting of germ cells, coelomic surface epithelium and mesenchyme. At this stage also internal Müllerian (paramesonephric) and Wolffian (mesonephric) ducts, a urogenital sinus and an undifferentiated external genitalia can be identified (Fig. 20.1). The subsequent sex-specific development of internal and external genitalia is primarily dependent on the karyotype, but is also influenced by the endocrine function of the gonads. It has long been known that presence of a Y chromosome is decisive for testicular differentiation. Recently, the essential DNA sequence on the short arm of the Y chromosome has been cloned and called the sex-determining region of the Y (Sinclair et al. 1990).

Testes

Seminiferous cords containing germ cells and Sertoli cells originating from invading coelomic surface cells appear at 6–7 weeks of gestation (Wartenberg 1989). Germ cells multiply by mitosis during fetal life and most actively during the first and second trimesters. At 7–8 weeks of gestation, numerous Leydig cells originating from mesenchymal cells can be seen in the interstitium (Kerr 1989). The Leydig cells secrete testosterone under the influence of human chorionic gonadotrophin from the placenta. After 10–12 weeks of gestation the hypothalamo–pituitary–gonadal axis is operating, and from this time testosterone biosynthesis is under the control of fetal luteinising hormone (Reyes et al. 1974; Clements et al. 1976). At this stage of fetal development, the level of testosterone in serum reaches its maximum and is as high as in the adult male. This is crucial for male differentiation of Wolffian ducts, urogenital sinus and external genitalia (Figs. 20.1 and 20.2a). During the second half of the first trimester the Sertoli cells secrete a peptide hormone, the Müllerian inhibiting substance (Josso 1986), which induces regression of the Müllerian ducts.

Ovaries

In the absence of the sex-determining region of the Y, the indifferent gonads develop into ovaries. Germ cells aggregate in the peripheral zone, which becomes the cortex. Thereupon, they enlarge and become oogonia. After rapid

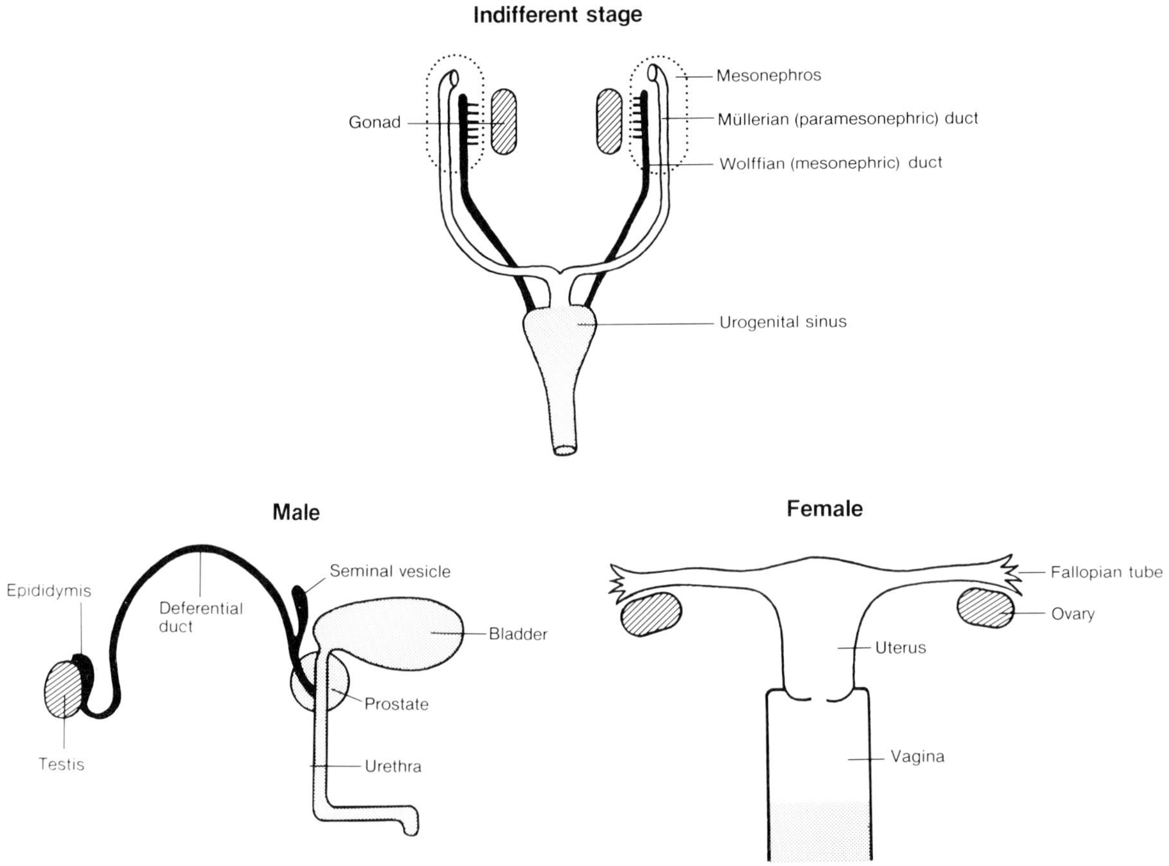

Fig. 20.1. Differentiation of the internal genitalia. The indifferent stage has paired Müllerian and Wolffian ducts, and a urogenital sinus. In the male the Wolffian ducts have developed into epididymis, deferential ducts and seminal vesicles. The urogenital sinus has become the prostate and urethra. The Müllerian ducts have regressed leaving only the appendix testis (not shown). After female differentiation, the Müllerian ducts have developed into paired fallopian tubes, uterus and upper vagina, whereas the Wolffian ducts have regressed. Possible remnants of the Wolffian ducts may be identified as epoophoron, paroophoron, and Gartner's duct. The urogenital sinus has become the lower vagina and the urethra (not shown).

mitotic proliferation, the oogonia enter the first meiotic prophase during 9–12 weeks of gestation to become primary oocytes (Byskov and Høyer 1988). Using a light microscope, these cells may be recognised by their prominent nuclei with condensed fibrillar chromatin. By mid-pregnancy the fetal ovaries contain 6–7 million of closely packed germ cells, but hereafter and for the rest of a female's life the number is constantly decreasing (Byskov and Høyer 1988). After 20 weeks of gestation, primitive granulosa cells derived from the coelomic surface epithelium surround the germ cells to form single-layered primordial follicles and, later, multilayered primary follicles. All germ cells rest in the first meiotic prophase until further differentiation after puberty or until follicular involution. It is not believed that the fetal ovary secretes hormones important for further development of the female ducts and external genitalia (Byskov and Høyer 1988). Thus, in the absence of active testicular tissue, internal and external genitalia are directed into female development (Fig. 20.2b).

Ducts

In both genetic sexes, the Wolffian ducts appear at about 4 weeks of gestation. Under the influence of testosterone secreted by the fetal testes, the Wolffian ducts differentiate into the epididymis, the deferential ducts and the

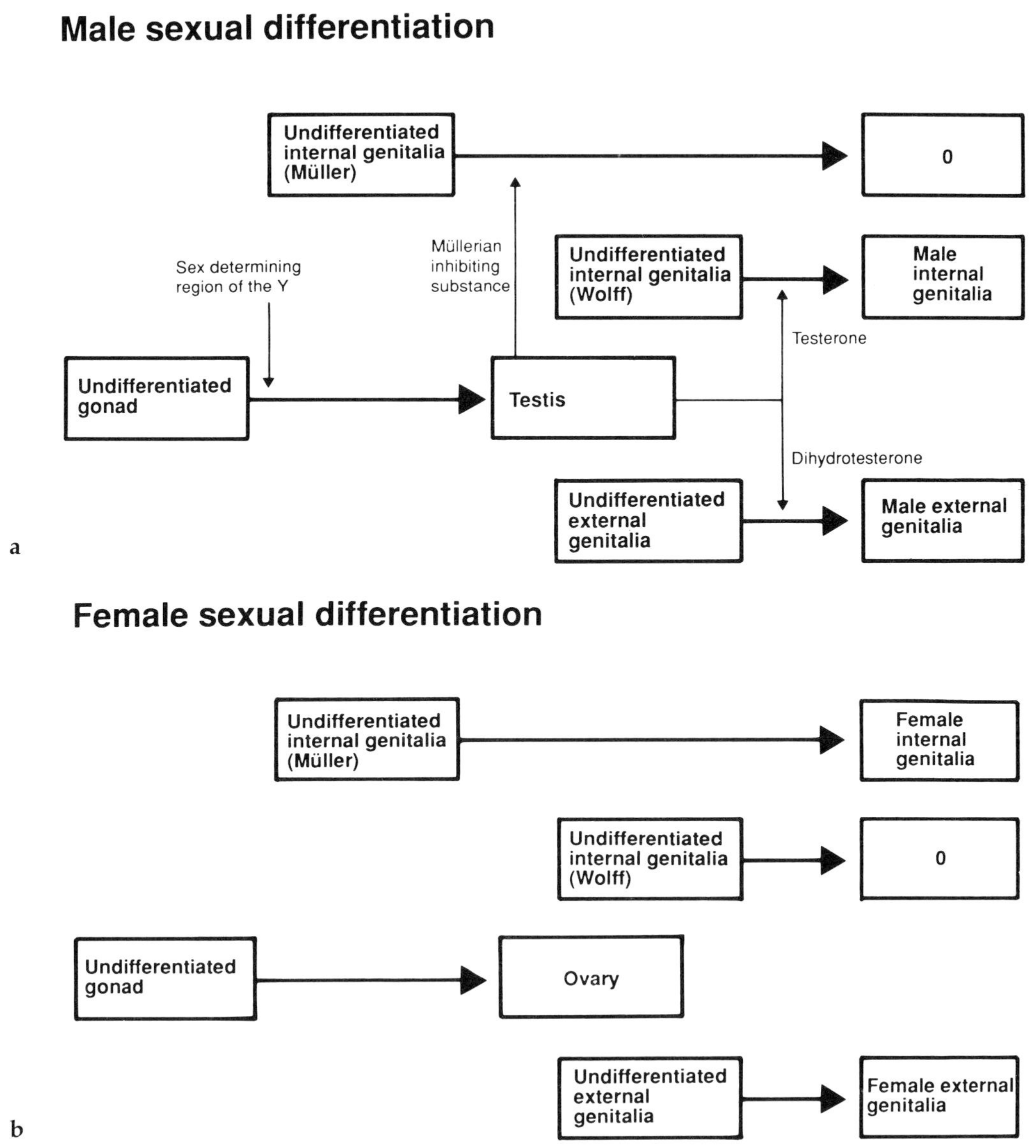

Fig. 20.2. Flow charts on sexual differentiation. **a** Male sexual differentiation. The presence of the sex-determining region of the Y causes the undifferentiated gonad to develop into a testis. The fetal testis secretes two hormones: testosterone and Müllerian inhibiting substance. Testosterone influences the Wolffian ducts to become epididymis, deferential ducts and seminal vesicles. The testosterone metabolite dihydrotestosterone is required for development of the male external genitalia including differentiation of the urethra and prostate. Müllerian inhibiting substance secreted by fetal Sertoli cells prevents development of the Müllerian ducts. **b** Female sexual differentiation. In the absence of the sex-determining region of the Y, the undifferentiated gonad develops into an ovary. The ovary has no significant hormone production during fetal life. Therefore, the Müllerian ducts develop into fallopian tubes, uterus and vagina. In the absence of androgens, the Wolffian ducts regress and the external genitalia become female in appearance.

seminal vesicles. The prostate develops from the urogenital sinus. The Müllerian ducts appear in both sexes at about 6 weeks of gestation. In the male fetus, regression of the Müllerian ducts begins at 8 weeks of gestation. It is induced by Müllerian inhibiting substance secreted by the Sertoli cells (Josso 1986). In the female, the absence of testosterone causes involution of the Wolffian ducts, and the Müllerian ducts, in the absence of Müllerian inhibiting substance, develop into the fallopian tubes, the uterus and upper third of the vagina (Figs. 20.1 and 20.2a,b).

External Genitalia

During the first 2 months of embryonic life, external genitalia are identical in both sexes. They consist of the genital tubercle, the paired lateral labioscrotal swellings and the urogenital sinus.

Masculinisation of the external genitalia takes place during 9–14 weeks of gestation under the influence of testosterone and its 5-alpha-reduced metabolite, dihydrotestosterone. Conversion of testosterone to dihydrotestosterone is an important step in male sexual differentiation. Males with 5-alpha-reductase deficiency are born with normal testes but ambiguous external genitalia, i.e. a small phallus and persistent urogenital sinus (Grumbach and Conte 1985).

Testicular descent takes place in two steps (Hutson and Donahue 1986). The transabdominal movement of the testis occurs during the first 12 weeks of gestation, at which time the gonads are located at the internal inguinal ring. This part of testicular descent seems to be possible even in the absence of androgen influence. Migration of the testis through the inguinal canal to the scrotum starts during the 7th and 8th months of gestation, and in most boys the process is completed at term. However, approximately 6% of all newborn boys have undescended testes (John Radcliffe Hospital Cryptorchidism Study Group 1988). By 3 months of age, the incidence of cryptorchidism has decreased to 1.6%. In boys born before 37 weeks of gestation, the frequency of cryptorchidism is higher (Morley and Lucas 1987). The mechanism of testicular descent is poorly understood. Both the gubernaculum and epididymis seem to play an important role (Wensing 1988), but the hormonal control of the process still remains to be clarified.

In the absence of testosterone and apparently without influence of the ovaries, the external genitalia feminise. The phallus remains small and bends ventrally to become the clitoris and the urethral groove remains open.

Intersex

Errors of Primary Sexual Determination

These disorders include sex chromosome abnormalities and/or defective gonad formation. True hermaphrodites are extremely rare and have both testicular and ovarian tissue. Internal and external genitalia may have all combinations of male and female appearance (Grumbach and Conte 1985). Abnormal pairing of the X and the Y chromosomes may result in either a 46XX phenotypic male containing the sex determining region of the Y on one X chromosome, or a 46XY phenotypic female without this DNA sequence (McLaren 1990). Such 46XY females have normal internal and external female genitalia, with the exception of dysgenetic gonads. The term dysgenetic is based on morphological criteria (Fig. 20.3). These include reduced numbers of germ cells, abnormal distribution of the cells, and increased amount of stromal tissue. In the case of 46XY females, the germ cells do not differentiate into oogonia, and they do not enter the first meiotic division. Thus primordial follicles are not formed, and it may be impossible to classify the gonad as either a testis or an ovary. The fetal dysgenetic gonad may contain areas resembling gonadoblastoma (Spear and Martin 1986). Chromosomal mosaicism such as 45X/46XY may result in the whole spectrum of external genital development, ranging from a normal male to a normal female phenotype. The histology of the gonads may also vary from typical testicular appearance to that of dysgenetic ovaries (Gantt et al. 1980). Individuals with a female phenotype or ambiguous genitalia and a karyotype including a Y chromosome are at increased risk of developing germ cell malignancies. Carcinoma-in-situ of the testis (Müller et al. 1985) and gonadoblastoma (Hung et al. 1981) may already be present in newborns. Pure 45X0 (Turner's syndrome) females have normal external and internal female genitalia, except for dysgenetic ovaries (see below).

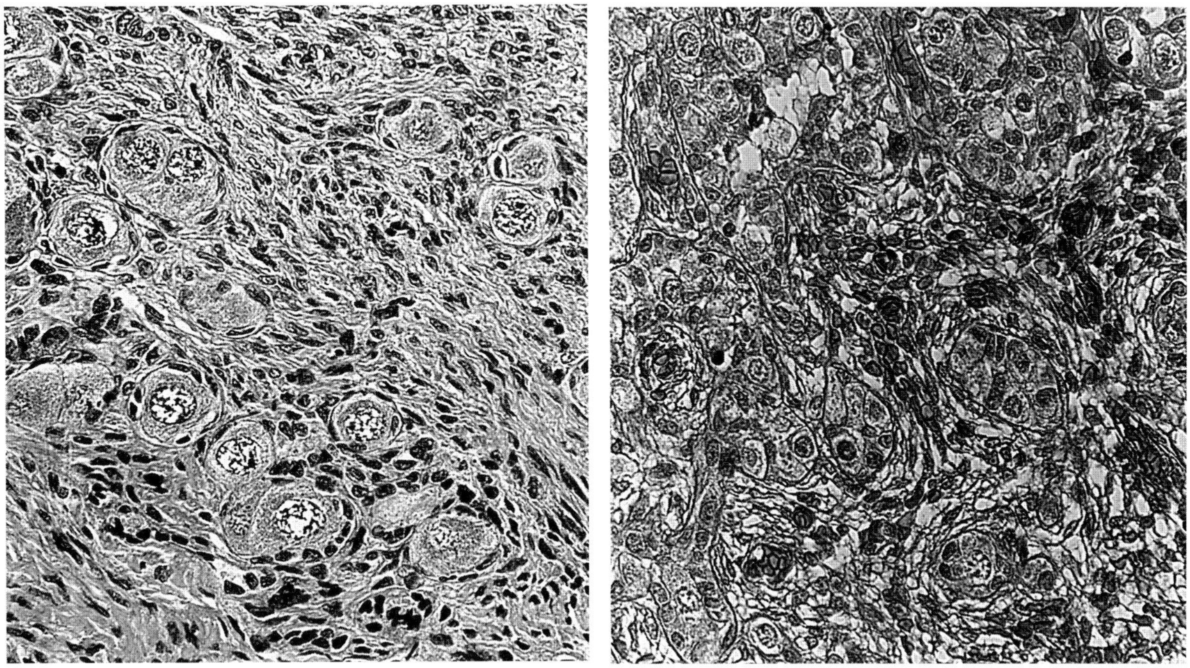

a b

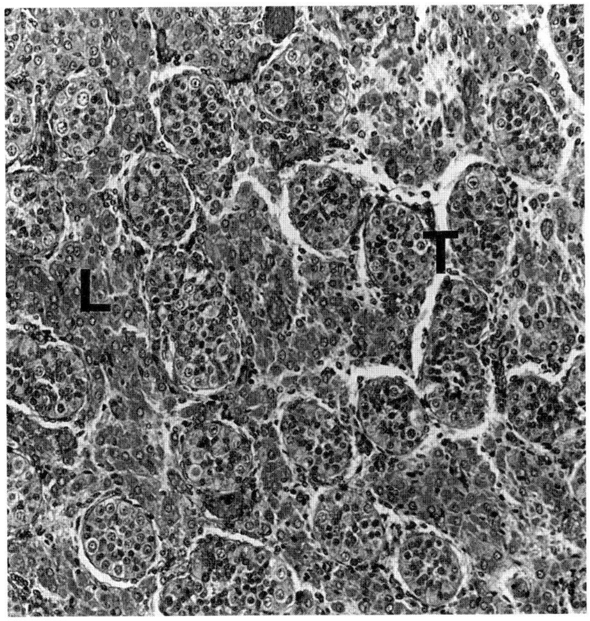

c

Fig. 20.3. Histology of fetal gonads. **a** Normal ovary from a fetus, 18 weeks of gestational age. The oocytes have entered the first meiotic division. (H&E ×225). **b** Dysgenetic gonad from a 19-week-old fetus with a 45X/46XY karyotype. The germ cells are smaller than normal and have not entered meiosis. (H&E ×235). **c** Testis from a 20-week-old fetus with a 47,XXY karyotype. Testicular histology is normal for the gestational age with abundance of Leydig cells (L), and seminiferous tubules (T) containing immature Sertoli cells and germ cells. (H&E ×93).

Errors of Sexual Differentiation

In these conditions, gonadal formation has occurred normally. However, abnormal differentiation of internal and/or external genitalia has taken place because of defective function of the gonad or other endocrine dysfunctions. The most common form of abnormal sexual differentiation is virilisation of a genetic female. This is called female pseudohermaphroditism and is most commonly related to congenital adrenal hyperplasia, which is described in Chap. 21. In 46XX individuals with congenital adrenal hyperplasia the phenotype may be that of a normal male with undescended testes (Fig. 20.4).

Defective genital virilisation, also called male pseudohermaphroditism, may be a result of absent or defective androgen receptors (Grumbach and Conte 1985). This is named

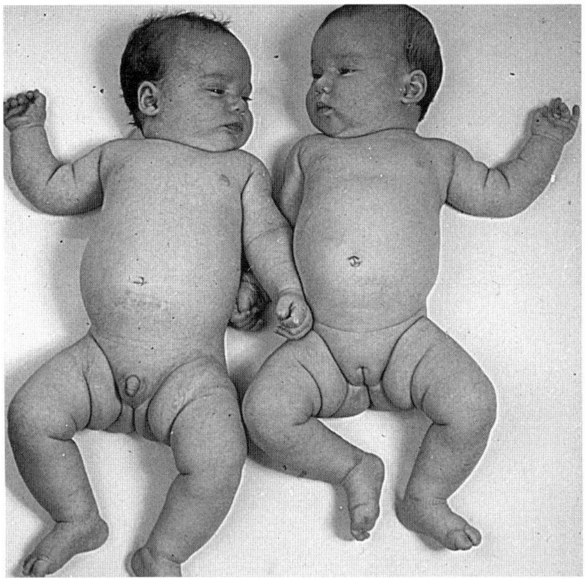

Fig. 20.4. Photograph of a pair of dizygous newborn twins, both with the karyotype 46XX. The twin to the left is completely virilised and has congenital adrenal hyperplasia. Penis is of normal size, the urethral orifice is normally located but the scrotum is empty. The twin to the right is a normal female.

androgen insensitivity syndrome or testicular feminisation syndrome. In its complete form a genetic male embryo develops into an individual with undescended, but otherwise normal testes, no Müllerian duct derivatives, and female external genitalia. These individuals also have increased risk of developing germ cell tumours and carcinoma-in-situ may be present at birth, although in most cases the testicular histology is unremarkable in the fetus and the newborn (Müller and Skakkebæk 1984). In the incomplete form of androgen insensitivity syndrome the phenotype may range from that of a slightly virilised female to that of a normal male. A 46XY individual with inborn errors of testosterone biosynthesis presents with a phenotype similar to that of a patient with the testicular feminisation syndrome (Grumbach and Conte 1985).

Hypospadias may be regarded as a mild defect of male sexual development. In most cases this is an isolated phenomenon without any demonstrable endocrine or genetic abnormality (Grumbach and Conte 1985). However, the possibility of hypogonadotropic hypogonadism, gonadal dysgenesis, androgen receptor defect, or an inborn error of testosterone biosynthesis should always be considered. Similarly, micropenis may occur as an isolated defect, but the condition may reflect an underlying endocrine or sex chromosomal disorder.

Unilaterally or bilaterally maldescended testes is a common finding, and the incidence may be increasing. In a large recent study, cryptorchidism was found in 5.9% of newborn boys. Three months later 1.6% still had undescended testes (Jackson 1988). In the majority of cases, cryptorchidism is an isolated phenomenon. Rarely, hypogonadotrophic hypogonadism and dysgenetic testes are underlying abnormalities.

Sex Chromosome Anomalies

Sex chromosome aneuploidy is not infrequent and usually compatible with life. In a screening of Danish newborns, Klinefelter's syndrome (47XXY karyotype) was found in 1.7 out of 1000 liveborn boys, and 47XYY individuals with a frequency of 1.1 per 1000 liveborn boys (Nielsen and Wohlert 1991). Testicular histology in fetuses and newborns with these syndromes is normal (Fig. 20.3), and degeneration of the germ cells and seminiferous tubules does not take place until later in childhood. In Turner's syndrome which has an incidence of 0.5 per 1000 liveborn girls (Nielsen and Wohlert 1991), gonadal histology develops normally until 14–16 weeks of gestation. From this time, germ cells degenerate rapidly and the ovaries are gradually replaced by connective tissue (streak gonads). In most girls with Turner's syndrome, only a few follicles are left at birth, but a wide variation exists and 5%–10% have spontaneous puberty.

Other Congenital Disorders of the Genitalia

Epispadias is rare. In these cases, the external urethral orifice is located on the dorsal side of the penis and the malformation is often combined with a defect in the abdominal wall and with bladder exstrophy.

Damage to the scrotum and the testis may occur after breech delivery, which may cause necrosis of testicular parenchyma and subsequent impairment of fertility (Tiwary 1989; see Chap. 14).

In the female, various abnormalities in the fusion of the paired Müllerian structures may be found as isolated phenomena (Simpson et al. 1976). Malformations of the internal and/or external genitalia may also be part of a major urogenital developmental defect including anal atresia. In these instances, underlying endocrine or chromosomal disorder is unusual.

Autosomal chromosomal disorders are rarely accompanied by malformations of the genitalia. However, in trisomy 13 syndrome, malformations of the Müllerian duct system, abnormal ovarian morphology, cryptorchidism, and hypoplasia of the external genitalia are frequent findings (Moerman et al. 1988).

References

Byskov AG, Høyer PE (1988) Embryology of mammalian gonads and ducts. In: Knobil E, Neill J, Ewing LL, Greenwald GS, Markert CL, Pfaff DW (eds) The physiology of reproduction, Raven Press, New York, pp 265–302

Clements JA, Reyes FI, Winter JSD, Faiman C (1976) Studies on human sexual development. III Fetal pituitary and serum, and aminotic fluid concentrations of LH, CG, and FSH. J Clin Endocrinol Metab 42: 9–19

Gantt PA, Byrd JR, Greenblatt RB, McDonough PG (1980) A clinical and cytogenetic study of fifteen patients with 45,X/46,XY gonadal dysgenesis. Fertil Steril 34: 216–221

Grumbach MM, Conte FA (1985) Disorders of sexual differentiation. In: Wilson JD, Foster DW (eds) Textbook of endocrinology, 7th edn. Saunders, Philadelphia, pp 312–401

Hung W, Randolph JG, Chandra R, Belman AB (1981) Gonadoblastoma in dysgenetic testis causing male pseudohermaphroditism in newborn. Urology 17: 584–587

Hutson JM, Donahue PK (1986) The hormonal control of testicular descent. Endocr Rev 7: 270–283

Jackson MB, John Radcliffe Hospital Cryptorchidism Study Group (1988) The epidemiology of cryptorchidism. Horm Res 30: 153–156

John Radcliffe Hospital Cryptorchidism Study Group (1988) Clinical diagnosis of cryptorchidism. Arch Dis Child 63: 587–591

Josso N (1986) AntiMüllerian hormone: new perspectives for a sexist molecule. Endocr Rev 7: 421–433

Kerr JB (1989) The cytology of the human testis. In: Burger H, de Kretser D (eds) The testis, 2nd edn. Raven Press, New York, pp 197–229

McLaren A (1990) What makes a man a man? Nature 346: 216–217

Moerman P, Fryns J-P, van der Steen K, Kleczkowska A, Lauweryns J (1988) The pathology of trisomy 13 syndrome. A study of 12 cases. Hum Genet 80: 349–356

Morley R, Lucas A (1987) Undescended testes in low birthweight infants. Br Med J 295: 753

Müller J, Skakkebæk NE (1984) Testicular carcinoma in situ in children with the androgen insensitivity (testicular feminisation) syndrome. Br Med J 288: 1419–1420

Müller J, Skakkebæk NE, Ritzén M, Plöen L, Petersen KE (1985) Carcinoma in situ of the testis in children with 45,X/46,XY gonadal dysgenesis. J Pediatr 106: 431–436

Nielsen J, Wohlert M (1991) Sex chromosome abnormalities found among 34910 newborn children: results from a 13-year incidence study in Århus, Denmark. In: Evans JA, Hamerton JL, Robinson A (eds) Children and young adults with sex chromosome aneuploidy. Wiley-Liss, New York, pp 209–223

Reyes FI, Boroditsky RS, Winter JSD, Faiman C (1974) Studies on human sexual development. II Fetal and maternal serum gonadotropin and sex steroid concentrations. J Clin Endocrinol Metab 38: 612–617

Simpson JL, Jirásek JE, Speroff L, Kase NG (1976) Disorders of sexual differentiation. Academic Press, New York, pp 341–359

Sinclair AH, Berta P, Palmer MS et al. (1990) A gene from the human sex-determining region encodes a protein with homology to a conserved DNA-binding motif. Nature 346: 240–244

Spear GS, Martin CG (1986) Fetal gonadoblastoid testicular dysplasia. Hum Pathol 17: 531–533

Tiwary CM (1989) Testicular injury in breech delivery: possible implications. Urology 34: 210–212

Wartenberg H (1989) Differentiation and development of the tests. In: Burger H, de Kretser D (eds) The testis, 2nd edn. Raven Press, New York, pp 67–118

Wensing CJG (1988) The embryology of testicular descent. Horm Res 30: 144–152

Chapter 21

The Endocrine System

Elizabeth S. Gray

Introduction

To understand the pathological lesions found in disorders of the endocrine system of the fetus and neonate it is necessary to have a knowledge of the interrelationships which exist within the developing endocrine system and its target tissues. Although the feedback and regulatory mechanisms are similar to those of the adult, the fetal endocrine system has also to incorporate an additional endocrine organ in the placenta, the steroidogenic zone in the adrenal cortex (fetal zone), and a contribution from the central nervous system, which in the fetus is probably capable both of the production of certain tropic hormones and of being a target organ for certain steroid hormones produced by the gonads, adrenal and placenta.

This complex endocrine system is developing and functioning within an organism in which cells of target organs are rapidly reduplicating, differentiating and maturing under the influence of tissue growth factors (the paracrine system). Thus, the effect of any fetal endocrine disorder is particularly far-reaching, e.g. fetal hyperadrenalism can cause gonadal intersex and possibly even alter sexual proclivity in adult life.

In the classic *endocrine system* specialised cells produce blood-borne hormones which act on distant target cells. They may be protein-polypeptides, amino acids, steroids or amines. They are produced by *endocrine glands*, i.e. hypothalamus, adrenal, pituitary, thyroid, parathyroid and pancreatic islets.

In the *paracrine system* a wide variety of cells produce peptides called tissue growth factors which act locally on adjacent cells (paracrine) or on secreting cells (autocrine). These peptides increase cell growth and stimulate protein, DNA and RNA synthesis through specific receptors on the target cell surface. Most fetal cells (Han et al. 1988) produce growth factors and have many more receptors than equivalent adult cells (Petraglia et al. 1990). These growth factors, structurally similar to viral oncogenes, are important to the growth, differentiation and modelling of fetal tissues. In this context insulin-like growth factors (IGFs) or somatomedins are particularly important. The *APUD system* is characterised by cells capable of *Amine Precursor Uptake* and *Decarboxylation*. These cells, whatever their site, show similar cytochemical and ultrastructural features and produce peptides or amines active as hormones or neurotransmitters. Many cells of the classic endocrine system are APUD cells, as are the argentaffin and argyrophil cells of the gut and lung. Pearse and Polak (1971), who coined the acronym APUD, proposed that they had all migrated from the primitive neural crest. However, delicate experiments (Le Douarin 1978) involving removal of the neural crest and transplanting neural crest between species showed that, while certain APUD cells, e.g. C cells of thyroid, definitely migrated from the neural crest, those of the digestive tract appeared to arise locally. Present opinion favours the suggestion that the digestive APUD cells are neuroendocrine-programmed cells of endodermal origin. Nonetheless, Pearse believes that migration occurs at a stage earlier than these neural crest experiments would detect; indeed, there is some evidence to support his view.

A brief outline of the development and function of the fetal endocrine system follows, together with an account of those abnormalities which present in the neonatal period. Certain clinical conditions, e.g. neonatal hypocalcaemia, which may mimic endocrine disease, will be briefly discussed.

Pituitary–Hypothalamic Axis

Ontogeny

The *hypothalamus* develops from a part of the diencephalon bulging into the third ventricle. Proliferation of neuroblasts in this area gives rise to the endocrine cells of the hypothalamus, those in the caudal region extending into the infundibulum and *neurohypophysis* to become modified neuroglia called pituicytes. The *adenohypophysis* is formed by ectoderm migrating upwards during the 3rd week of gestation (Rathke's pouch). The *pituitary portal system*, which forms the vascular connection between the hypothalamus and the adenohypophysis, develops from mesenchymal cells beside Rathke's pouch at about 7–8 weeks' gestation but is probably not fully functional until 18–20 weeks (Goodyer et al. 1979).

The *intermediate lobe* is poorly developed in humans and arises from the posterior portion of Rathke's pouch (pars intermedia). In the fetus it is more prominent than in the adult (Stark and Frantz 1983).

Hormone Production and Regulation

Although the hypothalamic/pituitary axis is not a functional unit until mid-gestation, individual hormones can be detected much earlier, at about 8–12 weeks. The *hypothalamus* secretes three types of hormones: monoamine neurotransmitters such as dopamine, noradrenaline and serotonin; the peptides, oxytocin and vasopressin, which are transported to the pituicytes of the *neurohypophysis*; and thirdly those polypeptide hormones acting as releasing factors with the adenohypophysis as their target organ.

The *adenohypophysis* secretes a range of hormones affecting both specific target organs, e.g. adrenal cortex, and metabolically active fetal tissues:

Growth hormone (GH) is controlled by a releasing factor and by a release inhibiting factor (somatostatin) from the hypothalamus. Its role in intrauterine growth is minimal: growth factors, insulin and fetal nutrition are all more important in maintaining fetal growth.

Prolactin (PRL) levels increase rapidly between 30 and 40 weeks' gestation, then fall after birth, reaching the normal prepubertal range by about 6 weeks of age. The role of prolactin in fetal life is unclear but it is reduced in the cord blood of infants who go on to develop respiratory distress syndrome (Smith et al. 1979).

Thyrotrophin (TSH) is first detectable at 12–14 weeks' gestation. It peaks at 20 weeks, by which time the hypothalamic/pituitary/thyroid axis is functional, and it is a prerequisite for fetal thyroid function, as maternal TSH does not cross the placenta. A placental thyrotrophin has been identified but cannot alone support normal fetal thyroid activity. There is a sudden increase in fetal TSH production at birth and increased thyroxine levels 1–2 h later. This increase occurs after caesarean and vaginal delivery. Histological changes also take place in the thyroid at this time (Sclare 1956).

Adrenocorticotrophin (ACTH). Pituitary ACTH is detectable from 7 weeks and peaks at 19 weeks' gestation. Although a placental ACTH exists, it appears from studies of the anencephalic fetus (Gray and Abramovich 1980; Young et al. 1989) that an intact hypothalamic pituitary adrenal axis is necessary to support the hyperplastic fetal zone (FZ) of the adrenal cortex from 16 weeks, and perhaps even 12 weeks.

Gonadotrophins (follicle-stimulating hormone and luteinising hormone) are also produced in utero.

The *intermediate lobe* responds to the stress of parturition by secreting endorphins which have opiate action (Facchinetti et al. 1989).

The Endocrine and Paracrine Systems and Fetal Growth

Although GH is essential for postnatal growth it does not control prenatal growth, a fact substantiated by the normal birthweights of infants born with GH deficiency.

Experimental systems show that the pituitary hormones GH, PRL and placental lactogen (hPL) have minimal growth effects mediated by stimulating the B cells of the endocrine pancreas. Insulin and paracrine growth factors, particularly IGFs, control embryonic and fetal growth (Milner and Hill 1987). IGFs promote cell growth, metabolism and division. Both experimental studies of the development and affinity of insulin receptors and observation of growth failure at about 28 weeks' gestation in the absence of the endocrine pancreas suggest IGFs are more important in early pregnancy, whilst insulin takes over in the third trimester. Adequate fetal nutrition and a normally functioning placenta are also essential for normal fetal growth.

The placenta influences both fetal and maternal metabolism. It produces hormones, neurohormones and tissue growth factors and has many receptors for insulin and IGFs. Recent evidence (Petraglia et al. 1990) indicates that both neuropeptides and growth factors stimulate the trophoblast to release hormones into the maternal circulation, where they promote metabolic and circulatory changes which favour fetoplacental growth. IGFs and insulin increase the uptake of nutrients by the placenta. In growth retardation the placenta has a reduced number of such receptors for both (Potau et al. 1981).

Pathology

Developmental Abnormalities of Structure

Isolated pituitary aplasia and *hypoplasia*, both rare, are due to a defect in the formation of Rathke's pouch which leads to total or partial absence of the adenohypophysis, but with an intact hypothalamus and neurohypophysis (Moncrieff et al. 1972). These normally grown infants present in the neonatal period with pro-

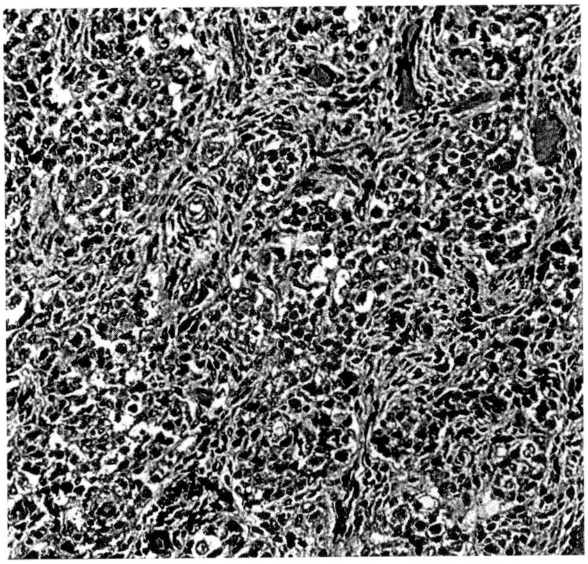

Fig. 21.1. Ovary. Neonate, alobar holoprosencephaly. Undifferentiated spindle cell stroma, poor primordial follicle formation. No oocytes. (H&E, ×180)

found hypoglycaemia; at necropsy the pituitary is small or absent. The adrenals are hypoplastic because of poor development of the fetal cortex, and the testes are small with absent Leydig cells. Both ovaries (Fig. 21.1) and thyroid appear inactive. Deficiency of pituitary function is more commonly associated with major cranial and facial deformities, i.e. alobar holoprosencephaly (see Chap. 23, p. 561), facial clefts, congenital cysts of Rathke's pouch (Cornelia de Lange's first syndrome), and anencephaly.

Anencephaly

Anencephaly is a neural tube defect, with a polygenic inheritance pattern (see Chap. 23, p. 553) in which the cephalad portion of the neural tube is grossly malformed with absence or disorganisation of much of the brain, including the hypothalamus and neurohypophysis.

Malfunction of the hypothalamic/pituitary axis throughout fetal life explains some of the findings in the *anencephalic syndrome*. Anencephalic pregnancies tend to be either abnormally short or abnormally long (Naeye and Blanc 1971). This is the only evidence that the human fetus can influence the time of parturition by hormone secretion. Naeye and Blanc also noted abnormal growth patterns in anencephalic fetuses, with the premature

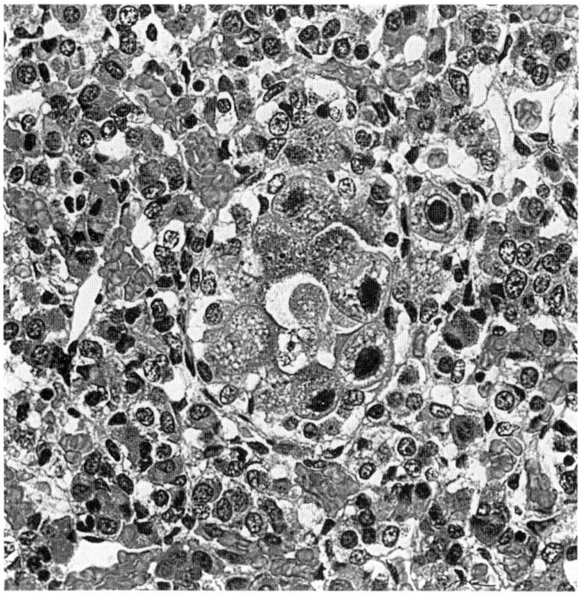

Fig. 21.2. Pituitary. Neonate with congenital CMV. CMV inclusions in acinar cells of adenohypophysis. (H&E, ×400)

group showing generalised growth retardation. This atrophy affects all organs except lymphoid tissue, the thymus being relatively large, an effect of reduced cortisol production by hypoplastic adrenals. In mature anencephalics, subcutaneous fat is frequently excessive. A similar finding in decapitated rabbit fetuses is due to increased insulin levels and abolished by ACTH (Jack and Milner 1975). Abnormal growth and excess fat have been attributed to a disorder of GH production but we now know that somatomedins and insulin, not GH, determine intrauterine growth. The suggestion that the growth disturbance is due to abnormal insulin production is interesting in view of disturbed carbohydrate handling and excess adiposity in mature anencephalics (Hayek et al. 1973).

The most constant feature in the anencephalic is severe *adrenal hypoplasia*; the glands weigh only 10% of normal at birth (see p. 505). The thyroid gland and gonads appear normal in anencephaly. The endocrine pancreas is normal, but if the mother is diabetic it may fail to develop the expected islet hyperplasia (Van Assche et al. 1969).

The relationship between the hypothalamic–pituitary axis and the function of the islet B cells is still not understood. Milner and Hill (1987) describe it as "the pea under the princess's mattress"!

Histological examination of the anencephalic pituitary shows an absent or abnormal hypothalamus and neurohypophysis (Salazar et al. 1969). The adenohypophysis is small with normal cell types. However, electron microscopy and immunocytological examination show that the corticotrophs are degenerate and decreased in number.

Idiopathic Pituitary Insufficiency

The term "idiopathic pituitary insufficiency" is used to describe those cases which have no anatomical or traumatic explanation.

In *isolated GH deficiency* birthweight is normal, as intrauterine growth is not GH dependent, and only those infants who develop severe neonatal hypoglycaemia present in the neonatal period. In about 3%–5% of cases it is an inherited condition, usually in autosomal-recessive fashion, but autosomal-dominant and X-linked recessive patterns are described. Isolated growth hormone deficiency is reported in congenital rubella (Preece et al. 1977) and Turner's syndrome (Faggiano et al. 1975). The anterior pituitary may be involved in congenital CMV infection (Fig. 21.2); functional impairment does not occur.

Multiple pituitary hormone deficiency is often related to traumatic or breech delivery, and is more likely to present in the neonatal period, sometimes with hypoglycaemic convulsions.

Adrenal Glands

Ontogeny

Adrenal glands comprise a *medulla* around which are layers of *cortex*. Cells which form the early *fetal zone* (FZ) of the adrenal cortex are first identified at 4 weeks' gestation, arising from a mesothelial zone medial to the urogenital ridge. By 7 weeks cells from the neural crest migrate into the centre of the early cortex to form the medulla. At about the same time a second migration of cells derived from coelomic epithelium envelop the entire gland. These cells later differentiate into the outer transitional zone of the FZ, and the *definitive zone* (DZ) or adult zone. During the first trimester the DZ is poorly formed and non-functional, while the FZ shows steroidogenic activity from the 7th week; this increases steadily through the first and second trimesters, and the FZ becomes large, comprising 80% of the entire adrenal cortex. From about the 25th week of gestation the DZ shows thickening and evidence of steroidogenic activity. During the last trimester FZ and DZ are fully developed. The FZ is formed by bulky polygonal cells with abundant eosinophilic cytoplasm, which continues to occupy 70%–80% of the adrenal cortex until birth, after which it shrinks progressively, to form only 50% of the gland at 6 weeks of age. Differentation of the DZ into the zona glomerulosa and zona fasciculata occurs between the 2nd and 4th week of postnatal life. The zona reticularis is slow to appear and is seen between 1 and 4 years of age.

Hormone Production and Regulation of the Adrenal Cortex

Although the DZ is capable of steroidogenesis in the latter half of gestation, it is the FZ, together with the placenta, which secretes the intrauterine steroid complement. Neither FZ nor placenta can do this alone as each lacks certain essential enzymes. In particular the FZ lacks 3β hydroxysteroid dehydrogenase (3βHSD), whilst the placenta has plenty (Buster 1980). The FZ extracts low-density lipoproteins from fetal blood and converts them, via cholesterol to Δ^5 pregnenolone sulphate, 17-hydroxy Δ^5 pregnenolone sulphate and dehydroepiandrosterone sulphate (DHEA-S) (Simpson et al. 1979). Because of the FZ deficiency of 3βHSD, these three steroids are secreted in large amounts to be used as substrates by 3βHSD in the placenta to synthesise progesterone and oestrogen. Progesterones are returned to the fetal circulation where the FZ uses them as substrates for conversion to the *glucocorticoids*. Placental oestrogen is secreted into both fetal and maternal circulations. Although the placenta and adrenal cortex cooperate to produce glucocorticoids, other organs can convert cortisol to cortisone and vice versa. This *peripheral steroid interconversion* occurs in the placenta, using maternal glucocorticoids. By altering the levels of maternal cortisol available to the fetus Pepe and and Albrecht (1990) postulate that tissue steroid interconversions stimulate the development of the fetal pituitary and adrenal cortex. The regulation of this mechanism is not understood. Conversions in later pregnancy are probably regulated by levels of placental oestrogen (Pepe et al. 1988).

Regulation of fetal adrenal steroidogenesis is not fully understood, but is reviewed by Pepe and Albrecht (1990). Study of the fetal adrenal cortex of anencephalics suggests that an intact hypothalamic/pituitary/adrenal axis is necessary for FZ maintenance after about 16 weeks' gestation (Gray and Abramovich 1980). Prior to this age, IGFs produced by the adrenal, peptides of placental origin, including hCG and a chorionic corticotrophin-like peptide, may be important for development of the fetal adrenal. Various pituitary peptides, particularly from the intermediate lobe, have been suggested as promoters of fetal adrenal function, but ACTH itself causes marked stimulation of fetal cortex in culture (Fujeida et al. 1981). Morever, in the presence of high levels of oestrogen from the placenta, ACTH promotes DHEA-S rather than cortisol production. The resulting low cortisol would then stimulate ACTH production (Fujeida et al. 1982) and cause the typical hyperplasia of the normal FZ.

At birth, loss of the placenta removes both the inhibitory influence of oestrogen and several steroid substrates, causing the FZ to shrink. Plasma ACTH also falls in the first few days of life. Circadian rhythms of ACTH and cortisol secretion are not achieved until 3–4 months of age.

The *adrenal medulla* is formed by neural crest cells which multiply to form neuroblastic islands. These cells mature and differentiate into catecholamine-secreting cells. The adrenal medulla is the major fetal source of catecholamines, and their production is controlled by glucocorticoids from the adjacent adrenal cortex. Catecholamines increase surfactant production in fetal lung and are probably important, along with thyroxine, for thermogenesis in the neonate (Artal 1980).

Pathology

Developmental Anomalies

Adrenal agenesis. This condition is extremely rare and, although previously reported in anencephaly, the finding reflects poor dissection. *Ectopic adrenals*, or ectopic adrenal cortical tissue seen as yellowish nodules is particularly common in organs of the urogenital tract including testes, ovaries, epididymis.

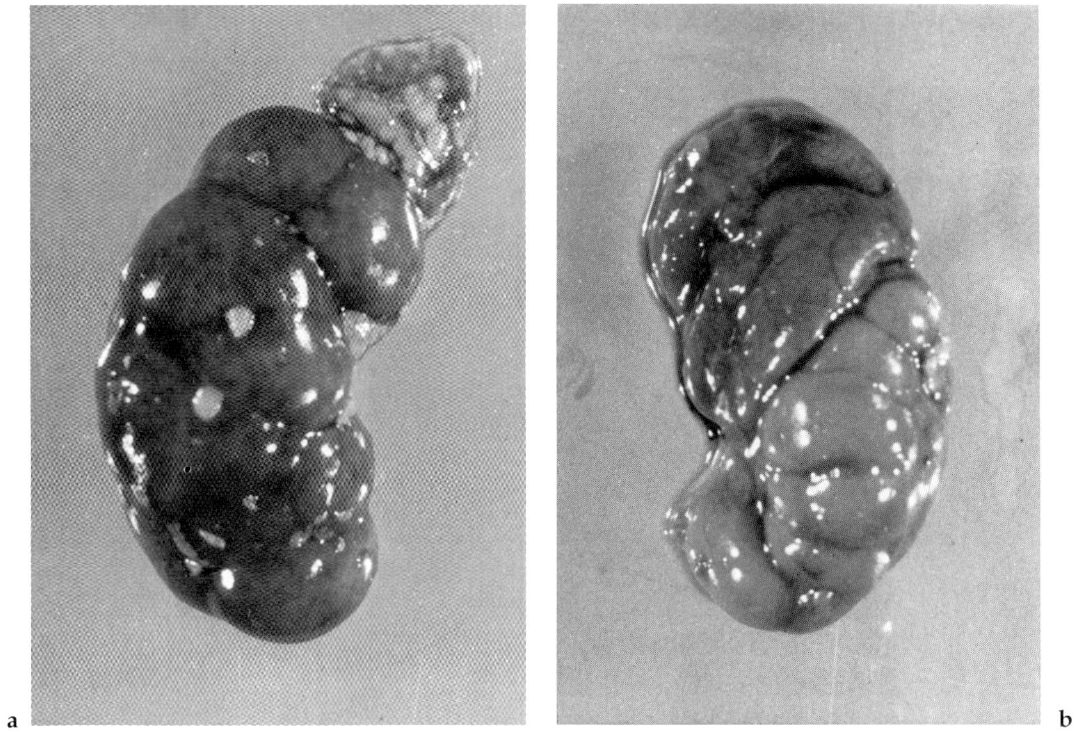

Fig. 21.3. Fetal kidney and adrenal gland. **a** Anencephalic fetus, 19 weeks: small yellow adult-shaped adrenal. (×3) **b** Normal fetus, 18 weeks: large pink adrenal. (×3)

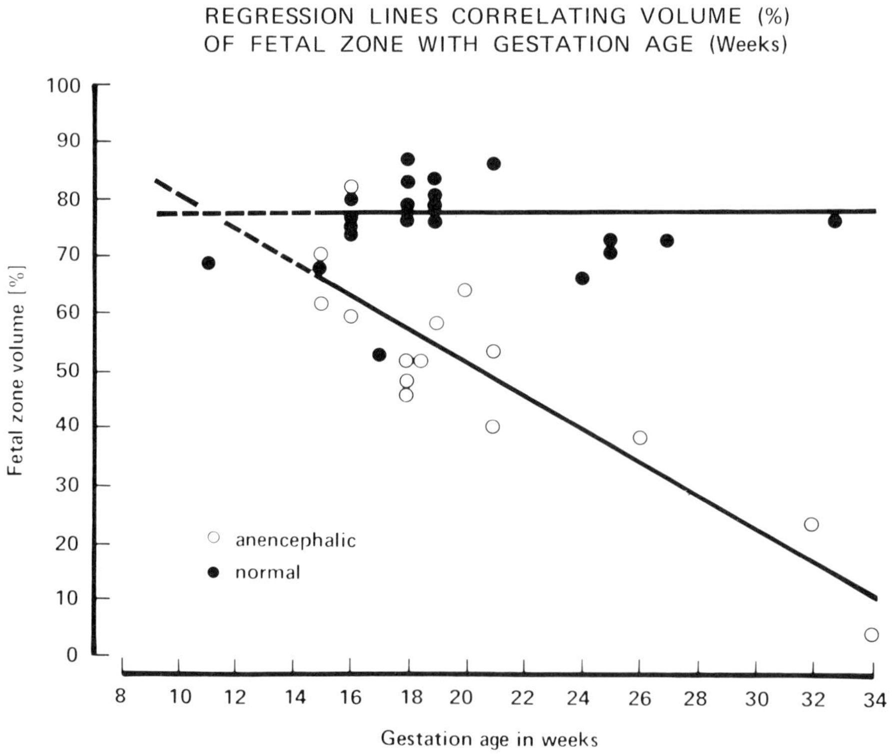

Fig. 21.4. There is a progressive diminution in the volume of FZ cortex in the anencephalic fetus

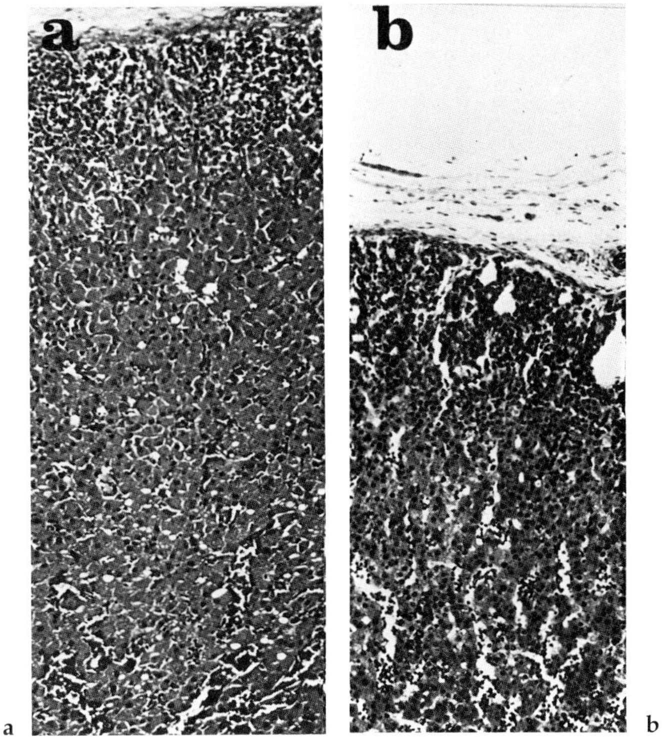

Fig. 21.5. Adrenal cortex at 19 weeks' gestation. **a** Normocephalic: FZ is 80% volume. **b** Anencephalic: FZ is 50% volume. (Both H&E, ×250)

Secondary adrenal hypoplasia. This condition occurs in alobar holoprosencephaly but most commonly in the *anencephalic syndrome* (see p. 553). In anencephaly the adrenal glands are smaller than normal from as early as 16–18 weeks' gestation and in shape come to resemble miniature adult adrenal glands (Fig. 21.3). At birth they weigh only 10% of the normal combined weight of 9 g. This hypoplasia is due to progressive shrinking (Fig. 21.4) of the FZ of the adrenal cortex (Fig. 21.5) from 80% of cortical volume to a mere 20% of cortical volume by 33 weeks' gestation (Gray and Abramovich 1980).

Idiopathic adrenal hypoplasia. This condition exhibits three histological patterns, of which the most common is the "anencephalic" pattern of FZ atrophy. Kerenyi (1961), who described only two patterns, believed that the anencephalic type was always due to a disorder of the pituitary or hypothalamus and therefore not truly idiopathic but secondary. Histology of type 2, *cytomegalic adrenal hypoplasia*, shows the adrenal cortex to be disorganised with marked cytomegaly of intensely eosinophilic cortical cells (Fig. 21.6); it is not associated with pituitary abnormality. Its aetiology is unknown, shows marked male predominance and may be X-linked. A third type in which both the FZ and DZ are proportionately reduced is described by Larroche (1977).

Partial adrenal hypoplasia. This condition occurs in some infants with trisomy 18. The glands show a reduction in the width of the FZ. This change in the FZ may be a reflection of the placental hypoplasia and hypofunction found in trisomy 18. A similar type of adrenal hypoplasia is associated with severe intrauterine growth retardation but its aetiology may be different.

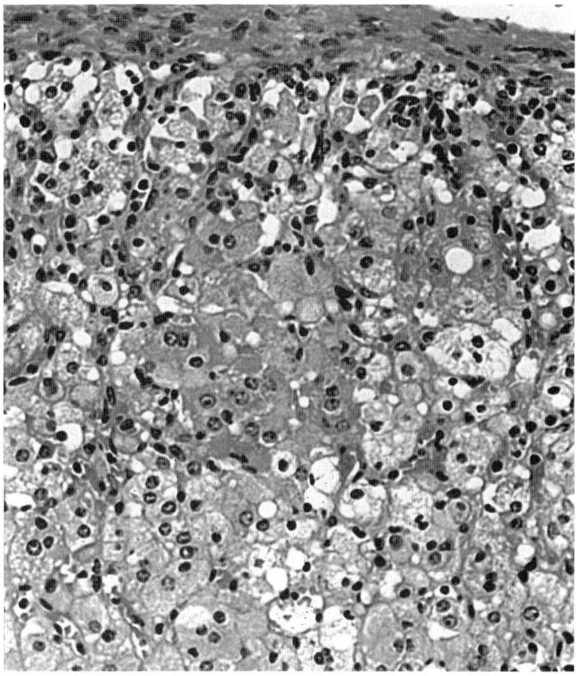

Fig. 21.6. Hypoplastic adrenal, male infant 4 months. X-linked form. Total adrenal weight = 0.29 g (normal 4.0 g). Cluster of eosinophilic cytomegalic cells in cortex. (H&E, ×192)

Fusion. The adrenal glands are occasionally seen to be fused in the midline in thoracolumbar spina bifida.

Acquired Pathology

Adrenal *haemorrhages* are not uncommon in infants with severe perinatal anoxia. The haemorrhages usually occur in the inner cortex and may be small, or massive and associated with extensive glandular necrosis (Fig. 21.7). Occasionally, haemorrhage may be subcapsular or predominantly periadrenal, spreading into retroperitoneal tissues.

Breech delivery, high birthweight and prolonged, difficult labour are associated with adrenal haemorrhage, often unilateral. They are also seen in premature infants without obvious trauma.

Adrenal *calcification* can occur in utero following infection, e.g. cytomegalovirus (Fig. 21.8) and toxoplasmosis. In such infections foci of calcification occur in other viscera, particularly liver, myocardium and brain. The identity of the infecting organism is often not established. Centrally placed microscopic foci of cal-

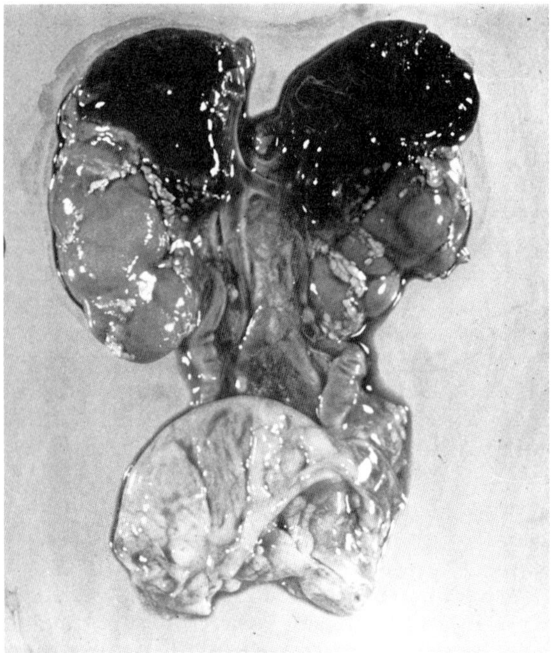

Fig. 21.7. Premature (30 weeks) neonate with respiratory distress syndrome. Massive bilateral adrenal haemorrhages. (×1.2)

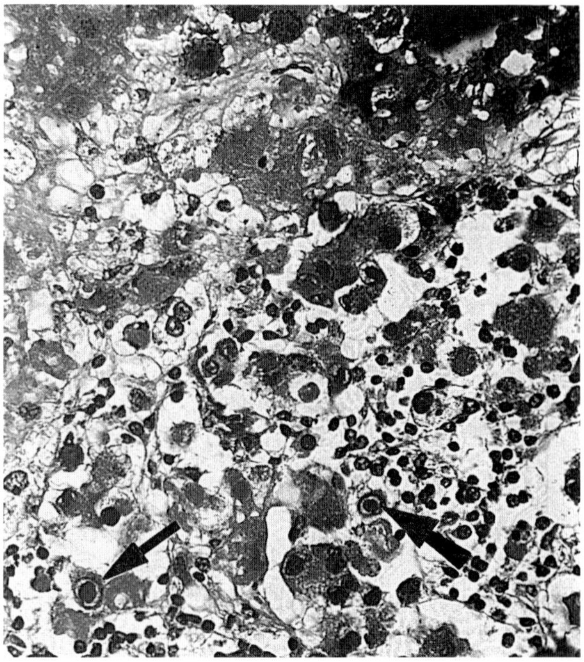

Fig. 21.8. Adrenal, neonate. Focal calcification, CMV inclusions (*arrows*) and lymphocytic infiltrate. (H&E, ×288)

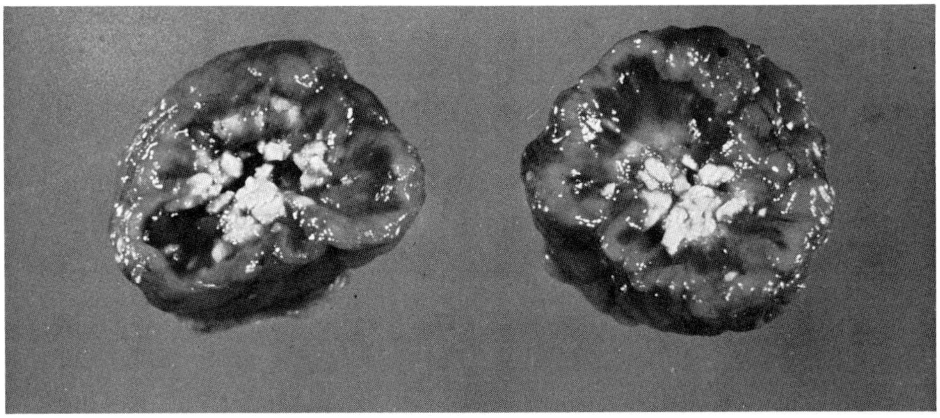

Fig. 21.9. Adrenal glands: mulberry-shaped glands with central calcification. Unknown aetiology, four affected siblings. (×2)

cification are found in the large fatty adrenals (see below) of hydrops fetalis, whether of immunological or non-immunological type. A similar calcification is found in the lipid-laden glands of Wolman's disease.

Extensive adrenal calcification in neonates and infants is usually the sequel of haemorrhagic necrosis caused by perinatal asphyxia. The calcification is usually in the inner portion of the cortex and the medulla, the outer cortex being well preserved. This dystrophic calcification can occur as early as 9 days post haemorrhage.

We have observed in two unrelated Scottish families with normal parents, four children with congenital nephrotic syndrome (Finnish type) who have also had massive congenital bilateral adrenal calcification. The adrenal glands in the affected children had an unusual mulberry shape (Fig. 21.9). None of the children showed clinical evidence of adrenal dysfunction, and all died in infancy of renal failure.

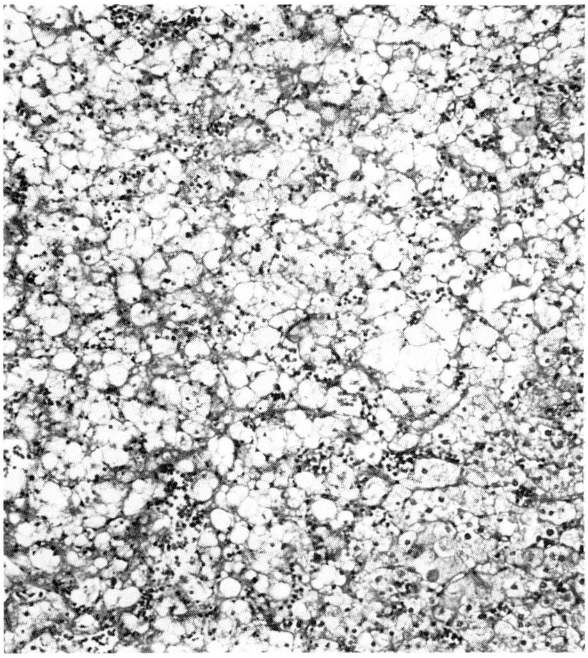

Fig. 21.10. Fetal adrenal cortex, immunological hydrops fetalis (26 weeks). Vacuolated lipid-rich cortical cells. (H&E, ×220)

Fatty adrenals. The fetal neonatal adrenal is normally pink and fleshy. When lipid content is increased the adrenal appears yellow, and on histological examination the FZ cells are clear and vacuolated (Fig. 21.10) and contain much stainable fat. Yellow, lipid-rich adrenals are a striking feature in some hydropic fetuses (Fig. 21.11). Larroche (1977) maintains that lipid-rich adrenals are specific to immunological (i.e. rhesus isoimmunisation) hydrops but we have frequently seen it in non-immunological hydrops fetalis. Sometimes these adrenals show microscopic foci of calcification. The accumulation of lipid is probably a non-specific response to prolonged intrauterine stress. Becker and Becker (1976) examined the amount and distribution of fat in the fetal cortex of stillborn infants. They describe three distinct histological patterns, each related to the duration of the intrauterine stress.

In *Wolman's disease* due to acid lipase deficiency massive amounts of neutral lipid are present in the enlarged, calcified adrenals as well as the liver and other organs. Deficiency of

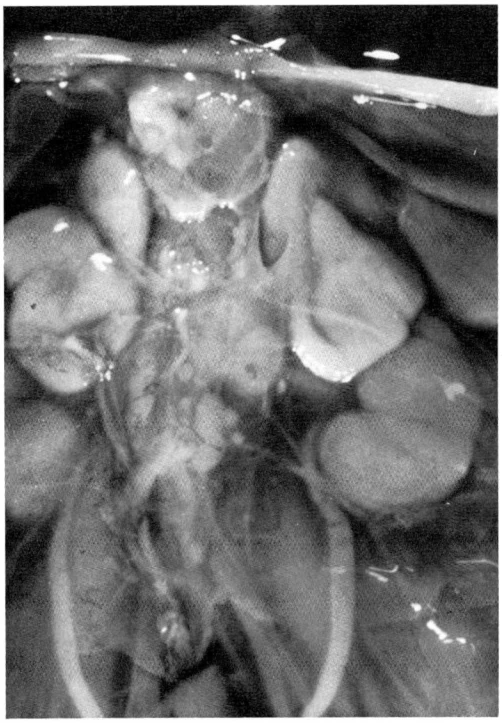

Fig. 21.11. Hydrops fetalis (same case as Fig. 21.10). Large pale-yellow adrenals. (×2.3)

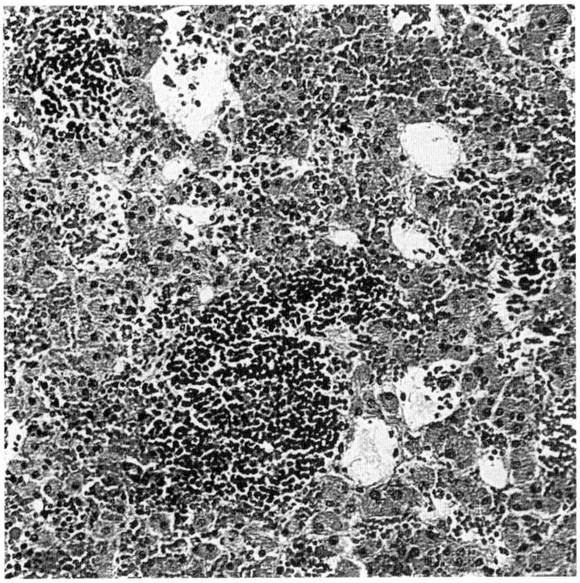

Fig. 21.12. Fetal adrenal at 28 weeks' gestation. Numerous aggregates of neuroblasts with some rosette formation. (H&E, ×170)

20–22 desmolase, an enzyme very early in steroid synthesis, will produce an accumulation of fat and cholesterol in enlarged hyperplastic adrenals.

Pathology of the Adrenal Gland: Microscopic

Neuroblastoma in situ. The adrenal medulla is formed from immature small dark cells called neuroblasts. Nodules of these cells may persist in the centre of the gland and be found incidentally on histological examination (Fig. 21.12). Some are quite large aggregates with rosette formation. They are more common in early than late gestation. The majority regress or mature, but some may be the nidus of malignant neuroblastoma (see p. 280). It is suggested that these nests of neuroblasts are more common in the anencephalic adrenals (Van Hale and Turkel 1979).

Haemopoietic activity. Foci of haemopoietic activity may be present in the adrenals of infants with no clinical evidence of increased haemopoiesis. In *leukaemoid reactions* (see p. 290) the adrenal is frequently infiltrated by cells of the myeloid series.

Adrenal cytomegaly. A frequent incidental finding at necropsy is adrenal cytomegaly, where some of the eosinophilic cells of the FZ show nuclear gigantism (Fig. 21.13); when severe, it is usually part of the Beckwith–Wiedemann syndrome (Fig. 21.14) (visceromegaly, exomphalos, hyperplasia of the islets of Langerhans, macroglossia and adrenal cytomegaly). In this condition it may be present as early as 20 weeks' gestation. Adrenal cytomegaly is also found in type 2 idiopathic adrenal hypoplasia but differs in that there is excess, glassy cytoplasm and normal-sized nuclei (Fig. 21.6).

Pseudocysts; pseudofollicular change. These are commonly found in the subcapsular adult cortex in aborted fetuses and neonatal deaths. The cells are arranged in a glandlike fashion, and eosinophilic fluid is generally present in the lumen (Fig. 21.15). These changes have been interpreted as a response to stress or anoxia (DeSa 1978) and are described in infection, premature rupture of membranes and following termination of pregnancy (Gaillard et al. 1990).

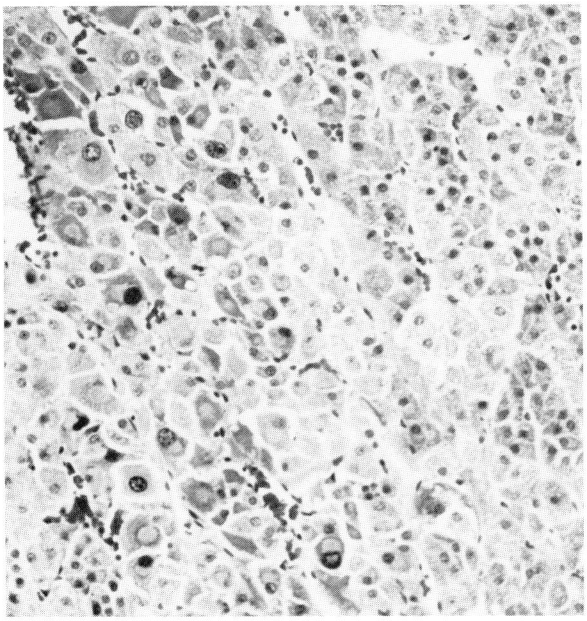

Fig. 21.13. Adrenal cortex, normal neonate. Focal cytomegaly with "inclusions" in cytoplasm. (H&E, ×140)

Other changes. As the result of *prolonged stress* other changes occur in the morphology of the adrenal gland. There may be reduction in the large pale FZ cells and an increase in the compact cells. Alternatively, the adrenals may be pale with increased lipid.

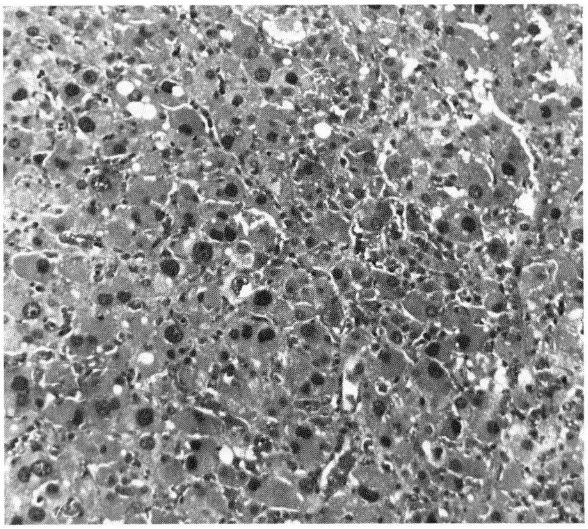

Fig. 21.14. Adrenal cortex, Beckwith–Wiedemann syndrome. Diffuse cytomegaly, no "inclusions". (H&E, ×180)

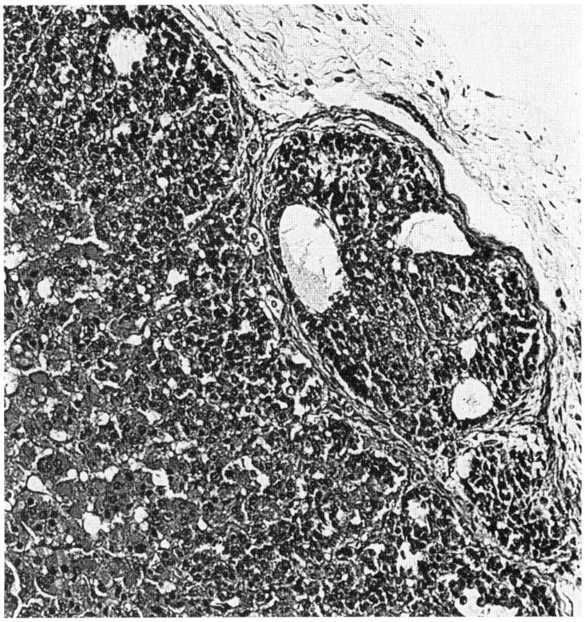

Fig. 21.15. Adrenal cortex, neonate (26 weeks) with respiratory distress syndrome. Pseudofollicular cysts in the definitive cortex. (H&E, ×250)

Functional Pathology

Congenital Adrenal Hyperplasia (Adrenogenital Syndrome)

Congenital adrenal hyperplasia is caused by an enzyme defect in cortisol synthesis; low cortisol levels cause excessive ACTH secretion. ACTH causes further stimulation of the adrenal cortex, but because of the blocking effect of the deficient enzyme, cortisol levels remain low and ACTH production is constantly switched on. The effect is adrenocortical hyperplasia and increased steroidogenesis with excessive production of androstenedione and so of testosterone and oestradiol. In 90% of cases the enzyme which is deficient is *21 hydroxylase*. As this enzyme is also necessary for the synthesis of aldosterone, complete deficiency will produce a salt-losing state, which can be fatal in the neonatal period.

If the enzyme defect occurs in a female fetus (80%), virilisation with ambiguous genitalia—female pseudohermaphrodite—is seen (Fig. 21.16). In the male without salt loss, the onset of precocious puberty first alerts clinicians to the possibility of congenital adrenal hyperplasia.

11β hydroxylase is much less commonly deficient and causes an excess production of

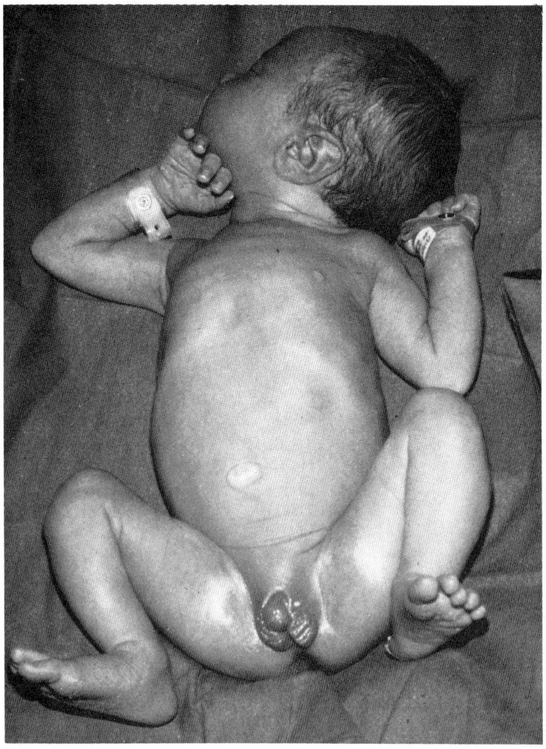

Fig. 21.16. Female infant with congenital adrenal hyperplasia. The clitoris is hypertrophied and the labia are rugose.

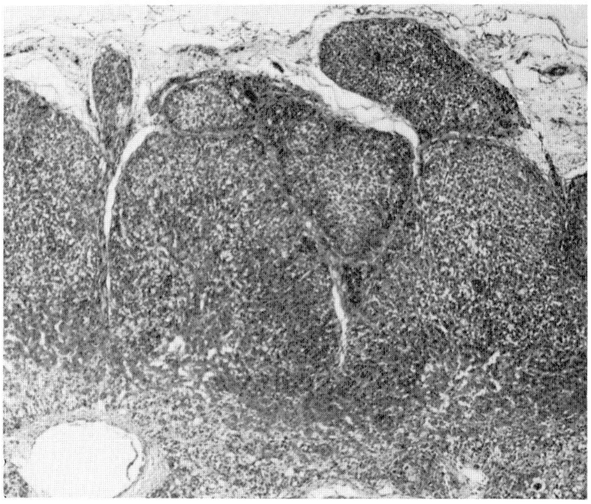

Fig. 21.18. Adrenal cortex, congenital adrenal hyperplasia. Irregular nodular hyperplasia of the cortex. (Courtesy of Prof. P.J. Berry, Bristol.) (H&E, ×60)

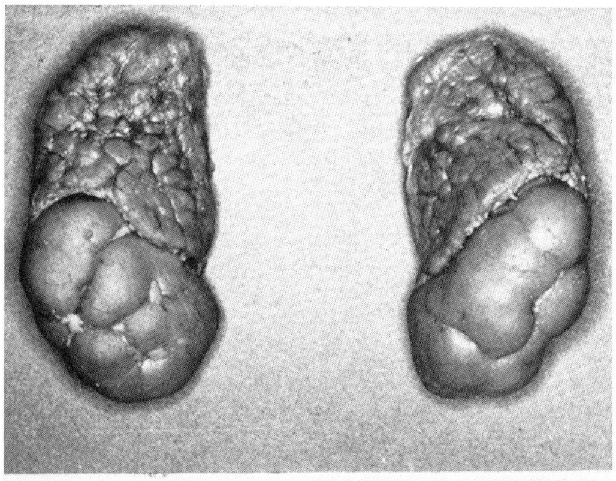

Fig. 21.17. Adrenal gland, congenital adrenal hyperplasia. Corrugated cerebriform surface. (Courtesy of Prof. P.J. Berry, Bristol)

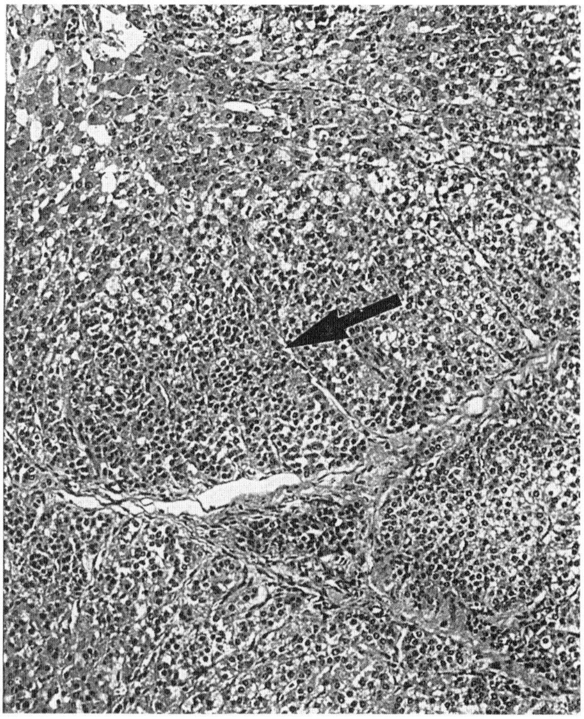

Fig. 21.19. Adrenal cortex, neonate (19 days) with congenital adrenal hyperplasia. Increased compact cells (*arrow*) extending focally to cortex. FZ cells also more eosinophilic than normal (*lower right* and *left*). (H&E, ×190)

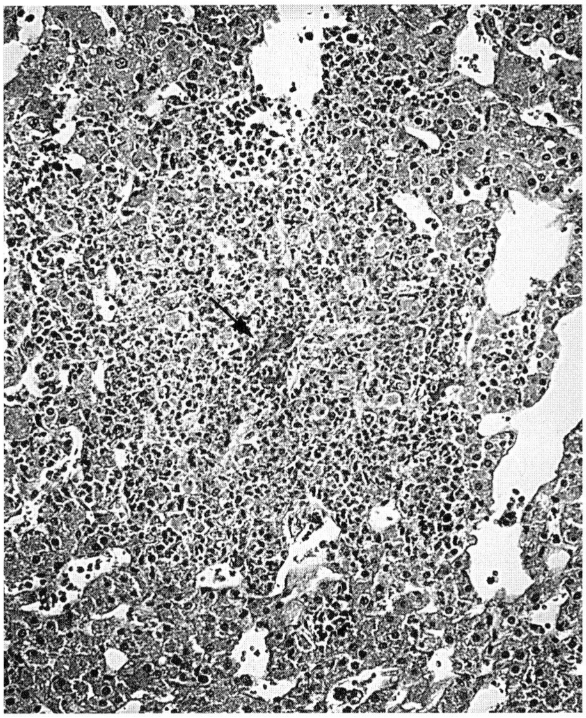

Fig. 21.20. Adrenal cortex, neonate (29 weeks) with generalised listeriosis. Typical "granuloma" with central fibrin (*arrow*), scanty polymorphs and monocytes. (H&E, ×130)

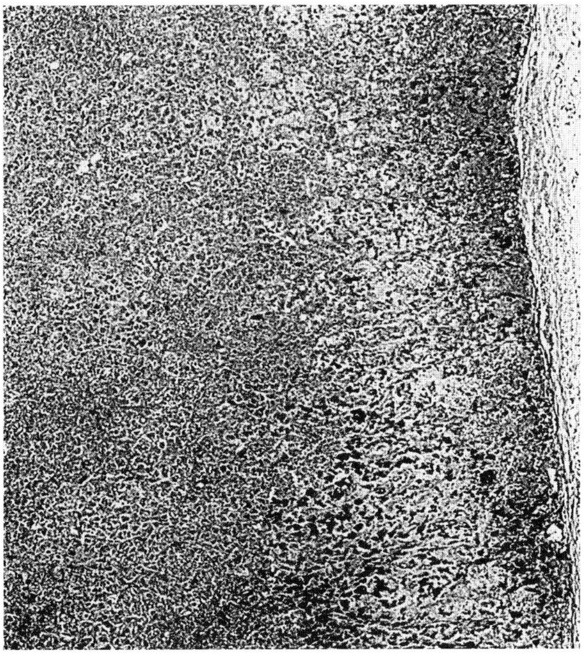

Fig. 21.21. Adrenal gland, neonate (10 days) with echo virus. Diffuse necrosis with haemorrhage (Courtesy of Dr. A. King, Cambridge.) (H&E, ×75)

aldosterone precursors as well as increased androgens. These infants have cardiomegaly and hypertension as a result of chronic sodium and water retention, in addition to virilisation. Because it affects a very early stage in steroid synthesis *3β hydroxylase* deficiency produces severe, often fatal salt loss with little virilisation.

These enzyme deficiencies are inherited in an autosomal-recessive pattern. The adrenals, in all forms, are greatly enlarged (average = 15 g) and have a corrugated "cerebriform" appearance (Fig. 21.17) and a brown cut surface. Histological examination (Fig. 21.18) shows nodular hyperplasia of the cortex with an increase in the active eosinophilic or compact cells which stream outwards towards the surface (Fig. 21.19). Lipid-containing cells of the zona fasciculata are greatly reduced.

Infections

In systemic listeriosis the adrenals are usually involved; white abscesses, the size of pin heads, with a characteristic histology are present (Fig. 21.20). Toxoplasmosis, echovirus (Fig. 21.21) and herpes infections (Fig. 21.22) produce typical changes. *Diffuse* necrosis with haemorrhage is typical of echovirus infection (Fig. 21.21) whilst in neonatal herpes there is *multifocal* punctate cortical necrosis with surrounding hyperaemia or haemorrhage (Fig. 21.22).

Tumours of the Adrenal Gland

Congenital neuroblastoma. Neuroblastoma is the most common congenital malignant tumour (Fig. 21.23; see also Chap. 12, p. 280). The tumour is composed of small cells with dark ovoid nuclei. The cytoplasm which is scanty has a fibrillary nature and the cells may form rosettes.

Adrenal cortical tumours. These are rare in childhood and show two incidence peaks, in infancy and adolescence. There is a marked female preponderance (female : male ratio of 2.5–5 : 1) and an association with the Beckwith–Wiedemann syndrome and hemihypertrophy. The majority of tumours are active, Cushing's syndrome and aldosteronism being common in benign tumours and virilisation (or feminisation) being more frequent in carcinomas. The histological criteria used to predict malignant behaviour in adults are not reliable in children.

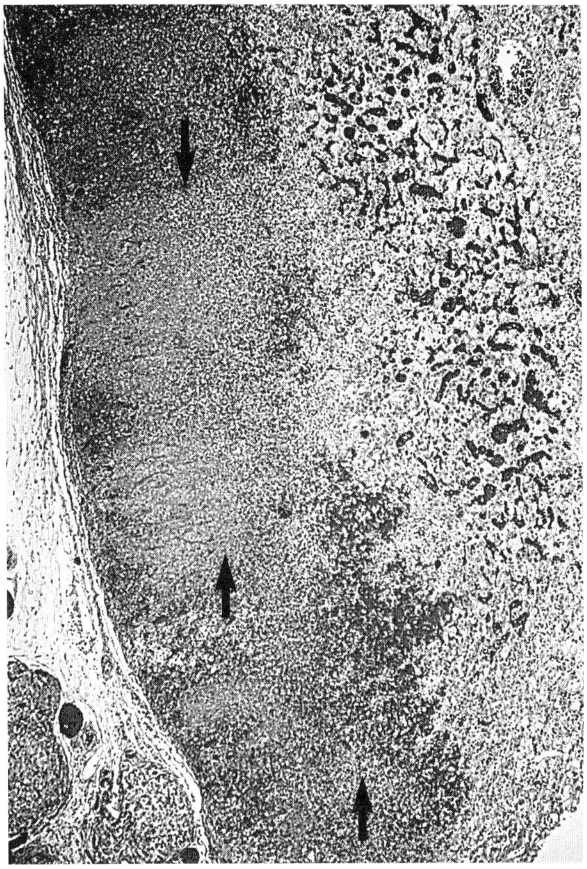

Fig. 21.22. Adrenal gland, neonate (12 days) with HSV1. Punctate necrosis, surrounding haemorrhage and hyperaemia, visible to naked eye. (H&E, ×50)

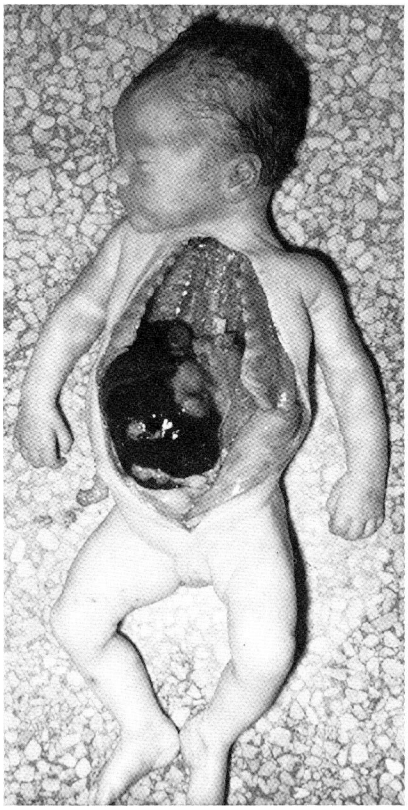

Fig. 21.23. Term neonate (8 h) with massive right congenital neuroblastoma.

Cagle et al. (1986) found that severe nuclear pleomorphism, mitotic activity, necrosis, fibrotic bands, capsular invasion and even invasion of smaller vessels did not necessarily predict malignancy in children. The only reliable predictor of behaviour was tumour size. All tumours <100 g were benign and all tumours >500 g were malignant.

Thyroid Gland

Ontogeny

The thyroid develops between the 2nd and 7th weeks from an outpouching in the floor of the mouth. This median portion travels caudally into the neck and is joined by contributions from the 4th pharyngeal pouch. By the 7th week the buccal connection with the median portion is severed. Between 8 and 11 weeks' gestation there occurs differentiation with follicle formation, concentration of iodine and formation of thyroxine. From this stage the fetal thyroid is vulnerable to damage by radioactive iodine. Although the different components of the hypothalamic/pituitary/thyroid axis are functioning by the 12th week, it is between 12 and 18 weeks that full regulatory interactions are established. After 20 weeks' gestation T_4 levels rise and thyroid-stimulating hormone (TSH) levels fall, indicating an effective feedback mechanism (Hobel 1980).

Maternal T_4 and T_3 can cross the placenta, but only in very small amounts unless maternal levels are abnormally high, i.e. thyrotoxicosis. Long-acting thyroid stimulator (LATS), an IgG immunoglobulin, crosses the placenta and stimulates the fetal thyroid.

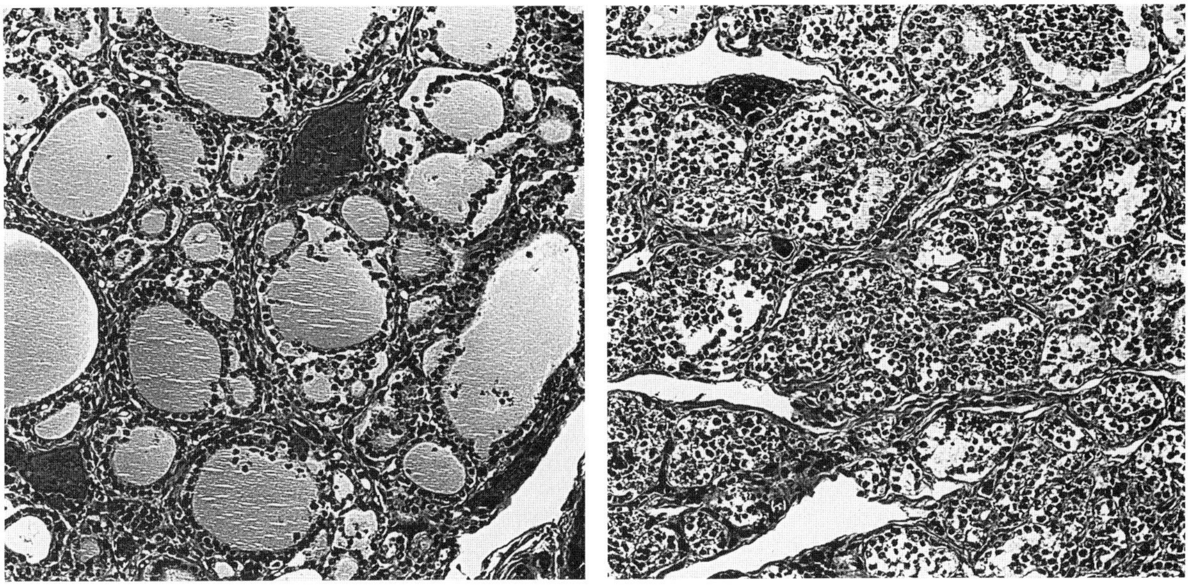

Fig. 21.24a,b. Neonatal thyroid showing different normal patterns **a** Follicles filled with colloid. **b** Follicles contain desquamated cells with pyknotic nuclei (both H&E, ×160)

In utero, fetal T_4 is converted to rT_3, not the active form T_3 (Hobel 1980). Just before birth a switch to T_3 production occurs to facilitate extrauterine survival. The mechanism is unclear, but there is a surge of fetal TSH at birth followed by an increase in T_3 and T_4 (Fisher and Odell 1969). A more chronic hypersecretion of TSH occurs in the first 24–48 h, and this can be significantly increased by cooling the infant. Perhaps this increased thyroid activity effects the histological changes found in the neonatal thyroid (see below).

The *parafollicular* (*C cells*) of the thyroid develop from the ultimobranchial arch and secrete calcitonin, which inhibits osteoclasts and stops dissolution of bone.

Histological Variation in Fetal and Neonatal Thyroid

Two histological patterns are seen in the neonatal thyroid (Fig. 21.24a,b). The more common is of small uniform follicles lined by cuboidal epithelium, containing a variable amount of colloid. The stroma is more abundant than in the adult thyroid. In the other, the centres of acini are filled by masses of cells. The second pattern was considered a post-mortem artefact (Potter and Craig 1976). However, Sclare (1956), Sagreiya and Emery (1970) and Larroche (1977), consider it physiological and labour-related, occuring in normal infants between the 2nd and 7th days. Our present, albeit incomplete, knowledge of the transition from intrauterine to neonatal thyroid function would support this pattern as functional rather than artefactual. In normal human neonates, born vaginally, there is a sharp rise in T_3 and T_4 levels 24–48 h postpartum, and TSH levels rise sharply at birth (Fisher and Odell 1969).

Pathology

Malformations

Thyroid agenesis and hypoplasia cause congenital hypothyroidism.

Ectopic thyroid gland. Thyroid tissue may be found at any point along the track followed by the thyroid in its migration from the posterior area of the tongue. Thyroid tissue at the base of the tongue is called a lingual thyroid. Thyroid tissue has been described at various sites within the mediastinum.

Congenital Hypothyroidism (Cretinism)

Congenital hypothyroidism may be associated with mental retardation and neurological defects including ataxia, spasticity, strabismus and poor muscle tone. Not all hypothyroid neonates have neuronal damage (cretinism) and Hetzel and Mano (1989) suggest that maternal thyroxine protects the early fetal brain. When the mother is hypothyroid, the risk of cretinism is higher.

Primary congenital hypothyroidism. There are three main causes of *primary hypothyroidism* in neonates: *thyroid dysgenesis* (1 in 5000 births), which may be due to agenesis or hypoplasia; a defect in *hypothalamic/pituitary function* (1 in 20000 births); and familial goitre or *thyroid dyshormonogenesis* (1 in 30000 births). This last condition, if associated with deafness, is called Pendred's syndrome.

Dyshormonogenesis rarely presents in the neonatal period, being more usual at puberty. Some cases have presented in utero with polyhydramnios (Perelman et al. 1990) and been successfully treated with intra-amniotic T_4. It is due to a defect in thyroid hormone biosynthesis secondary to a deficiency of one of the enzymes of which peroxidase, the enzyme responsible for the organic binding of iodide, is the most commonly involved. The enzyme defects are inherited in an autosomal-recessive fashion.

Secondary congenital hypothyroidism. The thyroid may be severely damaged in utero, either by toxic chemicals crossing the placenta (i.e. the antithyroid drugs thiouracil or methinazole) or radioactive iodine given after the 10th week of gestation. Topical iodine used during pregnancy can cause transient congenital hypothyroidism (Danziger et al. 1987).

Worldwide, secondary hypothyroidism is commonly caused by dietary lack of iodine—*endemic goitrous cretinism*. These infants are born in areas where adult goitre is endemic. Only a proportion of infants show features of cretinism, suggesting that maternal thyroid function and other factors, probably genetic, are also important.

The appearance and clinical findings of fetal hypothyroidism and neonatal cretinism are well known. In brief, the affected infant may be small for dates, fails to thrive and frequently suffers from prolonged physiological jaundice and constipation. Radiographs show delay in ossification centres with small and fragmented femoral epiphyses. Skin is dry, hair coarse and tongue protuberant (Fig. 21.25). Not all cases of hypothyroidism have this easily recognisable phenotype. TSH levels are raised in all cretins except those resulting from failure of hypothalamic/pituitary function. T_4 levels are always low. It is a relatively common disorder (1 in 4000 births; cf. PKU at 1 in 20000), which, if not treated early, can cause irreversible brain damage; thus there is a strong argument for mass neonatal screening.

The *size* of the *thyroid gland* in congenital hypothyroidism varies. In *thyroid dysgenesis*, irradiation damage and a minority of endemic cretins the thyroid is absent or very atrophic. In those *dyshormonogenetic* cases which present at birth, the thyroid is usually enlarged and nodular. Histological examination reveals nodular hyperplasia with small empty follicles

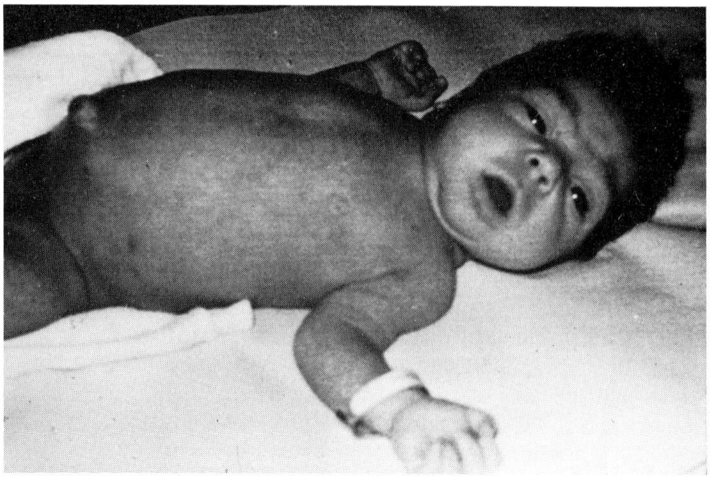

Fig. 21.25. Hypothyroid neonate. Coarse hair and facies; umbilical hernia.

lined by cells with focal nuclear pleomorphism and gigantism (Figs. 21.26, 21.27). This appearance has been mistaken for thyroid carcinoma.

The majority of *endemic cretins* have enlarged thyroids weighing 5–10 g (normals 1–3 g). Follicles are large and the amount of colloid increased. Some infants in areas of endemic goitre have large goitres but are euthyroid, i.e. not cretinous. Their large goitres have small follicles and hyperplasia of acinar cells.

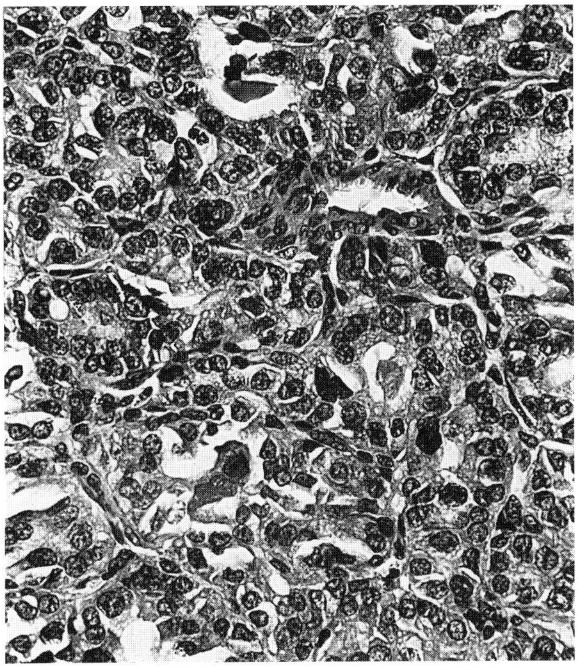

Fig. 21.26. Dyshormonogenetic thyroid gland. Hyperplastic nodule, small empty follicles, infolded lining cells showing nuclear pleomorphism. (H&E, ×284)

Congenital Thyrotoxicosis

Occasionally, thyrotoxic infants are born to mothers with thyrotoxicosis. As maternal TSH does not cross the placental barrier, the probable explanation is that maternal thyroid-stimulating IgG immunoglobulins are responsible. Histological examination shows a hyperplastic epithelium thrown into folds and colloid depletion. Affected infants are irritable, have diarrhoea and thyrotoxic cardiac failure. Twenty per cent die in the neonatal period.

Neonatal Goitres in Euthyroid Infants

Enlarged thyroids in euthyroid infants are a feature of thyroid dyshormonogenesis, some cases of environmental iodine deficiency (see above), and of certain iatrogenic disorders. *Congenital iodide goitre* is associated with prolonged use of *iodides* by the mother, as an expectorant in asthma and chronic bronchitis. Iodide crosses the placenta and inhibits peroxidase activity. Fetal T_4 levels fall and TSH levels increase. This causes hyperplasia of the gland, epithelial hyperplasia and varying degrees of colloid storage (Iancu et al. 1974). The gland may be so much enlarged that it causes respiratory obstruction in the neonate. *Para-amino salicyclic acid* for maternal tuberculosis may produce a similar type of congenital goitre.

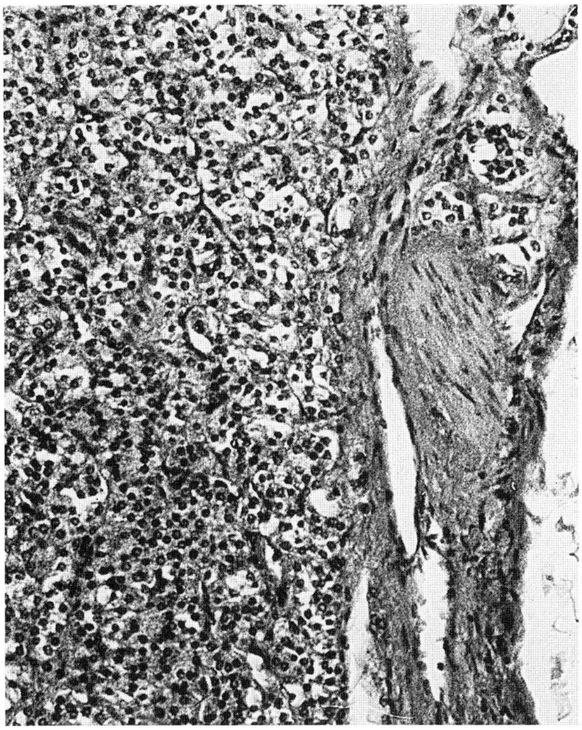

Fig. 21.27. Dyshormonogenetic thyroid gland. Marked nuclear pleomorphism with pseudomalignant capsular invasion. (H&E, ×315)

Tumours of the Thyroid

Teratomas are the most common neonatal thyroid tumour and may present with polyhydramnios.

Congenital carcinoma of the thyroid is extremely rare, and some of the cases reported were possibly examples of thyroid dyshormonogenesis.

Occult papillary carcinoma of the thyroid has been reported in a neonate (Mills and Allen, 1986).

Parathyroid Glands

Ontogeny

The parathyroids are variable in number and position, but usually number four. The superior pair are derived from the fourth pharyngeal pouch and lie close to the cricothyroid junction. The inferior pair, from the third pharyngeal pouch, are more variable in position but are usually posterolateral to the lower poles of the thyroid, although they may be found in the mediastinum within the thymus. Functionally there is only one cell type, which assumes three histological forms: chief cell (basic cell type), oxyphil cell and water clear cell. Only chief cells are found in the fetus and neonate. They secrete parathormone (PTH), which is controlled by the concentration of calcium ions in fluid perfusing the glands. Functional PTH can be detected in human fetal parathyroid from the 12th week, but blood levels are very low or undetectable because of suppression by the hypercalcaemic status of the normal fetus (Fleischman 1980).

Hypercalcaemia is achieved by an active placental pump of calcium from mother to fetus against a positive gradient; by this means the fetus will accrue 25–30 g of calcium by term. Calcitonin, secreted by parafollicular cells in the thyroid, inhibits bone dissolution, and its level in fetal serum is elevated above adult normal.

The combination of high calcitonin and hypercalcaemia enhances bone accretion and mineralisation of the fetal skeleton. Neither PTH nor calcitonin crosses the placenta, unlike the third hormone important in calcium homeostasis, 1,25 dihydroxycalciferol—vitamin D. Infants born with low levels of vitamin D, usually because of low maternal levels, have an increased incidence of early neonatal hypocalcaemia.

Pathology

Ectopia of the parathyroids, especially the inferior group, is common, and thymus and mediastinum are the usual sites. Ectopic parathyroid tissue has also been reported in the pericardium and in the wall of a thymic duct cyst.

Fetal and Neonatal Hypoparathyroidism

As PTH seems unnecessary for fetal calcium homeostasis and bone formation, deficient infants appear normal at birth. However, when falling blood calcium levels in the early neonatal period fail to trigger PTH secretion, severe hypocalcaemia develops with tetany and convulsions. There is hyperphosphataemia.

Primary hypoparathyroidism. This condition accompanies aplasia or hypoplasia of the parathyroid tissue in malformations involving the 3rd and 4th branchial clefts, e.g. in *Di George syndrome,* where there is associated thymic aplasia and malformation of the heart and aortic arch.

Idiopathic hypoparathyroidism. This condition rarely presents in the neonatal period. Some cases appear to have an X-linked recessive inheritance pattern (Peden 1960).

Secondary hypoparathyroidism. This condition occurs in babies of women with severe hypercalcaemia in pregnancy, usually complicating sarcoidosis, excessive vitamin D intake or hyperparathyroidism. Whatever the cause, maternal hypercalcaemia increases transport of calcium across the placenta, so that severe chronic fetal hypercalcaemia develops. This totally suppresses, and may even permanently damage, the infant's parathyroid function, so that neonatal hypocalcaemia develops.

Pseudohypoparathyroidism and *pseudopseudohypoparathyroidism.* The pseudo forms of hypoparathyroidism present in later childhood and are not due to parathyroid disorder.

Fetal and Neonatal Hyperparathyroidism

Hyperparathyroidism produces hypercalcaemia, which, in the neonate, presents with hypotonia, dehydration and respiratory distress. Generalised demineralisation of the skeleton, subperiosteal resorption, osteitis fibrosa cystica and even spontaneous rib cage fractures occur in severe untreated cases. The condition may be primary or secondary.

The only sure way to distinguish the primary and secondary fetal forms is by detailed study of the mother's own calcium status. This is very important for genetic counselling and management of future pregnancies.

Primary, familial hyperparathyroidism. Two main familial forms have been described: an autosomal-recessive type, *neonatal severe hyperparathyroidism (NSPH)* and an autosomal-dominant form which is usually part of the syndromes of multiple endocrine neoplasia (especially MEN 2) which presents in older children. In the cases of NSPH presented by Nishiyama et al. (1990) there was severe nephrocalcinosis and renal tubular acidosis.

Secondary fetal hyperparathyroidism. This condition, also known as neonatal rickets, occurs in infants as a response to chronic intrauterine hypocalcaemia. Fetal hypocalcaemia is due to diminished calcium transport across the placenta and is secondary to severe maternal hypocalcaemia. This may be caused by maternal hypoparathyroidism, severe dietary deficiency of vitamin D (as in Asian immigrants in the UK) and chronic renal failure.

Secondary neonatal hyperparathyroidism. Premature infants and neonates with malabsorption caused by biliary atresia may develop secondary hyperparathyroidism. The glands are only slightly enlarged and show uniform hyperplasia of the chief cells. Occasionally, nodular hyperplasia develops.

Early Neonatal Hypocalcaemia

Early neonatal hypocalcaemia occurs in approximately one-third of premature, sick neonates and is probably caused by failure of calcium homeostasis as a result of low vitamin D levels. Although the premature infant can eventually achieve adequate PTH levels, and has increased calcitonin levels, it frequently has decreased levels of 1,25 dihydroxycalciferol (vitamin D). This arrangement possibly tips the balance towards retaining calcium in the bone and diminishing the uptake from the gastrointestinal tract, so causing hypocalcaemia.

Early neonatal hypocalcaemia is more common after perinatal asphyxia or respiratory distress syndrome. It is a particular hazard for infants of diabetic mothers. The mechanism is not clear, but probably relates to the lower levels of 1,25 dihydroxycalciferol present in the serum of diabetic mothers at term. Hypocalcaemia is also found in hypomagnesia and hypoparathyroidism (see above).

Endocrine Pancreas

Ontogeny

The pancreas arises from two diverticula from the dorsal and ventral surfaces of the gut. As well as producing digestive enzymes (exocrine pancreas), the pancreas contains cells, mainly within the islets of Langerhans (endocrine pancreas), which produce a group of polypeptide hormones and are part of the APUD system. These peptide hormones are concerned with regulating the utilisation and storage of nutrients once they reach the bloodstream. There are four cell types in the endocrine pancreas: A cells produce glucagon, B cells produce insulin, D cells produce somatostatin and PP cells probably produce a variety of polypeptide hormones. G cells, which produce gastrin, may also occur in the pancreas.

The origin of these endocrine cells is controversial (see p. 499). A cells appear as early as 9 weeks and B cells at 10–11 weeks. They appear to develop in two generations (Liu and Potter 1962). The first generation comes from paratubular cell buds, later detaching and establishing the primary islets which continue to enlarge until 20 weeks' gestation, after which they disintegrate. From about 16 weeks the second generation of islets arises from terminal ducts and forms secondary islets which continue to increase in number and size to become typical adult islets. Because of this pattern of development the fetal and neonatal endocrine pancreas is much more diffuse and visibly occupies a higher proportion of the pancreatic volume than in older children and adults. It is important to remember this difference when assessing a neonatal pancreas for nesidioblastosis (excess endocrine tissue).

Insulin in B cells is detectable as early as 10 weeks, and prolonged hyperglycaemia will elevate fetal insulin levels (Obenshain et al. 1970), although less rapidly than certain amino acids (Milner et al. 1971). Glucagon in A cells appears at 8–9 weeks. In utero, glucagon shows no response to low glucose levels, adopting its regulatory role only after birth.

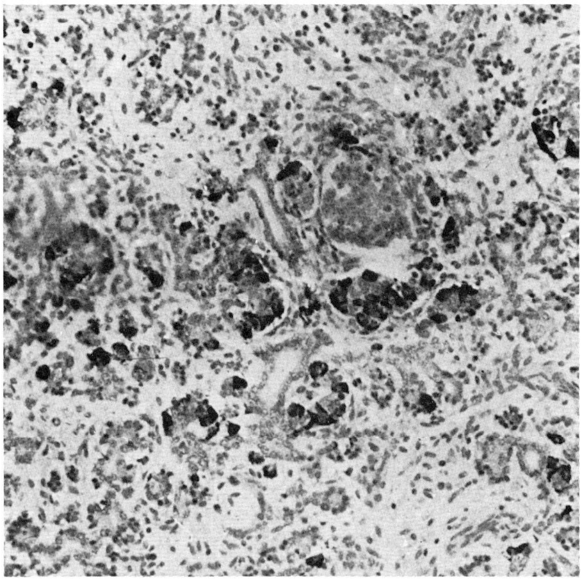

Fig. 21.28. Fetal pancreas, 14 weeks. Diffuse pattern of endocrine cells. Stained for human prealbumin, an APUD cell marker. (Gray et al. 1985.) (PAP, ×145)

However, glucagon levels are raised in fetal and perinatal distress (Hill 1980), and in erythroblastosis fetalis.

Histological study of the endocrine pancreas is more satisfactory if the tissue has been fixed in Bouin's solution. Although traditional stains can be used to differentiate the cell types, this is more reliably done by immunocytochemical techniques, and by electron microscopy.

Normal Histological Variations in the Fetal and Neonatal Pancreas

In the fetal and neonatal pancreas there is a variable but higher proportion of non-islet endocrine cells than in the adult (Fig. 21.28), and the percentage of pancreas occupied by endocrine tissue in the neonate (10%) (Jaffe et al. 1980) is much higher than in the adult (1%–2%). This diffuse involvement might suggest a pathological excess of endocrine tissue (diffuse nesidioblastosis, see p. 523), so it is most important in such cases to compare with several age-matched controls. There is also proportionately more endocrine tissue in the body and tail of the pancreas than in the head, so that sampling should also be comparable. Minor *cellular infiltrations* are relatively common. The infiltrate is usually of the erythromyeloid series and most marked in preterm infants. If myeloid, it may indicate a generalised leukaemoid reaction, as occurs in infection and trisomies 21 and 18. Occasionally, the infiltrate is predominantly lymphocytic. Liu and Potter (1962) found 50% of fetuses had a *lymphocytic infiltrate*, which was most marked between the 6th and 8th months, but present also at term. It has been postulated that this infiltrate is related to the natural degeneration of the primary islet tissue and of A cells in particular.

Pathology

Absence

Absence of the endocrine pancreas occurs in total *pancreatic agenesis*. Maternal insulin does not cross the placenta; thus these infants have total insulin deficiency. They are severely growth retarded, achieving only 28–30-week fetal size at term, lack fat deposition and have poor muscle development. Pancreatic agenesis is very rare and possibly has an autosomal-recessive inheritance.

Hyperplasia

A list of conditions in the fetus and neonate in which there is hyperplasia of the endocrine pancreas is given in Table 21.1.

Table 21.1. Conditions associated with hyperplasia of the endocrine pancreas

Infants of diabetic mothers (IDM)	
Erythroblastosis fetalis	
Beckwith–Wiedemann syndrome	
Zellweger syndrome (occasionally)	
Neonatal hepatitis (occasionally)	
Intrauterine growth retardation (occasionally)	
Persistent hyperinsulinaemic hypoglycaemia of infancy	diffuse nesidioblastosis, focal nesidioblastosis, adenoma

Infants of Diabetic Mothers

Infants of diabetic mothers (IDM) have many problems; the most fequent are increased somatic size (macrosomia) (Fig. 21.29), increased

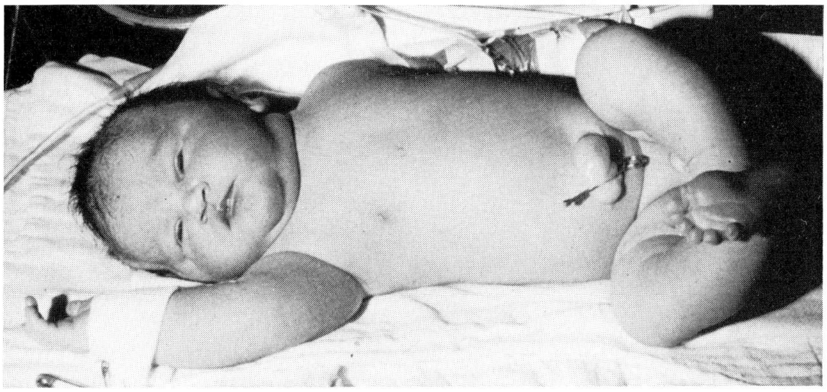

Fig. 21.29. Infant of diabetic mother. There is macrosomia and obesity.

incidence of perinatal death, increased frequency of malformation and hypertrophy of the islets of Langerhans, with B cell hyperplasia and hyperinsulinaemia. Morriss (1984), in an excellent review, explains many of these features, and many other clinical problems experienced by the IDM in the neonatal period, as the result of persistent maternal hyperglycaemia. However, maternal hyperglycaemia cannot be the only cause of islet hyperplasia, as both it and fetal hyperinsulinism have been found in IDM as early as 4 months' gestation, and the B cell is not responsive to glucose levels till after 24 weeks (Bloodworth 1982). Interestingly, ionic stimuli, leucine and arginine (Milner et al. 1971) are known to stimulate fetal B cells from 14 weeks onwards, and maternal hyperaminoacidaemia has been reported even in the mildest gestational diabetes (Milner 1979). This may explain the islet hyperplasia in some infants of prediabetic women (Fig. 21.30). The fetal hypothalamic–pituitary axis has an ill-understood role in B cell function: anencephalic infants of diabetic mothers fail to develop B cell hyperplasia (Van Assche et al. 1969).

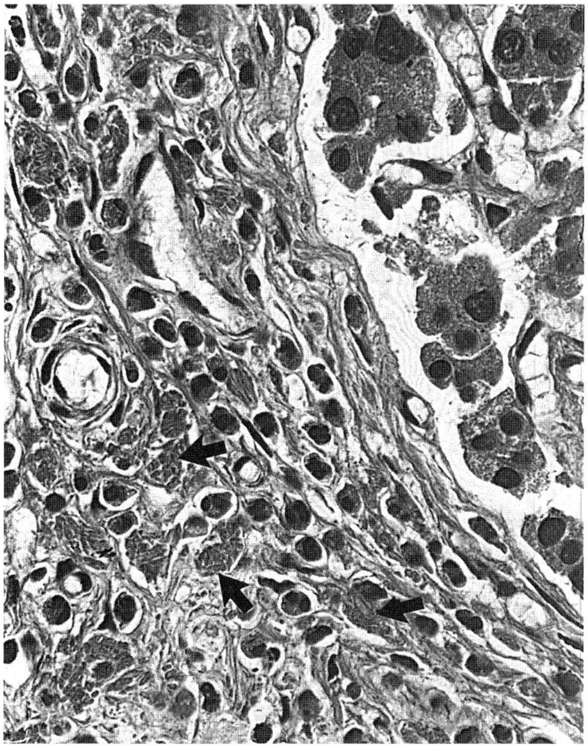

Fig. 21.30. Pancreas, neonate of prediabetic mother. Numerous eosinophils and Charcot-Leyden crystals (*arrows*). (H&E, ×292)

Histological examination of the pancreas in IDM shows an increased islet cell mass of about three times normal (Fig. 21.31a). This is due to hypertrophy of the islets (macronesia), neoformation of islets (polynesia), and hyperplasia of islet cells. The bulk of the increase is due to a great increase in B cells, but non-B cells are also increased. The B cells usually show nuclear pleomorphism and gigantism (Fig. 21.31b). In contrast the enlarged islets of erythroblastosis fetalis do not show this selective increase of B cells.

Numerous necropsy studies have shown that 34%–65% of IDM have cellular infiltration around, but not usually within, some hypertrophied islets (Fig. 21.32). Lymphocytes, histiocytes (occasionally with Charcot–Leyden crystals) and neutrophils are also present, but the eosinophilic infiltration is specific to IDM. Eosinophil insulitis is not found in erythroblastosis fetalis (see p. 523), the other condition

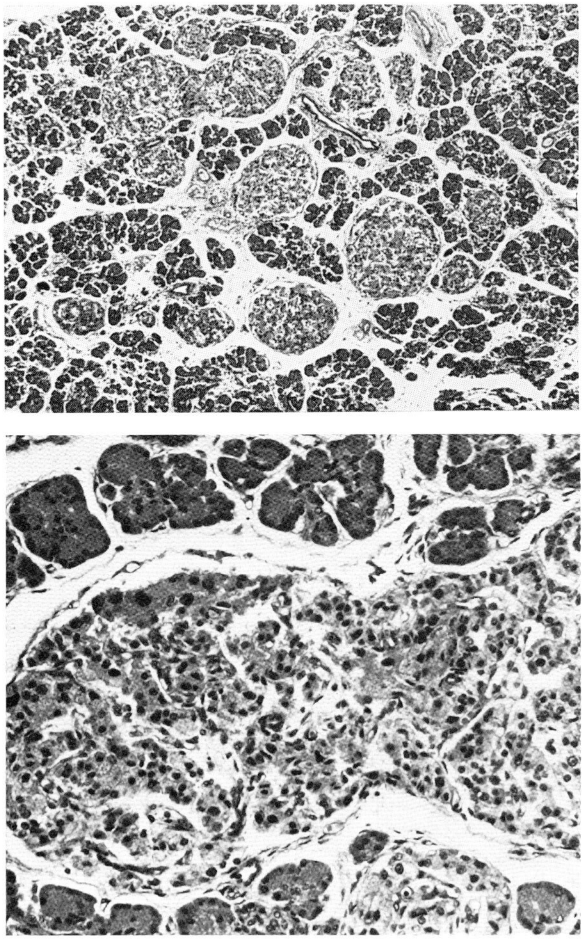
a
b

Fig. 21.31. a Pancreas of neonate (2.96 g): maternal diabetes. Increased islet size, no cellular infiltrate. ((H&E, ×50) b Nuclear pleomorphism and gigantism. (H&E, ×220.) (Both courtesy of Dr. A.M. Gibson, Glasgow.) (H&E, ×200)

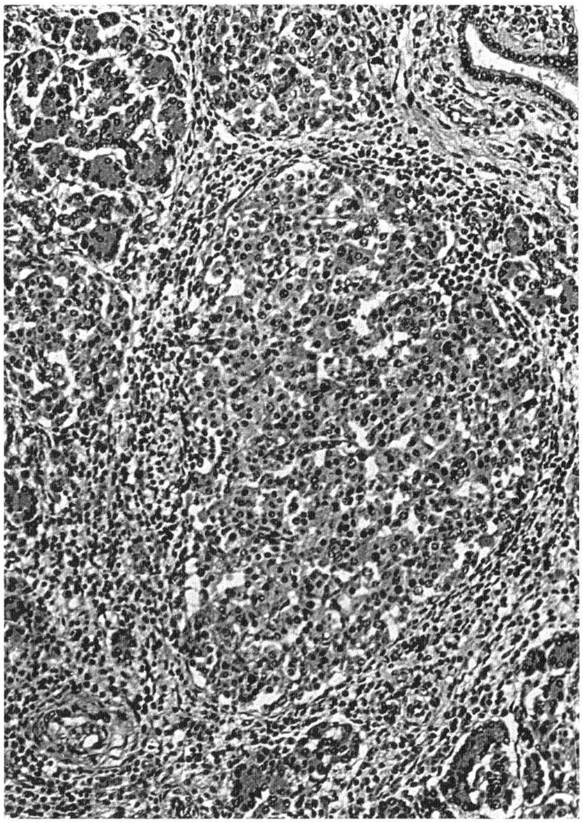

Fig. 21.32. Pancreas, neonate (5.2 kg): maternal glycosuria. Hypertrophied islets, nuclear gigantism, marked peri-insular cellular infiltration. (Courtesy of Dr. A.M. Gibson, Glasgow.) (H&E, ×236)

where islet hypertrophy is associated with cellular infiltration (Figs. 21.32, 21.33). It may, however, be seen in the pancreas in infants of prediabetic women (Fig. 21.30). Its presence and significance should be drawn to the attention of the obstetrician. Because eosinophilic infiltrates are not found in other viscera in IDM, its apparently organ-specific nature has caused speculation about a local immune reaction with maternal anti-insulin antibodies. There is considerable experimental and some clinical evidence to support this hypothesis, but the eosinophilic infiltrate has been found in IDM whose mothers have not had insulin (Silverman 1963) and moreover were considered to be non-diabetic at that time. This does not exclude the possibility of maternal IgG autoantibodies to insulin or islets crossing the placenta to localise in fetal islets. The eosinophil infiltration disappears a few days after birth.

From about 11 days onwards there may be fibrosis of the islets, affecting up to 20% of the islet mass (Nelson et al. 1977). It may be the sequel to cellular infiltration; it is not usually found in non-IDM infants, does not affect all islets, and may occur in IDM whose mothers do not receive insulin. These pancreatic changes are independent of the severity of the maternal diabetes and may be seen in infants whose mothers only exhibit diabetes many years later.

Hyperplasia of fetal B cells is associated with fetal hyperinsulinaemia, which may lead to neonatal hypoglycaemia.

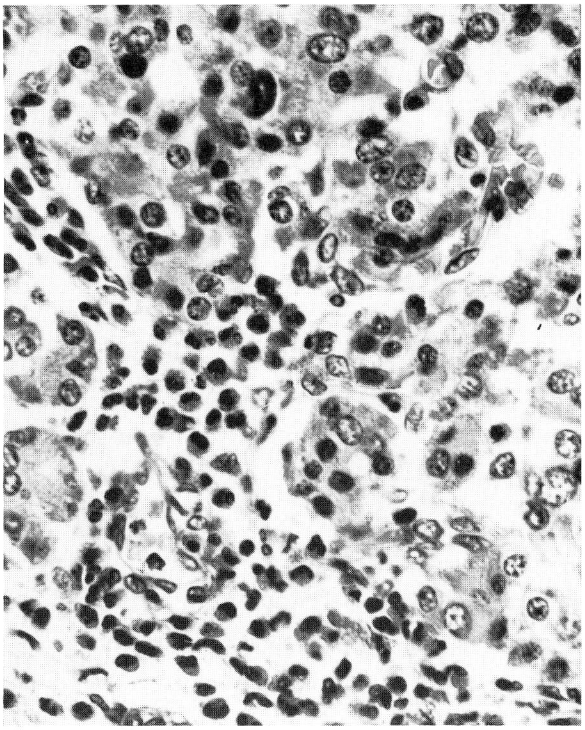

Fig. 21.33. Pancreas, same neonate as Fig. 21.32. Numerous eosinophils around and within islet. (Courtesy of Dr. A.M. Gibson, Glasgow.) (H&E, ×1250)

Table 21.2. The causes, at necropsy, of perinatal death in 50 IDM (Warren et al. 1966)

Unexplained[a]	36%
Prematurity[b]	26%
Hyaline membrane disease	16%
Birth injury (meningeal tears)	8%
Pneumonia	6%
Malformations	6%
Adrenal haemorrhage	2%

[a] Includes 11 macerated stillbirths.
[b] Defined as <32 weeks or <1500 g.

Table 21.3. Primary causes of neonatal death in 39 IDM compared with 70 non-IDM (Hubbell et al. 1965)

	IDM[a]		non-IDM (≤2500 g)	
	No.	%	No.	%
Extreme prematurity	1	2.5	7	10
Hyaline membrane disease (HMD)	18	46	23	33
Respiratory pathology (not HMD)	3	8	18	26
Congenital malformations	10	26	5	7
Infection (non-pulmonary)	6	15	1	1
Neurological (asphyxial)	0	0	10	14
Other	1	2.5	6	9
Total	39	100	70	100

[a] All deaths occurred to babies ≤37 weeks' gestation.

Increased perinatal mortality. A feature of the diabetic pregnancy is increased perinatal mortality (PNM). Before 1921 most babies and many diabetic mothers died in pregnancy. Rigorous control of maternal diabetes has reduced overall perinatal mortality to less than 2% (Somville 1990) but this is still two to three times higher than in non-diabetic pregnancies. The risk of fetal loss depends on the duration and severity of maternal diabetes and on the degree of uterine vascular damage. White (1965) defined five classes of maternal diabetes. In class A (gestational diabetes) the PNM was 16/1000, and class D (with diabetic vascular disease) PNM was >100/1000. The causes of perinatal and neonatal death in IDM are shown in Tables 21.2 and 21.3, respectively. The increase in PNM was due to an increase in both intrauterine and neonatal death. The increased risk of fetal death begins in the third trimester and increases gradually from the 30th to 40th weeks. Necropsy of stillborn infants usually fails to reveal a cause of death, although some will have malformations.

Experimental studies (Milley et al. 1981) have shown that fetal hyperglycaemia in lambs causes hypoxaemia, increased cardiac output, increased BMR and diminished cord blood flow. A similar pathophysiological state in humans may be the cause of unexplained intrauterine deaths in diabetic pregnancies. The stillbirth rate has been reduced dramatically by strict control of maternal hyperglycaemia.

Macrosomia. This condition is present in many IDM and consists of enlarged viscera, particularly liver, heart and adrenals, and adiposity. The brain is often smaller than normal. The thymus may show cortical involution.

The cause of macrosomia and adiposity is partly the combination of fetal hyperglycaemia and fetal hyperinsulinaemia (insulin does not cross the placenta), which results in glucose being converted to fat and protein. Macrosomia does not appear before 28 weeks' gestation, possibly because of low fetal tissue sensitivity to insulin action before this. Not all IDM are macrosomic and, if there is severe maternal vascular disease diminishing blood flow to the placenta, the fetus may show intrauterine growth retardation.

Macrosomia greatly increases the risk of shoulder dystocia and cephalopelvic disproportion, producing birth injury and intrapartum asphyxia. Although the incidence of macrosomia is reduced by good control of the diabetes, the condition can precede the onset of maternal diabetes, suggesting a more complex aetiology than fetal and maternal hyperglycaemia.

Cardiomegaly. Even in the absence of macrosomia, cardiomegaly occurs in IDM and 30% have transient hypertrophic cardiomegaly (Gutgesell et al. 1980) There may be generalised ventricular hypertrophy with asymmetric hypertrophy of the septum. If very severe, it may induce cardiac failure as the result of obstruction of the outflow (hypertrophic obstructive cardiomyopathy; HOCM). Histologically there is whorling and disorganisation of the muscle fibres in the septum and there may be foci of necrosis (Gutgesell et al. 1980), constituting cardiomyopathy.

The cause is not known but could be due to increased cardiac outflow in IDM or to direct action of insulin on fetal myocardium, which is very rich in insulin receptors.

Congenital malformations. There is an increased risk of most congenital malformations in diabetic pregnancies. A large prospective study has shown that infants of insulin-dependent diabetics are eight times more likely to have a major malformation (Becerra et al. 1990). Contrary to some earlier reports (Pedersen 1977) there is also an increase in minor malformations (Rosenn et al. 1990). An increase in anencephaly, spina bifida, hydrocephaly, coloboma, transposition of great vessels, ventricular septal defect, patent ductus arteriosus and limb flexion contractures is found (Becerra et al. 1990). Neave (1984) found an increased frequency of single umbilical artery and of microcephaly. Sacral dysgenesis and other caudal regression syndromes have been linked with IDM but Becerra et al. (1990) found only 2 of 9 cases of caudal regression had a history of maternal diabetes. A large study of limb reduction defects in Sweden between 1973 and 1986 showed no association with maternal diabetes (Kallen 1989).

Congenital malformations are more frequent amongst infants of women with poorly controlled diabetes (Miller et al. 1981). Studies of glycosylated haemoglobin, an index of long-term glucose control, have shown that elevated levels in the first trimester increase the risk of congenital malformations (Reece and Hobbins 1986; Rosenn et al. 1990). Malformation rates were related to the severity of diabetes using White's classification. However Damm and Molsted-Pedersen (1989) have shown a fourfold decline in major malformations in White Classes D and E between 1977 and 1986, with loss of the previously observed correlation between the severity of the maternal diabetes and the frequency of malformations. This probably reflects better diabetic control.

Placental pathology. The placenta in IDM tends to be heavy, but if there is maternal vascular disease the placenta is small and infarcts are present (see Chap. 2, p. 69). There is an increased incidence of single umbilical artery (3%–5%). Placental pathology in IDM is detailed by Fox (1978).

Other complications. Polyhydramnios is more common in IDM. In the neonatal period IDM are susceptible to *hypocalcaemia* (see p. 517), *renal vein thrombosis, hyperbilirubinaemia* and, most important, *respiratory distress syndrome.* This last condition, which was a major cause of death in IDM in the past, is possibly due to retarded production of one fetal lung phospholipid important for effective surfactant action (Cunningham et al. 1978).

Infants of maternal gestational diabetics. These infants may show some of the clinical features found in IDM but are usually less severely affected. Nonetheless, their metabolism is abnormal, producing hyperplasia of the islets of Langerhans. There is a significant increase in congenital heart disease in infants of women with gestational diabetes needing insulin during pregnancy.

Beckwith–Wiedemann Syndrome

The Beckwith–Wiedemann syndrome is characterised by exomphalos, macroglossia, visceromegaly, mild microcephaly, gigantism and hyperinsulinaemic hypoglycaemia. Histological examination shows islet cell hypertrophy, without a generalised pancreatic endocrine tissue increase and adrenal cytomegaly (see Fig. 21.14). That this condition may be due to an abnormality of fetal growth-regulating peptides is supported by the relative absence of somatostatin cells in the hyperplastic islets (Aynsley-Green 1982), and elevated levels of plasma GH and somatomedin at birth (Ashton and Aynsley-Green 1978).

The Beckwith–Wiedemann syndrome is inherited as an autosomal-recessive condition. There is an increased risk of nephroblastoma and other childhood tumours.

Erythroblastosis Fetalis

In severe erythroblastosis fetalis there is hyperplasia of the islets with cytomegaly, and the interstitium is infiltrated by erythropoietic cells (Fig. 21.34). The cause of islet hyperplasia is not known but it is functional, so that neonatal hypoglycaemia is a hazard in the newborn. Unlike the islet hyperplasia in IDM, where B cells predominate, normal distribution of insulin- and glucagon-secreting cells is maintained within the hyperplastic islets.

Islet Hyperplasia and Liver Disease

The Zellweger (cerebrohepatorenal) syndrome is characterised by abnormal facies, hypotonia, hepatic fibrosis, renal microcysts and abnormalities of the central nervous system. Several reported cases have shown hyperplasia of the islets of Langerhans. The syndrome is autosomal recessive and of uncertain aetiology.

Hyperplasia of the islets may be secondary to other liver disease; hyperplasia is found at necropsy in some neonates dying of neonatal hepatitis (Greco and Finegold 1973). The relationship between islet function and liver disease is unknown but could be due to elevated levels of amino acids which are tropic to fetal and neonatal islets (Milner 1979).

Persistent Hyperinsulinaemic Hypoglycaemia of Infancy: Nesidioblastosis

Many conditions produce transient or short-term hypoglycaemia in neonates, including the conditions causing islet hyperplasia already mentioned. In 20%–50% of cases, hypoglycaemia is persistent and severe and associated with inappropriately high insulin levels. If untreated, the infant dies; survivors may show permanent hypoglycaemic brain damage.

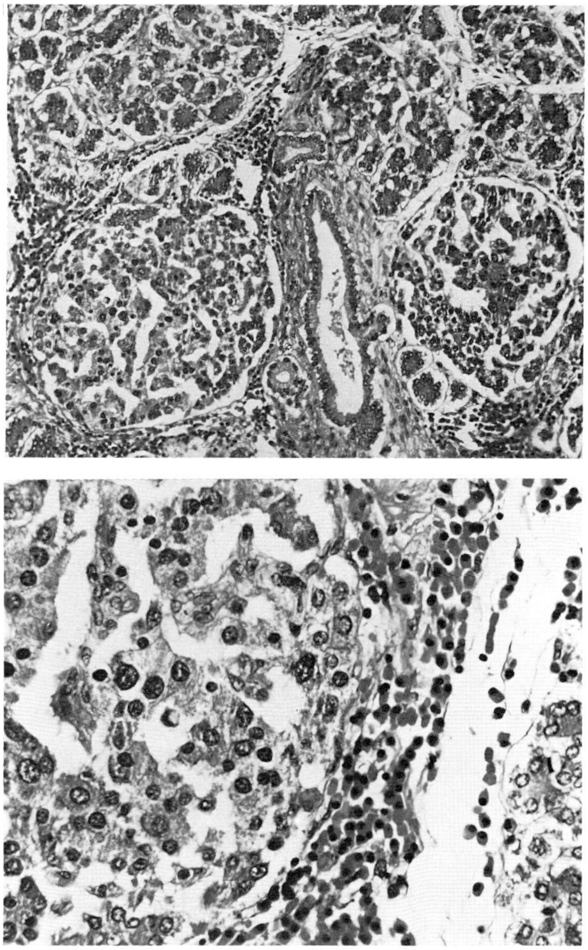

Fig. 21.34. Pancreas, term neonate: erythroblastosis fetalis (anti-Kell). **a** Hyperplastic islets, nuclear gigantism, interstitial infiltration (could be mistaken for IDM). (H&E, ×200.) **b** Infiltrate is erythropoietic (normoblasts). (cf. Fig. 21.33.) (H&E, ×800)

Familial forms exist and have an autosomal recessive inheritance pattern (Moreno et al. 1989)

In the majority of cases of persistent hyperinsulinaemic hypoglycaemia there is a morphological as well as a functional abnormality of the endocrine pancreas. This is commonly called *nesidioblastosis* (Laidlaw 1938). Because endocrine malfunction appears more important than morphology, other names, such as *nesidiodysplasia* (Gould et al. 1983) and *endocrine cell dysplasia* (Jaffe et al. 1980) have been suggested. Despite their logic neither term has been widely accepted to replace nesidioblastosis. Three forms of nesidioblastosis are described: *diffuse*, *focal* and, rare in infancy, *adenoma*.

a
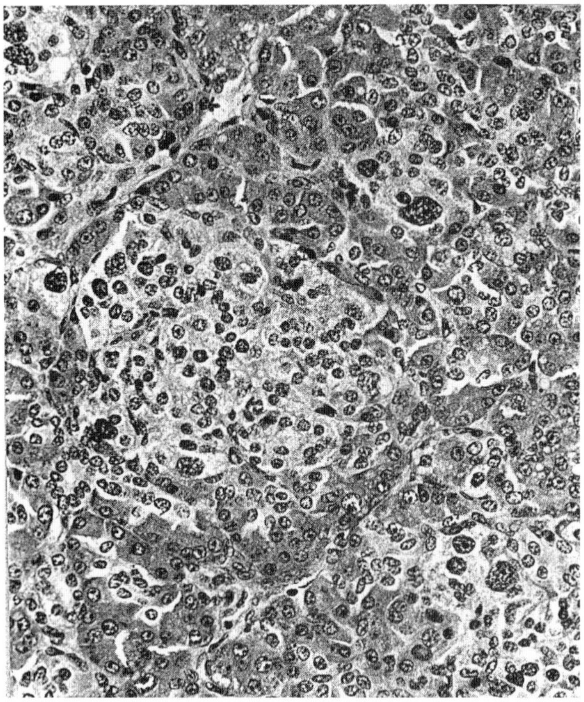

b
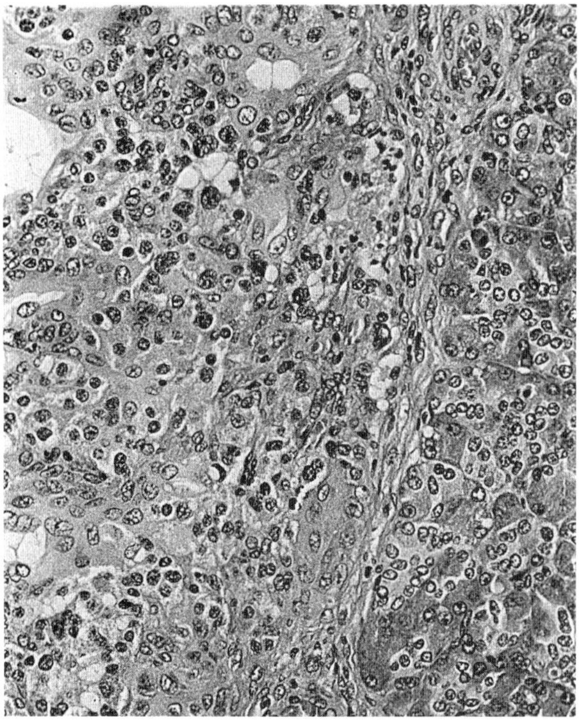

Fig. 21.35a,b. Pancreas, neonate with persistent hypoglycaemic hyperinsulinism. **a** Nuclear gigantism of both islet and non-islet endocrine cells. (H&E ×130). **b** Hyperplastic ducto-insular complex with squamous metaplasia and pleomorphism of endocrine cell component (H&E ×130). (Courtesy of Dr. A. Howatson, Glasgow).

In *diffuse nesidioblastosis* the pancreas is macroscopically normal. Histological examination shows an apparent increase in both islet and non-islet endocrine tissue. There is usually nuclear pleomorphism and gigantism of the insulin-producing B cells indicating hyperfunction (Fig. 21.35a). Ductuloinsular complexes may be hyperplastic with squamous metaplasia of ductular epithelium (Fig. 21.35b). Immunocytochemistry demonstrates all endocrine cell types and B cells may predominate. Not all cases of diffuse nesidioblastosis show hypertrophy of B cells and can thus be very difficult to distinguish from the normal perinatal pancreas with its high proportion (10%) of endocrine cells. Even quantitative studies (Jaffe et al. 1980; Gould et al. 1983) comparing total endocrine tissue and B cells in the pancreas of infants with persistent hypoglycaemia with normal controls found that the endocrine mass was not invariably higher in hypoglycaemic patients.

Focal nesidioblastosis and discrete *adenomas* are less of a diagnostic problem. One or more pale nodules 0.5–1.0 cm diameter may be visible.

In focal adenomatosis 40% of the affected area may be replaced by endocrine cells. They may be so densely packed that the admixed exocrine acini and ducts may be difficult to see so that the lesion mimics a true adenoma. Within focal nesidioblastosis the B cells may be very large with nuclear gigantism. Although all endocrine cell types are present, insulin cells predominate. In a true adenoma, no exocrine pancreas is present. It is composed entirely of B cells separated by fibrous septa. In a Belgian study (Goossens et al. 1989) of 24 neonates with hyperinsulinaemic hypoglycaemia 3 infants showed no B cell hypertrophy, 9 showed diffuse nesidioblastosis and 12 had focal lesions (Fig. 21.36).

In all cases of persistent hyperinsulinaemic hypoglycaemia in which any form of nesidioblastosis is suspected, immunohistochemical stains for insulin and other peptides should be carried out.

Rare causes of persistent neonatal hypoglycaemia are hypopituitarism, GH deficiency, hypomagnesia and glycogenosis types I and II.

Infection

CMV, mumps virus and the Coxsackie virus group can all infect the endocrine tissue. In

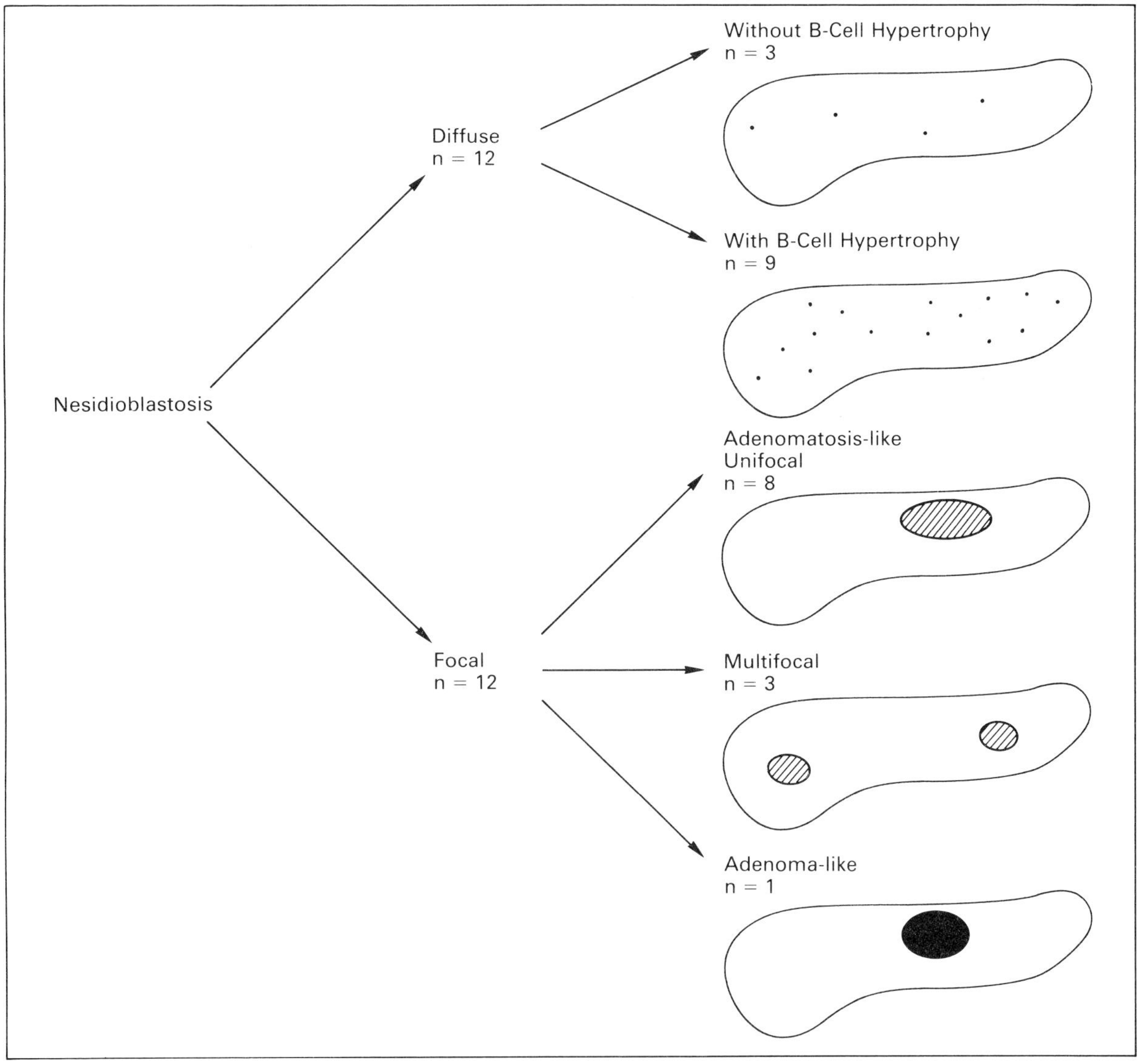

Fig. 21.36. Distribution of focal and diffuse nesidioblastosis in 24 infants with persistent neonatal hyperinsulinaemic hypoglycaemia (after Goosens et al. 1989).

CMV, typical "owl's eye" viral inclusions can be seen in islet cells (Fig. 21.37) but no inflammatory response is elicited and destruction of the islets does not appear to occur.

Mumps has not been shown to produce any specific lesion, but Coxsackie B viral infections do produce islet damage and for this reason have caused much interest as a possible environmental factor in the onset of diabetes mellitus.

Coxsackie B infections in neonates usually present as myocarditis, but occasionally there is involvement of the exocrine and endocrine pancreas. The histological picture is quite variable but the characteristic feature is a necrosis of many of the islet cells, the cytoplasm being intensely eosinophilic and the B cell nuclei pyknotic or even fragmented. The diagnosis may be easy to miss if there is not a significant accompanying inflammatory infiltrate (Fig. 21.38).

In our own case there was a generalised sparse interstitial lymphocyte infiltrate, but around the necrotic islets were numerous eosinophils (Fig. 21.39). Eosinophils are not described in a previous case (Yoon et al. 1979).

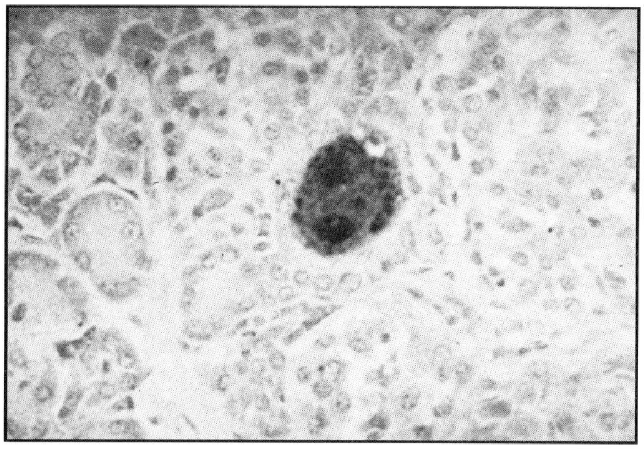

Fig. 21.37. Pancreas, stillbirth. CMV inclusion in islet cell. (PAP, ×1200)

The cells being destroyed are thought to be B cells; this was demonstrated in our case by immunohistochemical studies which showed total loss of insulin-containing cells.

The possible role of such viral infections of the endocrine pancreas in triggering insulin-

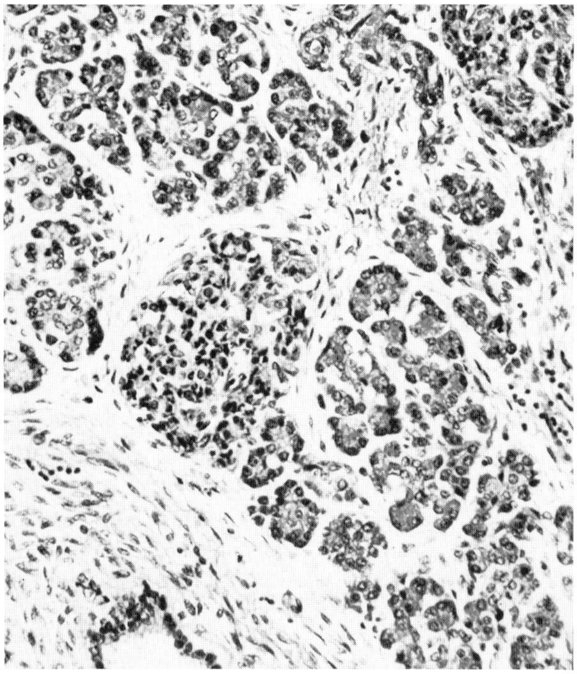

Fig. 21.38. Pancreas, neonate (3 days). Islet cells show eosinophilic shrinkage of cytoplasm, nuclear pyknosis and fragmentation. Probable Coxsackie infection. (Courtesy of Dr. A. King, Cambridge.) (H&E, ×200)

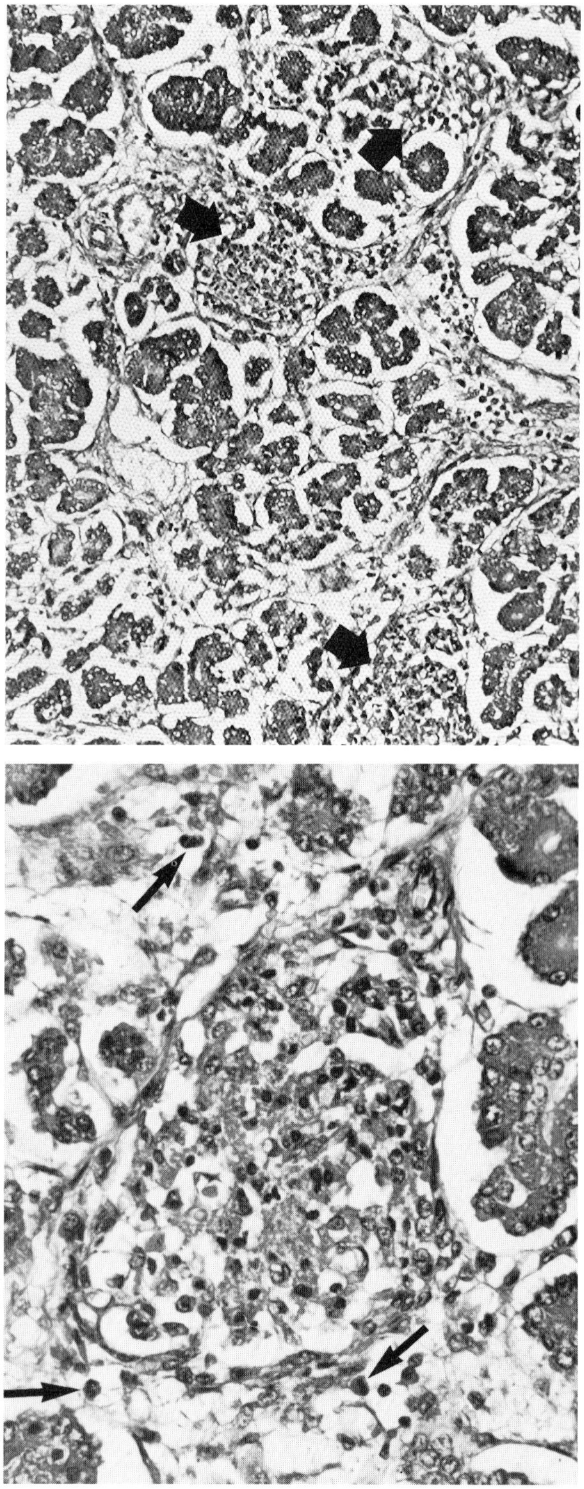

Fig. 21.39. Pancreas, neonate (9 days) with generalised Coxsackie B 3 infection. **a** Interstitial inflammatory infiltrate; severe necrosis of islets (*arrowed*). (H&E, ×125.) **b** Eosinophilic necrosis of islet cells; infiltrate of lymphocytes and eosinophils (*arrows*). (H&E, ×200)

dependent diabetes mellitus (IDDM) is controversial, but there are some human and animal studies implicating both mumps and Coxsackie. This topic as well reviewed by Klöppel (1984).

References

Artal R (1980) Fetal adrenal medulla. Clin Obstet Gynaecol 23: 825–836

Ashton IK, Aynsley-Green A (1978) Somatomedin in an infant with Beckwith's syndrome. Early Hum Dev 1: 357–366

Aynsley-Green A (1982) Hypoglycemia in infants and children. Clin Endocrinol Metab 11: 159–194

Becerra JE, Khoury MJ, Cordero JF, Erickson JD (1990) Diabetes mellitus during pregnancy and the risks for specific birth defects: a population based case-control study. Pediatrics 85: 1–9

Becker MJ, Becker AE (1976) Fat distribution in the adrenal cortex as an indication of the mode of intrauterine death. Hum Pathol 7: 495–504

Bloodworth JMB (ed) (1982) Endocrine pathology. Williams and Wilkins, Baltimore, p 625

Buster JE (1980) Fetal adrenal cortex. Clin Obstet Gynecol 23: 803–824

Cagle PT, Hough AJ, Pysher J et al. (1986) Comparison of adrenal cortical tumours in children and adults. Cancer 57: 2235–2237

Cunningham MD, Desai NS, Thompson SA, Greene JM (1978) Amniotic fluid phosphatidyl glycerol in diabetic pregnancies. Am J Obstet Gynecol 131: 719–724

Damm P, Molsted-Pedersen L (1989) Significant decrease in congenital malformations in newborn infants of an unselected population of diabetic women. Am J Obstet Gynecol 161: 1163–1167

Danziger Y, Pertzelan A, Mimouri M (1987) Transient congenital hypothyroidism after topical iodine in pregnancy. Arch Dis Child 62: 295–296

DeSa DJ (1978) Stress response and its relationship to cystic (pseudofollicular) change in the definitive cortex of the adrenal gland in stillborn infants. Arch Dis Child 53: 769–776

Facchinetti F, Lanzani A, Genazzani AR (1989) Fetal intermediate lobe is stimulated by parturition. Am J Obstet Gynecol 161: 1267–1270

Faggiano M, Minozzi M, Lombardi G, Carella C, Criscuolo T (1975) Two cases of the chromatin positive variety of ovarian dysgenesis (XO/XX mosaicism) associated with HGH deficiency and marginal impairment of other hypothalamic pituitary functions. Clin Genet 8: 324–329

Fisher DA, Odell WD (1969) Acute release of thyrotropin in the newborn. J Clin Invest 48: 1670–1677

Fleischman AR (1980) Fetal parathyroid gland and calcium homeostasis. Clin Obstet Gynecol 23: 791–802

Fox H (1978) Pathology of the placenta. Saunders, London, pp 223–230

Fujeida K, Faiman C, Reyes FI, Winter JSD (1981) The control of steroidogenesis by the human fetal adrenal cells in tissue culture, III. The effects of various hormonal peptides. J Clin Endocrinol Metab 53: 690–693

Fujeida K, Farman C, Reyes FI, Winter JSD (1982) The control of steroidogenesis by the human fetal adrenal cells in tissue culture, IV. The effects of exposure to placental steroids. J Clin Endocrinol Metab 54: 89–94

Gaillard DA, Lallemand AV, Moirot HH, Visseaux-Coletto BJ, Paradis PH (1990) Fetal adrenal development during the second trimester of gestation. Pediatr Pathol 10: 335–350

Goodyer GC, Guyda H, Giroud CJP (1979) Development of the hypothalamic-pituitary axis in the human fetus. In: Tolis G, Labrie G, Martin JB, Naftolin F (eds) Clinical neuroendocrinology: a pathophysiological approach. Raven, New York, pp 199–214

Goossens A, Gepts W, Saudubray JM et al. (1989) Diffuse and focal nesidioblastosis. A clinicopathological study of 24 patients with persistent neonatal hyperinsulinemic hypoglycemia. Am J Surg Pathol 13: 766–775

Gould VE, Dardi LE, Gould NS (1983) Nesidiodysplasia and nesidioblastosis of infancy: structural and functional correlations with the syndrome of hyperinsulinemic hypoglycemia. Pediatr Pathol 1: 7–13

Gray ES, Abramovich DR (1980) Morphologic features of the anencephalic adrenal gland in early pregnancy. Am J Obstet Gynecol 137: 491–495

Greco MA, Finegold MJ (1973) Familial giant cell hepatitis. Report of two cases and a review of the literature. Arch Pathol 95: 240–244

Gutgesell HP, Spear M, Rosenberg HS (1980) Characterisation of the cardiomyopathy of infants of diabetic mothers. Circulation 61: 441–450

Han VKM, Lund PK, Lee DC, D'Ercole AJ (1988) Expression of somatomedin/insulin-like growth factor messenger ribonucleic acids in the human fetus: identification, characterisation and tissue distribution. J Clin Endocrinol Metab 66: 422–429

Hayek A, Driscol SG, Warshaw JB (1973) Endocrine studies in anencephaly. J Clin Invest 52: 1636–1641

Hetzel BS, Mano MT (1989) A review of experimental studies of iodine deficiency during fetal development. J Nutr 119: 145–151

Hill DE (1980) Fetal endocrine pancreas. Clin Obstet Gynaecol 23: 837–847

Hobel CJ (1980) Fetal thyroid. Clin Obstet Gynecol 23: 779–790

Hubbell JP, Muirhead DM, Drorbaugh JE (1965) The newborn infant of the diabetic mother. Med Clin North Am 49: 1035–1052

Iancu T, Boyanower Y, Laurian N (1974) Congenital goiter due to maternal ingestion of iodide. Am J Dis Child 128: 528–530

Jack PMB, Milner RDG (1975) Effect of decapitation and ACTH on somatic development of the rabbit fetus. Biol Neonate 26: 195–204

Jaffe R, Hashida Y, Yunis EJ (1980) Pancreatic pathology in hyperinsulinic hypoglycemia of infancy. Lab Invest 42: 356–365

Kallen B (1989) A prospective study of some aetiological factors in limb-reduction defects in Sweden. J Epidemiol Community Health 43: 86–91

Kerenyi N (1961) Congenital adrenal hypoplasia. Report of a case of extreme adrenal hypoplasia and neurohypophyseal aplasia. Arch Pathol 71: 336–343

Klöppel G (1984) Islet histopathology in diabetes mellitus. In: Klöppel G, Heitz PU (eds) Pancreatic pathology. Churchill Livingstone, Edinburgh, pp 173–174

Laidlaw GF (1938) Nesidioblastoma, islet tumor of pancreas. Am J Pathol 14: 125–134

Larroche JC (1977) Developmental pathology of the neonate. Excerpta Medica, Amsterdam, p 220

Le Douarin NM (1978) The embryological origin of the

endocrine cells associated with the digestive tract; experimental analysis based on the use of stable cell marking technique. In: Bloom SR (ed) Gut hormones. Churchill Livingstone, Edinburgh
Lui HM, Potter EL (1962) Development of the human pancreas. Arch Pathol 74: 439–452
Miller E, Hare JW, Cloherty JP, Dunn PJ, Gleason RE, Soeldner JS, Kitzmiller JL (1981) Elevated maternal hemoglobin AIC in early pregnancy and major congenital anomalies in the infants of diabetic mothers. N Engl J Med 304: 1331–1334
Milley JR, Rosenberg AA, Jones MD, Simmons MA (1981) Circulating effects of hyperinsulinemia in the near term ovine fetus. Pediatr Res 15: 672 (abstract)
Mills SE, Allen MS (1986) Occult papillary carcinoma of thyroid gland. Hum Pathol 17: 1179–1181
Milner RDG (1979) Amino acids and beta cell growth. In: Merkatz IR, Adam PAJ (eds) The diabetic pregnancy: Grune and Stratton, New York. pp 145–153
Milner RDG, Hill DJ (1987) Interaction between endocrine and paracrine peptides in prenatal growth control. Eur J Pediatr 146: 113–122
Milner RDG, Barson AJ, Ashworth MA (1971) Human fetal pancreatic insulin secretion in response to ionic and other stimuli. J Endocrinol 51: 323–332
Moncrieff MW, Hill DS, Archer J, Arthur LJH (1972) Congenital absence of the pituitary gland and adrenal hypoplasia. Arch Dis Child 47: 136–137
Moreno LA, Turck D, Gottraud F, Fabre M, Manouvrier-Hanu S, Farriaux JP (1989) Familial hyperinsulinism with nesidioblastosis of the pancreas: further evidence for autosomal recessive inheritance. Am J Med Genet 34: 584–586
Morriss FH (1984) Infants of diabetic mothers. Fetal and neonatal pathophysiology. Perspect Pediatr Pathol 8: 223–234
Naeye RL, Blanc WA (1971) Organ and body growth in anencephaly. A quantitative, morphological study. Arch Pathol 91: 140–147
Neave C (1984) Congenital malformations in offspring of diabetics. Perspect Pediatr Pathol 8: 213–223
Nelson L, Turkel S, Shulman I, Gabbe S (1977) Pancreatic islet fibrosis in young infants of diabetic mothers. Lancet II: 362–363
Nishiyama S, Tomoeda S, Inoue F, Ohta T, Matsuda I (1990) Self-limited familial hyperparathyroidism associated with hypercalcemia and renal tubular acidosis in three siblings. Pediatrics 86: 421–427
Obenshain SS, Adam Paj, King KC, Teramo K, Raivo N (1970) Human fetal insulin response to sustained maternal hyperglycemia. N Engl J Med 283: 566–570
Pearse AGE, Polak JM (1971) Neural crest origin of the endocrine polypeptide (APUD) cells of the gastrointestinal tract and pancreas. Gut 12: 783–788
Peden VH (1960) True idiopathic hypoparathyroidism as a sex linked recessive trait. Am J Hum Genet 12: 323–327
Pepe GJ, Albrecht ED (1990) Regulation of the fetal adrenal cortex. Endocr Rev 11: 151–176
Pepe GJ, Waddell BJ, Stahl SJ, Albrecht ED (1988) The regulation of transplacental cortisol-cortisone metabolism by oestrogen in pregnant baboons. Endocrinology 122: 78–83
Perelman AH, Johnson RL, Clemens RD, Finberg HJ, Clewell WH, Trujillo L (1990) Intrauterine diagnosis and treatment of fetal goitrous hypothyroidism. J Clin Endocrinol Metab 71: 618–621
Petraglia F, Calza L, Garuti GC, Giardino L, De Ramundo BM, Angioni S (1990) New aspects of placental endocrinology. J Endocrinol Invest 13: 353–371
Potau N, Riudor E, Ballabriga A (1981) Insulin receptors in the human placenta in relation to fetal weight and gestational age. Pediatr Res 15: 798–803
Potter EL, Craig JM (1976) Pathology of the fetus and infant, 3rd edn. Year Book Medical Publishers, Chicago, p 326
Preece MA, Kearney PJ, Marshall WC (1977) Growth hormone deficiency in congenital rubella. Lancet II: 842–844
Reece EA, Hobbins JC (1986) Diabetic embryopathy: pathogenesis, prenatal diagnosis and prevention. Obstet Gynecol Survey 41: 325–335
Rosenn B, Miodovnik M, Dignan PStJ, Siddiqi TA, Khoury J, Mimouni F (1990) Minor congenital malformations in infants of insulin-dependent diabetic women: association with poor glycemic control. Obstet Gynecol 76: 745–749
Sagreiya K, Emery JL (1970) Perinatal thyroid discharge. A histological study of 1225 infant thyroids. Arch Dis Child 45: 746–754
Salazar H, Macaulay MA, Charles D, Pardi M (1969) The human hypophysis in anencephaly. Arch Pathol 87: 201–211
Sclare G (1956) The histological structure of the thyroid in the newborn. Scott Med J 1: 251–258
Silverman JL (1963) Eosinophil infiltration in the pancreas of infants of diabetic mothers. Diabetes 12: 528–537
Simpson ER, Carr BR, Parker CR, Milewich L, Porter JC, Macdonald PC (1979) The role of serum lipoproteins in steroidogenesis by the human fetal cortex. J Clin Endocrinol Metab 49: 146–148
Smith YF, Mullon DK, Hamosh M, Scolon JW, Hamosh P (1979) Serum prolactin and respiratory distress syndrome in the newborn. Pediatr Res 14: 93–95
Somville T (1990) Diabetes and pregnancy. Z Geburtshilfe Perinatol 194: 51–57
Stark RI, Frantz AG (1983) ACTH-ß-endorphin in pregnancy. Clin Perinatol 10: 653–657
Van Assche Fa, Gepts W, De Gasparo M (1969) The endocrine pancreas in anencephalics: a histological and biochemical study. Biol Neonate 14: 374–388
Van Hale HM, Turkel SB (1979) Neuroblastoma and adrenal morphologic features in anencephalic infants. Arch Pathol Lab Med 103: 119–121
Warren S, Le Compte PM, Legg MA (1966) The pathology of diabetes mellitus, 4th edn. Lea and Febiger, Philadelphia, pp 406–433
White P (1965) Pregnancy and diabetes: medical aspects. Med Clin North Am 49: 1015–1024
Yoon JW, Austin M, Onodera R, Notkins AL (1979) Virus induced diabetes mellitus. Isolation of a virus from a pancreas of a child with diabetic ketoacidosis. New Engl J Med 300: 1173–1179
Young MC, Laurence KM, Hughes IA (1989) Relationship between fetal adrenal morphology and anterior pituitary function. Horm Res 32: 130–135

Chapter 22

The Reticuloendothelial System and Blood

Colin L. Berry

Components of the Immune Response

Detailed accounts of the ontogeny of the immune response are available elsewhere (Pabst and Kreith 1980). However, it is worth considering the development of some immune functions as a way of understanding certain abnormalities of this system in childhood, in particular the development of the T lymphocyte series, the B lymphocyte series, the phagocyte series and the opsonic or complement system. An account of morphological development is given below.

The origin of all of these cell types is the fetal yolk sac, which is the source of circulating cells until around the 5th week of gestation, erythropoiesis having begun there at around the 14th day after conception; it is then superseded by the liver. The bone marrow does not assume a dominant role until the 5th month, although haemopoiesis can be found there at around 8–10 weeks. There is a differential distribution in skeletal sites, the clavicle, humerus, radius, tibia and ulna are colonised first (8–15 weeks), the vertebrae at the end of this time (15 weeks) and the sternum not until 20 weeks.

Recent studies suggest that the several populations of cells discussed here may be derived from embryonic stem cells at varying times under appropriate conditions (Wiles and Keller 1991). While some interactions are clearly necessary in immune system development (thymic epithelium/T lymphocyte) precision in dating a time of onset of abnormality based on morphological differentiation in the fetus may be less sustainable than has been thought in the recent past.

Morphological Development

Thymus

At the 10–12 mm stage in the human embryo the thymus begins to develop from the third and fourth endodermal pharyngeal pouches (6th week). The narrow caudal part of the third pouch supplies the caudal part of the thymus, which forms as the walls of the pouch thicken and its lumen is obliterated. At 20 mm, the parathyroid portion separates from the thymic part as the cell mass increases in size and moves caudally and medially, fusing with that from the other side and being included in the thorax. Changes accompanying development of the heart and lungs draw the thymus down into the developing thoracic cavity, with elongation of its cervical portion whose descent is variable.

At 35–37 mm a "glandular" structure develops as the epithelial mass is surrounded by a mesenchymal condensation, and a lobular

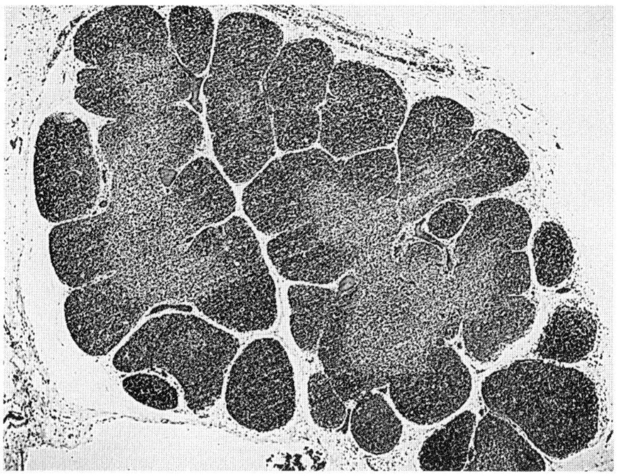

Fig. 22.1. Thymus of 120 mm embryo. Clear cortical and medullary demarcation is seen. (H&E, ×12)

pattern forms following vascular invasion. By 40 mm the thymic medulla and cortex can be distinguished; shortly thereafter, Hassall's corpuscles develop, as large cells with granular eosinophilic cytoplasm appear and aggregate (Figs. 22.1, 22.2). For details of electron microscopic appearances see Berry and Revell (1989).

Spleen and Lymph Nodes

The spleen appears in the dorsal mesogastrium at around the 10 mm stage, initially as a mesenchymal condensation supplied by a branch of the coeliac artery to the greater curve of the stomach. This will eventually become the splenic artery. An internal trabecular structure is evident by 30 mm, and haemopoiesis may be seen within this as early as the 80 mm stage.

Structures recognisable as lymph nodes are present in the cervical region at around 25 mm. There is sometimes evidence of haemopoiesis in these nodes for a brief period during development, but by 50 mm the cells populating the structures are entirely lymphoid.

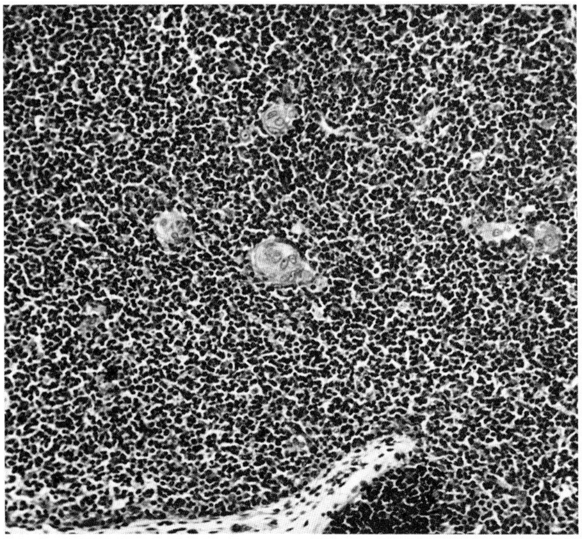

Fig. 22.2 Early Hassall's corpuscles in the thymus of 130 mm embryo. (H&E, ×90)

Cellular Development

"B" Lymphocyte Development

B lymphocytes originate in the fetal liver at around 8 weeks' gestation as large pre-B cells which lack surface antigen receptors and thus are able to develop independently of antigen and T cells. It is at this stage that clonal diversity may develop, for in the next stage, at 9 weeks, the cells acquire surface immunoglobulin, Fc receptors and antigen receptor sites. They will respond to exposure to antigen at this stage by becoming inactive or tolerant. Later (10–12 weeks' gestation), mature B cells appear, and by 15–16 weeks differentiation of the series is complete with expression of surface IgD and IgM and other receptors. There is evidence that several cycles of cell division are necessary before restricted production of a single type of immunoglobulin by individual cells is achieved; however, by 10–12 weeks these cells can synthesise IgM in response to antigenic stimulus.

A greater proportion of B cells have surface IgD in the neonate than in the adult, indicating a greater potential responsiveness to antigen. However, there is considerable suppression of B cell function by T cells in the neonate, and, in general, neonatal B cells are not good responders. Synthesis of immunoglobulin types other than IgM does not usually begin until well after birth. A detailed account of these changes is given by Lawton and Cooper (1980).

"T" Lymphocyte Development

At about 8–9 weeks of development a lymphocyte population appears in the thymic cortex and proliferates there. The origin of these cells is not clear; they may migrate from liver or bone marrow, but some support a local origin. The cells migrate to the medulla, where they subsequently proliferate slowly. During this process around 70% of the cells die, and it has been assumed that this represents the elimination of self-reactive clones. Thymic inducer hormones act on the cells in the medulla and they acquire their specialist functions there. Certain surface antigens are lost during development (T10) after a transient appearance, others, initially absent in fetal life (T1, T3) appear by term, when helper (T1, T3, T4) and suppressor (T1, T3, T5, T8) phenotypes are identifiable.

A mixed leucocyte response to allogenic cells can be demonstrated by 7.5 weeks, but from liver-derived mononuclear cells rather than T cells (Carr et al. 1973). Later studies have shown this to be a non-specific response caused by blastogenic substances in the stimulating T cells and involving no antigenic recognition. Response to phytohaemagglutinin (PHA) occurs from about 10 weeks with thymic cells and at 13–15 weeks with spleen cells. Specialist functions (helper, suppressor) are not really developed until a little after term, although antiviral mechanisms operate and fetal cells can induce graft versus host reactions.

Development of the Mononuclear Phagocyte System

Mononuclear phagocytes are derived from a bone marrow precursor and include macrophages in lymph nodes and bone marrow, Kupffer cells, alveolar macrophages and osteoclasts. In general, circulating mononuclear cells replenish this population in adult life. Deficiencies of the system have been well studied in animals where syndromes of failure of bone resorption mimic osteopetrosis and can be cured by transplantation, as in man.

Polymorphonuclear Phagocytes

The major acute phagocytic system of polymorphonuclear cells (PMNs) is derived from bone marrow stem cells which differ from the macrophage stem cell. However, mechanisms of phagocytosis and intracellular destruction are comparable in the two lineages. Neonatal PMNs show a number of relative deficiencies of function which make the diagnosis of abnormal states difficult, but some have been characterised and may depend on associated opsonising defects (see p. 532).

The Complement System

Colten (1977) has reviewed the development of the complement and properdin systems. Our knowledge of these systems has evolved using three routes of enquiry:

1. Using radioactive label incorporation techniques to determine the onset of synthesis of specific components in fetal material
2. Demonstration of discordance between maternal and fetal biochemical phenotype where polymorphism exists (C3)
3. Identification of genetic deficiencies of the systems in the mother with identification of the component in the fetus.

The complement series of proteins acts as a cascade system, like the proteins involved in coagulation. Activated complement components cause cytotoxic effects, often by cell lysis, and can alter cell surfaces in a way which facilitates phagocytosis. "Split" products of complement have histamine-releasing and chemotactic effects.

The family of proteins appears early in fetal life (Miller and Stiehm 1983). At 5–6 weeks of gestation C3 is synthesised in the liver (Gitlin and Biasucci 1969), C2 and C4 and synthesised in macrophages, while C3, C5, C6 and C9 are made in the liver. There is no evidence of maternofetal transmission of complement, despite higher than normal levels of maternal complement in pregnancy.

Functional Defects of Complement

Infants of less than 2000 g have serum which is deficient in opsonising powers. According to Miller (Miller and Stiehm 1983), fresh sera from full-term infants at birth yielded significantly less chemotactic activity towards Gram-negative bacteria, Gram-positive bacteria or antigen–antibody complexes than adult sera. The methodology of this type of investigation is difficult to standardise, but most investigators seem to find evidence of a functional deficit in this area in the neonate.

There are a number of clinical disorders of complement activity, although these may be difficult to detect because of the deficiencies described above. Leiner's disease (C5 deficiency) may present in the neonatal period as diarrhoea with failure to thrive, infection and a seborrhoeic dermatitis (Miller and Nilsson 1974).

Functional Aspects of Cellular Development

Immunoglobulins

IgM

Following stimulation from intestinal contents, IgM production is in progress by the end of the first week of postnatal life, irrespective of maturity. IgM levels rise rapidly for the first 3 weeks of life but do not reach more than 80% of adult levels by the end of the first year. Infection in the perinatal period will act as a powerful stimulus to IgM production, but because of the rapid "normal" rise a significant increment over controls is necessary for diagnosis. An IgM level above 50 mg/dl during the neonatal period is suggestive of systemic infection (see Kahn et al. 1969).

IgG

IgG is transferred across the placenta by an active mechanism involving Fc receptors on the trophoblast. This can be demonstrated by the end of the first 8 weeks of pregnancy, but significant transfer occurs only after around 32 weeks. Endogenous synthesis does not begin until around 18 weeks. By term, fetal serum levels of IgG usually exceed maternal levels by a small amount, but most are the result of placental transfer from the mother.

IgA

IgA, which like IgM does not cross the placenta, gradually increases in amount in the first year of life, although adult levels are not reached until adolescence. It first appears in the gut at about 1 month of age (Perkkio and Savilahti 1980) and is found in tears at 3 weeks of postnatal life.

The changes in immunoglobulin levels during fetal life and childhood are summarised by Chapel and Haeney (1984) (Fig. 22.3).

Cellular Immunity

T cells comprise a relatively smaller proportion of total lymphocytes at birth, although absolute numbers are close to adult levels because of the high lymphocyte count (Fleischer et al. 1975). There are some data to support a trend towards lower numbers in premature infants (Caul et al. 1978). Infants do not exhibit good responses to antigens that normally produce vigorous skin reactivity, although their lymphocytes respond well in vitro (Prindull 1974). Lymphokine production is also diminished according to some, but others have found normal values (Muller et al. 1976). Neonatal T cells are less effective as cytotoxic cells (Carne et al. 1973).

Phagocytic Cells

Neonatal PMNs are less responsive than adult PMNs towards a chemotactic stimulus and appear to be less motile in general (Christensen and Rothstein 1980). However, the phagocytic ability of the cells appears normal in serum, even in premature infants (see Miller and Stiehm 1983 for bibliography). Bactericidal activities also appear to be normal according to most workers, provided no metabolic abnormality is present.

Abnormalities of the Immunoreactive Cells and Tissues

Immune Neutropenia

In isoimmune haemolytic disease maternal antibodies against PMN-specific antigens may be formed and cause neutropenia. Affected infants have pyogenic infections, often involving the skin and including septicaemia, but the neutropenia clears spontaneously as maternal immunoglobulin disappears from the circulation (Boxer 1978).

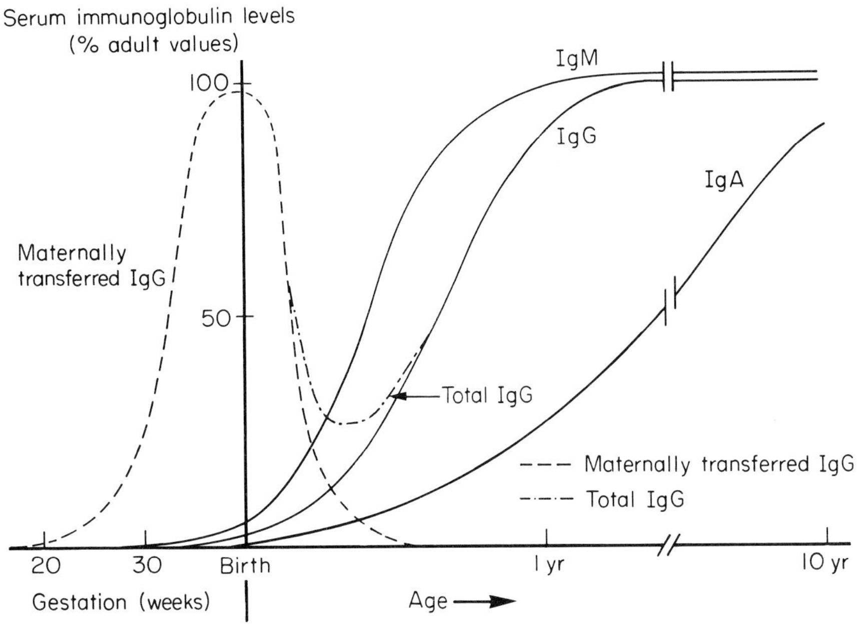

Fig. 22.3 Serum immunoglobulin levels and age (Chapel and Haeney 1984).

Chronic Neutropenia of Childhood

Chronic neutropenia of childhood apparently occurs as a result of varying patterns of inheritance, with autosomal-dominant and autosomal-recessive forms being reported (Pincus et al. 1976). The degree of neutropenia correlates poorly with clinical severity but there are few symptoms unless PMNs are fewer than $1500/mm^3$. The disease may be identified by routine examination in the neonatal period but rarely presents then. Recent studies suggest that the disorder is a heterogeneous collection of entities.

Infantile Agranulocytosis

Infantile agranulocytosis is a severe condition with leucocyte counts of less than $200/mm^3$ which often presents in the first month of life, with skin and respiratory involvement. It is apparently due to an arrest of development at the myelocyte stage (Kostmann 1975).

Chronic Granulomatous Disease

When a PMN leucocyte engulfs an organism, a phagolysosome is formed by fusion of lysosomes with the phagocytic vacuole. These are of two types, one containing lysozyme, peroxidase and cationic proteins, the other, which is smaller, containing alkaline phosphatase in addition to the other enzymes. Following this fusion there is a rapid increase in metabolic activity with an increase of two to three times in oxygen consumption. Hydrogen peroxide and other superoxides are formed and are bactericidal.

Chronic granulomatous disease is a group of conditions in which these processes are defective. Infants with the condition are particularly sensitive to catalase-positive non-hydrogen peroxide-producing bacteria such as staphylococci and enteric organisms. Although the disease rarely presents in the neonatal period, suppurative cervical lymphadenopathy may be seen (Fig. 22.4; see Berry and Revell 1989 for bibliography).

Thymus

Many of the consequences of abnormalities of thymic development are delayed, so that presentation after the neonatal period is usual. However, a number of forms of cellular or

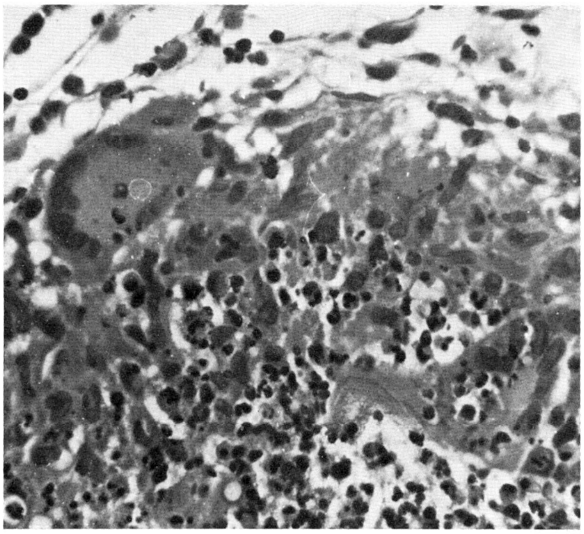

Fig. 22.4 Abscess in chronic granulomatous disease in a lymph node from a child dying at 5 weeks of age. (H&E, ×130)

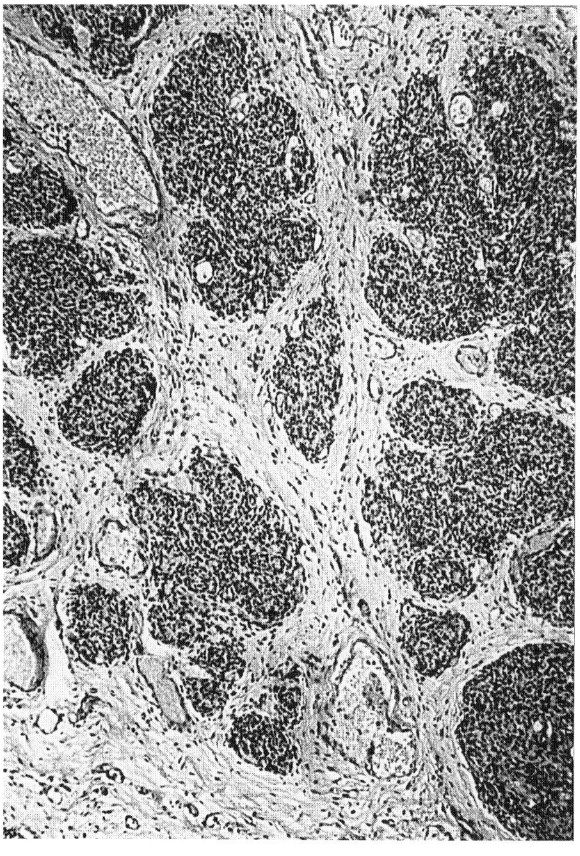

Fig. 22.5 Thymic dysplasia. The thymus consists entirely of medulla showing no evidence of cortical differentiation. No Hassall's corpuscles are seen. (H&E, ×84)

combined immune deficiency may be diagnosed sooner if actively sought.

Di George Syndrome

The Di George syndrome (thymic agenesis) is now known to have a much more variable expression than was originally thought: some patients have a small thymus and of the 19 cases of Lischner and Huff (1975), 12 had clearly identifiable thymic tissue. Parathyroid glands can be found where there is complete absence of thymic tissue and peripheral lymphoid tissue development is variable. The gene for the syndrome has been mapped to 22q11.21q11.23.

The syndrome may occur in either sex and is often associated with congenital heart disease, in particular with abnormalities of the aortic arches. The heart disease often provides the symptomatology leading to investigation, but I have seen a case where tetany occurred by 10 days of age. The presence of an associated tracheo-oesophageal fistula was a reason for early presentation in the case of Dische (1968).

There is a profound deficiency in T cell function with prolonged survival of allogenic skin grafts and a failure to become sensitised to powerful allergens such as dinitrochlorobenzine. The basic defect appears not to lie in the T cell lineage but in the absence of adequate functional activity of the thymic epithelium in "processing" T cells during their development.

In a recent paper, Chisaka and Capecchi (1991) have reported the production of athymic, aparathyroid mice with thyroid and submaxillary deficiencies, by the targeted disruption of the mouse homeobox gene Hox-1.5. Defects of the heart and arteries and of the face are also found. The similarity of this phenotype to the Di George syndrome is remarkable.

A fuller account is found in Berry and Revell (1989).

Thymic Dysplasia

I have used the term "thymic dysplasia" to describe an abnormality of thymic epithelial development resulting in gross reduction in the number of, or complete absence of, Hassall's corpuscles from the medulla (Fig. 22.5). Using this criterion, in a series of 1000 consecutive necropsies at the Hospital for Sick Children, Great Ormond Street, 18 cases of probable immune deficiency were identified with histories fitting a number of clinical syndromes (see Berry 1968). Subsequent studies have clearly indicated that a variety of clinical entities may present with this pivotal histopathological finding as a central feature, but the author is not convinced that division of the thymic appearances into categories as suggested by Gosseye et al. (1983) is a nosologically significant advance.

The thymus gland is small and is placed higher in the neck than normal, usually above the brachiocephalic vein. In sections a fetal appearance is preserved with a well-defined lobular pattern. These lobules are composed of connective tissue and vessels, and few lymphocytes are seen. Other lymphoid tissues are often lymphocyte depleted, and the paracortical area of the nodes is not developed (see Fig. 22.3). Follicular development is poor in the spleen, and the gut-associated lymphoid tissues are hypoplastic (nodes, Peyer's patches, tonsil; Fig. 22.6). Further details are found in Berry and Revell (1989).

Renal Disease in Immune Deficiency States

Mesangial sclerosis, tubular ectasia, tubular epithelial cell injury and dilatation of Bowman's space may all be found in the kidneys of children with severe combined immune deficiency; they are not specific for AIDS, as has been suggested.

Thymic Lymphocyte Depletion

In many infants the thymus appears to be grossly depleted of lymphocytes at necropsy. This depletion should not be confused with the changes seen in immune-deficient disease as the essential structure of the thymus is preserved. Thus, although the cortex is bare, the reticulin structure of this part of the gland persists in a collapsed form, and medullary lymphocytes are present, together with many Hassall's corpuscles, which often appear crowded together.

The significance of these changes is far from clear and they do not, in my view, permit any statements to be made about antemortem events, although Dourov (1982), in a study of stillbirths and neonatal deaths, was able to relate the histological appearance of the thymus to the length of postnatal survival. In the sequential study referred to above (Berry 1968), lymphocyte loss was evident in 616 cases but was not found in others with a comparable clinical course. At the time of writing, there have been no studies relating thymic lymphocyte depletion to antemortem cortisol levels or to the ratio of T and B lymphocytes in the circulating blood.

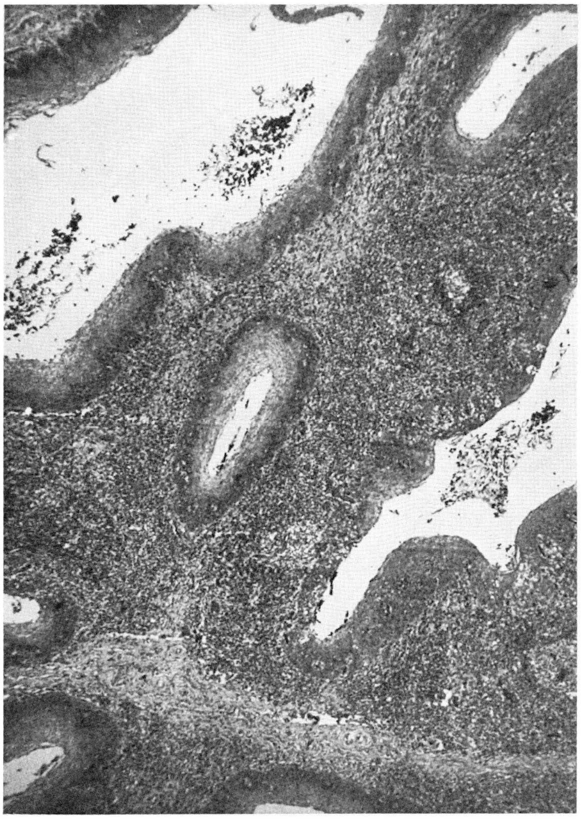

Fig. 22.6 Thymic dysplasia. The tonsillar epithelium has almost complete absence of follicular development. (H&E, ×70)

Spleen

Asplenia and Polysplenia

Asplenia is an important finding in a neonatal necropsy; it should alert the prosector to the probability of abnormal thoracic situs and abnormalities of the heart. Asplenia is almost always associated with bilateral symmetry of

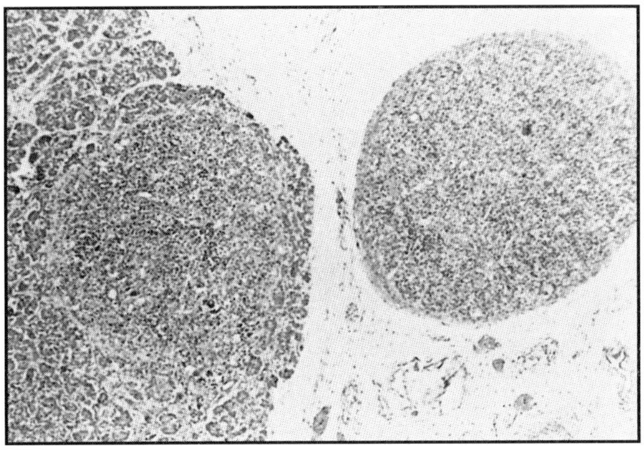

Fig. 22.7 Heterotopic splenic nodules adjacent to and within the tail of pancreas in trisomy 13.

the tracheobronchial tree with the presence of two eparterial main bronchi and two apparently right (trilobed) lungs. The bronchial findings in turn indicate that two right atria are present and that major cardiac anomalies are probable (see Becker and Anderson 1989). Associated abnormalities of mesenteric attachment may occur, and renal anomalies are common (Freedom 1972). The abnormality is commoner in males.

Honigman and Lanzkowsky (1979) have reported a case of overwhelming sepsis in an 8-week-old girl with isolated absence of the spleen diagnosed by CT scan and by the presence of Howell–Jolly bodies in the blood. (Review of the literature reveals only eight children with isolated asplenia, five from one family.) In general, asplenia from any cause is associated with an increased incidence of sepsis; causes include sickle cell disease and surgery. Asplenia may occur in Kartagener's syndrome.

Polysplenia

As with asplenia, polysplenia is a useful indicator of other abnormalities, although these may be less severe than with asplenia. The term should only be applied to cases where spleens are present on both sides of the mesogastrium; accessory spleens are always on the left of this structure. Both lungs are bilobed and have hyparterial bronchi. In simplistic terms, both are left lungs. Both atria have left-sided characteristics. This syndrome occurs with a similar frequency in both sexes.

Hamartomas and Heterotopia of the Spleen

It is important that the splenic nodules of hamartomas and heterotopia, which are usually less than 1 cm in diameter, should not be mistaken for more serious lesions. Hamartomas often consist of pancreatic tissue and fat (Butler 1984), but vascular lesions occur. Heterotopia with nodules of normal splenic tissue within the pancreas, adrenal gland or liver may be found in trisomy 13 (Fig. 22.7).

Splenomegaly

Splenomegaly is common in many neonatal infections, and in conditions associated with red cell haemolysis. Detailed pathological findings are available only for those conditions in which death is common. The spleen is commonly enlarged in congenital cytomegalovirus infection, and this may be the only abnormality evident at birth. A petechial rash may coexist with splenomegaly. Microscopically the typical inclusion bodies may be seen in the spleen, and the virus can be isolated from the parenchyma.

Splenomegaly is also common in toxoplasmosis. However, the organism is rarely seen in the tissue, and the only specific finding reported is an eosinophilic infiltrate (Frenkel and Friedlander 1952). The spleen is large in congenital syphilis but shows no distinctive features; the same is true of the organ in congenital tuberculosis. In listerosis, granulomas are commonly seen. Splenomegaly is usual in congenital leukaemia.

Lymph Nodes

Mesenteric lymph nodes are often enlarged and congested in cases dying from gastroenteritis. Histologically there is marked reactive change, but severe lymphoid depletion may also be seen and may not be related to the severity of the illness (Rho and Josephson 1967; Drucker et al. 1970).

The size of lymph nodes in the neonate is so variable that it is difficult to be certain of abnormality, but mesenteric nodes are usually clearly visible and may appear large to those performing neonatal necropsies infrequently.

Rhesus Isoimmunisation

Rhesus isoimmunisation is now uncommon as the result of a successful programme of administration of anti-D antibodies to at-risk mothers within 36 hours of delivery. A few women still become sensitised, despite appropriate administration of anti-D antibodies, probably because of unrecognised fetomaternal haemorrhage earlier in pregnancy. Some women become sensitised as a result of incompatible blood transfusion. These women can be treated by intensive plasmapheresis throughout their pregnancy, a course of management which requires careful monitoring for signs of fetal disease as rebound elevation of maternal antibodies can occur immediately after plasmapheresis. Amniocentesis, with the attendant risk of bleeding and further immunisation, should be monitored for its effect on maternal antibody levels and fetal wellbeing. The advent of successful intrauterine replacement transfusion and exchange transfusion both improve the chances of affected babies.

Incompatibility is seldom severe enough to necessitate exchange transfusion but fetal hydrops or intrauterine death may occur from Kell incompatibility.

Placenta and Central Nervous System

The placental changes are considered in Chapter 2 (p. 66) and kernicterus in Chapter 24 (p. 586). Hydrops is present in severely affected babies, and they become jaundiced after birth. The fluid in the body cavities is yellow in colour.

Liver

The appearances of the liver in rhesus-isoimmunisation depend on the extent of the extramedullary haemopoiesis, which is the fundamental pathological response to haemolysis. Thus in babies dying at or around birth the liver is a dusky red and is large and firm (Fig. 22.8). On histological examination massive haemopoiesis is seen in the sinusoids, and there may be visible iron deposits in hepatocytes, readily demonstrable with Perl's technique.

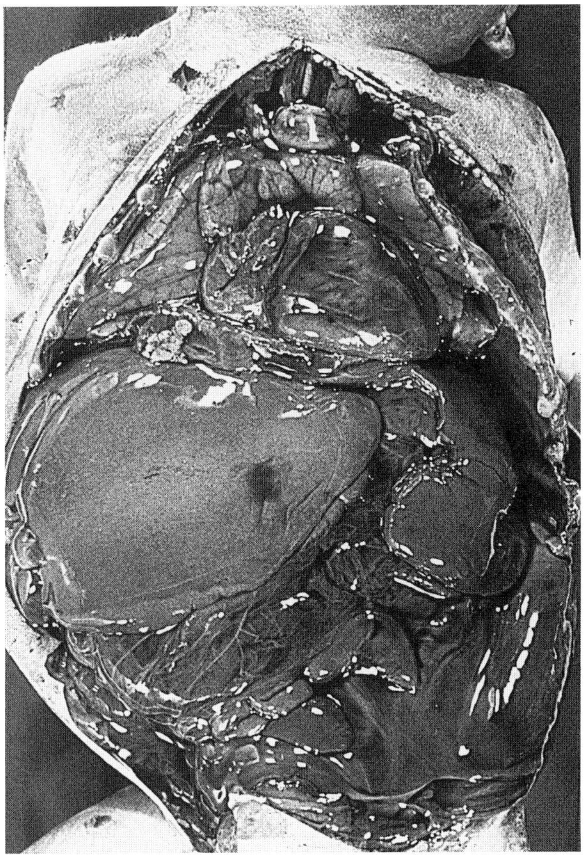

Fig. 22.8 Rhesus isoimmunisation. There is gross hepatosplenomegaly caused by increased erythropoiesis.

Although other diseases may result in persistent haemopoiesis (after 41 weeks) in the liver, the changes are seldom as marked. Later deaths are less distinctive because haemopoiesis will be less massive in extent and there may be bile visible in hepatocytes and canaliculi because of the hyperbilirubinaemia. The picture may then be confused with neonatal infection in the absence of an adequate history.

Spleen

As with the liver, the extent of extramedullary haemopoiesis is the principal determinant of the appearances seen. The organ is abnormally large, firm and dark-red, with a thin capsule and little evidence of a follicular pattern. Histologically there is haemopoiesis, and iron deposition may be seen, often less marked than in the liver. Haemophagocytosis and erythrocyte ghosts are common.

Other Organs

Foci of haemopoiesis may be found in many sites if sought; for instance, I have seen meningeal deposits. Pancreatic involvement is often found, but the supposed increase in islet size is not adequately documented. The adrenals may be extensively infiltrated by haemopoietic cells, and extensive lipid streaking is said to be common (Wigglesworth 1984).

Neonatal Isoimmune Throbocytopenia

Maternal immunisation by fetal platelets, resulting in the production of maternal antiplatelet antibodies, causes this disease. The responsible antigen (PLA-1) is almost ubiquitous in the population and the condition is thus rare; quoted figures of 1 in 5000 seem far too high to the author. In classic autoimmune thrombocytopenic purpura (ITP) maternal antibodies may cross the placenta and produce neonatal thrombocytopenia but the two conditions are easily distinguished serologically.

Anaemia in Infancy

In all infants the haemoglobin level falls rapidly in early postnatal life, dropping from around 19–21 g/100 ml to as low as 11–12 g/100 ml by 6–8 weeks, at the rate of 1% per day. This fall is exaggerated in the premature baby, where levels as low as 8 g may be found at 6–8 weeks post partum. This anaemia is normochromic but may become hypochromic during "recovery" if iron stores are low, a common event in prematurity.

In immature infants anaemia may also be due to haemolysis from glucose-6-phosphate dehydrogenase deficiency, from administration of sulphonamides, other antibiotics, certain vitamin K analogues, gluconuryl transferase deficiency and other defects of enzyme expression, or to functional immaturity of enzyme systems. Collectively this is an unimportant group of diseases with regard to red cell loss, but the hyperbilirubinaemia which ensues may be dangerous. Familial acholuric jaundice is rarely manifest in the neonatal period.

Haemorrhage

Haemorrhage is an important cause of anaemia in the fetus and neonate and may occur before, during or after birth. Fetomaternal haemorrhage is probably underdiagnosed except in the context of rhesus incompatibility. Twin–twin transfusion can result in profound anaemia in the donor twin (see Chap. 9, p. 225). Traumatic injury to the placenta and less commonly to the fetus or umbilical cord may complicate invasive prenatal investigation (see Chap. 4, p. 127). Haemorrhage from vessel disruption in vasa praevia is a serious complication of labour. In placenta praevia, haemorrhage from the fetal side of the placenta is an important cause of unexplained iron deficiency in the neonate, responding promptly to iron therapy. Significant fetal blood loss leading to anaemia can follow both placental abruption and placental incision during operative delivery. Traumatic fetal haemorrhage is discussed in Chapter 10, p. 246.

Postnatally, haemorrhage from the umbilicus, which may complicate cannulation of umbilical vessels, may be sufficient to result in anaemia. Haemorrhages into the cerebral ventricles or intestine are particular hazards for the preterm baby.

Repeated blood sampling for diagnostic purposes is an important cause of anaemia in the sick newborn.

Anaemia due to defects in coagulation is rare in the neonate. The only likely cause is congenital afibrinogenaemia, an autosomal-recessive characteristic, which may present as haemorrhage from the umbilical cord.

Rare Causes of Anaemia

In a number of syndromes an anaemia is part of the well-defined characteristics of the clinical entity. A brief description of these syndromes is given below.

Radial Aplasia/Thrombocytopenia Syndrome

Radial aplasia/thrombocytopenia syndrome (an autosomal-recessive condition) shows its most severe effects in early infancy. There is thrombocytopenia with absence or gross reduction in the number of megakaryocytes, a tendancy to leukaemoid reactions in bleeding episodes and anaemia out of proportion to the apparent blood loss. Eosinophilia occurs in the blood or bone marrow in around 50% of cases. Platelet levels tend to rise with age.

Associated anomalies include absent radii and shortened ulnar bones. The thumbs are normal, an important diagnostic point. Congenital heart disease is common (30% of cases) with Fallot's tetralogy and atrial septal defect the commonly associated lesions. Death may occur during infancy but as the condition improves in the first year of life vigorous supportive therapy is indicated (Smith 1982).

Aase Syndrome

Affected infants have a triphalangeal thumb, and a mild hypoplastic anaemia which improves with age. There is a variable leucopenia. Ventricular septal defect may occur (Jones and Thompson 1973).

Fanconi's Syndrome

Haematological problems in Fanconi's syndrome usually occur after the age of 5 years, but bone marrow hypoplasia may be evident on biopsy before this. Aspiration shows islands of haemopoiesis in a generally inactive marrow, some macrocytosis may be seen and fetal haemoglobin is present in large amounts.

Albers–Schönberg Disease

Pancytopenia is inevitable in the autosomal-recessive condition known as Albers–Schönberg disease, in which neonatal infection (often oral) may occur. Transplantation may improve the prognosis, and there have been recent successes.

Wiskott–Aldrich Syndrome

Wiskott–Aldrich syndrome and its variants often present as neonatal thrombocytopenia with adequate megakaryocytes and may mimic immune thrombocytopenia. The disease is now thought to be due in part to the production of abnormal amounts of lymphokines interfering with polymorph function. The thymus may be dysplastic.

References

Becker AE, Anderson RH (1989) Cardiac pathology. In: Berry CL (ed) Pediatric pathology. Springer, Berlin Heidelberg New York, pp 63–124
Berry CL (1968) The neonatal thymus and immune paresis. Proc R Soc Med 61(9): 867–871
Berry CL, Revell PA (1989) Spleen, lymph nodes and immunoreactive tissues. In: Berry CL (ed) Paediatric pathology. Springer, Berlin Heidelberg New York, pp 535–569
Boxer LA (1978) Immunologic function and leucocyte disorders in newborn infants. Clin Hematol 7: 123–146
Butler JJ (1984) Pathology of the spleen in benign and malignant conditions. Histopathology 7: 453–474
Carne S, Dewhurst CJ, Hurley R (1973) Rubella epidemic in a maternity unit. Br Med J 1: 444
Carr MD, Sites DP, Fudenberg HH (1973) Dissociation of responses to phytohemagglutinin and allogeneic lymphocytes in human foetal lymphoid tissues. Nature [New Biol] 241: 279
Caul EO, Hobbs SJ, Roberts PC, Clark S (1978) Revaluation of a simplified sucrose gradient method for the detection of rubella-specific IgM in routine diagnostic practice. J Med Virol 2: 153
Chapel HM, Haeney M (1984) Essentials of clinical immunology. Blackwell, Oxford
Chisaka O, Capecchi MR (1991) Regionally restricted developmental defects resulting from targeted disruption of the mouse homeobox gene Hox-1.5. Nature 350: 473–479
Christensen RD, Rothstein G (1980) Efficiency of neutrophil migration in the neonate. Pediatr Res 14: 1147–1149
Colten HR (1977) Development of host defenses: the complement and properdin systems. In: Cooper MD, Dayton DH (eds) Development of host defenses. Raven, New York, pp 165–173
Dische MR (1968) Lymphoid tissue and associated malformations in thymic agenesis. Arch Pathol 86: 312
Dourov N. (1982) L'examen microscopique du thymus au cours de la période périnatale. Ann Pathol 2: 255–261
Drucker MM, Polliack A, Yeivin R, Sacks TG (1970) Immunofluorescent demonstration of enteropathogenic *Escherichia coli* in tissues of infants dying with enteritis. Pediatrics 46: 855
Fleischer TA, Lucksen J, Rand Sabada A (1975) T and B lymphocyte subpopulations in children. Pediatrics 55: 162–165
Freedom RM (1972) The asplenia syndrome: a review of significant extracardiac structural abnormalities in 29 necropsied patients. J Pediatr 81: 1130–1132
Frenkel JK, Friedlander S (1952) Toxoplasmosis. Pathology of neonatal disease. Pathogenesis, diagnosis and treatment. Public Health Service Publication No 141. US Government Printing Office, Washington DC
Gitlin D, Biasucci A (1969) Development of gamma-G, gamma-A, gamma-M, beta 1C/beta 1A, C 1 esterase inhibitor, ceruloplasmin, transferrin, hemopexin, haptoglobulin, fibrinogen, plasminogen, alpha-1-antitrypsin, orosomucoid, beta-lipoprotein, alpha-2-

macroglobulin and pre-albumin in the human conceptus. J Clin Invest 48: 1422–1446
Gosseye S, Diebold N, Griscelli C, Nezelof C (1983) Severe combined immunodeficiency disease: a pathological analysis of 26 cases. Clin Immunol Immunopathol 29: 58–77
Honigman R, Lanzkowsky P (1979) Isolated congenital asplenia: an occult case of overwhelming sepsis. Am J Dis Child 133: 552–553
Jones B, Thompson J (1973) Triphalangeal thumbs associated with hypoplastic anaemia. Paediatrics 52: 609
Kahn WN, Ali RV, Werthmann M, Ross S (1969) Immunoglobulin M determinations in neonates and infants as an adjunct to the diagnosis of infection. J Pediatr 75: 1282–1286
Kostmann R (1975) Infantile genetic agranulocytosis. Acta Paediatr Scand 64: 362–368
Lawton AR, Cooper MD (1980) In: Steihm ER, Fulginiti VA (eds) Immunologic disorders in infants and children, 2nd edn. Saunders, Philadelphia, pp 36–51
Lischner HW, Huff DS (1975) T cell deficiency in Di George syndrome. In: Bergsama D, Good RA, Finstead JNW (eds) Immunodeficiency in man and animals. Sinaver, Sunderland, p 16
Miller ME, Nilsson UR (1974) A major role for the fifth component of complement (C5) in the opsonisation of yeast particles. Partial dichotomy of functional and immunohistochemical measurement. Clin Immunol Immunopath 2: 246–255
Miller ME, Stiehm ER (1983) Immunology and resistance to infection. In: Remington JS, Klein JO (eds) Infectious disease of the fetus and new-born infant. Saunders, Philadelphia, pp 27–68
Muller MR, Lazary S, Hitzig WH (1976) Production of migration inhibitory factor and blast cell transformation by cord blood lymphocytes. Int Arch Appl Immunol 50: 493–505
Pabst AF, Kreith HW (1980) Ontogeny of the immune response as a basis of childhood disease. J Pediatr 97: 519–534
Perkkio M, Savilahti E (1980) Time of appearance of immunoglobulin-containing cells in the mucosa of the neonatal intestine. Pediatr Res 14: 953–955
Pincus SH, Boxer LA, Stossal TP (1976) Chronic neutropenia in childhood. Am J Med 61: 849–861
Prindull G (1974) Maturation of cellular and humoral immunity during human embryonic development. Acta Paediatr Scand 63: 607–615
Rho Y, Josephson JE (1967) Epidemic enteropathogenic *Escherichia coli*, Newfoundland, 1963. Autopsy study of 16 cases. Can Med Assoc J 96: 392
Smith DW (1982) Recognisable patterns of human malformation. Saunders, Philadelphia, p 236
Wigglesworth J (1984) Perinatal pathology. Saunders, Philadelphia, p 341
Wiles MV, Keller G (1991) Multiple hematopoietic lineages develop from embryonic stem cells in culture. Development 111: 259–267

Chapter 23

Hydrocephalus and Malformations of the Central Nervous System

K. Michael Laurence

Development of the Central Nervous System

The central nervous system (CNS) is ectodermal in origin and is precocious in development. These are two fundamental facts in the development of the CNS. The ectoderm on either side of the midline in the bilaminar embryonic disc is destined, from an early stage, to form the nervous system ("neurectoderm"), and even before the disc becomes folded and begins to form an embryo the neurectoderm begins to sink below the surface as a result of the raising on either side of ridges—the neural crests. The summits of the neural crests begin to fuse in what eventually will become the neck region 22 days after fertilisation and fusion spreads cranially and caudally until the whole of the neurectoderm has sunk below the surface to form the neural tube; with the exception of the neuropores this closure is complete by the 28th day after conception. The neuropores close 1–2 days later. The cells at the summit of the neural crest separate off to develop into the posterior root ganglia, chromaffin cells of the sympathetic nervous system and various other cells. After the neural tube has developed, the mesodermal somites give rise to the bodies and neural arches of the vertebrae, the latter arching over the tube to meet in the midline behind it.

The neural tube extends the full length of the embryo and will become the brain and spinal cord. Since the spine grows faster than the spinal cord, the lower end of the cord retreats up the vertebral canal, reaching the level of about L-3 at birth and the lower border of L-1 in the adult. In both brain and spinal cord neural tube cells proliferate to form a lining ependymal layer and a thick mantle layer containing differentiating nerve and glial cells. Processes from the nerve cells form a marginal layer of axons on the surface.

In the brain, it becomes possible to distinguish forebrain, midbrain and hindbrain; these subdivisions became more obvious by day 36 with the formation of cervical and midbrain flexures, which are concave downwards, and a pontine flexure, which is convex downwards (Fig. 23.1).

Forebrain

At an early stage, the future cerebral hemispheres appear as outgrowths on either side of the forebrain. They are known as telencephalic vesicles, and the portion of the neural tube between them is the diencephalon (the "between brain"). The telencephalic vesicles grow very rapidly in all directions so that their anterior ends form the most anterior part of the brain, the original cranial end of the neural

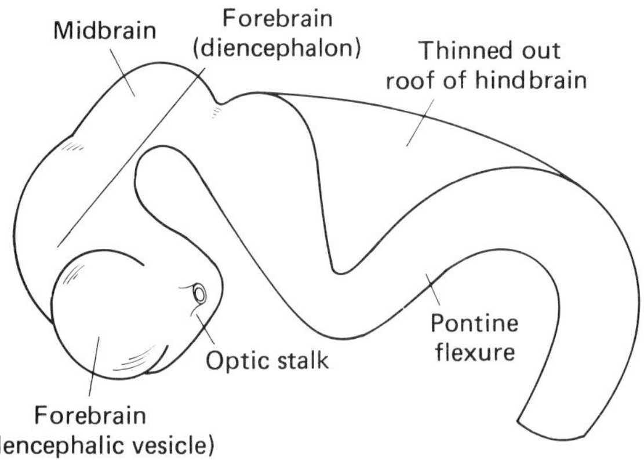

Fig. 23.1. The development of the pontine flexure forms an acute bend in the hindbrain. The telencephalic vesicle is an outgrowth from the midline portion of the forebrain.

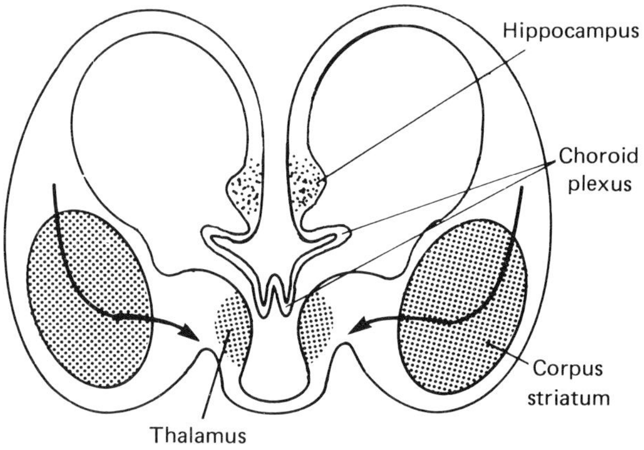

Fig. 23.3. Frontal section through the forebrain. The *arrows* show the pathway taken by projection fibres through the corpus striatum and into the diencephalon.

tube now being called the lamina terminalis (Fig. 23.2). A swelling in the lateral wall and floor of the telencephalic vesicle is the *anlage* of the corpus striatum, while another swelling in the lateral wall of the diencephalon forms the early thalamus. As can be seen from Fig. 23.2, the obvious pathway for commissural fibres to take is through (the upper part of) the lamina terminalis, while projection fibres from the developing cerebral cortex must pass down lateral to the thalamus.

The roof of the neural tube in the forebrain remains thin, as does a small area on the medial wall of the telencephalic vesicle. This ependymal layer, together with the overlying pia, becomes invaginated downwards to form the choroid plexus of the lateral ventricles (Fig. 23.3). The original sites of the outgrowth of the telencephalic vesicles become the interventricular foramina.

As projection fibres from the cortex increase in number and grow down into the brainstem, they divide the corpus striatum into caudate and lentiform nuclei and they themselves form the internal capsule (Fig. 23.4). They eventually become so numerous that they obliterate the narrow gap between the thalamus and the medial surface of the hemi-

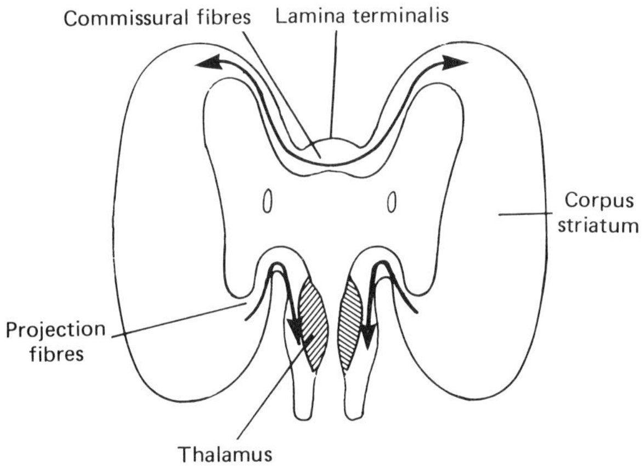

Fig. 23.2. Horizontal section through the forebrain to show how the commissural fibres use the lamina terminalis as a pathway while the projection fibres have to bend sharply round into the diencephalon.

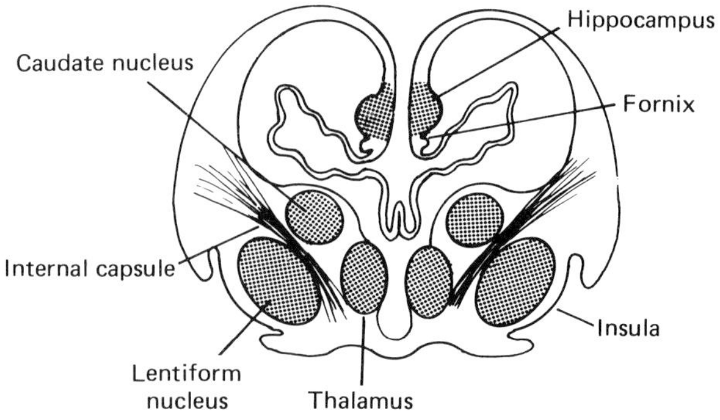

Fig. 23.4. Fusion has taken place between the lateral side of the diencephalon and the medial side of the telencephalon lateral to the thalamus. The corpus striatum has become divided into lentiform and caudate nuclei. Note also the choroidal fissure which is below the hippocampus and fornix.

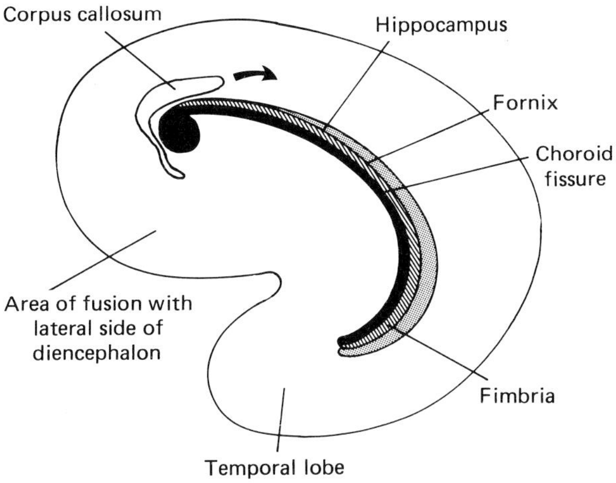

Fig. 23.5. Growth of the caudal part of the telencephalic vesicle has now formed the temporal lobe. The fornix lies above the choroid fissure, but its continuation, the fimbria, lies below the choroid fissure in the temporal lobe.

sphere (see Fig. 23.2) and the hemisphere fuses with the lateral surface of the diencephalon (see Fig. 23.2). Figure 23.3 also shows that above the invagination of choroid plexus into the lateral ventricle is a narrow band of fibres—the fornix—and above this again a mass of grey matter—the hippocampus. There is, as yet, no corpus callosum.

Figure 23.5 shows the medial surface of a detached telencephalic vesicle. It can now be seen that the invagination of the choroid plexus is slit-like and it is known as the choroid fissure. Above it are the fornix and the hippocampus. The telencephalic vesicle grows backwards and downwards so that the original posterior pole of the brain becomes the anterior pole of the temporal lobe and the structures on the medial wall of the hemisphere become C-shaped. This growth includes the lateral ventricle, so that its inferior horn develops, into which the choroid plexus is invaginated through the choroid fissure. The main bundle of commissural fibres begins to cross the midline in the upper part of the lamina terminalis to form the corpus callosum. This grows backwards above the fornix and causes degeneration of the upper part of the hippocampus, which is represented only by the thin indusium griseum on the upper surface of the corpus callosum. The lower part of the hippocampus, however, remains as a long swelling in the floor of the inferior horn of the lateral ventricle. The lower part of the fornix is known as the fimbria and lies above the hippocampus. The choroid fissure is below the fornix but above the fimbria (see Fig. 23.4).

Midbrain

The wall of the midbrain becomes greatly thickened in relation to the size of the lumen of the neural tube, which is represented in the adult by the aqueduct. Cells of the mantle layer aggregate to form various nuclei.

Hindbrain

In the roof of the hindbrain, mantle and marginal layers fail to develop so that only the ependymal layer is present. The formation of the pontine flexure causes the roof to expand, as can be seen in Fig. 23.1, and the ependyma, together with the overlying pia, forms the tela choroidea of the fourth ventricle. The tela becomes perforated in three places to form the foramina of Magendie and Luschka and becomes invaginated into the cavity to form the choroid plexus. The cerebellum develops later as an outgrowth from the dorsal surface of the cranial end of the hindbrain. The major enlargement concerns the neocerebellum, which grows backwards until the cerebellum, as a whole, completely covers over the roof of the fourth ventricle.

The very striking growth of the developing cerebral hemisphere is reflected in the C-shape of many structures in the brain, such as the lateral ventricle itself, the caudate nucleus, the cingulum and the fornix (whose name means an arch). The growth of the cerebral cortex in the human brain is accompanied by the backward growth of the neocerebellum and by the development of the basilar part of the pons, which contains the nuclei that relay fibres from the cortex to the cerebellum (Lemire et al. 1975; Beck et al. 1983).

It remains only to reiterate that the whole nervous system is precocious in development, compared with other parts of the body. The complement of neurons is almost complete by about 16 weeks, while the main growth spurt of the brain begins at about the 20th week and reaches its maximum at full term. At birth the brain has already reached 25% of its adult weight and by the age of 4, about 75%. Thus the vulnerability of the brain to undernutrition from any cause is greatest in late pregnancy and early childhood.

Hydrocephalus

Introduction

Hydrocephalus is best defined as the presence of excessive amounts of cerebrospinal fluid (CSF) within the cranial cavity. One form, "hydrocephalus ex vacuo", where CSF passively takes the place of atrophied or destroyed brain tissue and where there is generalised dilatation of the ventricular system in addition to enlargement of the extracerebral CSF spaces, will not be considered here.

Uncomplicated hydrocephalus (not associated with spina bifida) is an infrequent diagnosis in carefully conducted surveys, with reliable confirmatory evidence. A prevalence of 1 per 1000 births has been reported from the eastern USA (MacMahon et al. 1953), Hungary (Czeizel and Révész 1970) and Southampton (Williamson 1965); 0.7 per 1000 from Belfast (Adams et al. 1982); and less than 0.5 per 1000 from South Wales (Carter et al. 1968) and Sweden (Book 1951). Higher prevalences, such as those reported from Birmingham (McKeown and Record 1960) and Scotland (Record and McKeown 1949), probably result from heavy reliance on death certification without corroborative evidence.

Clinical Features

Hydrocephalus may develop early in the second trimester of pregnancy and can become so severe that it leads to death in utero. In some instances, severe head enlargement prevents engagement of the head and leads to breech presentation necessitating caesarean section; in others, a destructive operation is needed to effect delivery of the fetus, or severe birth trauma leads to perinatal death. More often, however, the head is not very enlarged at birth, even though there is marked ventricular dilation; hydrocephalus becomes progressively more obvious postnatally. The hydrocephalic head is rounded with a disproportionately large vault, with frontal and lateral bossing, large, possibly bulging fontanelles and dilated scalp veins (Fig. 23.6). The facies seem small with downward-turned eyes. In a proportion of cases hydrocephalus arrests spontaneously (Laurence 1958; Laurence and Coates 1962), but more usually the condition is progressive with raised CSF pressure, being fatal in months if not weeks unless the CSF is diverted by one of the various shunting operations now in use. Children in whom the condition arrests spontaneously or as a result of a shunt may be intellectually normal, but when it is not controlled, intellectual impairment is frequent, often with neurological deficit consisting of a combination of spastic paraplegia, affecting the legs more than the arms, and cerebellar ataxia (Laurence 1969). Hydrocephalus is now recognised in the second trimester of pregnancy both by ultrasound examination and when biochemical tests identify a concomitant neural tube defect. Problems related to the examination of these fetuses are discussed in Chapter 4, p. 129.

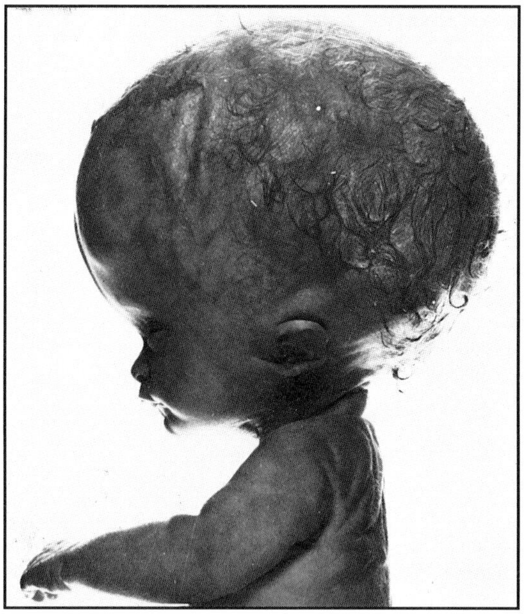

Fig. 23.6. Stillborn fetus with gross hydrocephalus; the vault is disproportionately large.

Types of Hydrocephalus

Theoretically, hydrocephalus may be caused by overproduction or underabsorption of CSF, or by a block in the CSF pathway (Table 23.1).

Table 23.1. Causes of hydrocephalus

Overproduction of CSF	Choroid plexus papilloma and villous hypertrophy
Defective absorption of CSF	?? Venous sinus thrombus
Obstruction to the CSF pathway	Within ventricular system: foramina of Monro, aqueduct, exit foramina
	Subarachnoid space: Arnold–Chiari malformation, basal cistern block
	Outside CNS: skull abnormalities

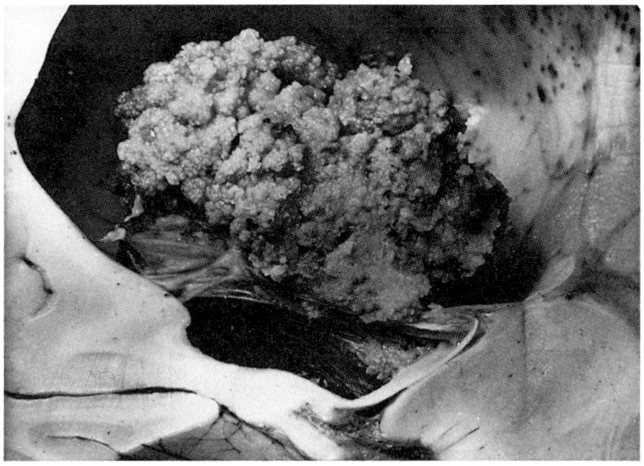

Fig. 23.7. Parasagittal section of a brain with hydrocephalus associated with a large choroid plexus papilloma situated in one lateral ventricle.

Overproduction of CSF

Choroid plexus papilloma is occasionally present at birth or develops soon after. It is a friable, vascular, cauliflower-like tumour attached to or replacing one of the choroid plexuses, situated in the posterior portion of one of the lateral ventricles (Fig. 23.7) or the fourth ventricle. Its microscopic structure resembles normal choroid plexus except that it is more vascular. It produces more CSF than can be absorbed. Absence of an obstruction to CSF flow has been demonstrated, but some cases undoubtedly have an associated basal cistern block, probably caused by repeated small haemorrhages from the vascular tumour or by the high protein content of the CSF (Laurence 1974).

Underabsorption of CSF

Theoretically, underabsorption should occur when there is obstruction of the intracranial venous system as in venous sinus thrombosis, preventing absorption of CSF into the venous circulation. However, this is not well authenticated and is probably not a cause of hydrocephalus.

Obstruction to the CSF Pathway

Obstruction to the CSF pathway is the only significant cause of hydrocephalus and is the main subject of a classic monograph by Dorothy Russel (1949). Hydrocephalus used to be divided into communicating and non-communicating varieties based on the appearance of dye injected into the lateral ventricle in the spinal subarachnoid space. Today it is classified according to aetiology or anatomical site of the blockage. In obstructive hydrocephalus the ventricular system becomes dilated proximal to the blockage. Thus if only one of the lateral ventricles is dilated, as happens rarely, then the respective foramen of Monroe is the likely site of the block. If, on the other hand, both lateral ventricles and the third ventricle are dilated, then the obstruction is within the aqueductal region (Fig. 23.8). When the whole of the ventricular system is dilated but basal cisterns are normal, then the abnormality is to be found in the exit foramina (of Magendie and Luschka) of the fourth ventricle

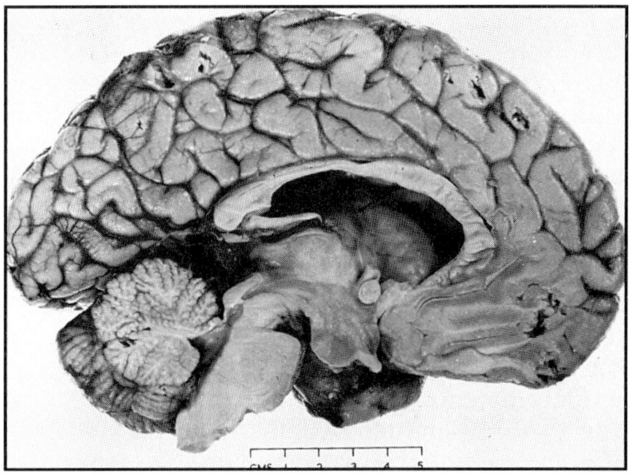

Fig. 23.8. Hemisected brain showing dilatation of the lateral ventricle (with the septum pellucidum dissected) and the third ventricle, which is ballooned out. There is a complete obstruction of the aqueduct of Sylvius. The fourth ventricle is normal in size.

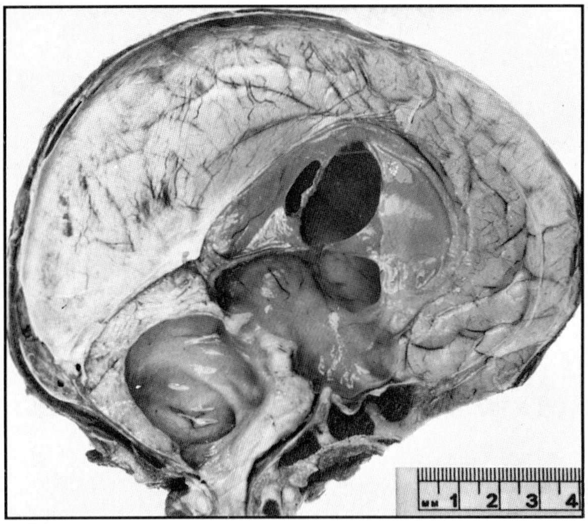

Fig. 23.9. Midline section of a brain within the skull, showing a hugely dilated ventricular system caused by an inflammatory block of the exit foramina of the fourth ventricle. The septum pellucidum is fenestrated, the foramen of Monroe is enlarged, the third and fourth ventricles are ballooned and the aqueduct is dilated and shortened.

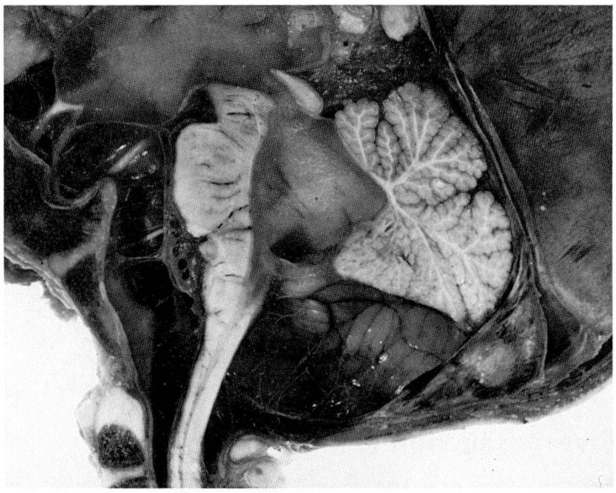

Fig. 23.10. Basal cistern block. Hemisected brain in situ, showing hugely dilated third and fourth ventricles, a dilated short aqueduct and an enormously distended cisterna magna traversed by fine fibrous strands. Dilatation of the interpeduncular cistern has led to elevation of the floor of the third ventricle and elongation of the pituitary stalk and optic nerves.

(Fig. 23.9). A basal cistern block (Fig. 23.10) causes dilation of the posterior fossa cisterns as well. As there are two pairs of choroid plexi, one in the lateral and third ventricles and the other in the fourth, dilatation may take place below an aqueduct block if an additional block is present in the fourth ventricle or in the basal cisterns, which may follow inflammation.

In infantile hydrocephalus, the cerebral hemispheres lying within a distensible calvaria rapidly become thinned as the lateral ventricles dilate. Thinning of the cerebral mantle is not uniform and tends to be most marked in the occipital and temporal lobes, with relative sparing of the frontal poles. It is largely due to atrophy of periventricular white matter (Fig. 23.11) as a result of ischaemia from compression of capillaries by elevated intraventricular pressure (Norman 1963) and rupture and destruction of nerve fibres. Until thinning is extreme, the brain, after removal of CSF, is actually heavier than normal. This is probably due to white matter oedema. The grey matter of the cerebral cortex is remarkably resistant, retaining its normal dimensions, perhaps because of its rich blood supply, though there is gradual unfolding of the convolutions. Cortical cytoarchitecture remains relatively normal even when the mantle is reduced to

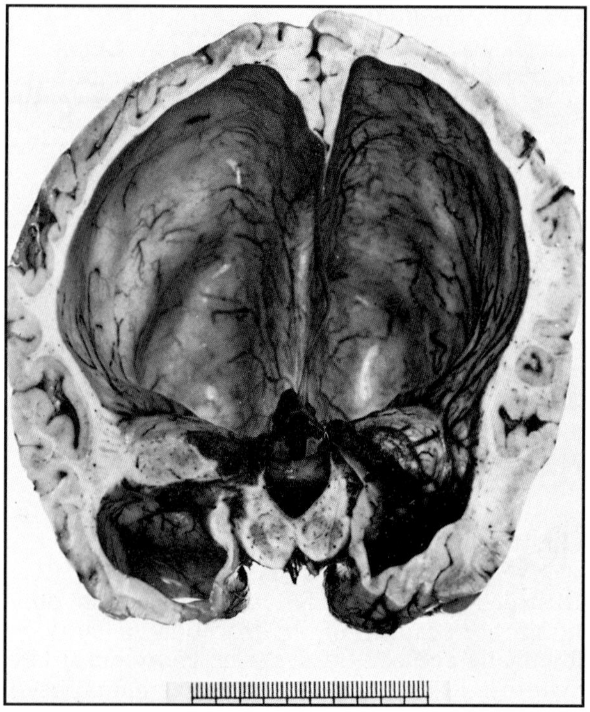

Fig. 23.11. Coronal section of a severely hydrocephalic brain showing thinning of the cortical mantle, with a relatively intact grey layer but virtual disappearance of the white matter. Note the atrophied septum pellucidum and the unfolding of the cerebral convolutions.

2–3 mm thickness and the white matter has all but disappeared. As the ventricles dilate, the ependyma first becomes discontinuous and then largely disappears to be replaced by glia, giving a granular appearance to the ventricular surface. At the same time, the septum pellucidum becomes thinned, fenestrated and finally destroyed, and the corpus callosum is elevated, stretched and thinned. The choroid plexi decrease in size and may eventually become quite sclerotic, especially when hydrocephalus has arrested spontaneously. The meninges may appear normal but adherent to the brain with compression of subarachnoid space. Meningeal vessels are initially increased, which may give a false impression of microgyria, but eventually become attenuated. The skull bones are often greatly thinned and may develop lacunae or even fenestration, allowing false encephaloceles to develop; later, wormian bones may develop within the enlarged fontanelles.

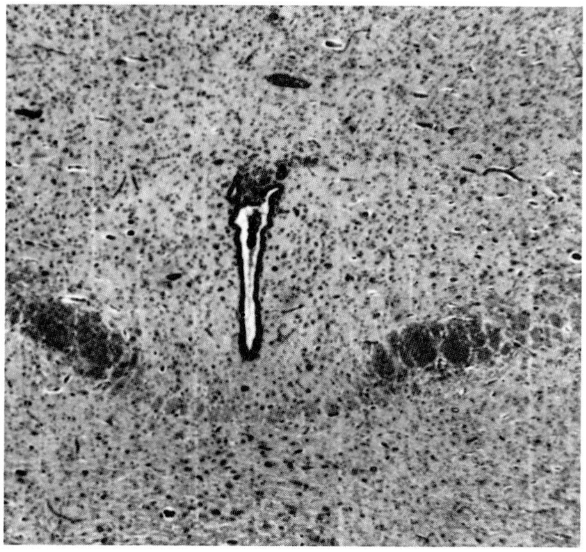

Fig. 23.12. Stenosis of the aqueduct showing one greatly reduced ependymal lined channel without gliosis in the surrounding midbrain. (H&E, ×52)

Malformations Leading to Hydrocephalus

Obstruction of the Aqueduct of Sylvius

At birth the aqueduct is a single channel linking the third and fourth ventricles; it is about 11 mm in length and has an average minimum cross-sectional area of 0.9 mm^2, with considerable variation. The aqueduct is lined by ependyma and surrounded by non-gliotic brain tissue. It is probable that obstruction at this level is not only due to reduction in the cross-sectional area of the aqueduct but also to its length, the viscosity of the CSF and the difference in pressure between the third and fourth ventricles (Alvord 1961).

Stenosis

Stenosis of the aqueduct is an uncommon condition which may be associated with other malformations such as spina bifida and the Arnold–Chiari malformation.

The normal contour of the aqueduct may be preserved but its diameter is markedly reduced; often it has a crenated and irregular outline. The ependymal lining remains intact and the surrounding brain tissue is normal and free from excessive gliosis (Fig. 23.12). A rare X-linked recessive variety of aqueduct stenosis is described by Bickers and Adams (1949) and Edwards and colleagues (1961); there is associated mental retardation and flexion abnormalities of the fingers. The hydrocephalus associated with this condition is usually not advanced by the time of birth.

Forking

Forking of the aqueduct is commonly found in association with the Arnold–Chiari malformation and spina bifida (Cameron 1957a). Here the aqueduct divides into several branches, often a larger dorsal channel and a number of smaller ventral ones, each with an irregular outline but with an intact ependymal lining and surrounded by non-gliotic brain tissue (Fig. 23.13). In this abnormality, probably caused by sideways compression (Emery 1974), one or more of these channels communicates with the third and the fourth ventricles but the cross-sectional area is greatly reduced, leading to at least partial obstruction.

Septum Formation

Septum formation is rare and usually found at the caudal end of the aqueduct. The septum is

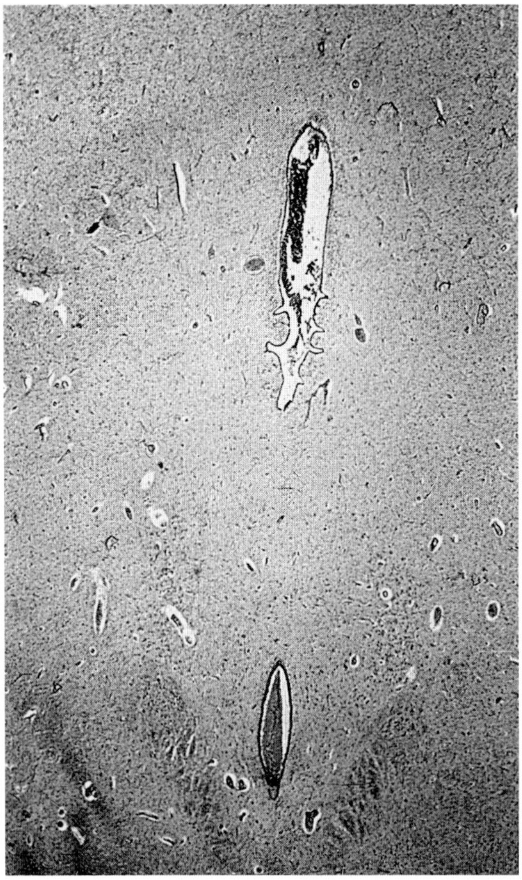

Fig. 23.13. Forking of the aqueduct with two relatively small channels lined by ependymal cells and no surrounding gliosis. (H&E, ×20)

composed of a thin neuroglial membrane. Its aetiology is unknown, but because it may be associated with granular ependymitis elsewhere in the ventricular system, intrauterine infection has been suggested as a possible causative factor (Russel 1949).

Gliosis

Gliosis of the aqueduct results in narrowing, subdivision or complete occlusion by an overgrowth of fibrillary neuroglia (Fig. 23.14). The original outline of the aqueduct is indicated by disorderly islets of ependymal cells within the gliosis. A central channel often remains but this rarely has an ependymal lining. This condition is rarely found in infancy; the hydrocephalus begins insidiously later in childhood. Its pathogenesis is obscure, but involutional hyperplasia of the subependymal glia, postinflammatory hyperplasia and a hamartomatous condition similar to von Recklinghausen's disease have been suggested (Laurence 1959).

Malformations of the Hindbrain

Arnold–Chiari Malformation

The Arnold–Chiari malformation is the commonest "cause" or association of congenital hydrocephalus in the UK, with its relatively high prevalence of spina bifida. Almost all cases of myelocoele (or myelomeningocoele) are associated with this anomaly, the only exceptions being some of those cases, where the spinal lesion is confined to the lower lumbar or sacral region (Cameron 1957a). This malformation, which may be apparent by the 10th week of gestation (Duckett 1966) and is well developed by 15 weeks (Laurence et al. 1983b) has cerebellar and pontomedullary components. The cerebellum usually appears

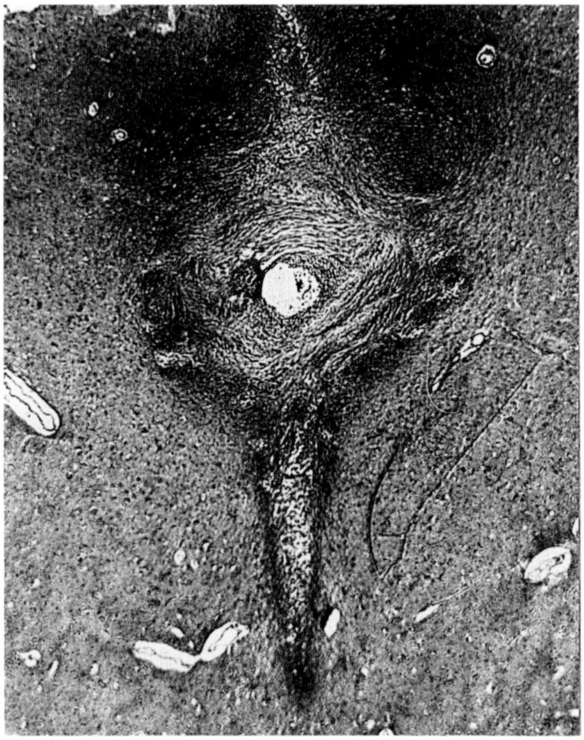

Fig. 23.14. Gliosis of the aqueduct, showing dense fibres in both the lumen and the area of original outline of the channel. (Mallory's phosphotungstic acid haematoxylin, ×24)

small, compact, poorly lobed, sometimes quite asymmetric and closely moulded to the contours of the posterior fossa and foramen magnum (Fig. 23.15). Posteriorly a midline tongue consisting of the vermis extends for a variable distance beyond the often funnel-shaped foramen magnum down the spinal canal, which may be wide. The medulla, and to some extent the pons, is displaced downwards beyond the foramen magnum and is thinned and distorted. Additionally, the medulla is frequently buckled backwards in the form of an S over the upper cervical spinal cord, which it compresses (Fig. 23.16). Lying between pons and medulla anteriorly and cerebellum posteriorly is an elongated, often narrow and compressed fourth ventricle, whose choroid plexus may form a compact congested mass near the tip of the cerebellar prolongation. The whole is covered by congested, often thickened meninges, which may be tightly bound to underlying structures. Internally, the cerebellum and medulla frequently show macroscopic and microscopic abnormalities and congestion of those portions situated below the foramen magnum (Cameron 1957a). The lower cranial nerves are considerably elongated and the upper cervical nerve roots run an upward course to gain their foramina because of downward displacement of the spinal cord. This malformation is extremely variable in extent and form. It may be relatively minor, with downward displacement of the vermis or medulla by only a few millimetres; occasionally, nearly the whole of the hindbrain lies in the cervical canal. Sometimes only the medulla is malformed. It may be distinguished from tonsillar herniation resulting from acutely raised intracranial pressure, when the cerebellar tonsils descend through the foramen magnum laterally without medullary displacement.

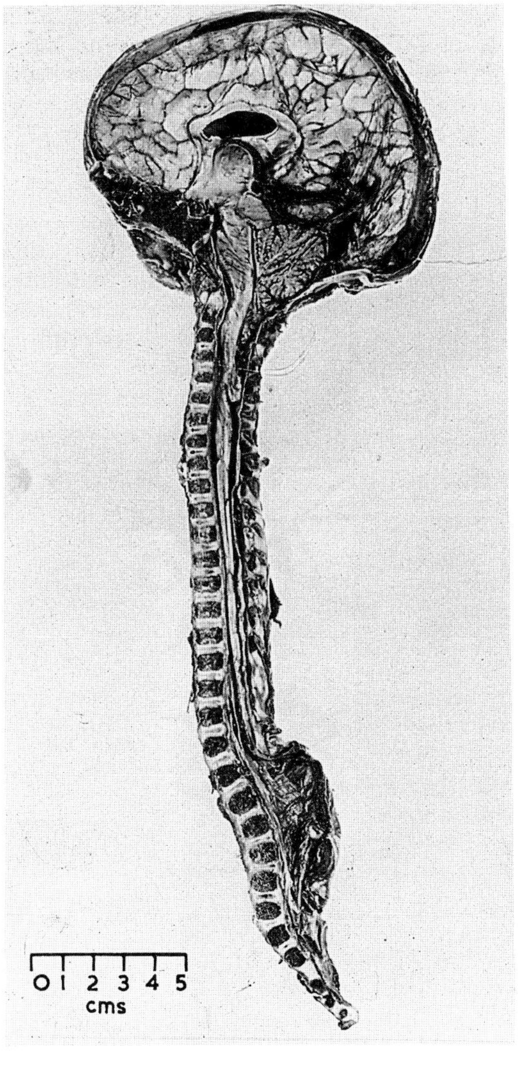

Fig. 23.15. Hemisected skull and spinal column showing the Arnold–Chiari malformation. The elongated medulla is not only largely intraspinal but is also kinked over the cord. The well-developed cerebellar tongue is well shown. A compressed elongated fourth ventricle lies between medulla and cerebellum. The myelocoele in the lumbosacral region is typical, with nerve roots leaving the neural plate to gain the root canals. The cord shows slight hydromyelia.

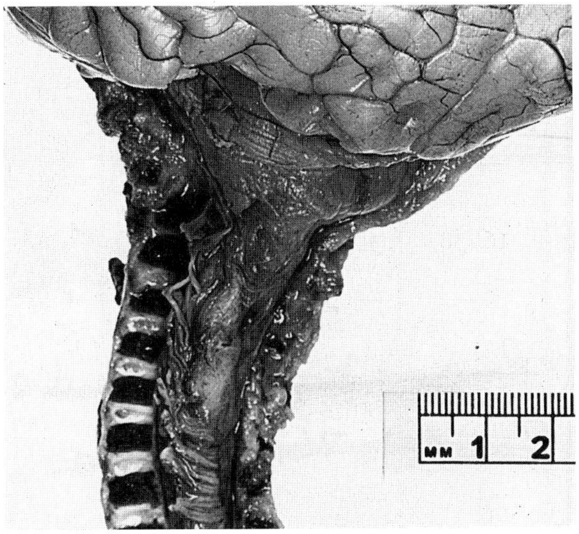

Fig. 23.16. An Arnold–Chiari malformation showing a moulded cerebellum with a cerebellar tongue, and an elongated medulla kinked upon the spinal cord lying almost entirely below the widened foramen magnum. Note the upward course of the cervical spinal nerve roots.

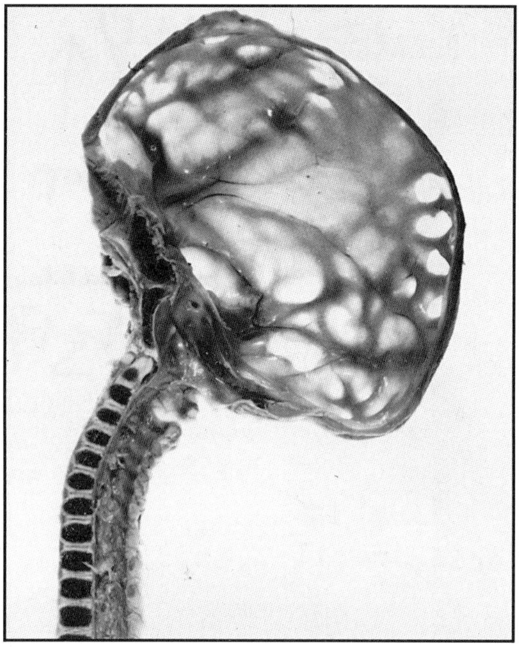

Fig. 23.17. Skull and upper vertebral column from an infant with a myelocoele and Arnold–Chiari malformation. Note the cranio-fenestra, the low insertion of the tentorium, the shallow posterior fossa and the wide foramen magnum.

This malformation, which usually lies in a small, shallow posterior fossa, with a narrow tentorium, often inserted low down and with a wide incisura, has had many aetiological explanations (Fig. 23.17). Tethering of the cord by the spina bifida (Penfield and Coburn 1938; Lichtenstein 1942), the pressure of the associated hydrocephalus (Gardener and Goodall 1950) and failure of the pontine flexure (Daniel and Strich 1958) have been suggested. The probable explanation is failure of the normal development of the posterior fossa in the presence of spina bifida, followed by the growth of the hindbrain structures in a restricted space (Marin-Padilla 1978). This abnormality alone will lead to obstruction of the CSF flow by compression of both the exit foramina and the subarachnoid spaces. Postnatally, inflammation, such as ascending meningitis from an open spinal lesion, will aggravate any obstruction.

Dandy–Walker Syndrome

In the Dandy–Walker syndrome the cerebellar hemispheres are widely separated caudally by a hugely enlarged fourth ventricle, the roof of which is covered by a bulging membrane of ependyma, neuroglia, connective tissue and blood vessels. The cerebellar vermis is small and poorly formed or absent (Norman 1963; Fig. 23.18). Usually the brain stem is flattened and anteriorly displaced, the fourth ventricular choroid plexus is small and basal cisterns are obliterated. In this abnormality, which may be well developed by 20 weeks' gestation, the foramina of Magendie and Luschka fail to develop at about 8–10 weeks.

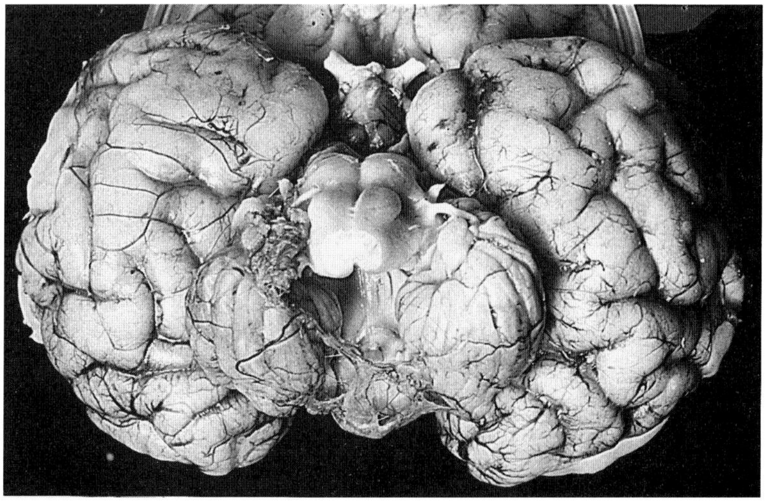

Fig. 23.18. Newborn infant with Dandy–Walker syndrome. The membrane roofing over the greatly distended fourth ventricle has been removed. Note the absence of the cerebellar vermis and the widely separated cerebellar hemispheres. (Courtesy of Dr. A. King, Cambridge)

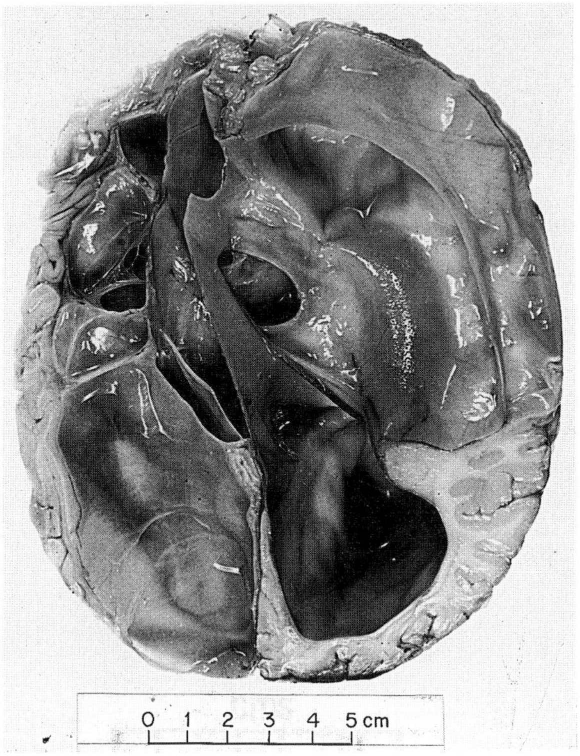

Fig. 23.19. Horizontal section through the cerebrum following *Escherichia coli* meningitis. The lateral ventricles have been converted into a series of intercommunicating cysts.

The Dandy–Walker syndrome, which probably accounts for no more than 5% of uncomplicated congenital hydrocephalus, is usually sporadic, but some cases are recessively inherited. It can be recognised by the characteristic radiographic appearances of an enlarged posterior fossa and high tentorium, torcula and transverse sinus (Taggart and Walker 1942). Sometimes the condition is complicated by other malformations both within the CNS and outside it.

Inflammation Causing Hydrocephalus

Post-inflammatory hydrocephalus in the newborn may follow either intrauterine or perinatal insult in the form of intracranial haemorrhage or infection. In the UK, post-haemorrhagic hydrocephalus usually affects preterm babies and is discussed in Chapter 24, p. 575, although in some parts of the world hydrocephalus is a well-recognised complication of traumatic haemorrhage.

Infections which give rise to hydrocephalus may be acute or chronic. They are usually bacterial and less frequently viral or protozoal in origin. Infections which are initially symptomless or of insidious onset so that treatment is delayed are more likely to have chronic sequelae than are acute infections. Meningitis is discussed in Chapter 24, p. 589.

A variety of pathological lesions may follow intracranial inflammation. The most severe effects, often resulting from an *Escherichia coli* meningitis, may lead to an organising pyocephalus (Fig. 23.19). Here, the whole ventricular system is converted into a series of intercommunicating cysts, and the foramina of Monro may become occluded. In less severe inflammation, the aqueduct, always a vulnerable structure in view of its site and size, may become blocked, either by pus or a small blood clot. Sometimes obstruction may follow damage to its ependymal lining; subependymal glia proliferates and may finally completely occlude the channel (Fig. 23.20). In the majority of cases, however, meningeal inflammation leads to occlusive fibrosis. This process blocks the exit foramina of the fourth ventricle, and the arachnoid may become bound down in their immediate vicinity (see Fig. 23.9). In other cases the foramina remain clear, but the arachnoid becomes bound down on the edge of the basal cisterns and thus gives rise to basal cistern block. The cisterns then dilate, compressing the cerebellum, elevating the floor of the third ventricle, or stretching the optic nerve and the pituitary stalk (see Fig. 23.10). Any combination of these post-inflammatory lesions may be present in a particular case, or may be superimposed on pre-existing malformations.

Tumours Leading to Hydrocephalus

Tumours are an uncommon cause of hydrocephalus in the perinatal period. They produce hydrocephalus either by compression and obstruction of the CSF pathway (Fig. 23.21) or as a result of haemorrhage from the tumour.

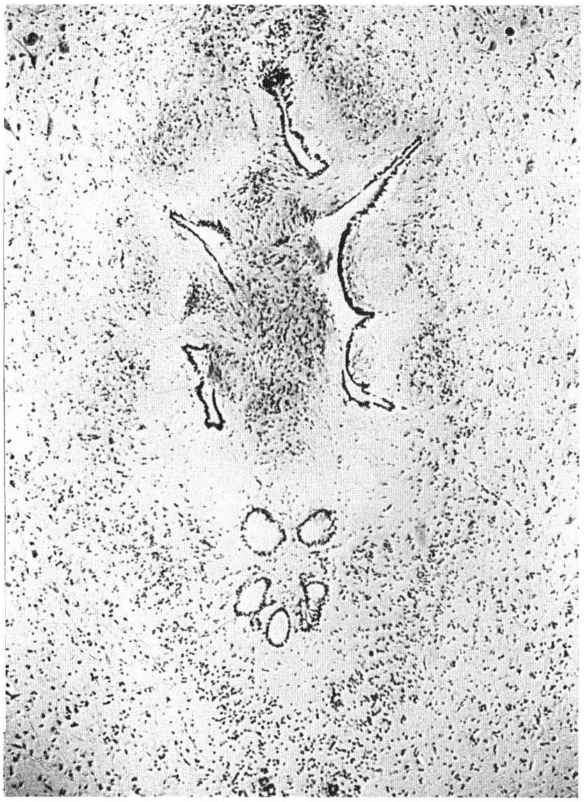

Fig. 23.20. Aqueduct with post-inflammatory gliosis, showing the numerous partially ependymal lined channels near the original outline of structure. The lumen is filled with organising exudate. (H&E, ×36)

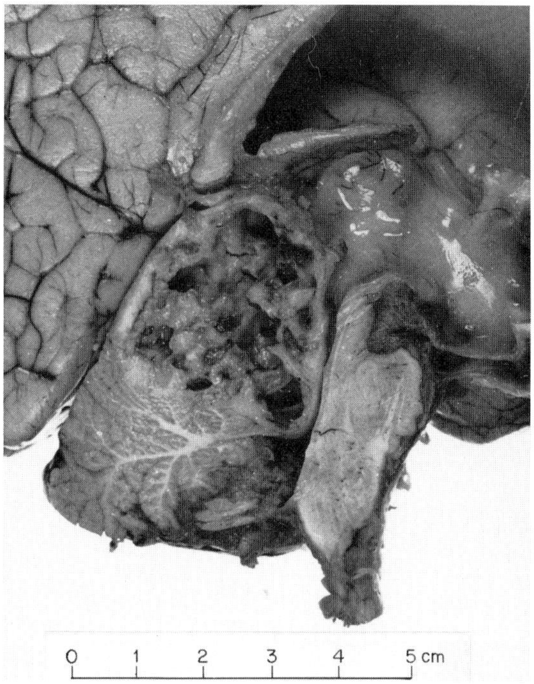

Fig. 23.21. Hemisected brain showing aqueduct compressed by an intrauterine cerebellar medulloblastoma causing dilatation of the lateral and third ventricles.

Neural Tube Defects

Introduction

Neural tube defects (NTDs) comprise a number of abnormalities of neural tube closure, anencephaly and its variants, encephalocoele and spina bifida cystica (or aperta), but not isolated hydrocephalus. The term "spina bifida" includes myelocoele (myelomeningocoele) where the spinal cord is involved, simple meningocoele involving only meninges, and "complicated" spina bifida occulta (Laurence 1990). This last disorder is usually excluded from NTD statistics because of diagnostic and definition problems (Fig. 23.22). These abnormalities are interrelated and may be found in siblings or extended family and almost

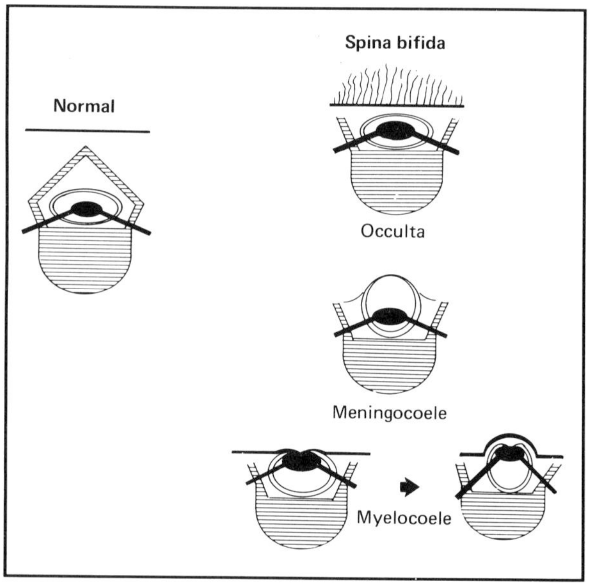

Fig. 23.22. Diagrammatic representation of the anatomy of the normal spinal column and of spina bifida.

certainly have a common, multifactorial aetiology (Carter 1974). The genetic component is polygenic and renders the developing embryo liable to interference to orderly closure of the neural tube by environmental trigger acting between 21 and 28 days after conception (Dekaban 1963; Lemire et al. 1965).

In most epidemiological studies about half the NTDs are anencephaly; myelocoeles account for most of the remainder (Laurence et al. 1968). Encephalocoeles are relatively uncommon and make up no more than 3% of the total (Laurence and Tew 1971), except in Thailand, where anterior encephalocoele is relatively frequently encountered. Meningocoeles are almost invariably over-reported; they comprise less than 5% of spina bifida cystica when careful pathological examination has been undertaken.

NTDs are one of the commonest serious malformations in the UK. Prevalence rates of over 10 per 1000 births were recorded from Northern Ireland, South Wales and south western Scotland (Elwood and Elwood 1980), but rates had fallen even before prenatal identification and selective abortion became available (Laurence 1989). Most parts of the UK now have pregnancy rates of 2 per 1000 or less, though the actual birth rates are very much less than that. High prevalence has also been reported in parts of northern India and Pakistan, in the Middle East and most recently in northern China (Ye 1986). In most of Europe, North America and Australia, the prevalence is only about 1 per 1000, whilst among orientals and blacks even lower prevalences are recorded. In most societies the prevalence is highest in the poorer section of society; seasonal and marked secular variations are found (Elwood and Elwood 1980). No convincing explanations have been found for the last, but maternal undernutrition could explain seasonal and social class differences. Genetic factors must underlie some of the racial differences.

Family studies carried out in the UK (Carter et al. 1968; Carter and Evans 1973) and elsewhere have shown that there is a high risk of recurrence and have produced data supporting a polygenic basis for the disorder, similar to most other common malformations. Although NTDs can be produced in susceptible experimental animals by a large number of different environmental agents (Elwood and Elwood 1980), few have been identified so far in man. Retrospective and prospective studies of maternal diet in South Wales women (Laurence et al. 1980; James and Laurence 1983; Laurence et al. 1983a) suggest that poor maternal nutrition may be one of the environmental triggers and that improvement of the diet with emphasis on the balance of food stuffs and inclusion of green vegetables can reduce the risk of recurrence. Intervention studies using a cocktail of vitamins (Smithells et al. 1980) or, more specifically, giving pharmacological amounts of folic acid preconceptionally, suggest that folic acid lack because of low intake, poor absorption or metabolic derangement is a significant if not the most important aetiological factor (Laurence et al. 1981; Laurence et al. 1983a; Laurence 1991; MRC 1991). Other factors such as sodium valproate and oral contraceptives and perhaps some virus infections may play a part in some cases. It is possible that preconceptional folic acid or vitamin supplementation can be used as a method of prevention in high-risk pregnancies. Since 1972, mid-trimester prenatal diagnosis of open NTD in high-risk pregnancies using alpha-fetoprotein levels in maternal serum and amniotic fluid, other biochemical markers and high-resolution ultrasonography has become common practice. Population screening programmes have been introduced. These measures have reduced the birth prevalence in many regions in the UK to considerably less than 1 per 1000 (Laurence 1989).

Anencephaly

Fetuses with anencephaly, the severest of the dysraphic NTDs, are either stillborn or die within a short time of birth. About half the pregnancies develop polyhydramnios during the third trimester, because of impaired fetal swallowing. Many are born prematurely because of polyhydramnios, but in some labour is difficult to initiate, probably because of abnormal fetal adrenal function. About three out of four anencephalics are female.

In this abnormality, which is equivalent to exencephaly in rodents, the cranial end of the neural tube fails to close, acrania (absence of the cranial vault) is usual with foreshortening of the anterior cranial fossa. The frontal bones are usually represented only by supraorbital ridges; the parietal bones are absent or represented by a narrow ridge; the occipital bone

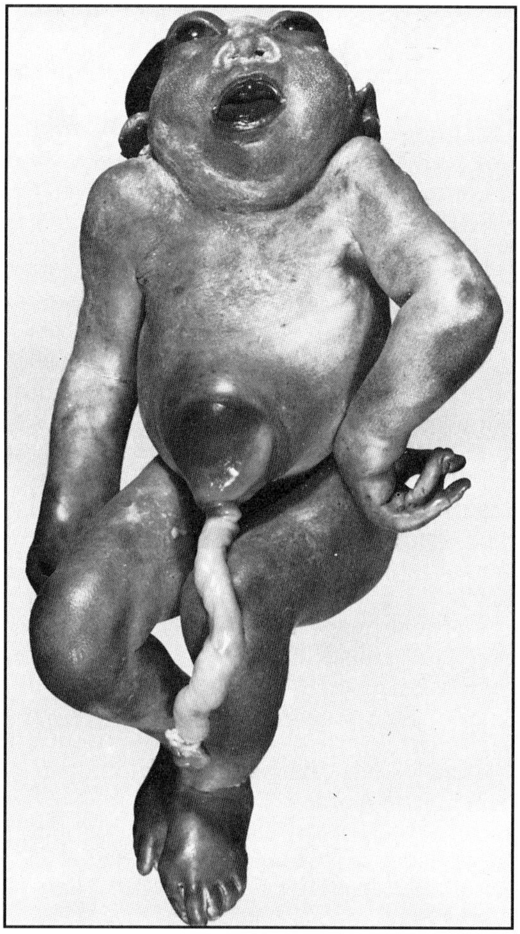

Fig. 23.23. Term anencephalic fetus with grotesque facies, short neck and a small omphalocoele.

is variably absent, its squamous part missing (Potter and Craig 1976). The pituitary fossa is usually flattened and empty. The whole of the base of the skull is covered by a congested mass of tissue of variable thickness (area cerebrovascularis) consisting of thin-walled vascular spaces, irregular brain tissue, sometimes with recognisable neurons, choroid plexus-like structures, glial nodules and ependyma. Recognisable cerebellar tissue may also be present and brainstem structures can often be found. Careful search will generally reveal anterior pituitary tissue, but no hypophysis. The whole area cerebrovascularis may be covered by a thin layer of squamous epithelium and occasionally by attenuated or normal skin.

The facies of an anencephalic are often quite grotesque (Fig. 23.23), with bulging eyes situated in shallow orbits, protuberant crumpled ears, flattened nose and a mouth with a prominent tongue. The eyes are well formed, except for absence of ganglia in the retina. The optic nerves end abruptly at the internal optic foramen. Other cranial nerves can be identified after painstaking dissection. The internal ear is generally normal.

In many instances there is no neck and the chin lies low over the sternum. In these circumstances the thorax is usually shortened; cervical vertebrae are abnormal or missing. Both exomphalos and club foot may be present. The palate is often high-arched, but cleft lip and palate is uncommon.

Internally, the most striking abnormality is the small size of the adrenal glands, which together usually weigh less than 1 g. In most instances, there is virtually no fetal zone (Anderson et al. 1969; Young et al. 1989) but the medulla is well developed (see Chap. 21, p. 504). The thyroid gland is well developed with colloid-full acina. The lungs are frequently hypoplastic, with interstitial haemorrhage. Coexistent malformations are diaphragmatic hernia, horseshoe kidney and occasionally renal dysplasia or agenesis. Cleft lip (with or without cleft palate) (Khoury et al. 1989), anal agenesis and exomphalos occur more frequently with anencephaly than would be expected by chance.

About 50% of cases of anencephaly have rachischisis (craniorachischisis) (Fig. 23.24), in which case there is no foramen magnum. The rachischisis may be short, but sometimes the whole length of the unclosed, often very thin, neural plaque representing the neural tube is exposed. It may be covered by a thin, delicate membrane.

Several defects related to anencephaly are recognised. The most common is iniencephaly (see Fig. 4.11, p. 130). This condition has some features in common with Klippel–Feil syndrome. The brain, enclosed by a cranial vault and covered by scalp, is severely disorganised. Severe abnormalities of the cervical vertebrae with reduction in number cause the head to be hyperextended so that the face points upwards. The remainder of the vertebral column is often abnormal and the trunk tends to be shortened. Umbilical hernia, diaphragmatic hernia and cardiac malformations may be present.

Other variants, exencephaly acrania, microcephalus acrania and microcephalus craniorachischisis, occasionally occur. In exencephaly acrania there is absence of the roof of the

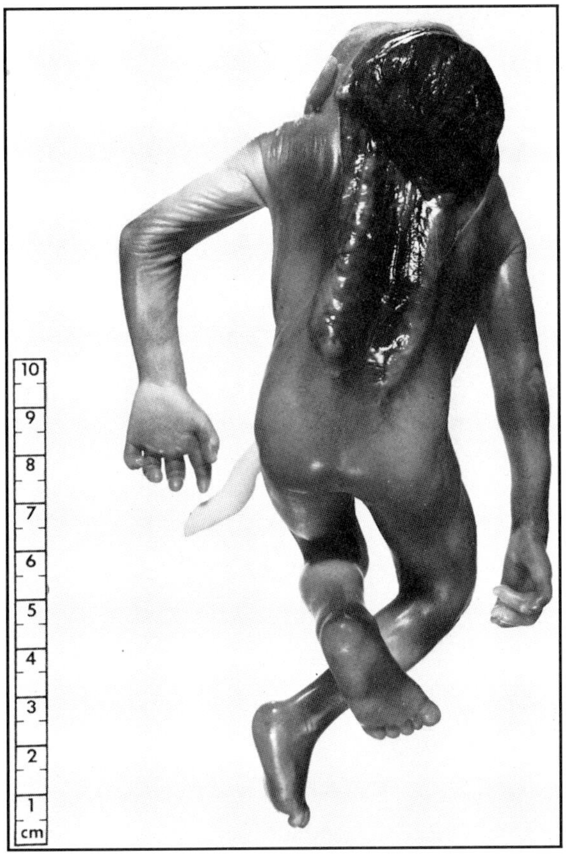

Fig. 23.24. An 18-week anencephalic fetus with a congested mass of disorganised brain tissue over the base of the skull and a rachischisis.

cranium and a massive herniation of a fluid-filled sac of brain tissue; the whole lesion is covered by normal scalp. Microcephalus acrania is anencephaly with disorganised brain tissue covered by vestigial skull bones and scalp giving a form of gross microcephaly. Microcephalus craniorachischisis is similar to the last condition but with a rachischisis and a tendency for the face to be upward-pointing as cervical and upper dorsal spine are grossly disorganised (Morison 1970).

The mid-trimester anencephalic differs from the nearer term because at this stage there is more neural tissue present and cerebral structures are recognisable (Bell 1982; Laurence et al. 1983b). Presumably much of this tissue degenerates between mid-trimester and term because of continuing exposure to amniotic fluid and minor trauma. Suprarenal glands at this stage of development are relatively larger than in the more mature fetus (Young et al. 1989).

Cranial Meningocele and Encephalocele

Cranium bifidum is a herniation of meninges or meninges and brain through a cranial defect. Over three-quarters of these occur in the occipital region; protrusions in the frontal, parietal, nasopharyngeal and orbital regions are very much less common. When there is protrusion of meninges only, even a large lesion may be almost asymptomatic, and surgical removal is successful unless there is an associated brain abnormality. When the defect includes brain tissue (encephalocoele), it is always a serious condition, and even with surgery there is usually severe mental defect and neurological abnormality, such as spasticity or blindness. However, such infants often survive as meningitis and hydrocephalus are infrequent complications. Surgical removal of a large lesion may often become a necessity to facilitate nursing.

A typical encephalocoele (Fig. 23.25) is situated in the occipital region and is usually totally covered by normal, sometimes hair-bearing skin, which may become thin or ulcerate. The skull defect, which is often quite small, lies in the squamous part of the occipital bone and may involve the foramen magnum and sometimes the posterior arch of the atlas, whilst the encephalocoele may be huge, larger than the skull, which is often microcephalic. The contents of the encephalocoele are variable (Fig. 23.26) and may include one or both occipital lobes with fairly normally laminated or microgyric grey matter and underlying white matter or part of the posterior horns of the lateral ventricles. Sometimes it contains cerebellum and brainstem. Often the brain contains glial scars or abnormal vessels, and is engorged or infarcted (Karch and Urich 1972; Urich 1976).

Anterior encephalocoeles (Fig. 23.27), most commonly found in the frontoethmoid junction, are rare in Europe but relatively common in southeast Asia. Encephaloceles may be detected in mid trimester by high-resolution ultrasonography, but as they are "closed" lesions they are not normally associated with elevated serum or amniotic alpha-fetoprotein levels (Laurence 1983).

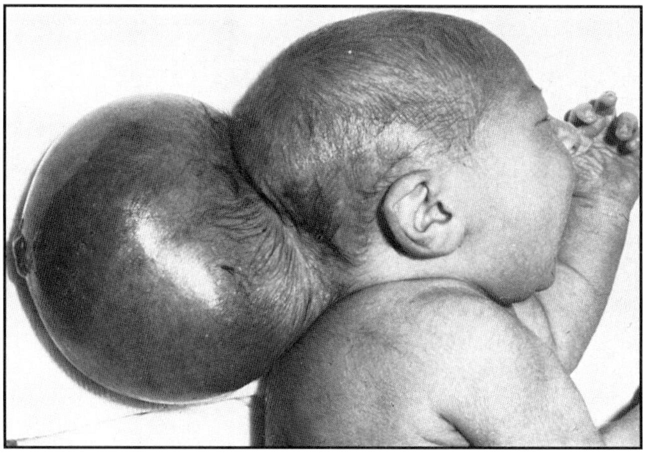

Fig. 23.25. Newborn infant with a large skin-covered occipital encephalocoele as large as the microcephalic head from which it has arisen.

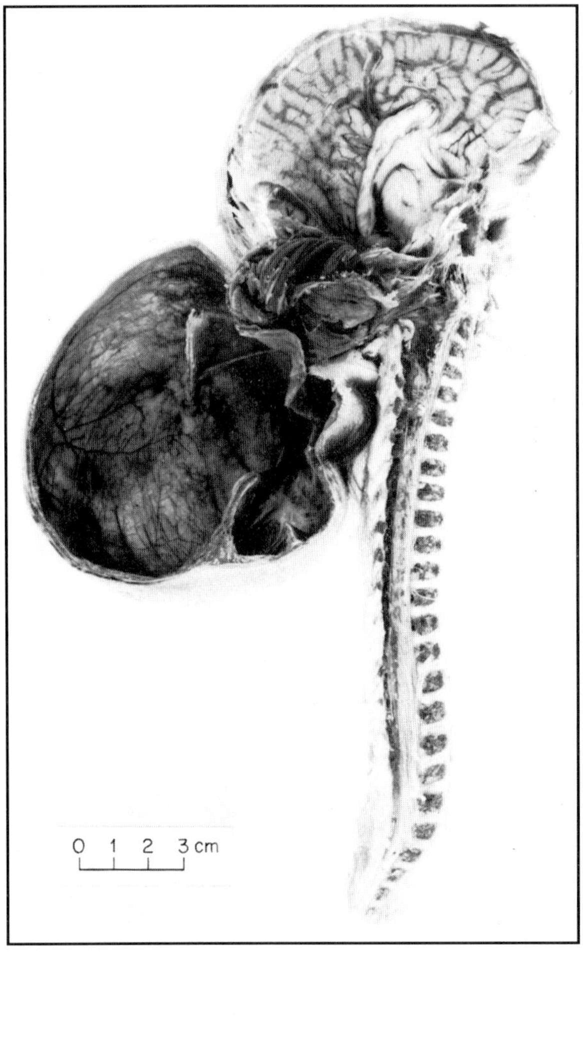

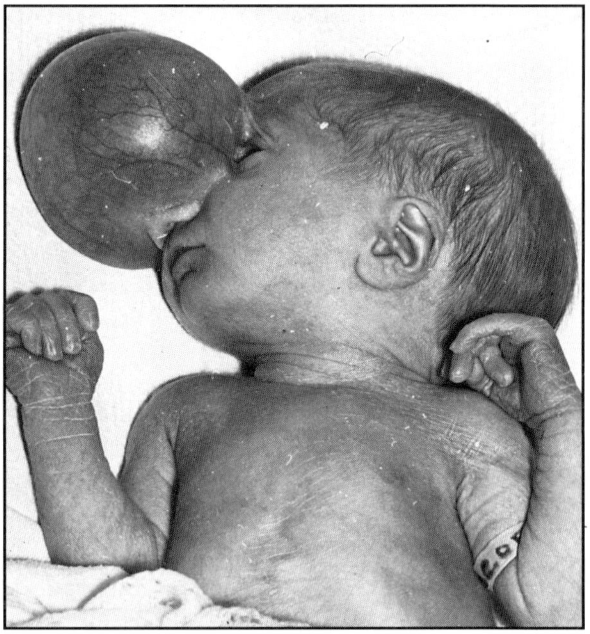

Fig. 23.27. Newborn infant with an anterior encephalocoele. This contained part of the anterior lobes of both cerebral hemispheres.

Fig. 23.26. Hemisected head encephalocoele and spinal column of the patient in Fig. 23.25, showing the relatively little brain protruding through the large skull defect involving the foramen magnum. In addition to part of the occipital lobes and posterior horns of the lateral ventricles, the sac contains a hugely expanded subarachnoid space and part of the cerebellum.

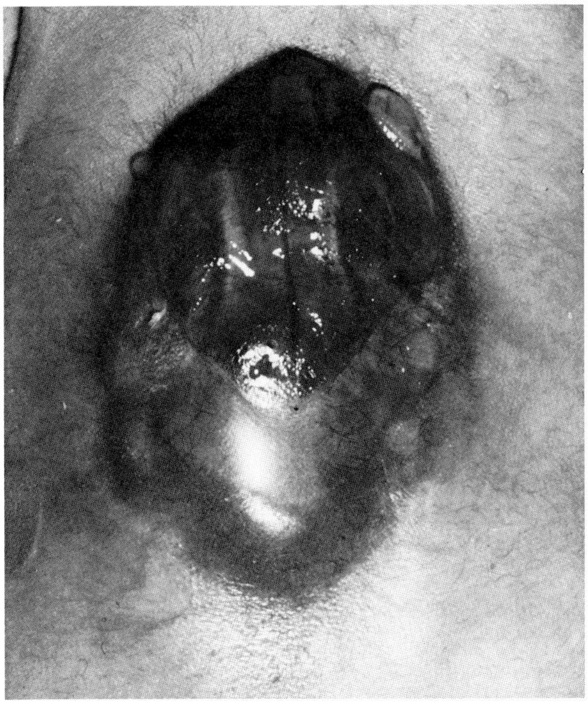

Fig. 23.28. Lumbar myelocoele in a newborn infant. The neural plaque can be seen covered by a very thin transparent membrane. Nerve trunks can be seen through the more peripheral thicker membrane, which blends peripherally with the skin of the back.

Myelocoele (Myelomeningocoele)

All cases of spina bifida cystica with nonclosure of the neural tube are, by definition, myelocoeles, though descriptive terms such as "myelomeningocoele" or "meningomyelocoele" are often used. Myelocoeles may be situated anywhere along the neuraxis but are most common in the lower dorsal, lumbar and upper sacral regions. They vary greatly in size and appearance, but a typical lesion (Fig. 23.28) consists of a flat, central zona vasculosa, the open exposed congested neural plate, often partially split longitudinally and onto which the central canal of the spinal cord may open at the upper end. The neural plate may be covered by a thin delicate membrane. It is surrounded by the zona membranosa, a semitransparent membrane representing meninges which merges peripherally with the skin of the back, which may be naevoid or hair bearing. Sometimes the whole is covered by normal skin and may be associated with a lipoma. In the newborn the neural plate is covered by ependyma and usually contains nerve bundles and well-organised nuclei with neurons. Spinal roots arise from the underside, traverse the spinal subarachnoid space and gain the root canals (Fig. 23.29). The spinal cord does not show the usual lumbar enlargement and may extend lower down the spinal canal than normal, always as far as the myelocoele. If the lesion is high up on the neuraxis, then the spinal cord beyond it is usually abnormal. Associated neural arches are widely splayed and vertebral bodies are abnormal, leading to kyphosis and sometimes scoliosis. Rib abnormalities are found with dorsal lesions. Above the myelocoele the spinal cord may show various abnormalities: there may be splitting of the cord with or without diastematomyelia, hydromyelia, diplomyelia or syringomyelia (MacKenzie and Emery 1971). Occasionally, dermoids, lipomas, enterogenous cysts or teratomas are present in the vicinity of the myelocele. Nearly all myelocoeles are associated with an Arnold–Chiari malformation (see Figs. 23.15, 23.16).

Over 80% of cases have well-established and sometimes severe hydrocephalus at birth, which may be due to the Arnold–Chiari mal-

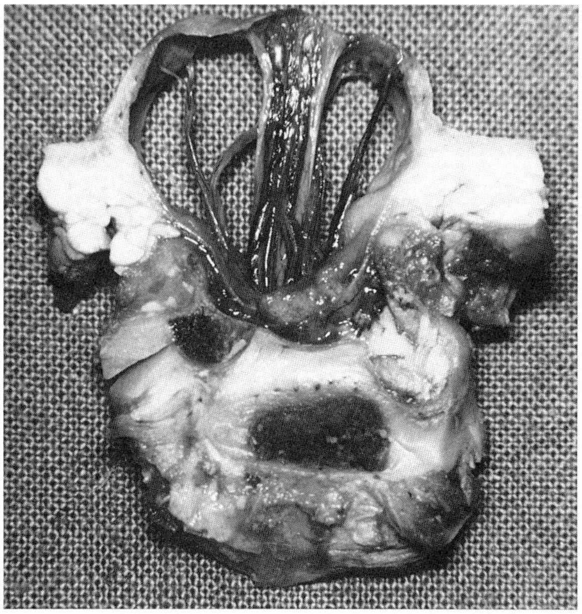

Fig. 23.29. Cross-section of the vertebral column at the level of a lumbar myelocoele. Nerve roots leaving the ventral surface of the thin neural plate traverse the subarachnoid space to gain the root canals.

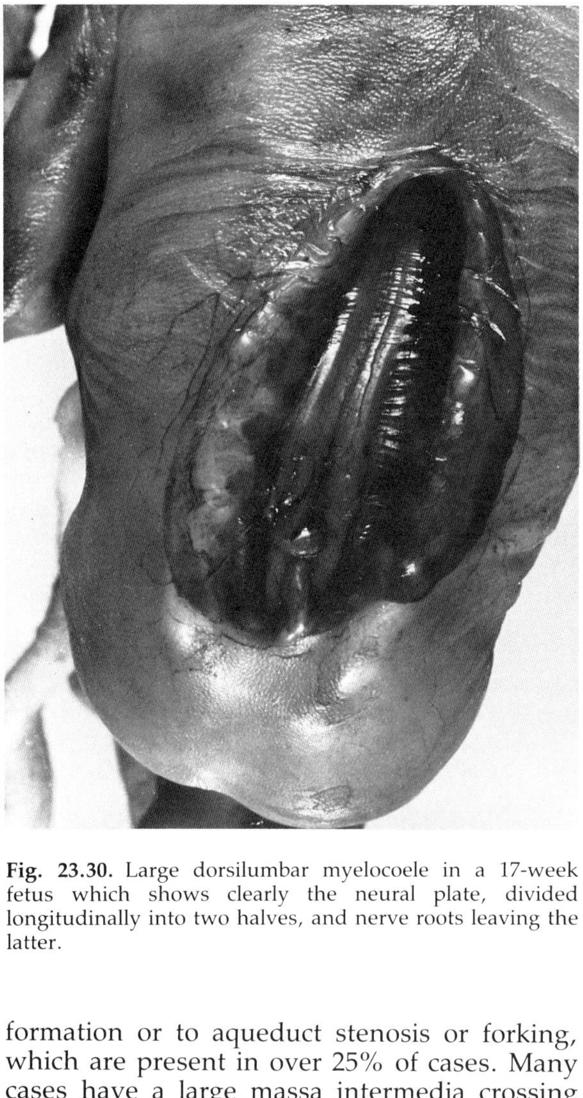

Fig. 23.30. Large dorsilumbar myelocoele in a 17-week fetus which shows clearly the neural plate, divided longitudinally into two halves, and nerve roots leaving the latter.

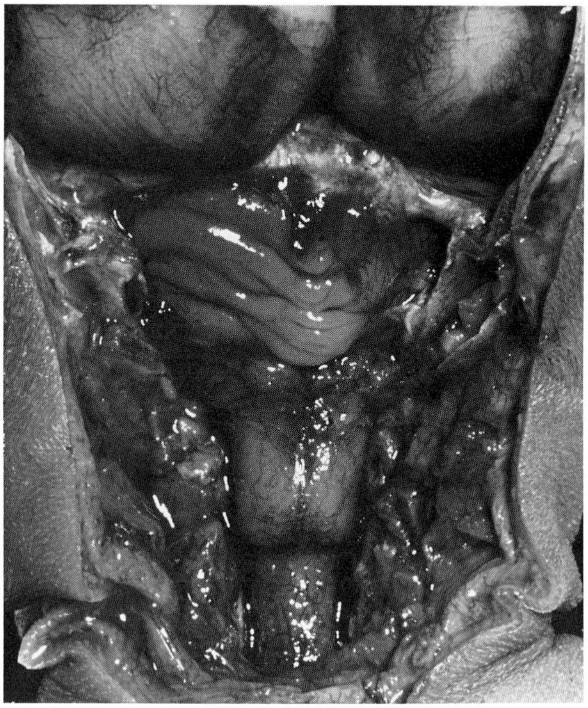

Fig. 23.31. Hindbrain dissection of an 18-week fetus with a lumbar myelocoele, showing a well-developed Arnold–Chiari malformation with a compressed abnormal cerebellum and a kinked medulla.

formation or to aqueduct stenosis or forking, which are present in over 25% of cases. Many cases have a large massa intermedia crossing the third ventricle or a hypoplastic falx cerebri allowing interdigitation between the two cerebral hemispheres. Sometimes there is heterotopic grey matter on the inside of the dilated cerebral hemispheres and there may be polymicrogyria.

Joint deformities or restriction of movement of lower limb joints are commonly associated with myelocoele. These abnormalities are due to absent or abnormal innervation of muscles as a result of the spinal malformation. Malformations of the renal system such as renal agenesis and dysplasia, horseshoe kidney, duplications and hydronephrosis are common (Cameron 1957b).

In the second trimester fetus, a myelocoele is usually better preserved than at term, with much more of the neural plate apparent (Fig. 23.30). An Arnold–Chiari malformation can almost always be identified (Fig. 23.31), and hydrocephalus is present in 90% of cases, often without accompanying head enlargement. Foot deformations are often well developed by this stage.

Some fetuses are stillborn; many infants die in the neonatal period or in infancy, first of brainstem failure or perinatal causes, then of ascending meningitis and progressive hydrocephalus. Only about 10% survive beyond 6 months without active treatment (Laurence 1974). Those that survive with the help of surgery and antibiotics, or because the lesion epithelialises over and the hydrocephalus arrests, may suffer intellectual deficit because of hydrocephalus or its complications. Nearly all have some degree of paralysis, often severe, usually with sphincter disturbance leading to incontinence; the pattern of disability is related to the level of the lesion.

Meningocoele

True meningocoele is uncommon and rarely comes to necropsy, but operative material may be submitted for pathological examination. The condition is often not detectable prenatally by elevated serum or amniotic fluid alpha-fetoprotein levels as it is a "closed" lesion, although the bony defect may be seen by ultrasonography. Meninges, dura and arachnoid fuse together into a relatively thick membrane and herniate through the bony defect (Fig. 23.32). The spinal cord remains within the spinal canal and is generally normal. Such infants have a good prognosis and rarely exhibit significant neurological deficit or develop hydrocephalus, and after surgical removal of the lesion develop normally, both physically and intellectually (Laurence and Tew 1971).

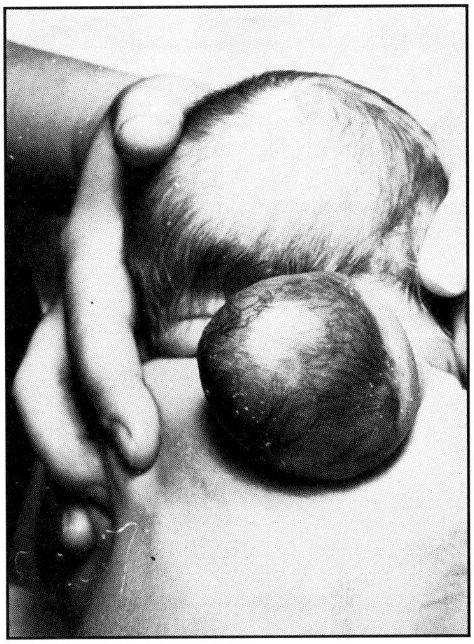

Fig. 23.32. Cervical meningocele in an infant, consisting of a CSF-filled sac covered by a thick membrane. After removal, this infant developed normally without physical or intellectual impairment.

Spina Bifida Occulta

Simple spina bifida occulta, comprising non-fusion of one neural arch, usually in the lower lumbar spine, and no other abnormality such as widening of the spinal canal, myelodysplasia neurological deficit or epidermal abnormalities, is seen in over 5% of the adult population. This is not part of the NTD spectrum of malformations but a normal variant and of no clinical importance.

Complicated spina bifida occulta, which rarely comes to pathological examination in the perinatal period, is relatively uncommon and must be regarded as part of the NTD spectrum (Laurence et al. 1971). The defect comprises non-fusion of more than two adjacent neural arches, involving widening of the spinal canal but no major neurological or other abnormality at one end of the continuum and extending to sacral agenesis with severe disability at the other.

When carefully examined, most cases have some neurological deficit, sphincter disturbance, lower limb asymmetry or orthopaedic abnormality, and severe cases may have unilateral or bilateral club foot. Many have a hairy patch or angioid malformation of the overlying skin or a sacrococcygeal dimple or sinus. The spinal cord may be dysplastic or contain a lipoma or dermoid.

Other Malformations of the Spinal Cord

Hydromyelia

Hydromyelia is congenital dilatation of the central canal of the cord most commonly found in association with a myelocoele. It may be an incidental finding, most commonly in the lumbar region, in an infant with no other CNS malformation. The canal may be lined by ependyma, or become replaced by glial tissue.

Diastematomyelia and Diplomyelia

Diastematomyelia and diplomyelia often coexist. Duplication of the central canal over a short distance may be an incidental finding. However, most duplications of the cord, each in its separate dural envelope, are found with a bony or fibrous diastematomyelia spur arising from the vertebral body (Fig. 23.33). This condition is found just caudal to a myelocoele or part of complicated spina bifida occulta. When duplication is not in conjunction with diastematomyelia, the two cords are generally within a single dural covering.

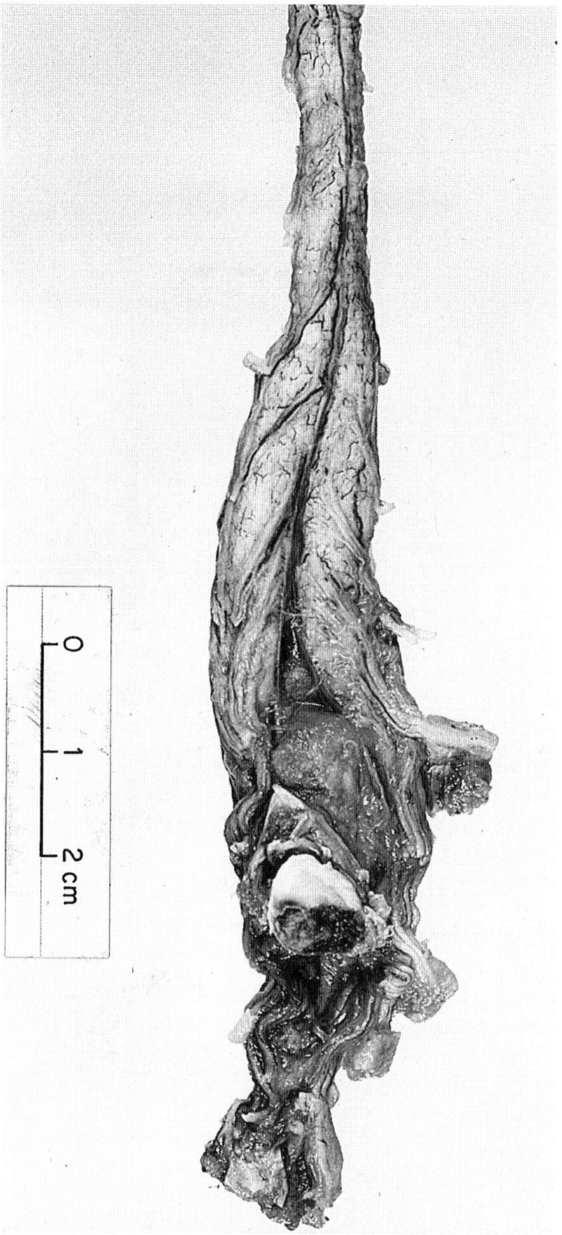

Fig. 23.33. Spinal cord split into two round a bony diastematomyelia spur that arose from a lumbar vertebral body in an infant with "complicated" spina bifida occulta who died of an unrelated cause. A small lipoma is also present.

Dermoid Cysts and Lipomas

Dermoid cysts and lipomas may be found in the distal end of the spinal cord, especially in cases of complicated spina bifida occulta and myelocoele.

Other Disorders with NTD as a Constant or Common Component

Fetal Disruption (Amniotic Band) Syndrome

Fetal disruption (amniotic band) syndrome may involve the head, leading to partial or total absence of the vault of the skull and the exposure of congested and grossly disorganised brain tissue, much of which will have degenerated by the end of the pregnancy or even in a mid-trimester abortus (Fig. 23.34). This open lesion may well resemble anencephaly and be identifiable on ultrasonography through raised serum and amniotic alphafetoprotein levels. However, other features such as facial disruption, involving mostly the eyes and mouth, amniotic bands on arms or legs and finger and toe amputations should help to identify the disorder, which unlike anencephaly, does not have a risk of recurrence (Smith 1982; see Chap. 4, p. 141).

Meckel–Gruber Syndrome

Meckel–Gruber syndrome (dysencephalia splanchnocystica) is an uncommon condition which has occipital encephalocoele as one of the more constant features, associated with polydactyly and polycystic kidneys (Fig. 23.35). Microcephaly, eye and orbital abnormalities, micrognathos, cleft lip and palate, cardiac defects, arhinencephaly and hydrocephalus are often present. The condition, which may be suspected because hydrocephalus, encephalocoele or large polycystic kidneys are detected on high-resolution ultrasonography, does not always show raised levels of alpha-fetoprotein. Few infants with this disorder survive more than a week or so. The importance of recognising this syndrome is the high risk of recurrence (one in four) in future pregnancies, as it is inherited as an autosomal recessive (Opitz and Howe 1969; Smith 1982).

Chromosome Abnormalities

Certain chromosome abnormalities, especially triploidy, trisomy 13, trisomy 18 and some-

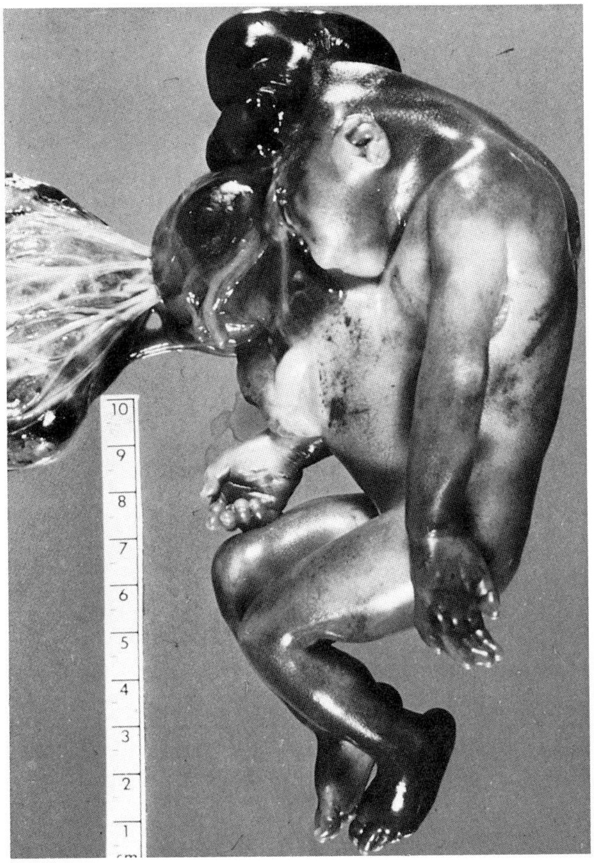

Fig. 23.34. A 20-week fetus with amniotic band syndrome, with a grossly disrupted head, showing absence of the cranial vault and an anencephaly-like brain, a disrupted face and an omphalocoele closely bound up with the membranes.

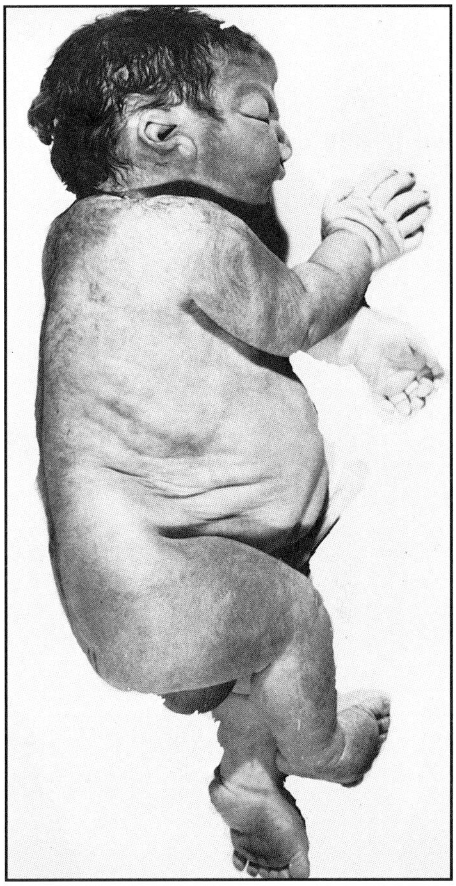

Fig. 23.35. Newborn with Meckel–Gruber syndrome. The abdomen is distended because of large polycystic kidneys; there is polydactyly of hands and feet and a dysmorphic facies. The encephalocoele in this case was small and there were no facial clefts.

times trisomy 21, commonly exhibit a myelocoele and, less commonly, encephalocoele or anencephaly. It would be wise to carry out chromosome investigations whenever an NTD seems to be part of a malformation syndrome. Positive findings might have implications for a future pregnancy, as the risks of recurrence and methods of prenatal detection for chromosome abnormalities are very different from those of NTDs.

Arhinencephaly

Arhinencephaly is a term coined by Kindrat in 1882 when he described the first case of what is now often called holoprosencephaly. In recent years the term "arhinencephaly" has been applied to a group of malformations, all of which have in common absence of the olfactory bulbs, tracts and trigones and abnormalities of the olfactory cortex. In holoprosencephaly, the severest malformation of this group, the brain is usually smaller than normal, in addition to the absence of the external olfactory structure; the cerebral hemispheres are represented by a single holosphere with simple macrogyric convolutions, including a median gyrus (Fig. 23.36). The cerebral mantle encloses a single ventricular cavity representing the two lateral and the third ventricles. There is no corpus callosum or septum pellucidum. At the posterior edge of the holosphere a telencephalic membrane roofs over this cavity. This membrane often bulges to form the cystic space occupying the posterior portion of the middle

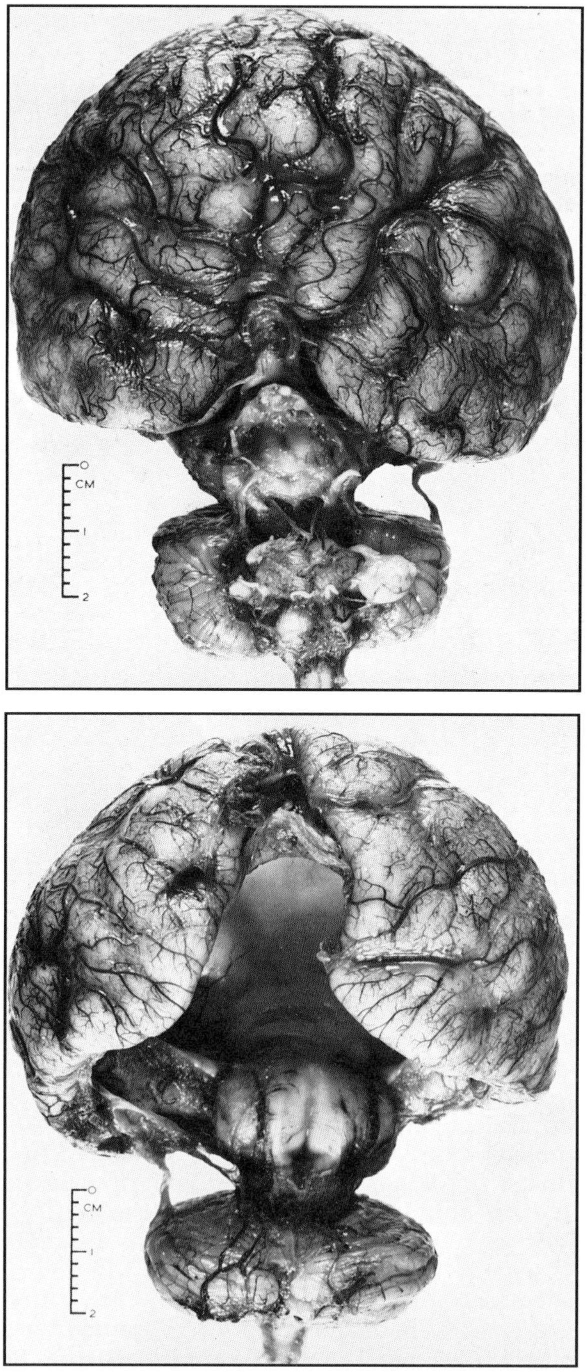

a

b

Fig. 23.36. Alobar holoprosencephaly: brain seen from the front (a) and the back (b). The undivided holosphere with macrogyric convolutions encloses a single ventricle representing the lateral and third ventricles. The telencephalic membrane has been removed. The mid- and hindbrain are relatively normal.

cranial fossa. There is generally a degree of hydrocephalus. In contrast to the severely abnormal forebrain the hindbrain is generally normal macroscopically. Neither sagittal sinus nor falx cerebri are present in this form of arhinencephaly.

In the least severe of this group of abnormalities, the only structures which are missing are the olfactory bulbs, tracts and trigones, while the rest of the brain, including the septum pellucidum and corpus callosum, is normal (Fig. 23.37). Usually the frontal lobe lacks the olfactory gyrus and sometimes the temporal lobes are large with extra convolutions. In between these extremes, all degrees of abnormality are found (Laurence and Bligh 1967), including partial division of the holosphere (Fig. 23.38) and partial or complete agenesis of the corpus callosum (see Fig. 23.43).

Strictly, however, the term "arhinencephaly" is a misnomer, for Yakovlev (1959), in a detailed anatomical study of ten arhinencephalic brains, has pointed out that even in the severest form not all rhinencephalic structures are missing. In each of the ten cases he was able to identify the praepiriform and hippocampal formations of the rhinic lobe, even though they were hypoplastic and dystrophic.

Arhinencephaly results from defective evagination of the paired olfactory buds, which should make their appearance at about the 36th day. Subsequently the forebrain (prosencephalon) fails to divide into mirror image cerebral hemispheres, which should be followed by lateral invagination and posterior rotation of the anterior portions. Any part of this process may be faulty, giving rise to the spectrum of abnormalities. The development of the neuroectoderm of the forebrain is influenced by that of the primitive foregut and the associated mesoderm, from which the nose and the mouth structures are derived, thus explaining the frequent association of arhinencephaly with facial clefts and a poorly developed nose. The close relationship between the development of the olfactory vesicles and the optic structures, which appear only very little later, would also be a reason for the associated anophthalmos, hypotelorism amounting in some instances to cyclopia, and the other eye abnormalities (Karseras and Laurence 1975). Indeed, these associations are so common that De Myer et al. (1964) suggested that it might be possible to predict the degree and type of brain abnormality from the facial appearances.

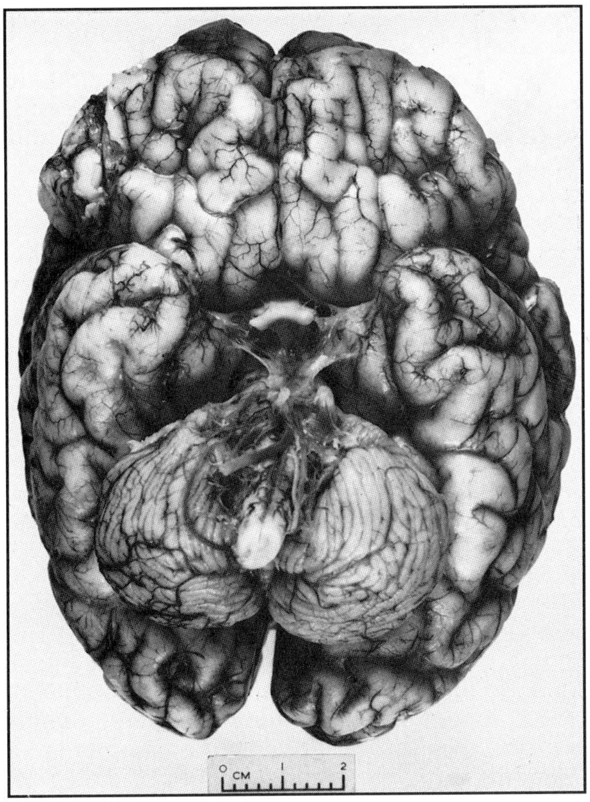

Fig. 23.37. Arhinencephaly, with absence only of the olfactory bulbs tracts, trigones and olfactory gyrus. On superficial examination, the brain seems normal.

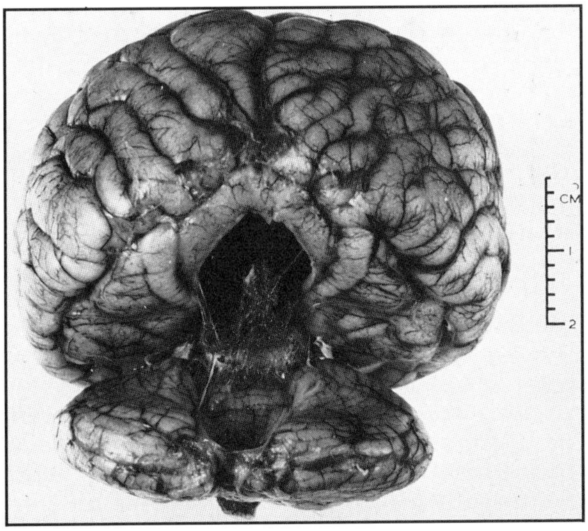

Fig. 23.38. Holoprosencephalic brain with partial division of the holosphere by a median sulcus.

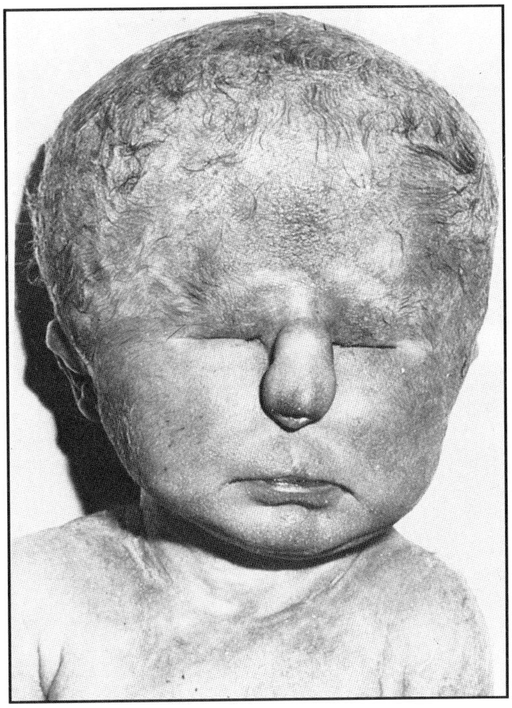

Fig. 23.39. Cebocephaly with a proboscis and narrowly spaced orbits with only vestigial eyes. This was associated with alobar holoprosencephaly and vestigial optic nerves.

Complete (alobar) holoprosencephaly is found with cyclopia or with gross eye abnormalities and a proboscis (cebocephaly) (Fig. 23.39). Partial separation of the holosphere is described with median cleft lip and palate (Fig. 23.40). Relationships between less severe forms of arhinencephaly and facial appearances are less predictable, but some form of facial dysmorphology is invariable.

Arhinencephaly has been produced experimentally by feeding pregnant sheep on the plant *Veratrum californicum*, in mice with vitamin A, in rabbits with alloxan and in rats with vincristine (De Myer 1966). In man, arhinencephaly, often of the milder variety, is found once in about 2500 births (Ishmael and Laurence 1965). There is an association with maternal diabetes mellitus (Dekaban and Magee 1958; Dekaban 1959) and a stronger one with trisomy of chromosome 13(D), triploidy and other chromosome abnormalities. Indeed, in nearly every reported case of trisomy 13 that has come to necropsy and where the brain has been examined carefully, arhinencephaly has been found (Laurence and Bligh 1967); however, about half of the infants with arhinen-

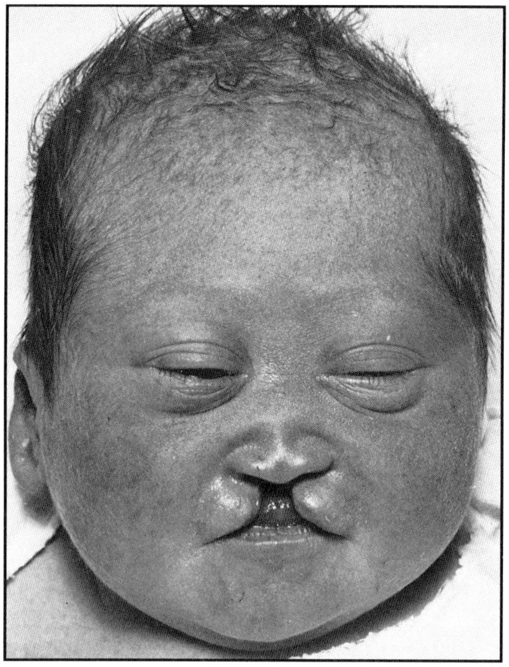

Fig. 23.40. Median cleft lip and palate, microcephaly and other facial abnormalities associated with alobar holoprosencephaly and D trisomy.

cephaly have a normal karyotype (Laurence 1966). Autosomal-recessive and autosomal-dominant forms not associated with other malformations have been reported. It is found as part of the Meckel–Gruber and other syndromes (Warkany et al. 1981). However, in many cases, no other malformations or aetiological factors are found. A good review is that of Gorlin et al. (1990).

Many of these pregnancies are complicated by polyhydramnios or intrauterine growth retardation. Those infants which have the severer forms of arhinencephaly, with chromosome abnormalities or associated visceral abnormalities are often stillborn or die in early infancy. However, some babies with the milder forms survive but are mentally retarded (Zellweger et al. 1962).

Hydranencephaly

Hydranencephaly is a rare abnormality occurring in less than 1 in 10 000 births. It has to be distinguished from gross hydrocephalus on the one hand and bilateral symmetrical schizencephaly on the other.

The majority of infants with hydranencephaly are born after an apparently normal pregnancy and seem unremarkable in the neonatal period; they have normal reflexes and responses, suck normally and have a normal reaction to light (Halsey et al. 1971). However, after a few weeks feeding difficulties are encountered, they ignore their surroundings, do not smile and may become spastic. Head enlargement begins, the skull transilluminates (Fig. 23.41) and an EEG over the vertex is entirely flat. Most do not survive beyond 3 months.

Post-mortem examination shows a balloon-like structure filling the cranial cavity, the wall being composed of the thin semitransparent membrane consisting of the leptomeninges and the gliotic molecular layer (Norman 1963), which may have focal calcification and brown staining.

There is no ependymal layer. The single ventricular cavity may be partially divided by the falx cerebri and filled with clear, possibly xanthochromic fluid containing an increased amount of protein. At the bottom of the cavity thalamic bodies stand out prominently; the basal ganglia are easily identifiable. Hippocampi and the lower portions of the occipital and temporal lobes are usually present. The demarcation between the structures and the thin membrane is abrupt (Fig. 23.42). The brainstem, the tentorium and the cerebellum are usually of normal appearance. The choroid plexi can be seen at the bottom of the cavity; the optic nerves are usually present but small. There is no corpus callosum. The aqueduct may be blocked. Histologically the cytoarchitecture of the preserved structures is abnormal with marked mineralisation and focal scarring. The carotid arteries are generally hypoplastic but the vertebral arteries are normal.

Hydranencephaly can be distinguished from extreme hydrocephalus where part of the cerebral mantle may well be reduced to a thin semitransparent membrane by the fact that the cerebral mantle does consist of a thinned-out layer of grey matter containing neurons and possibly a thin layer of white matter. There is no sudden demarcation between the thinned-out cerebral mantle and the basal nuclei, which are usually severely flattened. The differentiation from extensive bilateral or unilateral porencephaly may be difficult as occasionally hydranencephaly may be unilateral only.

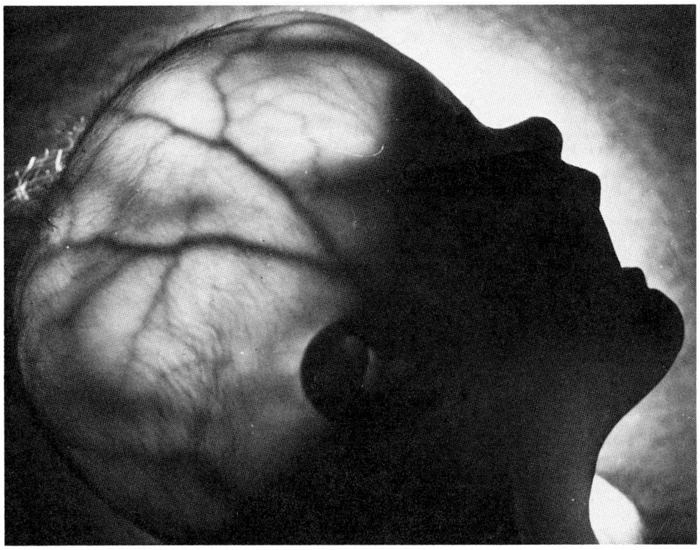

Fig. 23.41. Hydranencephaly. Transillumination causes the whole skull to light up "like a lamp" showing up the blood vessels in sharp relief. The vault of the skull is not unduly enlarged compared with the face.

The pathogenesis of hydranencephaly is a sudden destruction of the already formed brain in the second half of the pregnancy. This seems to be a vascular accident involving the internal carotid artery (Van Allen 1981), structures supplied by the vertebral artery being more or less preserved. A similar lesion can be produced experimentally in puppies (Becker 1949) and monkeys by tying the carotid arteries or obstructing them with paraffin. What causes this vascular occlusion in man is by no means clear. Hypoperfusion and hyperviscosity of the blood has been suggested (Lindenberg and Swanson 1967). An occasional case is associated with toxoplasmosis (Altshuler 1973) or cytomegalic inclusion disease, but in the majority of cases no aetiological factor can be identified.

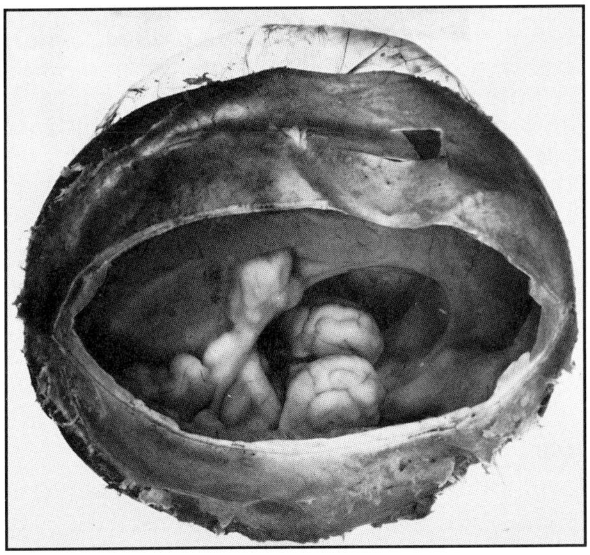

Fig. 23.42. Hydranencephaly. A post-mortem specimen with part of the skull and membranes cut away on the right side revealing the ventricular cavity, where it is possible to identify the basal ganglia masses, part of the occipital lobes, and the choroid plexus. Bone only was removed on the left, allowing the thin glial membrane with thin blood vessels coursing over it to bulge.

Agenesis of the Corpus Callosum

Agenesis of the corpus callosum is a rare finding in infancy, except when associated with other brain or visceral malformation, but is more frequently seen in brains from a mentally subnormal population. Clinically, it is an ill-defined condition usually presenting with mental retardation and convulsions that do not respond to therapy, but it may also be found incidentally in apparently normal subjects.

The brain often weighs less than normal and may show complete agenesis or only partial agenesis with the anterior portion intact but

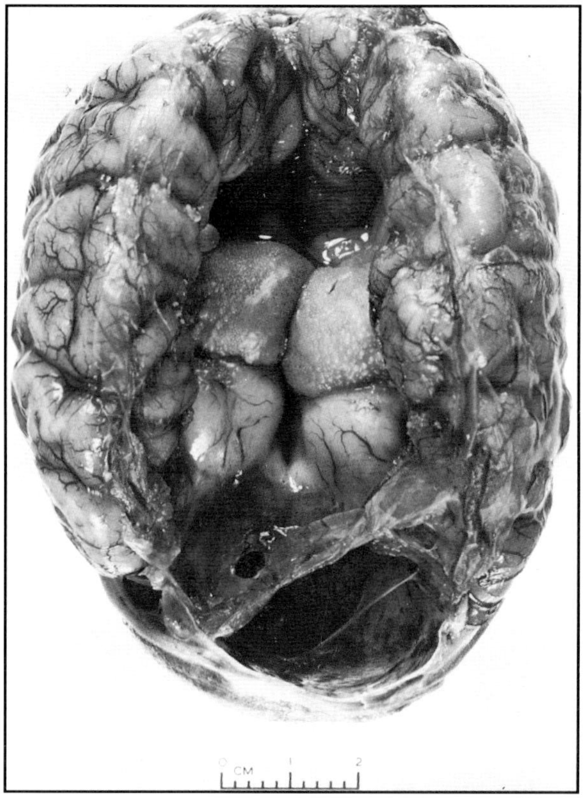

Fig. 23.43. Brain with complete agenesis of corpus callosum, seen from above after most of the "third ventricular" membrane had been removed.

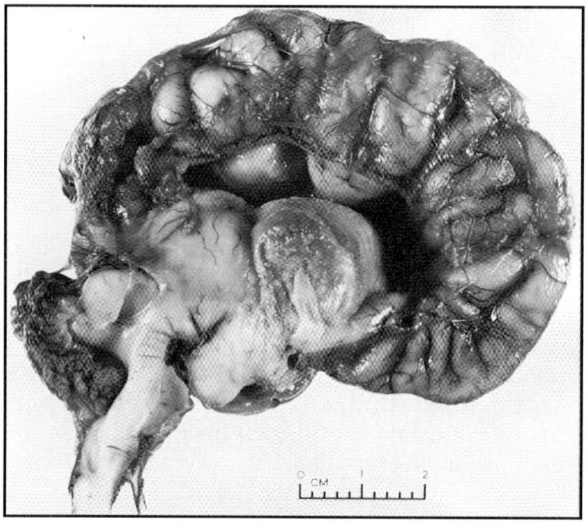

Fig. 23.44. Hemisected brain with agenesis of corpus callosum, showing radial arrangement of the medial gyri.

thin (Fig. 23.43). The gyri on the medial surface of the cerebral hemisphere have a radial arrangement with the cingulate gyrus buried below the surface (Fig. 23.44). The septum pellucidum is absent and the fornix is abnormal with a very large bundle of fibres, which probably represent those that normally cross over in the corpus callosum. The space between the hemispheres is generally occupied by a large "third ventricle" roofed over by a thin membrane, but occasionally a tumour may occupy the space.

The corpus callosum does not develop until the 12th week, when the first fibres appear anteriorly near the lamina terminalis. Fibres then cross further back and the structure is fairly complete by 22 weeks.

Interference with this process could readily account for all the features described. The cause of this disturbance is not known in man. It may occasionally be inherited as the only defect (McKusick 1983) but is more often found in association with arhinencephaly, facial clefts and chromosome abnormality (Warkany et al. 1981).

Cerebellar Malformations

Complete absence of the cerebellum occurs very rarely. Unilateral absence or hypoplasia, however, is more common. Other cerebellar malformations such as cerebellar rachischisis, caused by partial or complete aplasia of the vermis as in Joubert's syndrome (Joubert et al. 1969) and cerebellar microgyria, are sometimes encountered. These anomalies are normally seen in association with other severe brain malformations and are discussed by Larroche (1984).

Microcephaly

Microcephalic infants are born with either a normal or reduced head size, which subsequently fails to grow, whilst the face tends to develop at the normal rate producing a small head with a large face, a receding forehead and loose, often wrinkled scalp (Fig. 23.45). The fontanelles are usually small at birth and close

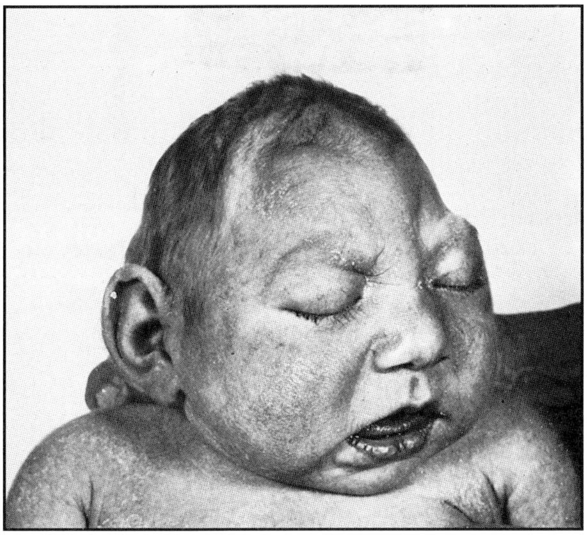

Fig. 23.45. Microcephaly. Typical example with a normal-sized face and small vault covered with loose-wrinkled scalp.

within a few weeks. The condition has been identified prenatally using ultrasonography but usually only in the third trimester.

Microcephaly may have many different causes. In most instances it results from an intrauterine, perinatal or early postnatal environmental problem such as an intrauterine infection with toxoplasma or a rubella virus, exposure to radiation or drugs, hypoxia or some destructive metabolic disorder. The other major group is where microcephaly is part of a malformation syndrome which may be chromosomal in origin. Only a small proportion of microcephaly is genetically determined. The condition, unassociated with other malformations, is recognised at birth in less than 2 out of 10000 births. In a large proportion of this group no aetiological factors can be found.

With such diverse aetiology the pathological findings are equally variable. The brain weighs less than 2.5 SD below the mean weight for the sex and maturity and may be only half the expected weight. The cerebral hemispheres are small but quite normally shaped and do not cover the cerebellum, which is usually relatively normal in size. The convolutional pattern tends to be simple, reminiscent of that of the anthropoid ape or a 5-month fetus. Microscopically, the cortical cells are relatively normal but tend to be arranged in cords. Some cases may show considerable arteritis with uligyria. Rarely, heavy calcium carbonate deposits are found in the cortex and nuclei together with myelin breakdown material reminiscent of a destructive process (Larroche 1984; Warkany et al. 1981).

Megalencephaly

Individuals with megalencephaly have very large brains weighing between 1600 and 2800 g in the adult (normal 1400 g). Although this weight is very occasionally associated with exceptional intelligence, nearly all these patients are mental defectives.

At birth the head of the megalencephalic, who is usually male, may be large, though as a rule not large enough to attract notice. The fontanelles are large and the sutures wide, and soon the skull begins to enlarge rapidly and assume a typical hydrocephalic shape, with the fontanelles and sutures remaining open. Mental and physical development is severely retarded and most babies suffer convulsions.

The brain is large, heavy (2–3 SD above the mean for age and sex) and firm, with convolutions more complex and larger than normal. Microscopically there is no evidence of degeneration, but in most cases the cortex shows numerous lamellae of well-formed neurons and broad zones of nerve fibrils. There is a great excess of glia, especially in the subcortical white matter. The brainstem and cerebellum show no obvious changes. Occasionally, one cerebral hemisphere only is affected (Laurence 1969).

Megalencephaly seems to be a heterogeneous condition. In many instances it is possible to obtain a family history of mental retardation, and sometimes there are several cases in one family. Some regard the condition as neoplastic. For further information, see Warkany et al. (1981).

Micropolygyria

Micropolygyria is a common malformation of the cerebral cortex, characterised by broad irregular granular gyri, with the grey matter extending in a festoon-like manner deep into the brain substance from the apex of the gyrus. The anomaly may be localised or involve the whole of one or both cerebral hemispheres. This has to be differentiated from what is sometimes called polygyria, where an excessive formation of secondary gyri may complicate an otherwise normal convolutional pattern. Microscopically, two main varieties of micropolygyria are recognised. In the first there is non-separation of the molecular layer between the folds and a failure of the molecular layer to be arranged in a laminar pattern. In the second variety the molecular layer is divided into four thick bands of nerve cells.

These patients show varying degrees of mental deficiency and may suffer from epilepsy. If the lesion involves the motor cortex, cerebral diplegia and hemiplegia may be present, as then the pyramidal tracts tend to be deficient. For further information, see Larroche (1984).

Porencephaly

Porencephaly is a circumscribed hemispheric defect occurring before development is complete and including both distortions of growth and destructive lesions. An abnormality which is probably developmental in nature is the bilateral symmetrical schizencephaly of Yakovlev, where a defect of the frontal and the parietal lobes in the region of the primary fissures involves the whole depth of the cortex. The cysts are often lined by heterotopic grey matter and there is no evidence of brain tissue destruction. It is probably due to localised agenesis before the end of the 2nd month of fetal life.

A different picture is seen in the more common localised, asymmetric, destructive lesion resulting from vascular occlusion or some encephalitic process occurring antenatally, or from birth injury. The position and extent of the lesion is variable. It does not often communicate with the ventricular system and is separated from it by ependyma and the subependymal glia. The overlying meninges are generally densely adherent. The cyst is often lined by a glial membrane and it contains yellow serous fluid. Altered blood may be found in it and haemosiderin within the wall. Further details are given by Larroche (1984) and Warkany et al. (1981).

Pachygyria, Lissencephaly and Agyria

From a neuropathological point of view, pachygria, lissencephaly and agyria are interrelated conditions in which there is reduction or absence of the secondary convolutions, over part or all of the cerebral hemispheres, together with an increase in the depth of the cortical grey matter. In an extreme case only the Sylvian fissure may be present, and the operculum may be poorly developed. Microscopically, abnormalities of the layers and immaturity of the neurons are found. This malformation is explicable on the basis of retardation of development at the 3rd or 4th month. For further information see Larroche (1984). There are several distinct malformation syndromes such as Miller–Dieker syndrome, often associated with chromosome 17 deletion, (Dobyns 1987) and Walker–Waarburg syndrome where lissencephaly is a constant feature.

Acknowledgements. I am grateful to Mr. R. Lunnon, of the Department of Medical Illustration, the Hospital for Sick Children, and Prof. R. Marshall, of the Department of Medical Illustration, University of Wales College of Medicine, for the illustrations and to Prof. D. Moffatt, of the Department of Anatomy, University College, Cardiff, for help with the embryological introduction.

References

Adams C, Johnston WP, Nevin NC (1982) Family study of congenital hydrocephalus. Dev Med Child Neurol 24: 493–498

Anderson ABN, Laurence KM, Turnbull C (1969) The relationship in anencephaly between the size of the adrenal cortex and the length of gestation. J Obstet Gynaecol Br Cmwlth 76: 196–199

Altshuler G (1973) Toxoplasmosis as a cause of hydranencephaly. Am J Dis Child 125: 251–252

Alvord EC Jr (1961) Pathology of hydrocephalus. In: Fields WS, Desmond MM (eds) Pathology of hydrocephalus. In: Disorders of the developing nervous system. Thomas, Springfield, Ill, pp 343–413

Beck F, Moffatt DB, Davies DP (1983) Human embryology, 2nd edn. Blackwell, Oxford

Becker H (1949) Uber Hirngefassausschaltungen: intrakranielle Gefassverschlusse; über experimentelle Hydranencephalie (Blasen hirn). Dtsch Z Nervenheile

161: 446–505
Bell JE (1982) The pathology of central nervous system defects in human fetuses of different gestational ages. In: Persaud TVN (ed) Advances in the study of birth defects, vol 7. MTP Press, Lancaster, pp 1–17
Bickers DS, Adams RD (1949) Hereditary stenosis of aqueduct of Sylvius as cause of congenital hydrocephalus. Brain 72: 246–262
Book JA (1951) Incidence of congenital disease and defects in a South Swedish population. Acta Genet (Basel) 2: 289
Cameron AH (1957a) The Arnold–Chiari and other neuroanatomical malformations associated with spina bifida. J Pathol Bacteriol 73: 195–211
Cameron AH (1957b) Malformations of the neuro-spinal axis, urogenital tract and foregut in spina bifida attributable to disturbances of the blastopore. J Pathol Bacteriol 73: 213–221
Carter CO (1974) Clues to the aetiology of neural tube malformations. Dev Med Child Neurol 16 (Suppl 16): 3–14
Carter CO, Evans K (1973) Spina bifida and anencephalus in Greater London. J Med Genet 10: 209–234
Carter CO, David PA, Laurence KM (1968) A family study of central nervous system malformations in South Wales. J Med Genet 5: 81–106
Czeizel A, Révész C (1970) Major malformations of the central nervous system in Hungary. Br J Prev Soc Med 24: 205–222
Daniel PM, Strich SJ (1958) Some observations on the congenital deformity of the central nervous system known as the Arnold–Chiari malformation. J Neuropathol Exp Neurol 17: 255–266
Dekaban AS (1959) Arhinencephaly in an infant born to a diabetic mother. J Neuropathol Exp Neurol 18: 620–626
Dekaban AS (1963) Anencephaly in early human embryos. J Neuropathol Exp Neurol 22: 533–548
Dekaban AS, Magee KR (1958) Occurrence of neurologic abnormalities in infants of diabetic mothers. Neurology (Minneap) 8: 193–200
De Myer W (1966) Production of major cerebral malformations by drugs with special reference to the holoprosencephalies (cyclopsia-arhinencephaly). In: Luthy F, Bishoff A (eds) Proceedings of the 5th international congress of neuropathology. Int Congr Ser No 100. Excerpta Medica, Amsterdam, pp 717–721
De Myer W, Zeman W, Palmer CG (1964) The face predicts the brain: diagnostic significance of median facial anomalies for holoprosencephaly (arhinencephaly). Pediatrics 34: 256–263
Dobyns WB (1987) Developmental aspects of lissencephaly and lissencephaly syndromes. Birth Defects 23(1): 225–241
Duckett S (1966) Foetal Arnold–Chiari malformation. Acta Neurol 7: 175–179
Edwards JH, Norman RM, Roberts JM (1961) Sex-linked hydrocephalus. Report of a family with 15 affected members. Arch Dis Child 36: 481–485
Elwood JM, Elwood JH (1980) Epidemiology of anencephalus and spina bifida. Oxford University Press, Oxford
Emery JL (1974) Deformity of the aqueduct of Sylvius in children with hydrocephalus and myelomeningocele. Dev Med Child Neurol 16 (suppl 32): 40–48
Gardener WJ, Goodall RJ (1950) Surgical treatment of Arnold–Chiari malformation in adults. Explanation of its mechanism and importance of encephalography in diagnosis. J Neurosurg 7: 199–206
Gorlin RJ, Cohen MM, Levin LS (1990) Syndromes of the head and neck, 3rd edn. Oxford University Press, Oxford, pp 573–582
Halsey JH, Allen N, Chamberlain HR (1971) Morphogenesis of hydranencephaly. J Neurol Sci 12: 187–217
Ishmael J, Laurence KM (1965) A probable case of incomplete trisomy of a chromosome of the 13–15 group. J Med Genet 2: 136–141
James N, Laurence KM (1983) Nutrition and the prevention of neural tube defects. In: Dodge JA (ed) Topics in paediatric nutrition. Pitman Medical, London, pp 225–236
Joubert M, Eisenring J-J, Robb JP, Andermann F (1969) Familial agenesis of the cerebellar vermis: a syndrome of episodic hyperpnoea, abnormal eye movements ataxia and retardation. Neurology 19: 813–825
Karch SB, Urich H (1972) Occipital encephalocele: a morphological study. J Neurol Sci 15: 899–112
Karseras A, Laurence KM (1975) Eyes in arhinencephaly syndromes. Br J Ophthamol 59: 462–473
Khoury MJ, Cordero JF, Mulinare J, Opita JM (1989) Selected midline defect association: a population study. Pediatrics 84: 266–272
Larroche JC (1984) Malformations of the nervous system. In: Hume-Adams J, Corsellis JNA, Duchen LW (eds) Greenfield's Neuropathology, 4th edn. Arnold, London, pp 385–450
Laurence KM (1958) The natural history of hydrocephalus. Lancet II: 1152–1154
Laurence KM (1959) The pathology of hydrocephalus. Ann Coll Surg (Engl) 24: 388–401
Laurence KM (1964) A case of unilateral megaloencephaly. Dev Med Child Neurol 6: 585–590
Laurence KM (1966) Discussion on arhinencephaly. In: Luthy F, Bishoff A (eds) Proceedings of the 5th international congress of neuropathology. Int Congr Ser No 100. Excerpta Medica, Amsterdam, pp 722–723
Laurence KM (1969) Neurological and intellectual sequelae of hydrocephalus. Arch Neurol 20: 73–81
Laurence KM (1974) The effect of early surgery for spina bifida cystica on survival and quality of life. Lancet I: 301–304
Laurence KM (1986) Prenatal detection and prevention of neural tube defects in South Wales. J Soc Health 106: 153–160
Laurence KM (1989) The declining incidence of neural tube defects in the UK. Z Kinderchir 41: 51
Laurence KM (1990) Genetics and prevention of neural tube defects and of "uncomplicated" hydrocephalus. In: Emery AEH, Rimoin DI (eds) Principles and practice of medical genetics, 2nd edn. Churchill Livingstone, Edinburgh, pp 323–346
Laurence KM (1991) Folic acid supplementation to prevent neural tube defect Lancet 338: 379 (letter)
Laurence KM, Bligh AS (1967) Radiological appearances in arhinencephaly. Clin Radiol 28: 383–393
Laurence KM, Coates S (1962) The natural history of hydrocephalus: detailed analysis of 182 unoperated cases. Arch Dis Child 37: 345–362
Laurence KM, Tew BJ (1971) The natural history of spina bifida cystica and cranium bifidum cysticum: the central nervous system malformations in South Wales Part IV. Arch Dis Child 467: 127–138
Laurence KM, Carter CO, David PA (1968) The major central nervous system malformation in South Wales. I. Incidence, local variations and geographical factors. Br J Prev Soc Med 22: 146–160
Laurence KM, Bligh AS, Evans KT, Shurtleff DB (1971) Vertebral abnormalities in parents and sibs of cases of spina bifida cystica and anencephaly. Proceedings 13th

Congress Paediatrics, vol V. Wiener Medizinischer Akademie, Vienna, pp 415–421
Laurence KM, James N, Miller M, Campbell H (1980) The increased risk of recurrence of neural tube defects to mothers on poor diets and the possible benefit of dietary counselling. Br Med J 4: 1592–1593
Laurence KM, James N, Miller MH, Tennant GB, Campbell H (1981) Double blind randomised controlled trial of preconceptional folate therapy to prevent recurrence of neural tube defects. Br Med J 2: 1509–1511
Laurence KM, Campbell H, James N (1983a) The role of improvement in the maternal diet and preconceptional folic acid supplementation in the prevention of neural tube defects. In: Dobbing J (ed) Prevention of spina bifida and other neural tube defects. Academic, London, pp 85–106
Laurence KM, Dew JO, Dyer C, Downey KH (1983b) Amniocentes is carried out for neural tube indications in South Wales 1973–1981: outcome of pregnancies and findings in the malformed abortuses. Prenat Diagn 3: 187–201
Lemire RJ, Shephard TH, Alvord EC Jr (1965) Caudal myeloschisis (lumbar spina bifida cystica) in a 5 mm (Horizon XIV) human embryo. Anat Rec 152: 9–16
Lemire RJ, Loeser JD, Leech RW, Alvord EC Jr (1975) Normal and abnormal development of the human nervous system. Harper and Row, Hagerstown, Md
Lichtenstein BW (1942) Distant neuroanatomic complications of spina bifida (spinal dysraphism). Arch Neurol Psychiatry (Chicago) 47: 195–214
Lindenberg R, Swanson PD (1967) Infantile hydranencephaly: a report of 5 cases of infarction of both cerebral hemispheres in infancy. Brain 90: 839–841
MacKenzie NG, Emery JL (1971) Deformities of the cervical spinal cord in children with neurospinal dysraphism. Dev Med Child Neurol 13 (Suppl 25): 58–61
MacMahon B, Pugh TF, Ingalls TH (1953) Anencephalus, spina bifida and hydrocephalus. Br J Prev Soc Med 7: 211–219
McKeown T, Record RG (1960) Malformations in a population observed for five years after birth. In: Wolstenholme GEW, O'Connor CMO (eds) Ciba Symposium: Congenital malformations
McKusick VA (1983) Mendelian inheritance in man, 6th edn. Johns Hopkins University Press, Baltimore
Marin-Pidella M (1978) Clinical and experimental rachischisis. In: Viulcen PJ, Bruyn GW (eds) Handbook of clinical neurology. Elsevier/North Holland, Amsterdam, pp 159–191
Morison E (1970) Foetal and neonatal pathology, 3rd edn. Butterworth, London, pp 468–470
MRC Vitamin Study Research Group (1991) Prevention of neural tube defects: results of the Medical Research Council vitamin study. Lancet 338: 131–137
Norman RW (1963) Malformations of the nervous system, birth injury and diseases of early life. In: Blackwood W, McMennemey WH, Meyer A, Norman RM, Russel DS (eds), Greenfield's neuropathology, 2nd edn. Arnold, London, pp 324–433
Opitz JM, Howe JJ (1969) Meckel syndrome (dysencephalia splanchnocystica, the Gruber syndrome). Birth Defects 5 (II): 167–179
Penfield W, Coburn DF (1938) Arnold–Chiari malformation and its operative treatment. Arch Neurol Psychiatry (Chicago) 40: 328–336
Potter EL, Craig JM (1976) Pathology of the fetus and the infant, 3rd edn. Year Book Medical Publishers, Chicago, pp 523–526
Record RG, McKeown T (1949) Congenital malformations of the central nervous system I. Survey of 930 cases. Br J Prev Soc Med 3: 183–219
Russel DS (1949) Observations on the pathology of hydrocephalus. Spec Rep Ser Medical Research Council No 265. HMSO, London
Smith DW (1982) Recognisable patterns of human malformation, 3rd edn. Saunders, Philadelphia
Smithells RW, Sheppard S, Schorah CJ, Nevin NC, Seller MJ, Harris R, Read AP, Fielding DW (1980) Possible prevention of neural tube defects by periconceptional vitamin supplementation. Lancet I: 339–340
Taggart JK, Walker AE (1942) Congenital atresia of the foramina of Luschka and Magendie. Arch Neurol Psychiatry 48: 583–617
Warkany J, Lemire RJ, Cohen MM (1981) Mental retardation and congenital malformations of the central nervous system. Year Book Medical Publishers, Chicago
Williamson EM (1965) Incidence and family aggregation of major central malformations of the nervous system. J Med Genet 2: 161–172
Urich H (1976) Malformation of the nervous system, perinatal damage and related conditions in early life. In: Blackwood W, Corsellis JAN (eds) Greenfield's neuropathology, 3rd edn. Arnold, London, pp 361–469
Van Allen MI (1981) Fetal vascular disruptions: mechanisms and some resulting birth defects. Pediatr Ann 10: 31–50
Yakovlev PI (1959) Patho-architectionic studies of the cerebral malformations. III. Arhinencephalies (holoprosencephalies). J Neuropathol Neurol 18: 22–55
Ye H (1986) THe strategy of risk approach in perinatal care in Shuniyi county of Beijing. Symposium on paediatrics in China and Africa. Royal Society of Medicine, London
Young MC, Laurence KM, Hughes IA (1989) Relationship between fetal adrenal morphology and anterior pituitary function. Horm Res 32: 130–135
Zellweger H, Milkamo K, Abbo G (1962) Two cases of multiple malformations with an autosomal aberration—partial Trisomy D? Helv Paediatr Acta 17: 290–300

Chapter 24

Acquired Diseases of the Nervous System

Marian V. Squier

Introduction

Acquired disorders of the nervous system are responsible for considerable perinatal mortality and for devastating chronic handicap in children.

Identification of acquired lesions and their distinction from malformations can be difficult because early damage to the brain disrupts the orderly and complex sequence of development and leads to structural abnormality. The hallmarks of a destructive process, such as scarring and gliosis, are not seen because of the limited responses of the immature brain. The earliest reported identification of reactive astrocytes is at 20 weeks of gestation by immunocytochemical methods (Roessmann and Gambetti, 1986); macrophages are seen from 28 weeks (Sherwood et al. 1978; Squier and Keeling 1991).

The distribution of acquired damage may give some clues to aetiology. Certain infectious agents show predilection for particular parts of the brain and ischaemic lesions may reflect vascular territories and watershed zones. The developing nervous system also shows changing patterns of susceptibility to hypoxic and ischaemic injury. Ischaemic damage to the white matter is characteristic of the preterm infant when the grey matter may escape unharmed, while at term the grey matter usually bears the brunt of injury.

Although these patterns of damage may provide clues to timing and nature of injury, the elapse of time between damage and death complicates the final picture because of superimposed secondary degenerative processes. So, for example, reduction in cerebral white matter results from loss of cortical neurons; similarly, the dentate and brainstem nuclei may degenerate following damage to the cerebellar cortex.

The commonest type of damage to the fetal and neonatal brain results from hypoxia/ischaemia. Unfortunately this is often thought to be linked to "birth asphyxia" or "perinatal damage", which might imply criticism of obstetric management. Increasing evidence from clinical, pathological and epidemiological studies shows that ischaemic and haemorrhagic brain damage not uncommonly occurs in the antenatal period and that the majority of severely handicapped children have no history of birth difficulties. The importance of careful macroscopic and histological examination of the brains of stillborn infants and early neonatal deaths cannot be overstressed. Only in this way can we hope to establish the timing and causes of acquired lesions which is essential for prevention of brain damage.

This chapter aims to give an account of the commoner acquired conditions likely to be encountered in routine post-mortem examination of infants and fetuses. Some knowledge of the normal development of the brain is important in understanding these conditions and excellent accounts are available in the work of Larroche (1977) and in the anatomical atlas *Development of the Human Foetal Brain* (Feess-Higgins and Larroche, 1987).

Haemorrhages

Subarachnoid Haemorrhage

Small subarachnoid haemorrhages are commonly encountered in the brains of neonates, especially those delivered preterm, and are probably related to mild hypoxia. Rarely, a subarachnoid haematoma may be confined to one lobe of the brain, associated with infarction of the underlying brain (Fig. 24.1a,b). Large collections of blood in the basal subarachnoid space usually accompany intraventricular haemorrhage.

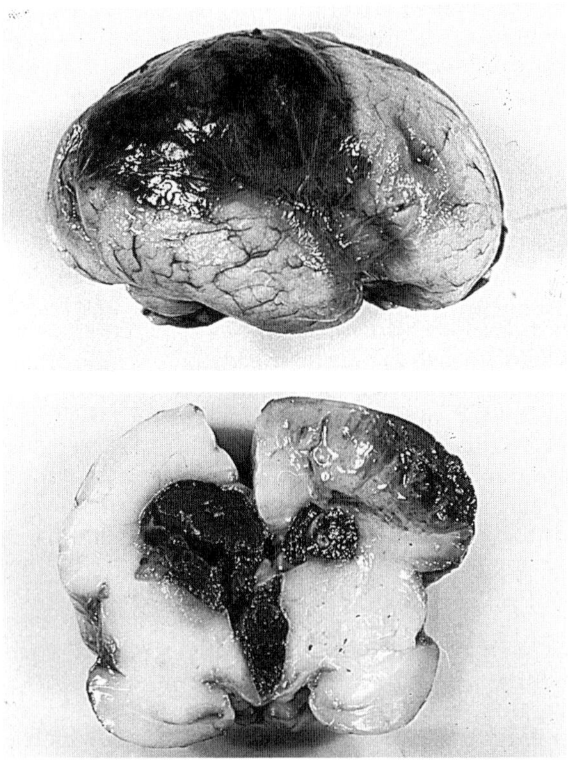

a

b

Fig. 24.1. a Subarachnoid haemorrhage overlying the parietal lobe in an infant born at 27 weeks' gestation and who survived for 6 days. **b** Coronal slice of the same brain shows the haemorrhage to overlie an area of infarction. There is a germinal matrix haemorrhage on the same side which has ruptured into the ventricular system.

Cerebellar Haemorrhage

Small subarachnoid haemorrhages over the cerebellum are not uncommon, and probably not of clinical significance. Parenchymal cerebellar haemorrhage occurs in 5%–14% of premature or sick infants (Larroche 1977; Rorke 1982). The pathogenesis is probably multifactorial but may involve trauma, hypoxia and prematurity (Volpe 1987).

Periventricular and Intraventricular Haemorrhage

Periventricular–intraventricular haemorrhage (PVH-IVH) characteristically occurs in the preterm infant. The incidence ranges from 60% in infants of less than 700 g to 20% in babies of 1000 g or more. Susceptible infants are usually sick and there is a strong association with respiratory distress syndrome (RDS) and its complications (Perlman 1989). The onset is usually between 12 and 72 h after birth (Wigglesworth 1989). Despite increased survival of low birthweight infants in recent years and the introduction of surfactant in treatment of RDS the incidence of PVH-IVH has not declined and remains the most important cause of morbidity and mortality in premature infants (Cooke 1991; Van de Bor et al. 1991).

Intraventricular haemorrhage usually arises from the vessels of the germinal matrix but bleeding from the choroid plexus has been identified in up to 61% of cases (Goddard-Finegold 1984; Armstrong et al. 1987), this being the most frequent site of origin in term infants (Donat et al. 1978).

The germinal matrix is a layer of densely packed immature cells found just beneath the ependymal epithelium and is thickest in the lateral walls of the lateral ventricles, where a prominent cushion pushes into the lateral ventricle at the level of the head of the caudate nucleus. The matrix is the site of active cell replication. During the first half of gestation neuroblasts develop and subsequently migrate out into the cerebral cortex. Later, glial cells are produced before the germinal matrix begins to involute and by 36 weeks only small groups of immature cells remain in the subependymal zone and clustered around vessels of the deep white matter. The matrix has a dense network of wide vascular channels lined by endothelium, but lacking muscle or collagen in their walls.

A clinical grading scheme for severity of haemorrhage has been devised based on CT scan appearances (Volpe 1987).

Grade I Small haemorrhages restricted to the germinal matrix or occupying less than 10% of the ventricular area.

Grade II Intraventricular haemorrhage occupying 10%–50% of ventricular area.

Grade III Intraventricular haemorrhage which occupies more than 50% of the ventricle and usually causes distension.

In previous grading schemes a fourth category was used for haemorrhages thought to extend into cerebral parenchyma, but this appearance is probably due to haemorrhagic infarction which has a separate pathogenesis and should not be classified with IVH.

Pathology of Germinal Matrix Haemorrhage

Germinal matrix haemorrhages may be single or multiple, unilateral or bilateral and are found in the lateral wall of the lateral ventricle (Fig. 24.2). Localisation is related to age; haemorrhage originates more frequently over the body of the caudate nucleus before 28 weeks of gestation, and further forward over the head of the caudate nucleus, close to the level of the foramen of Monroe after 29 weeks (Hambleton and Wigglesworth 1976; De Reuck 1984).

During fixation, blood pigments diffuse out of the clot into adjacent parenchyma which may give an initial impression of parenchymal involvement. Close inspection is usually sufficient to demonstrate integrity of the parenchyma but histological examination may be required to be certain.

The macroscopic appearance of fresh haemorrhage in the fixed brain is of a mass of deep red blood clot of uniform appearance. After some weeks the haemorrhage becomes paler in colour and begins to undergo lysis. In long-term survival the only evidence of previous haemorrhage may be a small residual, smooth-walled subependymal cyst.

Histology of fresh germinal matrix haemorrhage shows disruption of the matrix by blood cells. The capillary walls do not usually show

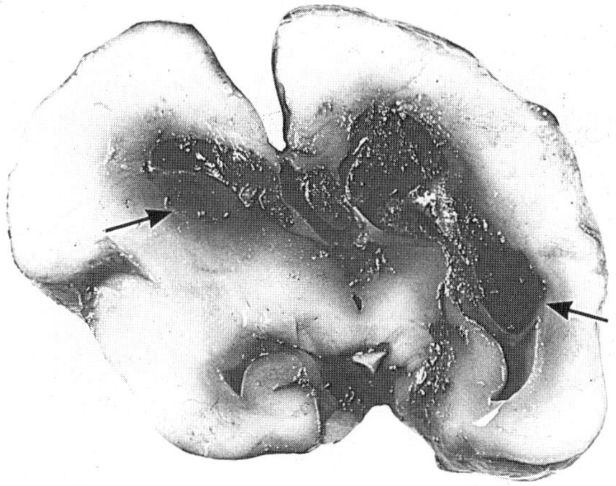

Fig. 24.2. Bilateral germinal matrix haemorrhages (*arrows*) with extension into the ventricular system. Infant 23 weeks' gestation, survived 3 days.

evidence of ischaemic damage and polymorph reaction is not seen. After 2–3 days large macrophages with red cells within their cytoplasm are seen in the region of the haemorrhage (Fig. 24.3) (Sherwood et al. 1978; Darrow et al. 1988). *Intraventricular extension* results

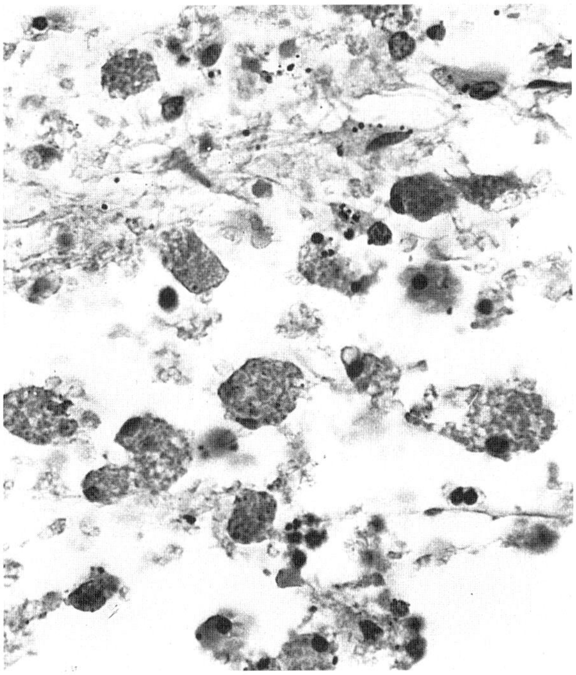

Fig. 24.3. Large macrophages stuffed with red cells and debris of necrotic cells in an area of infarction adjacent to a germinal matrix haemorrhage. Stillborn infant 33 weeks' gestation. (H&E, ×377)

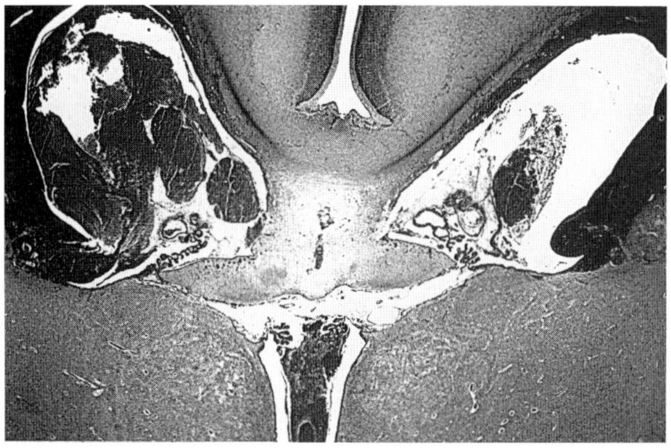

Fig. 24.4. Section of brain showing a germinal matrix haemorrhage on the left rupturing through the ependyma into the lateral ventricle. Blood is also present in the third ventricle. There is a small haemorrhage in the choroid plexus on the right side and an infarct in the midline septum. Fetus of 24 weeks gestation with listeriosis, died shortly after birth. (H&E ×5)

from rupture of the ependyma (Fig. 24.4) and blood clot is found in the lateral ventricles, often extending through the third ventricle, the aqueduct of Sylvius and the fourth ventricle. Escape of blood through the exit foramina of the fourth ventricle allows blood to collect in the basal cisterns around the brainstem and cerebellum, presenting a characteristic feature of IVH on the base of the uncut brain (Fig. 24.5a,b). Altered blood pigments cause brown discoloration of the entire ventricular system and meninges at the base of the brain.

The presence of blood in the ventricular system prompts a response in the ependymal lining and underlying tissues. Proliferating glial cells grow through and over the ependyma and form a thick layer. Fragments of ependyma persist as rosettes or isolated strips within this band of glial tissue, and groups of macrophages containing altered blood cells may be found on the surface or trapped within it (Fig. 24.6).

This ependymal and subependymal reaction is of significance when it occurs either in the cerebral aqueduct or in the outflow foramina draining the fourth ventricle. In these sites it can obstruct the flow of CSF, causing hydrocephalus. When the aqueduct alone is obstructed the lateral and third ventricles dilate, while obstruction of the outflow from the fourth ventricle causes the fourth ventricle and cerebral aqueduct to dilate as well.

Associated Brain Lesions

Up to 75% of babies with germinal matrix haemorrhage have damage to other parts of the brain. The most commonly found lesions are periventricular leucomalacia and pontosubi-

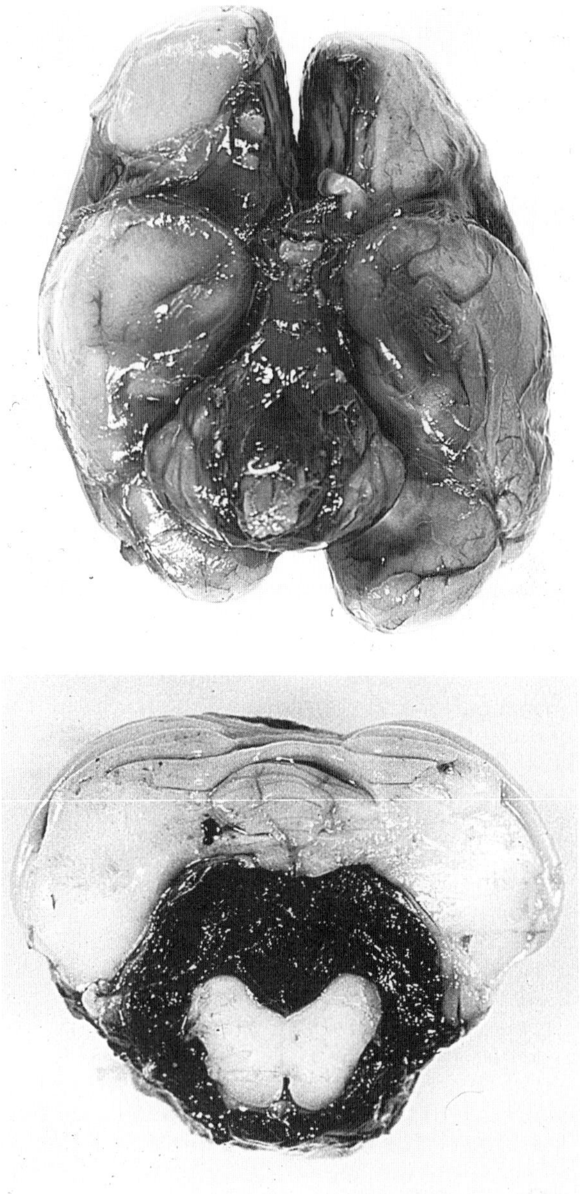

a

b

Fig. 24.5. **a** Intraventricular haemorrhage. Characteristic appearance of subarachnoid blood clot around the base of the brain of a 25-week gestation fetus. **b** Coronal slice through the hindbrain shows blood clot distending the fourth ventricle and escaping through lateral outflow foramina to fill the subarachnoid space around the medulla. 24-week gestation fetus.

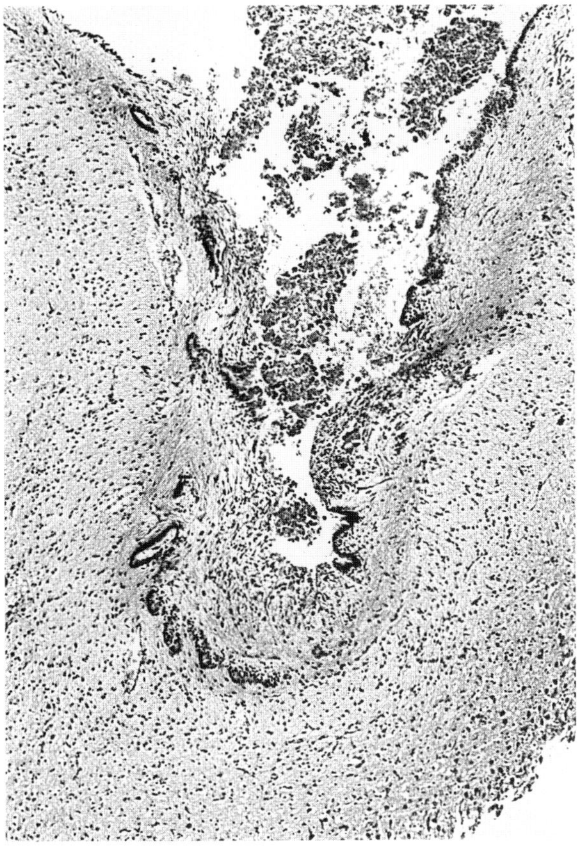

Fig. 24.6. Intraventricular haemorrhage in utero. Blood clot in the ventricles has caused reactive changes in the ependyma, remnants of which are seen as strips and rosettes buried in a dense band of gliosis. Infant delivered at 32 weeks' gestation for hydrocephalus. (H&E ×110)

cular necrosis. (Skullerud and Westre 1986; Armstrong et al. 1987)

Pathogenesis of Germinal Matrix Haemorrhage

The walls of the immature blood vessels of the germinal matrix are physically weak, lacking collagen or muscle. Involution of the germinal matrix towards the end of gestation reduces support offered by its closely packed cells leaving the vessels vulnerable to sudden haemodynamic changes. In common with other cerebral vessels the endothelial cells have large numbers of mitochondria (Oldendorf et al. 1977) implying high metabolic rate and susceptibility to oxygen deprivation.

The cerebral circulation of the preterm infant has only a limited capacity to react to changes in systemic blood pressure. Autoregulation of cerebral blood flow, which protects the capillary networks of the brain from large fluctuations in systemic pressure, is poorly developed in the preterm infant at birth, but has been shown to develop during the first week of extrauterine life (Ramaekers et al. 1990; Bignall and Rivers 1991). The cerebral circulation of the sick preterm infant is particularly susceptible to sudden changes in systemic blood pressure (Lou et al. 1979; Milligan 1980). Blood pressure swings which may occur during medical or nursing procedures or even seizures may be sufficient to rupture the delicate germinal matrix vessels in these infants (Van Bel et al. 1987; Volpe 1987; Van de Bor et al. 1991).

Increased venous pressure and carbon dioxide retention, either at birth or as a complication of respiratory disease have also been proposed as possible contributory causes. (Volpe 1987).

Parenchymal Haemorrhagic Infarction

Parenchymal haemorrhagic infarction occurs in 15% of infants with germinal matrix haemorrhage (Volpe 1989). It is usually unilateral and occurs at the angle of the lateral ventricle (Fig. 24.1b). Microscopic examination shows clusters of perivascular haemorrhages along the course of the veins fanning out into the centrum semiovale (Gould et al. 1987), suggesting venous haemorrhage into an area already damaged by ischaemia. Positron emission tomography has demonstrated reduced blood flow to an extensive area of the hemisphere around a matrix bleed which may precede the occurrence of the bleed, and persist for some time after it (Lou 1989; Volpe 1989).

Sequelae of Periventricular–Intraventricular Haemorrhage

The consequences of germinal matrix haemorrhage may be immediate or delayed.

The early consequences include haemorrhagic infarction of adjacent parenchyma where fibres from the motor cortex may be damaged in their course to the internal capsule and acute hydrocephalus due to obstruction of CSF flow by blood clot.

Hydrocephalus may also be a late complication due to the chronic reactive changes to blood in the ventricular system. Blood passing into the CSF around the brain may induce reactive fibrosis in the arachnoid granulations of the sagittal sinus and block CSF absorption. This results in increased volume of CSF both around the brain and within the ventricular system or "communicating hydrocephalus".

Neurological Sequelae

Small (Grade 1) haemorrhages are encountered frequently, may occur in the undamaged brain, and have an excellent prognosis (Lou 1989).

More than 50% of infants who have large haemorrhages are normal on follow-up (de Vries et al. 1985; Volpe 1987). The loss of germinal matrix cells which are a source of future glial cells, some of which will be responsible for myelin synthesis, does not appear to jeopardise future myelination (Johnson 1987; Van de Bor 1989). Other brain lesions found in association with germinal matrix haemorrhage may be responsible for greater morbidity. Parenchymal haemorrhagic infarction and post-haemorrhagic hydrocephalus both cause severe neurological handicap in the great majority of cases (Deonna et al. 1975; Volpe 1987; Leviton and Paneth 1989).

Brain Damage due to Hypoxia and Ischaemia

This is the commonest type of acquired brain damage in the fetal and neonatal brain. The pattern of injury is to some extent age-dependent but also varies with the degree of disruption of normal development and the nature, intensity and duration of the insult.

Clinical Manifestations of Hypoxic–Ischaemic Injury

Infants who have suffered severe asphyxia are extremely ill with coma, seizures, limb weakness, apnoeic attacks and a variety of other neurological signs. The clinical term used to describe this syndrome is hypoxic–ischaemic encephalopathy. In 35% there is a history of adverse intrapartum events, 35% have additional predisposing antepartum events and in 20% there is evidence that antepartum events alone are responsible (Volpe 1987).

Many factors operate in the aetiology of this syndrome: carbon dioxide retention, acidosis, circulatory arrest, hypotension and hypoglycaemia may all contribute. The relative contribution of these factors is poorly understood, but for brevity the term ischaemic damage will be used in the following text.

The Role of Birth in Ischaemic Damage

In 1861 Little described a series of children with spastic diplegia and attributed their condition to difficult birth. Since then there has been a tendency to regard chronic neurological handicaps in children (cerebral palsy) to birth injury. However, epidemiological studies over the last few years have shown that in only about 10% of cases of cerebral palsy is there a history of birth asphyxia (Freeman and Nelson 1988) and prenatal factors are more important as predictors of cerebral palsy (Nelson and Ellenberg 1986). In 1897 Freud pointed out that birth is not usually harmful and birth difficulties may be symptomatic of adverse conditions in utero. Indeed it can be shown that asphyxia may be present before birth in growth retarded fetuses (Soothill et al. 1987; Gudmundssen et al. 1990).

More recently, ultransound and CT scans have demonstrated acquired cerebral lesions of vascular origin in fetuses (Gunn et al. 1985; Larroche 1986; Stoddard et al. 1988; Tenorio et al. 1988).

Neuropathological study of the brains of stillborn infants and very early neonatal deaths has shown an incidence of antenatal damage in up to 44% (Sims et al. 1985; Roland et al. 1987; Ellis et al. 1988; Squier and Keeling 1991). It is obviously very important to identify cases of prenatal origin and to distinguish them from those arising during labour and delivery, not only for our further understanding of their causes and prevention but also for medicolegal reasons.

Patterns of Ischaemic Damage

Oedema seen in the acute phase of ischaemic damage in neonatal brains rarely causes flattening of the gyri as seen in older children and adults. Coronal slices of the fixed brain show compression of the lateral ventricles. The

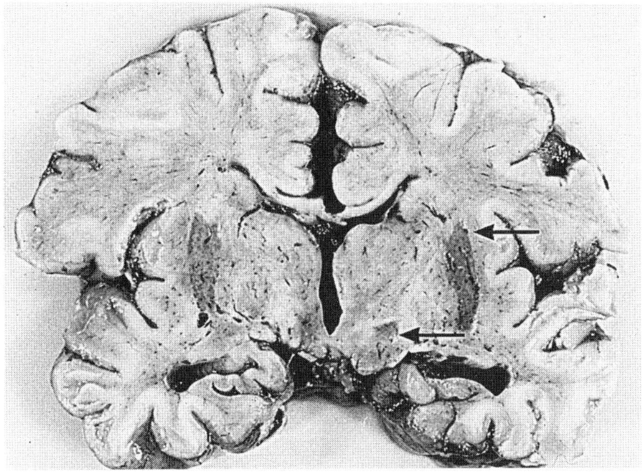

Fig. 24.7. Hypoxic–ischaemic encephalopathy. Coronal slice of the fixed brain of an infant who survived for 10 days following complicated delivery at 42 weeks. The brain is oedematous, the lateral ventricles are narrow and the cortex is a prominent white ribbon. There is recent infarction of the putamen and subthalamic nuclei (*arrows*).

cortex, usually not readily distinguished from white matter before myelination, stands out as a prominent white ribbon (Fig. 24.7). This contrasts with the translucent grey colour of the white matter which appears to sink back from the cortex. There may be a pink flush due to congestion of vessels in the white matter. Histologically, oedema produces widespread cytoplasmic vacuolation in the white matter where nuclei appear surrounded by a clear space. Vacuolation can be particularly conspicuous in myelinated fibre bundles.

Identifying the precise time sequence of cellular reactions to ischaemia in the immature brain is difficult, particularly in the antenatal period. There are few well-documented cases of single episodes of severe maternal hypoxia following trauma, hypotension or gas intoxication with subsequent examination of the fetal brain after a known period of survival (Larroche 1986). Single episodes of ischaemia are sometimes precisely timed when they occur postnatally and allow temporal evaluation of resulting damage (Janzer and Friede 1980). In most cases, however, the history is less clear. Accurate assessment of cellular reactions has been hampered by the assumption in many studies that birth has been solely responsible for asphyxia, without considering an earlier, prenatal onset.

Table 24.1 summarises the principal cellular reactions to ischaemic damage and their timing as derived from a number of accounts in the literature which is generally compatible with personal experience and provides a guide to histological assessment of acute ischaemic injury in the immature brain.

Table 24.1. Approximate timing of cellular responses to injury in the fetal and neonatal brain

Macrophages	
Microglial proliferation	3 h–3 d
Macrophages	4–5 d
Macrophages showing evidence of phagocytosis	4–6 d
Astrocytes	
Astrocyte proliferation	12 h–4 d
Astrocytes with cytoplasmic processes	3–11 d
Astrocyte fibillary gliosis	6 d
Capillaries	
Endothelial swelling	1–3 d
Endothelial reduplication	5 d
Coagulation necrosis	3 h
Retraction balls	3 h
Neuronal karyorrhexis	12–48 h
Mineralisation	8–14 d
Cysts	14–42 d

From Banker and Larroche (1972); Sherwood et al. (1978); Roessmann and Gambetti (1986); Armstrong et al. (1987); Darrow et al. (1988); Ellis et al. (1988); Lou (1989). *Abbreviations*: h, hours, d, days.

Ischaemic Damage to Grey Matter

Cerebral Cortex

Ischaemic lesions of the cerebral cortex characteristically occur in term infants (Larroche 1977; Volpe 1987). In the early stages, cortical lesions may be difficult to see macroscopically. Histology shows pallor of affected areas, neuronal karyorrhexis, macrophage infiltration and glial and endothelial proliferation in a sequence as indicated in Table 24.1. Karyorrhexis is a particularly prominent feature of early neuronal necrosis in the immature brain (Figs. 24.8, 24.9).

The distribution of neuronal necrosis is not uniform, affecting some areas preferentially (Larroche 1977). The hippocampus and subiculum are particularly often involved (Figs. 24.8a,b) and karyorrhectic nuclei can be found here in the least severely affected brains, making examination of a section of this region a particularly useful exercise in assessment of ischaemic brain damage.

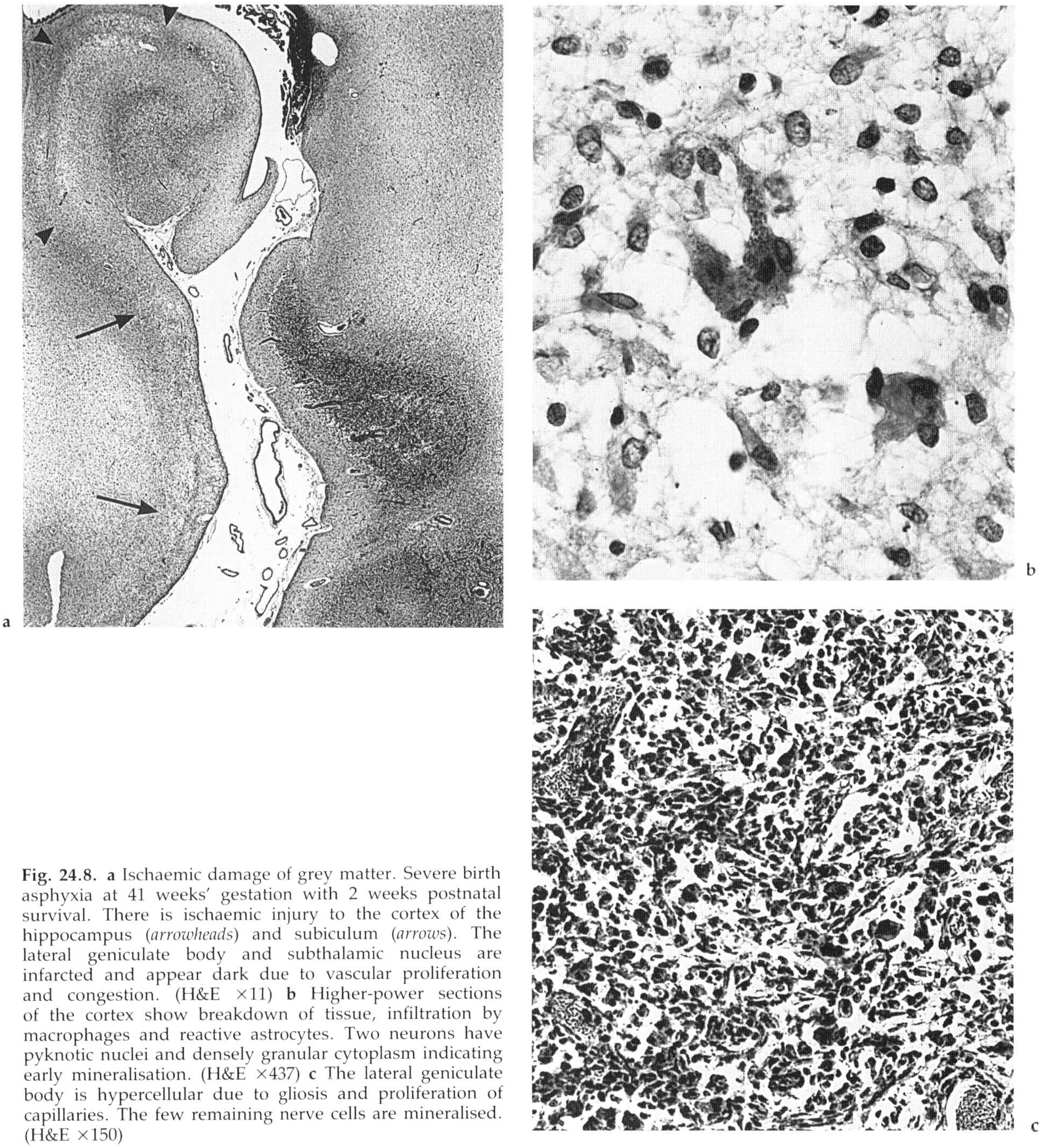

Fig. 24.8. **a** Ischaemic damage of grey matter. Severe birth asphyxia at 41 weeks' gestation with 2 weeks postnatal survival. There is ischaemic injury to the cortex of the hippocampus (*arrowheads*) and subiculum (*arrows*). The lateral geniculate body and subthalamic nucleus are infarcted and appear dark due to vascular proliferation and congestion. (H&E ×11) **b** Higher-power sections of the cortex show breakdown of tissue, infiltration by macrophages and reactive astrocytes. Two neurons have pyknotic nuclei and densely granular cytoplasm indicating early mineralisation. (H&E ×437) **c** The lateral geniculate body is hypercellular due to gliosis and proliferation of capillaries. The few remaining nerve cells are mineralised. (H&E ×150)

Damage to the parasagittal watershed areas of the cortex may be seen. Decreased cerebral blood flow to these areas has been demonstrated by positron emission tomography in term infants with hypoxic–ischaemic encephalopathy (Volpe 1989).

There are variations in the degree of damage within the cortex. Sometimes only the intermediate cortical layers are damaged resulting in laminar necrosis. More usual is damage to the depths of the cortical sulci with relative sparing of the crests of gyri.

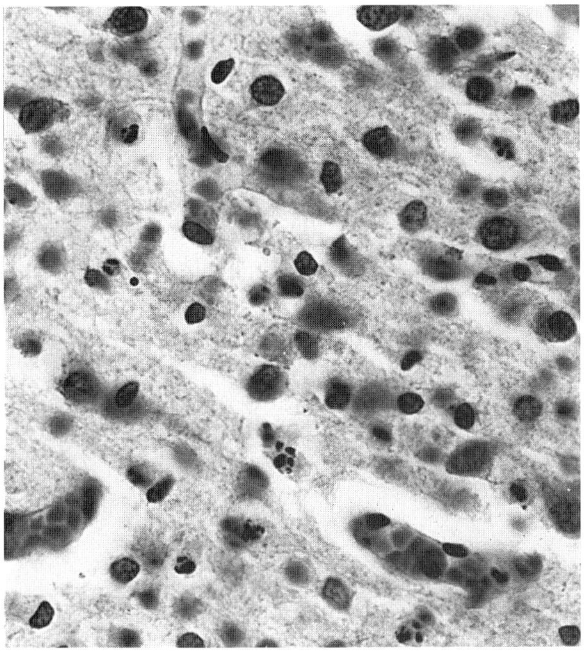

Fig. 24.9. Early neuronal necrosis. Section of the pons of an infant stillborn at 36 weeks' gestation. Many neuronal nuclei are undergoing karyorrhexis and appear as collections of small, densely basophilic, rounded granules. (H&E ×440)

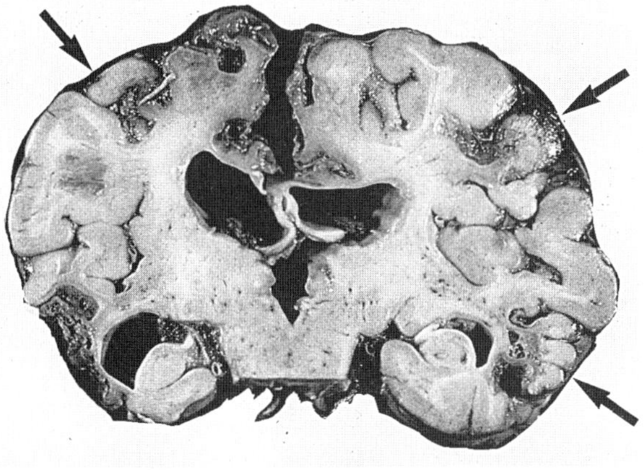

Fig. 24.10. Late effects of ischaemic damage. Coronal slice of the brain of a 5-year-old child with cerebral palsy, epilepsy and blindness. The lateral ventricles are dilated due to loss of tissue, the corpus callosum is thin. Areas of old cortical damage are seen as thinning of the cortex which is most marked on the medial surfaces of the hemispheres and in watershed areas. Here examples of ulegyria are seen (*arrows*) with more severe involvement of the deep sulcal cortex than the crests of gyri.

The long-term results of cortical necrosis are shrinkage and scarring by gliosis of the damaged zones. Where there has been preferential destruction of sulcal cortex the thin, scarred areas of the sulci contrast with the normal thick cortex over the gyral surfaces, producing a mushroom-like appearance described as ulegyria (Fig. 24.10).

Deep Grey Matter

The deep grey neurons most commonly involved by ischaemic damage are the thalamus, globus pallidus and the lateral geniculate bodies. Macroscopically there may be pink or brown discoloration, and histologically a pattern of nuclear karyorrhexis followed by glial and macrophage infiltration with marked vascular proliferation (Fig. 24.8c). In long-standing cases there is mineralisation of cells, diffuse proliferation of glial cells with an extensive fibrillary network (Fig. 24.11) and sometimes cyst formation.

Rarely, *status marmoratus* is seen. This is a macroscopic description of "marbling" of the

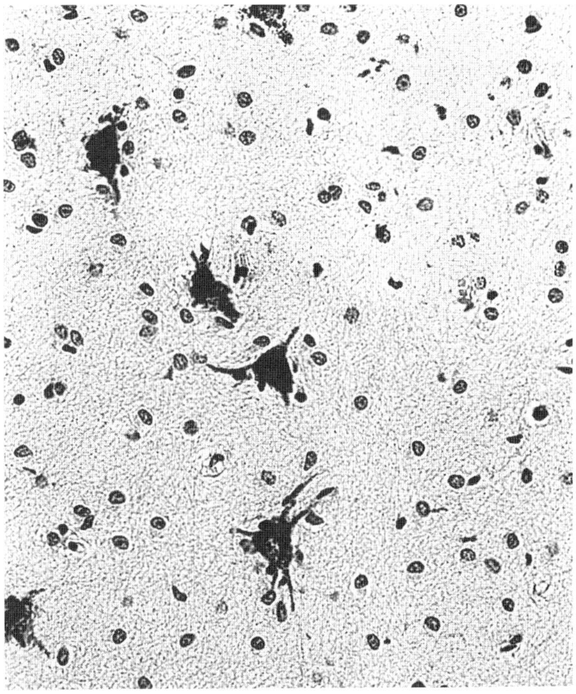

Fig. 24.11. Old ischaemic damage to deep grey nuclei. Thalamus of a child of 5 years with cerebral palsy. Almost all the nerve cells have disappeared except for a few mineralised neuronal cell bodies. There is intense gliosis. (H&E ×218)

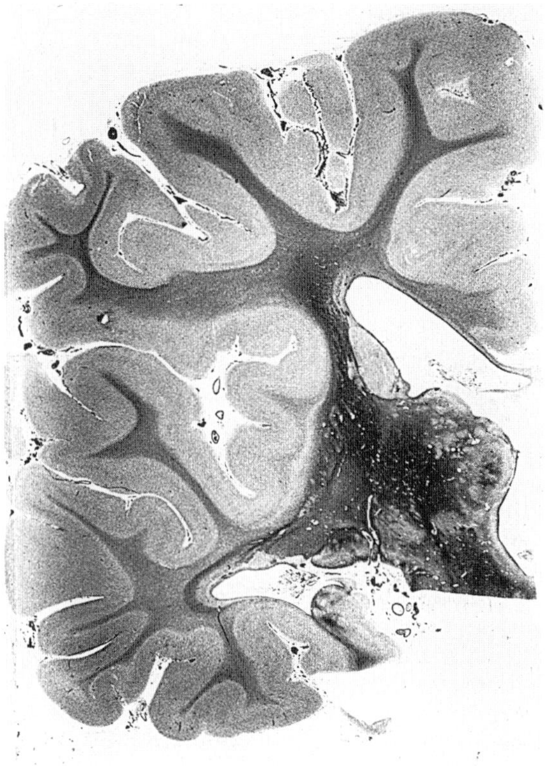

Fig. 24.12. Status marmoratus. Section of cerebral hemisphere of a child of 6 months with cerebral palsy. The thalamus shows abnormal, patchy myelination. (PTAH ×1.5)

basal ganglia due to aberrant bands of myelinated fibres (Fig. 24.12). The nature of these fibres is controversial: they may arise from myelination of glial fibres or from disorientation of bundles of myelinated nerve fibres secondary to neuronal loss. This condition is seen in infants surviving 6 months or more who may have had a history of complicated birth (Friede 1989).

Necrosis of basal ganglia causes choreoathetoid movement disorders which usually coexist with other severe handicaps.

Brainstem

Necrosis of brainstem nuclei following asphyxia is well recognised (Fig. 24.13). The inferior colliculi often show particularly severe damage but brainstem necrosis is rarely isolated and red nuclei, substantia nigra, thalamus and cerebral cortex are usually also involved. Brainstem and thalamic damage occurring after a single well-defined asphyxial episode or cardiac arrest has been called "cardiac arrest encephalopathy" (Leech and Alvord 1977; Janzer and Friede 1980). Although a similar pattern of injury occurs in the mature brain, it is much more frequent in infants. Brainstem necrosis has also been seen in fetuses who have suffered chronic intrauterine asphyxia (Dambska et al. 1987).

Infarction of cranial nerve nuclei is one of the underlying causes of Moëbius' syndrome (congenital facial diplegia).

Pontosubicular Necrosis

This is a well-recognised condition in which neuronal necrosis of the pontine nuclei, which are diffusely spread between the fibre bundles of the corticospinal tracts in the base of the

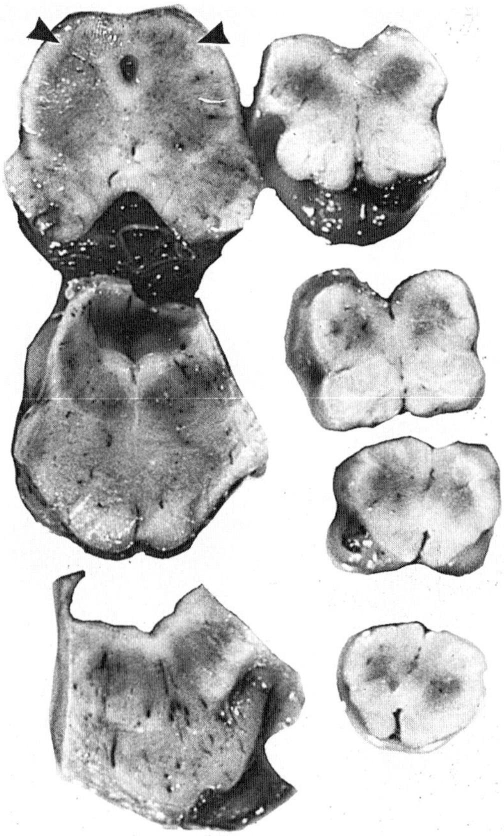

Fig. 24.13. Brainstem ischaemia. Slices of the brainstem of an infant who died 14 days after a complicated delivery at 42 weeks' gestation. There is dusky discoloration indicating recent infarction of neuronal groups in the brainstem tegmentum and inferior colliculi (*arrowheads*).

pons, coexists with necrosis of neurons of the subiculum, which is the cortex adjacent to the infolded area of the hippocampus. In the early stages, neuronal karyorrhexes are prominent, later there is atrophy with gliosis and sometimes cystic change.

Skullerud and Westre (1986) described pontosubicular necrosis in 59% of their series of preterm infants, where it was the most common type of brain damage. However it is rarely an isolated finding, almost always occurring in association with other forms of brain damage, for example germinal matrix haemorrhage (Armstrong et al. 1987).

Cerebellum

The cerebellum is frequently involved in ischaemic damage, usually in association with damage elsewhere. Conversely, the cerebellum may escape unharmed in cases of quite severe damage to cerebral hemispheres (Rorke 1982). The Purkinje cells and internal granular layer are particularly sensitive to hypoxia.

As a late result of ischaemic damage the cerebellum becomes shrunken, white and firm with increased space between the cortical folia. Occasionally old damage is manifest by selective sclerosis in the depths of the sulci bordering on central white matter (Fig. 24.14).

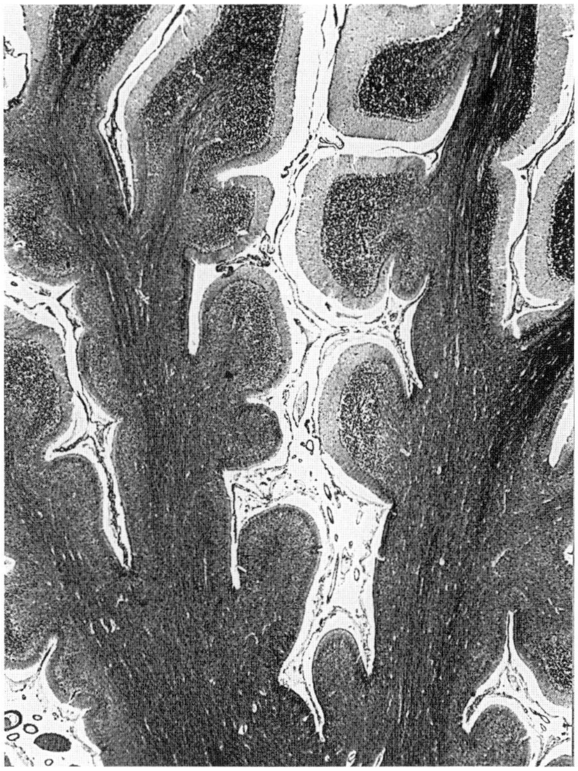

Fig. 24.14. Cerebellar ischaemia. Gliosis of the cerebellar cortex in a child of 6 months who suffered birth asphyxia at term. The superficial (molecular) layer of the cerebellar cortex is thin and gliotic in the depths of several sulci. The underlying granular layer is severely atrophic. Reactive gliosis stains darkly. (PTAH ×15)

Spinal Cord

Removal and examination of the spinal cord are often neglected. However, it is not infrequently the site of ischaemic damage. Destruction of anterior horn cells may be responsible for some of the motor deficits observed in infants with hypoxic–ischaemic encephalopathy (Clancy et al. 1989). Intrauterine ischaemic damage to anterior horn cells may cause arthrogyposis multiplex congenita (Horoupian and Yoon 1988).

Ischaemic Damage to White Matter

White matter infarction characteristically occurs in the immature brain. There may be surprisingly little associated neuronal damage. It has been recognised in neonates since Virchow's original description in 1867, but it was Banker and Larroche in 1962 who gave the first comprehensive account of tiny white spots of cystic necrosis in the deep white matter and introduced the term "periventricular leucomalacia".

White matter infarction is not only manifested by the white spots of periventricular leucomalacia. It may cause much more extensive diffuse gliosis (Leech and Alvord 1974; Dambska et al. 1989; Rodriguez et al. 1990) sometimes called "perinatal telencephalic leucoencephalopathy" (Gilles 1983b) or widespread multicystic destruction of the hemispheres.

There are several possible explanations for the specific vulnerability of the immature white matter to infarction. The vascular supply is from two sources, vessels which penetrate deeply from the surface of the brain and vessels which enter from the periventricular zone. Between these vessels is a relatively poorly perfused watershed area in the deep white matter, corresponding to the site of classic periventricular leucomalacia (De Reuck

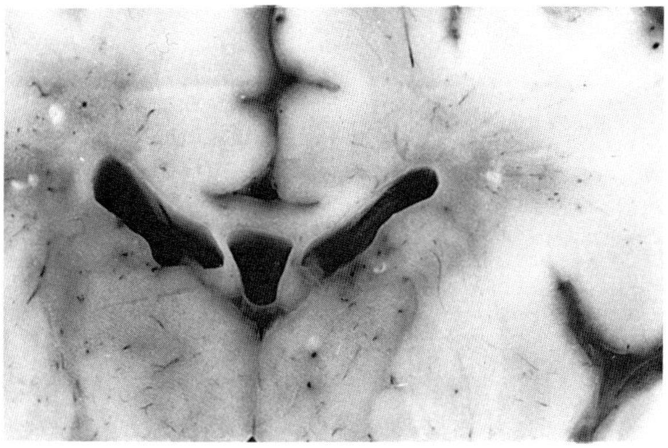

Fig. 24.15. Periventricular leucomalacia. Fixed brain slice showing the white spots of periventricular leucomalacia in the deep white matter adjacent to the angles of the lateral ventricles. Prenatal damage in an infant dying 30 minutes after birth.

et al. 1972). With increasing maturity the ventriculofugal vessels become longer and the vulnerable watershed zone moves outwards to the subcortical area (Takashima and Tanaka 1978). A second factor in the susceptibility of the white matter to infarction is its high metabolic rate in the second half of gestation due to active myelin synthesis. It is widely accepted that ischaemia is the underlying mechanism for periventricular leucomalacia (Larroche 1977; Norman 1978; Volpe 1987) but Gilles has proposed bacterial endotoxaemia as a cause (Gilles 1983a) and two studies of prenatal white matter damage in humans have shown an association with intrauterine infection (Sims et al. 1985; Bejar et al. 1988).

Periventricular Leucomalacia

The incidence of periventricular leucomalacia varies between 6% and 88% depending on the population studied. About 75% of cases are in premature infants (Banker and Larroche 1962; Shuman and Selednik 1980; Rorke 1982; Volpe 1987).

Coronal slices of the fixed brain show well-developed focal necroses as tiny white or yellow spots, several millimetres in diameter and sometimes centrally cavitated, in the deep white matter (Fig. 24.15). The original description of Banker and Larroche indicates three areas which are constantly involved, anterior to the anterior horn of the lateral ventricle; in the corona radiata adjacent to the lateral angle of the ventricles, and lateral to the temporal and occipital horns of the ventricles. Shuman and Selednik (1980) also found PVL in the deep white matter adjacent to the foramen of Monroe and in the occipital radiation at the trigonum, the latter site being involved in all cases. The deep white matter elsewhere usually has a light brown discoloration and radial vessels appear very prominent.

Histological appearance depends on the age of the lesions. In the early stages an irregular zone of coagulation necrosis is seen. Microglial reaction occurs early, followed by astrocytic proliferation and collections of macrophages (Fig. 24.16a). Retraction balls may be prominent. These are rounded eosinophilic masses, the swollen proximal ends of severed axons. Capillary endothelial reactions around the zone of necrosis may be very striking. The endothelial nuclei become plump and rounded and the endothelium thickens and may even be reduplicated. In our material, nuclear karyorrhexes are very common in capillary endothelium (Squier and Keeling 1991). One of the more eyecatching features of the older lesions is a peripheral zone of densely basophilic mineralisation in the form of sticks or balls, debris of old cells, axon stumps or capillaries (Fig. 24.16b).

Away from the focal necroses there are more diffuse and extensive changes in the white matter, with infiltration by macrophages and reactive astrocytes with ample eosinophilic cytoplasm and fibrillary processes. The capillary changes described above may also be prominent. Clusters of axon retraction balls may be seen.

Examination of the grey matter usually shows remarkably little change. There may be a few karyorrhectic neurons, usually in the subiculum, hippocampus, base of the pons or cerebellar internal granule layer (see Fig. 24.9).

Diffuse White Matter Ischaemia

Diffuse white matter ischaemic change is also seen alone without the focal necroses of periventricular leucomalacia. Although it probably represents a part of the same spectrum of damage it has attracted attention among paediatric and fetal neuropathologists and probably deserves clear definition as an entity.

The incidence is between 15% and 45% of low-birthweight or sick infants (Rorke 1982; Gilles 1983a; Paneth et al. 1990). The macroscopic changes may be subtle and easily con-

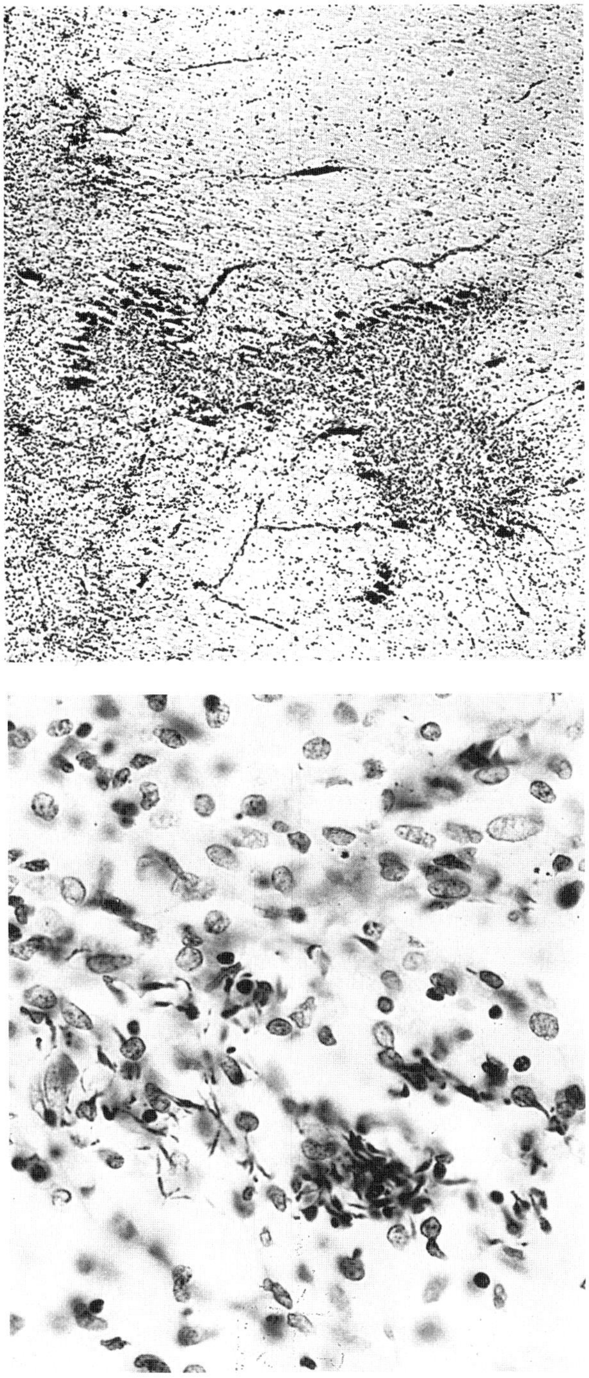

a

b

Fig. 24.16. a Periventricular leucomalacia. Low-power micrograph of periventricular leucomalacia with an infarct of the deep white matter infiltrated by reactive glial cells and macrophages. The edge shows focal mineralisation. (H&E ×42) **b** Higher-power micrograph shows mineralisation of necrotic cell bodies and processes. The cellular infiltrate in the infarcted area is seen on the left. (H&E ×423)

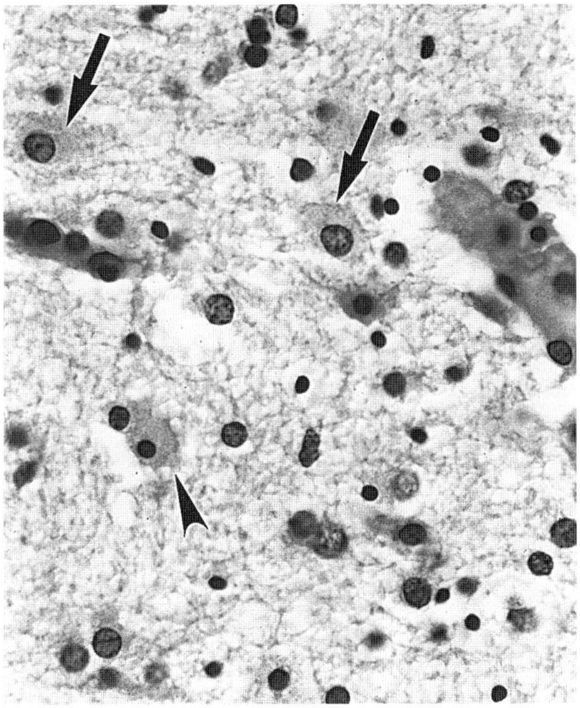

Fig. 24.17. Diffuse white matter ischaemic damage. Endothelial nuclei are prominent and plump. There are reactive astrocytes (*arrows*) and infiltration of the tissue by reactive macrophages (*arrowhead*). Infant of 35 weeks' gestation with oesophageal atresia who died within an hour of birth. (H&E ×437)

fused with fixation artefact. The deep white matter is grey or light brown and radial vessels are prominent. Yellow streaks may be seen around or adjacent to blood vessels. The histological changes are much the same as those seen in the white matter of infants with periventricular leucomalacia away from the focal necroses (Fig. 24.17). It is found throughout the cerebral white matter but most consistently in the occipital lobes. Examination of grey matter shows only a few karyorrhectic nuclei.

If this condition is to be considered part of the spectrum of ischaemic disease it is important that criteria of infarction are fulfilled, including reactive gliosis, macrophage infiltration, capillary reaction and presence of necrotic cells as manifest by karyorrhectic nuclei. The presence of large numbers of reactive astrocytes alone is not sufficient to constitute a diagnosis of ischaemic damage as these cells may be difficult to differentiate from the normal glia of myelination (Norman 1978;

Rorke 1982) and from the astrocytosis of metabolic disease (see Fig. 24.20).

Sequelae of White Matter Infarction

The increased use of ultrasound scanning, computed tomography and, more recently, magnetic resonance imaging has led to great advances in our understanding of the evolution of white matter ischaemic damage and its clinical consequences. The chronic stage of periventricular leucomalacia may manifest in two ways: either the development of clearly demarcated cysts in the deep white matter, or intense gliotic scarring of the centrum semiovale.

Sequential cranial ultrasound studies have shown that the cysts of periventricular leucomalacia may disappear after some weeks, leaving only ventricular dilatation. Examination of the brain at this stage shows dense periventricular gliosis in which collapsed cysts may be found as tiny spaces containing macrophages (Wigglesworth 1989; Rodriguez et al. 1990). In some cases there is no evidence of cysts but the white matter is intensely gliotic, particularly in the areas close to the lateral ventricles.

Neurological Sequelae of White Matter Infarction

Clinical follow-up of children with cystic lesions shows a very high proportion to have serious neurological handicaps including spastic quadriplegia, spastic diplegia, impairments of speech and vision and developmental delay (Weindling et al. 1985; Sinha 1990). Magnetic resonance imaging studies show delays in myelination following periventricular leucomalacia (Johnson 1987; van de Bor 1989). The clinical outcome of diffuse white matter ischaemia is less certain as the scan appearances correlating to this pathological change are unknown.

Cystic Cavitation of the Brain

Several patterns of cystic damage are described as the late results of a disturbance of cerebral blood supply during development.

Multicystic Encephalopathy

In this condition most of the cerebral white matter is replaced by multiple large cysts with smooth, clean walls (Fig. 24.18). Cysts may be found predominantly in the subcortical white matter or may extend to the lateral ventricles which are dilated due to tissue loss.

The cortex is gliotic and stretched over the cysts; deep grey matter and brainstem are shrunken, white and very firm. Tiny cysts a few millimetres in diameter may be seen in this gliotic grey matter. The cerebellum is atrophic.

Histology shows extensive fibrillary gliosis in the walls of the cysts with very little myelination in the cerebral hemispheres. Calcification is not marked. The grey matter is almost totally devoid of nerve cells and replaced by glial cells and small cystic cavities packed with macrophages which persist for many years.

This change is thought to be the end result of ischaemic injury and has similarities to the chronic cystic stage of periventricular leucomalacia. The location of cysts immediately below the cortex may be a reflection of the maturity at the time of insult (Takashima and Tanaka 1978). Multicystic encephalopathy was described by Larroche (1986) in four cases with well-documented episodes of maternal trauma, hypotension or hypoxia (due to butane intoxication) between 30 weeks of gestation and "a few weeks before term" and illustrate the vulnerability of the white matter at this stage of development.

Serial ultrasound scans of survivors show a much poorer neurological outcome in infants with subcortical cysts or a mixed pattern than in those with purely periventricular cysts (de Vries et al. 1987, 1988).

Porencephaly

This term is used for large cystic defects of the cerebral hemispheres, resulting from destruction of both cortex and underlying white matter. The cause may be ischaemia or haemorrhage.

Injury in the early months of gestation is indicated by irregularity of gyral arrangement or microgyria around the edge of the lesion.

The clinical manifestations depend on the site of the lesion, but a high proportion occur in the lateral part of the hemisphere (Friede

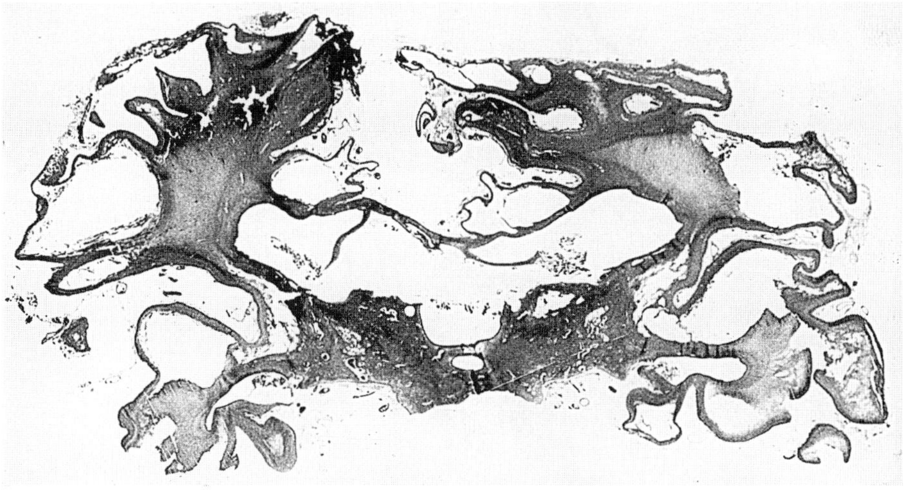

Fig. 24.18. Late effects of white matter ischaemia. Coronal section of brain shows multicystic encephalopathy. Large cysts are seen throughout both cerebral hemispheres, predominantly in the subcortical white matter; periventricular white matter is relatively intact. Smaller cysts are seen in deep grey matter. The corpus callosum is very thin. There is marked ventricular dilatation. Infant born at 34 weeks; survival 2 days. (LBCV)

1989) where motor cortex is likely to be damaged, causing hemiplegia. Occasionally, porencephalic cysts may enlarge progressively during life causing pressure symptoms and unilateral hydrocephalus (Tardieu et al. 1981).

Hydranencephaly

This term denotes bilateral destruction of the major part of both cerebral hemispheres which are each replaced by a thin-walled fluid-filled cyst. The membrane covering the cyst is made up of an outer layer derived from leptomeninges and an inner layer of glial tissue in which occasional neurons and clusters of macrophages, sometimes containing haemosiderin, are seen. The inferior aspects of the occipital lobes and temporal lobes, basal ganglia, brainstem and cerebellum are usually preserved, indicating that damage was due to failure of supply of the internal carotid arteries.

The history of the pregnancy usually reveals no clue as to an aetiology for such disastrous brain damage and many of these infants have normal deliveries with no evidence of neurological abnormality for weeks or even months after birth (Rorke 1982).

Although porencephaly and hydranencephaly are thought to result from vaso-occlusive conditions, examination of the cerebral arteries rarely reveals a specific lesion.

Subependymal Cysts

Small, rounded, well-demarcated cysts are not infrequently found close to the lateral walls of the lateral ventricles. Multiple bilateral cysts at the upper, outer angle of the ventricle are probably the result of previous white matter infarction (Friede 1989). Single, small, sometimes bilateral cysts may be found in the germinal eminence close to the ependyma. Histology shows gliotic walls which may contain clusters of germinal matrix cells but macrophages and blood pigment are not usually seen (Rorke 1982). The brain elsewhere is usually normal.

The origin of these cysts is uncertain but damage to the germinal matrix by haemorrhage or infection has been suggested (Larroche 1977; Rorke 1982; Friede 1989).

Vascular Malformations

Arteriovenous Malformations

These present rarely in neonates. Although correctly considered as malformations, they may damage the developing brain. The malformations may be small and suspected on clinical grounds of high-output cardiac failure and evidence of intracranial haemorrhage.

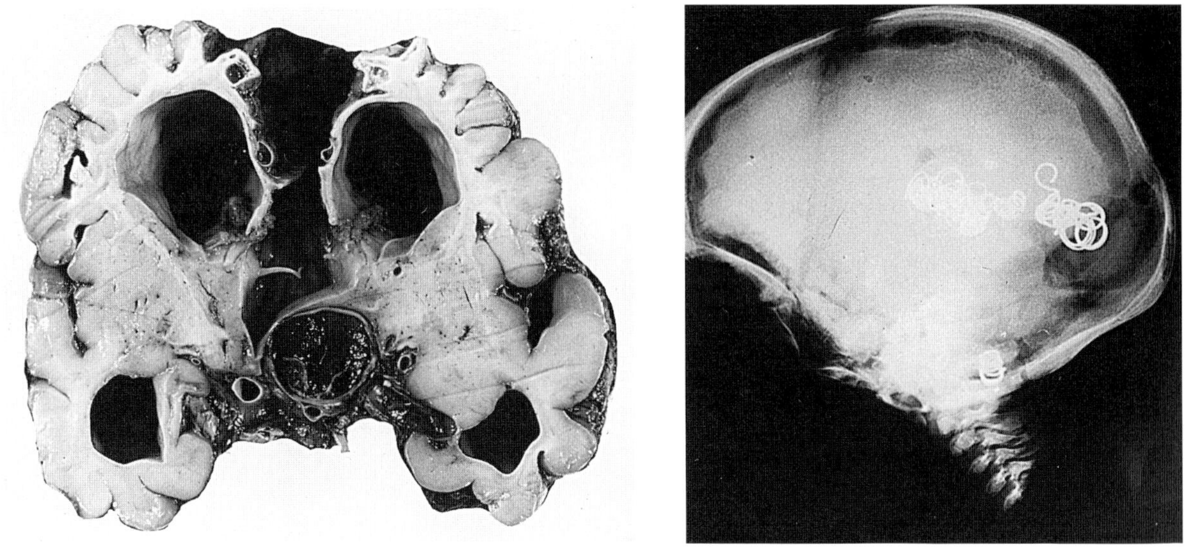

a b

Fig. 24.19. **a** Aneurysm of vein of Galen. Coronal slice of the fixed brain of an infant who died at 3 months. The dilated and thrombosed vein is distorting the third ventricle. There is dilatation of the ventricular system, atrophy of white matter and most marked on the medial surfaces of the cerebral hemispheres. There is dilatation of the ventricular system, atrophy of white matter and coflex, most marked on the medial surfaces of the cerebral hemispheres. **b** Lateral skull X-ray showing coils inserted into abnormal vessels to induce thrombosis. (Courtesy of Dr. Andrew Molyneux)

Examination of the brain shows massive dilatation of superficial vessels and wide draining and feeding vessels around the malformation.

The adjacent brain may be poorly grown and show areas of infarction due to diversion of its blood supply into the malformation.

Aneurysm of the Vein of Galen

This malformation results from direct shunting of blood from the main cerebral arteries into the vein of Galen which consequently dilates (Friede 1989). The dilated vein may compress the brainstem and produce hydrocephalus or cause venous infarction of the basal ganglia. Infarcts and poor growth of the cerebral hemispheres may result from vascular "steal".

The clinical manifestation is usually high-output cardiac failure which presents in the first weeks of life. Induced thrombosis of the malformation by insertion of coils may prolong life by some months (Fig. 24.19).

Metabolic Disorders

The neuropathology of metabolic disease is not strictly within the scope of this chapter, but a number of metabolic disorders, particularly those of amino acid metabolism, cause changes which enter the differential diagnosis of acquired disease, namely astrocytosis, spongy change of the white matter and reduction in amount of myelin (Martin and Schlote 1972). In others, malformation may be seen (Kolodny 1989).

Metabolic diseases may present at birth or in the neonatal period. In Leigh's disease (subacute necrotising encephalomyelopathy) the distinctive diagnostic features are of capillary proliferation and tissue rarefaction. However, there is diffuse but prominent astrocyte proliferation throughout the white matter. Englarged astrocytes with fibrillary processes are seen but none of the other features of white matter ischaemia (Fig. 24.20a–e).

Kernicterus. This is the selective pigmentation of basal ganglia and brainstem nuclei by bilirubin deposition causing subsequent degeneration. Due to improved control of rhesus incompatibility in pregnancy this condition is now seen very rarely. A detailed account is given by Friede (1989).

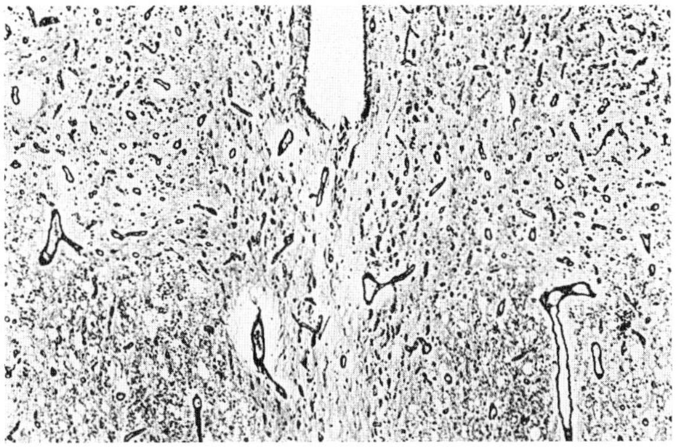
a

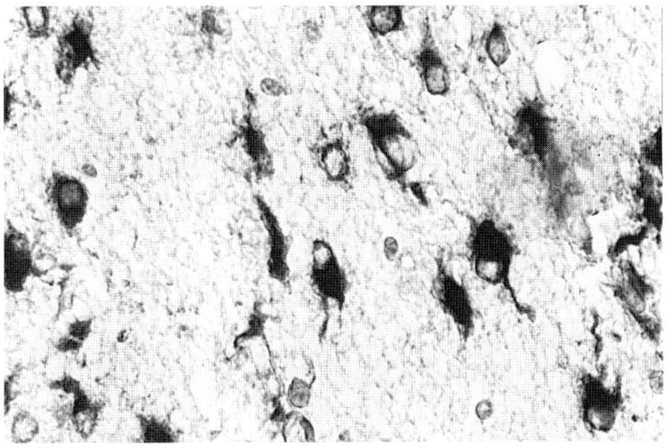
d

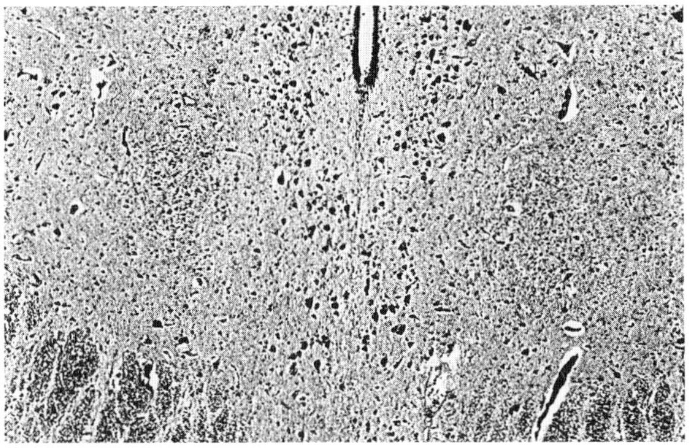
b

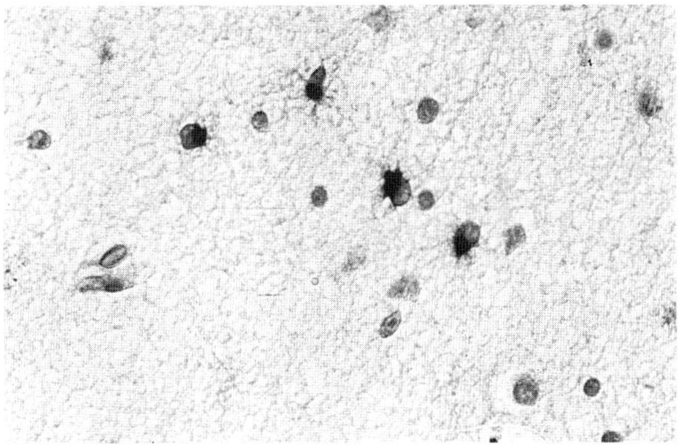
e

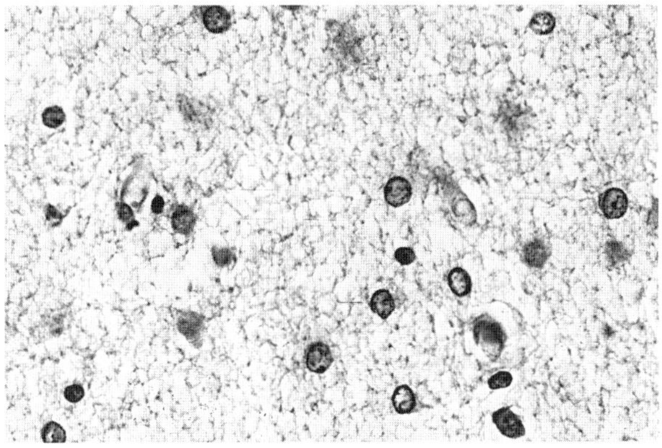
c

Fig. 24.20. a Leigh's disease. Section showing the periaqueductal grey matter of an infant of 6 weeks with Leigh's disease. There is marked capillary proliferation. (Reticulin ×28) **b** Control infant of similar age. (Reticulin ×26) **c** Sections of the cerebral white matter showing astrocytosis. (H&E ×290) **d** Antibodies to glial fibrillary acidic protein show the hypertrophic astrocytes with thick cytoplasmic processes. (GFAP ×290) **e** Control section from an infant of the same age. (GFAP ×410)

Viral Infections

Brain damage due to viral infections in the developmental period is well recognised. Some patterns of damage are characteristic of the infectious agent but most features are quite non-specific, for example microgyria, focal micronodular calcification and subependymal cysts. Demonstrating a viral aetiology may not be possible due to the immunological immaturity of the fetus at the time of infection. Routine serology is unhelpful before the humoral immune response develops in mid gestation, but cell-mediated responses develop earlier and may be abnormal in infants with malformations of the central nervous system (Thompson and Glasgow 1980).

Cytomegalovirus

This is the most common viral infection of the immature brain. The brain in the infected

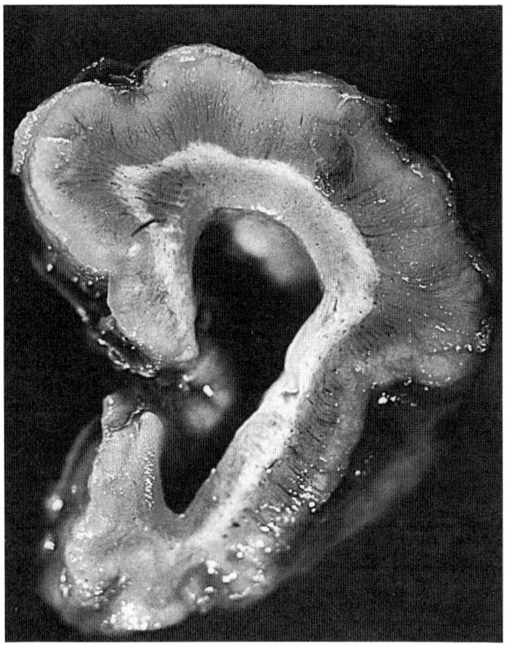
a

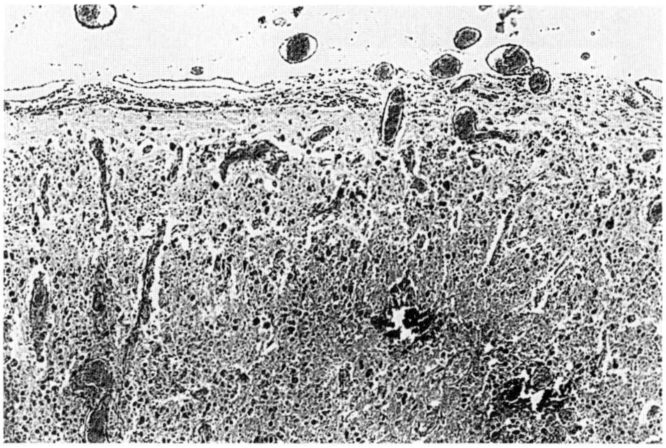
b

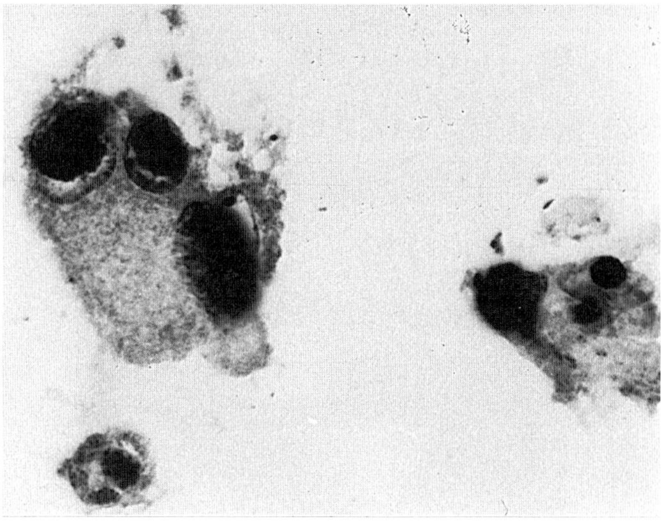
c

Fig. 24.21. **a** Cytomegalovirus. Coronal slice of the fixed brain of an infant of 39 weeks' gestation. There is a prominent band of calcification in the periventricular tissues. The brain is small with marked tissue destruction. Note the intense vascularity and congestion. **b** Section of the cerebral cortex. Loss of normal structure with infiltration by glial and inflammatory cells. Blood vessels are prominent. There is marked cellularity of the leptomeninges. Note calcification in the deep cortex. (H&E ×290) **c** Antibodies to cytomegalovirus demonstrate the typical intranuclear "owl's eye" inclusions in brain tissue. (Courtesy of Dr. Christine Morris.) (×750)

neonate is usually small with ventricular dilation due to tissue loss. It is deep brown in colour and periventricular calcification stands out as a prominent white band (Fig. 24.21a). Flecks of calcification also occur elsewhere throughout the cerebral tissue. About two-thirds of reported cases are microcephalic, some have polymicrogyria and a minority develop hydrocephalus (Marques Dias et al. 1984).

Histology shows predominant damage in the walls of the lateral ventricles. Cells containing inclusions occur singly or in small clusters with a variable glial response and associated calcification. Areas of tissue necrosis with calcification are most frequent in the subependymal region but also occur elsewhere (Fig. 24.21b).

The characteristic and diagnostic intranuclear inclusions are found in a variety of cell types including astrocytes, ependyma, microglia, leptomeningeal cells, vascular epithelium and occasionally neurons (Fig. 24.21c).

Acquired Immunodeficiency Syndrome

Transmission of human immunodeficiency virus (HIV) from seropositive mothers to their infants occurs transplacentally, at delivery and probably also via breast milk (European Collaborative Study 1992). By 18 months of age one-third of congenitally infected infants will be HIV positive or have AIDS and one-fifth of this group will have died (Blanche et al. 1989). Although the fetus may be infected in utero no cerebral manifestations of infection in the fetus have been described (Mulliez et al. 1989).

The incidence of encephalopathy in HIV-positive children is high. The pathological features are similar to those described in adults: generalised myelin pallor, microglial proliferation sometimes in focal collections (microglial nodules), multinucleate giant cells, calcification of basal ganglia and gliosis (Sharer 1986).

Rubella

Intrauterine rubella infection has a more dramatic effect on the eye and the ear than the central nervous system itself. Neuropathology in neonates shows focal tissue necrosis and discrete nodules of calcification close to vessel walls. Chronic inflammatory cells may be found in the leptomeninges and walls of the ventricular system. In older infants myelination is delayed. Malformations are described in congenital rubella syndrome including microcephaly, cerebellar hypoplasia and gyral abnormalities (Larroche 1977).

Herpes Simplex

Herpes simplex infection of the brain is rare. It is acquired at birth more commonly than by transplacental infection. Type II herpes is the virus usually involved (Friede 1989).

There is meningeal infiltration by lymphocytes, mononuclear cells and granulocytes with discrete proliferations of microglial cells and lymphocytes in the brain. Eosinophilic nuclear inclusions are seen in neurons and glial cells close to inflammatory foci. Definitive diagnosis is made by immunocytochemistry.

Protozoal Infections

Toxoplasmosis

Congenital toxoplasmosis usually causes hydrocephalus but this may not be present at the time of birth. It results from obstruction of CSF pathways due to ependymitis or from massive tissue destruction causing hydrocephalus *ex vacuo*. Less commonly, tissue destruction results in microcephaly.

The brain shows scattered soft yellow foci, sometimes cystic, and up to several centimetres in diameter. The ventricles are dilated and the walls irregular and necrotic. There may be obvious obstruction of the aqueduct by necrotic debris. Lesions involve cerebral hemispheres, brainstem and spinal cord but the cerebellum is relatively uninvolved.

Histology shows foci of necrosis containing macrophages and lymphocytes bordered by capillary and astrocytic proliferation. Calcification is obvious in the form of large granules or a fine basophilic dust. Inflammation and destruction of the ependyma is severe and may cause complete obstruction of the cerebral aqueduct either by plugging with necrotic debris or by intense reactive glial proliferation. The organisms may be encysted and cause little tissue reaction, or scattered individually when they induce granuloma formation. Microgyria and subependymal cysts may also be seen (Larroche 1977; Friede 1989).

Bacterial Infections

Bacterial infections of the brain cause meningitis and ventriculitis. Transplacental infection may occur but purulent leptomeningitis in utero is very rare.

The macroscopic features of purulent bacterial meningitis in the neonate are well known. In early cases the meninges may be infected but not purulent and the diagnosis may not be apparent. In the immature brain with shallow cerebral sulci the leptomeninges are readily torn off during removal and processing. A block for diagnosis should include the depths of a sulcus or the cerebellum, in which remnants of the meninges tucked deep into sulci survive processing (Fig. 24.22).

The brain is usually swollen and congested with narrowing of the ventricular system. In the first week polymorphs are prominent in the leptomeninges but later mononuclear cells predominate. Perivascular cuffs of inflammatory cells surround superficial vessels dipping into the cortex. Obstruction of superficial veins by thrombosis in the early stages of the disease causes haemorrhagic infarcts in 30% of cases (Friede 1989). Deep white matter infarcts due to thrombosis of subependymal veins are also seen. White matter necrosis may be particularly severe in Gram-negative bacterial infections (Larroche 1977). Meningeal inflammation may fill the sleeves surrounding cranial nerve roots causing compression and focal degeneration. In severe cases the infection spreads to involve

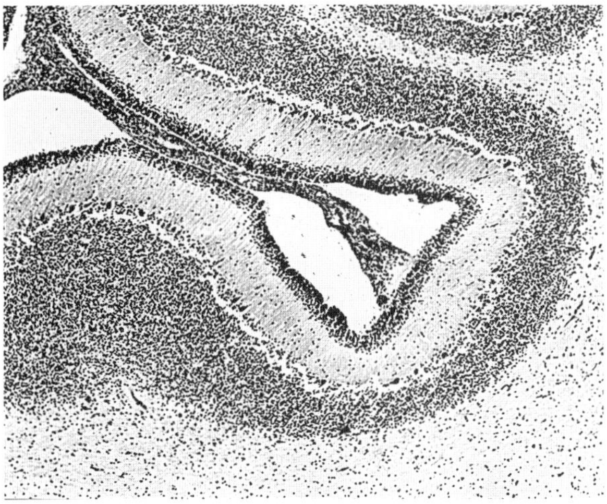

Fig. 24.22. Bacterial meningitis. Section of the cerebellum showing cellular infiltrate in the leptomeninges deep in a sulcus. In this site leptomeninges survive processing. (H&E ×36)

the lining of the ventricular system and choroid plexus.

The long-term complications of meningitis include hydrocephalus and multilocular cystic cavitation of the brain. Hydrocephalus follows fibrosis of the inflamed meninges which prevents drainage of CSF from the fourth ventricle and its resorption by arachnoid villi. Dilatation limited to the lateral and third ventricles results from obstruction of the cerebral aqueduct.

Listeria Meningitis

Listerial septicaemia acquired in utero usually involves the central nervous system causing meningoencephalitis. Granulomas form around blood vessels in the leptomeninges, in the ependyma and choroid plexus (Fig. 24.23a,b).

a

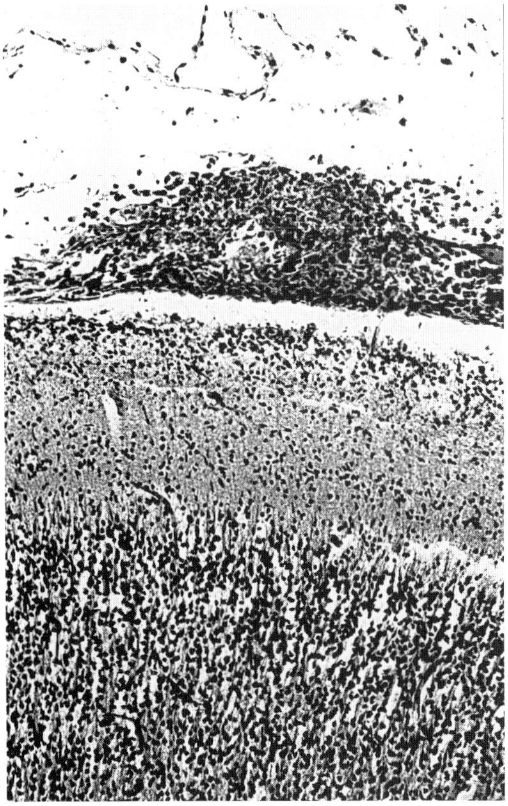

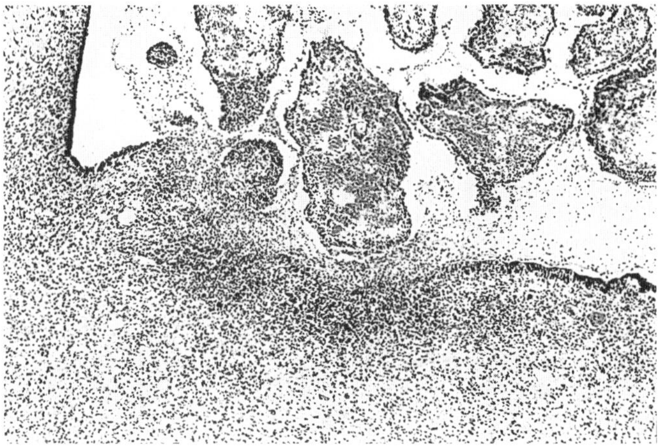

b

Fig. 24.23. **a** Listeriosis. Granulomatous reaction around a blood vessel in the leptomeninges of an infant of 24 weeks' gestation. (H&E ×104) **b** Granulomas and chronic inflammation in the ependyma and choroid plexus of the same case. (H&E ×33)

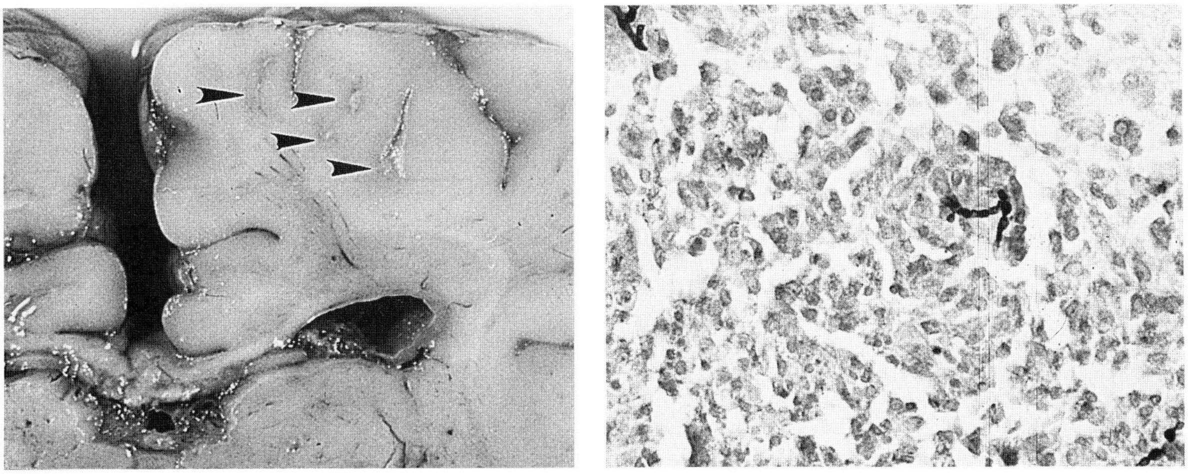

a b

Fig. 24.24. **a** Candidiasis. Coronal slice of fixed brain. Multiple lesions, some cavitated and slit-like, throughout the cerebral parenchyma of an infant of 38 weeks' gestation who survived for 22 days. **b** High-power micrograph of the same case shows the short budding hyphae of candida at the edge of a necrotic cerebral lesion. (PAS ×195)

The granulomas may be small and infrequent and examination of a large number of blocks is necessary to establish the diagnosis. In some cases small disseminated foci of necrosis are also found in the brain parenchyma.

Fungal Infections

Candidiasis

This is the most common bacterial infection of the brain in the neonatal period. There may be meningitis and ventriculitis or more widespread infection of the cerebral parenchyma. Multiple yellow lesions, sometimes cystic, are present throughout all areas of the cerebral parenchyma (Fig. 24.24a). Histology shows necrosis with a granulomatous response and reactive gliosis. Organisms are demonstrated in these lesions with PAS or Grocott stain and show small colonies of short budding hyphae (Fig. 24.24b).

References

Armstrong DL, Sauls CD, Goddard-Finegold J (1987) Neuropathologic findings in short-term survivors of intraventricular haemorrhage. Am J Dis Child 141: 617–621

Banker BQ, Larroche J-C (1962) Periventricular leucomalacia of infancy: a form of neonatal anoxic encephalopathy. Arch Neurol 7: 386–410

Bejar K, Wozniak P, Allard M et al. (1988) Antenatal origin of neurologic damage in newborn infants. Am J Obstet Gynecol 159: 357–63

Bignall S, Rivers RPA (1991) Pressure passivity of cerebral blood flow velocity in preterm infants in the first week of life. Early Hum Dev 25: 58

Blanche S, Rouzious C et al. (1989) A prospective study of infants born to women seropositive for human immunodeficiency virus type 1. N Engl J Med 320: 1643–1648

Clancy RR, Sladky JT, Rorke LB (1989) Hypoxic–ischemic spinal cord injury following perinatal asphyxia. Ann Neurol 25: 185–189

Cooke RWI (1991) Trends in preterm survival and incidence of cerebral haemorrhage 1980–89. Arch Dis Child 66: 403–407

Dambska M, Laure-Kamionowska M, Liebhart M (1987) Brainstem lesions in the course of chronic fetal asphyxia. Clin Neuropathol 6: 110–115

Dambska M, Laure-Kamionowska M, Schindt-Sidor B (1989) Early and late neuropathological changes in perinatal white matter damage. J Child Neurol 4: 291–298

Darrow VC, Alvord EC, Mack LA, Hodson WA (1988) Histologic evolution of the reactions to haemorrhage in the premature human infant's brain. Am J Pathol 130: 44–58

Deonna T, Payot M, Probst A, Prod'hom LS (1975) Neonatal intracranial hemorrhage in premature infants. Pediatrics 56: 1056–1064

De Reuck JL, Chatta AS, Richardson EP (1972) Pathogenesis and evolution of periventricular leukomalacia in infancy. Arch Neurol 27: 229–236

De Reuck JL (1984) Cerebral angioarchitecture and perinatal brain lesions in premature and full-term infants. Acta Neurol Scand 70: 391–395

de Vries LS, Dubowitz LMS, Dubowitz V et al. (1985) Predictive value of cranial ultrasound in the newborn baby. A reappraisal. Lancet 2: 137–140

de Vries LS, Dubowitz LMS, Pennock JM, Bydder GM

(1989) Extensive cystic leucomalacia: correlation of cranial ultrasound, magnetic resonance imaging and clinical findings in sequential studies. Clin Radiol 40: 158–166
de Vries LS, Connell JA, Dubowitz LMS, Oozeer RC, Dubowitz V, Pennock JM (1987) Neurological, electrophysiological and MRI abnormalities in infants with extensive cystic leukomalacia. Neuropediatrics 18: 61–66
Donat JF, Okazaki H, Kleinberg F, Reagan TJ (1978) Intraventricular hemorrhages in full-term and premature infants. Mayo Clin Proc 53: 437–441
Ellis WG, Goetzmann BW, Lindenberg JA (1988) Neuropathologic documentation of prenatal brain damage. Am J Dis Child 142: 858–866
European Collaborative Study (1992) Acquired immunodeficiency syndrome. Lancet 339: 1007–1012
Feess-Higgins A, Larroche J-C (1987) Development of the human foetal brain: an anatomical atlas. Masson, Paris
Freeman JM, Nelson KB (1988) Intrapartum asphyxia and cerebral palsy. Pediatrics 82: 240–249
Friede RL (1989) Developmental neuropathology, 2nd edn. Springer-Verlag, Berlin
Freud S (1897) Die infantile cerebrallahmung. In: Nothnagel J (ed) Spezialle pathologie und therapie. Vienna Band IX, ThIII, Holder, Vienna
Gilles, FH (1983a) Neurological damage: inconstancy during gestation. In: Gilles FH, Leviton A, Dooling EC (eds) The developing human brain, growth and epidemiologic neuropathology. Wright, Boston, pp 227–243
Gilles FH (1983b) Classification of the perinatal telencephalic leucoencephalopathies. In: Gilles FH, Leviton A, Dooling EC (eds) The developing human brain, growth and epidemiologic neuropathology. Wright, Boston, pp 244–250
Goddard-Finegold J (1984) Periventricular, intraventricular haemorrhages in the premature newborn. Arch Neurol 41: 766–771
Gould SJ, Howard S, Hope PL, Reynolds OR (1987) Periventricular intraparenchymal cerebral haemorrhage in preterm infants: the role of venous infarction. J Pathol 151: 197–202
Gudmundsson S, Lindblad A, Marsal K (1990) Cord blood gases and absence of end-diastolic blood velocities in the umbilical artery. Early Hum Dev 24: 231–237
Gunn TR, Mok PM, Becroft DMO (1985) Subdural haemorrhage in utero. Pediatrics 76: 605–610
Hambleton G, Wigglesworth JS (1976) Origin of intraventricular haemorrhage in the preterm infant. Arch Dis Child 51: 651–659
Horoupian DS, Yoon JJ (1988) Neuropathic arthrogryposis multiplex congenita and intrauterine ischaemia of anterior horn cells: a hypothesis. Clin Neuropathol 7: 285–293
Janzer RC, Friede RL (1980) Hypotensive brain stem necrosis or cardiac arrest encephalopathy. Acta Neuropathol (Berl) 50: 53–56
Johnson MA, Pennock JM, Bydder GM, Dubowitz LMS, Thomas DJ, Young IR (1987) Serial MR imaging in neonatal cerebral injury. Am J Neuroradiol 8: 83–92
Kolodny EH (1989) Agenesis of the corpus callosum: a marker for inherited metabolic disease? Neurology 39: 847–848
Larroche JC (1977) Lesions of ischaemic type, mainly arterial. In: Developmental pathology of the neonate. Excerpta Medica, Amsterdam, pp 399–445
Larroche JC (1986) Fetal encephalopathies of circulatory origin. Biol Neonate 50: 61–74
Leech RW, Alvord EC (1974) Morphologic variations in periventricular leucomalacia. Am J Pathol 74: 591–602
Leech RW, Alvord EC (1977) Anoxic–ischemic encephalopathy in the human neonatal period. The significance of brainstem involvement. Arch Neurol 34: 109–113
Leviton A, Gilles FH (1984) Acquired perinatal leukoencephalopathy. Ann Neurol 16: 1–8
Leviton A, Paneth N (1990) White matter damage in preterm newborns—an epidemiologic perspective. Early Hum Dev 24: 1–22
Little WJ (1861) On the influence of abnormal parturition, difficult labours, premature birth and asphyxia neonatorum on the mental and physical condition of the child, especially in relation to deformities. Transactions of the Obstetrical Society of London 3: 203–244
Lou HC (1989) Discussion. In: Evrard P, Minkowski A (eds) Developmental neurobiology. Nestlé Nutrition Workshop, Series 12. Raven Press, New York, p 239
Lou HC, Lassen NA, Friis-Hansen B (1979) Impaired autoregulation of cerebral blood flow in the distressed newborn infant. J Pediatr 94: 118–121
Martin JJ, Schlote W (1972) Central nervous system lesions in disorders of amino-acid metabolism. J Neurol Sci 15: 49–76
Marques Dias MJ, Harmant van Rijekevorsel G, Landrieu P, Lyon G (1984) Prenatal cytomegalovirus disease and cerebral microgyria: evidence for perfusion failure, not disturbance of histogenesis, the major cause of micropolygyria in CMV. Neuropediatrics 15: 18–24
Milligan DWA (1980) Failure of autoregulation and intraventricular haemorrhage in preterm infants. Lancet 1: 896–898
Mulliez N, Roume J et al. (1989) Etude de 62 foetus des mères HIV(+), aspects foetopathologiques. In: Azoulay M et al. (eds) SIDA: 1989; Transmission materno-foetale. Les editions INSERM 200: 105–114
Nelson KB, Ellenberg JH (1986) Antecedents of cerebral palsy. Multivariate analysis of risk. N Engl J Med 315: 81–86
Norman MG (1978) Perinatal brain damage. Perspect Paediatr Pathol 4: 41–92
Oldendorf WH, Cornford ME, Brown WJ (1977) The large apparent work capability of the blood–brain barrier: a study of the mitochondrial content of capillary endothelial cells in brain and other tissues of the rat. Ann Neurol 1: 409–417
Paneth N, Rudelli R, Monte W et al. (1990) White matter necrosis in very low birthweight infants: neuropathologic and ultrasonographic findings in infants surviving six days or longer. J Pediatr 116: 975–84
Perlman JM (1989) Intraventricular haemorrhage. Pediatrics 84: 913–915
Ramaekers V Th, Casaer P, Daniels H, Marchal G (1990) Upper limits of brain blood flow autoregulation in stable infants of various conceptional ages. Early Hum Dev 24: 249–258
Rodriguez J, Claus D, Verellan G, Lyon G (1990) Periventricular leucomalacia: ultrasonic and neuropathological correlations. Dev Med Child Neurol 32: 347–355
Roessmann U, Gambetti P (1986) Pathological reaction of astrocytes in perinatal brain injury. Acta Neuropathol (Berl) 70: 302–307
Roland EH, Norman MG, Hill A (1987) Antenatal periventricular white matter infarction. Ann Neurol 22: 423
Rorke LB (1982) Pathology of perinatal brain injury. Raven Press, New York Sharer LR, Epstein LG, Cho ES et al. (1986) Pathologic features of AIDS encephalopathy in children: evidence for LAV/HTLVIII infection of brain. Human Pathol 17: 271–284
Sherwood A, Hopp A, Smith JF (1978) Cellular reactions

to subependymal plate haemorrhage in the human neonate. Neuropath Appl Neurobiol 4: 245–261

Shuman RM, Selednik LJ (1980) Periventricular leucomalacia–a one-year autopsy study. Arch Neurol 37: 231–235

Sims ME, Turkel SB, Hatterman G, Paul RH (1985) Brain injury and intrauterine death. Am J Obstet 151: 721–723

Sinha SK, D'Souza SW, Rivlin E, Chiswick ML (1990) Ischaemic brain lesions diagnosed at birth in preterm infants: clinical events and developmental outcome. Arch Dis Child 65: 1017–1020

Skullerud K, Westre B (1986) Frequency and prognostic significance of germinal matrix haemorrhage, periventricular leucomalacia and pontosubicular necrosis in preterm neonates. Acta Neuropath (Berl) 70: 257–261

Soothill PW, Nicolaides KH, Campbell S (1987) Prenatal asphyxia, hyperlacticaemia, hypoglycaemia, and erythroblastosis in growth retarded fetuses. Br Med J 294: 1051–1053

Stoddard RA, Clark SL, Minton SD (1988) In utero ischemic injury: sonographic diagnosis and medicolegal implications. Am J Obstet Gynecol 159: 23–25

Squier MV, Keeling JW (1991) The incidence of prenatal brain injury. Neuropathol Appl Neurobiol 17: 29–38

Takashima S, Tanaka K (1978) Development of cerebrovascular architecture and its relationship to periventricular leukomalacia. Arch Neurol 35: 11–16

Tardieu M, Evrard P, Lyon G (1981) Progressive expanding congenital porencephalies: a treatable cause of progressive encephalopathy. Pediatrics 68: 198–202

Tenorio GM, Nazui M, Bickers GH, Hubbird RH (1988) Intrauterine stroke and maternal polydrug abuse. Clin Pediatr (Phila) 27: 565–567

Thompson JA, Glasgow LA (1980) Intrauterine viral infection and the cell-mediated immune response. Neurology 30: 212–215

Van Bel F, Van de Bor M, Stijnen T, Baan J, Ruys JH (1987) Aetiological role of cerebral blood flow alterations in development and extension of peri-intraventricular haemorrhage. Dev Med Child Neurol 29: 601–614

Van de Bor M, Guit GL, Schreuder AM, Wondergem J, Vielvoye GJ (1989) Early detection of delayed myelination in preterm infants. Pediatrics 84: 407–411

Van de Bor M, Ma EJ, Walther FJ (1991) Cerebral blood flow velocity after surfactant instillation in preterm infants. J Pediatr 118: 285–287

Virchow R (1868) Ueber interstitielle encephalitis. Archiv fur Pathol Anat 44: 472–476

Volpe JJ (1987) Neurology of the newborn. Major problems in clinical pediatrics, vol 22. Saunders, Philadelphia

Volpe JJ (1989) Intraventricular haemorrhage in the premature infant–current concepts part 1. Ann Neurol 25: 3–11

Weindling AM, Rochefort MJ, Calvert SA, Fok TF, Wilkinson A (1985) Development of cerebral palsy after ultrasonographic detection of periventricular cysts in the newborn. Dev Med Child Neurol 27: 800–806

Wigglesworth JS (1989) Current problems in brain pathology in the perinatal period. In: Pape KG, Wigglesworth JS (eds) Perinatal brain lesions. Contemporary issues in fetal and neonatal medicine, vol 5. Blackwell, Boston pp 1–23

Chapter 25

Skeletal Muscle and Peripheral Nerves

J. Patrick Barbet

Development of Skeletal Muscle

Skeletal muscle is a very specialised tissue made up of several different types of muscle fibres. These fibres differ both in their physical properties (speed of contraction, resistance to fatigue) and in the composition of their contractile proteins. Enzyme histochemical studies of oxidative enzymes and of myofibrillar ATPase and immunocytochemical studies using antibodies specific for different myosin isoforms have made it possible to characterise the slow (type I) and fast (type II- with two sub groups IIA and -IIB) contracting muscle fibres at light microscopic level.

The skeletal muscles originate from mesenchyme. The trunk musculature mainly derives from the paraxial mesoderm by way of the segmentally arranged somites, whereas the muscles of the head and neck arise from the presomitic mass or branchial arches (Hamilton and Mossman 1972). The limb muscles are formed from mesenchymal condensations near the base of each limb bud round the terminal ends of the spinal nerves: the question as to whether the muscle fibres differentiate in situ from the limb bud mesenchyme or whether there is a migration of myoblastic precursor cells from the somite into the limb bud has still not been resolved. However that may be, the formation of a skeletal muscle from undifferentiated cells occurs in three intricated phases: hyperplasia, metabolic differentiation and volumetric growth of the muscle fibres.

The initial phase of hyperplasia is characterised by the determination of undifferentiated muscle precursors into myoblasts, followed after several cycles of cell division by the fusion of the myoblasts into myotubes: elongated structures containing several centrally located nuclei and peripheral myofibrils, separated from the nuclei by an apparently empty halo (Fig. 25.1a). The myotubes are subsequently replaced by myofibres: elongated structures containing several peripheral nuclei and a homogeneous sarcoplasm filled with evenly dispersed myofibrils in the central portion (Fig. 25.1b). This replacement is completed between 18 and 20 weeks of gestation depending upon the muscle: in the quadriceps, myotubes can no longer be identified after 18 weeks. At this time the fibres have very irregular diameters and their subsequent development is accompanied by an increase in size which continues after birth until puberty. As early as 1937, Wohlfart demonstrated the existence of small and large diameter fibres in fetal muscle which he called respectively "a" and "b". At birth, all fibres have equivalent diameters and the Wohlfart "a" and "b" fibres can no longer be distinguished.

Enzyme histochemical studies have shown that during early fetal development all fibres

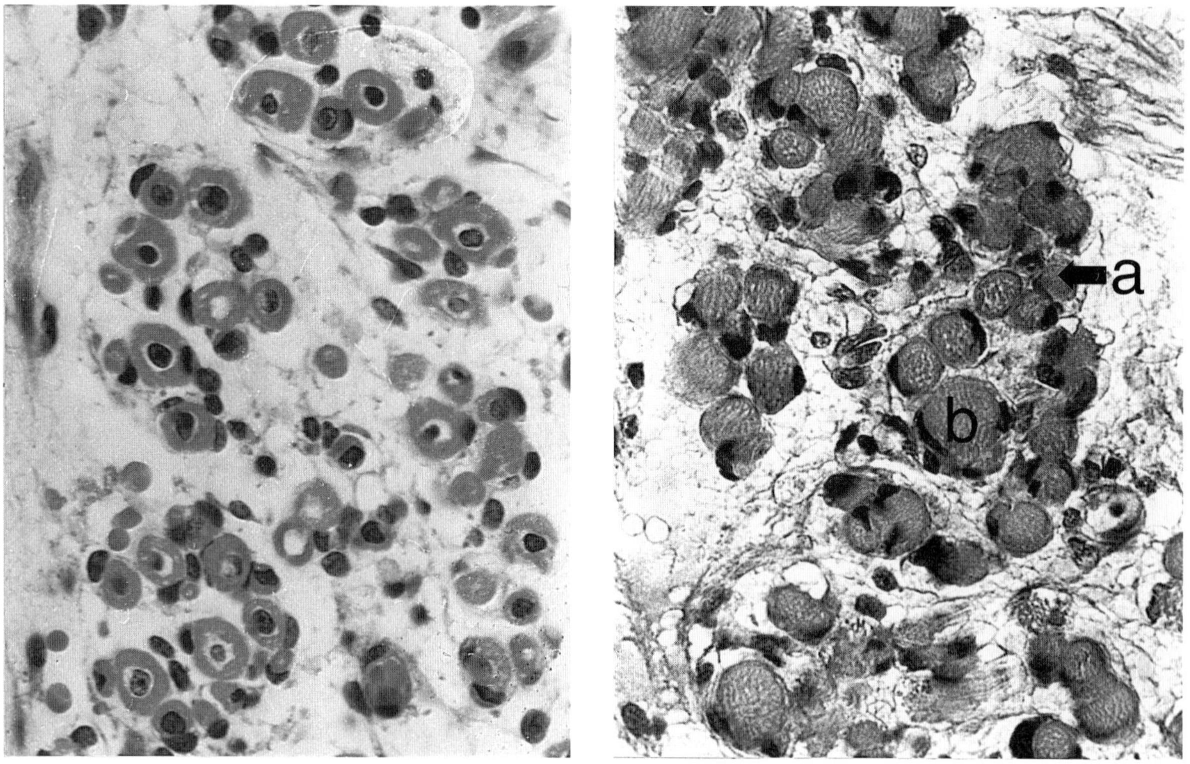

a b

Fig. 25.1. Normal fetal quadriceps. **a** At 12 weeks the muscle is composed only of myoblasts and of myotubes with central nuclei. **b** At 17 weeks myofibres of small and large diameter correspond respectively to Wohlfart type a and b fibres. (H&E, ×450)

are undifferentiated—type IIC, fetal fibres—and that these fibres are progressively replaced by mature type I and II fibres during pregnancy (Dubowitz 1965; Fenichel 1966; Farkas-Bargeton et al. 1977; Ringqvist et al. 1977; Colling-Saltin 1978; Kumagai et al. 1984). The histochemical differentiation begins with the appearance of the first type I fibres between 16 and 20 weeks depending upon the muscle and ends when the last type IIC fibres disappear soon after birth. In the quadriceps (Figs. 25.2 and 25.3), type I fibres become evident at 18 weeks and their number increases considerably after 30 weeks; type IIB fibres appear after 25 weeks and type IIA fibres after 35 weeks of gestation. The mature fibres increase in number during the last weeks of pregnancy and replace the type IIC fibres, so that at birth there are 40% type I and 60% type II fibres (and less than 10% type IIC). The largest diameter Wohlfart type "b" fibres always correspond to type I fibres whereas the smaller type "a" fibres correspond either to type II or to type I fibres. The evolution in the diameter of these type I and type II fibres during the development of the quadriceps muscle is shown in Fig. 25.4

The reactivities of the oxidative enzymes (NADH) also evolve during fetal development, due to the progressive organisation of the myofibrils and mitochondria. A particular feature of fetal fibres is the central reactivity associated with a peripheral halo devoid of reactivity (Fig. 25.5.). This aspect, corresponding upon ultrastructural analysis to a zone rich in glycogen and lacking myofibrils and mitochondria (Fig. 25.6), normally disappears before birth (Farkas-Bargeton et al. 1977).

The fibre types which differentiate during development are functionally specialised by virtue of the expression of genes coding for myosin and other muscle proteins. Several studies have recently been carried out on developing human muscle, mainly concentrating on the analysis of the myosin heavy chains (MHCs). Different adult isoforms of MHCs (slow and fast) have been identified (Billeter et al. 1981) and developing muscle

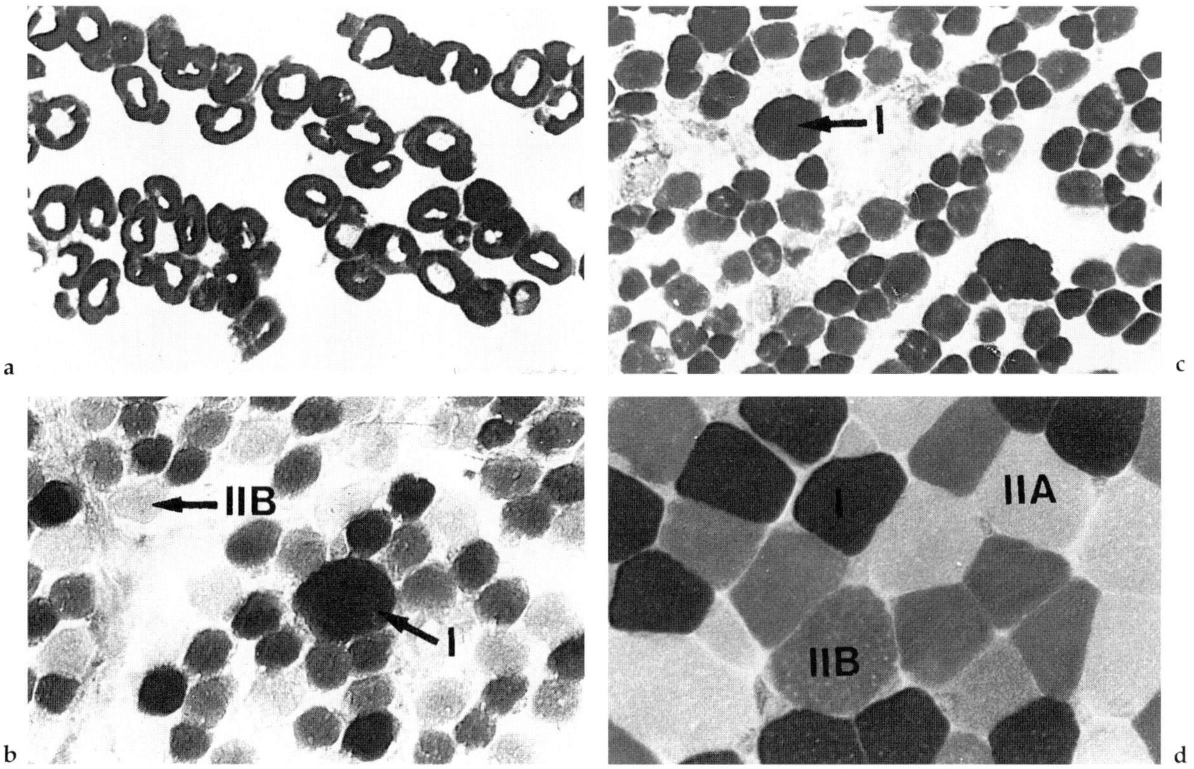

Fig. 25.2. Differentiation of fibre types in normal quadriceps at **a** 12, **b** 20, **c** 33 weeks of gestation and **d** in a 6-month-old child. **a** All fibres are of type IIC **b** Appearance of type I fibres **c** Appearance of type IIB fibres **d** mature pattern. ATPase following acid preincubations at pH 4.35 (**a**, **b**, **c**) and at pH 4.63 (**d**) ×350

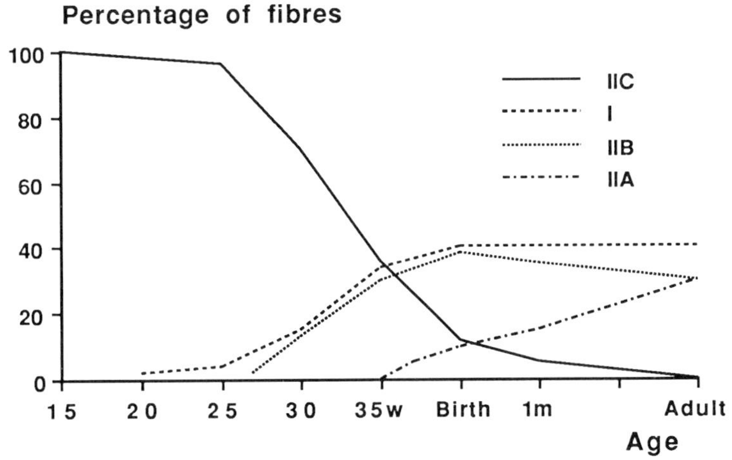

Fig. 25.3. Graphical representation of the evolution of fibre types during the development of the quadriceps.

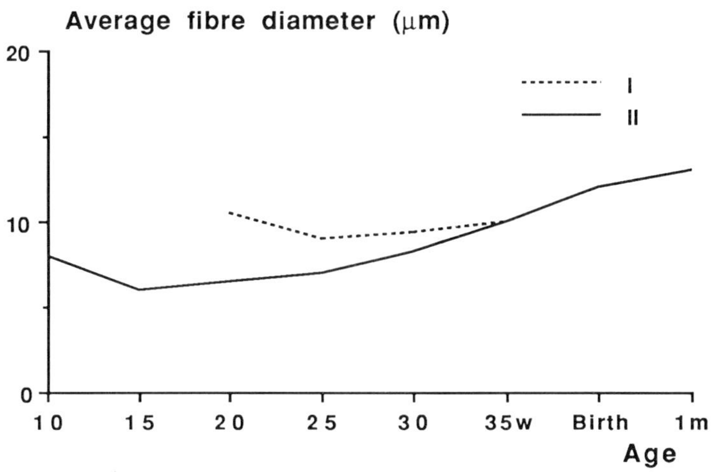

Fig. 25.4. Graphical representation of the average diameter of type I and type II fibres during the development of the quadriceps.

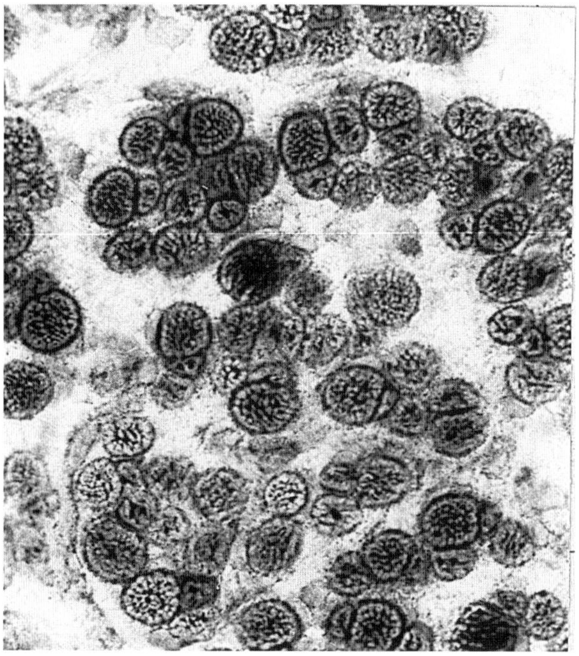

Fig. 25.5. Normal fetal quadriceps at 22 weeks. The strong central reactivity contrasts with the peripheral halo devoid of any reactivity present in all fibres. (NADH, ×342)

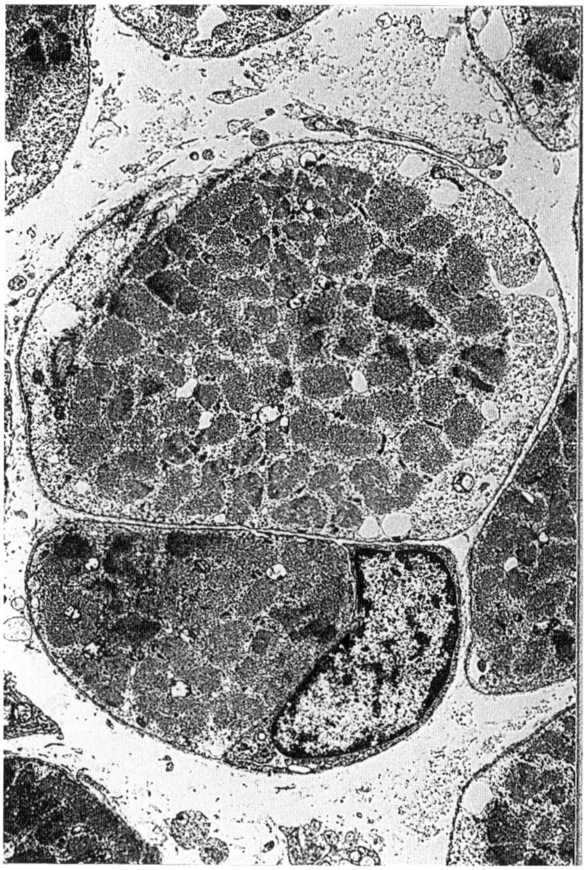

Fig. 25.6. Normal fetal quadriceps at 27 weeks. A peripheral halo lacking myofibrils and mitochondria is observed in the largest fibre (Electron microscopy ×4940)

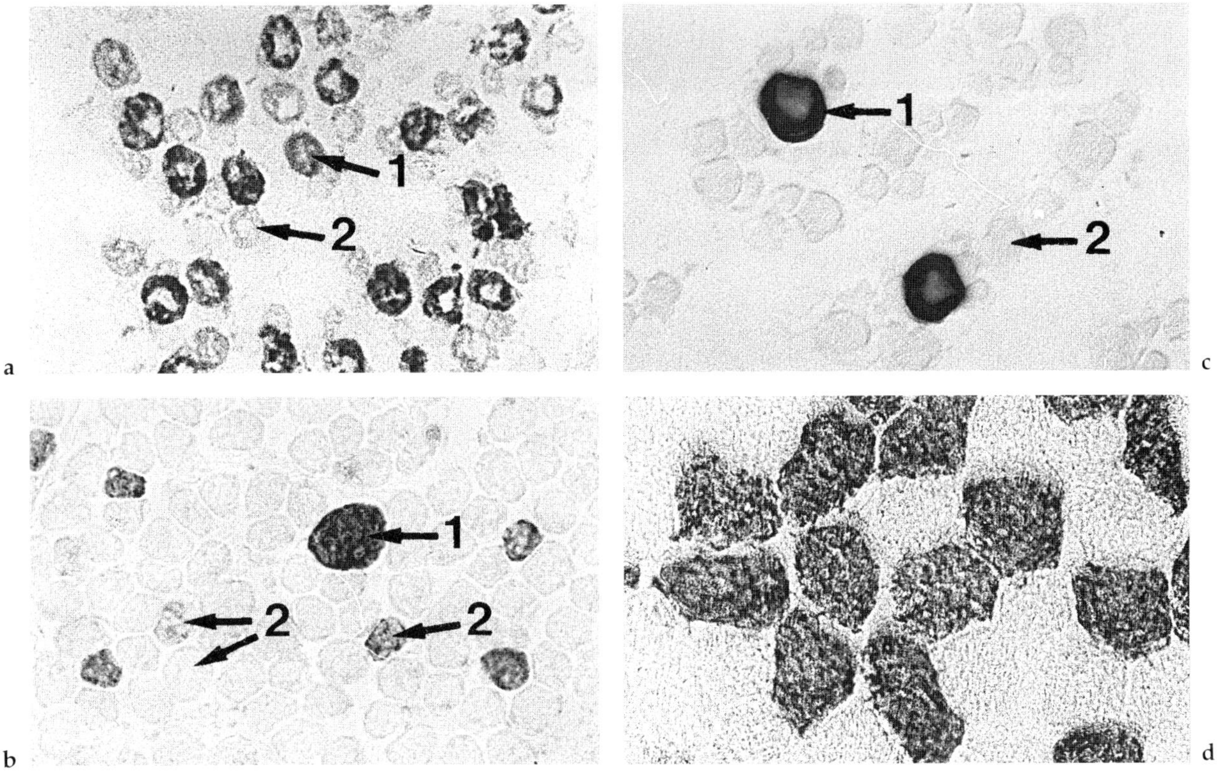

Fig. 25.7. Differentiation of slow fibres in the normal quadriceps at **a** 12, **b** 20, **c** 33 weeks of gestation and **d** in a 6-month-old child. All primary generation fibres (1) are slow whereas the secondary generation fibres (2) differentiate into slow (reactive) and fast (unreactive) fibres. Immunocytochemistry with an antibody specific for the slow myosin heavy chain, ×350.

expresses two additional embryonic and fetal isoforms (Whalen et al. 1981; Fitzsimons and Hoh 1981). All these isoforms are encoded by distinct MHC genes (Periasamy et al. 1985) and are developmentally regulated (Whalen et al. 1981; Lyons et al. 1983; Butler-Browne and Whalen 1984). Using immunocytochemical techniques with antibodies specific for the different MHCs, it has been possible to detect a heterogeneity in the reactivities of the muscle fibres as early as 14 weeks (Moore et al. 1984) and to demonstrate that at 15 weeks the larger diameter "b" fibres express the slow MHC whereas the smaller diameter "a" fibres do not (Thornell et al. 1984). It was also possible to demonstrate the replacement of fetal MHC by adult MHCs at the end of pregnancy (Pons et al. 1986). Subsequently Draeger et al. (1987) studied a series of 28 fetuses and suggested that human skeletal muscle is formed as three successive generations of muscle fibres: a first generation of fibres expressing the slow MHC from the beginning, a second and a third generation of fibres reacting differently with two antibodies directed against fast MHC. This finding was confirmed by Ecob-Price et al. (1989) on a series of six fetuses.

Similar studies carried out on the quadriceps muscle using biochemical and immunocytochemical techniques (Butler-Browne et al. 1990; Barbet et al. 1991) do not, however, confirm the existence of three generations of fibres. As in other animal species, the results clearly suggest the existence in man of two distinct generations of muscle fibres, each of which possesses a distinct pattern of expression of muscle specific proteins—especially of the slow MHC (Figs. 25.7 and 25.8).

First-generation fibres express the slow MHC almost as soon as they form (between 8 and 10 weeks), which is prior to any motor innervation, suggesting that in these first generation fibres the expression of slow MHC is independent of the effect of innervation.

Second-generation fibres form progressively and asynchronously around the primary fibres,

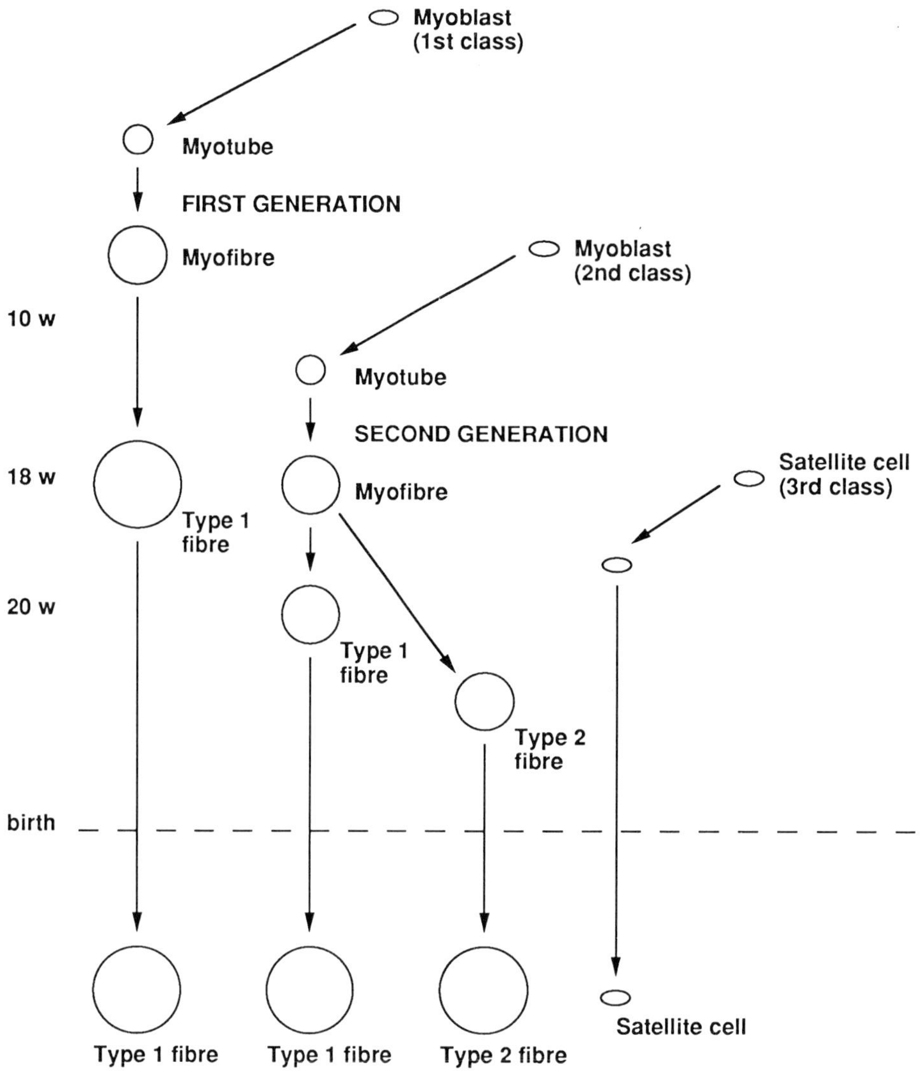

Fig. 25.8. Schematic representation of fibre formation in the quadriceps muscle.

do not initially express the slow MHC and give the muscle a very heterogeneous aspect between 10 and 18 weeks. By 20 weeks, the second-generation fibres become homogeneous, both in diameter and immunoreactivity and thereafter undergo a process of maturation when they eliminate the developmental MHCs to express either slow or fast MHC. Thus, second-generation fibres do not initially express the slow MHC but may express it secondarily (after 20 weeks and following motor innervation).

Apart from the expression of a predominant MHC isoform (slow or fast) in adult fibres, evolution of the profile of expression of other proteins probably corresponds to a process of maturation. The strong reactivity for embryonic and fetal MHCs, vimentin, desmin and sometimes fast MHC in recently formed myotubes/fibres, is probably due to the accumulation and disorganisation of these proteins. As the fibres increase in size, the proteins attain their ultimate organisation and their expression gradually decreases.

This maturation is terminated by about 18 weeks of gestation in the first-generation fibres, whereas the second-generation fibres mature later. When all second-generation fibres have attained the same diameter, the levels of immunoreactivity are homogeneous and only two different types of fibres can be distinguished in fetal quadriceps muscle:

Table 25.1. Correspondence between the enzyme histochemical and immunocytochemical reactivities of the primary and secondary generation fibres during development

Fibre	Type	ATPase reactivity			NADH reactivity	Slow MHC	Fast MHC	Vimentin	Desmin
		9.4	4.63	4.35					
1st generation									
immature	IIC	++	++	++	+	+	0	++	++
mature	I	+	++	++	++	+	0	0	+
2nd generation									
immature	IIC	++	++	++	+	0	+	++	++
mature slow	I	+	++	++	++	+	0	0	+
mature fast	IIA	+	0	0	+	0	+	0	+
	IIB	+	+	0	+	0	+	0	+

0 = unreactive, + = reactive, ++ = strongly reactive.

Table 25.2. Percentage and average diameter of the different fibre types in adult limb muscles

	Deltoid	Biceps	Quadriceps (vastus lateralis)	Tibialis anterior
Percentage (%)				
Type I fibres	55	45	40	70
Type II fibres	45	55	60	30
Diameter (μm)				
Type I fibres	50	52	48	55
Type II fibres	55	60	50	65

primary generation fibres have a larger diameter than secondary generation fibres and the fibres of these two generations correspond respectively to the fetal type "b" and type "a" fibres previously described by Wohlfart (1937). The first generation gives slow fibres in the adult muscle, whereas the second generation gives slow or fast fibres in the adult human muscle (Barbet et al. 1991). The reactivities of these different types of muscle fibres during development are summarised in Table 25.1.

At birth the majority of the muscles have attained their mature histochemical and immunocytochemical phenotype. The quadriceps, used as a reference muscle in pathology, is made up of fibres with a regular diameter of 12–15 μm. Enzyme histochemistry reveals that there are less than 10% type IIC fibres, that the Wohlfart "b" fibres can no longer be distinguished and that the halos lacking oxidative enzyme activity have disappeared. Immunocytochemistry reveals that the muscle fibres no longer express vimentin or embryonic MHC but do express either adult fast or slow MHC; only the few remaining type IIC fibres still express small amounts of fetal MHC.

The enzyme-histochemical and immunocytochemical maturation of the fibres is completed in the first few months after birth, resulting in a characteristic chequerboard pattern of the fibres of different types. The percentage of fibre types varies between the different muscles (Table 25.2).

Regulation of Muscle Development

In mammals and birds, each skeletal muscle has a distinct pattern of fibre types which has evolved to meet the functional requirements of that muscle in the locomotive or support system of the body. The development of this pattern is complex, usually involving distinct fibre fates within each generation (Condon et al. 1990a). Condon et al. (1990b) have shown in rats that primary and secondary generation myotubes will mature to become either fast or slow fibres in the adult, depending upon their location in the muscle. Many theories have been put forward to try to explain this diversity. The nerve is not required for the initial formation of slow and fast fibres (Miller 1991) and probably only serves in the final modulation of the fibre type pattern.

In man, the differentiation and maturation of the muscle phenotype probably also depend upon the motor innervation which develops in limb muscles after 10 weeks and becomes well established by 20 weeks when the active movements of the limbs develop (Butler-Browne et al. 1990). The innervation of these muscles is initially polyneuronal but subsequently becomes mononeuronal once the correct contacts have been established. Innervation is determining in the development of the slow phenotype in the second-generation fibres (Whalen et al. 1985; Barbet et al. 1991). Thyroid hormone regulates the accumulation of slow MHC and the transition of fetal to adult fast MHC in developing skeletal muscle, probably combining a direct effect on the accumulation of the fast MHC and an indirect effect on the maturation of fibre types due to a precocious neural maturation (Butler-Browne et al. 1990).

In man, as in animals, recent experiments support the idea that myoblasts can become determined before they fuse into myotubes (Hauschka 1974; Stockdale and Miller 1987; Vivarelli et al. 1988; Mouly et al. 1990) and that muscles can be formed from different classes of myoblasts with different intrinsic programmes. In addition to the two classes of myoblasts proposed to form the two generations of muscle fibres, a third type has been described as giving rise to the satellite cells appearing in the limbs after 16–18 weeks of gestation. These satellite cells normally remain quiescent but confer a regenerative capacity to skeletal muscle in case of damage. The formation of new muscle fibres by regeneration follows a pathway of differentiation and maturation very similar to that of the secondary fibres during normal myogenesis.

Investigation of Neuromuscular Disease

In the newborn infant suspected to be suffering from a neuromuscular disorder, examination of clinical (genetic survey), biological (serum creatine kinase) and electrophysiological data is essential and should avoid unnecessary biopsies. Whenever a muscle biopsy is indicated, it should be carried out on a muscle for which the normal histological pattern is readily available (quadriceps, tibialis anterior, deltoid, biceps brachialis). The choice of a muscle which is too severely affected (where end-stage lesions introduce difficulties in interpretation) or of a muscle which is only mildly affected (which may be histologically normal) should be avoided. Peripheral nerve biopsies should be considered exclusively in the investigation of confirmed peripheral neuropathies (Gherardi 1989).

If one considers the muscle biopsy itself, the classic histological technique following paraffin embedding often gives sufficient information for diagnostic purposes. However, it does not allow one to specify the morphology and exact physiological characteristics of the muscle fibres, which must be studied using enzyme histochemical or immunohistochemical techniques on frozen sections and occasionally by electron microscopy. Routine examination in cases of neuromuscular disorder should include techniques for the myofibrillar ATPase (at pH 9.4 and following acid preincubation), the mitochondrial enzymes (NADH, SDH) as well as the modified Gomori trichrome technique, the PAS and lipid stains (Esiri 1987). Immunocytochemical analysis of the expression of dystrophin is recommended to distinguish between Duchenne and other types of muscular dystrophy. These techniques have been described in detail elsewhere (Dubowitz 1985, Poirier et al. 1989; Johnson 1990).

Nerve biopsies must be fixed in glutaraldehyde prior to teasing and ultrastructural analysis (for details, see Schochet 1986).

The same techniques can be applied to necropsy material obtained from fetuses or newborn infants. It is useful to sample several muscles from different topographical sites (proximal or distal territory, face) or because of their clinical significance (diaphragm, intercostal muscles). Samples from the central nervous system (brain and spinal cord) complement those taken from the skeletal muscles and peripheral nerves.

The development of modern techniques of biological investigation means that it is often useful nowadays to sample for tissue culture (fibroblasts, myoblasts) or to freeze samples for biochemistry and molecular biology. If it is impossible to carry out or to store such biopsies, tissue which has been fixed in formalin or in paraformaldehyde and embedded in paraffin allows a certain number of molecular biological analyses (in situ hybridisation and polymerase chain reaction).

Generalised Abnormalities

Most of the true myopathies that present during fetal life or at birth are genetically determined and it is very important to determine exactly the type of disease in order to evaluate its evolution and/or to give accurate genetic counselling. Different general disorders (intrauterine growth retardation, etc.) can be accompanied by muscle weakness of varying severity, but usually of no diagnostic significance. Conversely, specific neuromuscular diseases may present different clinical pictures where hypotonia and muscle weakness are usually prominent (Dubowitz 1980).

Arthrogryposis is characterised by congenital fixation of joints, often mutiple (arthrogryposis multiplex congenita). This symptom can result from any affection immobilising portions of the developing fetus (Banker 1986). The main aetiologies include neurogenic disorders (central nervous system dysgeneses), usually as part of polymalformation syndromes, and primary muscular disorders (congenital muscular dystrophy, congenital myotonic dystrophy). External factors which produce an intrauterine constraint, such as oligohydramnios or uterine malformations, can also lead to arthrogryposis.

The term myotonia congenita (Oppenheim disease) has been applied to a syndrome of generalised muscular hypotonia and weakness with absent tendon reflexes, which is present at birth or manifest shortly after birth. Careful follow-up studies (Walton 1956) have shown that this syndrome occurs in diverse conditions, varying from Werdnig–Hoffmann disease to congenital myopathies and occasionally even to Duchenne muscular dystrophy. Conversely, no cause is found in many cases, which have been referred to as "benign congenital hypotonia" since they resolve completely in childhood (Dubowitz 1978).

Severe neuromuscular disorders presenting during intrauterine life often result in oligohydramnios and a decrease of fetal movements. At birth, severe hypotonia and muscle weakness are accompanied by respiratory distress and swallowing difficulties. Four main aetiologies should always be considered, which can usually be diagnosed clinically: congenital muscular dystrophy, Werdnig–Hoffmann disease, congenital myotonic dystrophy and the X-linked form of myotubular myopathy.

Muscular Dystrophies

Congenital muscular dystrophies (with or without involvement of the central nervous system) and, exceptionally, Duchenne muscular dystrophy can occur during fetal and neonatal life. The other forms of muscular dystrophy (Becker, limb-girdle, facioscapulohumeral, etc.) are not symptomatic in this age group.

Congenital Muscular Dystrophies

These are a heterogeneous group of affections which can occur in early life and result in variable dystrophic changes in the muscle. They have mostly an autosomal-recessive mode of transmission but the responsible gene or genes have not as yet been identified. In a few cases an intrauterine infection may have contributed to the disease.

The severe congenital forms of muscular dystrophy, present at birth, are characterised by generalised hypotonia and weakness of the face, trunk and limb muscles associated with variable difficulties in sucking, swallowing and breathing. Orthopaedic deformities and muscle retraction occur early in their evolution (Donner et al. 1975) and can lead to arthrogryposis in the newborn infant. Serum creatine kinase levels vary from being normal to moderately elevated; the electromyogram is myogenic.

Congenital muscular dystrophies without any involvement of the central nervous system have very variable patterns of evolution: the most severe forms begin in utero (polyhydramnios, poor fetal movements, arthrogryposis) and may eventually lead to fetal death or to neonatal death due to severe respiratory distress or to superimposed infection. Histological examination of the muscle shows typical dystrophic changes (Fig. 25.9) with an important proliferation of the endomysial connective tissue and a large decrease in both the number and diameter of the fibres (Zellweger et al. 1967). Necrosis and signs of regeneration are rare; round cell infiltration may be present. Enzyme-histochemical analysis often reveals a predominance of type I fibres. Immunohistochemical studies are important since they demonstrate a normal distribution of dystrophin (Fig. 25.10) whereas this protein is totally lacking in Duchenne muscular dystrophy (Patel et al. 1988). There does not seem to be any correlation between the evolution of congenital muscular dystrophy and the severity of the histological changes.

In some very severe forms of congenital muscular dystrophy, histological examination may be difficult because of the severity of

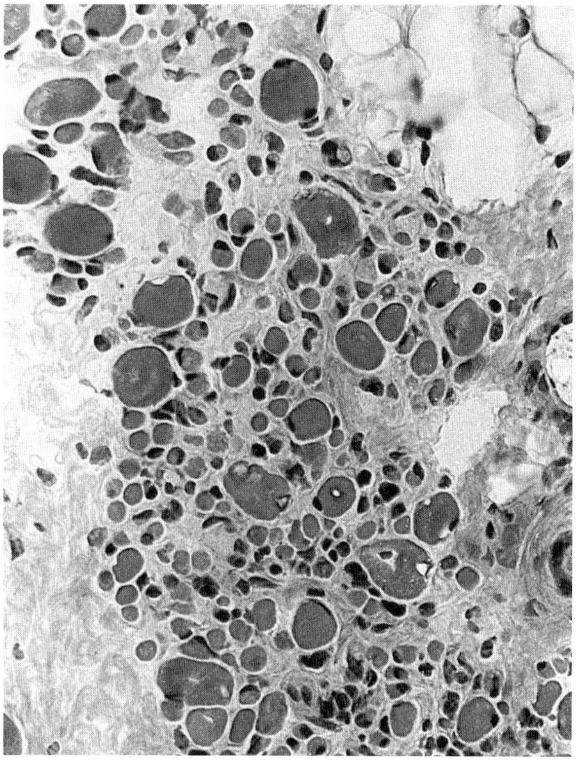

Fig. 25.9. Congenital muscular dystrophy in a 3-day-old infant. Marked atrophy of the fibres and proliferation of the endomysial connective tissue. (H&E, ×342)

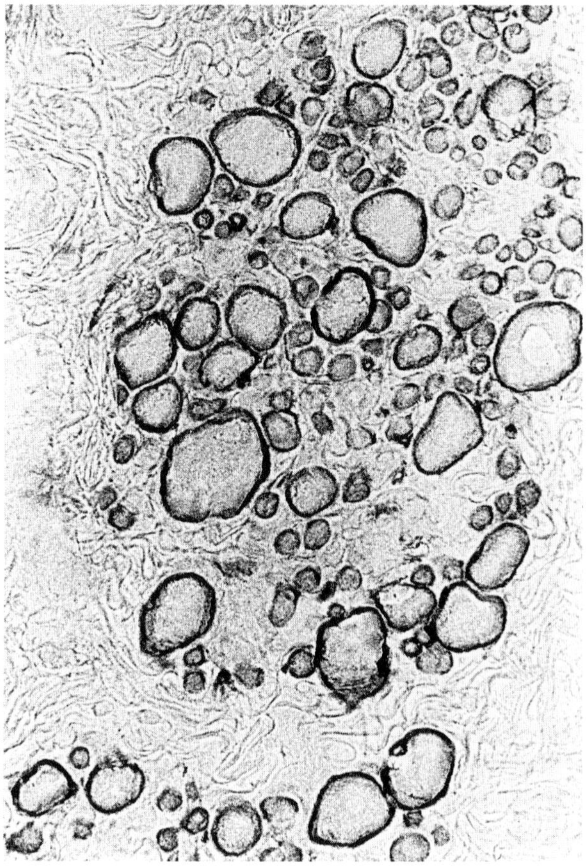

Fig. 25.10. Congenital muscular dystrophy in a 3-day-old infant. Dystrophin is expressed at the periphery of all the fibres, whereas it would have been absent in Duchenne muscular dystrophy. Immunocytochemistry with an antibody specific for dystrophin, ×400.

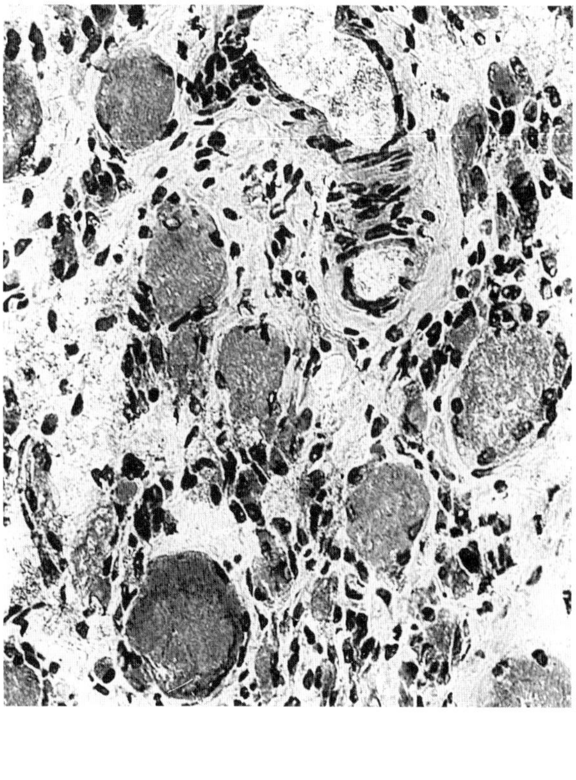

Fig. 25.11. Severe congenital muscular dystrophy in a 5-day-old infant. The important decrease in number and atrophy of the fibres is accompanied by marked connective tissue proliferation. (H&E, ×534)

the lesions (Fig. 25.11). These cases may be difficult to classify or to distinguish from severe neurogenic affections, emphasising the importance of carrying out complementary analyses (histological examination of the central and peripheral nervous system, biochemical analyses).

Congenital muscular dystrophies with involvement of the central nervous system also have variable prognoses. Only a few cases correspond to distinct pathological entities.

Fukuyama muscular dystrophy, frequent in Japan (Fukuyama et al. 1981) but only exceptionally found elsewhere (MacMenamin et al. 1982), may appear during the first few months after birth. This progressive muscular dystrophy is associated with cerebral abnormalities which develop very early in utero: polymicrogyria, pachygyria, lack of myelin (Takada et al. 1984).

Muscular dystrophies with hydrocephaly and ocular lesions do not seem to have any specific geographical distribution. In Walker–Warburg's syndrome, there is primarily a cerebral involvement (hydrocephaly, agyria, retinal dysplasia, Dandy–Walker's syndrome with or without occipital encephalocele = HARD ± E) and death usually occurs in the first few weeks after birth. Santavuori's syndrome probably corresponds to a similar though less severe disorder (Santavuori et al. 1977).

Duchenne Muscular Dystrophy

Duchenne muscular dystrophy is almost never detected in the neonatal period and the diagnosis should only be considered in exceptional cases.

This steadily progressive disease is X-linked recessive and occasionally associated with other anomalies linked to the X chromosome. Several male infants presenting in the neonatal period with adrenal hypoplasia have a muscle biopsy indistinguishable from Duchenne muscular dystrophy (Lake 1991). The gene localised to Xp21 codes for dystrophin, a protein which is totally absent in the disease.

When previous infants in a family are affected, the possibility of carrying out a diagnosis on the fetus or newborn infant has been attempted. An analysis of biopsies from presymptomatic infants (Bradley et al. 1972) only revealed focal lesions on routine histology before the age of 2 months. The muscles of fetuses identified by molecular biology as being affected by Duchenne muscular dystrophy do not have characteristic lesions and only a few cases seem to present a focal delay in maturation (Fig. 25.12). The expression of dystrophin is certainly impaired and has been found to be absent in at-risk fetuses (Patel et al. 1988) but it is not absolutely certain that the developing muscle fibres in Duchenne muscular dystrophy cannot express some form of dystrophin during early fetal life.

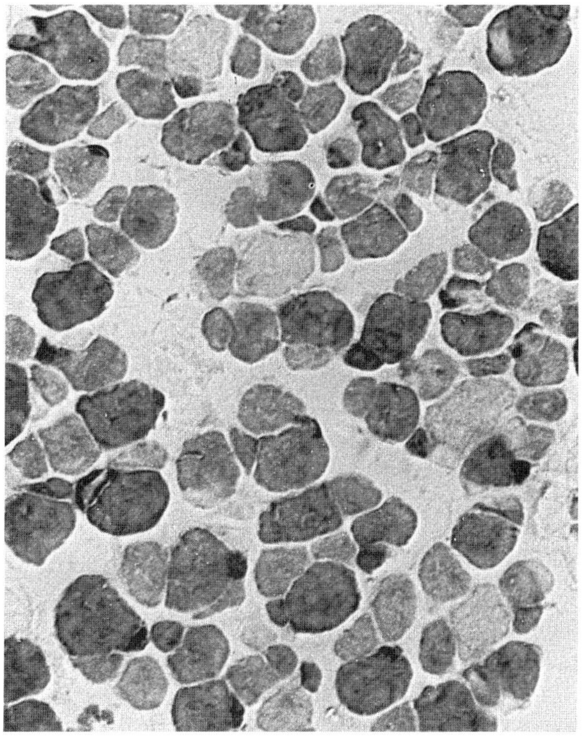

Fig. 25.12. 22-week-old fetus affected with Duchenne muscular dystrophy. Primary generation fibres are unreactive. Secondary generation fibres, reactive, show a marked dispersion in size suggesting a delayed development. Immunocytochemistry using an antibody specific for the fast myosin heavy chain, ×450.

Werdnig–Hoffmann Disease

Spinal muscular atrophy has an autosomal-recessive pattern of inheritance, the gene being located on chromosome 5. Cases presenting in the fetus or in the newborn are, by definition, included in the infantile group of spinal muscular atrophy, i.e. Werdnig–Hoffmann disease.

These neonatal forms, sometimes of acute onset (Dubowitz 1980), are characterised by a complete clinical picture: generalised hypotonia, severe limb and axial weakness, whereas the face is relatively spared, difficulties in sucking and in swallowing, absent tendon reflexes. The infants frequently have a characteristic frog posture and paralysis of the intercostal muscles is responsible for immobility of the thorax (which rapidly becomes bell-shaped) and for diaphragmatic respiration. Early onset fasciculations (tongue) are sometimes seem. The clinical diagnosis is in general evident, confirmed by electrophysiological

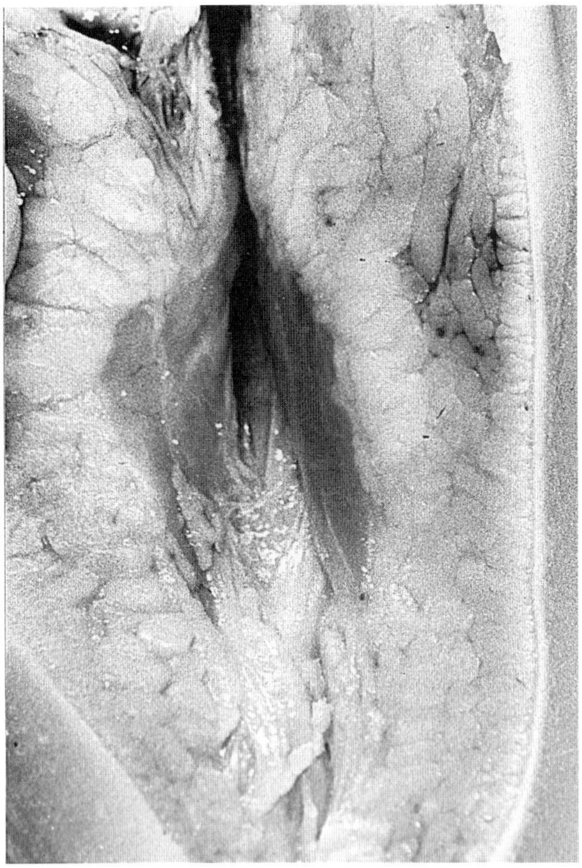

Fig. 25.13. Werdnig–Hoffmann disease in a 5-month-old baby. The dissection of the thigh shows severe atrophy of the muscle, which is replaced by fatty tissue.

demonstration of the homogeneous and severe affection of the motor peripheral nervous system. Despite its severity, the weakness is usually non-progressive but the children are very prone to respiratory infections and choking and eventually develop chronic respiratory insufficiency. Death usually occurs within 1 year.

Muscle biopsies, rendered difficult by the severe atrophy (Fig. 25.13), reveal neurogenic (group) atrophy as well as the presence of isolated or clustered hypertrophic muscle fibres (Fig. 25.14). These hypertrophic fibres are mainly of type I which, in addition to the fact that the atrophic fibres are rounded, is histologically in favour of a spinal origin for the neurogenic atrophy. The biopsy may show only minimal changes in early cases (Dubowitz 1980).

The primary lesions in the nervous system, i.e. degeneration of the anterior horn cells of the spinal cord with neuronal loss and foci of neuronophagia, can only be demonstrated when necropsy is eventually carried out. These lesions predominate in the cervical and lumbar regions of the spinal cord but are also observed in nuclei of the cranial nerves and of the thalamus (Gruner and Bargeton 1952). In a few cases, peripheral nerves may be affected by wallerian degeneration (Carpenter et al. 1978).

The pathogenesis of neuronal degeneration in Werdnig–Hoffmann disease is unknown. Recent studies suggest an intrinsic alteration in the metabolism of neurofilaments, leading eventually to cell death in certain neuronal subpopulations (Murayama et al. 1991). Several different hypotheses have been put forward to explain the mechanism by which the muscle is affected: the fact that the atrophic fibres are rounded (whereas denervated fibres are usually angular) has led to discussion of the possibility that these are immature fibres which have not received a proper neural input. Immunocytochemical studies (Sewry 1989; Sawchak et al. 1990) have demonstrated the presence of several types of fibres with different patterns of MHC expression, which is not in favour of a simple arrest of maturation of the fibres at a prenatal stage.

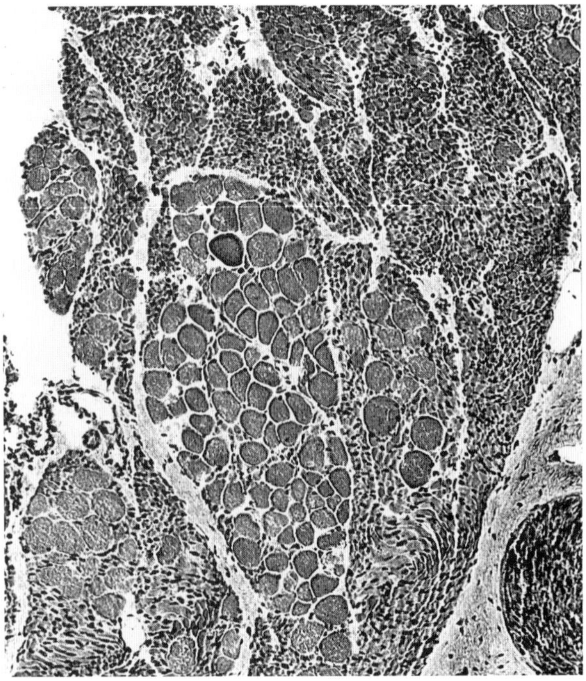

Fig. 25.14. Werdnig–Hoffmann disease in a baby 5 months of age. Fascicular (neurogenic) atrophy contrasts with the presence of hypertrophic fibres. (H&E, ×152)

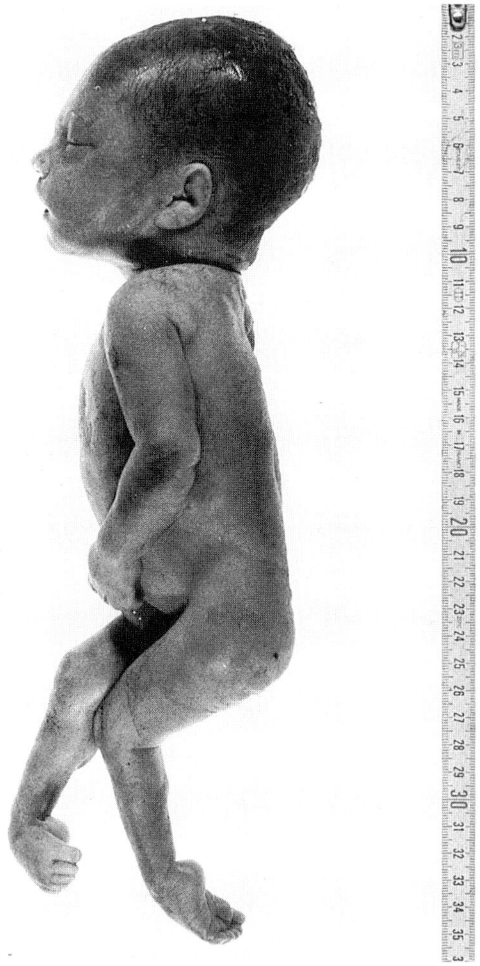

Fig. 25.15. Congenital myotonic dystrophy, 26-week-old fetus. Flexion deformities of lower limbs with talipes equinovarus.

Congenital Myotonic Dystrophy

Myotonic dystrophy is an autosomal-dominant inherited disease. In addition to the forms occurring in children and in adults, a severe congenital form was described by Vanier in 1960. Congenital myotonic dystrophy can be detected in utero (polyhydramnios, poor fetal movements) and is always present at birth. It is characterised by severe hypotonia, facial weakness and variable difficulties in breathing and swallowing. Intrauterine growth retardation, talipes equinovarus (Fig. 25.15) and other deformities which result from the posture in utero are present in more than 50% of severe cases.

The mortality rate is about 50% (Lake 1991) and the gravity of the prognosis is related to the number of signs which accompany the generalised hypotonia (Ferreira et al. 1989). In the most favourable cases, an improvement in respiratory function occurs during the first weeks and in the swallowing reflex in the first months after birth. The hypotonia gradually regresses and the prognosis of motor function is relatively good (Arthuis et al. 1990). Intellectual function is found to be impaired in about two-thirds of the cases, becoming evident with time as in the juvenile form of the disease. Myotonia does not appear before the age of 2 years.

Modifications in muscle morphology differ in many respects from those of the infantile and adult forms of myotonic dystrophy. A striking hypoplasia is evident in both limb and respiratory muscles, accounting for clinical features such as thin ribs and probably for the common occurrence of arthrogryposis (Harper 1989). The most characteristic pathological feature is a delay in muscle maturation accompanied by varying degrees of secondary degenerative changes (Farkas-Bargeton et al. 1974, 1977, 1988; Sarnat and Silbert 1976; Sahgal et al. 1983). Muscle immaturity is characterised at the light microscopy level by the abnormal presence of myotubes and by a delay in fibre type differentiation. Enzyme histochemistry shows, in most cases, hypotrophic changes of type I fibres but is frequently impaired by the irregular accumulation and distribution of myofibrils (Fig. 25.16). A peripheral rim devoid of oxidative enzyme reactivity in many fibres (Fig. 25.17) corresponds to a region devoid of mitochondria similar to that previously described in fetal fibres (Farkas-Bargeton et al. 1977). The essential ultrastructural characteristics are the relatively low abundance and disorganisation of myofibrils as well as the peripheral halo lacking both mitochondria and myofibrils (Fig. 25.18). Immunocytochemical analyses demonstrate a delay in the differentiation and maturation of the second-generation fast and slow muscle fibres (Fig. 25.19). This would suggest the implication of a defect in the nerve–muscle contact in the pathogenesis of the congenital form of myotonic dystrophy, confirming the hypothesis of Sarnat and Silbert (1976) that a primary lesion in the muscle membrane would produce a failure of the response to neural influences during development.

By increasing the time of survival, the muscle is able to gain a certain degree of maturity but never becomes normal and pro-

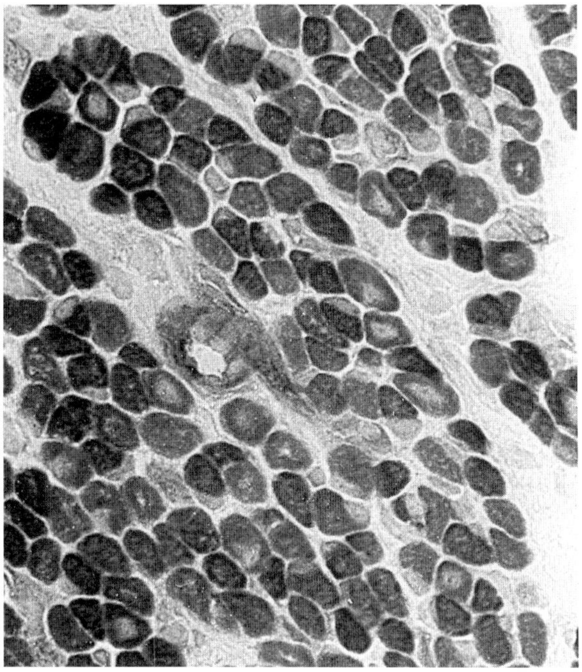

Fig. 25.16. Congenital myotonic dystrophy in a 26-week-old fetus. Small-sized myotubes and myofibres are almost undifferentiated. (ATPase at pH 9.4 ×342)

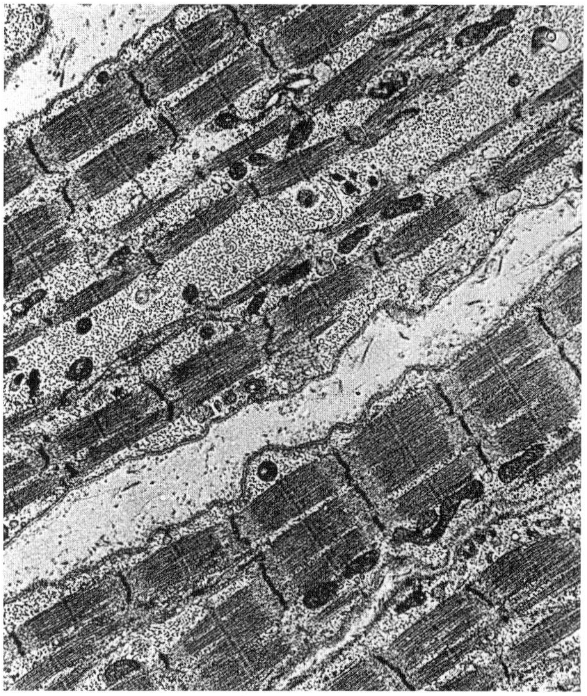

Fig. 25.18. Congenital myotonic dystrophy in a 33-week-old fetus. Immature fibres contain only scanty and sometimes poorly organised myofibrils. (Electron microscopy ×4940)

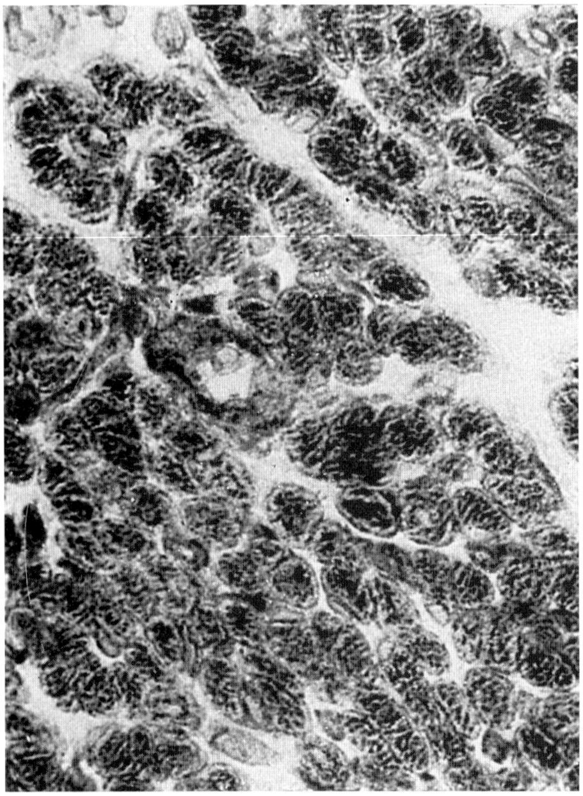

gressively shows the typical changes characteristic of adult myotonic dystrophy (Tanabe and Nonaka 1987; Farkas-Bargeton et al. 1988).

These severe congenital forms of myotonic dystrophy are always transmitted by the mother, which suggests the role of an environmental maternal factor (Harper and Dyken 1972; Farkas-Bargeton et al. 1988). The maternal affection may be only very slight, sometimes limited to an electrical myotonia, and thus care should be taken to carry out an accurate diagnosis (electromyogram,slit lamp). The risk for a mother with myotonic dystrophy of having a first child affected by the congenital form of this disease is 20%. This then increases to 50% in the second pregnancy if the first child was affected. The possibility of antenatal diagnosis is at present limited to the most severe forms where characteristic signs of

Fig. 25.17. Congenital myotonic dystrophy in a 26-week-old fetus. All myotubes/fibres have a marked peripheral halo lacking reactivity. (NADH, ×405)

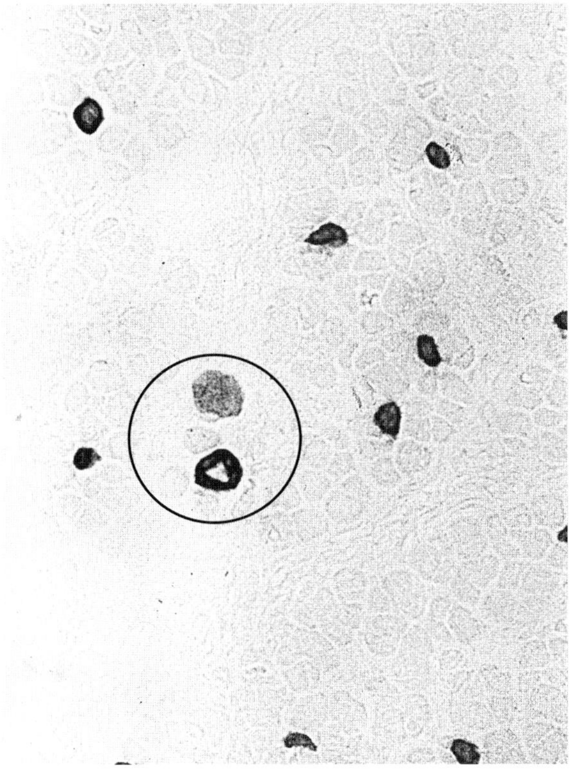

Fig. 25.19. Congenital myotonic dystrophy in a 26-week-old fetus. Apart for a muscle spindle (*circled*), the muscle is composed of small-sized primary (reactive) and secondary (non-reactive) fibres. The differentiation of the secondary fibres is delayed. (Immunocytochemistry with an antibody specific for the slow myosin heavy chain ×329)

the disease may be revealed by sonography, although at a rather late stage of pregnancy. The gene for the disease is located on chromosome 19 and more precise characterisation of this gene locus will most probably open up the possibility for earlier prenatal diagnosis in the near future.

Congenital Myopathies

Myotubular Myopathy (X-linked Form)

Myotubular myopathy was first described by Spiro et al. (1966) as the persistence of fetal muscle in a 12-year-old child. In 1967, Sher et al. described the familial occurrence of the disease and proposed the term centronuclear myopathy—not referring to a possible myogenic defect. Different clinical aspects have since been described, corresponding to distinct entities especially in terms of genetic transmission: severe neonatal form, common childhood form (sometimes presenting with mild hypotonia at birth), minor form occurring in late childhood or in adult life. In all these cases, histological examination reveals centrally located nuclei in a large number of muscle fibres.

The severe neonatal form of myotubular myopathy (Van Wijngaarden et al. 1969; Barth et al. 1975) is X-linked and often accompanied by polyhydramnios and decreased fetal movements during pregnancy. Severe asphyxia at birth with persistent respiratory distress is associated with hypotonia and opthalmoplegia. The disorder may be fatal during the first few weeks after birth, the prognosis being linked to the severity of respiratory distress and of the initial asphyxia.

This clinical presentation resembles congenital myotonic dystrophy but distinction can be made on examination of the mother, who will invariably show evidence of the disease in myotonic dystrophy (Heckmatt et al. 1985). It is important to make this distinction clinically since the muscle histology may be similar in the two conditions (Farkas-Bargeton et al. 1974).

On histological examination, the fibres are small (3–5 μm) and 5%–75% of them contain longitudinal chains of central nuclei (Fig. 25.20). These nuclei are separated by areas completely devoid of myofibrils but rich in mitochondria and glycogen, which explains the holes observed on the ATPases (Fig. 25.21) as well as the central aggregations of stain with NADH and PAS reactions. Both fibre types are differentiated and equally affected. A selective hypotrophy of type I fibres occurs occasionally (Engel et al. 1968) but this feature does not deserve to be distinguished as a separate entity. Ultrastructural analyses (Fig. 25.22) show myofibrillar disruption, Z-line streaming and signs of atrophy such as redundant basal lamina (Ambler et al. 1984). Unusual dense tubules have been observed in some cases (Sewry 1985) and may be formed from replicated triads that have lost their T-tubule component.

The pathogenesis of myotubular myopathy is unknown and the specificity of the lesions is disputed. The term myotubular postulated an arrest of muscle maturation at a fetal stage (Spiro et al. 1966) but many morphological findings are against this theory, especially the degree of enzyme histochemical differentiation, the degenerative changes in electron micro-

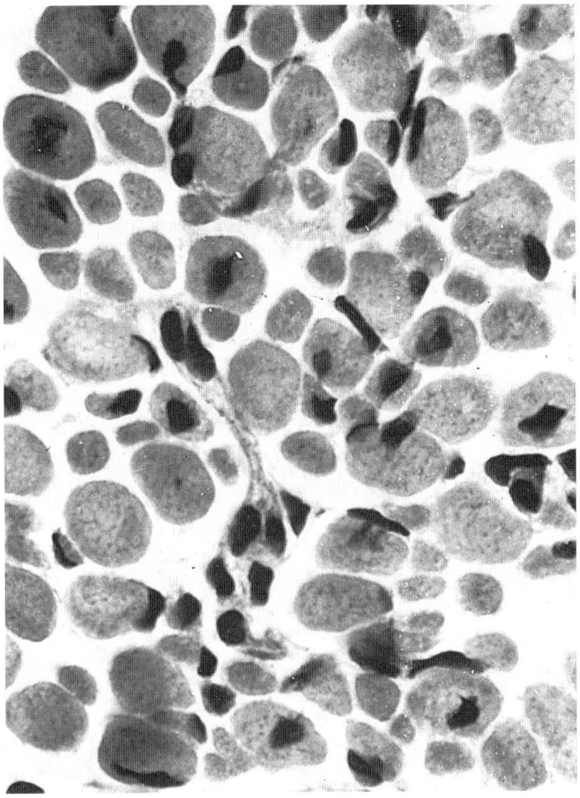

Fig. 25.20. X-linked myotubular myopathy in a 1-day-old infant. Marked discrepancy in fibre size and presence of central nuclei in about 20% of the fibres. (H&E, ×516)

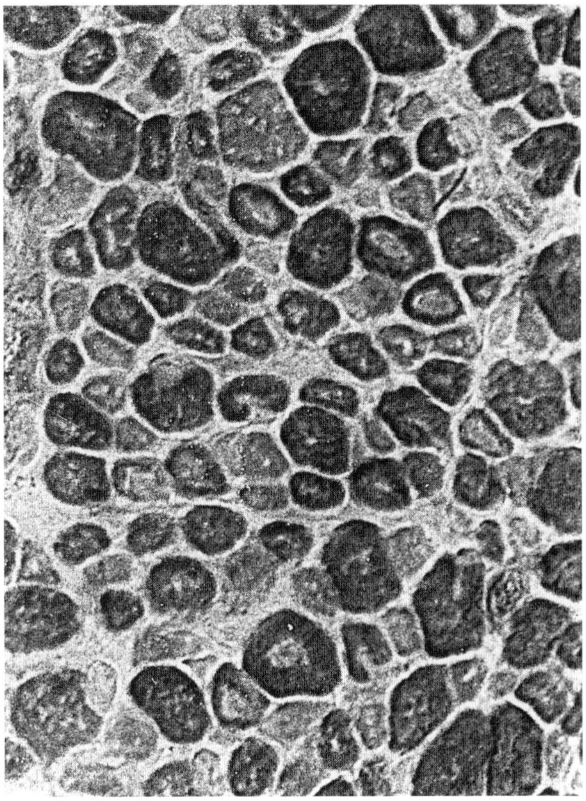

Fig. 25.21. X-linked myotubular myopathy in a 1-day-old infant. The central zone of the fibres is unreactive, like fetal myotubes. (ATPase at pH 9.4 ×540)

scopy and the immunocytochemical studies which demonstrate an almost normal expression of the adult MHCs by the fibres.

Nemaline Myopathy

Nemaline myopathy is a rare, usually nonprogressive, congenital myopathy defined by the presence of tiny rod-like structures in a varying number of muscle fibres (Shy et al. 1963). The genetic patterns of inheritance are diverse but fit best with an autosomal-dominant transmission with incomplete penetrance.

In the mild congenital form, the disease can start at any time between birth and adolescence. Hypotonia is associated with a nonprogressive or slowly progressive muscle weakness of variable severity.

The severe neonatal (fatal) form is characterised clinically by marked muscle hypotonia and weakness, respiratory distress and swallowing difficulties during the neonatal period (Korlin 1967). Affected children often present joint contractures and die before 1 year of age. Serum creatine kinase levels and electromyogram are normal. The diagnosis is based on the presence of small or large clusters of rod-like particles at the periphery of the fibres. The particles stain red on the modified Gomori trichrome (Fig. 25.23) and can be easily visualised by electron microscopy: they measure 2–5 μm in length and have characteristics of Z-bands with parallel filaments and regular cross-striations (Lake 1991). The rods are abundant in type I fibres which tend to be predominant and hypotrophic. As in other congenital myopathies, the rods may be associated with cores, minicores and focal loss of cross-striations (Bethlem et al. 1978), corresponding maybe to a common pathological process. The number of rods per fibre does not correlate with the clinical severity and muscle weakness probably results from an overall decrease in the total number of muscle

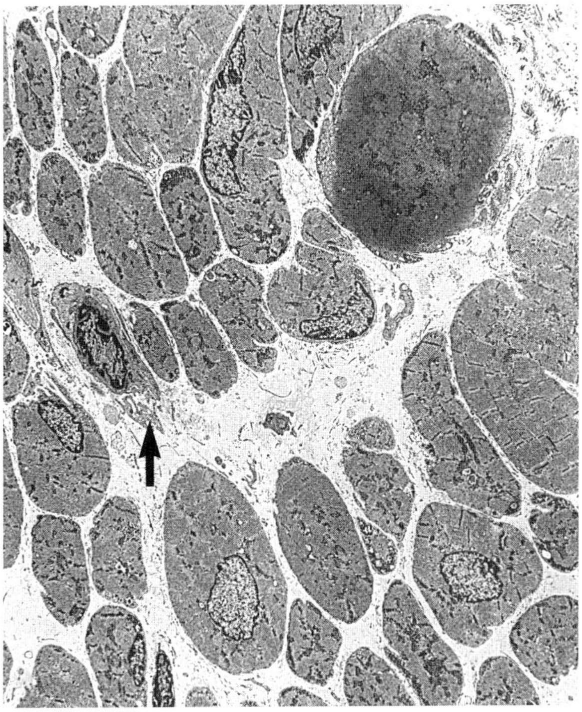

Fig. 25.22. X-linked myotubular myopathy in a 1-day-old infant. The fibres are irregular in size and show some degenerative changes (myofibrillar disruption, Z-line streaming). The presence of a redundant basal membrane (*arrow*) is indicative of an atrophic process. (Electron microscopy ×1520)

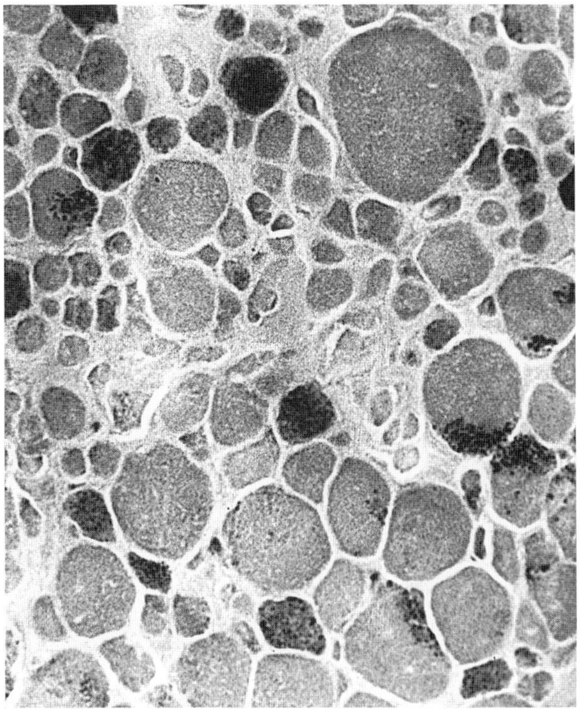

Fig. 25.23. Neonatal nemaline myopathy in a baby of 2 weeks of age. Discrepancy in fibre size and presence of characteristic nemaline bodies, which tend to predominate in the small fibres. (Modified Gomori trichrome ×456)

cells, an abnormal fibre type distribution and an immaturity of the muscle fibres (Shinomura and Nonaka 1989). Nemaline rods correspond to paracrystals of α-actinin and actin (Yamaguchi et al. 1978) and could result from a defective synthesis of myosin leading to a relative excess of α-actinin (Schmalbruch et al. 1987).

Other Congenital Myopathies

Congenital fibre type disproportion. This corresponds to a purely histological definition: small diameter type I fibres with a difference of more than 12% between type I and type II fibres (Brooke 1973). This histological picture has been observed in conditions varying from mild non-progressive muscle hypotonia and weakness to severe neonatal disease with associated skeletal abnormalities and early death. Some cases have an autosomal-dominant inheritance. The specificity of the selective hypotrophy of the type I fibres is questionable since it can also be observed in different circumstances, in particular in other congenital myopathies. Moreover, congenital fibre type disproportion could result from altered neural influences during fetal development (Argov et al. 1984) and the tendency for these type I fibres to be grouped has been reported in several cases (Fig. 25.24).

Minimal change myopathy—delayed muscle maturation. When minor non-specific changes such as excess in the proportions of fibre types occurs, Dubowitz (1980) has suggested the term "minimal change myopathy". Delayed muscle maturation can be defined in the neonatal period by (1) small size of the fibres, (2) persistence of Wohlfart type "b" fibres and (3) persistence of the peripheral halo devoid of reactivity for oxidative enzymes (Farkas-Bargeton et al. 1978). As for congenital fibre type disproportion, these minor abnormalities are not specific and correspond to different clinical situations. In some cases, the evolution

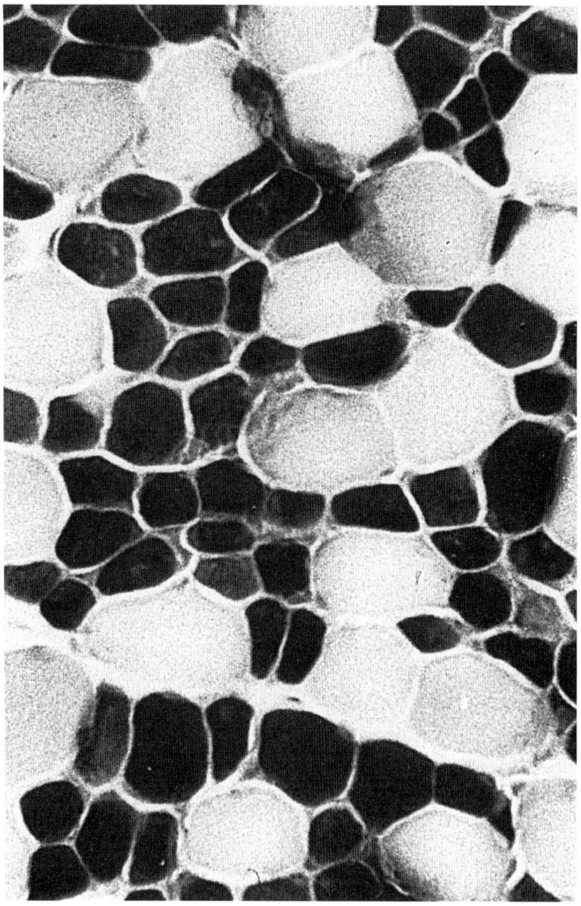

Fig. 25.24. Congenital fibre type disproportion in a 1-week-old infant. Type I fibres (reactive) are smaller than type II fibres (unreactive) and tend to form groups, suggestive of a neurogenic process. (ATPase following acid preincubation at pH 4.35 ×475)

is benign. In other cases, the evolution may be less favourable and progressive; structural changes may then appear in later years which allow one to fit the cases into one of the better characterised categories of muscle disease.

Other congenital myopathies, such as *central core disease* (Shy and Magee 1956) or *multicore disease* (Engel et al. 1971), are not symptomatic in the fetal or neonatal period. They have been described in detail in different reviews, including those of Dubowitz (1980) and Fardeau (1992).

Peripheral Neuropathies

Peripheral neuropathies rarely occur in fetal or neonatal life.

Trauma

Traumatic lesions induce wallerian degeneration of the nerve distal to the lesion. The most common nerve injury encountered in neonates is an avulsion injury produced by birth trauma. Anterior nerve roots at the junction with the spinal cord of those roots supplying the brachial plexus are most at risk (Esiri 1987).

Hereditary Motor and Sensory Neuropathies

The motor and sensory neuropathies lead to degeneration of both motor and sensory nerve fibres.

Dyck's classification (1984b) distinguishes three different types based on their electrical expression and genetic mode of inheritance: demyelination and autosomal-dominant transmission for type I, axonal involvement and variable genetic transmission although most frequently autosomal-dominant for type II, demyelination and autosomal recessive inheritance for type III. These forms normally occur in older children or even in adults and the diagnosis is based on electrophysiological studies and genetic enquiry. They are sometimes symptomatic in the neonatal period, which does not indicate a more severe evolvement (Arthuis et al. 1990). When the familial study is not clear, a biopsy may be necessary to establish the diagnosis.

In addition to these three forms, Lyon (1969) has described a group of specifically congenital forms of motor and sensory neuropathies with a variable transmission (autosomal dominant or recessive, sporadic). Severe hypotonia and muscle weakness are associated with distal amyotrophy, respiratory and swallowing difficulties. The evolution varies from a progressive improvement with severe motor handicap to neonatal death due to respiratory insuffficency. Histology shows a decreased density of the myelinated fibres and sometimes even a total lack of myelin. There is usually no significant Schwann cell reaction in these congenital forms of motor and sensory neuropathies.

Hereditary Sensory Neuropathies

The sensory neuropathies are characterised by sensory deficits and variable degrees of autonomic dysfunction.

Dyck's classification (1984a) distinguishes type I with a late onset and types II–V with a possible onset in the neonatal period. Types II, III and IV have an autosomal-recessive mode of inheritance. A more or less complete insensitivity to pain, responsible for cutaneous and bone trophic lesions, is associated with autonomic disturbances which may be severe (type III). Anhidrosis leads to severe hyperthermic episodes in type IV, which is often rapidly fatal. The electromyogram is normal whereas the speed of nerve conduction is very low (exception made for type V).

Histology is characterised at the structural level by a decreased number of myelinated fibres in types II, III and IV and by the small diameter of myelinated fibres in type V. In electron microscopy, the number of amyelinated fibres is significantly decreased in sensory neuropathies of types II and IV.

Myasthenia

Myasthenia is practically the only abnormality of the neuromuscular junction which manifests itself in the neonatal period. As in later presentations of this disorder, auto-immune myasthenia gravis should be distinguished from the congenitally inherited syndrome.

Transient Neonatal Myasthenia

Neonatal myasthenia is a transient disorder, occurring in 10%–20% of infants born to myasthenic mothers (Fenichel 1978) and lasting no more than a few weeks. It results from the transplacental passage of maternal antiacetylcholine receptor antibodies. There is no correlation between the severity of the disease in the mother and in the infant.

In the first few hours after birth, the baby has a weak cry as well as difficulties in breathing and sometimes hypotonia. The progressive clinical improvement is correlated with the disappearance of antiacetylcholine receptors antibodies from the baby's serum.

Congenital Myasthenia

Congenital myasthenia is a rare hereditary disorder with an autosomal-recessive pattern of inheritance. There is no single pathogenesis of this condition and there are most probably different types of congenital myasthenia due to diverse abnormalities, e.g. defective synthesis or lacking activity of acetylcholine, decreased number or defective function of acetylcholine receptors (Engel 1984).

Metabolic Myopathies

Myopathies in which specific metabolic disorders have been identified or suspected chiefly involve abnormalities of energy metabolism. They can be broadly subdivided into (1) primary disorders of glycogen metabolism, (2) biochemical mitochondrial defects leading to structural mitochondrial abnormalities and (3) primary disorders of lipid metabolism (Esiri 1987).

The majority of these affections do not occur during fetal and neonatal life.

Pompe's Disease

Pompe's disease is the severe neonatal form of type II glycogenosis, due to an acid maltase deficiency. This autosomal-recessive disease can be diagnosed prenatally on trophoblastic or amniotic cells.

Severe generalised hypotonia with no amyotrophy is associated with macroglossia and cardiomegaly. A positive diagnosis is made from the decreased acid maltase activity in the leucocytes. The child usually dies between 5 and 8 months of age from cardiorespiratory insufficiency.

All skeletal muscle and heart fibres are overloaded with glycogen, usually in the form of vacuoles. On routine stains, this vacuolisation is often so severe that only a small proportion of the sarcoplasm of each fibre remains (Fig. 25.25), giving the tissue a lace-like appearance (Johnson 1990).

Cytochrome Oxidase Deficiency

Mitochondrial myopathies, morphologically characterised by abnormal muscle fibres on mitochondrial enzyme reactions and by the presence of voluminous red granules on the

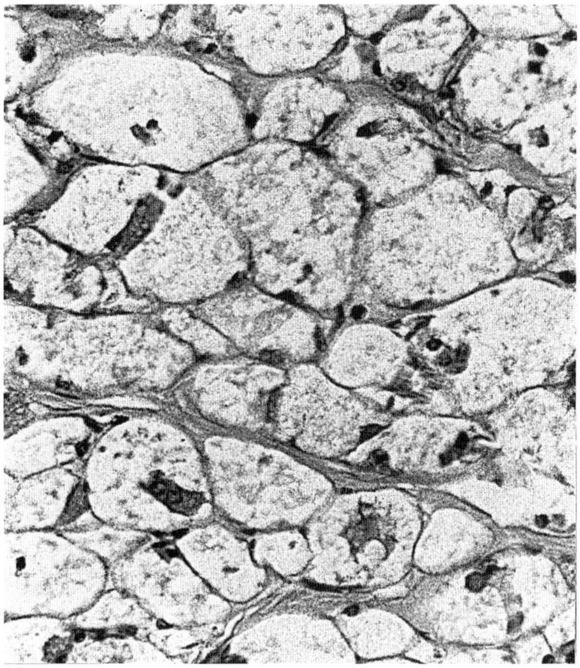

Fig. 25.25. Pompe's disease in a baby 1 month of age. Marked vacuolation of the fibres due to accumulation of glycogen. (H&E, ×490)

modified Gomori trichrome (red-ragged fibres) are not usually seen in the neonatal period. Nevertheless, as Lake (1991) pointed out, this diagnosis should be considered in any patient presenting with increased lactate levels.

The deficiency in cytochrome oxidase can occur as a fatal neonatal form, with severe generalised hypotonia and lactate acidosis developing during the first few weeks after birth (Nonaka et al. 1988). Progressive muscle weakness is occasionally associated with renal dysfunction and cardiomyopathy. Muscle fibres show increased NADH and SDH reactivities and clumps of finely granular red-staining material on the modified trichrome. Cytochrome oxidase activity is absent from all the fibres.

Other Metabolic Myopathies

Other defects of glycogen metabolism (phosphofructokinase deficiency, myophosphorylase deficiency) or mitochondrial myopathies are only very rarely detected in the newborn infant. These conditions have been recently reviewed in detail by Lake (1991).

Inflammatory Myopathies

Congenital Inflammatory Myopathy

Congenital inflammatory myopathy begins either in utero or just after birth. Hypotonia and muscle weakness with or without arthrogryposis are sometimes associated with microcephaly. Serum creatine kinase levels are elevated and the electromyogram is myopathic. Muscle biopsy shows the presence of inflammatory infiltrates (Fig. 25.26), muscle fibre damage and class I major histocompatibility complex products in the muscle sarcolemma (Shevell et al. 1990). Possible aetiologies include intrauterine viral infection or autoimmune process. Corticosteroid treatment may improve motor function but has no effect on the central nervous system. The clinical evolution is heterogeneous, sometimes suggestive of the development of a congenital muscular dystrophy syndrome.

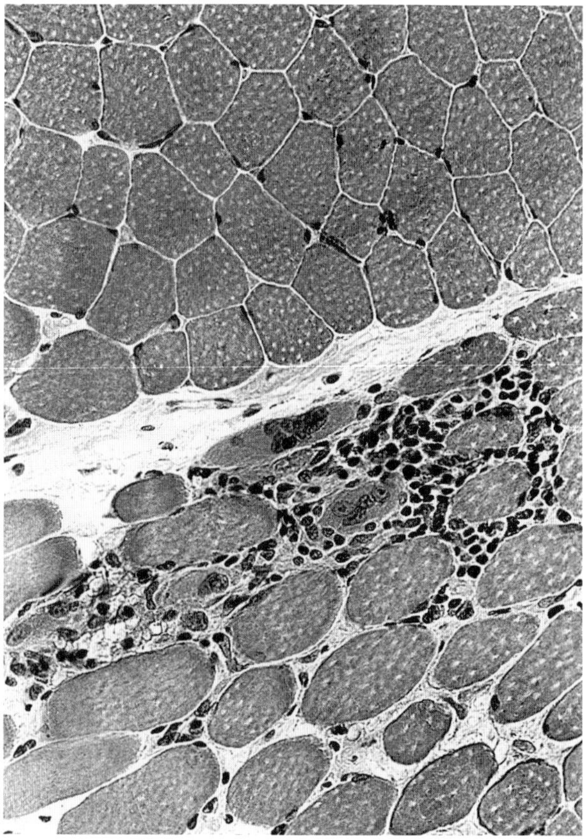

Fig. 25.26. Congenital inflammatory myopathy in a 1-week-old infant. Focal round cell infiltration and muscle fibre damage. (H&E, ×400)

Other Inflammatory Myopathies

Infantile myositis corresponds to the onset of polymyositis before the age of 1 year (Thompson 1982). It is exceptional in the newborn and should be distinguished from congenital inflammatory myopathy.

Viral or parasitic (toxoplasmic) myositis is only occasionally found and is usually of no clinical significance.

Localised Abnormalities

Malformations

Congenital localised absence of muscle (amyoplasia) most frequently involves the pectoralis muscle. The association with ipsilateral symbrachydactyly constitutes Poland syndrome, almost always sporadic.

Abnormalities of muscle development, varying from a simple delay in maturation to hypoplasia or aplasia, can be found as part of numerous malformations or malformative syndromes. It is often difficult to define the significance of the muscle defect (primary or secondary). One such example is the defective development of the rectus abdominis muscle, most probably secondary to severe distension of the urinary tract with which it is associated in the prune belly syndrome (Banker 1986).

Pseudo-tumours and Tumours

Sternocleidomastoid Tumour (Fibromatosis Colli)

Fibromatosis colli usually becomes apparent between 1 and 4 weeks after birth as a firm mass within the sternocleidomastoid muscle. This mass increases in size but then regresses spontaneously, and may result in a secondary shortening of the muscle and torticollis. The outcome is always favourable and the treatment is non-surgical. If it is removed, the tumour appears to be composed of fibrous tissue containing degenerate muscle fibres (Fig. 25.27).

The pathogenesis of this condition is still unclear. Birth trauma may be responsible for some cases. The hypothesis that the lesion may develop from a haematoma of the muscle has been discounted since it usually contains only small amounts of haemosiderin.

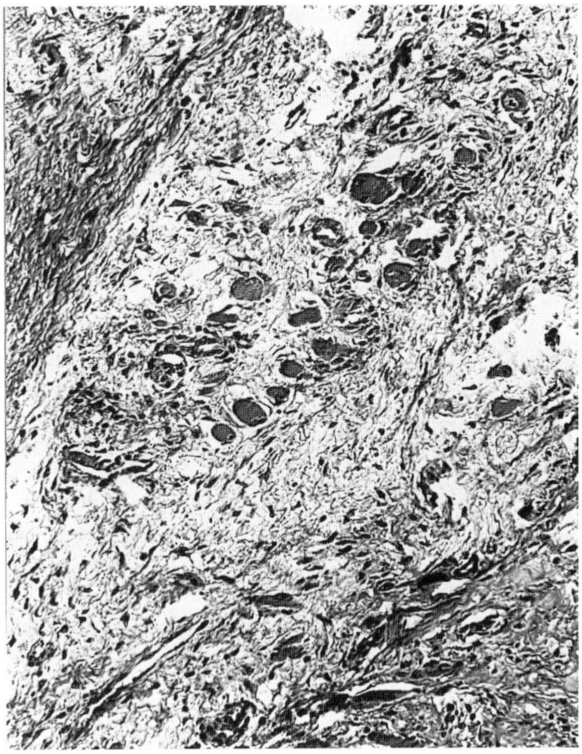

Fig. 25.27. Fibromatosis colli in a 2-week-old infant. Degenerative muscle fibres are dispersed in fibrous connective tissue. (H&E, ×152)

Fetal Rhabdomyoma

Fetal rhabdomyoma probably represents a skeletal muscle hamartoma rather than a true neoplasm. It is most frequently found as an isolated retroauricular mass but may also be found in the chest wall or in the perineum. The outcome is always favourable.

This tumour, well-limited though non-encapsulated, develops in the dermis and subcutaneous tissues which are replaced by lobular networks of muscle fibres. The presence of regular mononuclear cells between the well-defined muscle fibres is useful to distinguish fetal rhabdomyoma from rhabdomyosarcoma (Dehner 1987).

Congenital Rhabdomyosarcoma

Rhabdomyosarcoma is rare before 1 year of age, predominantly localised in the extremities

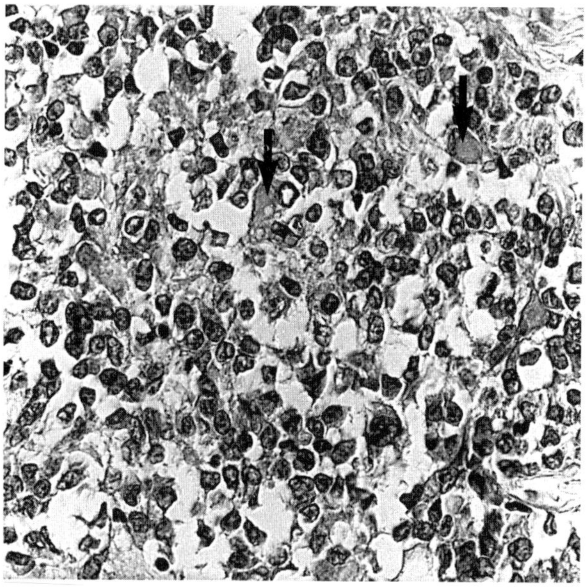

Fig. 25.28. Congenital alveolar rhabdomyosarcoma in a 1-day-old baby. Presence of differentiated tumoural muscle cells (*arrows*). (H&E, ×300)

and the urogenital tract, less commonly in the head or neck region. The embryonic (botryoid) and alveolar forms are the most frequent in this age group.

The congenital forms are exceptional and do not share the relatively favourable prognosis of other tumours (such as neuroblastoma or nephroblastoma) seen during the first few months of life. The evolution is often rapid and fatal (Barbet et al. 1989).

Histological diagnosis relies upon the identification of skeletal muscle differentiation in the tumour. In well-differentiated forms, this is obvious even on routine preparations (Fig. 25.28). In undifferentiated or poorly differentiated forms, muscle differentiation can only be ascertained by electron microscopy or by immunocytochemical analyses using antibodies specific for skeletal muscle proteins (desmin, titin, isoforms of the MHCs). The tumour cells follow a cycle of differentiation and maturation very similar to that observed during normal myogenesis (Barbet et al. 1989). By studying the different muscle markers, it is possible to evaluate accurately the degree of cytological differentiation and its evolution under chemotherapy (Molenaar et al. 1984; Barbet et al. 1989; Carter et al. 1990).

References

Ambler MW, Neave C, Singer DB (1984) X-linked recessive myotubular myopathy: II. Muscle morphology and human myogenesis. Human Pathol 15: 1107–1120

Argov Z, Gardner-Medwin D, Johnson MA, Mastaglia FL (1984) Patterns of muscle fiber-type disproportion in hypotonic infants. Arch Neurol 41: 53–57

Arthuis M, Pinsard N, Ponsot G (eds) (1990) Neurologie pédiatrique. Flammarion, Paris

Banker BQ (1986) Congenital deformities. In: Engel AG, Banker BQ (eds) Myology. McGraw-Hill, New York, pp 2109–2159

Barbet JP, Kurzenne JY, Butler-Browne GS, Mouly V, Laurent M, Gubler JP (1989) Rhabdomyosarcomes de découverte néonatale. Etude des marqueurs de différentiation musculaire. Ann Pathol (Paris) 9: 363–368

Barbet JP, Thornell L-E, Butler-Browne GS (1991) Immunocytochemical characterisation of two generations of fibres during the development of the human quadriceps muscle. Mech Dev: 3513–3521

Barth PG, Van Wijngaarden GH, Bethlem J (1975) X-linked myotubular myopathy with fatal neonatal asphyxia. Neurology 25: 531–536

Bethlem J, Arts WF, Dingemans KP (1978) Common origin of rods, cores, miniature cores, and focal loss of cross-striations. Arch Neurol 35: 555–566

Billeter R, Weber H, Lutz H, Eppenberger HM, Jenny E (1980) Myosin types in human skeletal muscle fibres. Histochemistry 65: 249–259

Bradley WG, Hudgson P, Larson PF, Papapetropoulos TA, Jenkison M (1972) Structural changes in the early stages of Duchenne muscular dystrophy. J Neurol Neurosurg Psychiatr 35: 451–455

Brooke MH (1973) Congenital fibre type disproportion. In: Kakulas BA (ed) Clinical studies in myology. Excerpta Medica, Amsterdam, pp 147–159

Butler-Browne GS, Whalen RG (1984) Myosin isozymes transitions occurring during post-natal development in the rat soleus muscle. Dev Biol 102: 324–334

Butler-Browne GS, Barbet JP, Thornell LE (1990) Myosin heavy and light chain expression during human skeletal muscle development and precocious muscle maturation induced by thyroid hormone. Anat Embryol 181: 513–522

Carpenter S, Karpati G, Rothman S, Watters G, Andermann F (1978) Pathological involvement of primary sensory neurons in Werdnig–Hoffmann disease. Acta Neuropathol (Berl) 42: 91–97

Carter RL, Jameson CF, Philp ER, Pinkerton CR (1990) Comparative phenotypes in rhabdomyosarcomas and developing skeletal muscle. Histopathology 17: 301–309

Colling-Saltin A-S (1978) Enzyme histochemistry on skeletal muscle of the human foetus. J Neurol Sci 39: 169–185

Condon K, Silberstein L, Blau HM, Thompson WJ (1990a) Development of muscle fiber types in the prenatal rat hindlimb. Dev Biol 138: 256–274

Condon K, Silberstein L, Blau HM, Thompson WJ (1990b) Differentiation of fiber types in aneural musculature of the prenatal rat hindlimb. Dev Biol 138: 275–295

Dehner LP (1987) Pediatric surgical pathology, 2nd edn. Williams Wilkins, Baltimore

Donner M, Rapola J, Somer H (1975) Congenital muscular dystrophy: a clinicopathological and follow-up study. Neuropädiatrie 6: 239–258

Draeger A, Weeds AG, Fitzsimons RB (1987) Primary, secondary and tertiary myotubes in developing skeletal muscle: a new approach to the analysis of human myogenesis. J Neurol Sci 31: 245–259

Dubowitz V (1965) Enzyme histochemistry on skeletal muscle. Part II. Developing human muscle. J Neurol Neurosurg Psychiatr 28: 519–524

Dubowitz V (1978) Muscle disorders in childhood. Saunders, London

Dubowitz V (1980) The floppy infant, 2nd edn. Heinemann, London

Dubowitz V (ed) (1985) Muscle biopsy. A practical approach. Baillière Tindall, London

Dyck PJ (1984a) Neuronal atrophy and degeneration predominantly affecting peripheral motor, sensory and autonomic neurons. In: Dyck PJ, Thomas PK, Lambert EH, Bunge R (eds). Peripheral neuropathy. Saunders, Philadelphia, pp 1557–1599

Dyck PJ (1984b) Inherited neuronal degeneration and atrophy affecting peripheral motor, sensory, and autonomic neurons. In: Dyck PJ, Thomas PK, Lambert EH, Bunge R (eds) Peripheral neuropathy. Saunders, Philadelphia, pp 1600–1655

Ecob-Price M, Hill M, Brown W (1989) Immunocytochemical demonstration of myosin heavy chain expression in human muscle. J Neurol Sci 91: 71–78

Engel WK (1984) Myasthenia gravis and myasthenic syndromes. Ann Neurol 16: 519–533

Engel WK, Gold GN, Karpati G (1968) Type I hypotrophy and central nuclei: a rare congenital muscle abnormality with a possible experimental model. Arch Neurol 18: 435–444

Engel WK, Gomez MR, Groover RV (1971) Multicore disease: a recently recognised congenital myopathy associated with multifocal degeneration of muscle fibres. Mayo Clin Proc 46: 666–681

Esiri M (1987) Skeletal muscle and peripheral nerves. In: Keeling JW (ed) Fetal and neonatal pathology. Springer-Verlag, Berlin, pp 509–527

Fardeau M (1992) Congenital myopathies. In: Mastaglia FL, Walton J (eds) Skeletal muscle pathology, 2nd edn. Churchill Livingstone, London, pp 237–281

Farkas-Bargeton E, Aicardi J, Fardeau M, Arsenio-Nunes ML, Dreyfus P, Diebler MF (1974) Histochemical and ultrastructural study of muscle biopsies in 3 cases of dystrophia myotonica in the newborn child. J Neurol Sci 21: 273–288

Farkas-Bargeton E, Diebler MF, Arsenio-Nunes ML, Wehrle R, Rosenberg B (1977) Etude de la maturation histochimique, quantitative et ultrastructurale du muscle foetal human. J Neurol Sci 31: 245–260

Farkas-Bargeton E, Aicardi J, Arsenio-Nunes ML, Wehrle R (1978) Delay in the maturation of muscle fibres in infants with congenital hypotonia. J Neurol Sci 39: 17–29

Farkas-Bargeton E, Barbet JP, Dancea S, Wehrle R, Checouri A, Dulac O (1988) Immaturity of muscle fibres in the congenital form of myotonic dystrophy. Its consequences and its origin. J Neurol Sci 83: 145–159

Fenichel GM (1966) A histochemical study of developing skeletal muscle. Neurology 16: 741–745

Fenichel GM (1978) Clinical syndromes of myasthenia in infancy and childhood. A review. Arch Neurol 35: 97–103

Ferreira O, Morvan J, Bernard AM, Verjut JP, Cleophax JP (1989) Maladie de Steinert néonatale. J Gynecol Obstet Biol Reprod 18: 349–354

Fitzsimons RB, Hoh JFY (1981) Embryonic and fetal myosins in human skeletal muscle. J Neurol Sci 52: 367–384

Fukuyama Y, Osawa M, Suzuki H (1981) Congenital progressive muscular dystrophy of the Fukuyama type—clinical, genetic and pathological considerations. Brain Dev 3: 1–29

Gherardi R (1989) Pathologie neuro-musculaire. In: Poirier J, Gray F, Escourolle R (eds) Manuel de neuropathologie, 3rd edn. Masson, Paris, pp 204–245

Gruner JE, Bargeton E (1952) Lésions thalamiques dans la myatonie du nourrisson. Rev Neurol 86: 236–242

Hamilton WJ, Mossman HW (1972) Human embryology, 4th edn. McMillan, London

Harper PS (1989) Myotonic dystrophy, 2nd edn. Saunders, London

Harper PS, Dyken PR (1972) Early-onset dystrophia myotonica. Evidence supporting a maternal environmental factor. Lancet 2: 53–57

Hauschka SD (1974) Clonal analysis of vertebrate myogenesis. IV. Developmental changes in the muscle colony-forming cells of the human fetal limb. Dev Biol 37: 345–368

Heckmatt JZ, Sewry CA, Hodes D, Dubowitz V (1985) Congenital centronuclear (myotubular) myopathy. A clinical, pathological and genetic study in eight children. Brain 108: 941–964

Johnson MA (1990) Skeletal muscle. In: Filipe MI, Lake BD (eds) Histochemistry in pathology, 2nd edn. Churchill Livingstone, Edinburgh, pp 129–157

Korlin IS (1967) Nemaline myopathy. A fatal case. Am J Dis Child 114: 95–100

Kumagai T, Hakamada S, Hara K et al. (1984) Development of human fetal muscles: a comparative histochemical analysis of the psoas and the quadriceps muscle. Neuropediatrics 15: 198–202

Lake BD (1991) Skeletal musculature. In: Wigglesworth JS, Singer BD (eds) Textbook of fetal and perinatal pathology. Blackwell, Oxford, pp 1221–1246

Lyon G (1969) Ultrastructural study of a nerve biopsy from a case of early infantile chronic neuropathy. Acta Neuropathol 13: 131–142

Lyons GE, Haselgrove J, Kelly AM, Rubinstein NA (1983) Myosin transitions in developing fast and slow muscles in the rat hind limb. Differentiation 25: 168–175

MacMenamin JB, Becker LE, Murphy EG (1982) Congenital muscular dystrophy: a clinicopathologic report of 24 cases. J Pediatr 100: 692–697

Miller JB (1991) Myoblasts, myosins, MyoDs, and the diversification of muscle fibers. Neuromusc Dis 1: 7–17

Molenaar WM, Oosterhuis JW, Oosterhuis AM, Ramakaers FCS (1984) Mesenchymal and muscle-specific intermediate filaments (vimentin and desmin) in relation to differentiation in childhood rhabdomyosarcomas. Human Pathol 16: 838–843

Moore GE, Hurko O, Walsh FS (1984) Immunocytochemical analysis of fibre type differentiation in developing skeletal muscle. J Neuroimmunol 7: 137–149

Mouly V, Lemonnier M, Libri D, Gros F, Fiszman MY (1990) Transformation and cloning of different types of myoblasts during avian development. In: Pette D (ed) The dynamic state of muscle fibre. W Gruyter, Berlin, pp 651–665

Murayama S, Boudin TW, Suzuki K (1991) Immunocytochemical and ultrastructural studies of Werdnig–Hoffmann disease. Acta Neuropathol (Berl) 81: 408–417

Nonaka I, Koga Y, Okino E, Kikuchi A, Fujisawa K, Miyabayshi S (1988) Defects in muscle fibre growth in fatal infantile cytochrome-C oxidase deficiency. Brain Dev 10: 223–230

Patel K, Voigt T, Dunn MJ, Strong PN, Dubowitz V (1988) Dystrophin and nebulin in the muscular dystrophies. J Neurol Sci 87: 315–326
Periasamy M, Wieczorek DF, Nadal-Ginard B (1985) Characterisation of a developmentally regulated perinatal myosin heavy chain expressed in skeletal muscle. J Biol Chem 259: 13573–13578
Poirier J, Gray F, Escourolle R (eds) (1989) Manuel de neuropathologie, 3rd edn. Masson, Paris
Pons F, Léger JOC, Chevallay M, Tomé FMS, Fardeau M, Léger J-J (1986) Immunocytochemical analysis of myosin heavy chains in human fetal muscles. J Neurol Sci 76: 151–163
Ringqvist M, Ringqvist I, Thornell L-E (1977) Differentiation of fibres in human masseter, temporal and biceps brachii muscles. J Neurol Sci 32: 265–273
Sahgal VS, Bernes S, Sahgal S, Lischwey C, Subramani V (1983) Skeletal muscle in preterm infants with congenital myotonic dystrophy. Morphologic and histochemical study. J Neurol Sci 59: 47–55
Santavuori P, Leisti J, Kruss S (1977) Muscle, eye and brain disease: a new syndrome. Neuropädiatrie 8: 550–553
Sarnat SB, Silbert SW (1976) Maturational arrest of fetal muscle in neonatal myotonic dystrophy. Arch Neurol 33: 466–474
Sawchak JA, Benoff B, Sher JH, Shafiq SA (1990) Werdnig-Hoffmann disease: myosin isoform expression not arrested at prenatal stage of development. J Neurol Sci 95: 183–192
Schmalbruch H, Kamieniecka Z, Arrøe M (1987) Early fatal nemaline myopathy: case report and review. Dev Med Child Neurol 29: 800–804
Schochet SS (1986) Diagnostic pathology of skeletal muscle and nerve. Appleton, Norwalk
Sewry CA (1985) Ultrastructural changes in diseased muscle. In: Dubowitz V (ed) Muscle biopsy. A practical approach. Baillière Tindall, London, pp 129–183
Sewry CA (1989) Contribution of immunocytochemistry to the pathogenesis of spinal muscular atrophy. In: Merlini L, Granata C, Dubowitz V (eds) Current concepts in childhood spinal muscular atrophy. A Gaggi, Bologna, pp 57–68
Sher JH, Rimalovski AB, Athanassiades TJ, Aronson SM (1967) Familial centronuclear myopathy: a clinical and pathological study. Neurology 17: 727–742
Shevell M, Rosenblatt B, Silver K, Carpenter S, Karpati G (1990) Congenital inflammatory myopathy. Neurology 40: 1111–1117
Shinomura C, Nonaka I (1989) Nemaline myopathy: comparative muscle histochemistry in the severe neonatal, moderate congenital, and adult-onset forms. Pediatr Neurol 5: 25–31
Shy GM, Magee KR (1956) A new congenital non-progressive myopathy. Brain 79: 610–620
Shy GM, Engel WK, Somers JE, Warko T (1963) Nemaline myopathy: a new congenital myopathy. Brain 86: 793–810
Spiro AJ, Shy GM, Gonatas NK (1966) Myotubular myopathy: persistence of fetal muscle in an adolescent boy. Arch Neurol 14: 1–14
Stockdale FE, Miller JB (1987) The cellular basis of myosin heavy chain isoform expression during development of avian skeletal muscles. Dev Biol 123: 1–9
Takada K, Nakamura H, Tanaka J (1984) Cortical dysplasia in congenital muscular dystrophy with central nervous system involvement (Fukuyama type). J Neuropathol Exp Neurol 43: 395–407
Tanabe Y, Nonaka I (1987) Congenital myotonic dystrophy. Changes in muscle pathology with ageing. J Neurol Sci 77: 59–68
Thompson CE (1982) Infantile myositis. Dev Med Child Neurol 24: 307–313
Thornell L-E, Billeter R, Butler-Browne GS, Eriksson P-O, Ringqvist M, Whalen RG (1984) Development of fibre types in human fetal muscle. An immunocytochemical study. J Neurol Sci 66: 107–115
Vanier TM (1960) Dystrophia myotonica in childhood. Br Med J ii: 1284–1288
Van Wijngaarden GK, Fleury P, Bethlem J, Meijer AEFH (1969) Familial "myotubular" myopathy. Neurology 19: 901–908
Vivarelli E, Brown WE, Whalen RG, Cossu G (1988) The expression of slow myosin during mammalian somitogenesis and limb bud differentiation. J Cell Biol 107: 2191–2197
Walton JN (1956) Amyotonia congenita: a follow-up study. Lancet i: 1023–1028
Whalen RG, Sell SM, Butler-Browne GS, Schwartz K, Bouveret P, Pinset-Harmström I (1981) Three myosin heavy chains appear sequentially in rat muscle development. Nature 292: 805–809
Whalen RG, Butler-Browne GS, Bugaiski LB, Harris JB, Herlicoviez D (1985) Myosin isozyme expression in developing and regenerating rat muscle. In: Strohman RC, Wolf S (eds) Gene expression in muscle. Adv Exp Med Biol 182: 193–199
Wohlfart G (1937) Über das Vorkommen verscheidener Arten von Muskelfasern in der Skelettmuskulatur der Menschen und einiger Säugetiere. Acta Psychiatr Neurol Scand 12 suppl: 1–119
Yamaguchi M, Robson RM, Stromer MH, Dahl DS, Oda T (1978) Actin filaments form the backbone of nemaline myopathy rods. Nature 271: 265–267
Zellweger H, Afifi A, McCormick WF, Mergner W (1967) Severe congenital muscular dystrophy. Am J Dis Child 114: 591–602

Chapter 26

The Skeletal System

Hans J. van der Harten

Introduction

The different phenotypes of disturbances of skeletal development have for centuries fascinated artists as well as medical men. As an example of achondroplasia, one may admire the painting *Don Sebastian de Mora* by Velasquez, in the Prado, Madrid. There are, at present, more than 500 disorders known in which the skeleton is involved. These are mostly congenital disorders and are, in part, genetic in nature. The birth prevalence of each disorder is low but, as a whole, they constitute a significant body of disease in childhood. Reliable estimates on their frequency are scarce. The overall frequency among stillbirths and liveborns has been estimated to be 1 per 4000 births and the frequency among perinatal deaths is 1 per 110 deaths (Camera et al. 1982; Orioli et al. 1986).

The recognition of congenital abnormalities and the classification of syndromes in general requires careful attention to detail. This is particularly true for the rare congenital skeletal dysplasias incompatible with life. Besides documentation of external abnormalities in such cases, radiographic examination of the skeleton before necropsy is essential (Winter et al. 1984). The diagnosis is made primarily on radiological features, although the remainder of the post-mortem examination is still important. Interpretation of the radiographs should be based on the knowledge of morphology and dimensions of the normal skeleton in all stages of development (van der Harten et al. 1990). Histological examination of cartilage and bone may clinch the diagnosis in some forms of dysplasia. In cases of suspected lethal bone dysplasia, the following radiograph examinations should be undertaken: anteroposterior view of the whole body (babygram); lateral view of the whole body; lateral view of the skull; hand and foot separately (Cremin and Beighton 1978; Kozlowski 1985). In order to demonstrate ossification in very young fetuses more clearly, the contrast in the radiographs is increased by immersion of the whole body overnight in a 0.5% aqueous solution of silver nitrate (O'Rahilly and Meyer 1956; Fig. 26.1).

Histological examination of cartilage and bone is primarily directed at the growth plate (Yang et al. 1976; Sillence et al. 1979; Gilbert et al. 1987).For adequate examination the head of humerus and femur are necessary, in addition to trachea, vertebrae and costochondral junction of a rib. The severity of radiographic abnormality of the metaphysis parallels the degree of disorganisation at the growth plate on histological examination.

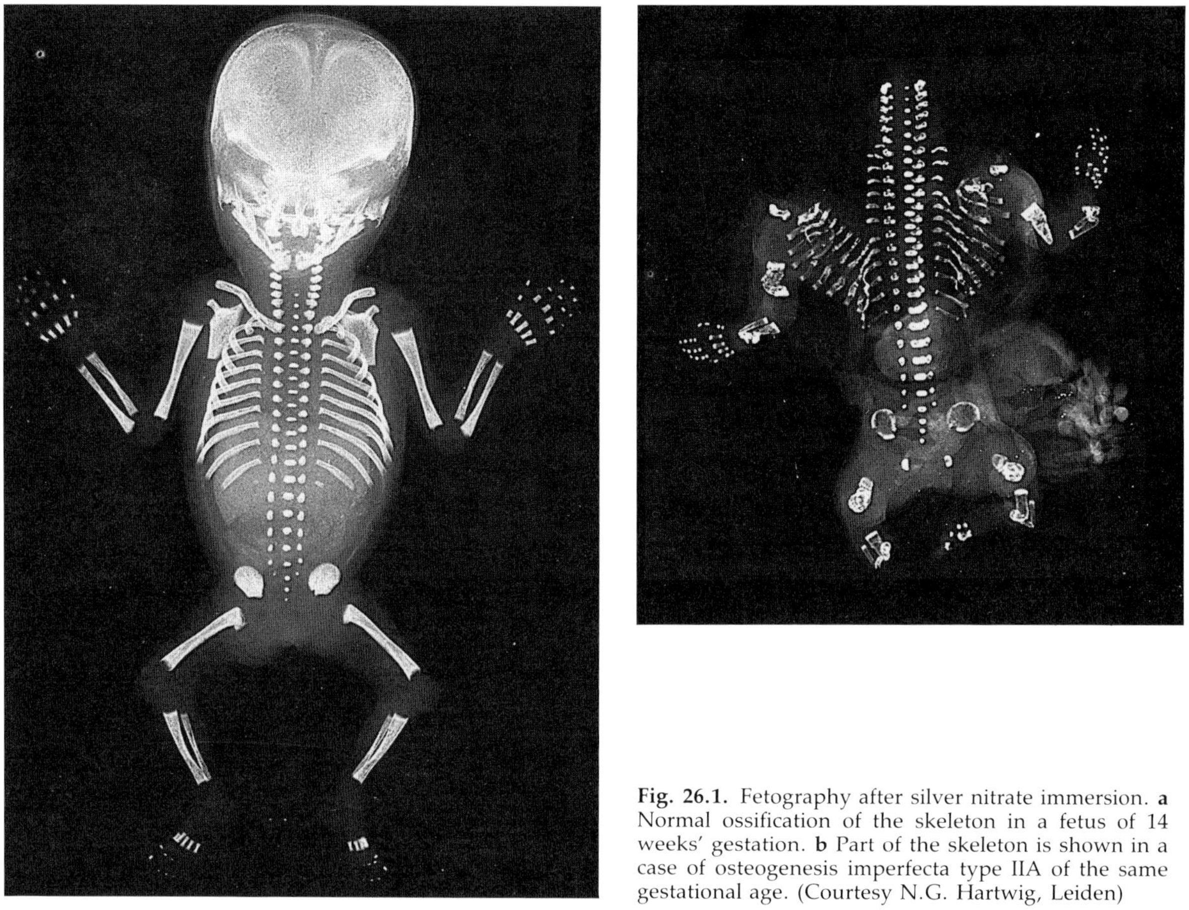

Fig. 26.1. Fetography after silver nitrate immersion. **a** Normal ossification of the skeleton in a fetus of 14 weeks' gestation. **b** Part of the skeleton is shown in a case of osteogenesis imperfecta type IIA of the same gestational age. (Courtesy N.G. Hartwig, Leiden)

Normal Development of the Skeleton

The skeleton develops in the embryo from mesoderm through the process of enchondral and intramembranous ossification. Consideration of endochondral ossification which takes place at the growth plate is particularly important in generalised skeletal dysplasias (Brighton 1984). This plate determines the longitudinal growth of long bones, and there are abnormalities in osteochondrodysplasia which may or may not be characteristic.

The transformation of cartilage into bone is a complicated and incompletely understood process in which collagen and the proteoglycans that give cartilage its tensile strength and elasticity, play an important role (Buckwalter 1983; Hunter 1991). In this chondro-osseous transformation, several layers with characteristic histological findings may be distinguished. Starting at the pre-epiphysial cartilage and moving towards the metaphysis the growth plate is made up of:

1. The reserve or resting cartilage in which cells are arranged in a regular fashion and embedded in a matrix of proteoglycans and collagen. A perichondrocyte lacunar space is present but is narrow compared with cells in other zones.
2. The proliferative cartilage in which cells are flattened and arranged in parallel rows that are separated by longitudinal and horizontal septa formed of matrix.
3. The hypertrophic cartilage, likewise arranged in columns, in which lacunae are expanded. In conventional histological sections the chondrocytes are shrivelled and appear degenerate. At the border of the metaphysis, calcium is precipitated in the longitudinal septa with formation of trabeculae (primary spongiosum). Osteoblast and osteoclast

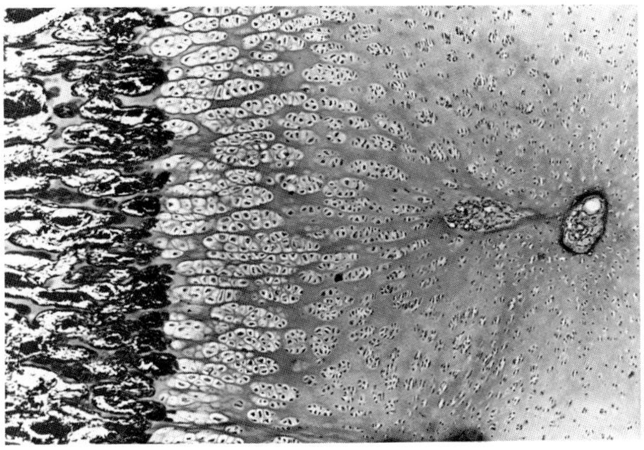

Fig. 26.2. Normal growth plate with resting, proliferative and hypertrophic cartilage and transformation of cartilage into bone. (Ladewig, ×33)

activity transform these trabeculae into trabecular bone (secondary spongiosum) (Fig. 26.2).

Osteochondrodysplasias

Osteochondrodysplasias are abnormalities of cartilage and of bone growth leading to faulty development of tubular bone and/or vertebrae. Before 1970, several classifications of the osteochondrodysplasias had been proposed because of confusion when different names were used by different authors for the same abnormality (Rubin 1964). Through the initiative of the European Society of Paediatric Radiology, a group of international experts convened in Paris in 1969 to formulate an acceptable nomenclature. Because of increasing interest in this field, which had led to the recognition of new types of dysplasia, this so-called Paris classification was revised in 1977 and again in 1983. The classification is based on clinical, radiological and anatomical criteria (Maroteaux et al. 1984); the first of the main subgroups, the osteochondrodysplasias, usually lethal before or shortly after birth (Table 26.1), is particularly important in the perinatal period and is the only group which will be considered in detail here. The correct diagnosis of lethal bone dysplasia is important because of the implications for parental counselling on the prospects for future pregnancies. Second trimester ultrasound diagnosis can be confidently offered in most cases (Hobbins et al. 1982; Wladimiroff et al. 1984; Brons et al. 1990; Romero et al. 1990). Diagnosis may follow the birth of an affected baby or the recognition of a complication of the pregnancy such as polyhydramnios, fetal hydrops or an inappropriately small uterine size for gestation. An increasing proportion of first affected babies are being identified during ultrasound examination in the second trimester of pregnancy for unrelated reasons. For this reason, too, the pathologist may find himself examining a fetus with a non-lethal type of dysplasia. Findings in other bone dysplasias are detailed by Beighton 1988.

Table 26.1. International nomenclature of constitutional diseases of bone (Paris Classification), first group. Mode of transmission has been noted only if well proven

Abnormalities of cartilage and/or bone growth and development	
Defects of growth of tubular bones and/or spine	
Identifiable at birth—Usually lethal before or shortly after birth	
Achondrogenesis type I (Parenti–Fraccaro)	AR
Achondrogenesis type II (Langer–Saldino)	
Hypochondrogenesis	
Fibrochondrogenesis	AR
Thanatophoric dysplasia	
Thanatophoric dysplasia with cloverleaf skull	
Atelosteogenesis	
Short rib syndrome (with or without polydactyly)	
type I (Saldino–Noonan)	AR
type II (Majewski)	AR
type III (lethal thoracic dysplasia)	AR

Abbreviation: AR, autosomal recessive

Achondrogenesis, hypochondrogenesis

Achondrogenesis was described for the first time in 1936 by Parenti under the name "anosteogenesis" because of the minimal ossification of the cartilaginous skeleton. In 1952 Fraccaro described an identical case under the name "achondrogenesis". In 1969, Langer et al. and in 1971, Saldino used this name for a lethal dysplasia whose skeletal abnormalities differed from the cases described by Parenti and Fraccaro. After several authors had used this name it was listed and two subtypes were accepted, type I (Parenti–Fraccaro) and type II (Langer–Saldino). Recently a division of achondrogenesis type I into subtypes IA and IB was proposed on clinical, radiographic and histopathological features (Borochowitz et al. 1988; van der Harten et al. 1988a). Types IA/IB

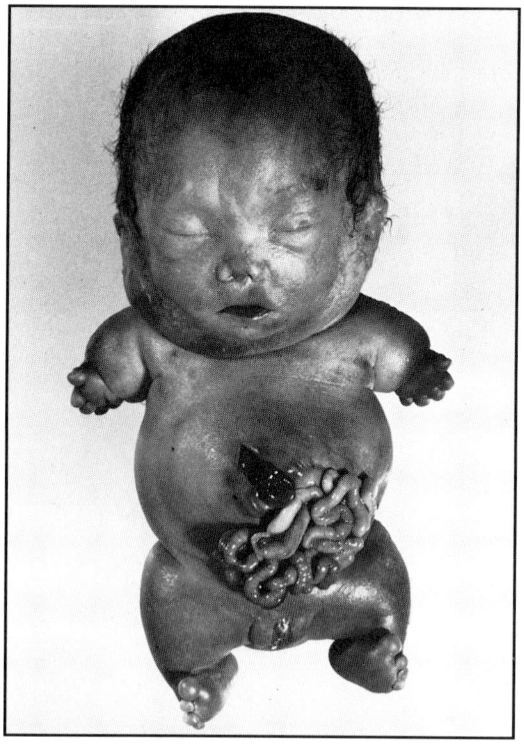

a

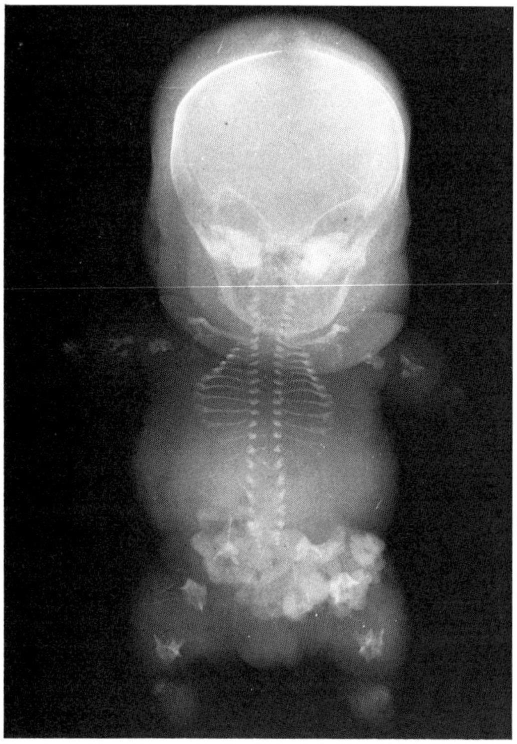

b

Fig. 26.3. **a** Achondrogenesis type IB (accidental rupture of abdominal wall during breech delivery) **b** Babygram illustrates cupped metaphysis with spiked spurs and lack of ossification of vertebral bodies.

and type II turned out to be histologically easily separable (Yang et al. 1976; Sillence et al. 1979a; Gilbert et al. 1987; van der Harten et al. 1988a). The transmission of types IA and IB has been shown to be autosomal recessive. Most cases of type II have been sporadic and are new dominant mutations (Godfrey and Hollister 1988).

Type I (Parenti–Fraccaro)

Type I achondrogenesis represents the most severe abnormality in the group of osteochondrodysplasias. It is lethal either before or shortly after birth. On external examination the extremely short limbs with very short hands and fingers, relatively large head, short trunk with protruding abdomen, and short neck are

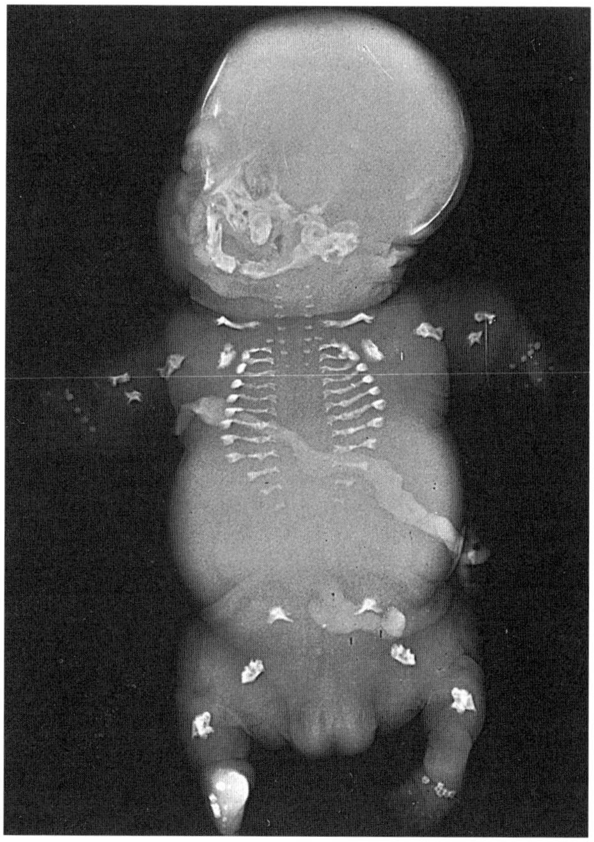

Fig. 26.4. Achondrogenesis type IA; in addition to Fig. 26.3b the babygram illustrates healing fractures of several ribs, nearly total absence of ossification of the spine and a partly ossified cranial fault. (Van der Harten et al. 1988a)

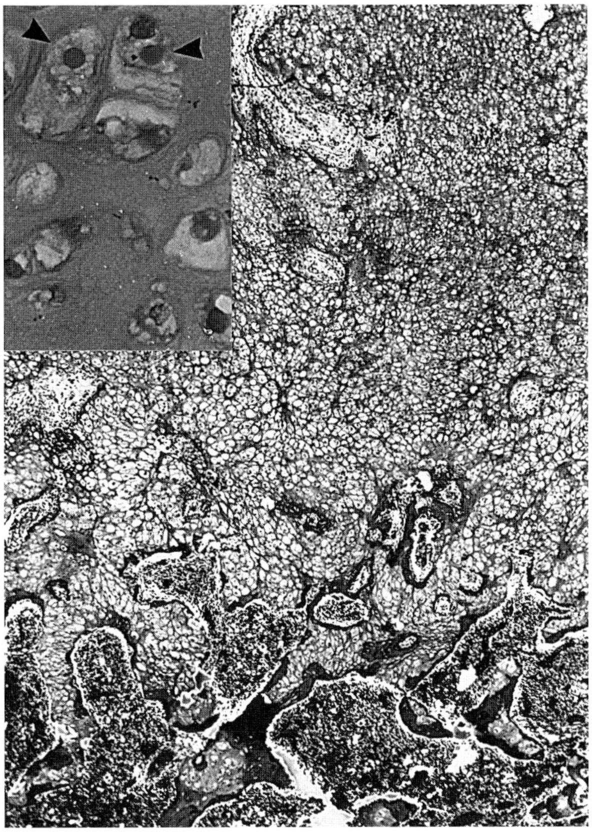

Fig. 26.5. Achondrogenesis type IA. The growth plate on the left shows marked disorganisation with total lack of columnisation of the chondrocytes. (Ladewig, ×24) (*Inset*) chondrocytes with dilated lacunae and intracytoplasmic inclusions "arrow heads". (PAS-diastase, ×380) (Van der Harten et al. 1988a)

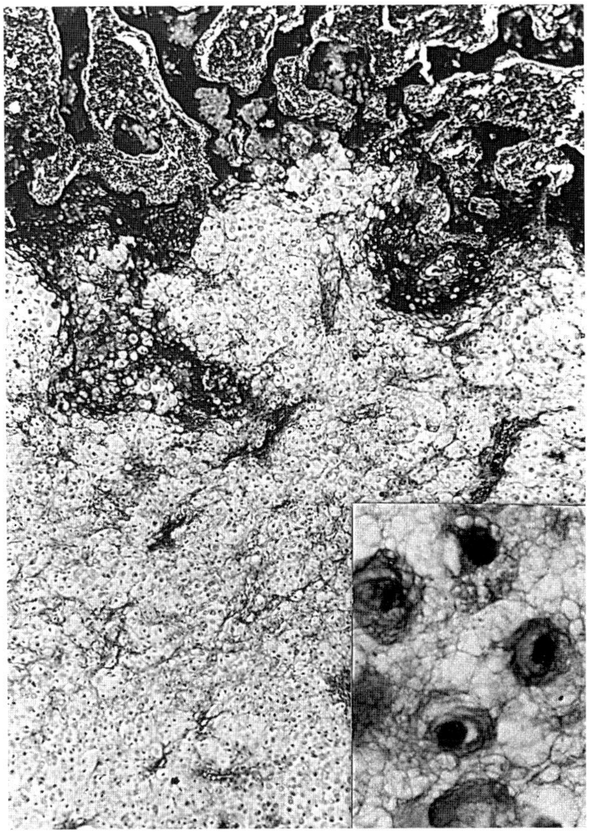

Fig. 26.6. Achondrogenesis type IB. The disorganised growth plate is comparable with Fig. 26.5. The cartilage matrix however is hardly stained. (Ladewig, ×30) (*Inset*) chondrocytes and intervening matrix with vacuolation, the lacunae are not dilated. Rings of condensed matrix surround the chondrocytes. (Ladewig, ×475) (Van der Harten et al. 1988a)

striking. Radiographically, extremely short tubular bones are seen in both types A and B, with metaphysial spikes or spurs in type B. The vertebrae show defective ossification, particularly in the cervical and lumbosacral region. The thorax is small and bell-shaped, the ribs show cupping of the metaphyses and, in type A, fractures of the diaphyses. Contrary to the normal ossification of the skull in type B, type A shows a membranous calvarium (Figs. 26.3 and 26.4).

At necropsy one seldom finds developmental anomalies of internal organs, but the lungs are hypoplastic.

Histological examination of the bones shows characteristic abnormalities. In both types endochondral ossification is disorganised. In type A the resting cartilage is hypercellular and the chondrocytes are clustered within a diffusely monochromatic matrix. These chondrocytes contain round or oval inclusions (Fig. 26.5). In type B the chondrocytes are vacuolated, more randomly dispersed and intracytoplasmic inclusions are not seen. The pericellular (territorial) matrix is condensed and forms rings around the chondrocytes. The intervening (interterritorial) matrix shows extreme vacuolation and is slightly stained (Figs. 26.6 and 26.7). The same appearances are seen in extraskeletal cartilage, e.g. the larynx. Because of the severe disturbances of the endochondral ossification of the long bones, the subperiosteal ossification is not limited to the upper border of the metaphysis, which explains the cupping seen on radiographs. In both types A and B, formation of columns in the proliferative and hypertrophic zones is barely present. Osseous trabeculae at the metaphysis are

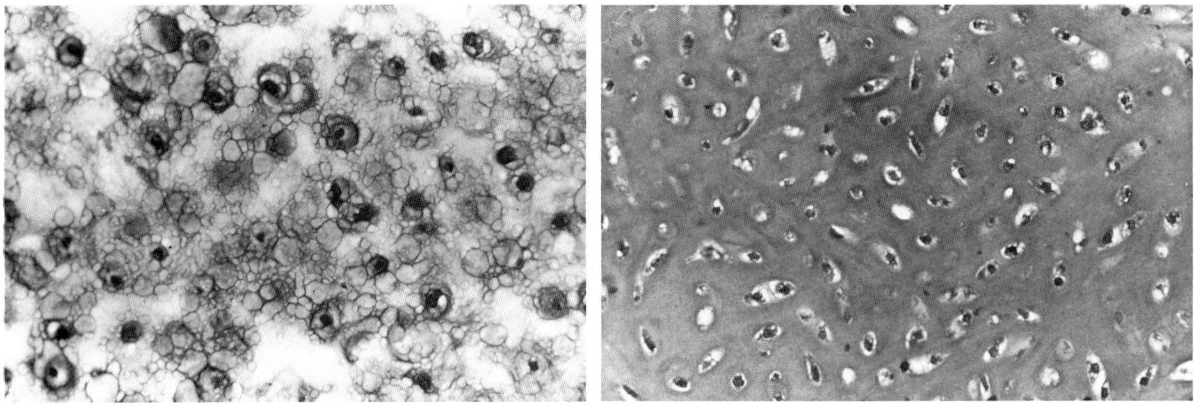

Fig. 26.7. **a** Achondrogenesis type IB. Resting cartilage with swollen chondrocytes and vacuolation of the intercellular matrix. (Alcian blue, ×211) **b** Resting cartilage from normal control of same gestational age. (Alcian blue, ×211)

irregularly arranged, broader than normal and extend in a transverse direction. Because of the extremely underdeveloped skeleton, the abnormalities are clearly visible by ultrasound early in the second trimester (Romero et al. 1990). It seems likely, that a basic defect in cellular function of the chondrocytes results in a deficient cartilage matrix and in disorganised endochondral ossification (van der Harten et al. 1988a).

Type II (Langer–Saldino)

The phenotype of type II achondrogenesis differs little from type I, but development of

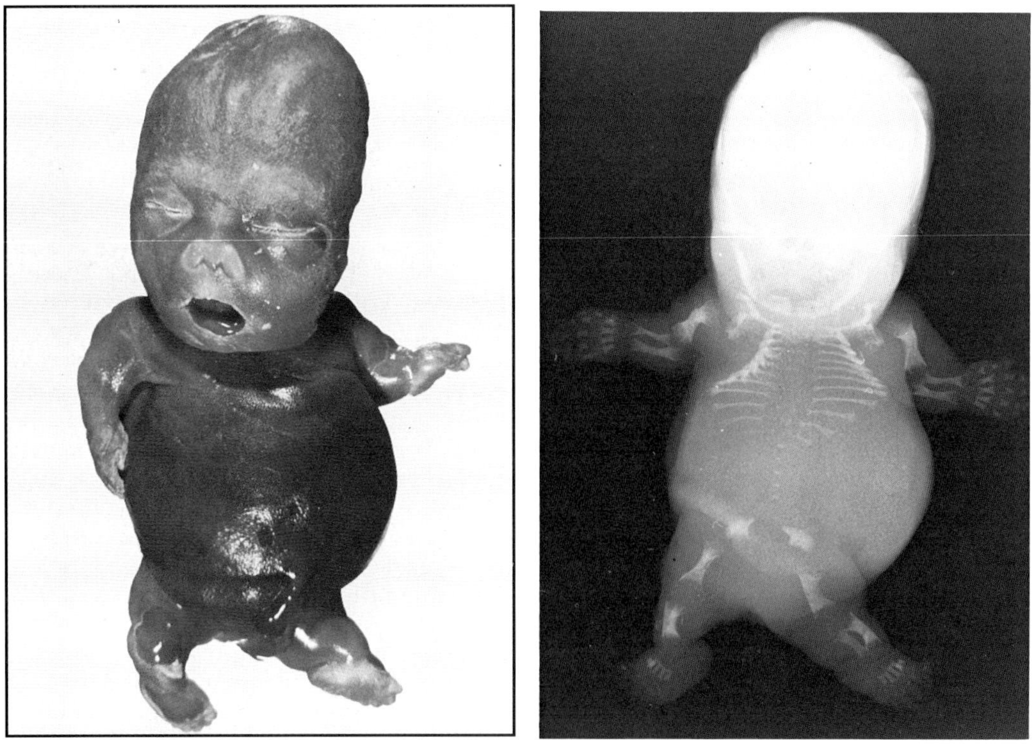

Fig. 26.8. **a** Achondrogenesis type II. **b** Babygram. The tubular bones are more developed than in type I. (Courtesy of Dr. J.C. den Hollander, Rotterdam)

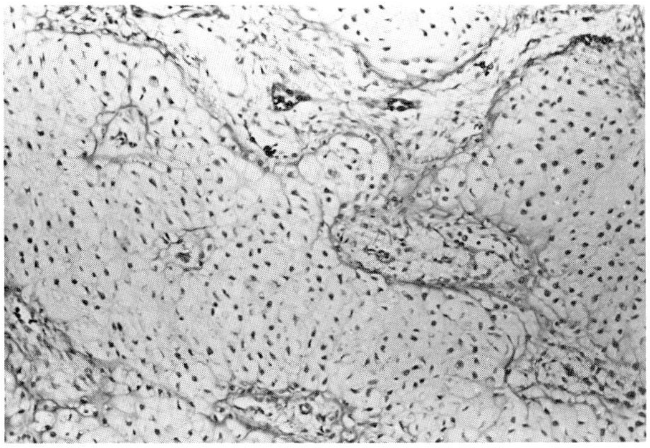

Fig. 26.9. Achondrogenesis type II. Resting cartilage of tubular bone with prominent vascular channels between swollen chondrocytes. (Ladewig, ×82)

hands and feet is better (Fig. 26.8). Radiographically, shortening of the tubular bones is not as marked as in type I, but disturbance of vertebral ossification is striking. There is seldom coexistent disturbance of organ development apart from pulmonary hypoplasia. The difference from type I is clear from the histological examination of resting cartilage. It is quite cellular and resembles fetal cartilage. Chondrocytes are swollen and matrix is reduced in volume. Most striking, however, are the large numbers of stellate vascular channels (Fig. 26.9) with abundant fibrous tissue (Stanescu et al. 1977; Chen et al. 1981). The disorganisation of the growth plate differs little from that of type I, but the formation of columns is focally distinct. Vascular channels are also found in the cartilages of larynx and trachea (Fig. 26.10). Even as in type I, the skeletal abnormalities are clearly visible by ultrasound early in the second trimester. In recent studies a defect in the biosynthesis of type II collagen and a decrease in the amount of proteoglycans e.g. chondroitin-4-sulphate have been found (Godfrey and Hollister 1988; van der Harten et al. 1988a; Feshchenko et al. 1989; Horton et al. 1989).

a

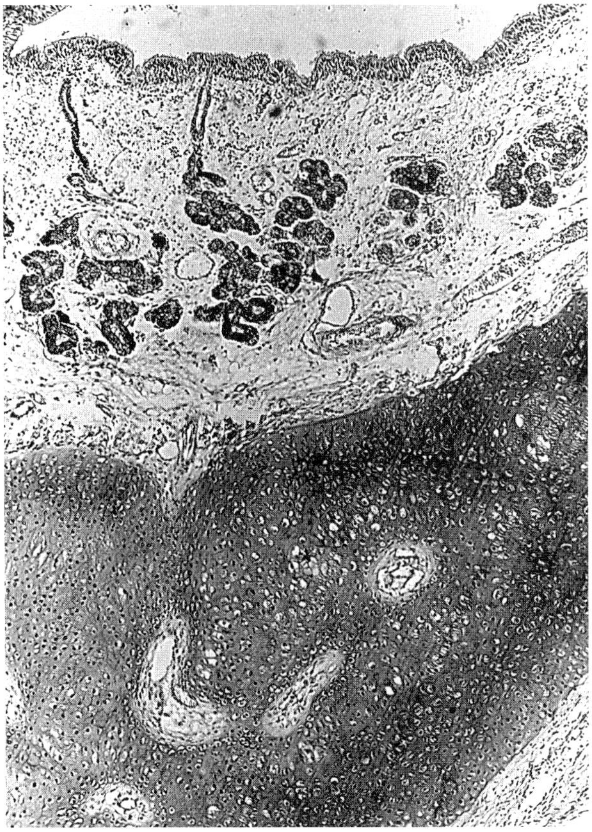

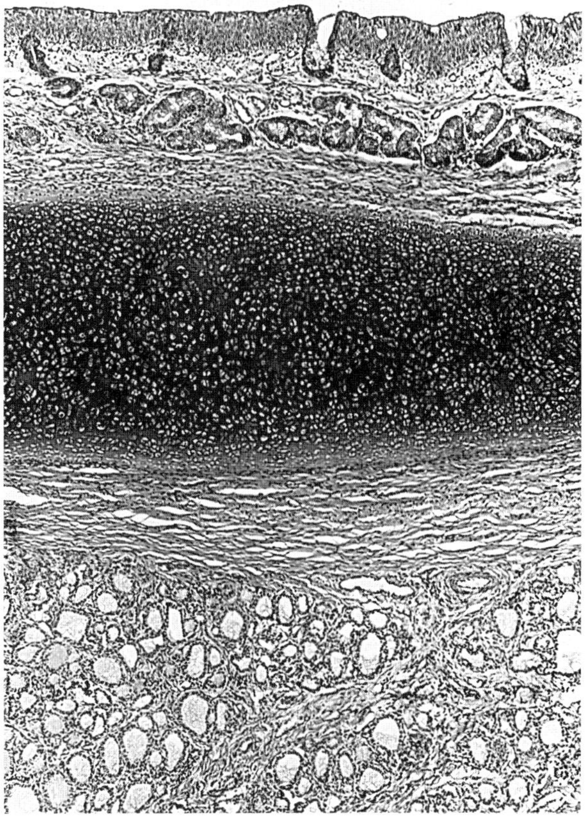

b

Fig. 26.10. a Achondrogenesis type II. Section of trachea with vascular channels in cartilage. (Ladewig, ×48) **b** Section of trachea from normal control of same gestational age. (Ladewig, ×46)

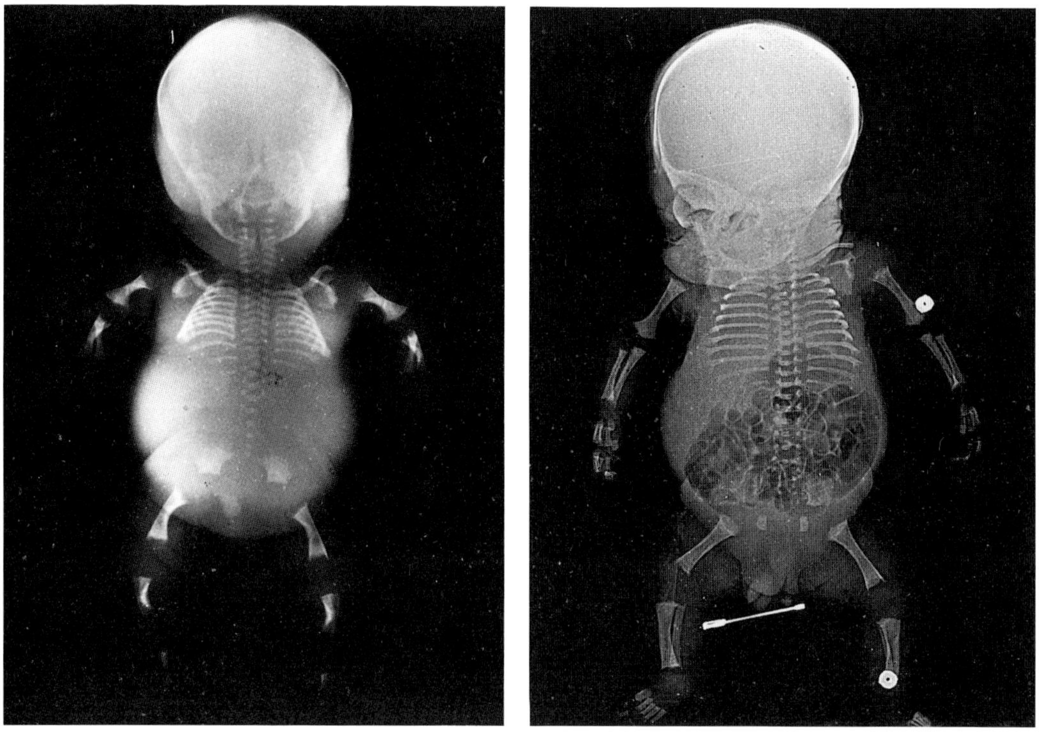

a b

Fig. 26.11. Achondrogenesis II/hypochondrogenesis. **a** Achondrogenesis type II, babygram transitional form. The limbs are not as short as in the severe form and the spine is more ossified than in Fig. 26.8. **b** Babygram hypochondrogenesis. The long bones are straight, the vertebral bodies more developed, except in the cervical and sacral regions. (Van der Harten et al. 1988a)

Hypochondrogenesis

The dysplasia known as hypochondrogenesis was officially accepted as an entity at the last revision of the Paris nomenclature in 1984. It is an example of phenotypic variability of expression which can exist within one dysplasia (Maroteaux et al. 1983). Hypochondrogenesis represents a mild form of type II achondrogenesis in which the skeleton is radiographically better developed (Fig. 26.11). The deficient ossification of the vertebral column, particularly of sacral and cervical vertebrae, is still distinct. At one end of the spectrum, distinction from type II achondrogenesis may be difficult (Borochowitz 1984). Whitley and Gorlin (1983) introduced the femoral cylinder index (maximum femoral length divided by the width at mid shaft). On this basis, four types of achondrogenesis can be distinguished; type IV is synonymous with hypochondrogenesis. Within the different groups, affected siblings are found to be concordant for phenotype.

As with type II achondrogenesis it is not yet certain that hypochondrogenesis is inherited in an autosomal-recessive manner or represents an autosomal-dominant mutation. At the other end of the spectrum it may be difficult to distinguish between hypochondrogenesis and spondyloepiphyseal dysplasia congenita (SEDC) in the neonatal period (McPherson and Wood 1980; Maroteaux et al. 1983). However, SEDC is generally compatible with life, whilst survival in hypochondrogenesis is usually short.

Histological examination of the growth plate is important in the differential diagnosis. In hypochondrogenesis, cartilage has the same characteristics as in type II achondrogenesis. Numerous dilated vascular channels dominate the picture and there is obvious perivascular fibrosis (Fig. 26.12). Disturbance in the formation of the growth plate is also present although not as obvious (Fig. 26.13).

Fibrochondrogenesis

Fibrochondrogenesis is a rare dysplasia which, besides the radiographic findings, can be

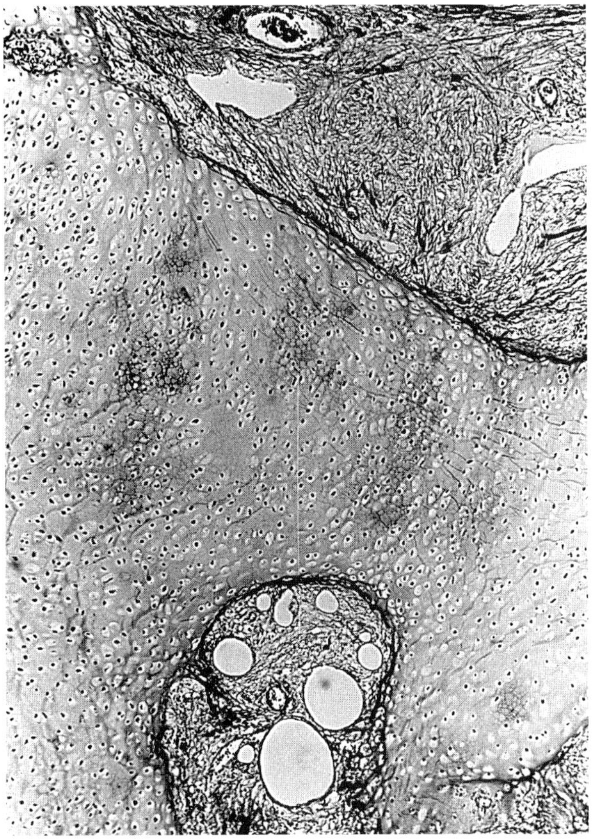

Fig. 26.12. Hypochondrogenesis. Resting cartilage with prominent vascular channels and abundant perivascular fibrosis. (Ladewig, ×49)

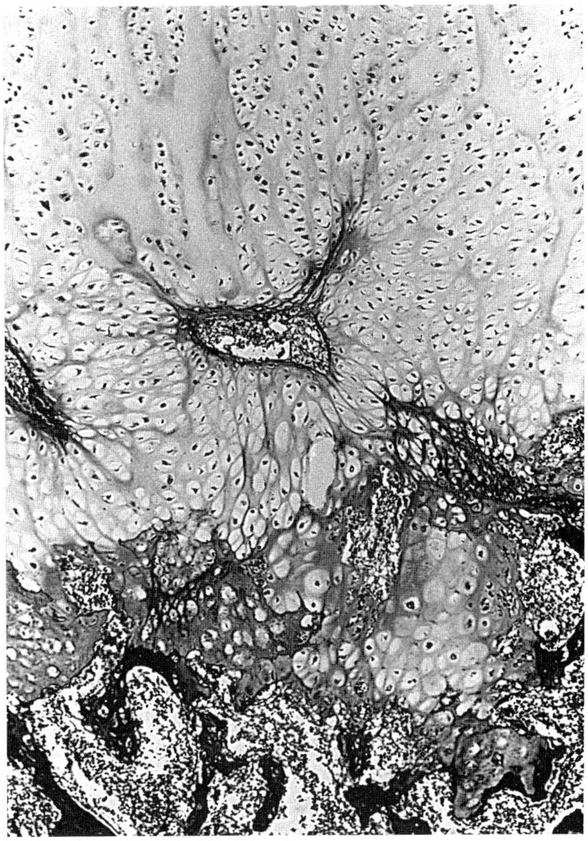

Fig. 26.13. Hypochondrogenesis. Growth plate with marked disorganisation, especially of the hypertrophic and transformation zones. (Ladewig, ×48)

distinguished with certainty from achondrogenesis by the histological appearance of resting cartilage. The chondrocytes are spindle shaped, resemble fibroblasts and are separated into groups by a meshwork of collagen fibres (Fig. 26.14). In the proliferative and hypertrophic zones, formation of irregular columns is seen (Lazzaroni-Fossati et al. 1978; Bankier et al. 1991). Occurrence in sibs suggests autosomal-recessive inheritance.

Thanatophoric Dysplasia

Thanatophoric dysplasia is the commonest type of lethal chondrodysplasia and was distinguished from classic achondroplasia by Maroteaux et al. in 1967. Unlike achondroplasia this dysplasia is not normally compatible with life (hence the name, derived from Greek *thanatos*, death and *phorus*, seeking). The longer survival of some patients reflects modern neonatal care (MacDonald et al. 1989). It is probably a sporadic dominant mutation as is usually the case in achondroplasia (Serville et al. 1984).

Classic Type

In contrast to the previously described dysplasias, in thanatophoric dysplasia the trunk is relatively long but the limbs are short with exo- or endorotation of legs and feet (Fig. 26.15). The head is relatively large with craniofacial disproportion. Radiographically the skeleton shows platyspondyly with U- or H-shaped vertebrae. The ribs are short, making the thorax narrow and pear or barrel shaped. The most striking radiographic characteristic is bowing of the shortened femur, the so-called telephone receiver (Fig. 26.16), with cupping and flaring of metaphyses. Variation of ex-

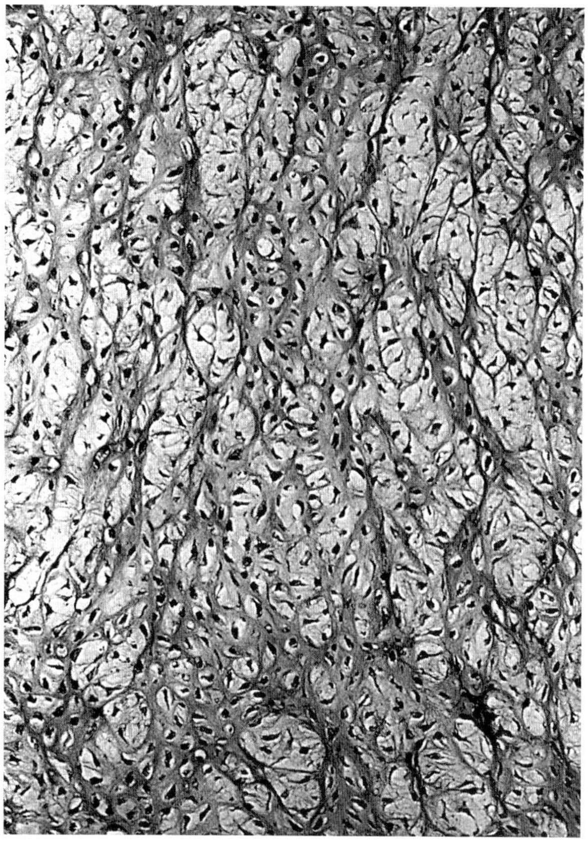

Fig. 26.14. Fibrochondrogenesis. Resting cartilage with spindle-shaped chondrocytes in a meshwork of collagen fibres. (Ladewig, ×120)

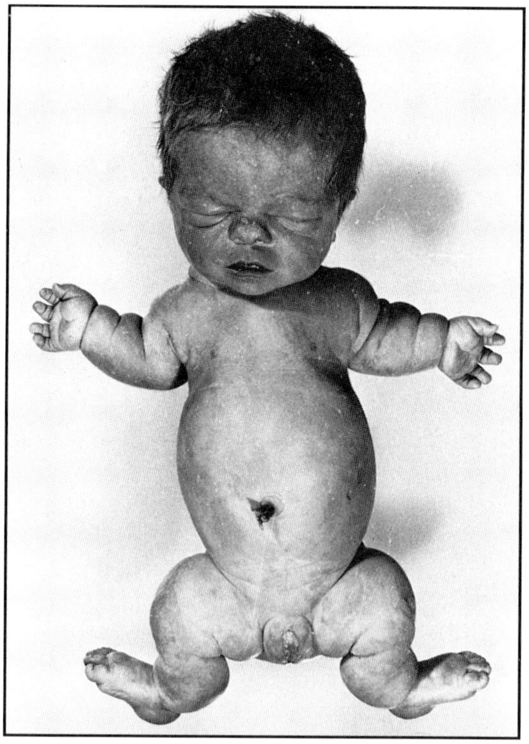

a

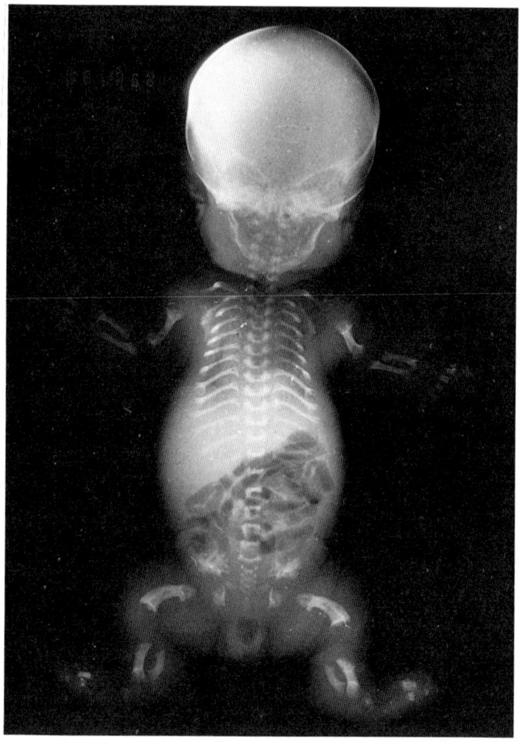

b

Fig. 26.15. a Thanatophoric dysplasia. Short limbs and relatively long trunk compared with achondrogenesis. **b** Babygram illustrates platyspondyly with U-shaped vertebrae, short ribs and typical bowing of femora.

pression, as seen in achondrogenesis and achondroplasia, is not observed in thanatophoric dysplasia; the underlying defect is so far unidentified.

Histologically, the resting cartilage has normal cellular density with an abundant homogeneous matrix. Enchondral ossification is severly disturbed (Fig. 26.17). Hypertrophic chondrocytes are recognisable but in disorderly arrangement. The most characteristic abnormality is hypertrophy of the perichondrial ring with penetration of the growth plate (Fig. 26.18) so that fibrous dysplasia with formation of plump haphazardly arranged bony trabeculae is apparent (Maroteaux et al. 1976; Ornoy et al. 1985a). This fibrous dysplasia of the growth plate is not uniform. Abnormalities in the central nervous system (CNS) have been described and mainly affect the temporal lobe (Wongmongkolrit et al. 1983; Ho et al. 1984; Knisely and Ambler 1988).

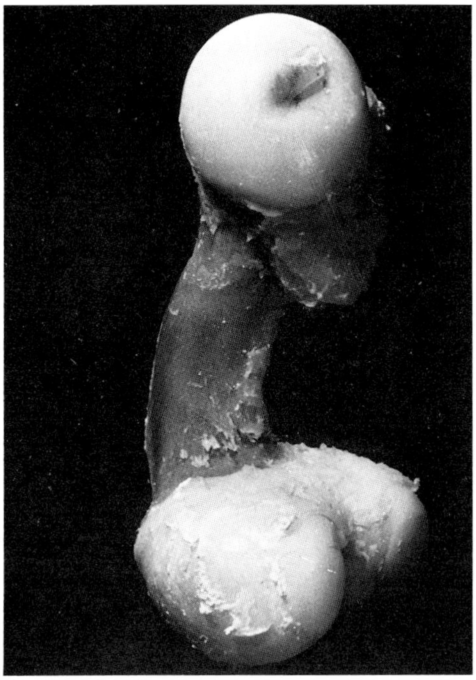

Fig. 26.16. Thanatophoric dysplasia. Femur with "telephone receiver" shape.

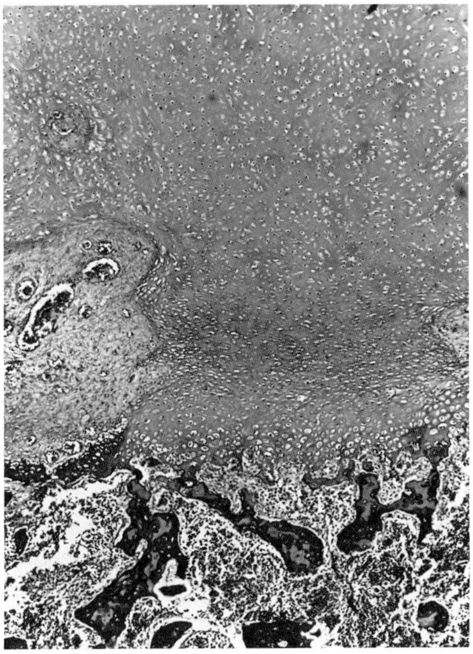

Fig. 26.17. Thanatophoric dysplasia. Growth plate with disturbed endochondral ossification. On the *left* a focus of fibrous dysplasia. (Ladewig, ×38)

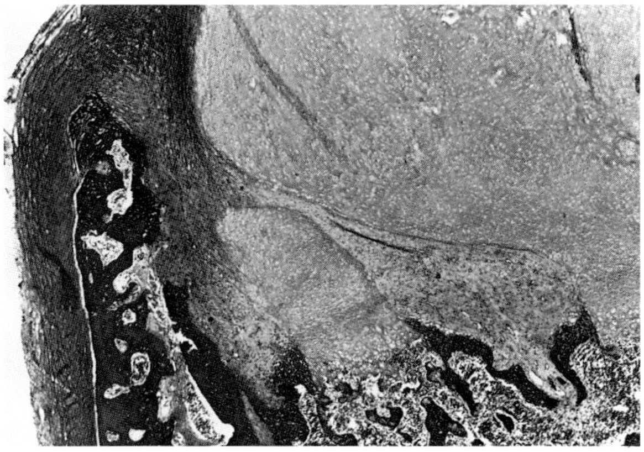

Fig. 26.18. Thanatophoric dysplasia. *Left*, overgrowth of subperiosteal ossification; *centre*, from *left* to *right*, fibrous tissue from the perichondreal ring penetrates the growth plate. (Ladewig, ×20)

Thanatophoric Dysplasia with Cloverleaf Skull

In 1960, Holtermüller and Wiedemann described a form of craniosynostosis with trilocular configuration of the cranium and severe internal hydrocephalus, under the name *Kleeblattschädel*. Thanatophoric dysplasia may be accompanied, rarely, by a mild type of cloverleaf skull (Fig. 26.19). The presence of two different abnormalities was shown by the report of identical twins who were concordant for thanatophoric dysplasia and discordant for the cloverleaf skull (Horton et al. 1983). The abnormalities of the remainder of the skeleton and the histological appearance of the growth plate are identical to those seen in thanatophoric dysplasia without craniosynostosis. Recently a different type of thanatophoric dysplasia has been described, the so-called generalised bone dysplasia, with straight femora and a cloverleaf skull that is usually severe (Langer et al. 1987).

Atelosteogenesis

Atelosteogenesis (AO) is a relatively new disorder which was first described by Kozlowski et al. in 1981 as a new form of lethal short limb skeletal dysplasia. Maroteaux et al. (1982) proposed the name "atelosteogenesis" (derived from Greek *ateles*, incomplete, +*osteon* +*genesis*, bone development) for six newly described cases; the term was accepted in the 1983 revision of international nomenclature. It is characterised by rhizomelic (proximal) micromelia,

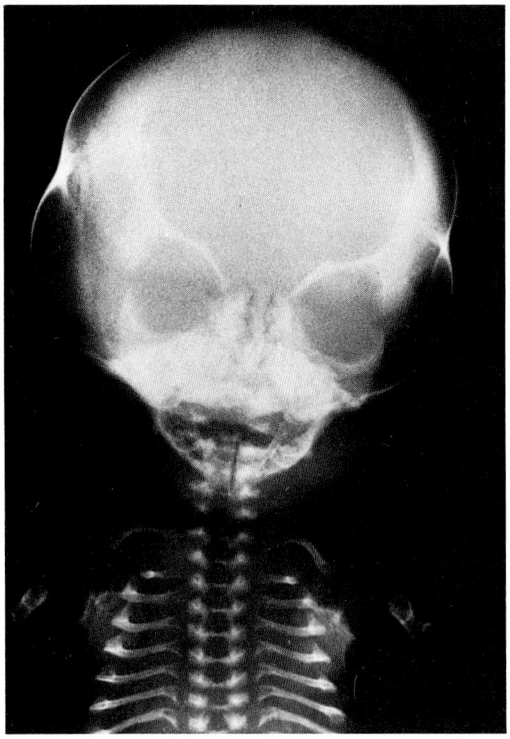

Fig. 26.19. Thanatophoric dysplasia with cloverleaf skull, craniosynostosis with trilocular configuration. (Courtesy of Dr. D. van Velzen, Delft)

bowing of the limbs together with subluxations of elbows, knees and ankles.

Radiographic examination is diagnostic. The most characteristic signs are distal hypoplasia and club-shaped femora and humeri together with hypoplastic/dysplastic changes in the hands and feet, which show lack of ossification of single phalanges and metacarpals. The fibula is hypoplastic or absent. Vertebral bodies show incomplete ossification with coronal clefts of lumbar vertebrae and hypoplasia of the upper vertebral bodies.

Histologically, resting cartilage shows focal hypocellular areas of matrix degeneration that extend into the growth plate with disruption of column formation. Giant, sometimes multinucleate chondrocytes have been described in the hypocellular areas in a few cases (Sillence et al. 1982) but they are not pathognomonic for this dysplasia (Hwang et al. 1982; Yang et al. 1983). Recently cases resembling AO but with distinctive radiographic and histopathological features were reported. In addition to the original description (AO I) the names AO II (Sillence et al. 1987) and AO III (Stern et al. 1990) have been proposed for these entities. Genotypic heterogeneity is present, since both AO I and III are sporadic, without reported recurrence and AO II has been reported in brothers, suggesting an autosomal-recessive trait.

Short Rib Polydactyly Syndromes

Short ribs are present in many different skeletal dysplasias, both lethal and non-lethal types, e.g. thanatophoric dysplasia, asphyxiating thoracic dysplasia (Jeune syndrome) and chondroectodermal dysplasia (Ellis–van Creveld syndrome). The distinction between asphyxiating thoracic dysplasia and the short rib syndromes is not precise and in practice depends on the size of the thorax and the length of the infant's survival. These conditions may belong to the spectrum of a pathogenetic entity (Yang et al. 1987). Classification is based on the radiographic appearance (Spranger et al. 1974; Yang et al. 1980, 1987). These syndromes are often accompanied by anomalies of other systems. Besides cardiovascular defects and renal cystic dysplasia, sexual ambiguity is frequently found. Death is due to pulmonary hypoplasia secondary to the extremely narrow thorax. All the cases so far described have exhibited autosomal-recessive inheritance.

Type I (Saldino–Noonan)

In the condition known as Saldino–Noonan thoracic dysplasia the narrow thorax, short limbs and postaxial polydactyly of hands and/or feet are striking. Radiographic examination of the skeleton shows extremely short, horizontal ribs and a barrel-shaped thorax, dysplastic pelvis, platyspondyly with distorted vertebral bodies and short tubular bones with very irregular metaphyses (Saldino and Noonan 1972).

In about one-half to one-third of the cases, congenital heart defect, renal cystic dysplasia and malformed genitals are found; cleft palate is an occasional association. At the growth plate, disorganisation of the proliferative and hypertrophic zones with irregular column formation is found on histological examination. The transitional zone from cartilage to bone is irregular with small groups of chondrocytes localised in the metaphysis and trabeculae of newly formed bone extending into the cartilage.

This reflects the irregular radiographic appearance of the metaphysis.

Type II (Majewski)

In addition to the narrow thorax and short limbs, a median cleft lip is usually present. Polydactyly is preaxial as well as postaxial. Radiographically, the ribs are very short but spine and pelvis are normal. Unlike type I, the short tubular bones have a smooth metaphysis while the tibia is dysproportionately short and oval (Fig. 26.20). Renal cystic dysplasia is found in 50% of cases but heart defects are rare (Majewski et al. 1971; Chen et al. 1980). Histologically, a regular chondro-osseous transformation zone is seen, which is in keeping with the smooth radiographic appearance of the metaphysis. The proliferating and hypertrophic zones are narrow and have irregular columns (Fig. 26.21).

a

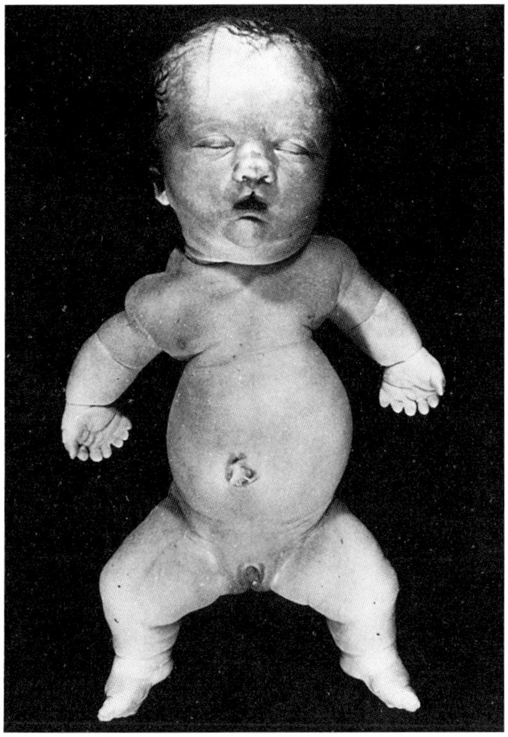

b

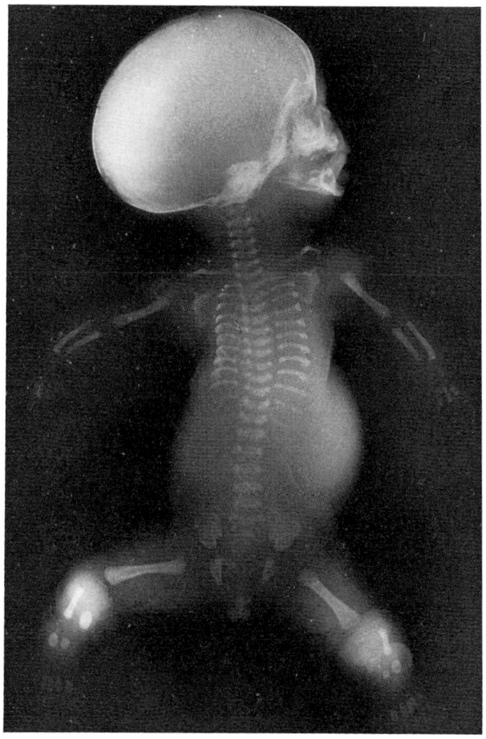

Fig. 26.20. **a** Short-rib syndrome with polydactyly type II. Note the characteristic median cleft lip. **b** Babygram illustrates marked short ribs, smooth metaphysis of the tubular bones, normal spine and pelvis. (Courtesy of Dr. Ph. Moerman, Leuven, Belgium)

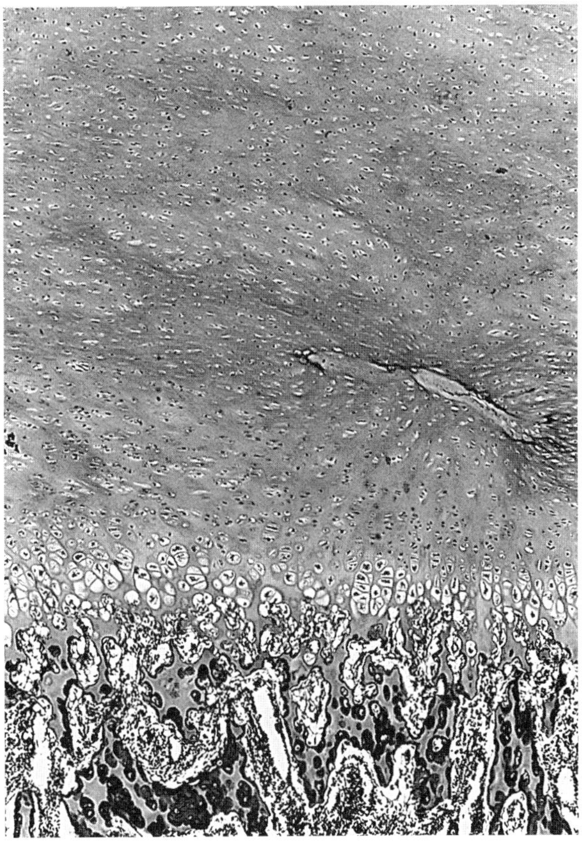

Fig. 26.21. Short-rib syndrome type II. Growth plate with narrow hypertrophic zone and irregular column formation. (Ladewig, ×47)

Type III (Lethal Thoracic Dysplasia)

Verma et al. (1975) and Naumoff et al. (1977) described several cases with short ribs and polydactyly which they considered distinct from type I on radiographic apearances. Doubt has been expressed about the appropriateness of such separation because of the substantial overlap between types I and III (Sillence 1980; Bernstein et al. 1985; Yang et al. 1987). Even polydactyly does not seem to be obligatory; cases have been described when all the radiographic criteria are met but polydactyly is absent (Sillence 1980; Beemer et al. 1983). In the International Nomenclature, type III has become a dustbin for all cases that do not fit into types I or II either phenotypically or radiographically. The histological appearance of the growth plate parallels metaphysial irregularity radiographically. Yang et al. (1980) described intracytoplasmic PAS-positive, diastase-resistant inclusions in the chondrocytes of type III, but they do not seem to be universally present (Sillence 1980).

Other Generalised Skeletal Abnormalities Associated with Perinatal Death

Many other skeletal dysplasias are recognisable before or after death; some of them must be mentioned briefly as they may be encountered at necropsy. Radiographic examination is important in the investigation of babies with these conditions. Many of these dysplasias are inherited in an autosomal-recessive fashion, so that all subsequent pregnancies are at risk and ultrasound monitoring is advisable.

Chondrodysplasia punctata, especially the rhizomelic type is a well-recognised disorder. It has to be differentiated from many other conditions in which stippled epiphyses are present (Sillence et al. 1979a).

Campomelic dysplasia is characterised by shortening and bowing (angulation) of the long bones. This syndrome is not yet clearly defined because increased curvature of the limbs may occur in many other bone dysplasias (Roth et al. 1982; Houston et al. 1983; Nogami et al. 1986; Roth et al. 1991). Affected males may have normal genitalia or female genitalia with streak-like gonadal rudiments, or any stage of male pseudohermaphroditism between these two extremes.

Curvature of long bones is also found when there is skeletal involvement in *cryptophthalmos (Fraser) syndrome* (Thomas et al. 1986; Fig. 26.22). Fraser (1962) described a combination of cryptophthalmos and syndactyly with additional anomalies including cleft lip and palate, laryngeal atresia or stenosis, renal, genital and anal abnormalities, inherited as an autosomal-recessive condition. The frequency of bilateral renal agenesis as part of this syndrome has been underestimated (Lurie and Cherstvoy 1984). In our experience, very marked shortening of all limbs may accompany renal agenesis, and a clinical diagnosis of short-limb dysplasia may be entertained.

Homozygous achondroplasia can only occur in the offspring of a couple of achondroplastic parents and is almost always lethal in early life.

In *diastrophic dysplasia,* characterised by short limbs and a short trunk, a typical "hitch hiker" thumb is present. This abduction deformity is caused by a shortened and abnormally shaped first metacarpal bone. The cartilage matrix shows cystic degeneration, the resting chondrocytes are irregular in distribution (Horton et al. 1979; Stanescu et al. 1984).

In *metatropic dysplasia* there are short extremities and the long bones show an enlarged metaphysis, the so-called barbell-like bones (Beck et al. 1983).

The differentiation of chondroectodermal dysplasia (Ellis–van Creveld) from asphyxiating thoracic dysplasia (Jeune) and from the short-rib syndromes may be difficult, even on radiological grounds (see p. 630).

In the group of congenital spondyloepiphyseal dysplasias an early lethal form has been described, resembling hypochondrogenesis. However, the growth plate abnormalities are less severe and the chondrocytes contain PAS-positive, diastase-resistant inclusions.

Kniest dysplasia and *dyssegmental dysplasia* are examples in which, apart from the radiological criteria, histological examination of the bone and cartilage may be helpful for diagnosis (Horton and Rimoin 1979; Greco et al. 1984).

Another example of a well-known generalised skeletal disorder is *osteogenesis imperfecta* (the brittle bone disease), of which different types and subtypes have been described (Sillence et al. 1979b, 1984; Maroteaux et al. 1986). The "Sillence classification" has gained wide usage. The classification describes four

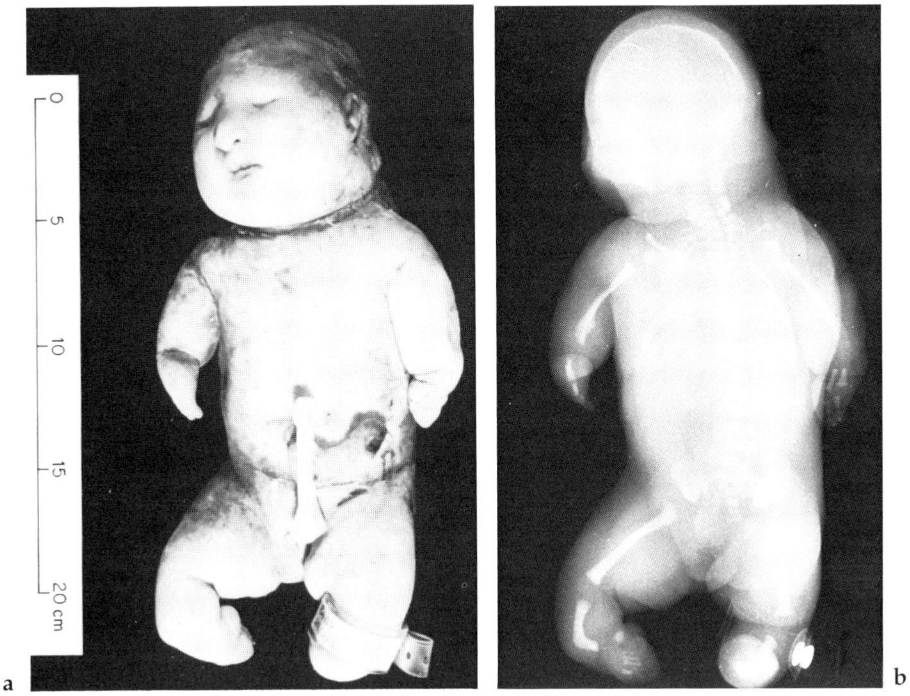

Fig. 26.22. Cryptophthalmos (Fraser) syndrome. **a** Broad nose, short forearm, syndactyly and bowed lower leg. **b** Babygram illustrates short radius and ulna, bowing of the tibia with absent fibula. (Courtesy of Dr. J.W. Keeling, Edinburgh)

categories of which type II is the perinatal lethal type. Within type II there are three separate variants, A, B and C, which can be distinguished by radiography. Formerly type II was thought to be autosomal recessively inherited but it is now clear that besides this type of transmission, many sporadic cases, especially of type II A, may be found and interpreted as new dominant mutations (Thompson et al. 1987; Young et al. 1987). The period of gestation during which a certain type of osteogenesis imperfecta may be demonstrated or excluded by ultrasound will vary according to the type of osteogenesis imperfecta. Type II A, for example, has been diagnosed as early as 15 weeks' gestation (Brons et al. 1988a). Although type III is usually non-lethal, it may be very difficult to separate from type II B on radiographs. In view of this, it has been postulated that type II B is the severe end of the type III spectrum. Type II A is the most severe form of osteogenesis imperfecta and characterised on radiographs by severe osteopenia and shortened, deformed bones, with "harmonica" shape caused by numerous fractures and contiguous beading of the ribs. The skull is soft due to reduction of ossification of the cranial vault (Fig. 26.23). Type II B and type III show wavy thin ribs and few fractures on the radiographs. The skull bones are recognisable with scattered small spots of ossification (Fig. 26.24). The characteristic differences between the long bones of types IIA and III are shown in Fig. 26.25. Type II C is rare and characterised by an extreme underossification of the cranial fault, thin ribs with contiguous separate fractures (beaded ribs) and multiple fractures of the long bones (Fig. 26.26). Histological examination of the growth plate cartilage shows no specific abnormalities in the different subtypes, but at the zone of chondro-osseous transformation the primary and secondary (osseous) trabeculae and the cortical bone are reduced in volume with thin osseous seams in types II A, II B and III (Fig. 26.27a). Type II C has a different histologic picture. The primary and secondary spongiosa of the metaphysis have a network of relatively broad and irregularly arranged cartilaginous trabeculae with many interconnections and thin osseous seams (Fig. 26.27b) (Van der Harten et al. 1988b). The healing fractures frequently show islets of metaplastic cartilage in the formation of hyperplastic callus (Fig. 26.28a).

Osteogenesis imperfecta is now recognised to represent a group of heritable disorders of

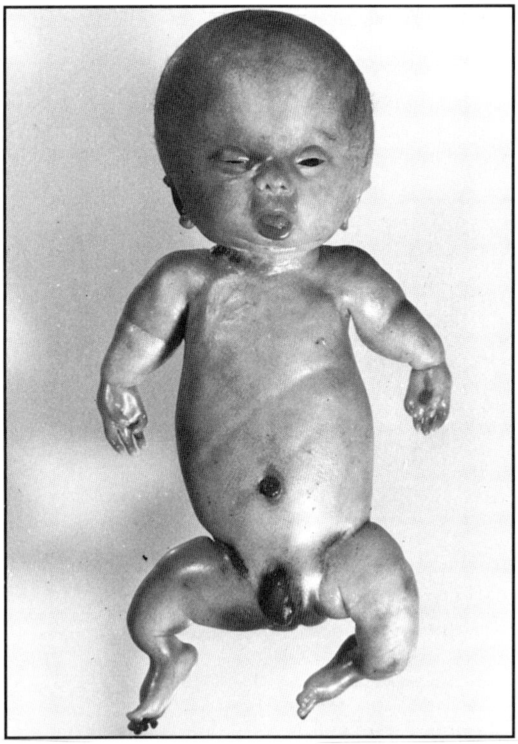

a

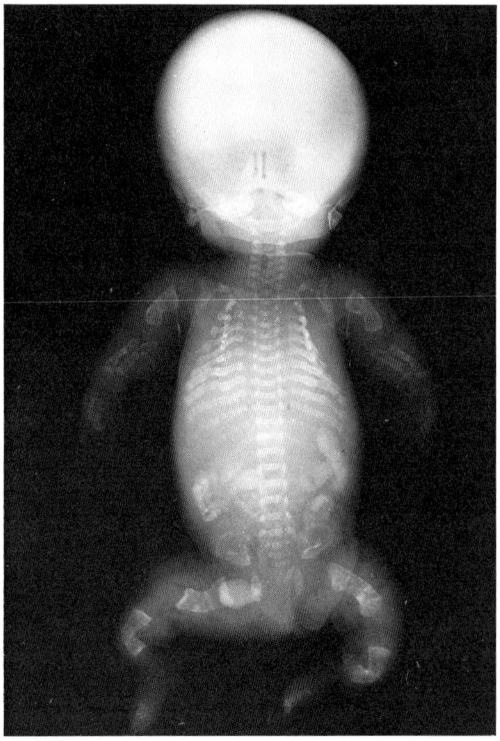

b

Fig. 26.23. Osteogenesis imperfecta type II A "Sillence classification". **a** Deformed shortened limbs and large soft head. **b** Babygram illustrates unossified cranial vault, crumpled long bones and ribs.

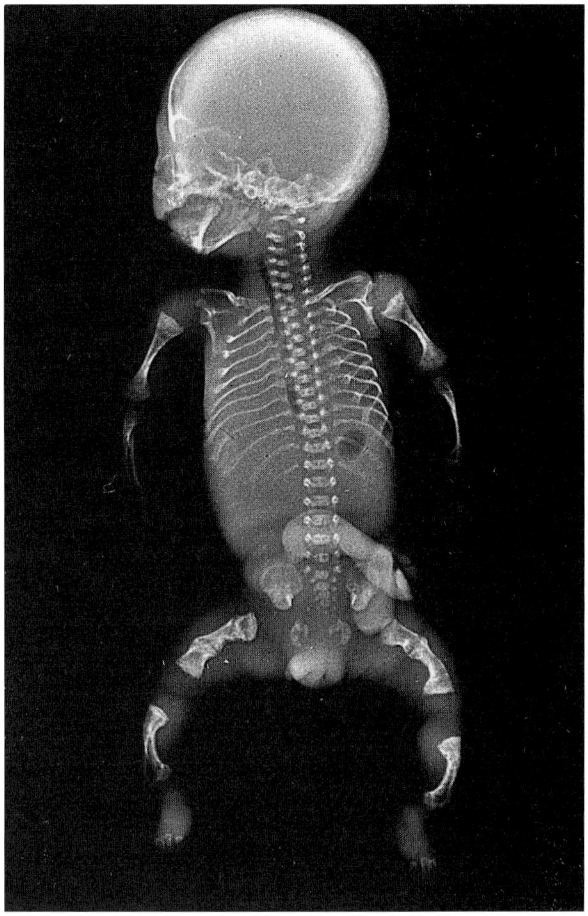

Fig. 26.24. Osteogenesis imperfecta type II B "Sillence classification". Babygram illustrates the wavy thin ribs without fractures, femora with healing fractures and bowing of the tibia. (Van der Harten et al. 1988b)

connective tissue and is currently the subject of biochemical studies. Based on a well-defined primary defect, a more detailed classification may be expected in the near future. With recent developments in collagen molecular biology, reliable prenatal diagnosis of the autosomal dominant and recessive forms has become a reality (Pope et al. 1985; Sykes et al. 1986; Byers et al. 1988).

In considering the diagnosis osteogenesis imperfecta, one should always keep in mind the diagnosis *hypophosphatasia*. Several forms of this primary metabolic disorder have been described (Caswell et al. 1989). They are characterised by a reduced activity of alkaline phosphatase in serum and various tissues, including cartilage and bone. The perinatal form has a mortality of 100%. As in the lethal form of osteogenesis imperfecta, the skull is

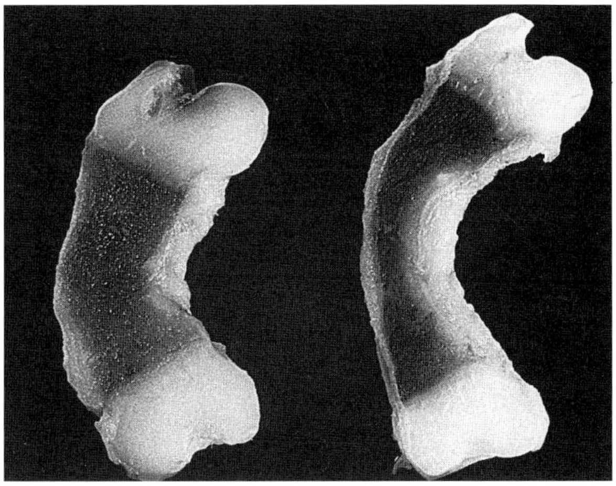

Fig. 26.25. **a** Osteogenesis imperfecta type IIA: short femur with broad diaphysis (27 weeks, gestation). **b** Osteogenesis imperfecta type III: femur with widened metaphysis (23 weeks, gestation). Both femora show bending (campomelia) and characteristic difference in length, despite the difference in gestational age.

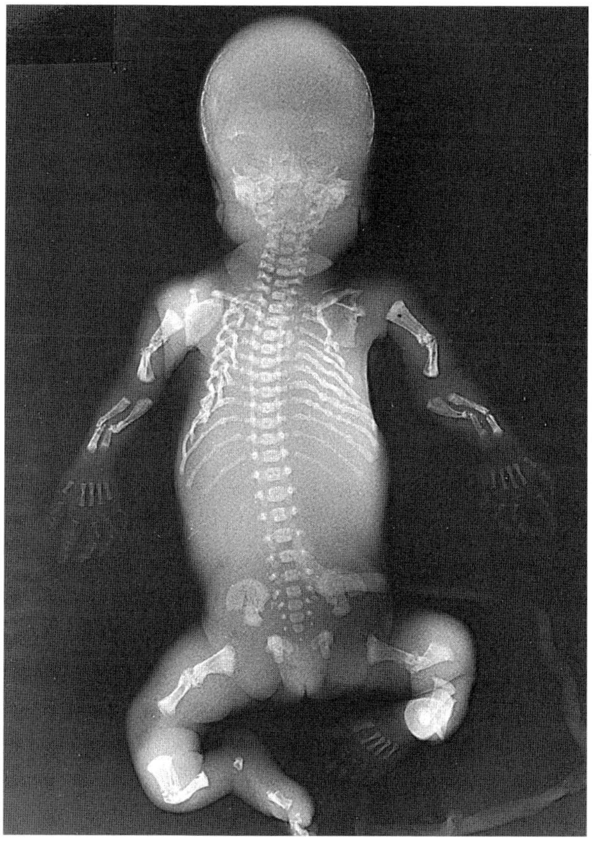

Fig. 26.26. Osteogenesis imperfecta type II C "Sillence classification". Babygram showing thin beaded ribs, long bones with multiple fractures and poorly mineralised cranial vault. (Van der Harten et al. 1988b)

soft because of the absence of ossification of the neurocranium. Radiographic examination shows undermineralisation of the skeleton and shortening and bowing of the long bones, with angulation and diaphyseal spurs and fractures. In some newborns almost no bone is formed. Both the lethal perinatal and the infantile forms have been described within one family (Wladimiroff et al. 1985; Macfarlane et al. 1992).

Histologically, the metaphysis shows irregular bone formation with foci of persisting cartilage islets (Fig. 26.28b). In the diaphysis and close to the metaphysis the bone trabeculae appear normal but are often lined by relatively wide, uncalcified osteoid seams. The picture resembles that of severe rickets (Ornoy et al. 1985b).

Other Skeletal Abnormalities

Skeletal abnormalities are common amongst perinatal deaths and may be sufficiently characteristic to indicate a likely diagnosis (Wiedemann et al. 1985; Brons et al. 1988b, 1988c; Jones 1988) and give a good return for routine radiographic examination as part of perinatal postmortem examination.

Fractures

Fractures of skull and long bones are recognised manifestations of birth trauma (see Chap. 10). Rib fractures may complicate nutritional rickets in preterm babies (Oppenheimer and Snodgrass 1980; see Fig. 14.21, p. 341).

Osteomyelitis

In the neonatal period osteomyelitis is a relatively uncommon complication of a sepsis that is usually caused by *Staphylococcus aureus* or haemolytic streptococci. Two recent studies suggest that *Haemophilus influenzae* type b and *Streptococcus pneumoniae* are also important causes (Faden and Grossi 1991; Jacobs 1991). Outstanding features that distinguish it from osteomyelitis in older children are benign onset

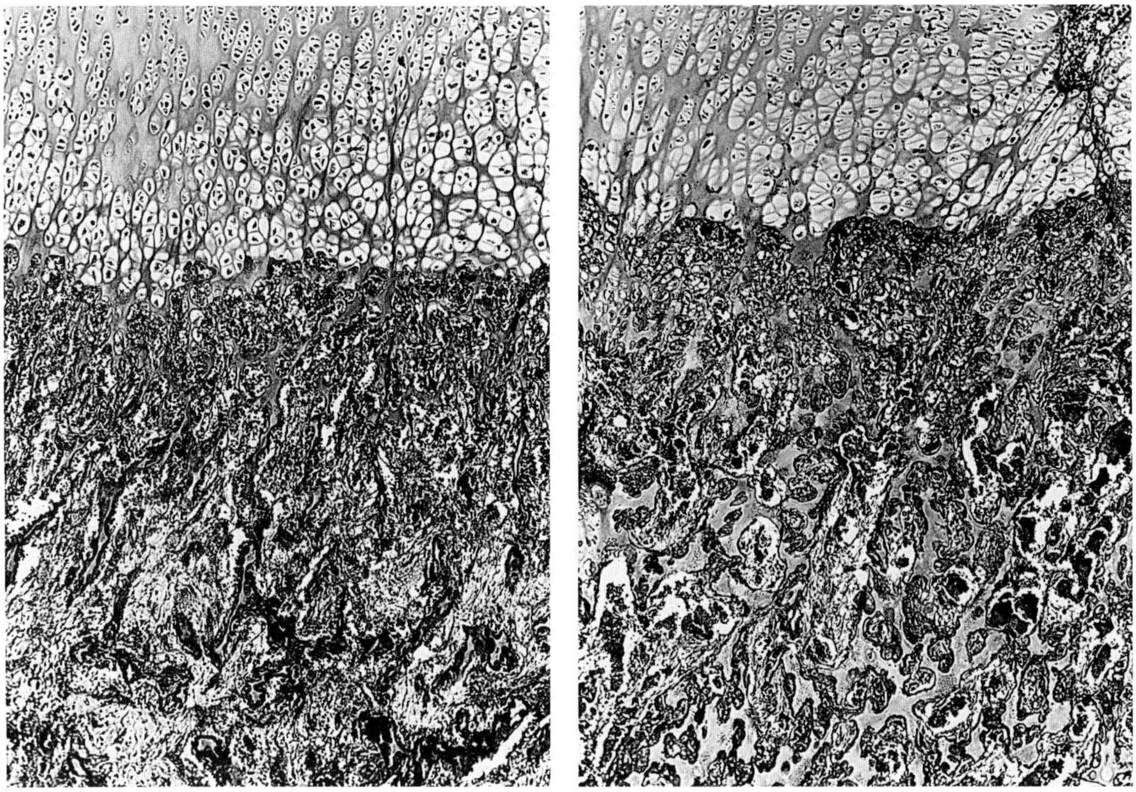

a b

Fig. 26.27. a Osteogenesis imperfecta type III. Growth plate with near normal columnisation of the chondrocytes and narrow bony trabeculae with thin osseous seams. The bone marrow shows fibrosis. (Ladewig, ×47) (Van der Harten et al. 1988b) b Osteogensis imperfecta type II C. Growth plate, the metaphysis shows a network of broad and haphazardly arranged trabeculae with thin osseous seams. (Ladewig, ×47) (Van der Harten et al. 1988b)

and course in most neonates, involvement of multiple foci and involvement of contiguous joints in cases with long bone infection (Fox and Sprunt 1978; Knudsen and Hoffman 1990). Predisposing factors are complications of pregnancy and delivery. The majority of the newborn have antecedent illnesses or were subjected to invasive procedures in the perinatal period (Weissberg et al. 1974).

Osteomyelitis of the lower extremity, secondary to catheterisation of the umbilical artery, is a well-known complication associated with ischaemic changes in the affected limb and infected catheter tip (Lim et al. 1977). Although rare, other modes of infection in neonates include osteomyelitis of the scalp secondary to fetal monitoring and osteochondritis of the calcaneus caused by repeated heel punctures for medical purposes. Osteomyelitis has a predilection for the metaphysis of long bones because bacteria precipitate from the capillaries draining along the cartilaginous growth plate into venous sinuses, rapidly spreading to the subperiosteal space. Early diagnosis is primarily clinical with supporting radiographic findings. When the infection is treated at an early stage, recovery is usually uneventful.

In overwhelming intrauterine infections such as listeriosis, tuberculosis, toxoplasmosis and candidiasis with intrauterine death, the bone marrow may be involved (Fig. 26.29). Congenital syphilis, a rare disorder that usually becomes manifest shortly after birth, is increasing (Toohey 1985). The pathologist would find more congenital syphilis than current figures indicate, if all fetuses, stillbirths and placentae were examined histologically (Oppenheimer and Dahms 1981). Characteristic findings include periostitis, metaphysitis and osteitis involving the long bones, with focal inflammation and fibrosis, the typical syphilitic granulation tissue. Adequate and early treatment provides prompt reversal of symptoms and radiographic findings (Ikeda and Jenson 1990).

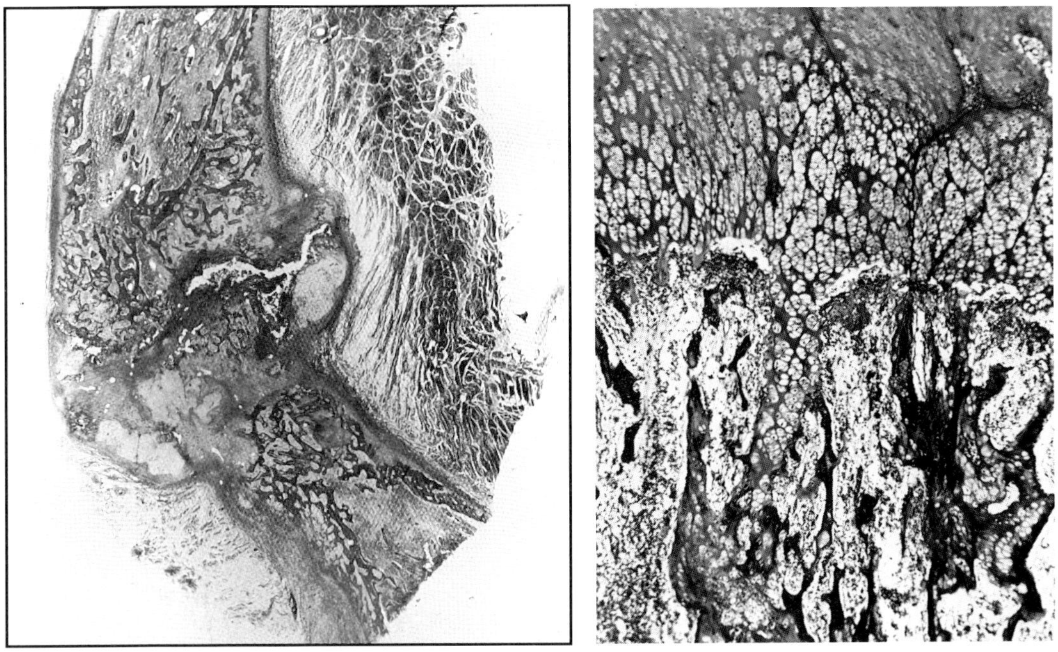
a b

Fig. 26.28. **a** Osteogenesis imperfecta type II C. Healing fracture of the shaft of the femur. Islets of metaplastic cartilage are present. (Ladewig, ×3.5) **b** Hypophosphatasia. Growth plate with irregular bone formation and foci of chondrocytes in the centre of the unmineralised spongiosa. (Ladewig, ×23)

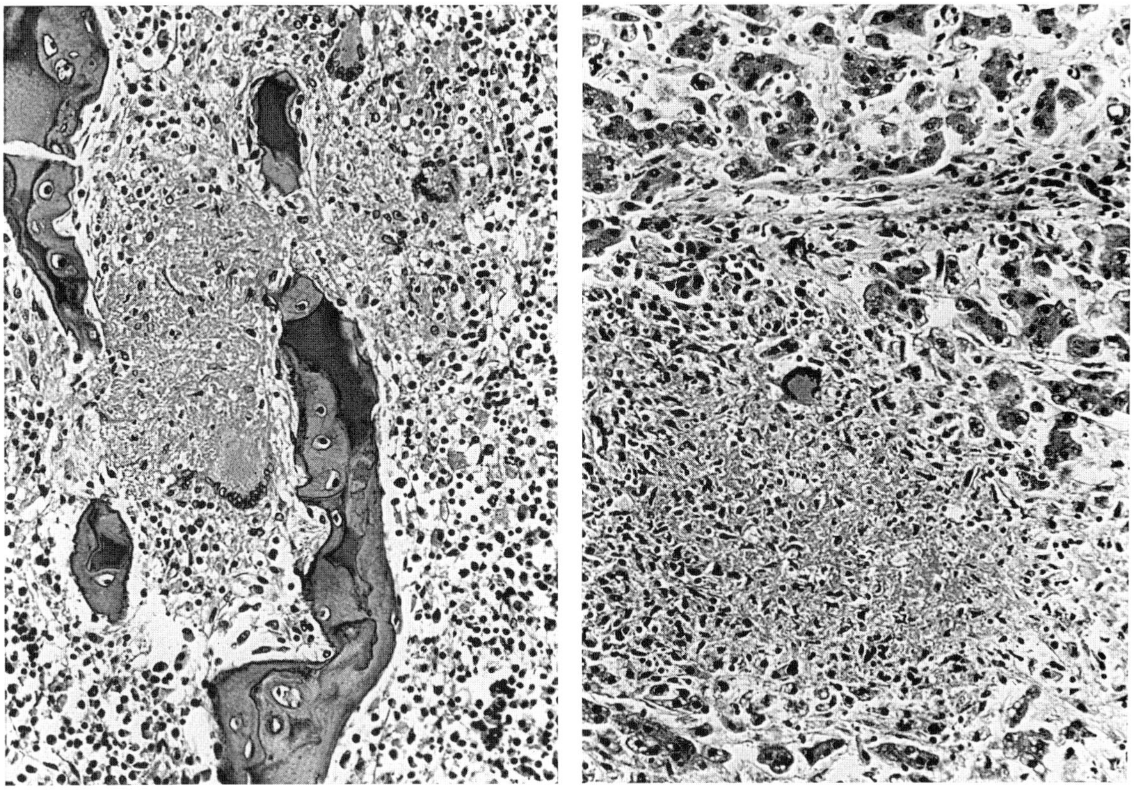
a b

Fig. 26.29. **a** Newborn with congenital tuberculosis; tubercle in bone marrow. (H&E, ×189) **b** Same case; tubercle in liver. (H&E, ×189)

References

Bankier A, Fortune D, Duke J, Sillence DO (1991) Fibrochondrogenesis in male twins at 24 weeks gestation. Am J Med Genet 38: 95–98

Beck M, Roubieck M, Rogers JG, Naumoff P, Spranger J (1983) Heterogeneity of metatropic dysplasia. Eur J Pediatr 140: 231–237

Beemer FA, Langer LO Jr, Klep-de Pater JM et al. (1983) A new short rib syndrome: report of two cases. Am J Med Genet 14: 115–123

Beighton P (1988) Inherited disorders of the skeleton. Churchill Livingstone, Edinburgh

Bernstein R, Isdale J, Pinto M, Du Toit Zaayman J, Jenkins T (1985) Short rib-polydactyly syndrome: a single or heterogeneous entity? A re-evaluation prompted by four new cases. J Med Genet 22: 46–53

Borochowitz Z, Ornoy A, Lachman R, Rimoin DL (1986) Hypochondrogenesis-achondrogenesis II-variability vs. heterogenecity. Am J Med Genet 24: 273–388

Borochowitz Z, Lachman R, Adomian GE, Spear G, Jones K, Rimoin D (1988) Achondrogenesis type I: delineation of further heterogeneity and identification of two distinct subgroups. J Pediatr 112: 23–31

Brighton CT (1984) The growth plate. Orthop Clin North Am 15: 571–595

Brons JTJ, van der Harten HJ, Wladimiroff JW et al. (1988a) Prenatal ultrasonographic diagnosis of osteogenesis imperfecta. Am J Obstet Gynecol 159: 176–181

Brons JTJ, van Geijn HP, Wladimiroff JW et al. (1988b) Prenatal ultrasound diagnosis of the Holt–Oram syndrome. Prenat Diagn 8: 175–181

Brons JTJ, van der Harten JJ, van Geijn HP et al. (1988c) Prenatal ultrasonographic diagnosis of radial-ray reduction malformations. Prenat Diagn 10: 279–288

Brons JTJ, van der Harten JJ, van Geijn HP et al. (1990) Ratios between growth parameters for the prenatal ultrasonographic diagnosis of skeletal dysplasias. Eur J Obstet Gynecol Reprod Biol 34: 37–46

Buckwalter JA (1983) Proteoglycan structure in calcifying cartilage. Clin Orthop Relat Res 172: 207–232

Byers PH, Tsipouras P, Banadio JF, Starman B, Schwartz RC (1988) Perinatal lethal osteogenesis imperfecta (OI type II): a biochemically heterogeneous disorder usually due to new mutations in the genes for type I collagen. Am J Hum Genet 42: 237–248

Camera G, Mastroacovo P (1982) Birth prevalence of skeletal dysplasias in the Italian Multicentric Monitoring System for birth defects. In: Papadatos CJ, Bartsocas CS (eds) Skeletal dysplasias New York, Liss, pp 441–449

Caswell AM, Russell RG, Whyte MP (1989) Hypophosphatasia: pediatric forms. J Pediatr Endocrinol 3: 73–92

Chen H, Yang SS, Gonzalez E, Fowler M, Al Saadi A (1980) Short rib-polydactyly syndrome Majewski type. Am J Med Genet 7: 215–222

Chen H, Liu CT, Yang SS (1981) Achondrogenesis: a review with special consideration of achondrogenesis type II (Langer–Saldino). Clin Genet 10: 379–394

Cremin BJ, Beighton P (1978) Bone dysplasias of infancy, a radiological atlas. Springer, Berlin Heidelberg New York

Faden M, Grossi M (1991) Acute osteomyelitis in children. Am J Dis Child 145: 65–69

Feshchenko SP, Rebrin IA, Sokolnik VP et al. (1989) The absence of type II collagen and changes in proteoglycan structure of hyaline cartilage in a case of Langer–Saldino achondrogenesis. Hum Genet 82: 49–54

Fox L, Sprunt K (1978) Neonatal osteomyelitis. Pediatrics 62: 535–542

Fraccaro M (1952) Contributo allo studio delle malattie del mesenchima osteopoietico l'acondrogenesi. Folia Hered Pathol 1: 190–207

Fraser CR (1962) Our genetic "load": A review of some aspects of genetic variation. Ann Hum Genet 25: 387–415

Gilbert EF, Yang SS, Langer L, Opitz JM, Roskamp JO, Heidelberger KP (1987) Pathologic changes of osteochondrodysplasia in infancy, a review. Pathol Annu 22: 283–345

Godfrey M, Hollister DW (1988) Type II achondrogenesis—hypochondrogenesis: identification of abnormal type II collagen. Am J Hum Genet 43: 904–913

Greco MA, Alvarez SP, Genieser NB, Becker MH (1984) Dyssegmental dwarfism: a histologic study of osseous and nonosseous cartilage. Hum Pathol 15: 490–493

Ho Kl, Chang CH, Yang SS, Chason JL (1984) Neuropathologic findings in thanatophoric dysplasia. Acta Neuropathol (Berl) 63: 218–228

Hobbins JC, Bracken MB, Mahoney MJ (1982) Diagnosis of fetal skeletal dysplasias with ultrasound. Am J Obstet Gynecol 142: 306–312

Holtermüller K, Wiedemann HR (1960) Kleeblattschädel syndrome. Med Monatsschr 14: 439–446

Horton WA, Rimoin DL (1979) Kniest dysplasia. A histochemical study of the growth plate. Pediatr Res 13: 1266–1270

Horton WA, Rimoin DL, Hollister DW, Silverberg R (1979) Diastrophic dwarfism: a histochemical and ultrastructural study of the endochondral growth plate. Pediatr Res 13: 904–909

Horton WA, Harris DJ, Collins DL (1983) Discordance for the Kleeblattschädel anomaly in monozygotic twins with thanatophoric dysplasia. Am J Med Genet 15: 97–101

Horton WA, Campbell D, Machado MA, Chou J (1989) Type II collagen screening in the human chondrodysplasias. Am J Med Genet 34: 579–583

Houston CS, Opitz JM, Spranger JW et al. (1983) The campomelic syndrome: review report of 17 cases, and follow up on the currently 17-year-old boy first reported by Maroteaux et al. in 1971. Am J Med Genet 15: 3–28

Hunter GK (1991) Role of proteoglycan in the provisional calcification of cartilage, a review and reinterpretation. Clin Orthop Relat Res 262: 256–280

Hwang WS, McQueen D, Monson RC, Reed MH (1982) The significance of cytoplasmic chondrocyte inclusions in multiple osteochondromatosis, solitary osteochondromas and chondrodysplasias. Am J Clin Pathol 78: 89–91

Ikeda MK, Jenson HB (1990) Evaluation and treatment of congenital syphilis. J Pediatr 117: 843–852

Jacobs NM (1991) Pneumococcal osteomyelitis and arthritis in children. Am J Dis Child 145: 70–74

Jones KL (1988) Smith's recognizable patterns of human malformation, 4th edn. Saunders, London

Knisely AS, Ambler MW (1988) Temporal-lobe abnormalities in thanatophoric dysplasia. Pediatr Neurosci 14: 169–176

Knudsen CJM, Hoffman EB (1990) Neonatal osteomyelitis. J Bone Jt Surg Ser B 72: 846–851

Kozlowski K (1985) The radiographic clues in the diagnosis of bone dysplasia. Pediatr Radiol 15: 1–3

Kozlowski K, Tsuruta T, Kameda Y, Kan A, Leslie G (1981) New forms of neonatal death dwarfism. Report of three cases. Pediatr Radiol 10: 155–160

Langer LO Jr, Spranger JW, Greincher I, Herdman RC (1969) Thanatophoric dwarfism: a condition confused with achondroplasia in the neonate, with brief comments

on achondrogenesis and homozygous achondroplasia. Radiology 92: 285–294
Langer LO Jr, Yang SS, Hall JG et al. (1987) Thanatophoric dysplasia and cloverleaf skull. Am J Med Genet (Suppl 3): 167–179
Lazzaroni-Fossati F, Stanescu V, Stanescu R, Serra G, Magliano P, Maroteaux P (1978) La fibrochondrogenèse. Arch Fr Pediatr 35: 1096–1104
Lim MO, Gresham EL, Franken EA Jr, Leake RD (1977) Osteomyelitis as a complication of umbilical artery catheterisation. Am J Dis Child 131: 142–144
Lurie IW, Cherstvoy ED (1984) Renal agenesis as a diagnostic feature of the cryptophthalmos-syndactyly syndrome. Clin Genet 25: 528–532
MacDonald IM, Hunter AGW, MacLeod PM, MacMurray SB (1989) Growth and development in thanatophoric dysplasia. Am J Med Genet 33: 508–512
Macfarlane JD, Kroon HM, van der Harten JJ (1992) Phenotypically dissimilar hypophosphatasia in two sibships. Am J Med Genet 42: 117–121
Macpherson RI, Wood BP (1980) Spondyloepiphyseal dysplasia congenita: a cause of lethal neonatal dwarfism. Pediatr Radiol 9: 217–224
Majewski F, Pfeiffer RA, Lenz W, Müller R, Feil G, Seiler R (1971) Polysyndactylie, verkürzte Gliedmassen und Genitalfehlbindungen, Kenzeichen eines neuen Syndroms? Z Kinderheilk 111: 118–138
Maroteaux P, Lamy M, Roberts JM (1967) Le nanisma thanatophore. Presse Med 75: 2519–2524
Maroteaux P, Stanescu V, Stanescu R (1976) The lethal chondrodysplasias. Clin Orthop Relat Res 114: 31–45
Maroteaux P, Spranger J, Stanescu V et al. (1982) Atelosteogenesis. Am J Med Genet 13: 15–25
Maroteaux P, Stanescu V, Stanescu R (1983) Hypochondrogenesis. Eur J Pediatr 141: 14–22
Maroteaux P, Beighton P, Cremin B et al. (1984) International nomenclature of constitutional diseases of bone. Ann Radiol 27: 275–280
Maroteaux P, Frézal J, Cohen-Solal L, Bonaventure J (1986) Les formes anténatales de l'osteogenèse imparfaite, essai de classification. Arch Fr Pediatr 43: 235–241
Naumoff P, Young LW, Mazer J, Amortegui AJ (1977) Short rib-polydactyly syndrome type 3. Radiology 122: 443–447
Nogami H, Oohira A, Kuroyanagi M, Mizutani A (1986) Congenital bowing of long bones: clinical and experimental study. Teratology 33: 1–7
Oppenheimer EH, Dahms BB (1981) Congenital syphilis in the fetus and neonate. In: Rozenberg HS, Bernstein J (eds) Perspectives in pediatric pathology, vol 6. Year Book Medical Publishers, Chicago, pp 115–138
Oppenheimer SJ, Snodgrass GJAI (1980) Neonatal rickets. Histopathology and quantitative bone changes. Arch Dis Child 55: 945–949
O'Rahilly R, Meijer DB (1956) Roentgenographic investigation of the human skeleton during early fetal life. Am J Roentgenol 76: 455–468
Orioli IM, Castilla EE, Barbosa Neto JG (1986) The birth prevalence rates for the skeletal dysplasias. J Med Genet 23: 328–332
Ornoy A, Adomian GE, Eteson DJ, Berguson RE, Rimoin DL (1985a) The role of abnormal mesenchyme-like tissue in the pathogenesis of thanatophoric dysplasia. Am J Med Genet 21: 613–630
Ornoy A, Adomian GE, Rimoin DL (1985b) Histologic and ultrastructural studies on the mineralization process in hypophosphatasia. Am J Med Genet 22: 743–758
Parenti GC (1936) La anosteogenesi: una varieta della osteogenesi imperfecta. Pathologica 28: 447–461
Pope FM, Nickolls AC, Mc Pheat et al. (1985) Collagen genes and proteins in osteogenesis imperfecta. J Med Genet 22: 466–478
Romero R, Athanassiadis AP, Jeanty Ph (1990) Fetal skeletal anomalies. In: Benacerraf BR (ed) Fetal ultrasound. Radiol Clin North Am 28: 75–99
Roth M (1991) Campomelic syndrome: experimental models and pathomechanism. Pediatr Radiol 21: 220–225
Roth SI, Jimenez JF, Husted S, Seibert JJ, Haynes DW (1982) The histopathology of camptomelia (bent limbs), a dyschondrogenesis. Clin Orthop Relat Res 167: 152–159
Rubin P (1964) Dynamic classification of bone dysplasias. Year Book Medical Publishers, Chicago
Saldino RM (1971) Lethal short-limbed dwarfism: achondrogenesis and thanatophoric dwarfism. Am J Roentgenol Radium Ther Nucl Med 112: 185–197
Saldino RM, Noonan CD (1972) Severe thoracic dystrophy with striking micromelia, abnormal osseous development, including the spine and multiple visceral abnormalities. Am J Roentgenol Radium Ther Nucl Med 114: 257–261
Serville F, Carles D, Maroteaux P (1984) Thanatophoric dysplasia of identical twins. Am J Med Genet 17: 703–705 (letter)
Sillence DO (1980) Invited editorial comment: non-Majewski short rib-polydactyly syndrome. Am J Med Genet 7: 223–229
Sillence DO, Horton WA, Rimoin DL (1979a) Morphologic studies in the skeletal dysplasias. Am J Pathol 96: 811–870
Sillence DO, Senn A, Danks DM (1979b) Genetic heterogeneity in osteogenesis imperfecta. J Med Genet 16: 101–116
Sillence DO, Lachman RS, Jenkins T, Riccardi VM, Rimoin DL (1982) Spondylohumerofemoral hypoplasia (giant cell chondrodysplasia): a neonatally lethal short-limb skeletal dysplasia. Am J Med Genet 13: 7–14
Sillence DO, Barlow KK, Garber AP, Hall JG, Rimoin DL (1984) Osteogenesis imperfecta type II, delineation of the phenotype with reference to genetic heterogeneity. Am J Med Genet 17: 407–423
Sillence DO, Kozlowski K, Rogers JG, Spraque PL, Cullity GJ, Osborn RA (1987) Atelosteogenesis: evidence for heterogeneity. Pediatr Radiol 17: 112–118
Spranger J, Grimm B, Weller M et al. (1974) About rib-polydactyly (SRP) syndromes, types Majewski and Saldino–Noonan. Z Kinderheilk 116: 73–94
Stanescu V, Stanescu R, Maroteaux P (1977) Etude morphologique et biochemique du cartilage de croissance dans les ostéochondrodysplasies. Arch Fr Pediatr [Suppl 3]: 1–80
Stanescu V, Stanescu R, Maroteaux P (1984) Pathogenic mechanisms in osteochondrodysplasias. J Bone Joint Surg [Am] 66: 817–836
Stern HJ, Graham JM Jr, Lachman S et al. (1990) Atelosteogenesis type III: a distinct skeletal dysplasia with features overlapping atelosteogenesis and oto-palato-digital syndrome type II. Am J Med Genet 36: 183–195
Sykes B, Wordsworth P, Ogilvie D, Anderson J, Jones N (1986) Osteogenesis imperfecta is linked to both type I collagen structural genes. Lancet II: 69–72
Thomas IT, Frias JL, Felix V, Sanchez de Leon L, Hernandez RA, Jones MC (1986) Isolated and syndromic cryptophthalmos. Am J Med Genet 25: 85–98
Thompson EM, Young ID, Hall CM, Pembrey ME (1987) Recurrence risk and prognosis in severe sporadic osteogenesis imperfecta. J Med Genet 24: 390–405

Toohey JS (1985) Skeletal presentation of congenital syphilis: case report and review of the literature. J Pediatr Orthop 5: 104–106
Van der Harten HJ, Brons JTJ, Dijkstra PF et al. (1988a) Achondrogenesis, hypochondrogenesis, the spectrum of chondrogenesis imperfecta: a radiologic, ultrasonographic and histopathologic study of 23 cases. Pediatr Pathol 8: 571–597
Van der Harten HJ, Brons JTJ, Dijkstra PF et al. (1988b) Perinatal lethal osteogenesis imperfecta: radiologic and pathologic evaluation of seven prenatally diagnosed cases. Pediatr Pathol 8: 233–252
Van der Harten HJ, Brons JTJ, Schipper NW, Dijkstra PF, Meijer CJLM, van Geijn HP (1990) The prenatal development of the normal human skeleton: a combined ultrasonographic and post-mortem radiographic study. Pediatr Radiol 21: 52–56
Verma IC, Bhargava S, Agarwal S (1975) An autosomal recessive form of lethal chondrodystrophy with severe thoracic narrowing rhizoacromelic type of micromelia polydactyly and genital abnormalities. In: Bergsma D (ed) Birth defects 11(6): 167–174
Weissberg ED, Smith AL, Smith DH (1974) Clinical features of neonatal osteomyelitis. Pediatrics 53: 505–510
Whitley CB, Gorlin RJ (1983) Achondrogenesis: new nosology with evidence of genetic heterogeneity. Radiology 148: 693–698
Wiedemann HR, Grosse KR, Dibbern H (1985) An atlas of characteristic syndromes. A visual aid to diagnosis. Wolfe Medical, London
Winter RM, Sandin BM, Mitchell RA, Price AB (1984) The radiology of stillbirths and neonatal deaths. Br J Radiol 91: 762–765
Wladimiroff JW, Niermeyer MF, Laar J, Jahoda M, Steward PA (1984) Prenatal diagnosis of skeletal dysplasia by real-time ultrasound. Obstet Gynecol 63: 360–364
Wladimiroff JW, Niermeyer MF, van der Harten JJ et al. (1985) Early prenatal diagnosis of congenital hypophosphatasia. Prenat Diagn 5: 47–52
Wongmongkolrit Th, Bush M, Roessmann U (1983) Neuropathologic findings in thanatophoric dysplasia. Arch Pathol Lab Med 107: 132–135
Yang SS, Heidelberger KP, Brough AJ, Corbet DP, Bernstein J (1976) Lethal short-limbed chondrodysplasia in early infancy. In: Rosenberg HS, Bolande RP (eds) Perspectives in pediatric pathology, vol 3. Year Book Medical Publishers, Chicago, pp 1–40
Yang SS, Lin CS, Al Saadi A, Nangia BS, Bernstein J (1980) Short rib-polydactyly syndrome type 3 with chondrocytic inclusions: report of a case and review of the literature. Am J Med Genet 7: 205–213
Yang SS, Roskamp J, Liu CT, Frates R, Singer DB (1983) Two lethal chondrodysplasias with giant chondrocytes. Am J Med Genet 15: 615–625
Yang SS, Langer LO Jr, Cacciarelli A et al. (1987) Three conditions in neonatal asphyxiating thoracic dysplasia (Jeune) and short rib-polydactyly syndrome spectrum: a clinicopathologic study. Am J Med Genet [Suppl] 3: 191–207
Young ID, Thompson EM, Hall CM, Pembrey ME (1987) Osteogenesis imperfecta type II A: evidence for dominant inheritance. J Med Genet 24: 386–389

Addendum

Since the preparation of this Chapter, The International Working Group on Constitutional Diseases of Bone has again amended the International Classification of Osteochondrodysplasias. Some of the lethal osteochondrodysplasias are reclassified.

Spranger J, for The International Working Group on Constitutional Diseases of Bone (1992) International classification of osteochondrodysplasias. Eur J Pediatr 151:407–415

Chapter 27

The Skin

Peter R. Millard

Development of the Skin

The development of the epidermis is outlined in Table 27.1

Periderm

This presents as large a surface area as possible to the amniotic fluid (Fig. 27.1). This and the pinocytic vesicles suggest a secretory or absorptive function, and it is interesting that the amniotic fluid composition changes coincidentally with the loss of the periderm and onset of keratinisation (Holbrook and Odland 1975). Prior to keratinisation, its composition resembles that of the fetal extracellular space. With keratinisation the permeability of the fetal skin is reduced and the fluid resembles fetal urine, with an increased concentration of urea and creatinine and a decrease in sodium and glucose (McCarthy and Saunders 1978).

Keratinisation

Tonofilaments, often mistakenly regarded as keratin fibrils, are synthesised by the epidermal cells together with sulphur-rich keratohyaline granules. Both increase in size as these cells become more superficial and the keratohyaline granules are aligned between and around the tonofilaments. The tonofibrils form the cytoskeleton of the keratinocytes and are pliable. The keratohyaline granules provide rigidity to these cells by contributing to the amorphous firm matrix of the cells, particularly those of the granular layer, but most especially the horny layer where keratinisation is complete (Elias 1989).

The intercellular keratinosomes or Odland bodies should not be confused with the intracellular keratohyaline granules. Odland bodies are lamellated masses that develop from the cell membranes of the granular and more particularly the horny layer cells and lie in the intercellular spaces. These regions are filled with lipids which are derived from the keratinosomes and limit water loss.

Melanocytes

Neural crest cells are recognisable at 18 days post fertilisation and seen as aggregates along the neural tube at 25 days. They migrate to the periphery and are found in the dermis around vessels and nerves. Non-keratinocytes were described by Breathnach and Robins (1969) in the germinative layer of a 6-week embryo. Melanosomes are recognisable in epidermal melanocytes at 8 weeks and melanin pigment at 10 weeks. Migration and maturation appears to occur slightly earlier in cranial than in caudal regions (Sagebiel and Odland 1970).

Similar numbers of peripheral melanocytes are present in pigmented races and Caucasians, but in the former they are more active (McDonald 1988). These differences do not affect the spectrum of cutaneous disorders

Table 27.1. Development of the skin

Conceptual age	Crown–rump length (mm)	Description	Ultrastructure[a]
<5 weeks	<10	Single layer of cells—ectoderm	Few small microvilli on free surface. No desmosomes
5–8 weeks	10–30	Bilaminar, upper periderm, lower germinative. Occasional non-keratinocyte	Microvilli and pinocytic vesicles on periderm surface. Immature desmosomes; no hemidesmosomes. Basal lamina present. Peripheral tonofilaments
8–11 weeks	30–65	Incomplete layer of interstitial cells. More melanocytes	Periderm large cells with central elevation. Many surface microvilli with surface fuzz of mucopolysaccharide
9–13 weeks	40–95	Trilaminar epithelium. Early hair germs	Periderm cells have large surface bulb covered by microvilli
12–16 weeks	80–140	Two or more layers of interstitial cells	Periderm cells stop dividing and expand laterally. Surface still has bulb, microvilli and pinocytic vesicles
13–17 weeks	95–150	As above	Periderm shows complex surface infoldings and protuberances. Interstitial cells accumulate tonofilaments
16–23 weeks	140–185	Four or more layers of interstitial cells. Keratinisation first seen around hair follicles	Many periderm cells lose nucleus and internal structure. Periderm begins to peel away. Upper interstitial cells contain keratohyalin
>23 weeks	>185	Appearance approaches adult epidermis	

[a] Hashimoto et al. (1966), Wessells (1967), Hoyes (1968), Breathnach and Robins (1969), Breathnach (1971), Holbrook and Odland (1975).

amongst black neonates (McLaurin 1988; Nanda et al. 1989).

Langerhans' Cells

Langerhans' cells are cells of the monocyte/macrophage series. They are potent antigen-presenting cells, able to stimulate T-cells, particularly in response to surface antigens on keratinocytes and melanocytes (Shimada and Katz 1988; Stingl and Steiner 1989). They form 2%–8% of the epidermal cells and occur in smaller numbers in the dermis. The cells are identified by characteristic rod or tennis racquet-shaped Birbeck granules and have been seen in the epidermis of a 12-week post-fertilisation embryo (Breathnach and Wylie 1965). The granules are lacking in otherwise similar forms, indeterminate cells. All cell forms are OKT6 and CD4 positive and express Class II antigens.

Dermis and Dermo-epidermal Junction

The dermis develops from loosely arranged mesenchymal cells at 5 weeks to a pattern mimicking the adult form, including appendages, by the end of the first trimester (Smith and Holbrook 1986). A smiliar pace of development occurs at the dermo-epidermal junction where the many basement membrane zone proteins are formed (Smith et al. 1988) (Fig. 27.2).

Skin Function

The functions of the skin of the neonate are identical to those of the adult but are modified in several important ways. Microbial colonisation begins at birth and is equivalent to that of the adult only after several weeks of life. The protective antagonism of the resident flora to microbial pathogens is consequently absent and different patterns of skin infection can be anticipated (Roth and James 1989). Exposure to other antigens has also not occurred and immune responses to environmental antigens are consequently not developed. A minority of infants will, however, have been exposed to harmful antigens in utero and may as a result manifest skin infections, neoplasms and immunologically mediated disorders at birth (Krusinski and Saurat 1989).

Heat loss is greater in the neonate because of the large surface area of the skin relative to volume, the small amount of subcutaneous

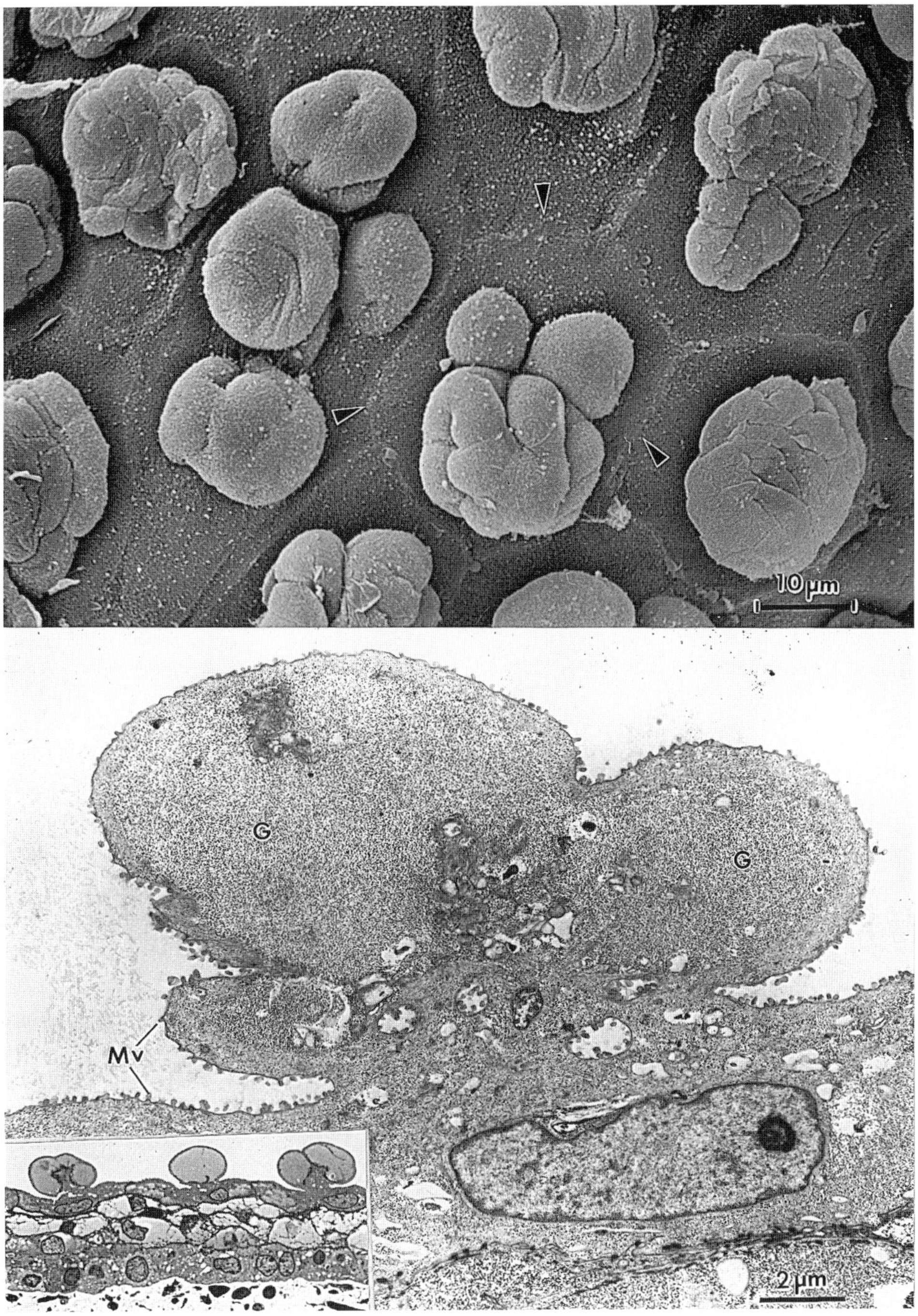

Fig. 27.1. Periderm of a 14-week fetus. *Top*: Scanning electron microscopy of the sole of the foot. Individual periderm cells with complex surface protuberances are evident, arrow-heads defining the cell margins. *Bottom*: Transmission electron microscopy of the same area with thin section light microscopy. *Insert*: Microvilli (MV) extend from the surface of the protuberance and glycogen (G) is abundant in the cytosol. The trilaminar epithelium supporting the protuberances is seen in the insert. (Courtesy of Dr. D. Ferguson, Oxford)

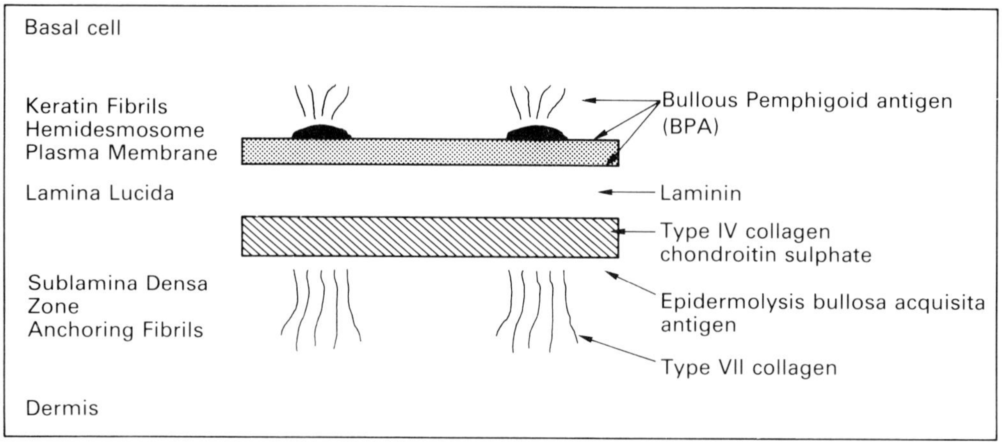

Fig. 27.2. Components of the dermal-epidermal junction and location of main proteins. Using antibodies to these proteins the site of some skin disorders can be localised (Eady 1987; Rasmussen et al. 1989).

fat and immaturity of vascular tone regulation. Conversely, the poor responses of the eccrine glands will preserve heat and even overheat the infant (Atherton and Rook 1986).

Disorders of Development

Amniotic Constriction Bands

If the amnion ruptures in the first half of pregnancy without rupture of the chorion, the exposed extraembryonic mesoderm can adhere to the embryo. Fibrous strings are sometimes formed which may encircle parts of the fetus and give rise to constriction bands. When circulation is seriously impaired, amputation of parts of limbs, syndactyly, cleft lip, anencephaly, encephalocoeles etc. may result (see also Chap. 4, p. 141). The reported incidence is 1:10000 of live births and 1:5000 total births and abortions. Amniocentesis may also result in amniotic constriction bands (Gellis 1977).

Small skin pits are occasionally encountered in the neonate, and some may arise from direct trauma during amniocentesis (Fig. 27.3).

Dermoid Cysts

These are congenital cystic structures with a wall of keratinising epithelium possessing adnexae and are thought to be a developmental abnormality occurring at sites of closure of development planes. Of congenital dermoid cysts 37% are in an orbital or periorbital site and 80% are on the face and neck (Pollard et al. 1976). The cysts may be large and may occasionally extend through the bone of the orbit or face.

Congenital sinus

Epithelial-lined sinus tracts are most commonly seen in the midline in the neck and the lumbosacral area tethered to the filum terminale. A hairy tail is occasionally present in the lumbosacral area (Fig. 27.4).

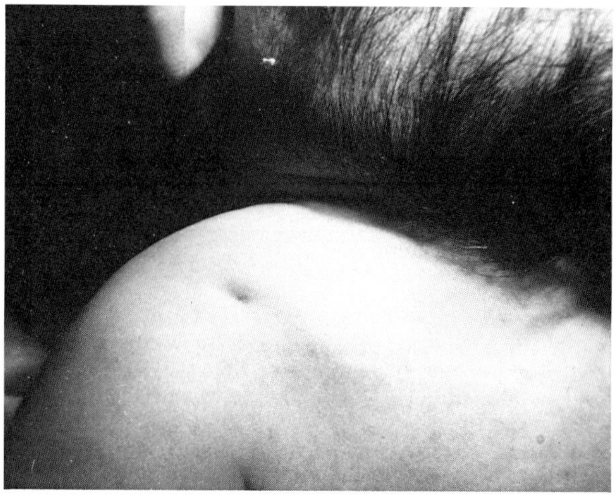

Fig. 27.3. Congenital dermal pit on the shoulder. (Courtesy of Drs. T.J. Ryan and R. Dawber, Oxford)

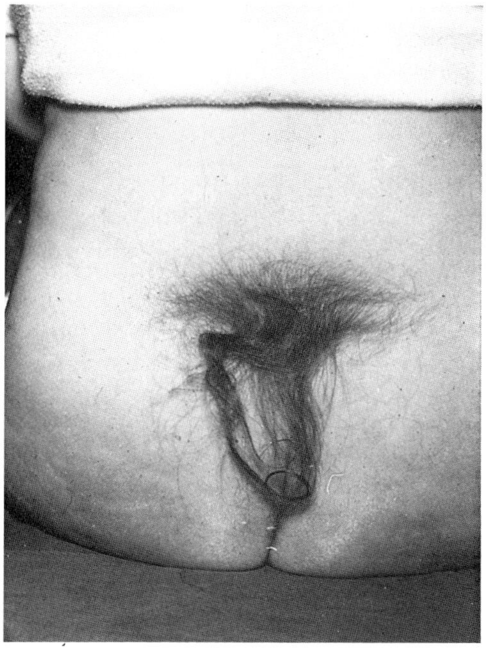

Fig. 27.4. Congenital hairy tail. These sometimes overlie spina bifida occulta. (Courtesy of Drs. T.J. Ryan and R. Dawber, Oxford)

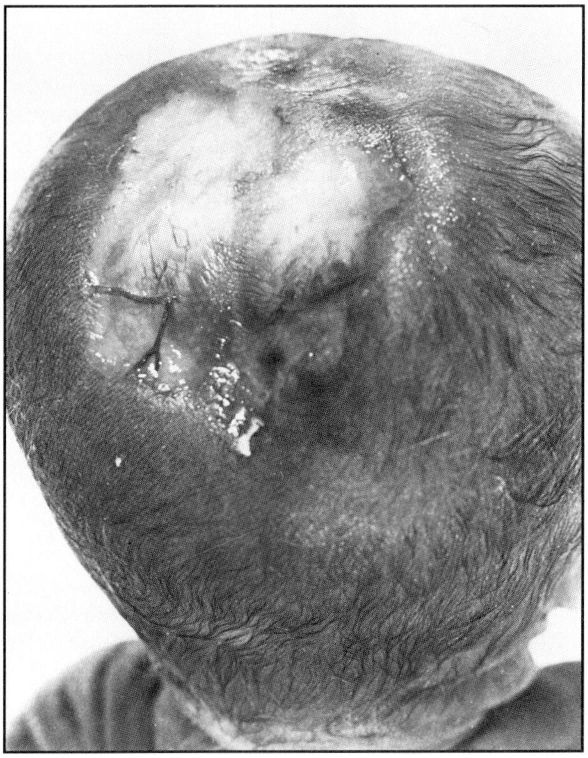

Fig. 27.5. Aplasia cutis congenita on the scalp in trisomy 13. Blood vessels are easily seen within the affected area.

Aplasia Cutis Congenita

This is a very rare, possibly autosomal-dominant disorder characterised by a localised absence of epidermis, dermis and subcutis, most usually on the scalp (Fig. 27.5). Healing of smaller lesions takes place with scarring and focal alopecia. A generalised form with widespread skin loss and autosomal-recessive inheritance is described. Some reports may actually be examples of recessive dystrophic epidermolysis bullosa with skin loss in utero (Fukamizu et al. 1983).

Ectodermal Dysplasia

Ectodermal dysplasia is a heterogeneous group of congenital developmental abnormalities of structures derived from ectoderm. All syndromes possess one or more abnormalities of epidermis or its appendages; they are generalised and non-progressive (Solomon and Keuer 1980). The best-defined is X-linked recessive anhidrotic ectodermal dysplasia (AED) in which there is failure to sweat, complete or partial anodontia, thin sparse growth of body and scalp hair and a characteristic facies with prominent forehead, brow ridges and a pointed chin. Sometimes there is nail dystrophy, hyperkeratosis of palms and soles, cleft lip and absence of the mammary glands. Female carriers show mild, patchy epidermal changes (Martin-Pascual et al. 1977). Histologically, there is a marked reduction in the numbers of eccrine glands, hair follicles and sebaceous glands (Martin-Pascual et al. 1977; Arnold et al. 1984). The disease can be diagnosed in male fetuses by prenatal skin biopsies (Arnold et al. 1984). Several biopsies must be taken, and although the normal development of sweat glands is not complete until 22–24 weeks, lack of normally developing hair follicles and sebaceous glands is diagnostic.

Another well-documented disorder is hidrotic ectodermal dysplasia (Clouston type) with autosomal-dominant inheritance, characterised by sparse, thin hair, hyperkeratosis of palms and soles, nail dystrophy with or without dental abnormalities, pigment disturbance and central nervous system involvement. There is a marked reduction in the numbers of hair follicles with abnormalities of existing hair bulbs and hyperkeratosis and acanthosis of the palms and soles (Pierard et al. 1979).

Rare ectodermal dysplasias are reviewed by Solomon and Keuer (1980) and Pinheiro and Freire–Maia (1983).

Dermal Developmental Disorders

Ehlers–Danlos Syndrome

Several inherited conditions referred to collectively as the Ehlers–Danlos syndrome show varying degrees of skin hyperextensibility, fragility, hypermobility of joints and aneurysm formation. They are all associated with abnormalities of collagen.

Collagen provides the mechanical scaffolding for many tissues and at least 11 types are described. The interstitial collagens are types I–III, of which type I is the most abundant and the major type in the adult dermis. Type III collagen is usually associated with type I and comprises 50% of the collagen of fetal dermis. After birth, less than 20% of the dermal collagen is type III. Type IV and VII are constituents of the basement membrane zones. The Ehlers–Danlos disorders are related to changes in the types I and III collagens or associated enzyme deficiencies (Pope and Nicholl 1986).

At least nine main variants of the disorder exist. Type IV Ehlers–Danlos syndrome, a severe disease with a high incidence of fatal rupture of large arteries, is due to a variable deficiency of type III collagen. This deficiency is associated with mutation of the type III collagen gene and may be recognised antenatally (Pope et al. 1988). It is type IV Ehlers–Danlos that can present in the neonatal period with skin, ocular and skeletal deformities. These are due to a deficiency of lysyl-hydroxylase, which converts lysine residues within the molecule to hydroxylysine, important for stable covalent cross-links between collagen molecules during fibre formation.

The skin bruises easily and is thinner than normal, often by as much as half, and collagen depleted. The collagen fibrils may be larger or smaller and mixtures are common (Sulica et al. 1979). Elastic fibres, because of the loss of collagen, falsely appear increased. Electron microscopy reveals alterations in collagen fibre diameters (Black et al. 1980; Holbrook and Byers 1982).

Cutis Laxa

The term "cutis laxa" covers a spectrum of rare conditions all of which possess loose and inelastic skin. The inheritance may be autosomal dominant, recessive or sex linked. Abnormally loose skin is sometimes apparent at birth, and the infant may develop systemic involvement including emphysema (Ledoux-Corbusier 1983). These babies may have lysyl oxidase deficiency and large collagen fibrils (Pope and Nicholl 1986). Holbrook and Byers (1982), however, proposed that there is a structural defect in elastic fibres with changes occurring in collagen as a secondary phenomenon. Elastic fibres in the skin are not necessarily depleted or absent.

Focal Dermal Hypoplasia

Focal dermal hypoplasia is rare, almost only found in females and characterised by multiple focal lesions in which the dermis is extremely thin. Many children have systemic abnormalities especially skeletal (80%) and ocular (40%). The skin lesions are apparent at birth as atrophic red scars and become worse with age. In places, subcutaneous fat protrudes through the deficient dermis. Histologically, the dermis is focally thin and the collagen fibres have smaller diameters but show normal striation. Connective tissue is reduced but fat cell content maintained (Lawler and Holmes 1989). The female preponderance raises the possibility of a dominant gene on the X chromosome that is usually lethal in males (Goltz et al. 1970; Gottlieb et al. 1973).

Developmental Abnormalities of Pigment

Albinism and Piebaldism

Oculocutaneous albinism is characterised by variable loss of skin pigmentation, translucent irides and hypopigmentation of the retina. The term encompasses a heterogeneous group. The incidence is 1:200000 in the USA but is much more frequent in some societies.

There are normal numbers of melanocytes with melanosomes but reduced or absent melanin production. There is an increased incidence of malignant skin tumours. Piebaldism, or partial albinism, has autosomal-dominant inheritance and shows well-circumscribed areas of depigmentation that often have a characteristic and almost symmetrical pattern. A lock of white hair on the forehead is commonly seen in this disorder. Melanocytes are absent in the epidemis and dermis of the affected areas and this may be due to a defect in development or migration of neural crest cells (Jimbow et al. 1975).

Common Neonatal Skin Conditions

Most of these conditions can be diagnosed clinically. Biopsy is rarely resorted to unless complications, principally infection, have developed. In these circumstances a small punch biopsy with multiple levels is often appropriate.

Erythema Toxicum Neonatorum

This is a diffuse rash of unknown cause which never affects palms and soles and occurs in 30% of mature babies. It is usually seen at age 2–3 days and is self-limiting with a blotchy erythema and superimposed pustules. The baby is well but a dermal infiltrate of eosinophils is seen, especially around hair follicles; the pustule is an intraepidermal bulla filled with eosinophils and close to one or more hair follicles. There is sometimes a peripheral blood eosinophilia (Luders 1960).

Nappy Rash

Nappy rash accounts for 20% of skin consultations in infants and young children (Honig 1983). The "primary irritant" type is caused by tight-fitting nappy and plastic pants leading to moist skin, maceration and friction damage exacerbated by the irritant effect of ammonia and proteolytic faecal enzymes. There are red, shiny, glazed areas sparing the inguinal folds (Fig. 27.6). Nappy rash caused or prolonged by *Candida albicans* consists of clusters of erythematous papules and pustules coalescing into a red rash (Fig. 27.7). Candida can be cultured from the skin in 40% of babies with nappy rash and rarely this is complicated by generalised plaques all over the body; the Id reaction. This reaction is thought to have an immunological basis, as candida cannot be cultured from lesions other than in the nappy area. Nappy rash is more common in bottle-fed babies and babies with a family history of atopic dermatitis

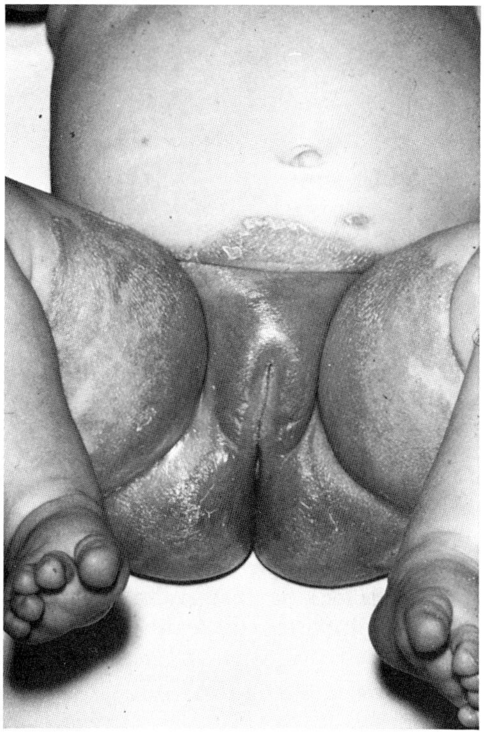

Fig. 27.6. Napkin dermatitis. There is scaling and red, shiny glazed areas. (Courtesy of Drs. T.J. Ryan and R. Dawber, Oxford)

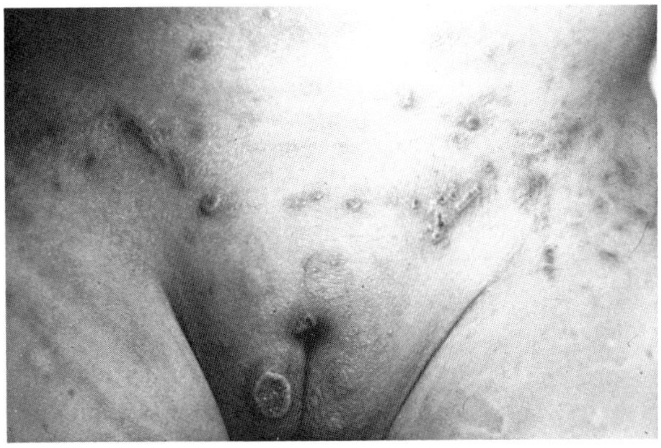

Fig. 27.7. Napkin dermatitis with raised circumscribed pustules and papules often associated with *Candida albicans* infection. (Courtesy of Drs. T.J. Ryan and R. Dawber, Oxford)

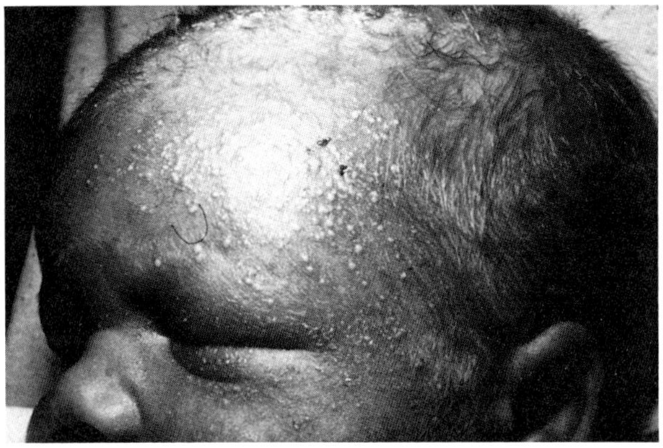

Fig. 27.8. Milia. Clusters of small white papules characteristically seen on the upper part of the face. (Courtesy of Drs. T.J. Ryan and R. Dawber, Oxford)

or seborrhoeic eczema. The differential diagnosis includes histiocytosis X, infantile psorasis (Farber et al. 1986), scabies and allergic contact dermatitis. Granuloma gluteale can be a complication (Walsh and Robson 1988).

Milia

These are tiny white papules seen on the forehead and face of up to 50% of infants (Fig. 27.8). They disappear during the first 4 weeks of life and are due to retention of keratin and sebaceous material within the pilosebaceous apparatus.

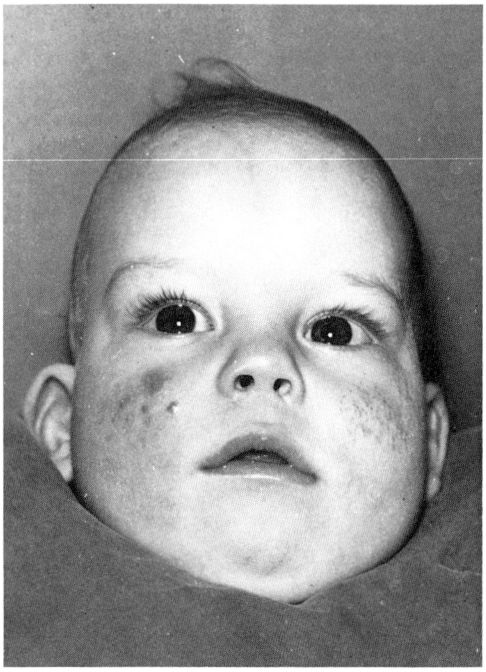

Fig. 27.9. Neonatal acne. Males are usually affected. (Courtesy of Drs. T.J. Ryan and R. Dawber, Oxford)

Neonatal Acne

This acne-like eruption develops within a few days of birth in 20% of neonates, almost always boys, and is confined to the face (Fig. 27.9). The spots disappear in the great majority of babies. The aetiology is unclear, but stimulation of facial pilosebaceous units by fetal androgen may be responsible.

Miliaria

Miliaria is very frequent in the neonate, particularly in a hot, humid environment, e.g. incubators. It is a symmetrical micropapular and vesicular rash occurring on the face, neck and trunk and clinically, taking two forms; sudamina and prickly heat. Recurrent crops develop and resolve after 2–3 days. Sweat retention from the relative immaturity of the eccrine glands and ducts is the cause.

Infantile Seborrhoeic Dermatitis

An erythematous scaly rash beginning on the scalp (cradle cap) in a neonate suggests infantile seborrhoeic dermatitis and is due, in part, to increased sebaceous gland activity (Fig. 27.10). The features are those of a subacute dermatitis. No relationship with the adult disorder is known.

Subcutaneous Fat Necrosis

This self-limiting disorder, usually resolving within 2–4 weeks of birth, is seen in full-term, often post-mature, babies. Single or multiple circumscribed indurated small nodules to large plaques, rarely painful, are evident on pressure areas. Within the involved fat is a lobular panniculitis with necrosis of fat cells, a lymphohistiocytic infiltrate and needle-shaped crystals within the fat and histiocytic cells (Friedman and Winkelmann 1989). Rarely, calcification and liquefaction supervene in which case scar-

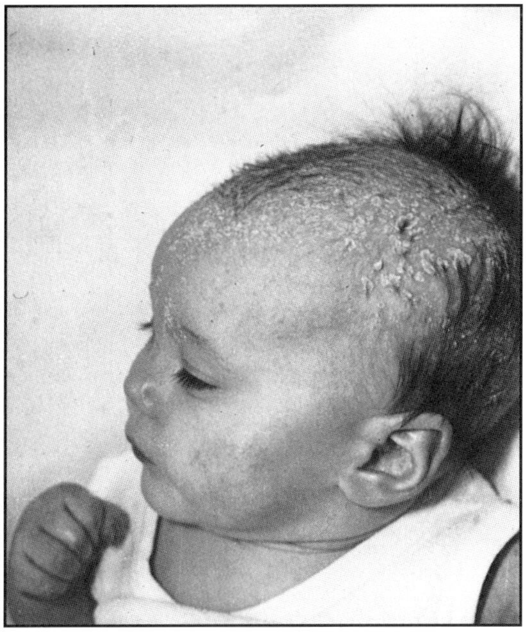

Fig. 27.10. Infantile seborrhoeic keratosis. There is extensive crusting of the scalp and some loss of hair. (Courtesy of Drs. T.J. Ryan and R. Dawber, Oxford)

ring will follow. Trauma, asphyxia, hypothermia and maternal diabetes have all been advanced as causative although these conditions may only serve to unmask a basic defect in the composition and metabolism of the fat (Friedman and Winkelmann 1989).

Sclerema Neonatorum

This condition holds a grave prognosis for the infant. It is seen in premature and debilitated neonates, often with congenital heart disease, sepsis or other severe illness. The skin is diffusely involved with a wax-like hardening comparable to that of the cadaver. The skin including the fat is oedematous but there is only rarely any inflammatory infiltrate. The child generally dies from the associated condition and no cause has been recognised.

Birthmarks

A birthmark is a cutaneous lesion present at birth which may persist, enlarge or regress with age. The terminology is confused but any form is often prefaced by either the cell type (melanocyte) or the tissue formed (vascular, lymphatic, organoid) or the epithelium involved (epidermis).

Pigmented Birthmarks

Mongolian Spot

This blue lesion presents over the sacrum and back in approximately 10% of white and up to 95.5% of black babies and tends to regress in childhood (Osburn et al. 1987; McLaurin 1988; Nanda et al. 1989; Gross et al. 1990). The diameter may extend from a few millimetres to several centimetres. Collections of pigmented melanocytes are located deep in the dermis, supporting the suggestion that migration arrest occurred during development.

Café au Lait Spots

These spots are well circumscribed and uniformly pale brown lesions, one or more of which can be found in 0.8% of newborn white babies and in 12% of black babies. Children have higher numbers probably because pigmentation is less developed in the neonate (Sigg et al. 1990). The majority occur in normal children, but just occasionally they are associated with systemic disorders such as von Recklinghausen's neurofibromatosis or Albright's syndrome. In the former, Crowe and Schull (1953) have suggested that six or more lesions greater than 1.5 cm in diameter in a child is presumptive evidence of neurofibromatosis. In Albright's syndrome a single large café au lait spot with an irregular edge is usually encountered. There is increased epidermal pigmentation without an increase in melanocytic cells.

Lentigines

These dark brown or black lesions are usually acquired during life in sun-exposed sites (solar lentigines). However, they may be present at birth, especially with certain systemic disorders, for example lentigines of the oral mucosa and lips in Peutz–Jeghers syndrome.

Gorlin et al. (1969) described a syndrome with autosomal-dominant inheritance and multiple lentigines. The mnemonic is LEOPARD: *L*entigines, *E*lectrocardiographic conduction defects, *O*cular hypertelorism, *P*ulmonary stenosis, *A*bnormalities of genitalia, *R*etardation of growth, and *D*eafness.

Lentigines have increased numbers of melanocytes disposed singly along the base of the epidermis and increased pigmentation of the basal epidermal cells.

Melanocytic Naevi

These lesions are formed by melanocytes and can involve the epidermis or the dermis, possibly reflecting their progress along the melanocytic developmental pathway (Cramer 1988). A variable histological pattern occurs amongst all melanocytic naevi although individual lesions maintain a consistent pattern (Nickoloff et al. 1986) and grow at the same rate as the child (Rhodes 1986). Clinically, congenital and acquired forms are recognised but histologically this distinction is not always possible (Rhodes et al. 1985; Nickoloff et al. 1986; Cramer 1988) and may in fact be false in that in some congenital lesions pigmentation has not developed at birth (Osburn et al. 1987). Consequently, under-reporting of incidence figures may result (Osburn et al. 1987; Sigg et al. 1990) and, more importantly, estimates of malignant potential (Rhodes 1986; Gari et al. 1988). The possibility of malignancy cannot be predicted histologically in the neonate (Rhodes 1986) but melanoma encountered at this time has followed transplacental spread from the mother (Krusinski and Saurat 1989).

Melanocytic naevi are present at birth in approximately 1% of white babies (Jacobs and Walton 1976; Rhodes and Melski 1982; Gross et al. 1990). They vary in size (Fig. 27.11) from tiny lesions to giant hairy pigmented lesions. The latter may show a dermatomal distribution on the trunk with sparing of the distal extremities (garment or bathing trunk naevi). Such naevi (i.e. greater than 10 cm in diameter) occur in less than 1 in 20 000 neonates.

Small melanocytic lesions are junctional or compound naevi histologically (Jacobs and Walton 1976). The larger lesions tend to involve the reticular dermis and subcutis, with naevus cells sometimes growing in an Indian file or neurofibroma-like pattern (Mark et al. 1973). A characteristic is growth along and within epidermal adnexal structures; collections of naevus cells are sometimes present beneath the endothelium of dermal veins (Figs. 27.12 and 27.13).

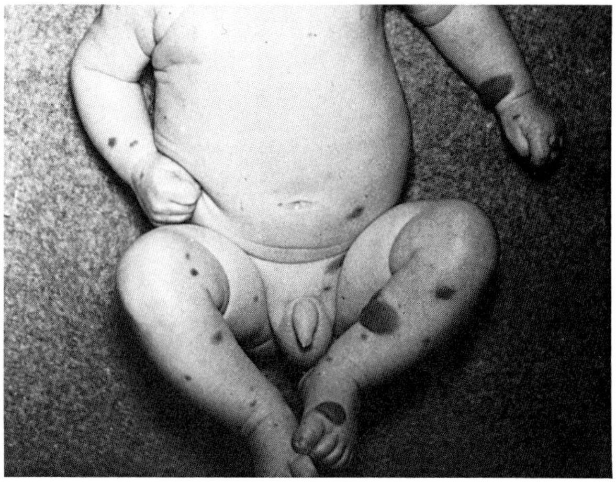

Fig. 27.11. Multiple congenital pigmented naevi. (Courtesy of Drs. T.J. Ryan and R. Dawber, Oxford)

Giant naevi have a recognised malignant potential (Gari et al. 1988). Estimates of the relative risk are complicated by definitions, age of referral and previous surgery. An estimate of the lifetime probability of developing melanoma in a giant naevus is 6.3% which is 16.6 times the risk to a normal person (Rhodes 1986).

Small melanocytic naevi may also carry a risk of malignant change. Rhodes and Melski (1982) examined 134 patients with melanoma and found that 15% described a pigmented lesion present since birth. Examination of 234 melanomas revealed a melanocytic naevus in contiguity with melanoma in 64, and 19 of these patients described a congenital naevus. Others have found similar histories of pre-existing naevi, as reviewed by Rhodes (1983).

Other Melanocytic Birthmarks

A rare congenital melanocytic lesion is the naevus of Ota, usually seen in female oriental children. There is unilateral patchy discoloration in the region of the second division of the trigeminal nerve (Rhodes 1983). Two-thirds of patients have involvement of the sclera and malignancy can develop (Dompmartin et al. 1989). The naevus of Ito is similar but is more extensive, involving the shoulder as well.

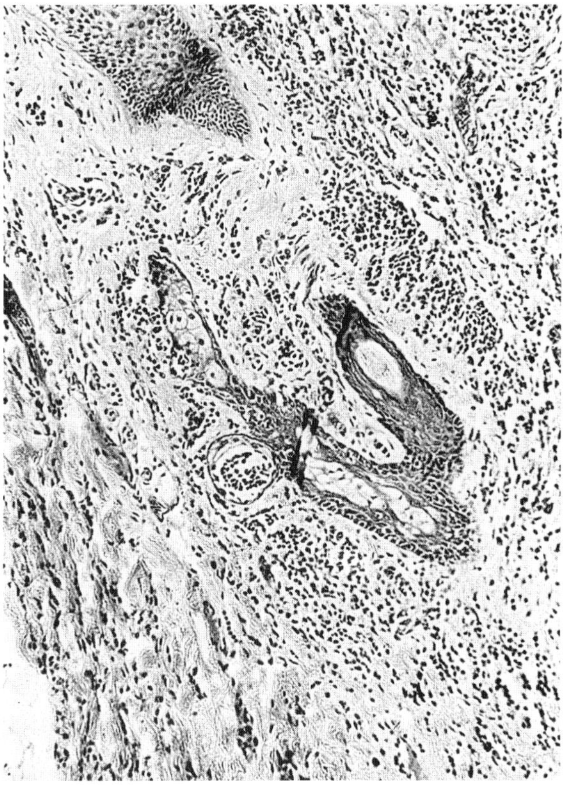

Fig. 27.12. Congenital pigmented naevus. There is junctional activity associated with the pilosebaceous unit. Nests and groups of naevus cells are present within the surrounding dermis. (×41)

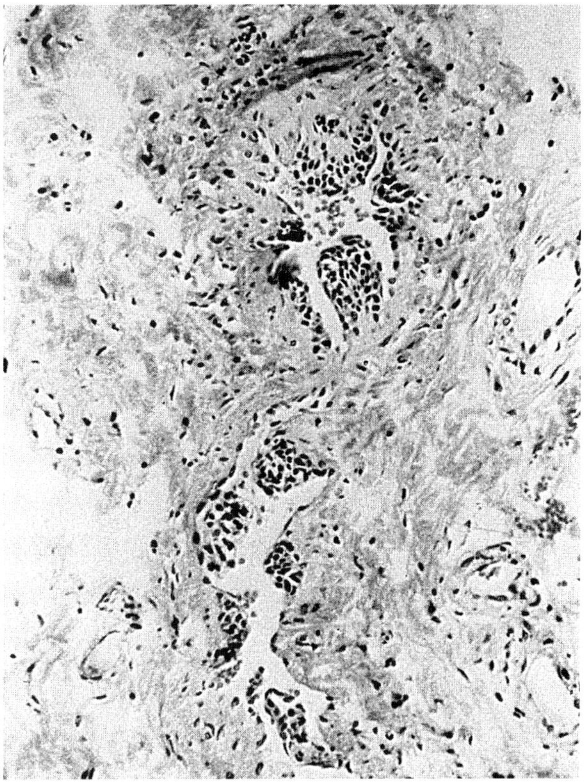

Fig. 27.13. Congenital pigmented naevus. Groups of naevus cells are apparent beneath the endothelium of a dermal vein and protrude into its lumen. (×108)

Congenital Vascular Abnormalities

Lesions present at birth or shortly thereafter which are due to a vascular ectasia or proliferation are quite common. Of these, the most frequent are capillary or strawberry haemangiomas (Osburn et al. 1987).

Strawberry Naevus

Present in 1.1%–2.6% of neonates and seen in 10% of children between the ages of 1 month and 1 year, strawberry naevi are raised deep-red lesions which invariably regress spontaneously (Fig. 27.14), especially the smaller examples (Salmon patches). They may be heralded at birth by a flat area of telangiectasia which rapidly changes into a typical lesion. This change follows canalisation between ectopic islands of vascular tissue and the dermal vessels. Any part of the body may be affected. Most are less than 5 cm in size but occasionally very large examples may result in significant arteriovenous shunting. Similar and sometimes fatal shunting can complicate diffuse haemangiomatosis (Held et al. 1990).

These naevi consist of proliferation of ectatic blood-filled vascular spaces lined by endothelial cells. Ectatic vessels in the deep dermis or subcutaneous tissue may have smooth muscle fibres in their walls, and those with a significant deep component may be called cavernous haemangiomas (Figs. 27.15, 27.16).

Regression is seen as a blue discoloration of the overlying skin, and histologically there is thrombosis and fibrosis of the ectatic vessels culminating in scar tissue. By the age of 7 years, 70% of haemangiomas have regressed. The smallest lesions (salmon patches) found in 44% of neonates of either sex can all be expected to have disappeared by 6 years of age. Those at the nape of the neck (stork bite

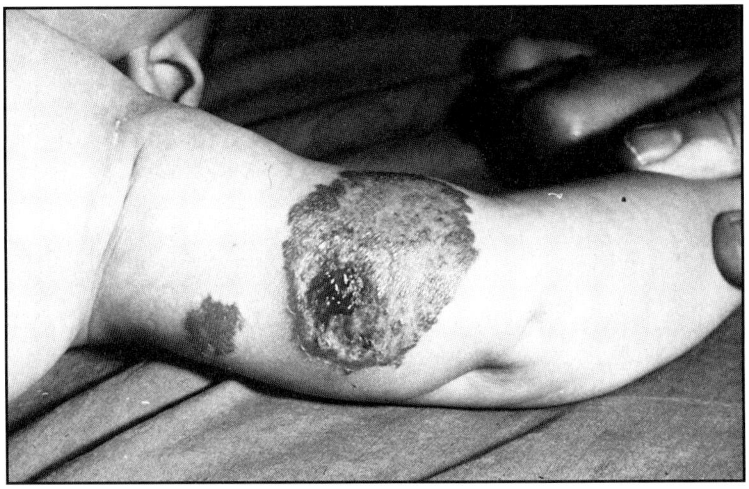

Fig. 27.14. Capillary haemangiomas on the arm of an infant. The larger lesion shows surface ulceration. (Courtesy of Drs. T.J. Ryan and R. Dawber, Oxford)

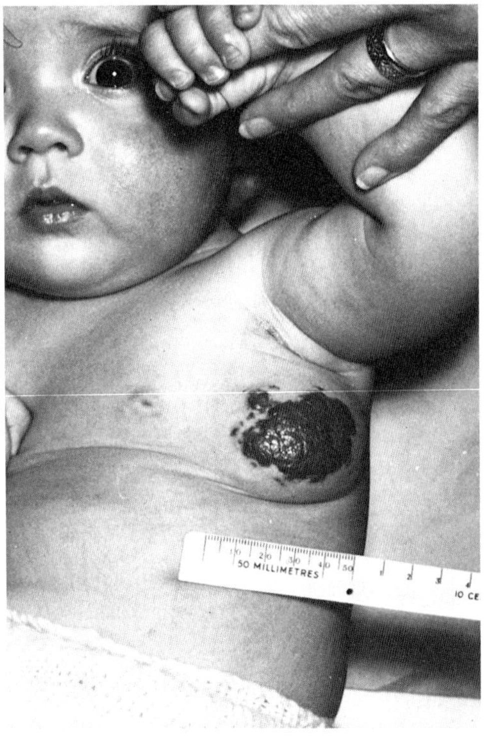

Fig. 27.15. Cavernous haemangioma. There is soft tissue involvement extending beyond the margin of the superficial skin lesion.

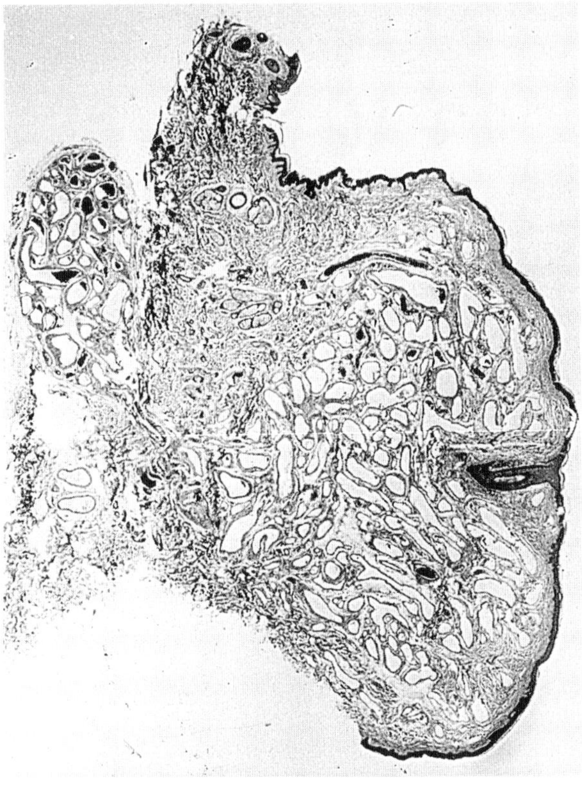

Fig. 27.16. Cavernous haemangioma with subcutaneous and dermal vessels; those more deeply placed have thicker walls containing smooth muscle. (×9)

mark) will take the longest time (Leung and Telmesani 1989).

Port Wine Stain

This flat pink lesion is present in 0.3% of neonates. It does not involute but grows with the child. It is often unilateral and may follow a dermatomal distribution. There is no histological abnormality in the neonate, but in an older child dermal capillaries are dilated but not increased in number (Jacobs 1983; Finlay et al. 1984).

A port wine stain in the distribution of the first division of the trigeminal nerve may be a manifestation of the Sturge–Weber syndrome. Concurrent, ipsilateral leptomeningeal angiomatosis results in focal seizures. Approximately 45% of babies also have ipsilateral congenital glaucoma indicating involvement of the maxillary and ophthalmic divisions of the trigeminal nerve.

Lymphangiomas

These malformations are characterised by dilated lymphatic vessels lined by endothelium. Distinction from haemangiomas is not always easy since bleeding into some occurs and no good antibody marker for lymphatic endothelium has been developed. The hypothesis that lymphatics and capillaries can be distinguished by a double-staining technique with Ulex europaeus 1 lectin (marking endothelial cells) and anti-Type IV collagen antibody (marking basal lamina) (Fallowfield and Cook 1990) rests upon the absence of basal lamina in many small lymphatics and requires further evaluation. Lymphangioma circumscriptum is the commonest form in the neonate. This is present at birth or develops in early infancy and persists with a predilection for neck, shoulders, proximal limbs, perineum and mouth. Multiple small vesicles are seen on one or more circumscribed areas of skin filled with clear or blood-stained fluid. The vesicles are ectatic lymphatic spaces within the papillary dermis and deep to this are dilated lymphatics, some with smooth muscle in their walls (Fig. 27.17). The high incidence of recurrence after excision, together with lymphangiographic observations led Whimster (1976) to propose that the primary abnormality was one or more lymph cisterns deep in the subcutis and not in continuity with the main lymphatic system. The cisterns give rise to the dermal ectatic vessels and are not affected by superficial excision.

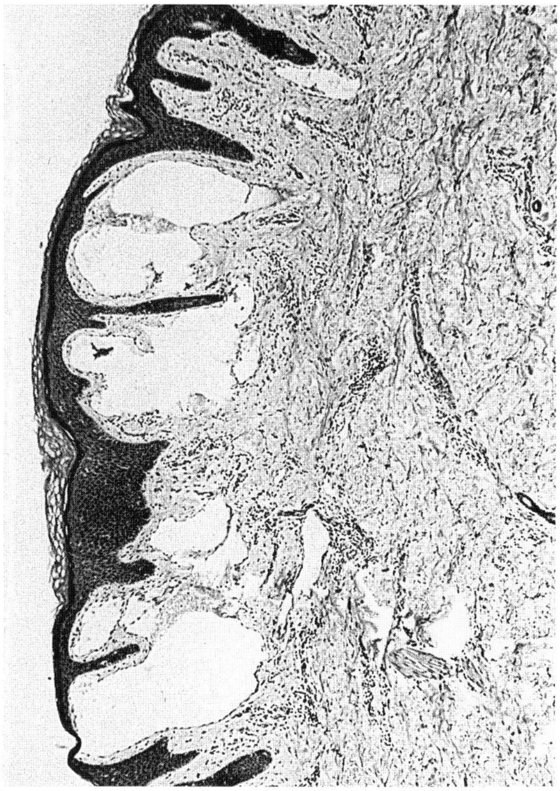

Fig. 27.17. Lymphangioma: ectatic lymphatics are present in the papillary dermis. (×24)

Another type (which may have a similar histogenesis) is the cavernous lymphangioma or cystic hygroma. This comprises one or more large cystically dilated spaces in the dermis, subcutis or intermuscular septum. They tend to occur on the neck, in the axilla, groin or popliteal fossa.

Other Birthmarks

Epidermal Naevi and Organoid Naevi

Localised malformations of the epidermis or skin appendages had an incidence of 0.2% in one neonatal survey (Jacobs and Walton 1976). The epidermal naevus appears darker than the surrounding skin, can occur anywhere on the body, has a warty or granular surface and may be single and localised or linear and extensive. Sometimes, spiral streaks are seen. The epidermal naevus is papillomatous and hyperkeratotic with irregular acanthosis. Extensive bilateral epidermal naevus may mimic the histology of epidermolytic hyperkeratotic ichthyosis and in such a case is referred to as ichthyosis hystrix (Hurwitz 1983; Fig. 27.18).

The organoid or sebaceous naevus characteristically occurs on the scalp as a flat yellow-pink hairless plaque. There is hyperkeratosis, irregular acanthosis and papillomatosis; skin appendages are malformed and irregular. At puberty apocrine glands are a prominent feature. During a lifetime, 10%–15% of organoid naevi are said to undergo neoplastic proliferation, usually giving rise to basal cell carcinoma and occasionally to syringocystadenoma papilliferum or other adnexal tumour.

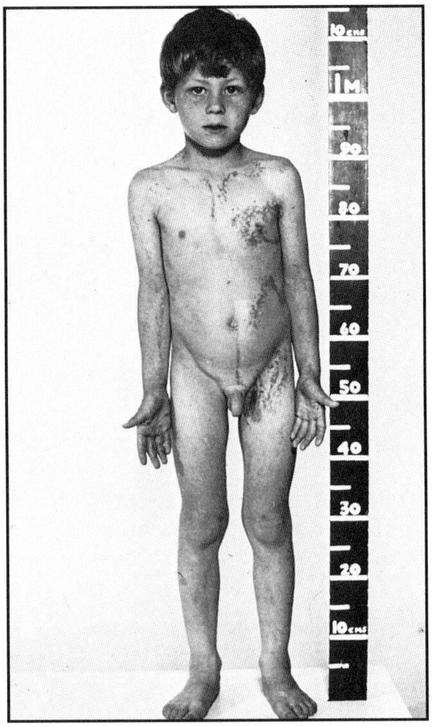

Fig. 27.18. Ichthyosis hystrix. The lesions are often linear and asymmetrically distributed. (Courtesy of Drs. T.J. Ryan and R. Dawber, Oxford)

Congenital Infections with Skin Manifestations

Viral Infections

These may be transmitted across the placenta, from the birth canal or from lesions on the mother or medical staff. The diagnosis may be reached from examination of neonatal and also maternal tissues including serum and this can be aided in biopsy material by labelled antibodies and molecular biology techniques. Not all such viral infections will declare themselves in the neonatal period, most notably human immunodeficiency virus (Straka et al. 1988; Lim et al. 1990). Others such as cytomegalovirus will manifest themselves in different forms in the neonate to those found in older infants (Sandler and Snedeker 1987).

Cytomegalovirus, Rubella

Congenital infections such as cytomegalovirus (CMV) or rubella sometimes exhibit a generalised rash at birth which is maculopapular and purpuric and occasionally includes Blueberry muffin lesions. These are magenta, 2–7 mm and have a raised indurated character and persist for 3–6 weeks. They comprise foci of erythrocyte precursors within the dermis and subcutis especially around eccrine adnexae. As dermal erythropoiesis is normal in embryos of crown–rump length less than 50 mm, they are thought to be due to persistence of erythroblastic elements rather than an infiltrative process (Brough et al. 1967). Similar lesions are occasionally seen other viral disorders in the neonate as well as in congenital toxoplasmosis (Krusinski and Saurat 1989).

Herpes Viruses

Congenital herpes simplex infections are usually due to type II virus and acquired from active maternal genital disease. Occasionally transplacental spread of virus, type I or II, occurs and, a few infections have resulted from home or hospital contacts (Francis et al. 1975). Over half of affected neonates have vesicles on the scalp and face erupting between the fourth and tenth days of life. There may be a conjunctivitis, or generalised eruption. Systemic disease follows rapidly.

Congenital varicella syndrome, in which infection occurs in the first trimester, includes abnormalities of limbs, eyes, brain and skin.

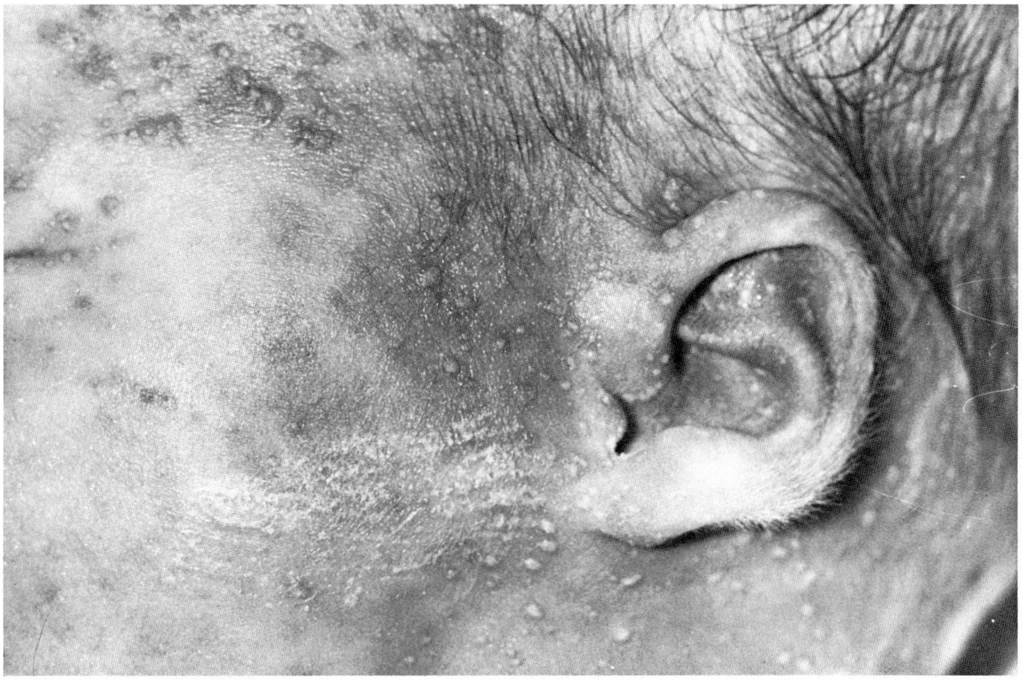

Fig. 27.19. Congenital chickenpox. Infection acquired in late pregnancy during overt maternal infection. Multiple small papules and vesicles are present.

Skin lesions heal leaving cicatricial scars at birth. Hyperplasia or absence of digits is sometimes observed. Varicella infection acquired shortly before delivery resembles postnatal infection (Fig. 27.19), but haemorrhagic pneumonitis is a serious and sometimes fatal complication in the neonatal period.

Bacterial Infections

Group A β-haemolytic Streptococcus

Neonates may acquire the highly contagious impetigo which is caused by a group A β-haemolytic streptococcus. Predisposing factors include a warm humid atmosphere and poor hygiene. Infants are also at risk of streptococcal cellulitis or erysipelas, which is a rapidly spreading superficial infection of skin precipitated by minor trauma including needle puncture and circumcision.

Staphylococcus aureus

Bullous impetigo is due to *Staphylcoccus aureus* and may be passed to a neonate from an attendant carrier producing infection in the nappy area or umbilicus. The causative organism is a phage group II staphylococcus, most commonly type 71 (Tunnessen 1983). A staphylococcus may also be responsible for neonatal cellulitis.

Staphylococcal Scalded Skin Syndrome

This syndrome affects neonates, infants and small children, and is due to an epidermolytic exotoxin produced by phage group II staphylococci. An affected baby may appear well despite an extensive erythematous exfoliative rash with a predilection for the face, upper trunk and groin areas (Fig. 27.20). There is a split in the epidermis at the level of the granular layer without a significant inflammatory infiltrate. The staphylococci producing the toxin are often found in the pharynx (Elias et al. 1977; Hansen 1983).

Congenital Syphilis

This disorder continues to appear and may be increasing. Affected neonates can be seronegative at birth despite positive serology in the mother and both baby and mother can be negative at the time of the birth (Dorfman and Glaser 1990). The skin involvement is most usually a diffuse macular papular eruption but atypical presentations are seen and in all examples there is systemic involvement. If there is a biopsy, demonstration of treponema with silver preparation confirms the diagnosis.

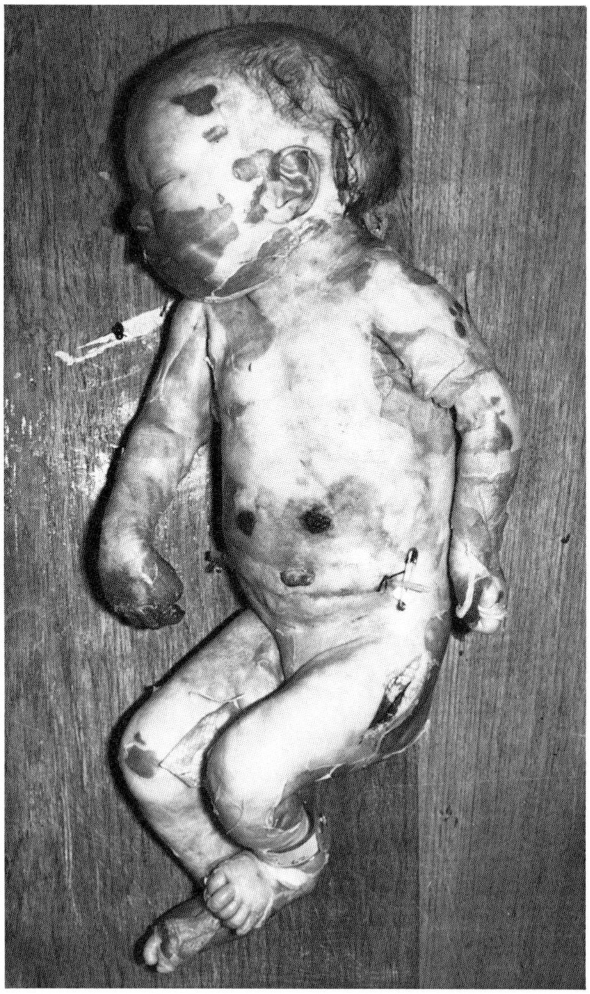

Fig. 27.20. Staphyloccocal scalded skin syndrome. Exfoliation of the epidermis affecting the face, shoulders, hands and feet. (Courtesy of Dr. A. King, Cambridge)

Congenital Genetically Determined Diseases

Disorders of Keratinisation

There are several congenital disorders of keratinisation. All are inherited and a classification is presented in Table 27.2.

Collodion Baby

At birth, a baby may be covered by a tight shiny collodion-like membrane (Fig. 27.21). Within a few days this membrane detaches, leaving the underlying skin red and scaly. The collodion membrane consists of orthokeratin (De Dobbeleer et al. 1982). Most collodion babies have lamellar ichthyosis, but occasionally the subsequent clinical picture resembles X-linked ichthyosis or ichthyosis vulgaris.

Lamellar Ichthyosis

This presents at birth either as a collodion baby or with generalised large epidermal scales 0.5–1.5 cm in diameter (Figs. 27.22, 27.23).

There is moderate thickening of the epidermis, uniform marked hyperkeratosis with focal parakeratosis, a prominent granular layer, moderate papillomatosis and a mild patchy chronic inflammatory infiltrate within the dermis (Frost and van Scott 1966). Keratinosomes are prematurely formed and synthesis of keratohyalin granules within the stratum spinosum is reduced. Nucleated cells and cell organelles are seen high in the granular layer. Hyperkeratosis may be due to a combination of the increased epidermal proliferation, abnormal keratin formation and increased adhesiveness of the upper epidermis, possibly mediated by keratinosomes.

The term "lamellar ichthyosis" embraces a heterogeneous group of abnormalities with two distinct subtypes. The first, lamellar ichthyosis, has the histological features described above; the second, non-bullous ichthyosiform erythroderma, has more marked acanthosis and only moderate hyperkeratosis, more rapid cell turnover and focal parakeratosis. Epidermal scales are smaller and finer than classic lamellar ichthyosis, and erythroderma is common (Hazell and Marks 1985; Williams and Elias 1985).

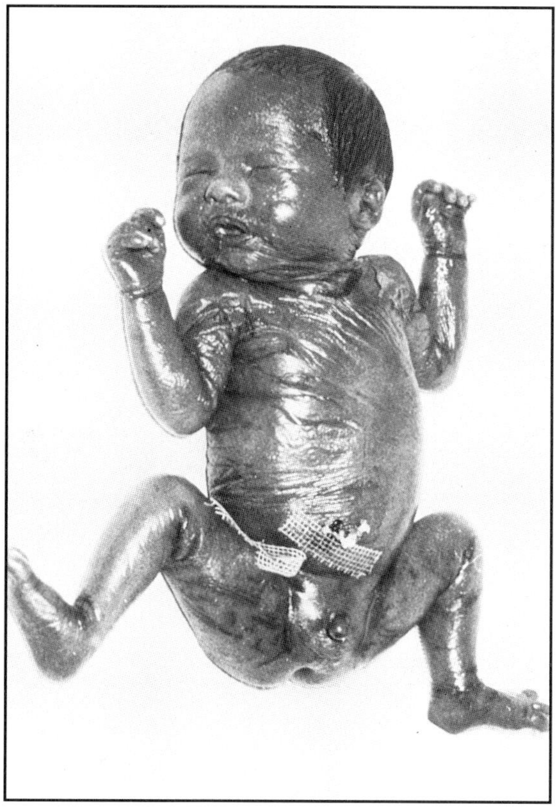

Fig. 27.21. Collodion baby. There is a tight shiny membrane involving the entire surface. (Courtesy of Prof. R. Marks, Cardiff)

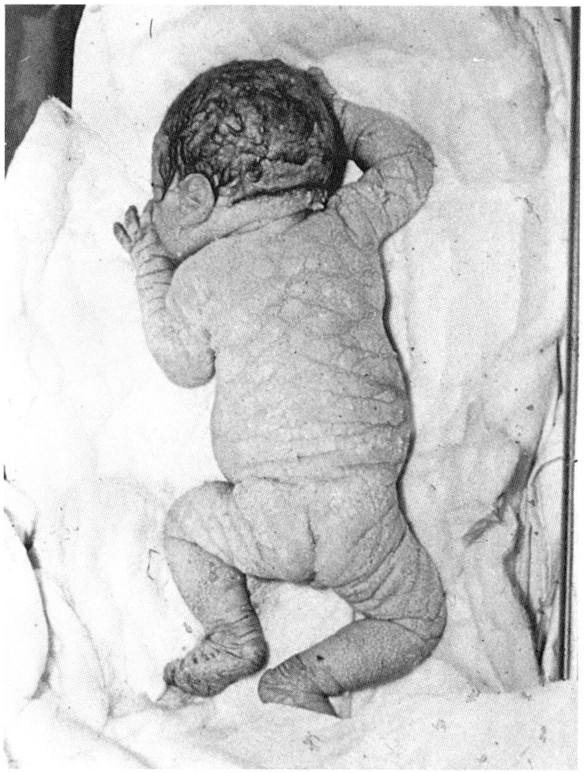

Fig. 27.22. Lamellar ichthyosis. (Courtesy of Drs. T.J. Ryan and R. Dawber, Oxford)

Harlequin Fetus

Harlequin fetus is a very rare recessive disorder in which the neonate is covered with thick plates of stratum corneum at birth. Affected babies usually die from sepsis within the first 2 weeks of life. A range of histological abnormalities is described, from hyperkeratosis with a normal granular layer to parakeratosis with an absent granular layer. Different X-ray diffraction patterns between patients suggests that the clinical presentation comprises more than one histogenetic entity (Baden 1982; Dale et al. 1990).

X-linked Ichthyosis

At birth this is only occasionally present as generalised mild scaling, more rarely as a collodion baby. The disease is due to a deficiency of steroid sulphatase in fetal epidermal

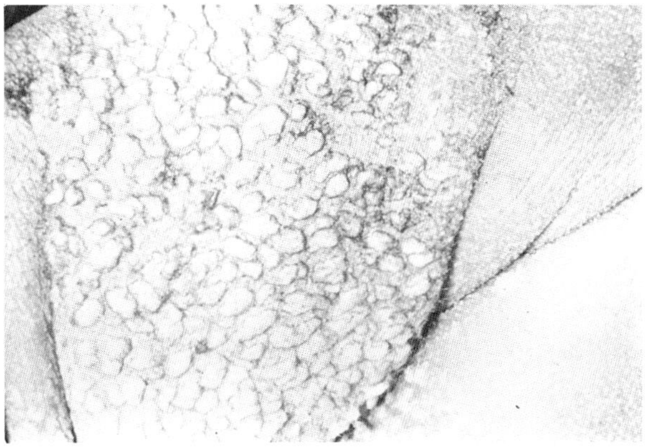

Fig. 27.23. Lamellar ichthyosis. Same patient as Fig. 27.22. High-power view of back of thigh. Individual scales are clearly seen. (Courtesy of Drs. T.J. Ryan and R. Dawber, Oxford)

Table 27.2. Congenital disorders of keratinisation in the neonate

Name	Genetics	Present at birth	Frequency	Histopathology	Turnover	Histogenesis	References
X-linked ichthyosis	X-linked recessive	Rarely Collodion baby	1:6000	Hyperkeratosis. Granular layer normal or slightly thick. Epidermis slightly thick	Normal	Steroid sulphatase deficiency	Epstein et al. (1981) Shapiro et al. (1978) Rehfield et al. (1988)
Lamellar ichthyosis	Autosomal recessive	Usually. Collodion baby or generalised ichthyosis	Rare 1:3 000 000	Hyperkeratosis. Normal or thick granular layer. Moderate acanthosis	Increased	Increased intercellular cement. Reduced synthesis of keratohyalin granules	Vandersteen and Muller (1972)
Epidermolytic hyperkeratosis (Bullous ichthyosiform erythroderma)	Autosomal dominant	Generalised erythema Blisters	Rare <1:100 000	Hyperkeratosis. Thick epidermis. Vacuolation of stratum spinosum and granular layer	Increased	Premature keratohyalin granules. Clumped tonofilaments interfering with desmosomes	Anton-Lamprecht (1983)
Harlequin fetus	Autosomal recessive	Thick plates of stratum corneum	Very rare	Variable; ortho- and sometimes parakeratosis	Unknown	Stratum corneum proteins abnormal	Baden (1982) Dale et al. (1990)
Non-bullous ichthyosiform erythroderma	Autosomal recessive	Generalised ichthyosis; fine scales and erythema. Collodion baby	Rare	Prominent acanthosis. Moderate hyperkeratosis. Focal parakeratosis	Increased	Unknown	Williams and Elias (1985) Hazel and Marks (1985)

Table 27.3. Neonatal forms of epidermolysis bullosa

Name	Genetics	Present at birth	Incidence	Level of blister	Antigen mapping		Electron microscopy
					Blister base	Blister roof	
Non-scarring							
Epidermolysis bullosa simplex	Autosomal dominant	Sometimes	1:50 000	Intraepidermal	BPA Laminin Type IV/VII collagen		Vacuolation of basal cells
Junctional epidermolysis bullosa (Herlitz)	Autosomal recessive	Yes	Very rare	Junctional	Laminin Type IV/VII collagen	BPA	Decrease and hypoplasia of basal hemidesmosomes
Scarring							
Dominant dystrophic epidermolysis bullosa	Autosomal dominant	Usually late infancy	1:100 000 to 1:50 000	Subepidermal	Type VII collagen	BPA Laminin Type IV collagen	Reduction of anchoring fibrils
Recessive dystrophic epidermolysis bullosa	Autosomal recessive	Yes	1:3 000 000	Subepidermal			Absence of anchoring fibrils

Eady 1987; Rasmussen et al. 1989. BPA, Bullous pemphigoid antigen (Fig. 27.2)

cells; cultured fibroblasts and placenta also show the defect (Shapiro et al. 1978). The result is a high concentration of cholesterol sulphate in the stratum corneum and hyperkeratosis. (Honour et al. 1985; Rehfield et al. 1988).

Epidermolytic Hyperkeratosis

Alternatively known as congenital bullous ichthyosiform erythroderma, this is a rare autosomal-dominant condition which may present at birth with generalised erythema, vesicles and bullae with subsequent development of thick brown scales. Localised forms sometimes resemble linear naevi. There is inter- and intracellular oedema within the upper stratum spinosum and stratum granulosum, a thick granular layer with irregular keratohyalin granules, and hyperkeratosis (Frost and van Scott 1966; Figs. 27.24, 27.25). Cell turnover is increased. The tonofibrils of the suprabasal epidermal cells are clumped, thereby reducing the effectiveness of desmosomal junctions resulting in separation and bulla formation. Anton-Lamprecht (1983) suggests that the increased cell turnover and hyperkeratosis are secondary reaction mechanisms.

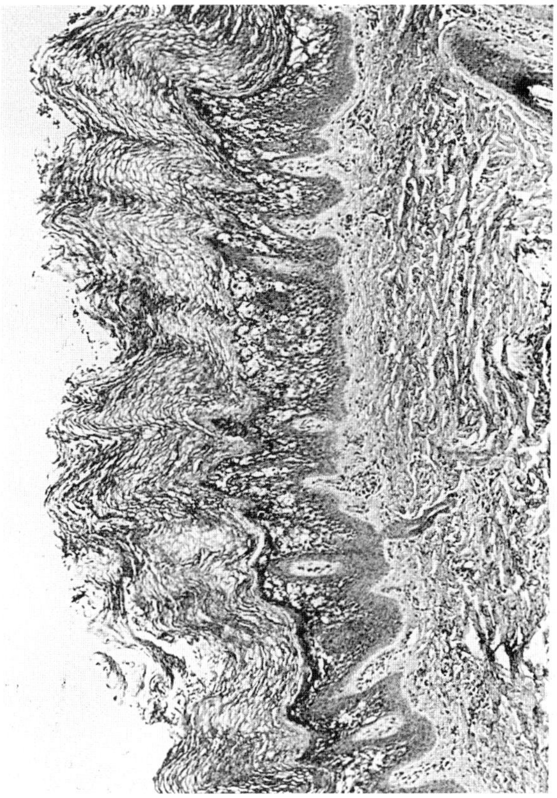

Fig. 27.24. Epidermolytic hyperkeratosis. There is uniform hyperkeratosis, vacuolation within the upper epidermis and irregular clumping of keratohyalin granules. (Courtesy of Dr. J. Mahood, Northampton.) (×41)

Blistering Disorders

A wide range of these are encountered in neonates, although fortunately most are uncommmon and innocuous (Frieden 1989). They may be subdivided clinically into overlapping groups, those in which the main lesions are pustules or vesicles (predominantly infective conditions); bullae (sucking blisters, epidermolysis bullosa, etc.); or erosive ulcerated lesions (staphylococcal scalded skin, toxic epidermal necrolysis, etc.). A fairly common finding is that the distribution of the lesions is often to those areas most exposed to mechanical stress such as the shoulders, elbows and heels. The infective conditions have the distinction that therapy is often available and that diagnosis can be made from appropriate swab and culture specimens. The much rarer genetic causes will often require electron microscopy and immunocytochemistry or immunofluorescent mapping (Fine et al. 1987) to define the level of blister formation in the dermo-epidermal junction, e.g. epidermolysis bullosa (Table 27.3), while others will involve biochem-

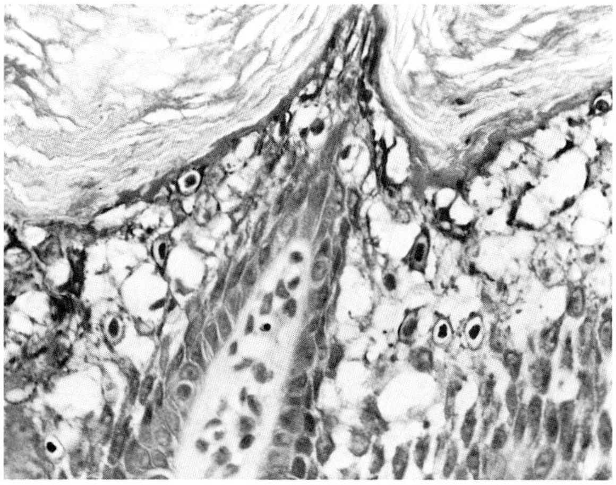

Fig. 27.25. Epidermolytic hyperkeratosis. (Courtesy of Dr. J. Mahood, Northamptom.) (×225)

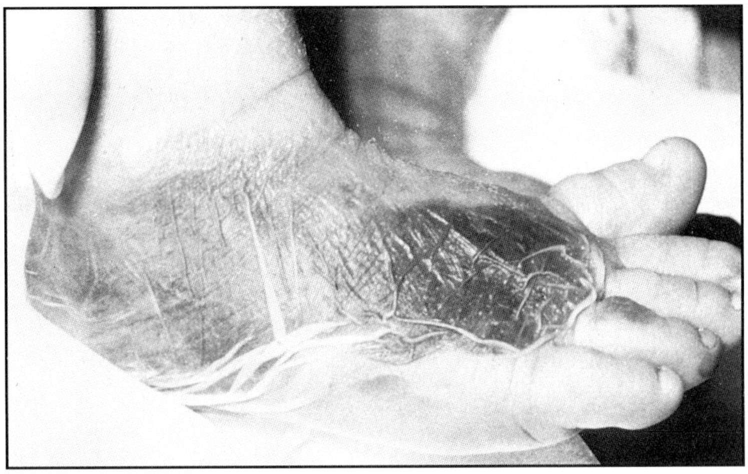

Fig. 27.26. Epidermolysis bullosa, non-scarring. There is loss of the epidermis over the foot. (Courtesy of Prof. R. Marks, Cardiff)

ical investigations, e.g. acrodermatitis enteropathica (zinc deficiency) and erythropoietic porphyria.

Epidermolysis Bullosa Simplex

Blistering occurs in the first few minutes of life from gentle trauma and is most often seen on the extremities (Fig. 27.26). Mucous membrane involvement may occur and blisters heal without scarring. The disorder improves before adolescence.

Junctional Epidermolysis Bullosa (Herlitz)

Neonates with this autosomal-recessive condition are born with erosions and bullae and minimal trauma promotes blistering. A similar tendency for mucosal separation is seen in the gastrointestinal, genitourinary and respiratory tracts (Schachner et al. 1977). Although the prognosis is poor with death from sepsis in the first years, survival into adulthood is becoming possible with the use of corticosteroids. Pregnancy and oral contraceptive agents are also described as beneficial. A diagnosis can be made prenatally by means of a fetal skin biopsy. If the basal epidermal hemidesmosomes are normal by 18–20 weeks' gestation, junctional epidermolysis bullosa can be excluded (Anton-Lamprecht 1983).

Dystrophic Epidermolysis Bullosa

Bullae are large and rupture, leaving deep ulcers (Fig. 27.27) which heal by scar formation. The disease is more severe in the recessive

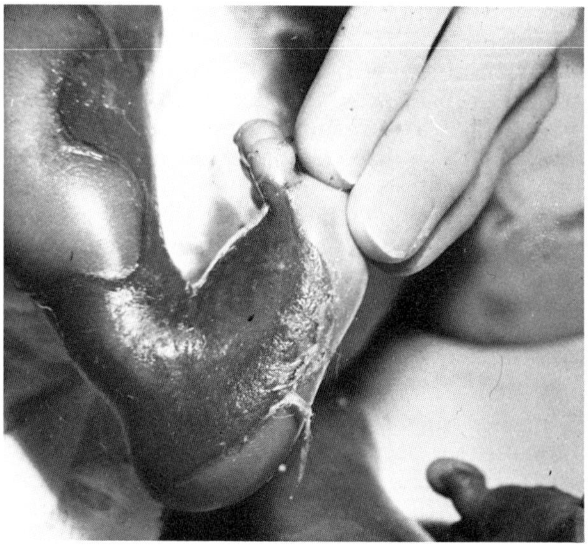

Fig. 27.27. Dystrophic epidermolysis bullosa. Rupture of bullae leaves extensive, well-defined, deep ulcers. (Courtesy of Drs. T.J. Ryan and R. Dawber, Oxford)

form with greater mucosal involvement, reduced lifespan and an increased incidence of basal and squamous carcinoma of the skin.

Anton-Lamprecht and Schnyder (1973) reported an absence of anchoring fibrils in patients with dominant scarring epidermolysis bullosa. Briggaman and Wheeler (1975), using an elegant experiment involving recombination of epidermis and dermis from normal patients and patients with the recessive disorder, found that there is absence of dermal anchoring fibrils. Recombination of the abnormal epidermis with normal dermis resulted in the formation of anchoring fibrils, while the reverse did not. Recent observations confirm the absence of anchoring fibrils associated with the absence of type VII collagen (Bruckner-Tuderman et al. 1989; Rusenko et al. 1989) as well as chondroitin sulphate (Fine and Couchman 1989) and may imply that there is a genetic defect in the synthesis of these proteins.

Incontinentia Pigmenti

This rare disorder, almost exclusive to girls, is possibly X-linked and dominant. Systemic changes including CNS, skeletal, dental and particularly ocular abnormalities (Francois 1984) are invariably present and are the cause of morbidity. In a study of 455 patients with incontinentia pigmenti, 34 were blind at the time of examination (Carney 1976). The skin lesions occurs as a series of stages, not always in the same sites of the body. The first stage is present at birth of within the first days of life as a linear erythematous vesicular lesion on the trunk and extremities. There may be a peripheral eosinophilia accompanying an interepidermal eosinophilic spongiosis. The second stage occurs within weeks as verrucous growths, often on the extremities and characterised by acanthosis, papillomatosis and hyperkeratosis. Later, these subside and linear whorls and streaks of pigmentation appear, especially on the trunk. At this stage melanin from melanocytes within the basal epidermis is present within dermal macrophages. All stages include dyskeratotic cells within the epidermis, some being phagocytosed by macrophages. Gradually the pigmented lesions fade to leave atrophic or depigmented areas (Guerrier and Wong 1974; Carney 1976).

The pathogenesis is unknown, though Schamburg-Lever and Lever (1973) have suggested that dyskeratosis promotes macrophage migration into the epidermis and incontinentia pigmenti results from subsequent macrophage elimination to the dermis.

Skin Disorders with Disordered Immune Responses

The immune responses of the neonate are incompletely developed and are also affected by those of the mother (Chap. 2). The effect of the latter will be to mask the appearance of primary immunodeficiency states in the neonate and the appearance of skin disorders associated with such conditions. If, however, the mother's immune responses are abnormal, skin disorders may be transmitted to the fetus and some may be declared in the neonate (Krusinski and Saurat 1989). Herpes gestationis and lupus erythematosus are rare examples while pemphigus vulgaris, although similarly transmitted, is not evident until later childhood (Paltzik and Laude 1978). The common denominator for these disorders is circulating maternal autoantibodies.

Neonatal Lupus Erythematosus

Although the mother has systemic lupus erythematosus she may be asymptomatic during pregnancy and the condition is unsuspected. Circulating RO (SSA) antibodies will nonetheless be found in her serum and that of the neonate. The infant may be small for dates and have a scaly annular erythematous and papular rash mainly on the head and scalp. Any sun or UVL exposure will exacerbate the rash. Examination of the skin reveals the changes associated with lupus erythematosus in adults, namely hyperkeratosis, epidermal atrophy, basal cell liquefaction and periappendageal mononuclear cell infiltrates. Remission with or without mild scarring is the usual outcome within a 6-month period (Watson and Provost 1987). Other features of lupus may be evident, the commonest being congenital heart block. Indeed the heart condition may dominate the clinical state and is probably a cause for an underestimate of the incidence of this condition (Olson and Lindsley 1987).

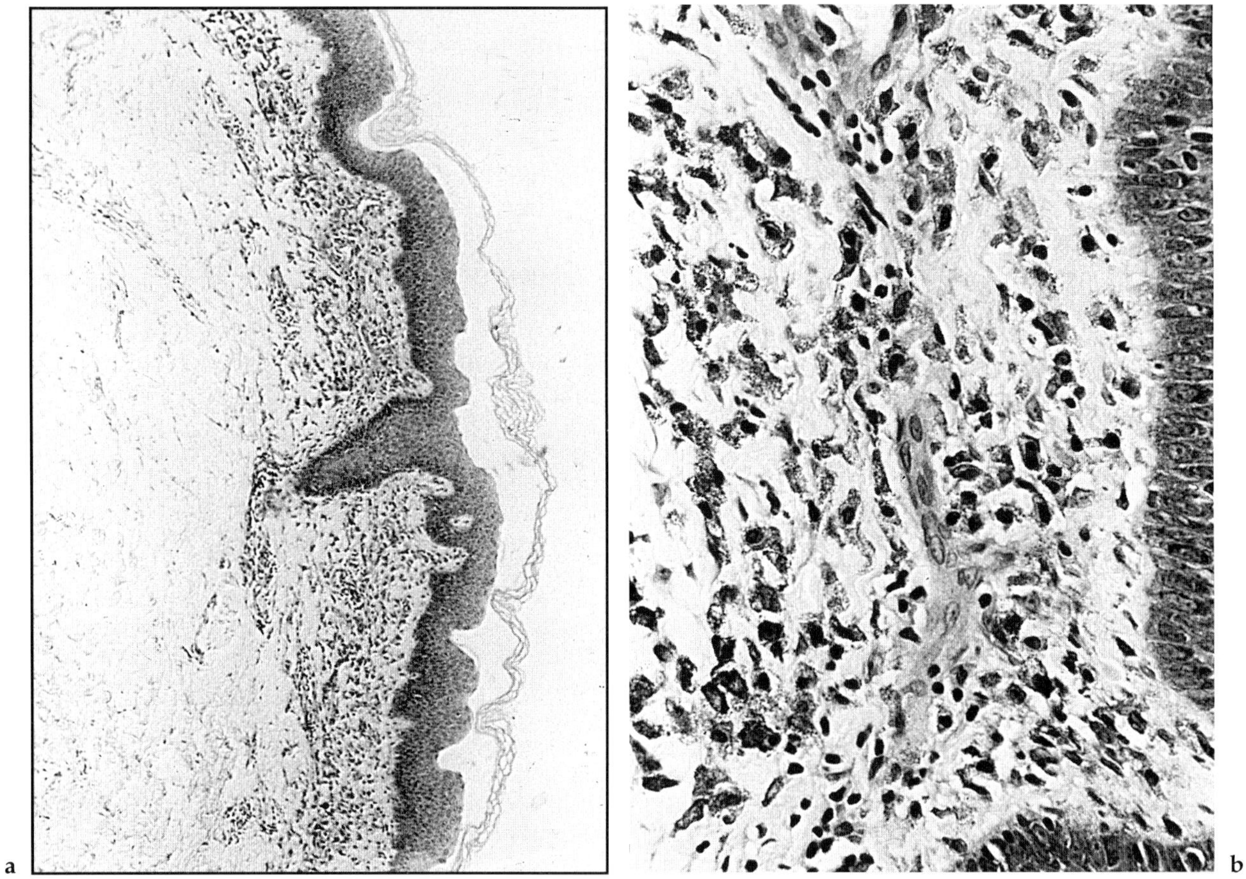

Fig. 27.28. Urticaria pigmentosa. **a** Numerous mast cells are present in the papillary dermis beneath a hyperpigmented epidermis. (Toluidine blue, ×49.) **b** At high power the mast cell granules are clearly seen. (Toluidine blue ×289)

Skin Infiltrations and Tumour-like Lesions

Urticaria Pigmentosa and Diffuse Cutaneous Mastocystosis

Urticaria pigmentosa usually begins in the first year of life as a pigmented maculopapular or nodular rash, most often on the trunk, and occasionally present at birth. There is mast cell proliferation within the superificial dermis and increased melanin pigmentation of basal cells of the overlying epidermis (Fig. 27.28). The skin urticates on stroking and uninvolved skin often shows dermatographism with a mild generalised increase in dermal mast cells. In most babies, the condition remains confined to the skin and improves gradually with ultimately complete resolution, though sometimes over several years. In a few, the condition remains active for many years, although only very rarely progressing to systemic mastocytosis (Klaus and Winkelmann 1962).

A less common variant is solitary mastocystosis (mast cell naevus) in which only one or a few individual lesions are found. Slightly elevated plaques or nodules are evident, often at birth, with histology similar to that of the diffuse condition.

Diffuse cutaneous mastocytosis in infancy is much less common than urticaria pigmentosa and presents as a widespread, diffuse infiltrate of mast cells in the dermis, sometimes with bulla formation. Systemic symptoms of histamine release are present and there is usually other organ involvement. (Travis et al. 1988).

Histiocytosis X

A persistent rash may be the initial manifestation in early infancy of the form of histiocytosis X known as Letterer–Siwe disease. The rash may be generalised or localised to the perineum, resembling nappy rash, or the scalp, masquerading as seborrhoeic dermatitis. Onset is usually during the first year of life, and signs of involvement of the bone marrow and reticulo-endothelial system follow. Rarely, the disease in infants appears confined to the skin (Wolfson et al. 1981). A dense infiltrate of cells with eosinophilic cytoplasm and convoluted nuclei is found in the dermis (Fig. 27.29). Scattered mitotic figures are seen and there is extension of cells into epidermis with occasional ulceration. A few eosinophils are present, but there are few or no multinucleate cells, lymphocytes or foamy cells, unlike other forms of histiocytosis X. Electron microscopy of infiltrating cells (Fig. 27.29), enzyme histochemistry and immunohistochemistry support a Langerhans' cell origin (Bos et al. 1984; Groh et al. 1988). The prognosis is difficult to assess. Spontaneous remission occurs (Lee et al. 1988) but, with generalised involvement of haemopoietic tissue, a fatal outcome can result.

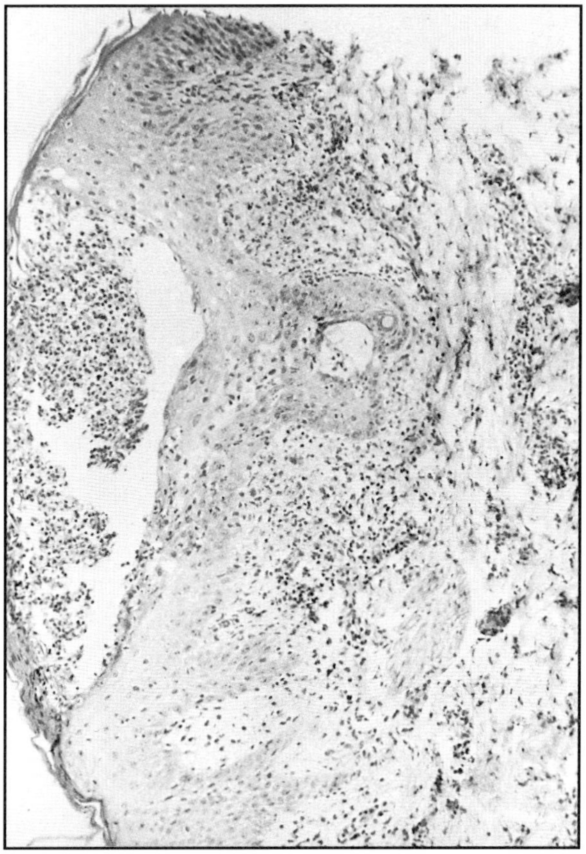

a

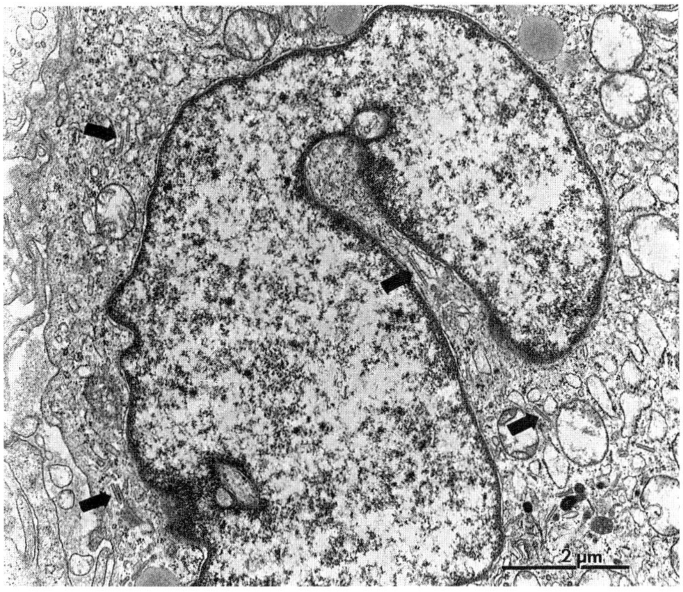

b

Fig. 27.29. Histiocytosis X. **a** There is a dense cellular infiltrate within the dermis and epidermis. **b** Ultrastructural appearances of the infiltrating cells. Typical Birkbeck granules are evident within many parts of the cytoplasm (*arrow*) and the nucleus is indented (Courtesy of A.J. Skinner, Oxford.)

References

Anton-Lamprecht I (1983) Genetically induced abnormalities of epidermal differentiation and ultrastructure in ichthyoses and epidermolyses: pathogenesis, heterogeneity, fetal manifestations and prenatal diagnosis. J Invest Dermatol 81: 1495–1565

Anton-Lamprecht I, Schnyder UW (1973) EB dystrophica dominant, a defect in anchoring fibrils. Dermatologica 147: 289–298

Arnold ML, Rauskolb R, Anton-Lamprecht I, Schnizel A, Schmid W (1984) Prenatal diagnosis of anhidrotic ectodermal dysplasia. Prenat Diagn 4: 85–98

Atherton DJ, Rook A (1986) The newborn. In: Rook A, Wilkinson DS, Ebling FJG, Champion RH, Burton JL (eds) Textbook of dermatology, 4th edn. Blackwell Scientific Publications, Oxford, pp 229–230

Baden HP (1982) Keratinisation in the harlequin fetus. Arch Dermatol 118: 14–18

Black CM, Gathercole LJ, Bailey AJ, Beighton P (1980) Ehlers–Danlos syndrome: an analysis of the structure of the collagen fibres of the skin. Br J Dermatol 102: 85

Bos JD, Sillevis-Smith JH, Krieg SR, Bakker PM, Vos GD, van Zaane DJ (1984) Acute disseminated histiocytosis X. J Cutan Pathol 11: 59–64

Breathnach AS (1971) The Herman Beerman lecture: embryology of human skin. J Invest Dermatol 57: 133–143

Breathnach AS, Robins J (1969) Ultrastructural features of epidermis of a 14 mm (6 weeks) human embryo. J Dermatol 81: 504–516

Breathnach AS, Wylie LM (1965) Electron microscopy of melanocytes and Langerhans' cells in human fetal epidermis at 14 weeks (menstrual dates). J Invest Dermatol 44: 51–60

Briggaman RA, Wheeler CE (1975) EB dystrophica recessive. A possible role of anchoring fibrils in the pathogenesis. J Invest Dermatol 65: 203–211

Brough AJ, Jones D, Page RH, Mizukami I (1967) Dermal erythropoiesis in neonates. A manifestation of intrauterine viral disease. Pediatrics 40: 627–635

Bruckner-Tuderman L, Mitsuhashi Y, Schnyder UW, Bruckner P (1989) Anchoring fibrils and Type VII collagen are absent from skin in severe recessive dystrophic epidermolysis bullosa. J Invest Dermatol 93: 3–9

Carney RG (1976) Incontinentia pigmenti—a world statistical analysis. Arch Dermatol 112: 535–542

Cramer SF (1988) The melanocytic differentiation pathway in congenital melanocytic nevi: theoretical considerations. Pediatr Pathol 8: 253–265

Crowe FW, Schull WJ (1953) Diagnostic importance of café au lait spot in neurofibromatosis. Arch Intern Med 91: 758–766

Dale BA, Holbrook KA, Fleckman P, Kimball JR, Brumbaugh S, Sybert VP (1990) Heterogeneity in harlequin ichthyosis, an inborn error of epidermal keratinisation: variable morphology and structural protein expression and a defect in lamellar granules. J Invest Dermatol 94: 6–18

De Dobeler G, Heenen M, Song M, Achten G (1982) Collodion baby skin. Ultrastructural and autoradiographic study. J Cutan Pathol 9: 196–202

Dompmartin A, Leroy D, Labbé D, Letessier JB, Mandard JC (1989) Dermal malignant melanoma developing from a nevus of Ota. Int J Dermatol 28: 535–536

Dorfman DH, Glaser JH (1990) Congenital syphilis presenting in infants after the newborn period. N Engl J Med 323: 1299–1302

Eady RAJ (1987) Babes, blisters and basement membranes: from sticky molecules to epidermolysis bullosa. Clin Exp Dermatol 12: 161–170

Elias PM (1989) The stratum corneum as an organ of protection: old and new concepts. In: Fritsch P, Schuler G, Hintner H (eds) Immunodeficiency and skin. Current problems in dermatology 18th edn. pp 10–21

Elias PM, Fritsch P, Epstein EH (1977) Review: staphylococcal scalded skin syndrome. Arch Dermatol 113: 207–219

Epstein EJ, Williams ML, Elias PM (1981) Editorial: steroid sulphatase, X linked ichthyosis and stratum corneum cell cohesion. Arch Dermatol 117: 761–763

Fallowfield ME, Cook M (1990) Lymphatics in primary cutaneous melanoma. Am J Surg Pathol 14: 370–374

Farber EM, Mullen RH, Jacobs AH, Nall L (1986) Infantile psoriasis: a follow up study. Pediatr Dermatol 3: 237–243

Fine J, Couchman JR (1989) Chondroitin-6-sulphate proteoglycan but not heparin-sulphate proteoglycan is abnormally expressed in skin basement membrane from patients with dominant and recessive dystrophic epidermolysis bullosa. J Invest Dermatol 92: 611–616

Fine J, Hintner H, Katz SI (1987) Immunofluorescent studies in epidermolysis bullosa utilising polyclonal and monoclonal antibodies. In: Beutner EH, Chorzelski TP, Kumar V (eds) Immunopathology of the skin, 3rd edn. John Wiley and Sons, Chichester, pp 399–405

Finlay JL, Noe JM, Arndt KA, Rosen S (1984) Port wine stains. Arch Dermatol 120: 1453–1455

Francis DP, Herrmann KL, MacMahon, JR, Chaviguy KH, Sanderlin KC (1975) Nosocomial and maternally acquired herpes virus hominis infections. Am J Dis Child 129: 889–893

Francois J (1984) Incontinentia pigmenti and retinal change. Br J Ophthalmol 68: 19–25

Frieden IJ (1989) Blisters and pustules in the newborn. Curr Probl Pediatr 19: 551–614

Friedman SJ, Winkelmann RK (1989) Subcutaneous fat necrosis of the newborn: light, ultrastructural and histochemical microscopic studies. J Cutan Pathol 16: 99–105

Frost P, van Scott EJ (1966) Ichthyosiform dermatoses. Arch Dermatol 94: 113–126

Fukamizu H, Matsumoto K, Inoue K, Moriguchi T (1983) Familial occurrence of aplasia cutis congenita. J Dermatol Surg Oncol 9: 712–713

Gari LM, Rivers JK, Kopf AW (1988) Melanomas arising in large congenital nevocytic nevi: a prospective study. Pediatr Dermatol 5: 151–158

Gellis SS (1977) Constrictive bands in the human. Birth Defects XIII(1): 259–265

Goltz RW, Henderson RR, Hitch JM, Ott JE (1970) Focal dermal hypoplasia. Arch Dermatol 101: 1–11

Gorlin RJ, Anderson RC, Blaw M (1969) Multiple lentigines syndrome. Am J Dis Child 117: 652–662

Gottlieb SK, Fisher BK, Violin GA (1973) Focal dermal hypoplasia, 9 year follow-up. Arch Dermatol 108: 551–553

Groh V, Gadner H, Radaszkiewicz T et al. (1988) The phenotypic spectrum of histiocystosis X cells. J Invest Dermatol 90: 441–447

Gross BD, Forman D, Ansell PE et al. (1990) The prevalence and characteristics of congenital pigmented lesions in newborn babies in Oxford. Paediatr Perinat Epidemiol 4: 448–457

Guerrier CJW, Wong CK (1974) Ultrastructural evolution of

the skin in incontinentia pigmenti. Dermatologica 149: 10–22
Hansen RC (1983) Staphylococcal scalded skin syndrome, toxic shock syndrome and Kawasaki disease. Pediatr Clin North Am 30(3): 533–544
Hashimoto K, Gross BG, DiBella RJ, Lever WF (1966) The ultrastructure of the skin of human embryos. IV Epidermis. J Invest Dermatol 47: 317–335
Hazell M, Marks R (1985) Clinical, histologic, and cell kinetic discriminants between lamellar ichthyosis and nonbullous ichthyosiform erythroderma. Arch Dermatol 121: 489–493
Held JL, Haber RS, Silvers DN, Grossman ME (1990) Benign neonatal hemangiomatosis: review and description of a patient with unusually persistent lesions. Padiatr Dermatol 7: 63–66
Holbrook KA, Byers PH (1982) Structural abnormalities of the dermal collagen and elastic matrix from the skin of patients with inherited connective tissue disorders. J Invest Dermatol 79: 7s–16s
Holbrook KA, Odland GF (1975) The fine structure of developing human epidermis: light, scanning and transmission electron microscopy of the periderm. J Invest Dermatol 65: 16–38
Honig PJ (1983) Diaper dermatitis. Postgrad Med 74(6): 79–84
Honour JW, Goolamali SK, Taylor NF (1985) Prenatal diagnosis and variable presentation of recessive X-linked ichthyosis. Br J Dermatol 112: 423–430
Hoyes AD (1968) Electron microscopy of the surface layer (periderm) of human foetal skin. J Anat 103: 321–336
Hurwitz S (1983) Epidermal nevi and tumours of epidermal origin. Pediatr Clin North Am 30(3): 483–494
Jacobs AH (1983) Vascular nevi. Pediatr Clin North Am 30(3): 465–482
Jacobs AH, Walton RG (1976) The incidence of birthmarks in the neonate. Pediatrics 58: 218–222
Jimbow K, Fitzpatrick TB, Szabo G, Hori Y (1975) Congenital circumscribed hypomelanosis; a characterisation based on electron microscopic study of tuberous sclerosis, nevus depigmentosus and piebaldism. J Invest Dermatol 64: 50–62
Klaus SN, Winkelmann RK (1962) Course of urticaria pigmentosa in children. Arch Dermatol 86: 68–71
Krusinski PA, Saurat J (1989) Transplacentally transferred dermatoses. Pediatr Dermatol 6: 166–177
Lawler F, Holmes SC (1989) Focal dermal hypoplasia syndrome in the neonate. J R Soc Med 82: 165–166
Ledoux-Corbusier M (1983) Cutis laxa, congenital form with pulmonary emphysema; an ultrastructural study. J Cutan Pathol 10: 340–349
Lee CW, Park MH, Lee H (1988) Recurrent cutaneous Langerhans' cell histiocytosis in infancy. Br J Dermatol 119: 259–265
Leung AKC, Telmesani AMA (1989) Salmon patches in Caucasian children. Pediatr Dermatol 6: 185–187
Lim W, Sadick N, Gupta A, Kaplin M, Pahwa S (1990) Skin diseases in children with HIV infection and their association with degree of immunosuppression. Int J Dermatol 29: 24–30
Luders D (1960) Histologic observations in erythema toxicum neonatorum. Pediatrics 26: 219–224
Mark GJ, Mihm MC, Liteplo MG, Reed RJ, Clark WH (1973) Congenital melanocytic naevi of small and garment type; clinical, histologic and ultrastructural studies. Hum Pathol 4: 395–418
Martin-Pascual A, de Unamuno P, Aparicio M, Herreros V (1977) Anhidrotic (or hypohidrotic) ectodermal dysplasia. Dermatologica 154: 235–243
McCarthy T, Saunders P (1978) The origin and circulation of the amniotic fluid. In: Fairweather DVI, Eskes TKAB (eds) Amniotic fluid research and clinical application, 2nd edn. Excerpta Medica, Amsterdam, pp 1–17
McDonald CJ (1988) Structure and function of the skin: are there differences between black and white skin? Dermatol Clin 6: 343–368
McLaurin CI (1988) Pediatric dermatology in black patients. Dermatol Clin 6: 457–473
Nanda A, Kaur, S, Bhakoo ON, Dhall K (1989) Survey of cutaneous lesions in Indian newborns. Paediatr Dermatol 6: 39–42
Nickoloff BJ, Walton R, Pregerson-Rodnan K, Jacobs AH, Cox AJ (1986) Immunohistologic patterns of congenital nevocellular nevi. Arch Dermatol 122: 1263–1268
Olson NY, Lindsley CB (1987) Neonatal lupus syndrome. Am J Dis Child 141: 908–910
Osburn K, Schosser RH, Evertt MA (1987) Congenital pigmented and vascular lesions in newborn infants. J Am Acad Dermatol 16: 788–792
Paltzik RL, Laude TA (1978) Childhood pemphigus treated with gold. Arch Dermatol 114: 768–769
Pierard GE, van Neste D, Letot B (1979) Hidrotic ectodermal dysplasia. Dermatologica 158: 168–174
Pinheiro M, Freire-Maia N (1983) Dermoodontodysplasia: an eleven member, four generation pedigree with an apparently hitherto undescribed pure ectodermal dysplasia. Clin Genet 24: 58–68
Pollard ZE, Harley RD, Calhoun J (1976) Dermoid cysts in children. Pediatrics 57(3): 379–382
Pope FM, Narcisi P, Nicholls AC, Liberman N, Oorthuys JWE (1988) Clinical presentation of Ehler–Danlos syndrome type IV. Arch Dis Child 63: 1016–1025
Pope FM, Nicholl AC (1986) Collagen genes and proteins in human diseases. In: Chapman RH (ed) Recent advances in dermatology. Churchill Livingstone, London, pp 23–52
Rasmussen HB, Teisner B, Chemnitz J, Rasmussen JM, Brandrup F (1989) Localisation of fetal antigen 2 (FA-2) in fetal and adult human skin. Br J Dermatol 121: 433–442
Rehfield SJ, Plachy WZ, Williams ML, Elias PM (1988) Calorimetric and electron spin resonance examination of lipid phase transitions in human stratum corneum: molecular basis for normal cohesion and abnormal desquamation in recessive X-linked ichthyosis. J Invest Dermatol 91: 499–505
Rhodes AR (1983) Pigmented birthmarks and precursor melanocytic lesions of cutaneous melanoma identifiable in childhood. Pediatr Clin North Am 30(3): 435–463
Rhodes AR (1986) Congenital nevomelanocytic nevi: histologic patterns in the first year of life and evolution during childhood. Arch Dermatol 122: 1257–1262
Rhodes AR, Melski J (1982) Small congenital nevocellular nevi and the risk of cutaneous melanoma. J Paediatr 100: 219–224
Rhodes AR, Silverman RA, Harrist TJ, Melski JW (1985) A histologic comparison of congenital and acquired nevomelanocytic nevi. Arch Dermatol 121: 1266–1273
Roth RR, James WD (1989) Microbiology of the skin: resident flora, ecology, infection. J Am Acad Dermatol 20: 367–390
Rusenko KW, Gammon WR, Fine J, Briggaman RA (1989) The carboxyl-terminal domain of type VII collagen is present at the basement membrane in recessive dystrophic epidermolysis bullosa. J Invest Dermatol 92: 623–627
Sagebiel RW, Odland GF (1970) Ultrastructural identifica-

tion of melanocytes in early human embryos. J Invest Dermatol 54: 96 (abstract)
Sandler A, Snedeker JD (1987) Cytomoegalovirus infection in an infant presenting with cutaneous vasculitis. Pediatr Infect Dis J 6: 422–423
Schachner L, Lazarus GS, Dembitzer H (1977) Epidermolysis bullosa hereditaria letalis: pathology, natural history and therapy. Br J Dermatol 96: 51–58
Schamburg-Lever G, Lever WF (1973) Electron microscopy of incontinentia pigmenti. J Invest Dermatol 61: 151–158
Shapiro LJ, Weiss R, Webster D, France JT (1978) X linked ichthyosis due to steroid sulphatase deficiency. Lancet I: 70–72
Shimada S, Katz SI (1988) The skin as an immunologic organ. Arch Pathol Lab Med 112: 231–234
Sigg C, Pelloni F, Schnyder UW (1990) Frequency of congenital nevi, nevi spili and café-au-lait spots and their relation to nevus count and skin complexion in 939 children. Dermatologica 180: 118–123
Smith LT, Holbrook KA (1986) Embryogenesis of the dermis in human skin. Pediatr Dermatol 3: 271–280
Smith LT, Sakai LY, Burgeson RE, Holbrook KA (1988) Ontogenesis of structural components at the dermal–epidermal junction in human embryonic and fetal skin: the appearance of anchoring fibrils and type VII collagen. J Invest Dermatol 90: 480–485
Solomon LM, Keuer EJ (1980) The ectodermal dysplasias. Problems of classification and some newer syndromes. Arch Dermatol 116: 1295–1299
Stingl G, Steiner G (1989) Immunological host defence of the skin. In: Fritsch P, Schuler G, Hintner H (eds) Immunodeficiency and skin. Current problems in dermatology, 18th edn. pp 22–30
Straka BF, Whitaker DL, Morrison SH, Oleske JM, Grant-Kels JM (1988) Cutaneous manifestations of the acquired immunodeficiency syndrome in children. J Am Acad Dermatol 18: 1089–1102
Sulica VI, Cooper PH, Pope FM, Hambrick GW, Gerson BM, McKusick VA (1979) Cutaneous histologic features in Ehlers–Danlos syndrome: study of 21 patients. Arch Dermatol 115: 40–42
Travis WD, Li C, Bergstralh EJ, Yam LT, Swee RG (1988) Systemic mast cell disease: analysis of 58 cases and literature review. Medicine 67: 345–368
Tunnessen WW (1983) Cutaneous infections. Pediatr Clin North Am 30(3): 515–532
Vandersteen PR, Muller SA (1972) Lamellar ichthyosis. Enzyme histochemical, light and EM study. Arch Dermatol 106: 694–701
Walsh SS, Robson WJ (1988) Granuloma gluteale infantum: an unusual complication of napkin dermatitis. Arch Emergency Med 5: 113–115
Watson RM, Provost TT (1987) Neonatal lupus erythematosus. In: Beutner EH, Chorzelski TP, Kumar V (eds) Immunopathology of the skin, 3rd edn. Wiley, Chichester, pp 583–602
Wessels NK (1967) Differentiation of epidermis and epidermal derivatives. N Engl J Med 277(1): 21–33
Whimster IW (1976) The pathology of lymphangioma circumscriptum. Br J Dermatol 94: 473–486
Williams ML, Elias PM (1985) Heterogeneity in autosomal recessive ichthyosis. Arch Dermatol 121: 477–488
Wolfson SL, Botero F, Hurwitz S, Pearson HA (1981) "Pure" cutaneous histiocytosis X. Cancer 48: 2236–2238

Chapter 28

The Special Senses

Brendan McDonald

Introduction

The special senses are specially adapted extero-receptor organs which receive and transduce stimuli from the external environment. They are capable of transducing physical and chemical stimuli into nerve impulses which are transmitted via cranial nerves to the brain for integration and conscious perception. The special senses and their cranial nerves are: olfactory epithelium (olfactory nerve), eye (optic nerve), taste buds (trigeminal, glossopharyngeal and vagus nerves) and vestibulocochlear apparatus (vestibulocochlear nerve).

The Eye

Embryology

Major stages in ocular development are summarised in Fig. 28.1. For a more detailed description of the embryological development of the eye the reader should consult Mullaney (1982).

The eyes start to develop following fusion of the neural folds, on day 23 of gestation, as paired indentations of neuroectoderm covered by surface ectoderm, known as the optic sulci on the anterolateral surface of the developing diencephalon (Fig. 28.1). The sulci develop evaginations with distal bulbous expansions, the optic vesicles. The proximal portion forms the optic stalk. The optic vesicles develop cup-shaped invaginations, commencing inferolaterally and extending into the optic stalk forming the fetal fissure, a longitudinally orientated cleft which permits mesodermal tissue to enter. The perimeter of the fissure undergoes closure by day 42, enclosing the mesoderm.

At this stage of embryogenesis all the major tissue progenitors are present permitting completion of oculogenesis. The neuroectoderm develops into the optic nerve fibres, the retina, pupillary sphincter muscles and surface epithelium of the iris and ciliary body. The surface ectoderm forms the lens and epithelial components of the cornea, conjunctiva, eyelids, lacrimal glands and their ducts. The mesoderm differentiates into the hyaloid vessels, extraocular muscles and fibrovascular tissue of the cornea, iris, ciliary body, choroid and sclera.

The development of the individual structural elements of the eye will now be described in more detail.

The Lens

The embryonic lens commences development on day 27 from an area of condensed surface

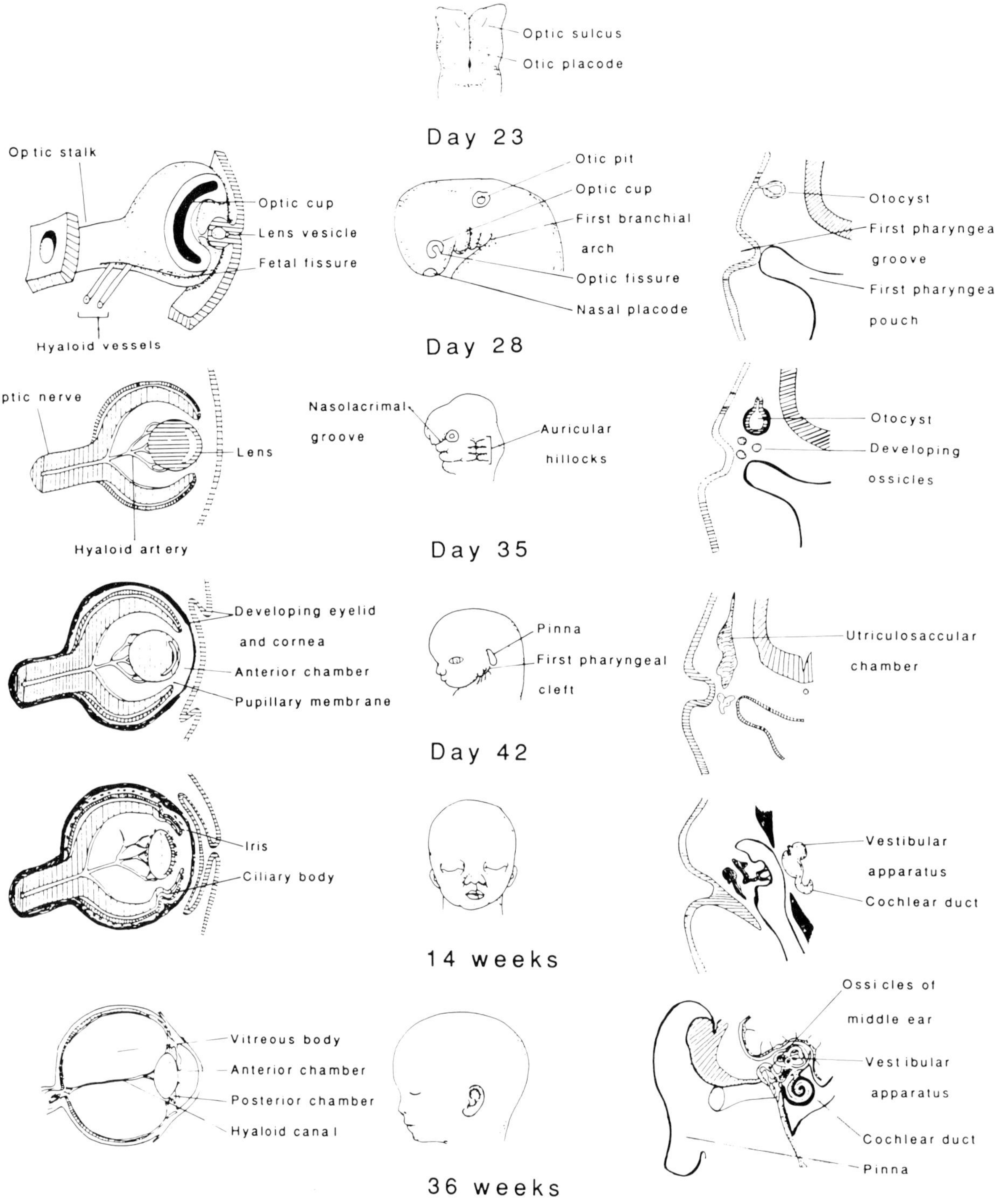

Fig. 28.1. Diagram summarising the major stages in ear and eye development. (Illustration by H. Mellor)

ectoderm, the lens placode, which overlies the optic vesicle. The lens placode invaginates, separating from the surface ectoderm during the 6th week to form the lens vesicle which is initially composed of a single cell layer surrounded by a basal lamina. The vesicle expands, developing a central cavity with an anterior wall of cells which will form the anterior lens epithelium and a posterior wall formed by the primary lens fibres which elongate and obliterate the vesicle cavity. The nuclei of the lens fibres are lost by day 44, increasing their transparency. Later, secondary lens fibres form at the lens equator by division of the anterior epithelial cells.

The lens vesicle gradually becomes invaginated into the optic cup, taking with it a layer of mesoderm which forms the lens capsule.

Growth and development of the lens are facilitated during the 12th to 28th weeks by a blood supply from the tunica vasculosa lentis, a branch of the hyaloid artery. Between the 28th and 38th weeks this degenerates. The lens is then entirely dependent upon a supply of nutrients from the flow of aqueous humour across its surfaces. Embryological remnants of the tunica vasculosa lentis, known as Mittendorf's dots, may be detected during fundoscopic examination of the eye.

The Retina

As a consequence of invagination by the optic vesicle to form the optic cup, a double layer of neuroectoderm is formed; the outer layer is composed of a single layer of columnar cells, the melanin synthesising retinal pigment epithelium which develops during the 6th to 12th weeks. The inner layer becomes the multilayered neural retina, initially composed of two layers, becoming trilayered by the 3rd month. Differentiation commences at the posterior pole. The trilayered retina consists of an outer neuroblastic, middle inner neuroblastic and innermost non-nucleated inner fibre layers. During the 3rd to 6th months there is extensive development of the outer neuroblastic layer which differentiates into the horizontal and bipolar cells, rod and cone photoreceptors. The inner neuroblastic layer differentiates into the amacrine and Müller cells. By the 22nd week the retina is composed of 10 layers similar in structure to that in the adult. These layers include: an outer nuclear layer of rod and cone photoreceptor nuclei, an outer plexiform layer of pigment containing photoreceptor processes and bipolar cells that form synaptic connections with the photoreceptor processes, an inner nuclear layer containing bipolar cells and an inner plexiform layer of synaptic processes connecting the bipolar cells to the ganglion cell layer. The innermost retinal layer is the optic nerve fibre layer formed by ganglion cell axons that merge to form the optic nerve, exit the eye at the optic disc, partially decussate at the optic chiasm and project in a precise retinotopic pattern in the lateral geniculate body.

Further retinal and optic nerve maturation occurs during the first year of life and is described in the section dealing with postnatal development.

The retinal vascular supply is derived from two sources; the outer nucleated photoreceptor-containing lamina receives its supply indirectly from the choroidal capillaries by active transport across the retinal pigment epithelium; the inner laminae are supplied by the central retinal vessels (which originate from the hyaloid vessels) and vascularise the inner retina in a radial pattern. The peripheral portion of the temporal retina is the last area to become vascularised by the central retinal vessels, only reaching completion around the 8th month of gestation (Ashton et al. 1954). This is of clinical significance in the pathogenesis of retinopathy of prematurity in preterm infants, which will be discussed later.

The Ciliary Body and Iris

The mesoderm situated on the margin of the optic cup opening, anterior to the lens after it has been invaginated, undergoes anterior growth and differentiation during the 10th week, forming the smooth muscle and connective tissue of the ciliary body and suspensory ligaments of the lens. Neuroectoderm at the margin of the optic cup migrates onto the posterior surface of the ciliary body, then over the pupillary membrane (formed by condensation of the lens anterior surface mesenchyme) forming the epithelium of the ciliary processes, the pigment-containing cells, stroma and pupillary smooth muscles of the iris. The anterior stroma of the iris is derived from the optic cup anterior mesoderm that migrates across the pupillary membrane. The pupillary membrane acts as a matrix for iris development

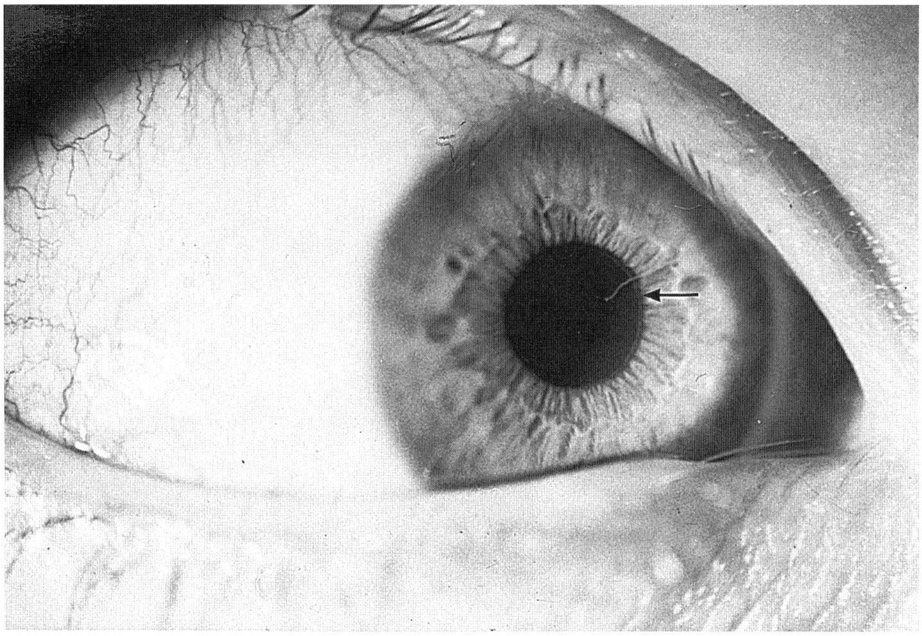

Fig. 28.2. Persistent pupillary membrane (*arrow*). (Courtesy of Mr. G.A. Shun-Shin, Oxford)

and undergoes degeneration during the 8th month, although remnants can frequently be observed during fundoscopic examination (Fig. 28.2).

The Cornea, Anterior and Posterior Chambers

The mesoderm on the anterior margin of the optic cup also coalesces to form the substantia propria, Bowman's and Descemet's membranes and the endothelium of the cornea. This is initially in continuity with the iris anterior stroma, until a clefted space develops permitting separation of these structures and formation of the anterior chamber and drainage angle. The endothelium extends laterally to line the canal of Schlemm and an interrupted plexus, the trabecular meshwork (McMenamin 1989).

The corneal epithelium is derived from the surface ectoderm.

The posterior chamber develops from a cleft-shaped split between the posterior surface of the pupillary membrane and the anterior capsular surface of the lens.

The chambers gradually fill with aqueous humour and communication is established between the two chambers via the pupillary aperture. The drainage angle apparatus starts to absorb aqueous humour by the 17th week (Pandolfi and Astendt 1971).

The Vitreous Body

The vitreous body develops during the 5th week within the cavity defined by the posterior surface of the lens and the interior surface of the optic cup, as the primary vitreous formed from a vascular matrix of fibrils originating from the retinal neuroectoderm and lens ectoderm. The secondary vitreous develops during the 9th week after encapsulation of the lens, from a retina-derived gelatinous acellular matrix which is rich in proteoglycans and collagen fibrils. This results in central and anterior displacement of the primary vitreous which normally undergoes degeneration and resorption during the second trimester. Persistence of the primary vitreous causes visual impairment and will be discussed later.

The interface between the retina and the secondary vitreous body is demarcated by the internal limiting membrane composed of condensed vitreous fibres.

The tertiary vitreous develops during the 24th week as anterior condensations of collagen fibrils which form the zonular fibres that attach the lens capsule to the ciliary body processes.

The Hyaloid Vessels

The hyaloid artery and vein provide the blood supply for development of the lens vesicle and the primary vitreous body. When the development of these structures is achieved, around day 64, the hyaloid vessels undergo degeneration, leaving a vestigial remnant, the acellular canal of Cloquet, which may be visible at birth.

The Choroid and Sclera

The choroid develops from the mesoderm surrounding the optic vesicle. The sclera is formed by condensation of the mesoderm surrounding the choroidal mesoderm, forming a tough fibrous connective tissue capsule.

The Extraocular Muscles

The extraocular muscles are derived from mesodermal preotic myotomes and subsequently receive nerve innervation from the third, fourth and sixth cranial nerves.

The Eyelids

The eyelids develop peripheral to the optic vesicle as folds of surface ectoderm during the 7th week and grow centripetally to fuse by the 9th week, enclosing a cleft-shaped space, the conjunctival sac, anterior to the cornea. The lids separate between the 5th and 7th months.

The Accessory Ocular Glands

Development of the nasolacrimal duct, lacrimal and eyelid accessory glands occurs whilst the eyelids are fused, from surface ectoderm.

Postnatal Development of the Eye

A full-term infant can distinguish between light and darkness and reflexly close the eyes to bright light. There is incoordination of eye movement because, at birth, development of the anterior focusing apparatus and the fovea, the region of the retina where sharpness of focusing is greatest, is incomplete. Growth and further maturation continues during the first year, with the fovea maturing during the first 4 months by peripheral displacement of the inner retinal layers, thereby providing maximum exposure of incident light to the photoreceptors. The size of the anteriorly located focusing apparatus increases in size by differential growth relative to the remaining eye structures during the first year. The intensity of pigmentation of the iris and retina also increases and myelination of the optic nerve fibres is incomplete until the 3rd month.

The structural and consequent functional changes after full-term birth are of particular significance when clinical assessment of preterm infants is attempted, since normal intrauterine development will be incomplete, depending on the degree of prematurity. In addition a small number of term infants show functional delay of visual maturation (Beauvieux 1947; Illingworth 1961), in isolation from other neurological abnormality. This often shows good spontaneous recovery, attributed by Lambert et al. (1989) to immaturity of the visual association areas. Tresidder et al. (1990) have recently reported that infants with delayed visual maturation as an isolated abnormality, in a cohort of 26 infants prospectively studied because of delayed visual maturation, showed recovery of visual deficit from week 8 onwards, which coincides with the period of postnatal development when binocular vision starts to become established (Braddick et al. 1983) due to maturation of cortical visual pathways (Atkinson 1984).

Synopsis of Eye Structure on Completion of Development

On completion of ocular development, (Fig. 28.1) the eye can be considered to be composed of:

(a) Two functional compartments: (i) *The anterior compartment* which is subdivided into two chambers—the anterior formed by the cornea, drainage angles and iris, and the posterior formed by the iris, ciliary body, suspensory ligament and lens. The two chambers communicate via the pupillary

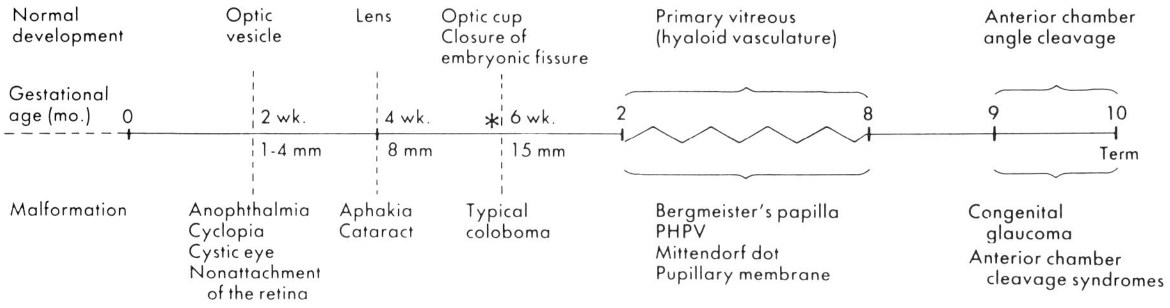

Fig. 28.3. Diagram correlating selected congenital ocular anomalies with gestational age. (Reproduced with permission from Apple, D.J. and Rabb, M.F.: Ocular Pathology, Clinical Applications and Self-assessment, 4th edn. Mosby, St. Louis, 1991)

aperture. The anterior compartment structures are responsible for focusing the image and regulating the intensity of light entering the posterior compartment. (ii) *The posterior compartment* contains the vitreous body and photosensitive retina.

(b) Three structural and functional layers: *outer*—corneoscleral, transparent anteriorly, remainder opaque and fibrous; *middle*—uveal tract (iris, ciliary body and choroid); *inner*—retina.

Histological Processing of Fetal and Neonatal Eyes

The removal, processing, cutting and staining of fetal and neonatal eyes lie outside the scope of the present text. For technical information the reader should consult Harry (1990).

Developmental Abnormalities of Oculogenesis

Major malformations of ocular development most commonly result from interference with the developmentally sensitive period of major organogenesis occurring during weeks 4–8. Because of the complexity of developmental changes occurring during this period a variety of other organ system malformations often coexist. Anomalies of ocular development arising later in fetal development usually cause more discrete changes, confined to defined ocular structures. The relationship of the sequence of organogenesis to a selection of ocular malformations is represented diagrammatically in Fig. 28.3.

Conditions Causing Absence or a Reduction in the Number of Eyes

Anophthalmos (absence of eye). This is usually a bilateral condition resulting from either failure of optic vesicle development or regression after initiation of vesicle development. In the former instance there is failure of eye, lens, optic nerve and optic chiasm development. When regression is the cause, vestigial remnants of oculogenesis may be detectable on histological examination.

Cyclopia. This is a rare consequence of anomalous development of a single optic vesicle.

Synophthalmia. This is a commoner event than cyclopia, resulting from varying degrees of fusion of the paired optic vesicles (Fig. 28.4).

Both cyclopia and synophthalmia are associated with severe neural tube malformations that are incompatible with fetal survival, such as the severe end of the spectrum of holoprosencephalic malformations (see Chap. 23).

Cryptophthalmos (covered eye). The condition includes failure of eyelid separation resulting in absence of the palpebral fissure and eyelashes, with resultant external absence of eye development which may be uni- or bilateral and is frequently associated with other developmental anomalies, particularly in the kidneys, for

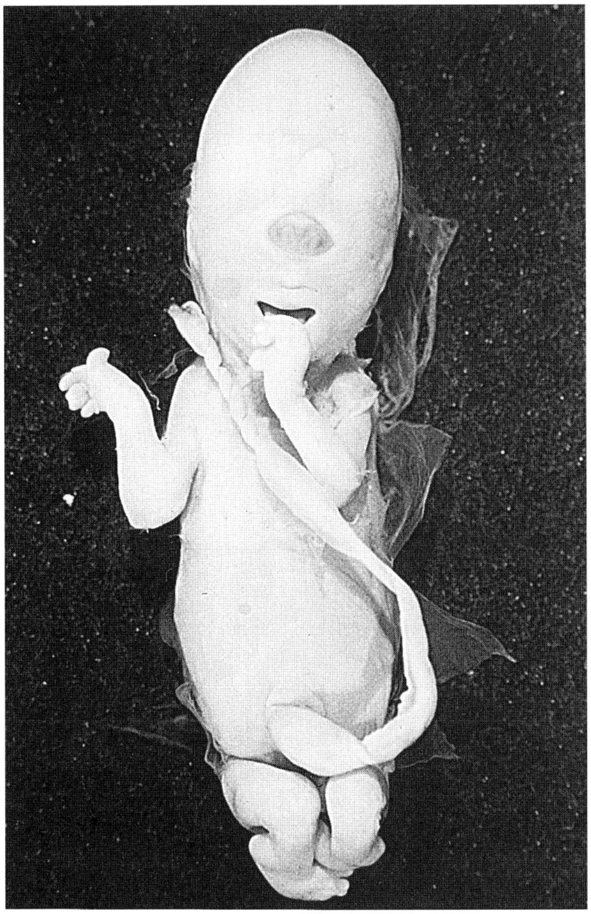

Fig. 28.4. Synophthalmia in trisomy 13.

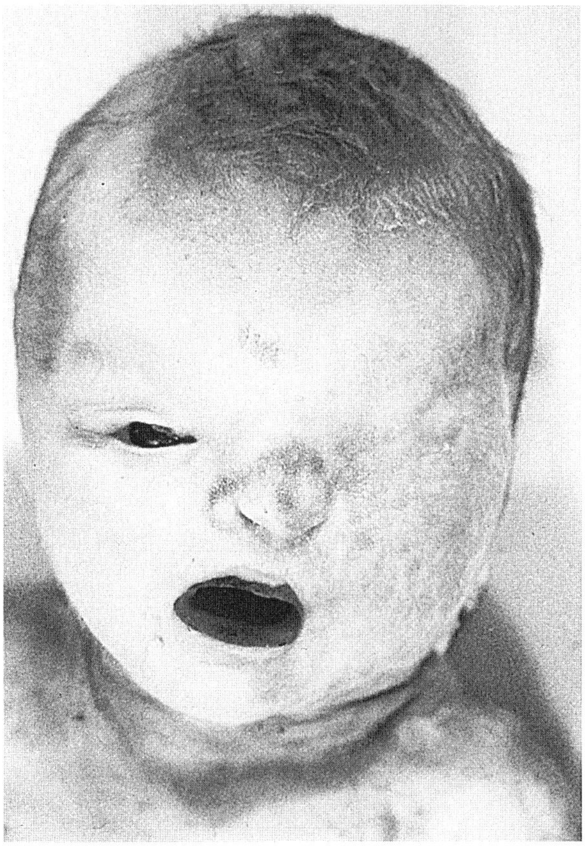

Fig. 28.5. Unilateral cryphthalmos in a case of Fraser's syndrome.

example Fraser's syndrome (Boyd et al. 1988) (Fig. 28.5). Examination of the underlying orbit may reveal a variety of ocular malformations ranging from anophthalmia to normal eye development.

Conditions Causing Alteration in Eye Size

Decreased Eye Size

Nanophthalmia. This refers to an eye in which there is proportional decrease in size of all the internal architectural structures. Infants born with a nanophthalmic eye are at increased risk of developing glaucoma and functionally the eye shows hypermetropia (farsightedness) due to reduction of the eye's axial dimension.

Microphthalmia (small eye). This refers to an eye measuring less than 15 mm maximum diameter at birth (Fig. 28.6). The eye may show a range of changes from mild size reduction without significant structural distortion (nanophthalmia) through to significant size reduction and structural distortion within the range seen in anophthalmia. Microphthalmic eyes may have coexistent colobomas.

Globe Enlargement

Eye enlargement (macrophthalmia) may occur with buphthalmos (Fig. 28.7) or without (simple myopia) an increase in the normal neonatal corneal diameter of 12 mm.

Coloboma

The majority, referred to as "typical" colobomas result from the persistence of a cleft-shaped

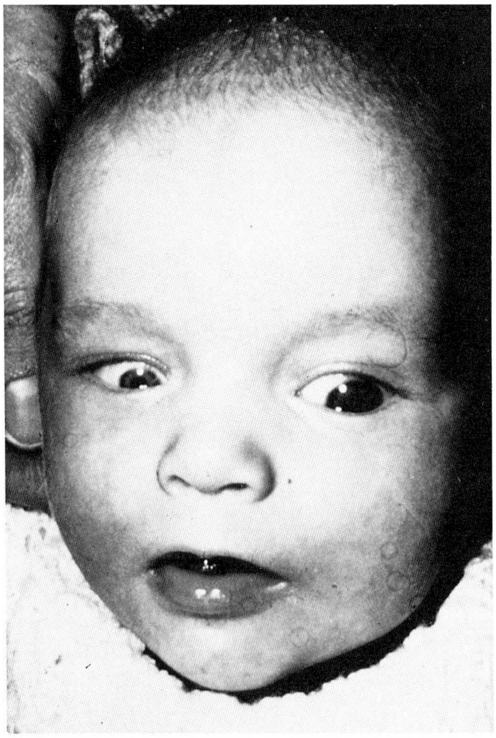

Fig. 28.6. Unilateral congenital microphthalmos.

fissure situated on the *inferonasal* aspect of the eye, resulting from incomplete fusion of the fetal fissure during the 6th week of development. The defective closure of the fissure can effect the eyelid (Fig. 28.8), iris (Fig. 28.9), ciliary body, retina (Fig. 28.10), choroid or optic nerve. The majority occur as sporadic abnormalities; there is an increased incidence of colobomas associated with trisomy 13 (Patau syndrome), intrauterine exposure to thalidomide and D-lysergic acid diethylamide (LSD).

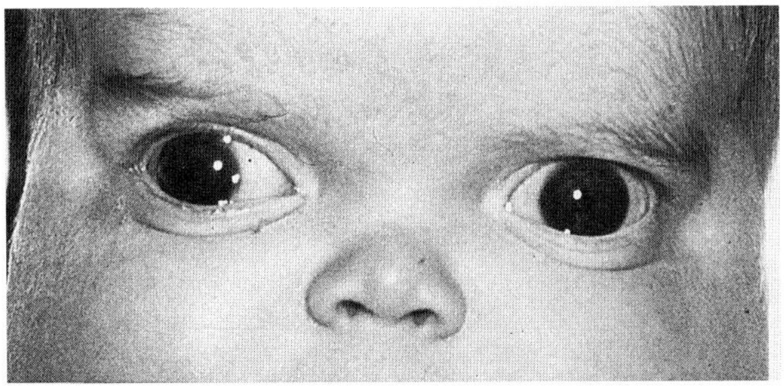

Fig. 28.7. Buphthalmos. (Courtesy of Mr. G.A. Shun-Shin, Oxford)

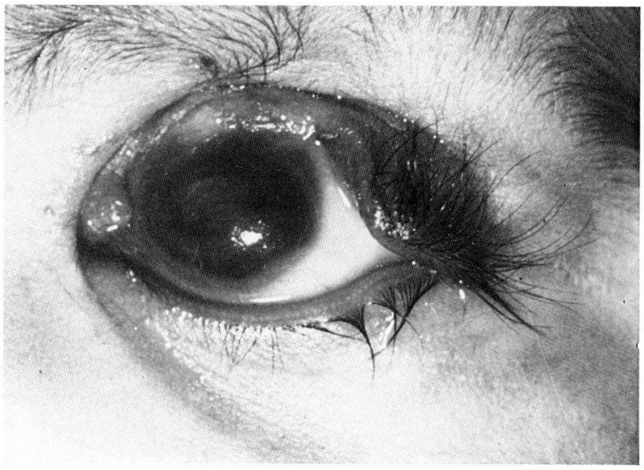

Fig. 28.8. Congenital coloboma of the upper eyelid.

The term "atypical" coloboma refers to a cleft-shaped defect occurring in any other eye quadrant. Vestiges of the anterior hyaloid vessels and pupillary membrane often occur in association with these defects and in fact it may be their persistence that impairs the normal ocular development in the quadrant affected.

Colobomas may occur in association with defective development in other organs, notably the CHARGE syndrome (Duval et al. 1987) where *C*olobomas occur in association with *H*eart anomalies, choanal *A*tresia, developmental *R*etardation, *G*enital hypoplasia and *E*ar malformations.

Developmental Abnormalities of the Cornea

Developmental anomalies of the cornea include:

Microcornea. A cornea measuring less than 10 mm diameter at birth predisposes to a shallow anterior chamber and angle closure glaucoma.

Megalocornea. A cornea measuring more than 12 mm diameter in a neonate.

Sclerocornea. Opacification of the peripheral cornea.

Dermoids. These may be central or limbal in location (Fig. 28.11). They are hamartomas arising due to arrested migration of ectoderm at the corneoscleral junction (limbus), most commonly on the temporal aspect. Corneal

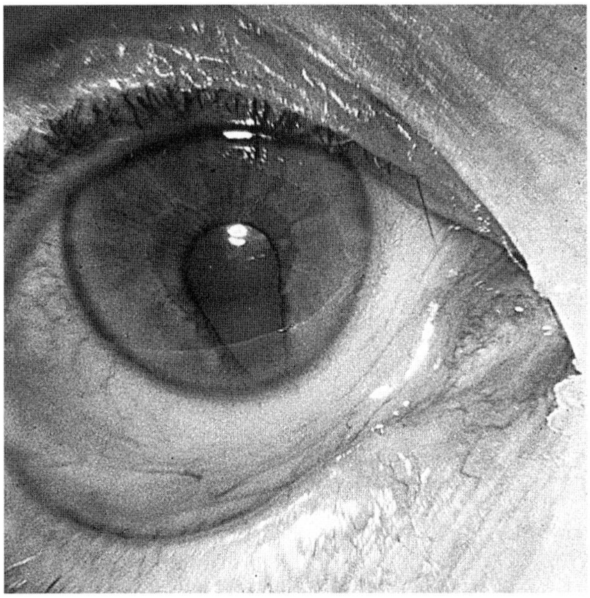

Fig. 28.9. "Typical" iris coloboma involving the inferonasal aspect. (Courtesy of Mr. G.A. Shun-Shin, Oxford)

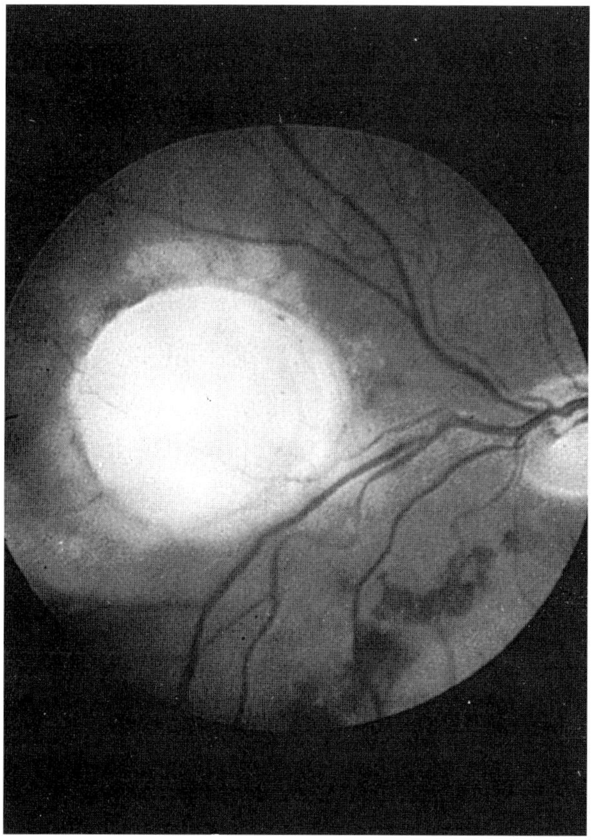

Fig. 28.10. Retinal coloboma. (Courtesy of Mr. G.A. Shun-Shin, Oxford)

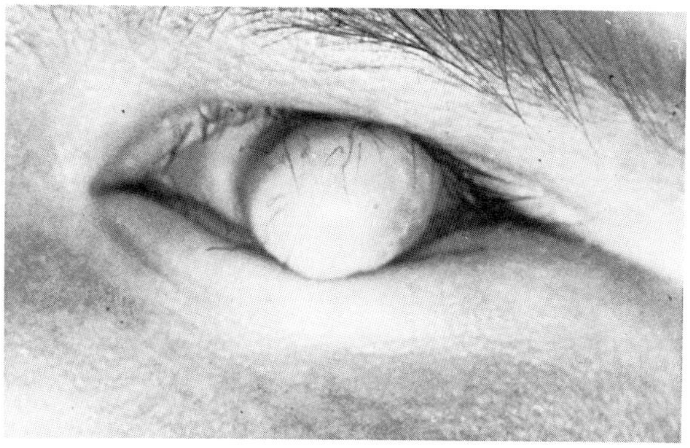

Fig. 28.11. Large central corneal congenital dermoid.

dermoids are one of the features of Goldenhaar's syndrome (Goldenhaar 1952).

Congenital hereditary corneal dystrophy. There are autosomal dominant and recessive variants. Corneal clouding is present from birth due to oedema of the basal layer of the epithelium, subepithelial fibrosis, reduction of the thickness of Bowman's membrane and central attenuation of the endothelial cell density (Kirkness et al. 1987).

Anterior Chamber Abnormalities

The anterior chamber cleavage syndrome comprises incomplete separation between the cornea, lens and iris causing distortion of the anterior chamber architecture and filtration angle apparatus. This predisposes the eye to the development of primary congenital glaucoma (Reese and Ellsworth 1966; Waring et al. 1975).

Defective anterior chamber separation can occur in isolation or in association with other congenital malformations, including those associated with trisomies of chromosomes 13, 18 and 21 and partial deletions of chromosomes 3, 10, 11, and 18 (Broughton et al. 1981; Bateman 1983). Three conditions are particularly associated with Axenfeld's anomaly, Peter's anomaly and Reiger's syndrome (also referred to as the mesodermal dysgenesis syndromes).

Axenfeld's anomaly. This refers to the persistence of strands of iris processes extending peripherally towards a prominent Schwalbe's line (the peripheral termination of Descement's membrane; also referred to as posterior

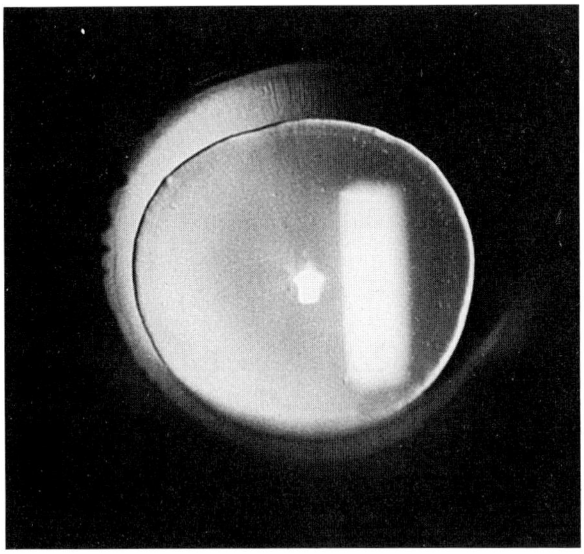

Fig. 28.12. Slit-lamp examination demonstrating iris hypoplasia (aniridia). (Courtesy of Mr. G.A. Shun-Shin, Oxford)

embryotoxon). The condition is not usually associated with congenital glaucoma, but raised intraocular pressure may develop during infancy.

Peter's anomaly. Commonly, this bilateral condition results in central opacification of the cornea due to a defect in Descemet's membrane with or without adhesion to the iris or lens. The anomaly is secondary to arrested separation of the lens vesicle from the overlying ectoderm and is associated with congenital glaucoma in up to half the individuals effected.

Reiger's syndrome. Usually this is a bilateral condition with corneal and drainage angle abnormalities, similar to those in Axenfeld's anomaly, but with additional adhesion of the peripheral portion of the iris (peripheral anterior synechiae) and pupillary aperture distortion due to hypoplasia of the iris. Congenital glaucoma is present in up to half the individuals affected.

Congenital Glaucoma

In *primary congenital glaucoma* raised intraocular pressure is present at birth or develops in the neonatal period and is due to structural abnormalities which impede flow of aqueous humour. Both eyes are usually affected and presenting features include photophobia, lacrimation, buphthalmos (globe and corneal enlargement, Fig. 28.7) and eye rubbing. The condition is usually autosomal-recessive inherited with a male preponderance, affecting 1 in 10 000 livebirths. Structural abnormalities predisposing to the development include: microcornea, abnormal anterior chamber angle cleavage, Barkan's membrane (a mesodemal membrane covering and occluding the drainage angles) and insertion of persistent fetal iris processes above the scleral spur.

In *secondary congenital glaucoma* raised intraocular pressure presents after the neonatal period. Causes include the rubella syndrome, aniridia (autosomal-dominant, Fig. 28.12), Lowe's syndrome (sex-linked recessive), Sturge–Weber syndrome, mesodermal dysgenesis syndrome (Peter's anomaly and Reiger's syndrome), persistent hyperplastic primary vitreous and retinopathy of prematurity.

Developmental Abnormalities of the Iris

Some of the commoner iris developmental anomalies include:

Aniridia. This refers to hypoplasia rather than aplasia of the iris (Fig. 28.12) and may occur sporadically or as an autosomal-dominant disorder. It predisposes to the development of secondary congenital glaucoma, congenital cataract, macular aplasia and is associated with increased risk of a Wilm's tumour (nephroblastoma) developing (Miller's syndrome).

Iris coloboma. See section on colobomas.

Developmental Abnormalities of the Lens

Abnormalities of the crystalline lens which may present at birth or in the neonatal period include:

Congenital absence of the lens. This rare condition is due to failure of lens vesicle formation or degeneration after the vesicle develops. It is associated with microphthalmos and coloboma.

Abnormalities of lens shape. In lenticornus there is a conically shaped anterior or pos-

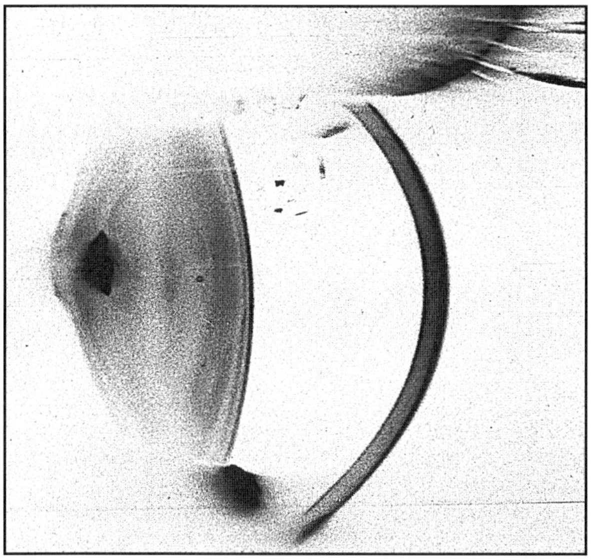

Fig. 28.13. Slit-lamp examination of a lens demonstrating conical distortion of the posterior surface (posterior lenticonus). (Courtesy of Mr. G.A. Shun-Shin, Oxford)

terior surface of the lens (Fig. 28.13). Anterior lenticonus is associated with cataract formation and Alport's syndrome. In lentiglobus the lens is hemispherically shaped.

Abnormalities of lens size. Microphakia—small sized lens. Associated with Lowe's syndrome. Microspherophakia—small spherical lens. Associated with hyperlysinaemia, Marfan's and Weill–Marchesani syndrome.

Abnormalities of lens position. Ectopia lentis results from zonular rupture, causing lens dislocation or subluxation. It causes secondary congenital glaucoma and is associated with hyperlysinaemia, sulphite oxidase deficiency, homocystinuria, buphthalmos, Marfan's, Weill–Marchesani and Ehlers–Danlos syndromes.

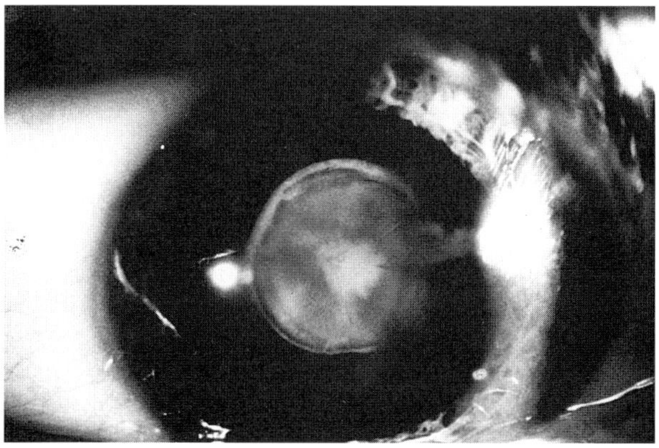

Fig. 28.14. Slit-lamp examination of the crystalline lens in a case of congenital polar lens opacity. (Courtesy of Mr. G.A. Shun-Shin, Oxford)

Congenital cataracts. The lens is opacified (Fig. 28.14); up to a quarter of cases have a hereditary component (most commonly autosomal-dominant inheritance). Congenital cataract may occur in isolation or associated with other intraocular anomalies (aniridia, persistent hyperplastic primary vitreous and vitreoretinal disease), or other systemic abnormalities (congenital rubella and cytomegalovirus infection, trisomy 21).

Persistence of the Primary Vitreous

The primary vitreous, as previously described, is a gelatinous matrix derived from mesoderm and includes the hyaloid vessels. The primary vitreous normally undergoes degeneration and resorption during the second trimester. However, mesodermal remnants may persist either anteriorly (most commonly) or posteriorly, within the posterior compartment. The presence of such remnants has been termed persistent hyperplastic primary vitreous (PHPV) by Reese (1955) and can be defined as an idiopathic persistence and proliferation of the normally transient primary vitreous vasculature and matrix leading to formation of a retrolental (arising behind the lens) mass with subsequent visual impairment (Apple and Rabb 1991).

The condition is usually sporadic and unilateral, presenting in the neonatal period as a small (microphthalmic) eye with a white pupillary reflex (leukocorea) and a funnel-shaped retrolental mass with its apex attached to the optic disc. Histological examination of enucleated eyes show that the retrolental mass contains remnants of the hyaloid vessels.

Other ocular abnormalities, in addition to microphthalmos that may coexist with PHPV include microcornea, shallow anterior chamber, ectropion uvea, atypical iris coloboma, pupillary membrane remnants, lens coloboma, cataract and retinal detachment.

Localised persistence of the primary vitreous remnant on the posterior aspect of the lens capsule is recognised clinically as Mittendorf's dot and hyperplastic posterior vascular remnants, which may or may not be accompanied by glial proliferation on the optic disc, as Bergmeister's papilla.

Developmental Abnormalities of the Retina

A variety of developmental disorders can affect retinal morphology and function including:

Congenital abnormalities of retinal photoreceptors. The most notable are congenital achromatopsia (monochromatism). Two variants are recognised:

(a) Complete rod monochromatism (autosomal recessive), when there is complete absence of cone photoreceptor development.

(b) Cone monochromatism, when the rod photoreceptor cells are morphologically and functionally normal; only one subtype of functionally active cone photoreceptor cell develops.

Leber's congenital amaurosis. This is an autosomal-dominant disorder in which the infant is born blind or with severe visual impairment, is deaf and has renal tract abnormalities. Other ocular defects may be present including keratoconus (central thinning of the cornea), cataract and variable degrees of retinal pigmentation. The condition is regarded as a variant of retinitis pigmentosa and arises due to either failure of normal development of the outer rod and cone photoreceptor segments or degeneration subsequent to initial retinal development.

Retinal dysplasia. This condition can occur in isolation in an otherwise normal eye or as part of a syndrome, for example, Norrie's disease, trisomy 13, incontentia pigmenti, Peter's anomaly, cyclopia, synophthalmia, maternal D-lysergic acid diethylamide (LSD) consumption and the HARD+/−E syndrome. The disorder is characterised by the presence of tubular retinal folds which on histological examination can be shown to be composed of rosettes formed from one or more cell layers of photoreceptors arranged around a central lumen, at the perimeter of which is a structure similar to the retinal external limiting membrane (Fig. 28.15).

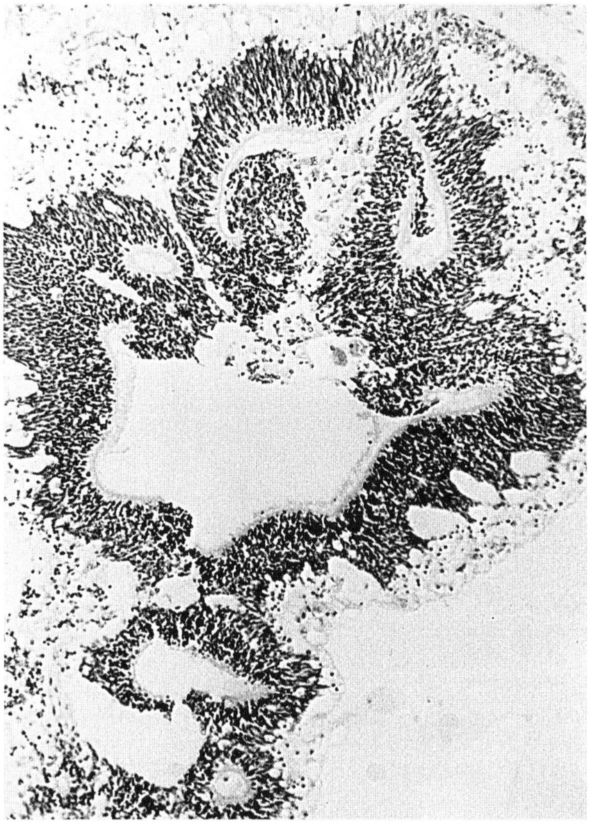

Fig. 28.15. Retinal dysplasia in trisomy 13 showing rosette formation.

Congenital non-attachment of the retina. In this rare disorder there is either partial or complete failure of fusion of the inner and outer layers of the optic vesicle with the intervening void forming a congenital subretinal space.

Congenital falciform retinal fold. This occurs as both a sporadic and an autosomal-recessive disorder in which a fold of retina extends from the optic nerve head anteriorly towards the ciliary body. The fold most commonly occurs in the inferior temporal quadrant and may be associated with persistence of remnants of the hyaloid vessels. Histological sections through the fold show the presence of dysplastic retinal rosettes.

Macular coloboma. These are usually sporadic, although an autosomal-dominant variant is recognised which shows bilateral exaggerated depression of the macula (the area of the retina containing the fovea). The coloboma therefore causes severe visual impairment.

Lange's retinal fold. This artefact of histological preparation in the eyes of fetuses and infants

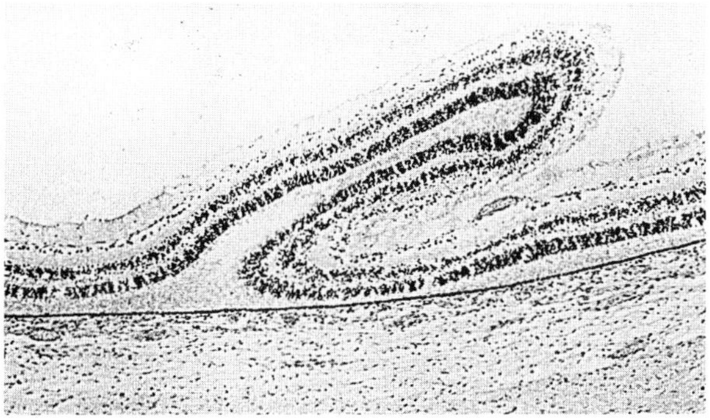

Fig. 28.16. Lange's retinal fold—an artefact of processing, commonly located close to the ora serrata.

is due to detachment of the peripheral retina, close to the ora serrata, between the outer photoreceptor layer and the pigment epithelium (Fig. 28.16).

Retinopathy of Prematurity (Retrolental Fibroplasia)

Retinopathy of prematurity (ROP) is the condition occurring in preterm infants where there is abnormal vascular proliferation affecting the retina. The clinical and pathological features of the disorder were first described in 1942 by Terry who introduced the term retrolental fibroplasia, indicating the presence of a gliotic mass behind the lens in end-stage disease (Fig. 28.17). Since earlier stages in the process are now recognised both clinically and pathologically (Reese et al. 1953; Garner 1984), the term retinopathy of prematurity is used in preference. The development of ROP appears to be related to the ambient oxygen concentration being breathed by the infant (Campbell 1951; Kinsey 1956).

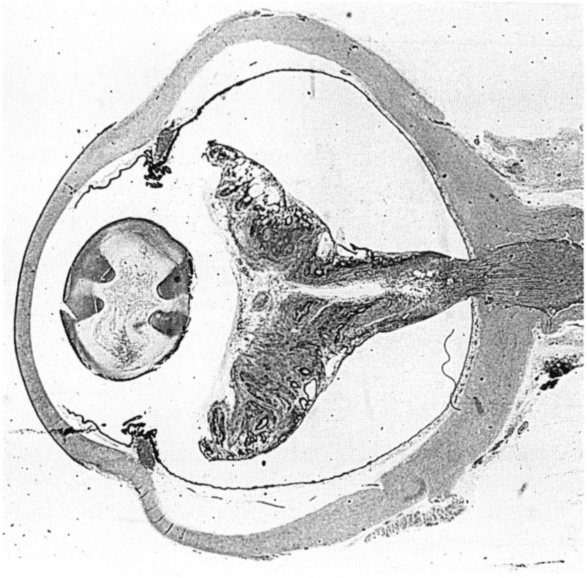

Fig. 28.17. Section through an eye showing retinal detachment and gliosis, forming a retrolental mass in retinopathy of prematurity.

The vascular supply of the inner retinal layers is provided by the central retinal vessels (which are derived from the hyaloid vessels). Completion of retinal vascular circulation development, notably in the temporal quadrant, occurs during the last month of gestation. In preterm infants born before 36 weeks' gestation, development of the retinal vascular circulation is incomplete.

The administration of high ambient oxygen concentrations to preterm infants because of respiratory distress syndrome appears to further inhibit development of the vasculature, causing vasoconstriction of the immature angioblastic tissue. Subsequent exposure of the infant to an atmosphere containing a lower ambient oxygen concentration, such as room air, removes the inhibitory effect, resulting in renewed and excessive proliferation of the vascular primordia, which may breach the internal limiting membrane of the retina with invasion of the vitreous. Thus, the retinas of preterm infants afflicted by ROP appear normal at birth, but subsequently develop retinal changes which can be graded clinically and pathologically during both active and cicatricial stages of the disorder (Reese et al. 1953; Garner 1984). Sequelae of ROP include microphthalmia, cataract and secondary angle glaucoma.

Following recognition of the association between development of ROP and exposure to high ambient oxygen concentrations, the incidence of ROP decreased following the introducton of oxygen concentration monitoring. However, in recent years there has been a resurgence of the disorder in many developed countries which appears in part to be due to the improved survival of preterm infants of less than 30 weeks' gestation and very low birthweight. A possible explanation may be that these infants, even when breathing room air, are experiencing hyperoxaemia relative to the partial pressure of oxygen to which they

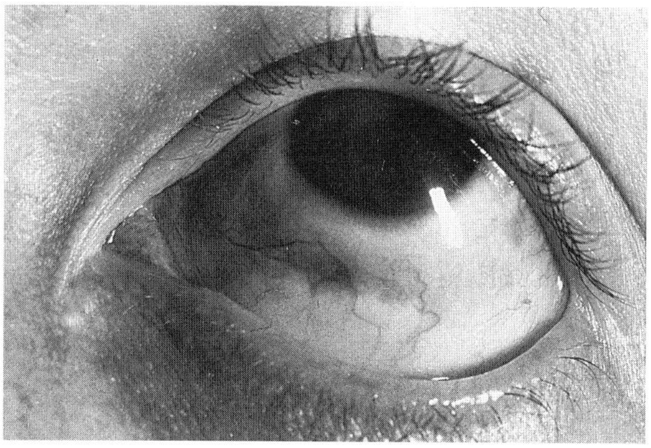

Fig. 28.18. Naevus of Ota in an adult showing melanin pigmentation of the sclera and periorbital skin. (Courtesy of Mr. G.A. Shun-Shin, Oxford)

would have been exposed if they were still in utero (MacMahon et al. 1986). Recent studies in Britain by Ng et al. (1988) indicate an association between short duration of gestation, low birthweight and Asian ethnic origin. Forty-nine per cent of preterm infants weighing under 1700 g at birth showed evidence of acute ROP, but none subsequently became blind. In other studies (Phelps 1981; Saigal 1984; Darlow 1988) it was estimated that 8% of preterm infants of birthweight <1000 g who survived subsequently became blind.

Vitreoretinal Disorders

Sex-linked recessive retinoschisis (congenital vascular veils in the vitreous) is a disorder resulting in schisis (splitting) of the retina between the ganglion and nerve fibre layers, resulting in vitreous veils and haemorrhages. There are two variants, the foveal and peripheral types. Only the peripheral variant presents in the neonate, most frequently in the inferotemporal retina. The condition is often bilateral and in a minority of cases there is coexistent retinal detachment. Prenatal, intrapartum and neonatal trauma to the face and eye can result in extensive vitreous haemorrhage, which, following organisation, exerts traction on the retina causing detachment and subsequent gliosis, originally described as massive gliosis of the retina (Friedenwald 1926). This condition may clinically and radiologically mimic retinoblastoma.

Disorders of Ocular Pigmentation

The melanin pigment-containing cells of the iris and retinal pigment epithelium may give rise to localised pigmentary conditions or form part of the spectrum of systemic disorders of pigmentation. Since the intensity of pigmentation of the iris and retina continues to deepen postnatally, only those conditions which may be clinically apparent at birth or during the neonatal period will be considered.

Disorders Resulting in Localised Increased Ocular Pigmentation

Congenital ocular melanosis. This neural crest disorder affects melanocytes which may result in either focal or diffuse increased pigmentation of the sclera, conjunctiva, iris and ciliary body. The condition may also include the skin, when it is known as naevus of Ota (Fig. 28.18).

Disorders Resulting in Reduced Ocular Pigmentation

Reduced intensity of ocular pigmentation of the iris and retina may occur in isolation as sex-linked recessive ocular albinism or as part of the spectrum of changes seen in generalised oculocutaneous albinism (tyrosine-negative and -positive variants) which is inherited as an autosomal-recessive trait.

It is noteworthy that in partial albinism, (autosomal-dominant) there is normal development of ocular pigmentation, presumably because the disorder does not affect melanin pigment produced by cells originating from the optic vesicle, in contrast to those derived from the neural crest.

Disorders of Optic Nerve Development

Optic nerve aplasia. This rare condition causes blindness because there is failure of development of the optic disc and retinal vasculature.

Optic nerve hypoplasia. This rare sporadic abnormality causes a variable degree of visual

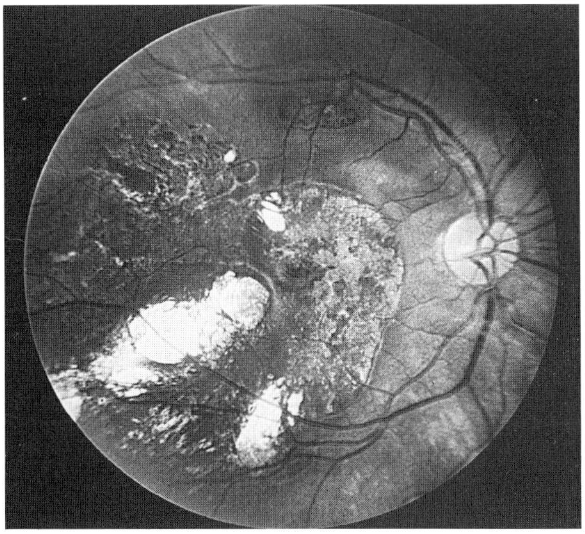

Fig. 28.19. The fundus in quiescent, congenitally acquired toxoplasmosis. (Courtesy of Mr. G.A. Shun-Shin, Oxford)

loss and field defects. The condition shows a male preponderance and fundoscopy reveals a small optic disc surrounded by a corona of pallor, the so-called "double ring sign". Other ocular abnormalities may coexist, including microphthalmos, aniridia and optic nerve hypoplasia which are features of de Morsier's septo-optic dysplasia syndrome.

Optic nerve coloboma. The optic nerve is a relatively common site in the eye for colobomas to occur, usually causing deep excavation of the optic nerve head (in contrast to the cupping resulting from glaucoma). Variants of "typical" optic nerve colobomas include the congenital tilted disc and morning glory syndromes. "Atypical" colobomas of the optic nerve include the optic disc pit.

Infection and the Eye

The eye is susceptible to infection by a range of micro-organisms. It may be infected by maternal viral infections if they occur during the period of organogenesis. During later intrauterine development the eye is susceptible to maternal systemic infections such as *Toxoplasma gondii, Treponema pallidum* and ascending infection.

Vaginal delivery places the neonate at risk of acquiring conjunctival infections from the maternal genital tract, including *Staphylococcus aureus, Escherichia coli, Haemophilus influenzae, Chlamydia trachomatis, Neisseria gonorrhoeae, Candida albicans* and herpes simplex type II. In the neonatal period, the conjunctiva remains susceptible mainly to bacterial infections owing to immaturity of both the immune and lacrimal systems. Both preterm infants and those born with immune deficiency syndromes are prone to intraocular as well as conjunctival infections, including *Candida albicans* infection. The increasing number of infants born to mothers infected with the human immune deficiency virus (HIV), may well show an increased susceptibility to ocular infections, both in utero because of maternal immune deficiency and post-partum, especially if the neonate has congenitally acquired HIV.

Important ocular infections are discussed below.

Intrauterine Ocular Infections

Viral chorioretinitis. This necrotising chorioretinitis is associated with congenital viral infections, most notably cytomegalovirus, herpes simplex and herpes zoster. Histologically there is extensive retinal and choroidal necrosis without significant inflammation. Viral particles are demonstrable by electron microscopy, viral capsid proteins by immunocytochemistry and viral nucleic acid by in situ hybridisation and polymerase chain reaction.

Toxoplasma gondii chorioretinitis. The retina may be affected in isolation or accompanied by other visceral organ involvement in intrauterine acquired toxoplasma (Fig. 28.19) infection. Histologically there is severe granulomatous retinal necrosis with associated vitreoretinal exudate (Fig. 28.20).

Congenital rubella infection. The cytopathic effects of rubella infection occurring before the 12th week of gestation include necrotising chorioretinitis and nuclear cataract. The association was first established in Australia by Gregg (1941), following a rubella outbreak which principally affected young adults including pregnant women. The cataractous lens is characterised by the retention of nuclei by the primary lens fibres (Fig. 28.21). Other ocular abnormalities that occur as part of the syn-a 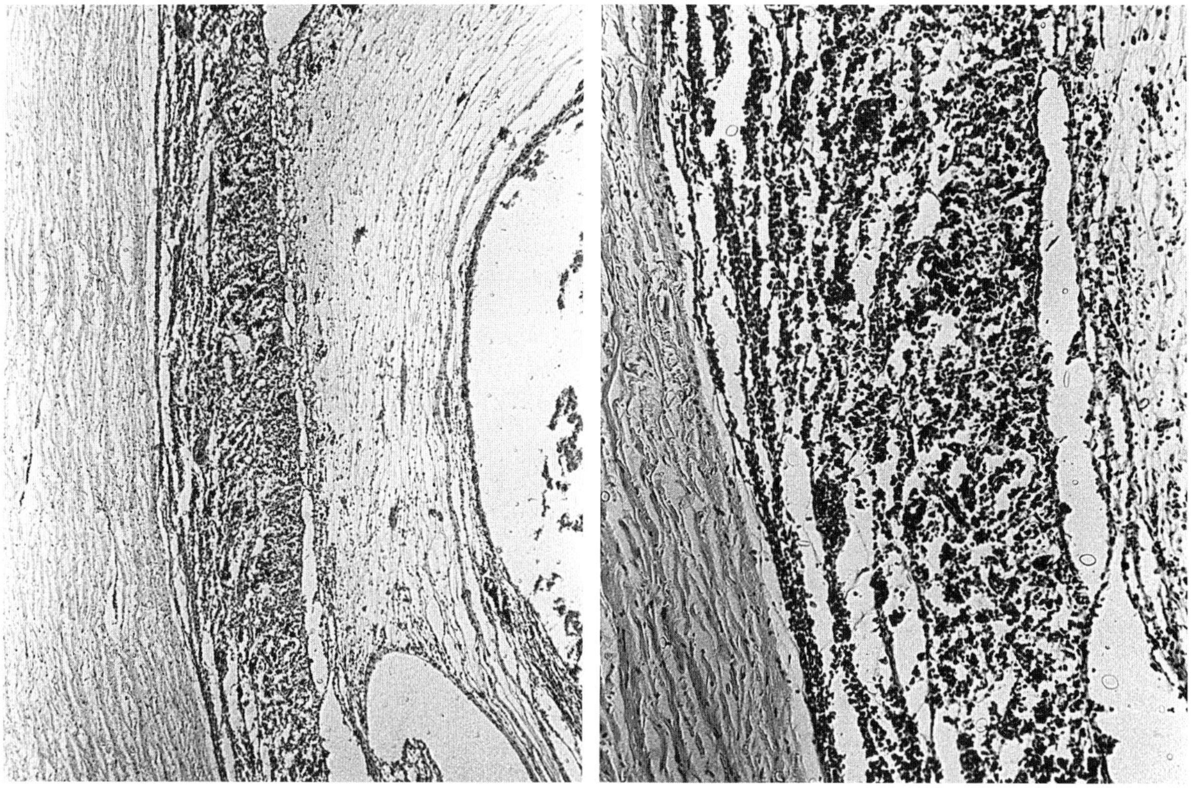 b

Fig. 28.20a,b. Retinal necrosis in congenital toxoplasmosis. (Courtesy of the late Dr. A.D. Bain, Edinburgh) **a**×43, **b**×107

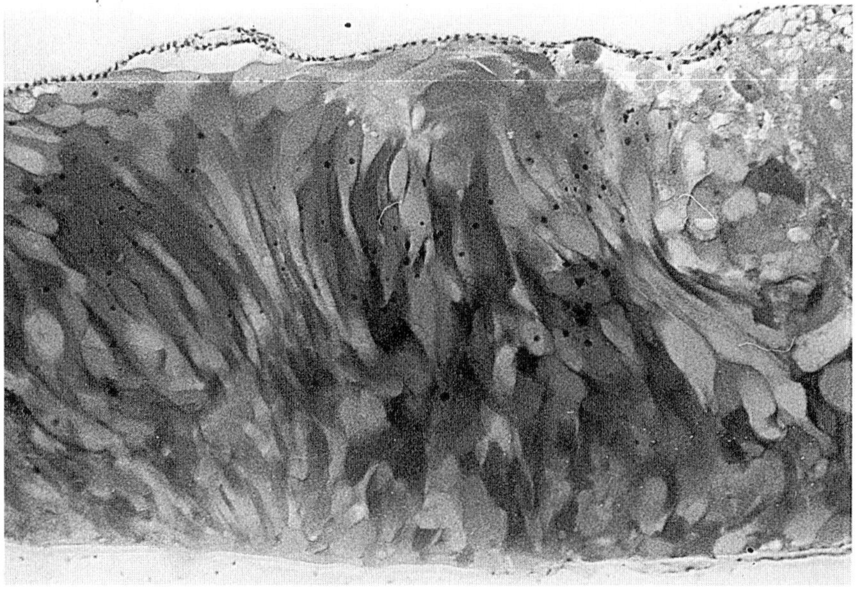

Fig. 28.21. Cataract due to congenital rubella infection. Note the disruption of the lens fibre orientation and the primary lens fibres showing retention of their nuclei. (×117)

Table 28.1. Common chromosomal abnormalities which affect ocular development

Chromosome	Disorder	Ocular abnormalities	Reference
13	Trisomy 13 (Patau's syndrome)	Synophthalmia, microphthalmia, corneal opacity, coloboma, anterior chamber malformations, cataract, PHPV, retinal dysplasia, retrolental mesodermal mass	Apple et al. (1970)
18	Trisomy 18 (Edwards syndrome)	Exophthalmos, microphthalmos, corneal opacity, cataract, anterior segment malformation, iris and ciliary process abnormalities, coloboma, retinal folds, retinal dysplasia	Ginsberg et al. (1971) Mullaney (1973)
21	Trisomy 21 (Down's syndrome)	Cataract, Brushfield's spots on iris, Ectropian uvea, optic nerve hypoplasia	Ginsberg et al. (1977)
13	Deletion of the long arm of chromosome 13 (del 13q)	Retinoblastoma	Stallard (1962)
11	Partial deletion of short arm of chromosome 11 (del 11p)	Corneal opacity, aniridia, cataract, macular hypoplasia, optic nerve hypoplasia	Burck et al. (1982)

drome include microphthalmia and secondary congenital glaucoma. Congenital deafness is the most common congenital abnormality, but often coexists with ocular changes and congenital heart disease.

Congenital HIV infection. There are no reports of ocular effects of congenital HIV infection. The experience of eye disease reported in adults with acquired immune deficiency syndrome, suggests that candida, cryptococcus, toxoplasma and pneumocystis might be expected to cause eye infection in the neonatal period.

Maternal Drugs and the Eye

Some maternally ingested drugs may have a teratogenic effect on the developing eye. Alcohol has been demonstrated to cause ocular abnormalities in mice during studies on the fetal alcohol syndrome (Cook et al. 1987). Chloroquine and streptomycin cause corneal opacities (and congenital deafness), lysergic acid (LSD) and thalidomide exposure increases the incidence of coloboma development.

Effect of Chromosomal and Genetic Disorders on Oculogenesis

Ocular developmental abnormalities are associated with chromosomal disorders, particularly autosomal trisomies and partial deletions. Some of the commoner examples are listed in Table 28.1. Other autosomal chromosome deletions associated with ocular abnormalities include those affecting chromosomes 2, 4, 5, 7, 9, 12, 14, 15 and 22.

Sex-linked and autosomal inheritable conditions that particularly have an effect on oculogenesis and present around the time of birth include those in Table 28.2.

The Ear

The structures forming the ear act as specially adapted mechanoreceptors which are sensitive to the stimulus of sound waves (hearing) and gravitational force (balance). The organs responsible are the organ of Corti in the cochlea and the vestibular apparatus, which are both situated in the inner ear. Functionally the ear is composed of three compartments: (1) the external ear formed from the sound-collecting pinna and the auditory canal, (2) the middle ear which converts sound waves into mechanical energy, and (3) the inner ear containing the vestibulocochlear apparatus.

Embryology

Due to the compartmentalisation of the ear, its embryogenesis which involves structures

Table 28.2. Genetic disorders where disordered oculogenesis is usual

Disease	Inheritance	Ocular changes	Reference
Norrie's disease	X-linked recessive	Shallow anterior chamber, cataract, iris—atrophic or ectropian uvea, retrolental mesodermal mass, disorganised retina, atrophic optic nerve	Apple et al. (1974)
Type I generalised form of gangliosidosis	Autosomal recessive	Macula—cherry red spot at birth Retinal cells contain cytoplasmic deposits of glycolipid	Emery et al. (1971)
Walker–Warburg syndrome	Autosomal recessive	Retinal dysplasia (may form part of a syndrome involving hydrocephalus, agyria, retinal dysplasia +/− encephalocoele)	Donnai and Farndon (1986)

originating from surface ectoderm, mesoderm, endoderm and the first two branchial arches, is most easily understood by considering the development of each compartment separately (see Fig. 28.1).

The inner ear. The sensory apparatus of the inner ear develops from paired otocysts around day 25 following invagination of a thickened area of surface ectoderm, the otic placode, that develops during day 22 at the level of the hindbrain. The majority of the otocyst forms the utriculosaccular chamber from which, by the 6th week, the dorsal portion starts to form the semicircular canals of the vestibular apparatus and the ventral portion, the cochlear duct, within which develops the auditory organ of Corti, during week 11.

The vestibulocochlear ganglion, the progenitor of the eighth cranial nerve develops during the 4th week, between the otocyst and the developing hindbrain. This provides innervation for the sensory mechanoreceptors of the inner ear.

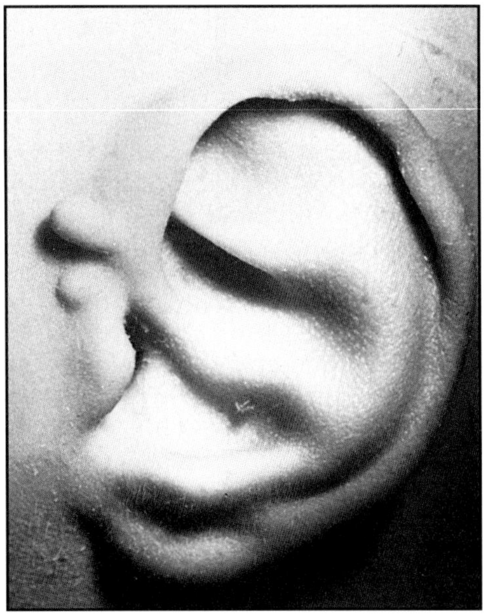

Fig. 28.22. Malformed auricle including preauricular vestigial tag, due to incomplete fusion of the auricular hillocks.

The middle ear. The middle ear structures develop during the 4th to 6th weeks in the first pharyngeal pouch. The ossicles are derived from cartilage of the first two branchial arches, whilst the tympanic membrane develops from the first pharyngeal membrane.

The external ear. The auricle develops during the 5th week from fusion of six auricular hillocks which arise at the margin of the first branchial groove.

Developmental Abnormalities of the Ear

The external ear. Minor degrees of abnormality in the shape of the auricle and the presence of accessory auricular tags due to incomplete fusion of the auricular hillocks are quite common. They are usually considered to be of cosmetic rather than of functional significance (Fig. 28.22). Malformed low-set ears are often associated with chromosomal abnormalities e.g. trisomies such as Patau syndrome (trisomy 13), Edward syndrome (trisomy 18) (Fig. 28.23), triploidy and some autosomal deletion syndromes. Malformed auricles are recognised as part of many malformation syndromes, and deformity is severe in mandibulofacial dysostosis (Treacher Collins syndrome). Many

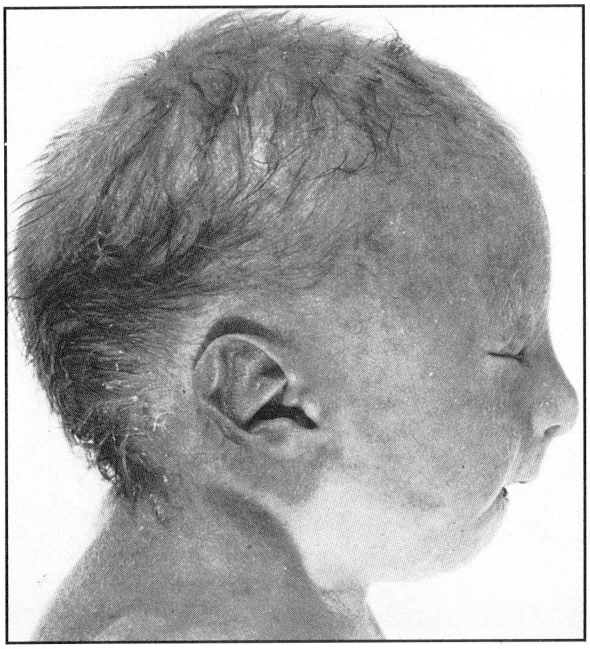

Fig. 28.23. Low-set malformed auricle in trisomy 18.

types of auricular deformity are illustrated in *Smith's Recognizable Patterns of Human Malformations* (Jones 1988). Absence of the auricle (anotia) is very rare.

Congenital atresia of the external auditory canal is rare, affecting 1 in 10 000 infants (Maniglia 1981). The atresia may be associated with the first arch syndrome. Partial duplication of the external auditory canal may predispose to later development of branchial cleft cysts and fistulae.

Defective development of the first pharyngeal pouch predisposes to atresia of the external auditory meatus and canal or malformations of the tympanic cavity and middle ear.

The middle and inner ear. Conductive and sensorineural deafness result from abnormal development of the ossicle or organ of Corti or its neural innervation. Isolated congenital deafness is most commonly due to an autosomal-recessive inheritance. Other causes include intrauterine rubella infection before the 19th week (Brookhouser and Bordley 1973; Smithells et al. 1990), congenital cytomegalovirus infection, maternal ingestion of streptomycin and thalidomide, severe intrapartum birth asphyxia and post-partum hyperbilirubinaemia. Very low birthweight infants are at increased risk of deafness due to haemorrhage around the eighth cranial nerve (Michaels et al. 1985). More detailed classifications of inner ear malformations are provided by Ormerod (1960) and Suehiro and Sando (1979).

Michaels (1987) provides a very useful alphabetical index of inner ear malformations and other associated conditions.

Examination of the Middle and Inner Ear

The technical approach to examining the middle and inner ear structures lies beyond the scope of the present chapter; for technical information the reader is advised to consult Michaels et al. (1985).

Syndromes Affecting Oculogenesis and Otogenesis

Oculogenesis and otogenesis occur during the critical period of organogenesis when teratogenic effects of both environmental and genetic disorders may cause severe derangement of both eye and ear development. Conditions in which congenital abnormalities of these special senses coexist include Alport's syndrome, Alstrom's syndrome, Crouzon's (craniofacial dysostosis) syndrome, Goldenhaar's syndrome, Hallgre's syndrome, Leber's congenital amaurosis, Norrie's disease, Usher's syndrome, Wallenburg syndrome and the congenital rubella syndrome.

Olfaction

The special sense of olfaction is a phylogenetically ancient chemoreceptor-mediated function of specially adapted bipolar cells situated in the nasal mucosa.

Embryology

The olfactory bipolar chemoreceptors develop from surface ectoderm as areas of thickening referred to as the nasal placodes, which migrate towards the superior region of the developing nasal cavities where they form the olfactory pits from which further differentiation of the ectoderm occurs, forming the pseudostratified columnar ciliated olfactory epithelium. The olfactory bipolar cells develop synapses via their axons, with the olfactory bulbs. At birth, the olfactory neuroepithelium is present between the upper half of the nasal septum, the superior turbinate and the roof of both nasal cavities. Between infancy and adulthood the extent of distribution of the neuroepithelium becomes more restricted (Nakashima et al. 1984).

Congenital Disorders of Olfaction

Histopathological studies on olfactory deficits are rare. However Douek et al. (1975) described histological changes in the olfactory mucosa in a variety of conditions causing anosmia, including congenital anosmia. In this condition they described incomplete or incorrect synapse formation between the olfactory bipolar neurons and the olfactory bulb. Igarashi et al. (1986) in a case of Kallmann syndrome and Yamagishi et al. (1988) in two cases of congenital anosmia, described the complete absence of olfactory bipolar cells from the olfactory mucosa. In utero, *Treponema pallidum* infection may cause extensive disruption of nasal development, including the olfactory mucosa.

Examination of the Nose

A technical description of examination of the nose and paranasal sinuses at autopsy is provided by Michaels (1987).

Taste

At birth the taste buds are present as specialised chemoreceptors formed by modification of the oral cavity surface epithelium, with the highest density of taste receptors present on the anterior two-thirds of the tongue. Lower densities are also distributed over the posterior third of the tongue, the inferior surface of the soft palate, the epiglottis and oropharynx. The epithelium is mainly derived from the endoderm covering the medial aspect of the four pharyngeal arches. The developing taste receptors establish synaptic connections with the following nerves depending on their location and the pharyngeal arch the endoderm originated from: the lingual branch of the trigeminal nerve (anterior two-thirds of the tongue, first arch), the inferior ganglion of the glossopharangeal nerve (third arch derived endoderm) and the inferior ganglion of the vagus (fourth arch derivatives).

Unlike the olfactory chemoreceptors, the specialised taste receptor cells are continually being desquamated and replaced. The density of taste-sensing cells is greatest in infancy and diminishes with advancing age.

References

Apple DJ, Holden JD, Stallworth B (1970) Ocular pathology of Patau's syndrome with an unbalanced D/D translocation. Am J Ophthalmol 70: 383–391

Apple DJ, Fishman GA, Goldberg MF (1974) Ocular histopathology of Norrie's disease. Am J Ophthalmol 78: 198–03

Apple DJ, Rabb MF (1991) Ocular pathology, clinical applications and self-assessment, 4th edn. Mosby Year Book, St Louis

Ashton N, Ward B, Serpell G (1954) Effect of oxygen on developing retinal vessels with particular reference to the problem of retrolental fibroplasia. Br J Ophthalmol 38: 397–432

Atkinson J (1984) How does infant vision change in the first three months of life? In: Prechtl HER (ed) Continuity of neural functions. Clin Dev Med 94: 159–178

Bateman JB (1983) Genetics in paediatric ophthalmology. Paediatr Clin North Am 30: 1015–1031

Beauvieux M (1947) La cecite apparence chez le nouveau-né: la pseudoatrophie grise du nerf optique. Arch d' Ophthalmol 7: 241–249

Boyd PA, Keeling JW, Lindenbaum RH (1988) Fraser syndrome (cryptophthalmos-syndactyly syndrome): a review of eleven cases with post mortem findings. Am J Med Genet 31: 159–168

Braddick OJ, Atkinson J, Waltham-Bell J, Day J (1983) The onset of binocular function in human infants. Hum Neurobiol 2: 65–69.

Brookhouser PE, Bordley JE (1973) Congenital rubella deafness. Pathology and pathogenesis. Arch Otolaryngol 98: 252–257

Broughton WL, Fine BS, Zimmerman LE (1981) Congenital glaucoma associated with a chromosomal defect. A histologic study. Arch Ophthalmol 99: 481–486

Burck U, Held KR, Hamann K-U, Domarus D von (1982) Aniridia-Wilms' tumour syndrome with deletion of the short arm of chromosome 11. Ophthalmic Paediatr Genet

1: 183
Campbell K (1951) Intensive oxygen therapy as a possible cause of retrolental fibroplasia: a clinical approach. Med J Aust ii: 48–50
Clinch TE, Duker JS, Eagle RC, Calhoun JH, Augsburger JJ, Fischer DH (1989) Infantile endogenous candida endophthalmitis presenting as a cataract. Surv Ophthalmol 34: 107–112.
Cook CS, Nowotny AZ, Sulik KK (1987) Fetal alcohol syndrome: eye malformations in a mouse model. Arch Ophthalmol 105: 1576
Darlow BA (1988) Incidence of retinopathy of prematurity in New Zealand. Arch Dis Child 63: 1083–1086
Donnai D, Farndon PA (1986) Walker–Warburg syndrome (Warburg syndrome, HARD+/− E syndrome). J Med Genet 23: 200–203
Douek E, Bannister LH, Dodson HC (1975) Recent advances in the pathology of olfaction. Proc Roy Soc Med 68: 467–470
Duvall J, Miller SL, Cheatle E, Tso MOM (1987) Ocular changes in a syndrome of multiple congenital anomalies. A histopathological study. Am J Ophthalmol 103: 701–705
Emery JM, Green WR, Wyllie RG (1971) GM1-gangliosidosis. Ocular and pathological manifestations. Arch Ophthalmol 85: 177–187
Friedenwald JS (1926) Massive gliosis of the retina. In: Contributions to ophthalmic science. Banta Publishing Co, Wisconsin
Garner A (1984) An international classification of retinopathy of prematurity. Br J Ophthalmol 68: 690–697
Ginsberg J, Bove K, Nelson R, Englender GS (1971) Ocular pathology of trisomy 18. Ann Ophthalmol 3: 273–279
Ginsberg J, Bofinger MK, Roush JR (1977) Pathologic features in Down's syndrome with relationship to other chromosomal abnormalities. Am J Ophthalmol 83: 874–880
Goldenhaar M (1952) Associations malformations de l'oriel et de l'oreille en particular le syndrome dermoide epibulbaire-appendices auricularies-fistula auris congenita et ses relations avec la dysostose mandibulfaciale. J Genet Hum 1: 243–282
Gregg NM (1941) Congenital cataract following German measles in the mother. Trans Ophthalmol 3: 35–46
Harry J (1990) The eye and associated structures. In: Weller RO (ed) Systemic pathology, vol 4, 3rd edn. Churchill Livingstone, Edinburgh pp 673–375
Igarashi Y, Oka Y, Ishizuka Y (1986) Electron microscopic observations of the nasal olfactory area in Kallmann syndrome. Pract Otol (Kyoto) 79: 2041–2048
Illingworth RS (1961) Delayed visual maturation. Arch Dis Child 34: 407–409
Jones KL (1988) Smith's recognizable patterns of human malformations. Saunders, Philadelphia
Kinsey VE (1956) Retrolental fibroplasia: co-operative study of retrolental fibroplasia and the use of oxygen. Arch Ophthalmol 56: 481–543
Kirkness CM, McCartney A, Rice NC, Garner A, Steele McG (1987) Congenital hereditary corneal oedema of Maumenee: its clinical features, management and pathology. Br J Ophthalmol 71: 130–144
Lambert SR, Kriss A, Taylor D (1989) Delayed visual maturation: a longitudinal clinical and electrophysiological assessment. Ophthalmology 96: 524–528
MacMahon P, Fleming PJ, Speidel BD, Dunn PM (1986) Low inspired oxygen concentrations in very low birthweight infants needing ventilatory support: an approach to the prevention of retrolental fibroplasia. Br J Obstet Gynaecol 93: 361–363
Makley TA (1955) Posterior lenticonus: report of a case with histopathological findings. Am J Ophthalmol 39: 308
Maniglia AJ (1981) Embryology, teratology and arrested developmental disorders in otolaryngology. Otolaryngol Clin North Am 14: 25–39
McMenamin PG (1989) A morphological study on the inner surface of the anterior chamber angle in pre- and postnatal human eyes. Curr Eye Res 8: 727–739
Michaels L, Gould SJ, Wells M (1985) The microslicing method in the study of temporal bone changes in the perinatal period: an interim report. Acta Otolaryngol [suppl] (Stockholm) 423: 9–14
Michaels L (1987) Ear, nose and throat histopathology. Springer Verlag, Berlin
Mullaney J (1973) Ocular pathology in trisomy 18 (Edwards' syndrome). Am J Ophthalmol 76: 246–254
Mullaney J (1982) Normal development and developmental anomalies of the eye. In: Garner A, Klintworth G (eds) Pathobiology of the eye. Dekker, New York
Ng YK, Fielder AR, Shaw DE, Levene MI (1988) Epidemiology of retinopathy of prematurity. Lancet ii: 1235–1238
Nakashima T, Kimmelman CP, Snow JB (1984) Structure of human fetal and adult olfactory neuroepithelium. Arch Otolaryngol 110: 641–646
Ormerod F (1960) The pathology of congenital deafness. J Laryngol Otol 74: 919–950
Pandolfi M, Astendt B (1971) Outflow resistance in the foetal eye. Acta Ophthalmol 49: 344–350
Phelps D (1981) Retinopathy of prematurity: an estimate of vision loss in the United States—1979. Paediatrics 67: 924–926
Reese AB (1955) Persistent hyperplastic primary vitreous. Jackson Memorial Lecture. Trans Am Acad Ophthalmol Otolaryngol 59: 271–286
Reese AB, Ellsworth RM (1966) The anterior cleavage syndrome. Arch Ophthalmol 75: 307–318
Reese AB, King MJ, Owens WC (1953) A classification of retrolental fibroplasia. Am J Ophthalmol 36: 1333–1335
Saigal S, Rosenbaum P, Stoskopf B, Sinclàir JC (1984) Outcome of Infants 501–1000 g birth weight delivered to residents of the McMaster health region. J Pediatr 105: 969–976
Smithells R, Sheppard S, Holzel H, Jones G (1990) Congenital rubella in Great Britain 1971–1988. Health Trends 22: 73–76
Stallard HB (1962) The conservative treatment of retinoblastoma. Doyne Memorial Lecture. Trans Ophthalmol Soc 83: 473–535
Suehiro S, Sando I (1979) Congenital anomalies of the inner ear. Introducing a new classification of labyrinthine anomalies. Ann Otol Rhinol Laryngol 88 [Suppl 59]: 1–24
Terry TL (1942) Extreme prematurity and fibroblastic overgrowth of persistent vascular sheath behind the crystalline lens. Am J Ophthalmol 25: 203–204
Tresidder J, Fielder AR, Nicholson J (1990) Delayed visual maturation: opthalmic and neurodevelopmental aspects. Dev Med Child Neurol 32: 872–881
Waring GO, Rodrigues MM, Laibson PR (1975) Anterior chamber cleavage syndrome: a stepladder classification. Surv Ophthalmol 20: 3–27
Yamagagishi M, Hasegawa S, Nakano Y (1988) Examination and classification of human olfactory mucosa in patients with clinical olfactory disturbances. Acta Otorhinolaryngol 245: 316–320

Subject Index